Edited by

WALTER F. BALLINGER, II, M.D.

*Bixby Professor of Surgery and Head of the Department,
Washington University School of Medicine, St. Louis;
Surgeon-in-Chief, Barnes Hospital, St. Louis.*

ROBERT B. RUTHERFORD, M.D.

*Associate Professor of Surgery,
University of Colorado School of Medicine*

GEORGE D. ZUIDEMA, M.D.

*Warfield M. Firor Professor and Director,
Section of Surgical Sciences, The Johns Hopkins University
School of Medicine;
Surgeon-in-Chief, The Johns Hopkins Hospital*

The Management of Trauma

Second Edition

W. B. SAUNDERS COMPANY
Philadelphia • London • Toronto

W. B. Saunders Company: West Washington Square
Philadelphia, PA 19105

12 Dyott Street
London, WC1A 1DB

833 Oxford Street
Toronto, Ontario M8Z 5T9, Canada

The Management of Trauma ISBN 0-7216-1521-X

 Library of Congress catalog card number 73-77933.

Print No: 9 8 7 6 5 4 3 2

CONTRIBUTORS

CHARLES B. ANDERSON, M.D. Assistant Professor of Surgery, Washington University; Attending Surgeon, Barnes and Allied Hospitals and St. Louis City Hospital

VIRGINIA M. BADGER, M.D. Assistant Professor of Orthopedic Surgery, Washington University; Attending Surgeon, Barnes and Allied Hospitals, Shriner's Hospital and St. Louis City Hospital

WALTER F. BALLINGER, II, M.D. Bixby Professor of Surgery and Head of the Department, Washington University; Surgeon-in-Chief, Barnes Hospital, St. Louis

DONALD W. BENSON, M.D., Ph.D. Professor of Anesthesiology, The Johns Hopkins University; Anesthesiologist-in-Charge, The Johns Hopkins Hospital

PERRY BLACK, M.D., C.M. Associate Professor of Neurological Surgery, The Johns Hopkins University

JOHN FRANCIS BURKE, M.D. Associate Professor of Surgery, Harvard University; Chief of Staff, Shrine Burns Institute, Boston; Visiting Surgeon, Massachusetts General Hospital

JOHN L. CAMERON, M.D. Assistant Professor of Surgery, The Johns Hopkins University; Attending Surgeon, The Johns Hopkins Hospital; Visiting Surgeon, Baltimore City Hospitals

JOHN A. COLLINS, M.D. Associate Professor of Surgery, Washington University; Attending Surgeon, Barnes and Allied Hospitals and St. Louis City Hospital

MARSHALL B. CONRAD, M.D. Assistant Professor of Orthopedic Surgery, Washington University; Attending Surgeon, Barnes and Allied Hospitals and St. Louis City Hospital

RAYMOND M. CURTIS, M.D. Associate Professor of Plastic Surgery and Associate Professor of Orthopedic Surgery, The Johns Hopkins University; Plastic Surgeon, The Johns Hopkins Hospital; Visiting Hand Surgeon, Union Memorial Hospital and The Children's Hospital, Baltimore; Consultant in Hand Surgery and Surgeon General of the Army

JAMES J. DELANY, M.D. Associate Clinical Professor of Obstetrics and Gynecology, University of Colorado

MILTON T. EDGERTON, Jr., M.D. Professor and Chairman, Department of Plastic Surgery, University of Virginia; Plastic Surgeon-in-Chief, University of Virginia Medical Center, Charlottesville, Virginia

JARED M. EMERY, M.D. Assistant Professor of Ophthalmology, Baylor University; Chief of Service, Ben Taub General Hospital, Houston; Attending Surgeon, Methodist Hospital, Houston

RAINER M. E. ENGEL, M.D. Associate Professor of Urology, The Johns Hopkins University; Attending Urologist, The Johns Hopkins Hospital and Columbia Hospital and Clinic, Columbia, Maryland; Consulting Urologist, Good Samaritan Hospital and Baltimore City Hospitals

MARGARET M. FLETCHER, M.D. Assistant Professor of Laryngology and Otology, The Johns Hopkins University; Attending Otolaryngologist, The Johns Hopkins Hospital

MELVIN FRIEDMAN, M.D. Instructor in Orthopedic Surgery, The Johns Hopkins University

J. ALEX HALLER, Jr., M.D. Robert Garrett Professor of Pediatric Surgery, The Johns Hopkins University; Children's Surgeon-in-Charge, The Johns Hopkins Hospital

JOHN E. HOOPES, M.D. Professor of Plastic Surgery, The Johns Hopkins University; Plastic Surgeon-in-Charge, The Johns Hopkins Hospital; Chief of Plastic Surgery, Children's Hospital and Baltimore City Hospitals

JAMES LANGSTON HUGHES, Jr., M.D. Assistant Professor of Orthopedic Surgery, The Johns Hopkins University; Attending Surgeon, The Johns Hopkins Hospital, Children's Hospital, Good Samaritan Hospital and Baltimore City Hospitals

MICHAEL E. JABALEY, M.D. Associate Professor of Surgery and Chief of Plastic Surgery, University of Mississippi; Consultant in Plastic Surgery, Veterans Administration Hospital and Mississippi Baptist Hospital, Jackson

THOMAS J. KRIZEK, M.D. Associate Professor of Surgery (Plastic) and Chief, Section of Plastic and Reconstructive Surgery, Yale University; Attending Surgeon, Yale-New Haven Hospital

EDWARD R. LAWS, Jr., M.D. Assistant Professor of Neurosurgery, Mayo Medical School; Staff Neurosurgeon, Mayo Clinic, St. Mary's Hospital and Rochester Methodist Hospital, Rochester, Minnesota

CHARLES B. MANLEY, M.D., F.A.C.S. Associate Professor of Genitourinary Surgery, Washington University; Assistant Professor of Pediatric Urology, St. Louis Children's Hospital; Director, Division of Urology, Jewish Hospital, St. Louis

J. DONALD McQUEEN, M.D. Associate Professor of Neurology, The Johns Hopkins University; Neurosurgeon-in-Charge, Baltimore City Hospitals and Loch Raven Veterans Administration Hospital; Attending Neurosurgeon, The Johns Hopkins Hospital

DAVID PATON, M.D., F.A.C.S. Professor and Chairman, Department of Ophthalmology, Baylor University; Chief of Ophthalmology, Methodist Hospital, Texas Medical Center; Consultant, Veterans Administration Hospital; Senior Attending Physician, Ben Taub General Hospital, Texas Children's Hospital, St. Luke's Hospital, Houston

CHARLES D. RAY, M.D., F.A.C.S., F.R.S.H. Clinical Associate Professor of Neurology, University of Minnesota; Attending Neurologist, Northwestern-Abbott Hospital, Children's Health Center and Sister Kenney Rehabilitation Institute, Minneapolis

FRED C. REYNOLDS, M.D. Professor of Orthopedic Surgery, Washington University; Attending Surgeon, Barnes and Allied Hospitals, St. Louis

ALAN M. ROBSON, M.D., M.R.C.P. Associate Professor of Pediatrics and Director of Pediatric Nephrology, Washington University; Attending Pediatrician, St. Louis Children's Hospital

MARTIN C. ROBSON, M.D. Assistant Professor of Surgery (Plastic), Yale University

RONALD E. ROSENTHAL, M.D. Associate Professor of Orthopedic Surgery, Washington University; Attending Surgeon, Vanderbilt University Hospital, Nashville, Tennessee

ROBERT B. RUTHERFORD, M.D. Associate Professor of Surgery, University of Colorado Medical Center, Denver

GERHARD SCHMEISSER, M.D. Professor of Orthopedic Surgery, The Johns Hopkins University; Chief of Orthopedic Surgery, Baltimore City Hospitals; Attending Orthopedic Surgeon, The Johns Hopkins Hospital

ARTHUR H. STEIN, JR., M.D. Professor of Orthopedic Surgery, Washington University; Attending Surgeon, Barnes and Allied Hospitals, St. Louis

JAMES L. TALBERT, M.D. Professor of Pediatrics and Surgery, University of Florida; Chief Pediatric Surgeon and Medical Director of Emergency Services, W. A. Shands Teaching Hospital and Clinics, Gainesville, Florida

GEORGE B. UDVARHELYI, M.D. Professor of Neurological Surgery, The Johns Hopkins University; Attending Neurosurgeon, The Johns Hopkins Hospital; Visiting Neurosurgeon, Baltimore City Hospitals

A. EARL WALKER, M.D. Professor Emeritus of Neurosurgery, The Johns Hopkins University; Visiting Professor of Neurosurgery, University of New Mexico; Attending Neurosurgeon, The Johns Hopkins Hospital and Bernalillo County Hospital, Albuquerque, New Mexico

ROBERT CHRISTIE WRAY, JR., M.D. Assistant Professor of Plastic and Reconstructive Surgery, Washington University; Assistant Professor of Surgery, Barnes Hospital; Assistant Surgeon, Barnes and Allied Hospitals and St. Louis Children's Hospital; Chief of Plastic Surgery, St. Louis County Hospital

JACK M. ZIMMERMAN, M.D. Associate Professor of Surgery, The Johns Hopkins University; Chief of Surgery, Church Home and Hospital, Baltimore

GEORGE D. ZUIDEMA, M.D. Warfield M. Firor Professor and Director of the Department of Surgery, The Johns Hopkins University; Surgeon-in-Chief, The Johns Hopkins Hospital

PREFACE

The battleground, with its insistent pressure for immediate yet thoughtful and considered management of injury, has traditionally been a rich medium for development of surgical principles and procedures. The progressive decrease in the mortality rate of the wounded from World War I, World War II, the Korean War and the Vietnam conflict offers striking evidence of advantages, not only in the surgical management of trauma but also in general supportive care and rapid means of transportation to centers where definitive management is possible.

But just as disease patterns and epidemiology change with the passage of time, so has the spectrum of trauma altered in recent years. We can now speak of the epidemiology of trauma with at least as much assurance as of the epidemiology of hepatitis, and we can state with precision that since the turn of the century the contribution of motor vehicles to the annual accidental death rate has steadily risen to the point where it now exceeds 45 per cent. As a result, blunt trauma, frequently producing multiple injuries, has taken a dominant position in our accident wards and, therefore, in the surgeon's training and experience.

While our methods of treatment have improved and continue to improve, our means of producing injury are also being perfected. Ever increasing horsepower, coupled with an unchanging degree of human error, has exceeded the rate of our willingness or ability to incorporate safety features into our automobiles. Furthermore, new weapons and changing methods of waging war continue to demand much of our resources. In our opinion, these factors provide clear evidence of the large and continuing need for investigation of the mechanism of injuries and for a methodology for their prevention and management.

Although impressive progress has been made recently in a number of dramatic areas, such as organ transplantation, mechanical cardiopulmonary assistance and prosthetic valves and vessels, we have not paid sufficient attention to another area—one which involves the death or disability of large numbers of our population every year. The following statistics bear sobering insight into the serious impact of trauma in this country. Accidents injure more than 50 million people and kill more than 100,000 in the United States each year. Trauma is exceeded only by cardiovascular disease and cancer as a cause of death in this country, and it is the leading cause of death among persons between the ages of 1 and 37. Thus, in terms of productive man-years lost, trauma can be considered our leading "killer." Moreover, for every person killed accidentally, approximately 100 suffer a temporarily disabling injury, and 10 to 15 require hospitalization. Accident patients occupy 12 per cent of the total general hospital space, requiring more hospital bed days than all heart patients and four times more than all cancer patients.

The challenge is obviously great.

We have asked many of the authors of the first edition of this text to update their original contribution. In addition, we have received valued additions from others, expert in the field of the management of trauma. We have considered trauma as a continuum from the moment of injury to the operating theater and beyond. It is most important to remember that, in any severe illness, there is a beginning but never a definable end.

However, in order to confine the almost limitless scope of trauma, from injury through rehabilitation, we have urged our associates to stress the principles and techniques of early management as opposed to those of late reconstructive care. We have asked them to pay special attention to interpretation of the constellation of physiologic disturbances which inevitably accompany serious injury, and to describe the ways they have found effective for restoring body functions quickly and gently to a normal pattern.

To each of the contributors the editors owe their sincere appreciation, as well as to Ms. Patricia Ingram, Ms. Karma Berry, Mr. David Zimmerman and the many others who aided the authors and editors in making this second edition possible.

WALTER F. BALLINGER
ROBERT B. RUTHERFORD
GEORGE D. ZUIDEMA

CONTENTS

chapter

1

INITIAL EVALUATION AND TREATMENT OF THE INJURED PATIENT

George D. Zuidema, M.D., and John L. Cameron, M.D.

GENERAL PRINCIPLES

There is no task in surgery more difficult or more important than the initial evaluation of a trauma victim. When dealing with acute trauma it is often impossible to separate diagnostic and therapeutic measures; in fact, it is improper to attempt to dissociate them. The care of the acutely injured patient imposes certain important time restrictions upon the physician. He must not only carry out his usual diagnostic evaluation, but must also attend to the urgent therapeutic needs of his patient. It is frequently impossible and impractical to obtain a detailed history. He is forced to rely heavily on physical findings for diagnosis, and the initial examination may well be performed with an agitated, uncooperative patient making the task even more difficult.

The proper evaluation of an acutely injured patient hinges on several urgent determinations. It is essential to assure airway patency and to insert an endotracheal tube if called for, to start central intravenous lines capable of monitoring central venous pressure and carrying large-volume infusions if necessary, and to control significant hemorrhage. Other pressing needs are analysis of the patient for spinal cord injury, presence of fractures, and thoracic or acute intra-abdominal injury. The urinary tract must be evaluated and the integrity of peripheral nerves established.

When immediate life-threatening situations have been controlled, complete patient evaluation is essential to assess the full extent of injury. This is also the time to elucidate any preinjury conditions that may influence and modify management. Following severe trauma there are only a few situations that are reversible but produce death within minutes if left unattended. The first of these is inadequate ventilation;

the second is hypoxia resulting from circulatory insufficiency; and the third, which often accompanies the second, is rapid, continuing bleeding. Other types of reversible injury lead to slower deterioration of the patient's condition and, therefore, are not given the same priority for emergency management.

Inadequate Ventilation

Inadequate ventilation leads immediately to hypoxemia and insufficient oxygen delivery to tissues. This state is tolerated poorly and if complete asphyxia follows, the brain suffers irreversible anoxic damage within five minutes. If ventilation is to be re-established, it must be done quickly.

Inadequate ventilation can result from several sources, but in acute trauma upper airway obstruction is the most common. If obstruction is complete, all methods of resuscitation fail until the obstruction is removed. Frequently, such obstruction can be relieved simply. In an unconscious, apneic patient obstruction is frequently caused by the relaxation of the soft tissue of the pharynx, the falling back of the tongue, or blockage of the upper airways by mucus, blood or vomitus. If foreign material is discovered in the mouth or oropharynx, suctioning should be performed immediately. The head should be tilted backward so that the jaw is pointing upward, and the jaw should be pushed or pulled into a jutting position. This maneuver relieves obstruction in the airway by moving the base of the tongue away from the back of the throat. If these measures fail to restore adequate ventilation—if the patient remains apneic or cyanotic, displays retractions of the chest with ventilatory effort, or has only shallow and inadequate respiratory movements—the cause is probably not simple upper airway obstruction. Such a situation occurs in severe neurological damage, in obstruction of the trachea below the glottis, in flail chest injury, in bilateral pneumothorax and in laryngeal fracture. Precise diagnosis is often impossible in the short time allowed to restore adequate ventilation and therefore should not delay treatment. An oral or nasal endotracheal tube should be inserted immediately and positive pressure ventilation instituted with a compressible bag. Only in the case of direct laryngeal trauma will an endotracheal tube be inadequate. A direct tracheal airway should then be established. This can be done most quickly by creating a temporary opening in the subcutaneously located cricothyroid ligament in the midline of the neck. The classic tracheostomy performed below the cricothyroid ligament is too time-consuming in real emergency situations. The introduction of large bore needles into the cricothyroid membrane has been recommended, but these needles are frequently not available. Resuscitation by this technique can be continued until an artificial respiratory apparatus becomes available. At this point, with an endotracheal or tracheostomy tube in place, chest tubes can be inserted if part of the ventilatory inadequacy is secondary to intrapleural air or blood.

Circulatory Insufficiency

Primarily, two varieties of circulatory insufficiency are seen with acute trauma. The first is associated with marked hypovolemia secondary to blood loss, resulting in inadequate delivery of oxygen to tissues, and the second is cardiac arrest. Hypovolemia, when present, has to be attended to as soon as an adequate airway is achieved if only one physician is present, or concurrently, if more than one physician is available for the resuscitative effort. At least one central venous line inserted through the external jugular vein, or via the subclavian route if the jugulars are collapsed, is essential. Peripheral lines should also be used. If chest trauma is present, at least one of the intravenous routes should be through a lower extremity in case a superior vena caval injury is present. The rapid administration of electrolyte solutions and plasma substitutes is adequate for short periods until blood is available. In most instances, if heart action is still present by the time a trauma victim reaches an emergency room, the restoration of blood volume should be possible if care is efficiently and rapidly delivered.

The diagnosis of cardiac arrest is made initially by the detection of pulselessness. It can be confirmed by cardiac auscultation or an electrocardiogram. Usually, however, resuscitative efforts are begun without EKG confirmation. Since ventilatory insufficiency is always an accompanying condition, its treatment is an integral part of the management of circulatory arrest. External cardiac massage is the best way to restore the circulation immediately. Circulation without ventilation is useless. The treatment of circulatory arrest, therefore, involves two features: restoration of both ventilation and circulation. This resuscitative effort can be performed by a single operator who alternates every fourth manual compression of the chest with a single mouth-to-mouth positive pressure breath. Such an effort, however, is tiring and cannot be continued for a long period of time. A more satisfactory approach is resuscitation by two operators—one performing artificial ventilation by mouth-to-mouth positive pressure breathing, or preferably by the use of a compressible bag and an endotracheal tube, and the other performing artificial circulation by closed heart massage. The latter technique is performed with the patient lying supine on an unyielding surface. The operator kneels to one side of the patient or straddles him and rhythmically compresses the lower end of the sternum against the spine. This is done with the heel of the hand or with the clenched fists pressed against the lower end of the sternum. Compression should be carried out at a rate of 80 times per minute. The effectiveness of the effort can be monitored by the palpation of pulses in the groin or in the neck.

In the absence of intrinsic cardiac disease, there are a few situations in which such a resuscitative effort will be unsuccessful. These include bilateral tension pneumothorax and severe injury to the thoracic wall that renders it incapable of rebound when compressed. In these situations circulation can be restored by emergency thoracotomy and direct manual massage of the heart. As long as positive pressure ventilation, external cardiac massage, and blood volume support are continued, life can be supported for long periods of time. It is possible to transport patients during these resuscitative efforts to an area where definitive therapeutic measures are available. The most important aspects of emergency treatment of respiratory and circulatory failure are immediate recognition of the problem and the instantaneous application of simple therapeutic measures. This condition must be assessed and treated where it occurs, whether on the highway, in a casualty clearing station or in the emergency ward of a hospital.

Bleeding

The final situation that has to be controlled within a very short time is continuing rapid bleeding. In the past a great deal was taught about the application of tourniquets and the use of pressure points to control arterial bleeding. Both of these techniques are more cumbersome than necessary, and much misunderstanding has resulted from their use. External bleeding can almost always be adequately controlled by direct pressure over the bleeding site. Any clean cloth will do in providing this pressure. Unfortunately, patients are still brought into the hospital with proximal tourniquets in place and continued bleeding that can easily be stopped by removal of the tourniquet, which has impeded venous return and produced excessive venous bleeding. Occult bleeding will be discussed completely under the diagnosis of hypovolemia.

Rapid Estimation of the Extent of Injury

When ventilatory and circulatory competence are assured and external bleeding sources have been controlled, rapid evaluation of the patient's injuries is necessary to determine what precautions are necessary in the subsequent handling and moving of the patient. Movement of the patient should be accomplished with great care. Simple splinting of limb fractures is advisable to prevent more serious compounding of these injuries. Medications to relieve pain should not be given before a more detailed examination is performed.

As soon as an injured patient has been stabilized as regards his respiratory and circulatory function, a complete and rapid survey of the possible sites of injury must be carried out. Such a survey can usually be accomplished within a matter of minutes. It serves two purposes: first, to direct the course of therapy and, second, to establish a base line to which changing signs and symptoms can be compared. To omit a rapid survey for additional injuries in eagerness to treat an obvious one is an error that often leads to catastrophe. Most medical institutions have insisted that major trauma cases be supervised by general surgeons, hoping that they would be less prejudiced toward a specific organ system. Only rapid overall evaluation of the patient will avoid such disasters as a patient overwhelmed by an incipient cardiac tamponade during evaluation of a minor cerebral injury or irreversible shock produced by intra-abdominal hemorrhage during operative repair of a long bone fracture. Brief but accurate and thorough records of the initial evaluating examination should be kept for later comparison. Changes in vital signs or late appearance of abdominal tenderness when the initial examination showed none is evidence of progressive injury. The following brief outline is a reliable guide for such a rapid survey of injuries:

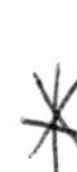

1. Examination of the head will determine the state of consciousness. The skull should be palpated for evidence of laceration and fractures. The nose and ears should be inspected for evidence of oozing blood or fluid. The size and symmetry of the pupils should be ascertained and noted. The neck should be palpated to determine the position of the trachea and to ascertain the presence of air in the soft tissues.

2. Examination of the chest will disclose any thoracic wounds. Wounds of the thorax should be covered immediately with petrolatum gauze. Auscultation will determine whether breath sounds can be heard on both sides of the chest. The thoracic cage should be compressed to determine whether rib fractures have occurred. The quality of heart sounds and the pulse rate should be noted.

3. The abdomen should be examined for evidence of muscle spasm and abdominal tenderness. Wounds that have permitted herniation of abdominal contents should be covered with moist packs.

4. The patient should be asked to move all parts of his extremities. If he is unable to cooperate, the extremities should be gently moved and palpated for evidence of fracture.

5. The wings of the ilium should be compressed to discover whether the pelvis has been fractured.

6. The legs should be separated. The perineum should be inspected for evidence of extravasated blood and urine.

7. The patient should be moved sufficiently to inspect the back and buttock areas for previously undisclosed wounds.

8. The extremities should be examined for temperature and color. The quality and rate of the peripheral pulse should be determined bilaterally and in all extremities.

9. A record of serially determined blood pressure, pulse, respiration and level of consciousness should be started immediately and maintained until it has become clear that the patient's condition is stable.

From this point the initial evaluation of the injured patient is determined by the results of the rapid survey of injuries and by the condition of the patient. The more detailed evaluation of specific injuries is now begun and carried on simultaneously with specific therapy for already discovered injuries.

SPECIAL PROBLEMS IN DIAGNOSIS AND MANAGEMENT

Hypovolemia

Injury is almost always associated with the loss of some fluid from the fluid-containing compartments of the body. Hemorrhage at a wound site is a simple and classic example of rapid fluid loss. Even in the absence of hemorrhage, however, and without disruption of the integrity of the vascular system, tissue injury produces a sequestration of fluid into the area of the wound. Such sequestered fluid is, of course, derived from the fluid-containing compartments of the body, which are in dynamic equilibrium. The amount of fluid that is lost into a wound depends upon the size of the wound, the extent of tissue damage produced and the type of tissue injured. Whenever the fluid lost into the wound is of sufficient magnitude, depletion of all the fluid compartments of the body results. The distribution of the loss between intracellular, extracellular and intravascular compartments probably also depends upon the magnitude and severity of the wound, the type of wounded tissue, and the interval between time of injury and commencement of replacement therapy. The complex syndrome of physiological derangement resulting from the sudden loss of fluid from the fluid-containing compartments of the body has been called hypovolemic shock. Before discussion of the signs, symptoms and function tests that are useful in the evaluation of the hypovolemic state, it is necessary to consider the pathological physiology that results from the acute loss of body fluids. Although a complete discussion of the shock state follows in a later chapter, basic information is pertinent here.

Compensatory Mechanisms. Following an acute injury fluid is lost first from the vascular space. This is true whether the fluid is whole blood, as in the severance of a major artery, or interstitial fluid flowing into an extensive burn area and producing edema. The initial response to such a loss is a fall in the pressure within the cardiovascular system. Such a response is immediately monitored by a complex baroreceptor system in the aortic arch and carotid sinus and relayed to the medullary vasomotor center. Reflexes then effect changes that restore the pressure to its normal level. In general, this effect is mediated through the sympathetic nervous system and is achieved by arterial constriction that raises the peripheral resistance in the vascular system and by an increase in the cardiac output resulting from an increase in the force of cardiac contraction and an increase in the heart rate. An additional effect is constriction within the venous portion of the vascular system, mobilizing blood from reservoirs to the central portion of the vascular system. During these sympathetically induced restorative efforts, blood is mobilized from the extremities, the intestine and the kidney to provide sufficient volume for the heart and brain. This set of reactions reduces the size and changes the shape of the vascular compartment.

Other responses act to restore the plasma volume to the vascular compartment. Small increases in the osmolarity of the blood plasma are detected in the hypothalamic region; this stimulates the release of antidiuretic hormone and this, in turn, influences the kidney to conserve both water and sodium. It has been postulated that the juxtaglomerular apparatus in the kidney is also stimulated, possibly by a narrowing of the pulse pressure, to release renin which, in turn, releases an octapeptide, angiotensin, from plasma protein precursors to stimulate the adrenal cortex to release aldosterone. This also has the effect of producing water and sodium conservation by the kidney. Further shifts of fluid between the vascular compartments are dictated by tension at the capillary level.

A fall in pressure in an arteriole produces a reduction of transmural capillary pressure so that extracellular fluid is moved into the capillary to restore blood volume. However, following the sympathetic response when venoconstriction has been established, the pressure relationships at the capillary level are such that in areas where constriction is prominent, plasma is lost from the capillary into the extracellular space. The inadequate perfusion following hypovolemia produces an elevation of carbon dioxide tension in the blood and a fall of the oxygen tension with a rise in hydrogen ion concentration. These chemical changes are immediately sensed by chemoreceptors located in the carotid and aortic bodies, which signal the respiratory center. The response is hyperpnea, which is effective in reducing the carbon dioxide tension and returning pH values toward normal.

All of these compensatory mechanisms function as an emergency reaction to preserve life. When hypovolemia is not corrected and these compensatory changes are allowed to persist, they themselves produce irreversible damage. The heart will eventually fail under these circumstances. Studies in experimental shock indicate that left atrial pressure rises after severe hypotension even when the blood volume has been restored. In the shock-dog preparation following the reinfusion of blood, cardiac output can be sustained only by progressive increase in the left atrial pressure. It has been a clinical finding with patients in advanced shock that intravenous infusion sometimes results in a rapid rise of central venous pressure without a concomitant increase in the cardiac output. The pulmonary edema characteristic of advanced shock has been attributed to progressive left heart failure and also to the redistribution of blood volume in which the pulmonary circulation is regarded as preferential circulation. It has also been attributed to the destructive action of certain humoral agents released into the blood stream which alter the permeability of lung capillaries.

Recently it has been suggested that certain phospholipid substances having surface-active properties are diminished in prolonged hypovolemia. These phospholipid substances are known to be of importance in maintaining the patency of pulmonary alveoli. Evidence bearing upon the impairment of renal function during prolonged hypovolemia has been obtained from experimental shock preparations. This information indicates that the renal vascular constrictive response that results in a high renal vascular resistance may continue inappropriately after the restoration of depleted blood volume. The renal cortical circulation, which under normal circumstances is rapid and requires a high oxygen concentration, may be especially impaired by the constrictive response. Thus, renal function may remain impaired long after the successful restoration of hemodynamic variables.

The profound gastrointestinal alterations which have been noted frequently in shock-dog preparations have never been an important feature of profound hypovolemic shock in patients. It is probable, however, that the function of almost all organ systems is affected by the changes resulting from inadequate tissue perfusion in hypovolemia and from the compensatory mechanisms called into play to preserve life.

The Diagnosis of Hypovolemia

Systemic Blood Pressure. Systemic hypotension is still frequently regarded as essential for the diagnosis of shock. In order to evaluate a single pressure recording as hypotensive it is necessary to know previous levels. Patients who normally function with a severe hypertension may be profoundly hypotensive with a blood pressure that would generally be regarded as normal. Because a fall in blood pressure is rapidly compensated by sympathetic responses, it is a poor indication of the severity of shock. Serial determinations of the systemic blood pressure, however, do reflect the course of developing hypovolemic shock in relationship to compensatory mechanisms. It is for this reason that the blood pressure should be monitored during the evaluation of a patient with suspected hypovolemia at no more than 15-minute intervals. The data should be evaluated in relationship to other data such as pulse rate, central venous pressure and urine production.

Signs of Increased Sympathetic Activity. As noted, the earliest compensatory mechanism following the loss of a significant amount of fluid from the vascular space is a profound sympathetic one. For this reason detection of sympathetic activity forms the most reliable basis for the early diagnosis of hypovolemic shock. Evidence includes pallor of the skin and mucous membranes, coolness of extremities, increased sweating, anxiety, collapse of veins on the dorsum of the hand and in the neck, tachycardia, and a reduction in the pulse pressure. The combination of these two produces what has become known as the rapid, weak and thready pulse. These signs should be observed at periodic intervals and an appropriate record kept. Following the institution of therapy, color and warmth return to the skin, anxiety disappears, the pulse rate reduces, and the pulse pressure widens.

Central Venous Pressure. In hypovolemic shock the central venous pressure is low but can be raised by an infusion of saline. The heart will respond to such an infusion with an increased cardiac output. At the beginning of this century, Yandall Henderson insisted that observation of the central venous pressure was a reliable guide to the treatment of shock. At the present time there is considerable enthusiasm for the wide use of venous pressure measurements. The technique can be easily performed and is an effective guide for the measurement of fluid replacement in the therapy of shock. An improvement in systemic blood pressure with no rise in the central venous pressure strongly suggests that a hypovolemic state still exists. In general, it is safe to continue therapy under close observation until a rapid rise in the venous pressure indicates that the heart is loaded to its capacity. Failure to detect this rise may result in dangerous overloading. It must also be pointed out that venous pressure is determined not only by the volume on the venous side but also by the contractile force of the heart; at the stage at which myocardial failure complicates hypovolemia, the measurement fails as an indicator of volume deficits.

Hyperpnea. The hyperventilation seen in hypovolemia is an important compensatory mechanism and a good indication of hypoxia as well as possibly a developing metabolic acidosis. It has been suggested that the hypocapnea resulting from hyperventilation may have injurious effects by producing increased fatigue and decreased myocardial function.

Oliguria. Because of the renal vasoconstriction which is part of the compensatory mechanism in shock, a diminution of urinary output is noted. Periodic measurements of urinary output are a helpful guide to the course of hypovolemic shock and efficacy of therapy. An indwelling urinary catheter provides for hourly determinations of volume and specific gravity. A urinary output of less than 30 milliliters per hour is generally accepted as indicating an inadequate renal blood flow.

Chemical Measurements. As noted, chemical determinations are static, whereas responses to hypovolemia, both untreated and during therapy, are dynamic. For that reason, chemical determinations have little value unless repeated frequently. Techniques are now available for measuring blood volume with the aid of albumin labeled with radioactive iodine or red blood cells tagged with radioactive chromium. The chief objection to these techniques is that they are time consuming, and there is some difficulty in obtaining consistent and reproducible determinations. The hematocrit is not a reliable test of volume but indicates only the concentration of red blood cells. Its value in acutely developing hypovolemia is sharply restricted, but it has considerable value in slowly developing hypovolemia in which shifts of fluid between compartments gradually compensate for the loss of whole blood. The determination of oxygen tension in mixed venous blood is helpful in predicting low cardiac output with a high extraction of oxygen by the tissues. The degree of cellular hypoxia and respiratory compensation can be determined by measurements of arterial pH and arterial pCO_2. A precise measurement of cellular hypoxia can be obtained by direct determination of the serum lactate level.

SUMMARY

The proper diagnosis of hypovolemia in an injured patient depends upon the continuous monitoring of a variety of signs related to volume deficit and of a series of compensatory mechanisms that attempt to protect the patient. Because of the dynamic nature of these mechanisms, estimates of loss and simple replacement are not adequate. A graphic record of variables providing continuous evaluation permits adequate therapy. In advanced shock many organ systems are damaged and demonstrate extreme malfunction. The primary aim of therapy in hypovolemic shock is to restore tissue perfusion and thereby restore function. However, such therapy becomes extremely complicated since it depends on the time and course of development of the hypovolemia, the type of fluid loss, the degree of organ damage and the advancement of compensatory mechanisms. The therapy of acute hypovolemia will be discussed in a later chapter.

The Evaluation of Thoracic Injuries

Careful evaluation of patients with thoracic injuries is important since apparently insignificant injuries are potentially lethal. Injuries of the chest may be obvious because of position of the wound or the complaints of the patient or, especially in a severely injured patient, may be obscure. A history of the nature of the injury is extremely important; the approach to a penetrating injury of the thoracic cage differs from that to a blunt injury without penetration. The proper evaluation and successful management of various thoracic injuries depend upon an understanding of physiological aberrations that result from the different types of wounds. Diagnosis is made largely by observation of the patient and a satisfactory x-ray examination of the chest. In evaluating thoracic trauma an upright x-ray, if the patient is able to stand, is much preferable to one obtained flat. The established techniques of physical diagnosis for detection of thoracic abnormalities (percussion and auscultation) are probably less valuable than a satisfactory x-ray examination. The most important part of a good evaluation for thoracic injury is the physician's awareness of the potential of all thoracic wounds and systematic elimination of such potential damage.

Injury of the Thoracic Wall without Penetration. Injury to the thoracic wall without penetration usually results from a blow, a contusion or a crush injury. Such injuries have become common as the result of deceleration injuries. The automobile steering wheel is a special offender.

Rib Fractures. Rib fractures may be single or multiple. They may occur spontaneously in the presence of osteal disease but usually are the result of a fall or a blow on the chest. Patients complain of pain in the region of the fracture. This pain is aggravated by deep inspiration, and there is usually an associated voluntary restriction of respiratory activity on the side of the rib fracture. The patient should be stripped to the waist, examined and the painful site carefully palpated. A crunchy sensation of air in the subcutaneous space is sometimes detected and movement of the fractured rib fragments produces exquisite pain. Identification of the injured rib is made by counting ribs. The recommended techniques are identification of the second rib at the angle of Louis with downward counting or identification of the twelfth rib where it is palpable with upward counting. On occasion, fractures of the ribs are occult and, in such cases, the diagnosis usually can be made by gently compressing the chest in the antero-posterior direction, which usually elicits pain at the site of the rib fracture. A fracture of the rib may be associated with significant intrathoracic damage as the result of lacerations of the lung or tears of intercostal vessels. A remarkable degree of hemothorax may be produced by a single rib fracture; therefore, percussion and auscultation of the chest should be carried out to detect the signs of pneumothorax and pleural effusion. Every patient with suspected rib fracture should have an x-ray of the chest to rule out the presence of air or fluid within the pleural space.

Multiple rib fractures which result from severe compression injuries of the chest frequently show two fracture sites for each rib and result in a complete separation of a portion of the chest wall, producing loss of stability. This condition is known as traumatic flail chest. The mobile portion of the chest wall moves paradoxically, being sucked in with inspiration and expanding outward with expiration. Thus, expired air from the lung within the undamaged hemithorax passes into the lung on the injured side, increasing the amount of dead space and decreasing the effectiveness of ventilation. Patients with flail chest injuries usually complain of great pain. Respiration is difficult, and cyanosis frequently develops. On close inspection the paradoxical movement of the chest cage is obvious. However, patients with this injury who appear to be quite well may develop an insidious hypercapnia, resulting in sudden cardiac arrhythmias and death. Because of the severe injury necessary to produce such a flail chest, underlying pulmonary damage is a frequent complication; and the development of bronchial spasm, excessive bronchorrhea and mucosal edema results in a situation known as traumatic wet lung and further interferes with adequate ventilation. Traumatic flail chest therefore becomes a surgical emergency requiring immediate treatment.

Adequate stabilization of the chest can sometimes be accomplished with sandbags. Techniques of external fixation of separated portions of the chest wall have been largely abandoned in favor of tracheostomy and artificial ventilation. The former reduces dead space and permits an adequate clearing of accumulated secretions; the latter encourages adequate ventilation. Separation of the costochondral junction is frequently an occult injury that cannot be detected by x-ray or definite physical signs and is usually detected by careful palpation and gentle compression of the costochondral areas.

Still another injury that can result from a blow of great violence is fracture of the sternum. This injury produces extreme pain in the region of the sternum. The patient breathes shallowly and assumes a characteristic posture in which the head and neck are held forward rigidly. Inspection of the sternal area may reveal evidence of depression and ecchymosis over the fracture site. The diagnosis of sternal fracture is established by palpation in the region of the injury and detection of movements of the ends of the bone. X-ray examination of the sternum with special views makes possible a definite diagnosis. It has frequently been noted that patients with sternal fractures are subject to severe cardiac contusion, with the development of sudden cardiac arrhythmias.

Injuries to the Chest Wall with Penetration. In civilian practice penetrating injuries of the chest are usually produced by stab wounds or by gunshot wounds. The evaluation of such wounds depends upon information concerning the damage most frequently produced by various weapons. Stab wounds are usually made with knives, daggers or ice picks. Most of the weapons are short and narrow and cause minimal destruction. However, the external appearance of a wound may be misleading since it does not reflect the degree of damage within the chest. In general, the wider the blade, the greater the possibility of severe injury. Ice pick wounds have a tendency to seal off quickly and, even when they penetrate the lung, they usually do not produce a severe air leak. The angle of entry should be determined and a search made for a site of exit. In general, women tend to stab downward whereas men tend to stab in an upward direction. When the line of entry points toward the diaphragm the possibility of intra-abdominal damage should be considered; when an abdominal site of entry points upward, there is the possibility of intrathoracic damage. It is well recognized that high thoracic wounds can penetrate the diaphragm if the injury was produced during deep expiration.

Civilian gunshot wounds are usually caused by revolvers, high velocity rifles or shotgun pellets. A variety of high velocity industrial accidents simulate shotgun injuries, notably the propulsion of fragments by the blades of a rotary mower. The path of a missile injury is usually in a straight line, although deflection by various tissues, particularly bone, is not uncommon. Bullet wounds penetrate more deeply than stab wounds and produce an area of damage around the track of the bullet resulting from compression injury within the tissue. A jacketed slug produces less damage than a soft-nosed slug, which has a tendency to produce ragged tears within the tissue. A complication of missile injuries occurs when fragments of wadding and clothing are carried inward with the missile. Shotgun injuries received at close range produce injury by blast as well as by the penetrating missile.

The Pathophysiology of Penetrating Wounds of the Thorax. A wound that permits an open communication between the pleural space and the exterior atmosphere causes collapse of the lung as air under atmospheric pressure enters the chest. With inspiration, additional air is drawn into the chest, producing further collapse of the lung and a shift of the mediastinum toward the uninjured side. With expiration, the mediastinum is pushed toward the injured side and air passes from the lung on the uninjured side to the lung on the injured side. Some air is then forced by partial inflation of the collapsed lung out through the open wound. Such to-and-fro movement of the mediastinum is known as mediastinal flutter.

The movement of air from one lung to the other has been referred to as "Pendelluft," and the situation is known to be extremely deleterious and often lethal. Such an inefficient movement of air reduces tidal exchange by a volume equal to that entering and escaping through the wound in the chest wall. There is then an inefficient exchange of oxygen and carbon dioxide. Open wounds that produce mediastinal flutter and "Pendelluft" have been referred to as sucking wounds. It is important to recognize that all wounds of the chest have the potential to produce this abnormality. No effort should be made to determine whether a significant collapse of the lung has occurred or whether there is significant mediastinal flutter but, rather, all wounds of the chest should be immediately closed with a sterile dressing. The closure of a large sucking wound must be regarded as an emergency procedure; in desperate cases the wound should be closed with any available material without regard for sterility.

In the most extreme situations a sucking wound of the chest produces the following picture: The patient is in considerable distress with signs of asphyxiation. His respirations are labored and his expiratory efforts seem forced. He may be cyanotic and hypotensive. Tachycardia is usually present. Frothy material may appear with expiration, and the sound of air rushing in and out of the wound can usually be detected. If there has not been significant injury to the lung, the patient's condition should stabilize when a sucking wound of the chest has been closed. His respiration will improve, and diagnosis and evaluation may proceed at a more leisurely pace. If a sucking wound of the chest has been complicated by the penetration of the underlying lung with a leak of air from pulmonary tissue, closure of the sucking wound will permit more rapid development of two other severe complications. The most important of these is tension pneumothorax. The other is the development of subcutaneous and mediastinal emphysema.

Tension Pneumothorax. In the presence of a significant parenchymal leak of air and maintained integrity of the chest wall, air is drawn from the lung into the pleural space with each inspiration and trapped there. As more air is drawn into the pleural space, collapse of the injured lung occurs and the mediastinum begins to shift toward the uninjured side. This reduces the function of the uninjured lung as well. As it becomes increasingly severe, it produces collapse of the major veins in the thorax. Many wounds of the lung stabilize without the development of these lethal abnormalities, but it is important to recognize that every patient with a penetrating wound of the chest that has been closed may develop tension pneumothorax. In the most severe form of tension pneumothorax, the patient is markedly dyspneic and appears to be suffocating. Cyanosis may be produced, and there is vascular collapse resulting from the cardiac embarrassment that occurs when there is prevention of an adequate venous return to the heart. This results in systemic hypotension, tachycardia and a reduction in the pulse pressure, which is easily confused with hypovolemic shock.

The diagnosis of tension pneumothorax is made by the detection of the physical signs of pneumothorax as well as by tracheal shift and displacement of the apical heart beat. Tracheal shift is discovered by simple palpation of the trachea in the neck just above the thoracic inlet. The diagnosis can be made with certainty by an x-ray examination of the chest, which will demonstrate pulmonary collapse and mediastinal shift. However, it is important that patients be positioned properly for this examination since rotation of the patient will produce confusing x-rays that obscure the diagnosis. Recognition of developing tension pneumothorax requires immediate aspiration of trapped air from the pleural space.

PHYSICAL SIGNS OF PNEUMOTHORAX. Physical signs of pneumothorax depend upon its extent and are minimal when only a small amount of air is trapped in the pleural space. Consequently, radiographic examination of the chest is a more reliable diagnostic tool than physical examination. The physical signs described here are those seen with extensive pneumothorax. Inspection of the patient reveals diminished respiratory excursion of the chest wall on the affected side. There is usually an increase in ventilatory rate. The patient complains of pain in the chest and, frequently, of shortness of breath. Percussion reveals hyperresonance and tympany and, if done with care, a mediastinal shift. Tactile fremitus is absent. Various signs of air and fluid in the pleural space have been described, including the "coin" test in which a coin is laid against the chest wall and tapped with another. This produces a particular metallic sound. In addition, one can frequently hear a succussion splash in which fluid in the pleura space moves about when the patient is moved. In addition to these signs, tension pneumothorax will produce mediastinal shifts and tracheal deviations.

Subcutaneous Emphysema and Mediastinal Emphysema. The combination of a chest wall wound and an underlying lung wound permits air under pressure in the pleural space to dissect into the tissue planes about the wound, especially when there is no open external communication. The presence of air in the subcutaneous tissues is called subcutaneous emphysema. The classic situation in which this condition develops is a compression injury of the chest producing fractures of the ribs that may result in stab wounds of the lung at a moment of extreme thoracic pressure. Air is then injected into the tissues about the fractured ends of the ribs. Mediastinal emphysema occurs most commonly when there is a rupture of the pulmonary parenchyma without significant damage to the visceral pleura. Air can leak along the peribronchial planes during inspiration, enter the mediastinum and travel toward the superior outlet of the thorax, continuing as subcutaneous emphysema that spreads over the neck, face, chest and the anterior abdominal wall. When fully developed the condition produces a frightening appearance but is usually not serious. On occasion, mediastinal emphysema has produced compression of mediastinal structures and has required cervical mediastinotomy for its relief. The physical signs of subcutaneous and mediastinal emphysema are swelling and crepitation in the subcutaneous tissues; frequently, it can be diagnosed before it progresses to cervical subcutaneous emphysema by the detection of a so-called crunching sound on auscultation over the sternum.

Hemothorax. In addition to pneumothorax and subcutaneous emphysema, penetrating wounds of the chest frequently produce hemothorax because of associated injuries to blood vessels in the lung or chest wall. Hemothorax, of course, occurs as a complication of injuries that do not destroy the integrity of the chest wall such as severe crushing injuries in which fractured ribs damage the underlying pleura and the lung parenchyma. When hemothorax occurs as a complication of a penetrating wound, pneumothorax is usually associated—a combination known as hemopneumothorax. The extent of bleeding within the pleural space depends upon the type of injury. When major vessels have been damaged, bleeding may be massive and death may occur quickly; lacerations of the lung, however, do not usually produce excessive bleeding. Blood pressure in the pulmonary circulation is low and the elastic qualities of pulmonary tissue allow for collapse and vessel retraction in areas of injury. Rapidly developing hemothorax usually indicates damage to a small systemic vessel or an intercostal artery. Blood in the pleural space, like air, produces collapse of the lung and eventual shifting of the mediastinum so that signs of respiratory embarrassment are combined with the signs of developing hypovolemia and also include percussion dullness and diminished or absent breath sounds. In cases of hemopneumothorax the signs of the pneumothorax tend to dominate, and rather extensive collections of blood within the pleural space produce a minimal physical sign. Consequently, the most reliable tool in the diagnosis of hemothorax as well as pneumothorax or hemopneumothorax is x-ray examination.

Penetrating Wounds of the Mediastinum. All penetrating wounds of the chest must be regarded as possible penetrating wounds of the mediastinum. Damage to the major airways, major vessels, esophagus and heart can occur, and such injury can be surprisingly occult. Mediastinal hemorrhage can be contained temporarily in a hematoma, but rupture may later produce fatal exsanguination. Undetected esophageal injuries can produce fatal mediastinitis, and major airway injuries produce rapidly developing and fatal mediastinal emphysema if not relieved by proper venting. Penetrating injuries of the heart with contained bleeding in the pericardium produce cardiac tamponade which results in progressive compression of the heart and obstruction of the great veins with diminished cardiac output and ultimate death. The most reliable sign of developing cardiac tamponade is a rise in the central venous pressure. In the evaluation of a patient with a penetrating wound of the chest, therefore, serial monitoring of venous pressure is essential.

A variety of other signs produced by cardiac tamponade either are unreliable or are also produced by other injuries. Examination for mediastinal widening is not reliable, for example, because rapid effusions may occur that do not appreciably enlarge the area of cardiac dullness or significantly change the size of the cardiac shadow on an x-ray examination. Dyspnea and pallid cyanosis, which occur in cardiac tamponade, are also complications of hemopneumothorax and tachycardia; systemic hypotension and diminution of the pulse pressure also appear in hypovolemia. Pulsus paradoxus, in which the systolic blood pressure falls with each inspiration, is a difficult physical sign to detect and so is considerably less reliable than serial monitoring of the venous pressure. Whenever mediastinal injury is suspected, a gastrograffin swallow should be obtained to rule out injury to the esophagus. Serial x-rays should be obtained to follow any changes in the contour of the mediastinal shadows. Foreign bodies lodged within the mediastinum should be observed fluoroscopically for evidence of movement; if it is noted, the relationship between such foreign bodies and the great vessels within the mediastinum should be determined through angiocardiography.

The management of cardiac tamponade and other mediastinal injuries is discussed in a later chapter.

Intrathoracic Injury with No Visible Evidence of Chest Wall Damage. Frequently, decelerating and crushing injuries produce intrathoracic damage without any visible evidence of chest wall damage. Such injury should always be suspected in the case of high velocity accidents and fall and crush injuries.

Lacerations of the Aorta. A syndrome of aortic laceration following deceleration is now well recognized. This laceration usually occurs at points of fixation of the aorta, most notably at the level of the left subclavian artery. The injury can be occult, at first producing only a small hematoma, but if unrecognized will lead to fatal exsanguination or formation of a traumatic aortic aneurysm. The diagnosis is suspected from observation of abnormal contours of the mediastinal shadows on roentgenographic examination and is confirmed by aortography.

Contusion of the Lung. Contusion injuries of the lung without evidence of chest wall damage produce intrapulmonary hemorrhage with dyspnea and hemoptysis. Physical signs are those of localized consolidation with diminished breath sounds and crepitant rales.

Contusion of the Heart. Contusion injury of the myocardium with intramyocardial hemorrhage occurs following blunt trauma to the chest. Such injury may be followed by cardiac arrhythmias and sudden death. When this condition is suspected, the patient should be followed with serial electrocardiograms to determine the presence of injury currents.

The Diagnosis of Intra-abdominal Injury

Intra-abdominal injury may be produced by blunt trauma or by a penetrating wound of the abdomen. When external wounds are evident, the examiner should immediately consider the possibility of intra-abdominal injury.

Closed Abdominal Injuries. The spleen, liver, stomach, intestines and pancreas are vulnerable to blunt injury. This may occur when the viscus is crushed against the vertebral column or is violently displaced on its mesenteric attachments. It is not unusual to have little or no evidence of intra-abdominal injury at the time of primary examination. Frequent examination of the abdomen is essential to discover early signs of injury. If there is reasonable doubt about the possibility of intraperitoneal injury, exploratory celiotomy is indicated. However, the severity of associated injuries must be weighed against the possibility of a negative exploration. It must be further recognized that the duration of the period of anesthesia and the postoperative recovery combined with analgesics may make it difficult to evaluate the extent or progression of other injuries. An alternative approach to routine, early celiotomy in cases of questionable intra-abdominal injury involves the use of peritoneal lavage. By instilling saline into the peritoneal cavity through a peritoneal dialysis catheter, and subsequently siphoning it back, very small amounts of hemorrhage can be detected. In addition, the retrieved fluid can be sent for a leukocyte count and an amylase determination, and can be examined for vegetable fibers under the microscope. Difficult cases can be observed with more confidence in the face of a negative lavage, while other cases can be brought to surgery earlier if the lavage is positive.

Injuries to the intra-abdominal viscera usually fall in certain general groups. One of these is laceration of the liver, resulting in intraperitoneal hemorrhage. The extent of hemorrhage varies widely, but if extensive—involving the major hepatic or portal veins—exsanguination and death may ensue. Minor degrees of laceration may produce bile peritonitis with serious consequences. In either instance, the physical signs shown by the patient are those of peritoneal irritation, possibly with shifting dullness, rebound tenderness and generalized peritonitis.

Splenic rupture is a very common injury and should be suspected when patients report blows on the left flank or left lower chest. The ribs overlying the area may or may not be fractured. Early physical signs may be unimpressive and feature only tachycardia and minimal abdominal tenderness. Later, abdominal pain may be severe and associated with shock and referred pain in the left shoulder. Physical examination usually reveals some indication of peritoneal irritation, which is most marked in the left upper quadrant. Diaphragmatic irritation may contribute to dyspnea. When there are minor lacerations of the spleen and continued slow bleeding, diagnosis may be difficult; continuing careful clinical evaluation is essential.

Mild degrees of trauma may produce subcapsular hematoma of the spleen, which may rupture several days or weeks later. Lateral abdominal x-rays may aid in differentiating this from retroperitoneal tumor masses, and an upright film of the abdomen after injection of a small amount of air through a nasogastric tube may reveal irregular margins of the hematoma in the gastrosplenic ligament. Recently, splenic scans and celiac axis arteriography have been of great help in making this difficult diagnosis. It is often helpful to know whether the patient had some pre-existing disease such as malaria, leukemia, infectious mononucleosis or other hematological disorder in which splenomegaly may be a prominent feature. In such patients splenic rupture may occur spontaneously or accompany minor degrees of trauma.

Compression of the intestine, particularly when filled with fluid, may lead to its rupture. The small intestine is more frequently involved than the large; and the commonest locations for perforation are at the ligament of Treitz, the terminal ileum, or at a point where an adhesion is present from previous surgery. These points are related to areas of fixation, which presumably limit the mobility of the bowel and contribute to the rupture. The duodenum and pancreas lie anterior to the spine and may be involved in a crushing injury against this bony structure. Pancreatic and duodenal injuries commonly occur together and carry a very high mortality. Laceration of the duodenum permits bowel contents to leak posteriorly into the retroperitoneum. Associated physical signs, such as spasm and abdominal rigidity, may be delayed.

Rupture of the large intestine is infrequently encountered. Lacerations of the large bowel mesentery may occur, however, resulting in hemorrhage, necrosis and gangrene. Patients with this type of injury may have considerable abdominal pain without early signs of peritonitis, and this diagnosis may be particularly difficult to make preoperatively.

Penetrating Wounds of the Abdomen. All patients with penetrating wounds of the abdominal wall caused by missiles that could have entered or traversed the peritoneal cavity require surgical exploration. This is not true, however, for stab wounds. With a high degree of accuracy it is possible to demonstrate penetration of the peritoneal cavity by the injection of radiopaque contrast material into the wound tract under local anesthesia. This technique permits one to rule out superficial, nonpenetrating stab wounds and possibly avoid unnecessary operation. If penetration is demonstrated, however, early operation is recommended. An alternative approach, called selective conservatism, requires admission to the hospital of all patients with abdominal stab wounds. Vital signs, the abdominal examination and the leukocyte count are monitored closely. If changes occur that suggest intraperitoneal injury, the patient is explored. Otherwise, in 24 to 48 hours the patient is discharged.

In performing the abdominal examination on a patient with a penetrating injury, several points are worth noting. When there are multiple wounds it is easy to overlook small wounds of entrance. It should be routine to inspect carefully the buttocks, perineum and anal canal as well as the obvious areas of the back, abdomen and flanks. Under certain circumstances the appearance of the wound and a discharge from it may provide information regarding the nature of the injury; the presence of intestinal contents or bile denotes specific visceral injury and indicates the need for prompt exploration. Small wounds of entrance necessitate a search for minor degrees of peritoneal irritation, including careful examination of the rectum and, when necessary, sigmoidoscopy without the use of air insufflation. The examiner must coordinate abdominal findings with those of the neurological examination since spinal cord injuries may either obscure or produce abdominal pain, rigidity and hypotension.

The development of pallor, sweating, restlessness and thirst following injury is significant, for it may indicate intra-abdominal hemorrhage resulting from laceration of the liver, spleen, mesenteric vessels or retroperitoneum. Other physical signs include the development of hypotension, rapid pulse rate with thready quality, dyspnea or "air hunger," shifting dullness and rebound tenderness. When there is massive hemorrhage the abdomen becomes progressively dull and distended. When the rate of hemorrhage is slower, normal blood pressure may be maintained for several hours. It is obviously important to follow pulse pressure and pulse rate with great care and not to be completely dependent upon the absolute systolic and diastolic arterial pressures. The course of the indices and physical signs is more significant in most instances than the actual initial value. With slow, continued bleeding, for instance, progressive abdominal tenderness and spasm may be evident.

Perforation of a hollow viscus is associated with abdominal rigidity, tenderness and absence of bowel sounds; it may be accompanied by abdominal pain and vomiting. These features tend to become more prominent as time elapses following injury. It is possible to overlook early signs of visceral perforation in the presence of multiple injuries and when analgesics or sedatives have been administered. When shock develops eight to 12 hours after injury, generalized peritonitis must also be considered as a cause. In this instance tachypnea and the characteristic anxious facies may be present.

Continuing blood loss with or without peritonitis may lead to "irreversible shock." The examiner should not be too quick to pronounce the hypotension irreversible, for he may simply be underestimating fluid losses. It is true, however, that failure of vital signs to return to normal after what appears to be adequate replacement transfusion carries with it a poor prognosis. One must be certain that a remediable lesion is not contributing to the patient's deteriorating clinical condition. Tension pneumothorax or cardiac tamponade may easily occur in association with intra-abdominal injury. Continual re-evaluation of the patient is required to be certain that the working diagnosis is accurate.

The Evaluation of Arterial Injury

The diagnosis of injury to a major artery is not usually a problem since such injury frequently produces a pulsatile hemorrhage or obvious acute ischemia in the part supplied by the damaged vessel. However, this is not always the case; the injury to a major vessel may sometimes be occult, with no or only slowly developing signs of ischemia and without much evidence of severe external hemorrhage. It is no longer a tenable view that the primary concern in major artery injury is the adequate control of hemorrhage. With the development of adequate techniques for arterial reconstruction, it has become increasingly important to make an early and accurate diagnosis of arterial injury so that circulation can be completely restored. Pulsatile and excessive wound hemorrhage should be controlled with pressure until an appropriate exploration of the wound can be performed under operating room conditions. Major vessels that can be reconstructed should never be blindly clamped and sutured.

In the absence of pulsatile hemorrhage, the most accurate sign of major vessel damage is distal pulselessness. For this reason an important part of the physical examination of the acutely injured patient is an examination of the pulses bilaterally in the neck and in the upper and lower extremities. Although it is true that in the absence of pre-existing arterial disease pulselessness is a definite sign of acute arterial injury, such injury may occur without the development of the pulselessness. It is even possible to have a completely severed artery and maintenance of distal pulses, and thus it is important that pulses be compared with their opposite member. Ischemia of a part produces pallor or pallid cyanosis and changes in temperature, with the ischemic part being cooler than the perfused part. In the conscious patient pain is a prominent symptom of ischemia; in time, associated neurological ischemia will produce sensory changes of paresthesia and anesthesia as well as motor changes of weakness and paralysis.

Major arterial damage occurs in a variety of ways, including laceration without loss of substance, laceration with loss of substance, external compression when an artery is impinged upon by a bony fragment or occlusion without loss of continuity due to subintimal hemorrhage or fracture of the vascular intima with arterial dissection. These latter two types of injury were formerly frequently attributed to arterial spasm and treated inappropriately.

Because of the occult nature of major vascular injuries, the suggestion has been made that all wounds in the vicinity of major vessels deserve a surgical exploration. Such a policy is at times impractical, and with the availability of arteriography is usually unnecessary. It is certainly true, however, that all wounds with pulsatile hemorrhage, rapidly expanding hematomas or pulsatile hematomas deserve surgical exploration. It is also true that the finding of pulselessness with signs of distal ischemia is an indication for surgical exploration. When the diagnosis of major vessel damage is in doubt, serially recorded observations related to the quality of pulse, temperature, color and sensory and motor activity of the affected part should be made. Arteriography has a definite and important part to play in the evaluation of arterial injury. It provides a certain diagnosis without long observation, precise localization of the wound and an estimate of collateral circulation. False negative results in arteriographic evaluation of vascular injury have been noted, but they are extremely rare. The technique has the disadvantage of being somewhat time consuming but when properly performed carries with it little hazard.

Initial Evaluation of the Burned Patient

A later chapter in this text is concerned with the complex subject of the management of the burned patient. The successful management of such a patient can be carried out only with the aid of repeated evaluation of the patient's wound and the burn shock that it has produced. The initial evaluation of such a patient, which is only the first of many evaluations, has two main functions. It must first be established whether the burn has produced respiratory injury. This is done by examining the nasal and oral airways for evidence of burn and by detecting evidence of hoarseness, crowing, coughing or ventilatory abnormality. When a severe burn has been sustained in a closed space and when there are significant burns of the face, head or neck, such respiratory damage must be anticipated. The diagnosis of respiratory burn alerts one to the possible need for tracheostomy.

The other objective of the initial examination is to estimate the severity of the burn. It must be remembered that all burns of the hands, feet or face, all burns of the aged and the very young, and all burns that involve more than 10 per cent of the body area must be considered serious and therefore require hospitalization. A record of the seriously burned patient's vital signs should be established early in the period of evaluation. This should include the pulse rate, rate of respiration, blood pressure and weight when they can be obtained. In planning and initiating treatment of burn shock, an estimate of the percentage area of the body burned and of the depth of burn are valuable. The "rule of nines" by which portions of the body are assigned 9 or 18 per cent is a helpful and adequate technique for quickly estimating the area of the burn.

The depth of the burn is considerably more difficult and is likely to be underestimated. Flame burns may be assumed to be full thickness. Full thickness burns may assume a variety of appearances, including a brown color with a leathery charred appearance, white and cadaveric, oily and transparent with the obvious thrombosed vessel or with large broken blisters. Blister formation, which was considered characteristic of second degree burns, is frequently seen with deeper burns. The fluid shifts accompanying burns may be rapid and extensive. The dynamics involved in their estimation and correction are those associated with hypovolemia.

The situation is further complicated by infection and by heat, water and energy losses through the damaged skin. Detailed consideration of these special problems is included in Chapter 20.

Diagnosis of Neurological Injury

A thorough history of the circumstances surrounding craniocerebral trauma and the postinjury behavior of the patient often provide information significant in diagnosis and treatment. Witnesses of the accident or people who have observed the patient immediately after injury should be carefully questioned regarding his state of consciousness, duration of unconsciousness, ability to move his extremities, ability to speak, confusion or disorientation and the presence of convulsions.

It is obvious that complete evaluation of the patient's physical condition is necessary and that initial treatment must be instituted as indicated. Patients with craniocerebral trauma frequently have associated airway obstruction or difficulties with ventilation that require primary attention. Once the pressing demands for evaluation of the patient's over-all condition and emergency treatment of life-threatening injury are cared for, neurological examination may be performed. This type of emergency neurological examination has three objectives: to obtain base line neurological information for later comparison, to establish the diagnosis of the existence of a head injury and to determine the need for emergency surgical intervention.

A few carefully selected neurological studies will often offer sufficient information to permit adequate initial treatment. A time-consuming and detailed neurological examination is not appropriate for the early care of head injury patients. The state of consciousness should be carefully evaluated, as well as the patient's response to painful stimulation. This may be obtained by noting response to supra-orbital pressure, pinprick or pressure on the sternum. The relative size, equality and response to light of the pupils of the patient's eyes should be observed early and carefully recorded. Small, contracted pupils that do not respond to light may be associated with midbrain damage. The administration of medication or the patient's recent consumption of alcohol may render this sign misleading. The presence of dilated fixed pupils usually indicates a poor prognosis. Inequality of the pupils may reflect local brain damage. Unilateral dilatation of the pupils, particularly when it occurs under observation, is strongly suggestive of intracranial hemorrhage.

The character of respiration may assist in diagnosis, since irregular or depressed respirations frequently accompany severe intracranial injury. If respiratory alterations persist with an adequate airway, the prognosis is grave.

The degree of the patient's motor activity should be evaluated. If the patient is conscious, this is easily appraised by having him squeeze the examiner's hands or by testing his ability to resist passive motion of the extremities. In the comatose patient this should be tested by determining the degree of flaccidity by lifting the extremity slightly and letting it drop. It should be emphasized that both sides of the patient should be tested. This permits comparison and provides base line information that is helpful as observation of his condition continues. Extensor rigidity of the extremities also carries a poor prognosis. Alcoholism or drug intoxication may confuse this issue, but complete flaccidity and areflexia are usually indications of severe central nervous system damage.

Body temperature should be recorded early and followed with care. When associated with evidence of intracranial injury, the development of hyperthermia is of significance. Fever in excess of 103° Fahrenheit indicates a bad prognosis.

Simple evaluation of the deep tendon reflexes is adequate for the initial examination. The triceps, biceps, radial-periosteal, plantar, knee and ankle reflexes, with a test for the presence of ankle clonus, should be sufficient for initial evaluation and later comparison.

One should be particularly cautious in handling a patient who is able to move his arms but whose legs are immobile. He should be regarded as having a fractured spine and spinal cord injury until it is proved otherwise. Evaluation of the level of injury should include determination of a sensory level and response to painful stimuli. X-rays of the spine should be included among the diagnostic procedures, and care should be exercised that manual traction is applied to the neck and feet to avoid flexion of the spine during movement.

The patient's head should be carefully inspected and palpated for lacerations and depressions in the skull. Bleeding from the ear without an obvious source of laceration strongly suggests basilar skull fracture involving the temporal bone. The eardrums should be inspected routinely for the presence of blood in the middle ear. Bleeding from the nose, often due to local trauma, may also indicate involvement of the paranasal sinuses by a fracture. Many of these fractures are difficult to visualize on skull films, and one should be acutely aware that a blood or cerebrospinal fluid leak into the middle ear or the sinuses provides ready access for invasion of the subarachnoid spaces, leading to meningitis or brain abscess. Consequently, antibiotic coverage is indicated in patients with these findings.

The significance of a simple linear skull fracture as seen on x-rays of the skull depends on possible injury to the central nervous system, signs and symptoms of which would be present in the individual patient. This finding should not in itself alter the over-all program of management. A depressed skull fracture is a result of direct trauma with an instrument or missile of some kind. The resulting brain damage may be extremely variable and, again, the importance of the finding depends on the neurological signs and symptoms present in that individual patient. One should, however, suspect a depressed skull fracture in all patients with lacerated or contused wounds of the scalp. The diagnosis of a depressed skull fracture is usually an indication for prompt surgical intervention. Failure to do so may result in progressive neurological deterioration or infection.

Penetrating wounds of the skull may be particularly misleading. Extensive intracranial injury may be associated with a very small wound of entrance obscured by hair. Early surgical exploration and debridement are indicated.

Cerebral concussion is associated with loss of consciousness and, often, memory loss regarding the time of the accident. Although the patient may appear to be well when first seen, careful, repeated observation is of vital importance because the possibility of delayed intracranial hemorrhage is always present.

Intracranial hemorrhage may be either extradural or subdural in location. Characteristically, a brief period of unconsciousness may be noted, followed by a "lucid interval," then confusion, drowsiness and progressive coma. When the hemorrhage is extradural in location, the sequence of events tends to be fairly rapid—often developing over a period of minutes or hours. With the development of a subdural hemorrhage the course may be extended over several weeks or even months. In either event, the presence of lateralizing neurologic signs, asymmetrical dilatation of the pupils and alteration in the deep tendon reflexes and motor responses should be sufficient to prompt neurosurgical diagnostic and operative steps.

Attention is often so focused on a head injury that associated injuries such as those of the cervical, dorsal or lumbar spine may be overlooked. A thorough evaluation is essential to the patient's over-all well-being. Fractures or fracture dislocations of the spine usually result from violent trauma and may occur independently or in association with head injury. Evaluation of suspected spine injury must be completed without disturbing the patient. This applies to his initial evaluation and transportation from the scene of the injury as well as to his diagnosis and therapy upon entrance into the hospital. Failure to observe this rule may result in irreversible injury to the spinal cord. The cervical spine, because of its mobility, is particularly susceptible to injury, and it is essential that gentle traction be exerted on the head and the long axis of the spine whenever a patient with a suspected spinal injury is moved. Flexion of the neck or any portion of the spine must be avoided. In general, the patient should be permitted as little motion as possible and transported in the prone or supine position without rotation, flexion or extension of the spine.

Injury of the spinal cord may be evaluated by asking the patient to move his legs and toes. If he can do this, he has escaped major cord damage. If the legs are paralyzed but the patient is able to move his hands, the spinal cord injury is located below the cervical region. If arm function is faulty, cervical spine involvement is likely. More precise localization of cord injury may be obtained by testing for loss of sensation to pinprick.

DIAGNOSIS OF PERIPHERAL NERVE INJURIES

Extensive wounds of the soft tissues and long bones of the extremities occur in both military and civilian life. Peripheral nerve injuries frequently accompany these injuries; the radial nerve, for example, may be injured if there are fractures about the elbow. Common peroneal nerve involvement may occur with fractures, soft tissue wounds or tight casts that produce pressure about the knee; and the sciatic nerve may be damaged by dislocations or fractures of the hip. Lacerations about the wrist may produce damage to median or ulnar nerves, and traction on the upper extremity may result in damage to the brachial plexus.

Peripheral nerve damage involves lower motor neuron axons as well as sensory nerves. The result is a flaccid type of paralysis. Early diagnosis may depend on loss of voluntary muscle power or absence of perception of pinprick. Inadequate treatment produces such late results as muscular atrophy, sensory loss and autonomic changes. Distally, the skin becomes thinned and smooth, often pale or mottled. Sweating is absent and fingernails and toenails become brittle.

Partial damage to a peripheral nerve may result in causalgia, which develops soon after injury or requires several days to make its appearance. This condition is characterized by constant, intense, burning pain and is worsened by touching or moving, minor trauma, excitement or temperature change. The sciatic and median nerves are those commonly involved. Characteristically, in this lesion peripheral nerve injury is incomplete, although the skin often tends to be shiny and glossy. Blocking the related sympathetic pathways may produce prompt relief of the pain of causalgia, and this observation may assist in making the diagnosis.

Diagnosis of Musculoskeletal Injury

Injuries to the musculoskeletal system are among the most common encountered in emergency services. Fractures make up the bulk of these injuries, often including joint involvement. Certain general physical signs, including local tenderness, deformity, loss of function, abnormal range of motion and crepitus, are common to all fractures. There may be additional physical findings associated with injury to soft tissue, peripheral nerves and blood vessels. In many instances, diagnosis will be apparent on the basis of simple physical examination. If this is the case, it is unnecessary, and indeed contraindicated, to demonstrate such physical signs as abnormal range of motion or crepitus. To do so may simply cause the patient extreme discomfort and increase local soft tissue damage. Prompt x-ray examination is of much greater value in determining the extent of the injury.

Fractures should be splinted before the patient is moved from the scene of the accident. If standard external splints are not readily available, improvised splints may be prepared from pillows, boards or doors. Early splinting minimizes discomfort, limits local extravasation and loss of blood and prevents the secondary damage that may occur from displacing fracture fragments, with associated laceration of blood vessels, nerves or other soft tissues. Careful evaluation of the patient for fractures should be included as a part of the general evaluation of the patient upon his arrival on the emergency service. Detailed description of diagnosis and treatment of fractures is included in Chapter Sixteen.

Injury of the Urinary Tract

Upper urinary tract injuries primarily involving the kidney are usually encountered with either blunt or penetrating abdominal trauma. Renal injuries may vary from simple contusion to severe laceration of the renal parenchyma. The latter may also involve extensive damage to the vascular pedicle of the kidney. In adults the kidney is protected to some degree from direct trauma. The bony chest cage, the lumbar spine and the vertebral muscles as well as the perinephric fat and Gerota's fascia offer protection. In infants and children the kidney occupies a lower position and is less well protected by perirenal fat and a poorly developed Gerota's fascia. As a result, children are more susceptible to renal injury. Renal trauma in adults is more often seen in men because of their greater exposure to automobile injury, athletic activities and industrial accidents.

Renal trauma can usually be detected by the presence of flank pain and hematuria. The amount of blood loss is variable but it is rarely exsanguinating. This obviously depends on the extent of the renal injury, whether parenchymal damage is accompanied by laceration of the renal capsule and the extent of involvement of the vascular pedicle. When parenchymal damage is associated with damage to the collecting system, hematuria and sometimes extravasation of urine into the renal fossa and flank result. The combination of hemorrhage and urinary extravasation may produce muscle spasm, tenderness and flank dullness. A mass may be palpable and, in some instances, detectable on inspection. Additional physical signs include ecchymoses in the flank, nonshifting flank dullness, and a positive psoas sign produced by extravasation of blood and urine over the psoas muscle.

Renal trauma is often associated with injury of the spleen or liver. If it can be accomplished with safety, an intravenous pyelogram is of great assistance in evaluating the patient's condition. This furnishes information regarding the extent of injury to the involved kidney, as well as evidence of the functional state of the kidney on the uninvolved side. If the contrast medium is injected intravenously into a femoral vein at the same time a flat abdominal x-ray is obtained, additional information about the state of the inferior vena cava can be obtained. The need for direct surgical intervention depends on the extent of the injury involved. The presence of an enlarging renal mass associated with signs of blood loss may make operation necessary but requires careful evaluation and is somewhat dependent upon the patient's condition. Recently, arteriography has been vitally important in evaluating the extent of renal injury, and is essential if attempts are to be made to preserve renal mass by partial nephrectomies. The presence of extravasated urine makes surgery mandatory to provide adequate drainage and conservation of renal tissue.

Injuries to the lower urinary tract are usually associated with fractures of the pelvis. Rupture of the bladder is the most common injury of the lower tract and is present in about 10 per cent of cases of pelvic fracture. In most instances, rupture of the bladder is of the extraperitoneal type, although in about 20 per cent the rupture is intraperitoneal. Extraperitoneal rupture is usually produced by chips of bone perforating the bladder wall and is associated with extravasation of urine into the extraperitoneal tissues, causing infection. Intraperitoneal rupture of the bladder is associated with a laceration of the dome of the bladder due to sudden compression of the full viscus; this, too, is associated with serious infection. The diagnosis is usually not difficult; the patient is unable to void or perhaps voids only a few drops of bloody urine. If the patient successfully voids clear urine after the accident, it is reasonably safe to assume that no serious injury to the lower urinary tract has resulted. Physical findings include deep tenderness, spasms of the lower abdominal muscles and peritoneal irritation, usually with rebound tenderness. Rectal examination demonstrates diffused tenderness with a normal prostate and membranous urethra. Catheterization should be performed early, and if bloody urine is obtained, urinary tract damage should be suspected. A cystogram should be performed in the anteroposterior and, in some instances, lateral positions. Intravenous pyelography should be performed if the initial evaluation and treatment indicate absence of other critical injury.

Injury of the bladder neck or membranous urethra is also common. The membranous portion of the urethra is particularly prone to injury at the level at which the urethra perforates the triangular ligament. Fractures of the pubic bone frequently disrupt this ligament and result in displacement of the proximal and distal segments of the lacerated urethra. This injury results in extravasation of urine into the tissues surrounding the bladder and lower abdominal wall. The extravasation extends laterally and the area is markedly tender; rectal examination is helpful in localizing the area of injury. When the prostatic urethra is damaged, the prostate gland is surrounded by a boggy tender mass. With laceration of the urogenital diaphragm, urine and blood are extravasated into the perineum. These physical findings are indications for early surgical intervention involving suprapubic exploration to permit re-establishment of urethral continuity.

Rupture of the vesicle neck and prostatic urethra combine the physical findings of both rupture of the bladder and rupture of the urethra. Since injuries of the lower urinary tract occur in conjunction with pelvic fractures, simple testing for lateral compression of the pelvis is useful in diagnosis. Once fracture of the pelvis is suspected, diagnostic measures to determine the extent of urinary tract injury should be undertaken.

THE SEARCH FOR OCCULT INJURY

Certain regions of the body do not readily permit usual techniques of physical examination. These may include the cranium, the vertebral column and the bony thorax. Under certain circumstances these protective bony envelopes or their contents may be injured without demonstrating classic clinical signs. For example, linear skull fractures or compression fractures of the spine may not be accompanied by neurological changes; in other instances, x-ray examination is much more accurate and effective in detecting subtle pulmonary mediastinal or cardiac changes than are the usual techniques of percussion and auscultation. Reference has been made to selected x-ray studies in relation to a variety of injuries. Certain general examinations are of considerable value and, as a general rule, should be obtained. Common sense should dictate when radiological studies will contribute to successful management. Under certain urgent circumstances, operative intervention is more important than obtaining a complete set of films. In situations of this kind only films that vitally affect important decisions are indicated.

With this understanding it is clear that the standard-sized chest film is of great value in providing accurate information about the condition of the heart and lungs. If the clinical situation permits, the film should be obtained in the upright position. A flat film of the abdomen is important if abdominal trauma has occurred. Free air from a perforated viscus may be detected by an upright or a lateral decubitus film. Intraperitoneal or retroperitoneal fluid may be detected by local loss of the psoas shadow. Pleural effusion may indicate subdiaphragmatic irritation, and so on.

X-ray examination of the skull is an important part of the evaluation of patients with head injury. It should be emphasized, however, that proper timing is important. To obtain satisfactory films of good quality, the cooperation of the patient is essential; and this is frequently impossible early after injury when manipulation of the patient may be hazardous. Skull films should be obtained when the patient's condition is stable, but since their principal value lies in the recognition of skull fractures that require specific treatment, these studies should be completed as soon as the general condition permits. It should also be recognized that the types of intracranial hemorrhage requiring prompt surgical intervention will be detected by observation of vital signs and neurologic examination rather than on the basis of an x-ray study alone.

It should be noted that radiologists are frequently helpful consultants in the diagnosis and management of injured patients. On many occasions the radiologist can recommend the films and techniques that will be of greatest value with least risk to the patient. Whenever possible, the case should be discussed with him for suggestions for obtaining the most meaningful data. Failure to enlist the cooperation of the radiologist may result in much wasted time and effectiveness at the expense of the patient's welfare.

chapter

2

THE PATHOPHYSIOLOGY OF TRAUMA AND SHOCK

Robert B. Rutherford, M.D.

TRAUMA

The term "trauma" encompasses a wide range of insults to the body. Even individual wounds take a wide variety of forms—a crushing blow, a jagged laceration, a missile penetration, a burn, a bite. It is natural to consider trauma primarily as the result of the body's striking, or being struck by, some object; but one must also consider injuries inflicted by chemical, electrical or thermal insult and those caused by changes in environmental pressure or gravitational force. Some injuries have diffuse systemic effects; others mainly involve one or two organ systems. Considerable variation is possible even among wounds of the same type. For example, the local damage from a gunshot wound depends on the mass and particularly the velocity of the missile; the degree of burn varies with the temperature and duration of contact with the burning agent; and deceleration injuries are largely determined by the victim's mass, the rate of deceleration and the surface area of the body over which the energy is dissipated. Finally, the effects of an injury may be modified significantly by personal and environmental factors such as age, sex, nutritional status, intercurrent disease, local contamination, ambient temperature, and so forth.

It is not possible to incorporate such an array of variables into a simple, uniform description of the effects of trauma on the body. In this chapter, emphasis is placed only on the general, local and systemic effects and responses to trauma. The specific effects of other contributing factors will be discussed in the presentation of the injuries to which they pertain.

LOCAL RESPONSE—THE WOUND

As Rhoads and Howard have emphasized, "It is incorrect to assume (after the initial wounding) that the injury has now been inflicted."[118] The injury will continue being inflicted until its components have been corrected or arrested. The major components of injury are tissue destruction, blood loss, mechanical defects and superimposed infections. Their local effects can be better appreciated if one first considers the events that normally occur in healing a simple, clean incision—a wound in which the contributions of these components are minimal.

Phases of Healing. The initial phase of wound healing is the period before tensile strength develops in the wound—the "lag" phase. However, it is by no means a quiescent period. There is increased vascularity with an outpouring of plasma and a diapedesis of leukocytes and macrophages into the wound area. Trauma always invokes a true inflammatory reaction which is at least initially indistinguishable from that caused by bacterial infection or physical or chemical agents. Damaged tissue is broken down and removed. Hexosamines derived from plasma glycoproteins accumulate locally and, in turn, are converted into a mucopolysaccharide ground substance by a process that appears to involve mast cells and requires methionine.[63] Because of these activities, this period has been called the "inflammatory," "catabolic," or "substrate" phase.

The second phase, called the "collagen," "productive" or "fibroblastic" phase, is characterized by the deposition of collagen and a progressive increase in the tensile strength of the wound. Fibrin deposition in the injured area provides the lattice-work for the invasion of fibroblasts derived from neighboring, undifferentiated mesenchymal cells. It is thought that the mucopolysaccharide ground substance provides the medium in which procollagen, a protein component of the fibroblast, is converted into collagen fibrils.[44] This process can be quantitated by the hydroxyproline content of the wound.

Hydroxyproline is found, ostensibly, only in collagen and its precursors. It is not incorporated into the collagen molecule as such. Rather, proline is first incorporated and is later hydroxylated as the molecule is being built up into triple helical coils held together by hydrogen bonds.[6, 160] Hydroxyproline and hydroxylysine are important factors in the stability of this helical structure. This ability to hydroxylate proline and lysine appears to be limited to fibroblasts, and this process appears to be the site of the essential action of ascorbic acid (vitamin C) in wound healing. The reaction also requires ferrous ion and alpha-ketoglutarate as well as molecular oxygen. The collagen content begins to level off at 10 to 12 days, and tensile strength reaches a temporary plateau by 10 days to two weeks.

In the final phase, there is a maturation of the collagen into a strong weave by a process of remolding and inter- and intramolecular cross-linkages. This is more important than the amount of collagen itself in determining the final tensile strength of the wound for, as Douglas has shown, the wound's tensile strength at the end of two weeks is only one-fifth its eventual maximum.[42] This maturation process may take six weeks or more.

Adverse Influences. The major components of injury—tissue destruction, blood loss, mechanical defects and superimposed infection—all influence wound healing adversely. Destroyed tissue delays wound healing because of the additional time required for its catabolism and clearance. It serves, along wilth extravasated blood plasma, as an ideal medium in which bacteria can multiply beyond the body's first line of defense. The pressure effects of hematomas and seromas are greater than generally appreciated and, along with the mechanical effects of tissue disruption, interfere significantly with wound healing. Avoiding tension is, of course, one of the cardinal rules in promoting wound healing. Extravasated blood has been shown to have a synergistic effect on the activity of certain bacteria, particularly *Escherichia coli*. Furthermore, if enough blood is lost so that shock ensues, the body's defense mechanisms against bacterial invasion may be greatly impaired.[111]

Simple bacterial contamination of the wound is not, in itself, a significant deterrent to normal wound healing. It occurs to some degree in nearly all "clean" surgical wounds.[23] However, in the presence of a dead space, foreign body, extravasated blood or devitalized tissue, bacterial multiplication will occur. This not only perpetuates the inflammatory phase of wound healing but delays the accumulation of factors essential to wound healing, since these factors also serve as bacterial substrates.

Local vascularity normally influences the rate of wound healing, as contrasted in the healing rates of facial and extremity wounds. Similarly, any factor that interferes with circulation to the wound, from arterial occlusion to anti-inflammatory drugs, will retard healing. The vascular bed in the area of the wound may be damaged directly by a sharp blow, a crushing injury or a burn, or be compromised later by the pressure of extravasated blood and edema. Similarly, a laceration may interrupt a significant portion of the circulation to the wound area. This is particularly true of oblique lacerations and partial avulsions. Interruption of the major arterial supply to the wound area, even if it does not produce actual ischemia, may impede the vascular response that assembles the elements necessary for wound healing at the wound site. Experience with pedicle flaps has shown that impaired venous outflow with secondary edema is equally harmful.

Because of difficulties in controlling the various components of injury independently and because the underlying mechanisms of wound healing have not yet been fully elucidated even in the simplest of wounds, very little actual investigation into the healing of wounds of violence has been made. Although it is clear that the cumulative effects of these components of injury are a significant deterrent to wound healing and, in turn, magnify and prolong the systemic effects of injury, we do not yet have any quantitative estimates of these effects on which to base our care of such wounds (e.g., the proper time for suture removal, for resumption of normal use of the injured part, and so on).

Certain drugs and a few disease states may have an adverse influence on wound healing.[63] Among the most important of these are cortisone therapy, some cancer chemotherapy and immunosuppressive drugs, diabetes, congestive heart failure, uremia,[108] scurvy and severe hypoproteinemia. More remarkable, however, is how little systemic conditions interfere with wound healing. "The primacy of the wound," the ability to heal a wound even while the body is in a continued state of catabolism, is still one of the great wonders, and mysteries, of the body.

THE SYSTEMIC EFFECTS OF INJURY

Just as there are gradations in the severity of the wound itself, so there are corresponding variations in its systemic effects. Following Churchill's concept that the severity of a wound is the sum of all factors acting in the direction of deterioration, Moore and Ball used a scale of ten in grading various forms of trauma (mainly operative procedures) according to severity.[101] Howard and Ladd devised a point system in evaluating battle casualties of the Korean War based on the injury itself, treatment delay and response to therapy.[71] Recently, the A.M.A.'s Committee on the Medical Aspects of Automotive Safety have developed a more comprehensive rating system, an abbreviated outline of which is presented in Table 2–1. Such systems are valuable in correlating studies on systemic responses to trauma but are of only relative value in quantitating the response of an individual patient to trauma.

Metabolic Response to Injury. Systemic or metabolic effects of trauma are commonly described in terms of

TABLE 2–1 INJURY DESCRIPTION

Injury Category *Severity Code*	GENERAL	HEAD AND NECK	CHEST	ABDOMINAL	EXTREMITIES
No Injury 0	None	None	None	None	None
Minor 1	Minor lacerations, contusions and abrasions. All 1°, small 2° and 3° burns.	Cerebral injury without loss of consciousness. "Whiplash" without vertebral damage. Ocular abrasions and contusions.	Minor chest wall contusions, abrasions.	Muscle contusions; seat belt abrasion.	Minor sprains and fractures, and/or dislocation of digits.
Moderate 2	Extensive contusions, abrasions; large lacerations; avulsions (<3" diameter) 10-20% 2° or 3° burns.	Cerebral injury with <15 minutes unconsciousness; no amnesia. Undisplaced skull or facial bone fractures. Eye lacerations, retinal detachment. "Whiplash" with vertebral injury.	Simple rib or sternal fractures. Major contusions of chest wall without hemo- or pneumothorax, or respiratory embarrassment.	Major contusion of abdominal wall without intraabdominal injury.	Compound fractures of digits or nose. Undisplaced long bone or pelvic fractures. Major joint sprains.
Severe 3 (not life-threatening)	Extensive contusions or abrasions; large lacerations or avulsions (>3" diameter). 20-30% 2° or 3° burns.	Cerebral injury with unconsciousness >15 minutes without severe neurologic signs; <3 hours post-traumatic amnesia. Displaced closed skull fractures without signs of intracranial injury. Loss of eye, or avulsion of optic nerve. Facial bone fractures, displaced or without antral or orbital involvement. Cervical spine fractures without cord damage.	Multiple rib fracture without respiratory embarrassment Simple hemo- or pneumothorax. Rupture of diaphragm. Moderate pulmonary contusion.	Contusion of abdominal organs. Extraperitoneal bladder rupture. Retroperitoneal hemorrhage. Avulsion of ureter. Laceration of urethra. Thoracic or lumbar spine fractures without neurologic involvement.	Displaced simple long bone fractures, and/or multiple hand and foot fractures. Single open long bone fractures. Pelvic fractures with displacement. Dislocation of major joints. Lacerations of major nerves or vessels of extremities.
Severe 4 (Life-threatening, survival probable)	Severe lacerations and/or avulsions with dangerous hermorrhage. 30-50% 2° or 3° burns.	Cerebral injury with or without skull fracture, with unconsciousness of >15 minutes with definite abnormal neurologic signs; post-traumatic amnesia 3-12 hours. Compound skull fracture.	Open chest wounds; flail chest; pneumomediastinum; myocardial contusion and pericardial injuries without circulatory embarrassment.	Minor lacerations of intra-abdominal viscera including kidney, spleen and tail of pancreas. Intraperitoneal bladder rupture. Avulsion of genitals. Dorsal and/or lumbar spine fractures with paraplegia.	Multiple closed long bone fractures. Amputation of limbs.
Critical 5 (Survival uncertain)	Over 50% 2° or 3° burns.	Cerebral injury with unconsciousness of >24 hours; post-traumatic amnesia >12 hours; intracranial hemorrhage; signs of increased intracranial pressure. Cervical spine injury with quadriplegia. Major airway obstruction.	Chest injuries with major respiratory embarrassment (laceration of trachea, hemomediastinum, etc.). Aortic laceration. Myocardial rupture or contusion with circulatory embarrassment.	Rupture, avulsion, or severe laceration of abdominal vessels or organs, except kidney, spleen or ureter.	Multiple open limb fractures.

fluid and electrolyte shifts, endocrine activity, nitrogen balance and weight change. Most investigators in this field, with certain justification, equate operative and non-operative trauma and, for the sake of simplicity, concentrate on responses to common surgical procedure to obtain reasonably comparable data.

Most traumatic states are not suitable for this type of study, not only because of problems in quantitating the severity of the injury but also because of the lack of baseline values and the variable nature of measures required in resuscitation and definitive treatment. The other important distinction is that operative trauma, particularly abdominal procedures, causes a greater degree of interference with alimentation than non-operative trauma. Nevertheless, the basic patterns that have been observed after operation are felt to be reasonably representative of post-traumatic states as well. Moore's description of the sequence of systemic events characterizing the response to trauma forms the basis for much of the discussion that follows.[99]

Initial Phase. During the initial phase after injury there is increased adrenergic activity, reflected by increased urinary excretion of catecholamines and their breakdown products and by elevation of blood glucose and free fatty acid levels. Clinically, this adrenergic response may be evident in the patient's sweating, restlessness, tachycardia and vasoconstriction—signs that may be mistaken for impending shock. These effects rarely persist beyond the second day.

Heightened adrenocortical activity is expected after such stress, and both blood and urine steroid levels are elevated for three to four days. Adrenocortical activity is thought to have an important supporting or permissive function since adrenalectomized animals tolerate stress and trauma poorly, but the exact mechanisms involved have not been elucidated. Increased capillary permeability and negative nitrogen balance characterize this period and can be ascribed, in part, to this steroid activity. However, the negative nitrogen balance, signifying a degree of catabolic imbalance, also reflects the breakdown of injured tissues, decreased oral intake and immobilization. Potassium is lost along with nitrogen, in excess of the ratio lost with simple protein catabolism. This may be a reflection of the changes in the efficiency of the cell membrane ion pump or merely represent increased aldosterone secretion. Aldosterone activity also leads to the retention of sodium and water, a response that may be marked after injury. Additional sodium-free water is often retained because of activity of the antidiuretic hormone of the posterior pituitary hypothalamic axis. Even in the absence of skeletal trauma, calcium is mobilized, probably in response to the patient's immobilization. Magnesium, like sodium, tends to be retained, and chloride is thought to shift in the same direction but to a lesser degree.

Except for sodium and potassium, these ion shifts are rarely reflected by changes in their serum levels. Even serum sodium and potassium levels may be misleading. After major trauma, sodium is retained by the kidneys and even shifts into the cell, so that the total body sodium may be quite high; yet because of additional water retained or, as is more often the case, administered intravenously, the serum sodium may be low. Similarly, the converse applies in that if there is a significant antidiuresis, potassium may be released from the tissues faster than it can be excreted, so that the serum potassium may be high despite a negative potassium balance.

After trauma, the levels of inorganic phosphate rise consistently. Several factors are involved here—diminished renal clearance, the release of phosphate from tissue breakdown and the mobilization of bone salts and, possibly, in the severely traumatized or shocked patient, the breakdown of energy-rich phosphate compounds.

Glycosuria often develops after injury, and a diabetic-like glucose tolerance curve, as well as resistance to insulin, has been demonstrated. These effects are proportional to the severity of the injury and may persist for a week. They appear to represent more than the hyperglycemic effects of increased adrenal activity. During the post-traumatic period, the major source of energy for the body continues to be fat despite a relative and absolute increase in glycogen and protein breakdown and utilization.

During the initial post-traumatic

period, there is usually some weight loss. However, depending on the severity of the injury and the tendency to retain salt and water, the actual loss of body tissue may be overshadowed by edema fluid and cellular swelling so that, at first, weight is gained. Eventually, unless renal shutdown occurs, there will be a period of consistent weight loss, the length of which is proportional to the severity of injury. The usual rate of loss is about 0.5 kg./day. The patient is ordinarily anorexic during the early part of this phase, and both gastrointestinal propulsion and absorption are reduced. However, this weight loss is not solely dependent on decreased alimentation, although loss of weight and tissue nitrogen can be minimized by forced intake or intravenous hyperalimentation. Even if oral intake is not curtailed, weight loss may be assured by the fluid loss associated with recumbency and the musculoskeletal breakdown that accompanies inactivity.

THE TURNING POINT. After a variable period, related to the severity of the injury, a turning point is reached and the above changes are reversed toward normal. The reversal may be abrupt, but the rate of return to normal is usually much more gradual than the initial deviation. This point is usually marked by a subjective feeling of improvement on the part of the patient. Thus, adrenal cortical and medullary overactivity subsides; urinary nitrogen losses decrease; sodium is more normally excreted; and the tendency to water retention wanes. If oral intake is still restricted, the nitrogen balance will continue to be negative and there will be a further depletion of the body's fat stores. This, along with a compensatory diuresis, may prolong the period of weight loss. However, in spite of the continued loss of weight and a negative nitrogen balance, protein synthesis and a gain in lean tissue may occur during this period. Eventually, as oral intake is resumed, nitrogen and weight losses will diminish steadily until a state of positive balance is reached. Potassium uptake regularly precedes the nitrogen gain, and the replenishment of potassium may be brisk during this second phase.

EARLY RECOVERY. There follows a much longer period, after the acute changes in endocrine activity (fluid and electrolyte shifts, etc.) have returned to normal, during which nitrogen balance remains positive, potassium uptake continues (at a normal N:K ratio) and there is a slow but steady weight gain. This is a purely anabolic phase during which muscle and other tissue masses are being repleted. Subjectively, the patient notes a steady increase in muscular strength and vigor over this period, which may last from three to five weeks rather than an equivalent of the number of days consumed by the first two phases.

LATE RECOVERY. Finally, there is a fourth or final phase of weight gain during which the body's fat deposits are restored. Little is known of this stage of convalescence, which may take months, because patients are no longer in the hospital where metabolic studies can be carried out.

SHOCK

The largest portion of this chapter is devoted to shock. The intense investigative and clinical interest in this condition demands this greater coverage. Despite great advances made in this century in understanding the pathophysiology of shock, the refractory state that develops during protracted shock still remains the greatest single barrier to the successful resuscitation of severely traumatized patients.

Definition. The term "shock" embraces a group of conditions with grossly similar physiologic derangements but a wide variety of inciting causes. Originally, it was represented in the English language by the word "collapse" from the Latin *conlapsus*. This connotation persists in the descriptive German word *Zusammenseukung*. The word "shock" itself first appeared in English medical literature in a 1743 translation of LeDran's "Reflection Drawn from Experiences with Gunshot Wounds," in which it implied a sudden violent impact. Its present connotation did not develop until the mid-nineteenth century.[37]

The earliest definitions of shock were descriptive expressions, such as Gross's "a rude unhinging of the machinery of life," and Warren's "a momentary pause in the act of death."[56] There followed many attempts to define it in precise terms. These usually failed to encompass its many facets or were too complex to be generally adapted. For this reason, it is expedient to define shock simply as *a generalized state of severe circulatory inadequacy.* It should be noted that this definition avoids reference to blood pressure or volume deficits, since *inadequate tissue perfusion,* which is the essence of shock, may occur when either of these parameters is within generally accepted normal limits.

Historical Background

Until the advent of the era of experimental physiology at the end of the nineteenth century, our concept of shock was based almost entirely on clinical description. Under the influence of the then popular spheres of physiologic interest, there followed periods of emphasis on the nervous, toxic, hemodynamic and metabolic aspects of shock. Many of the impressions of the pioneers in this field are interesting today because their significance was not fully appreciated at the time and has only recently been popularized by new and independent observations.

Early in this century, physiological studies on the neural control of circulation spawned the concept that shock represented an inhibition of the vasomotor center, producing weakened heart action and peripheral pooling of blood. In 1914, George W. Crile, one of the first to carry out extensive experiments on shock, stated: "There is a group of organs whose function is the conversion of potential to kinetic energy. This kinetic system includes the brain, thyroid, suprarenals, muscle and liver. If the stimuli are overwhelmingly intense, the kinetic system, particularly the brain, is exhausted, even permanently injured. This condition is acute shock."[33]

The concept of exhaustion of the central nervous system and its vasomotor control was one of the earliest physiological explanations of the mechanisms of shock. However, its popularity waned after evidence indicated that, if anything, vasomotor activity was heightened in response to hypovolemia. Nevertheless, vasomotor tone *is lost* late in shock. However, the mechanisms involved appear to be intrinsic or humoral, rather than of central nervous origin. As for Crile's "kinetic systems," a modern parallel can be found in current work on the effects of shock on the energy-producing intracellular enzyme systems.

Crile did much work in support of the use of saline as a temporary replacement for blood. Even earlier, in 1901, Roswell Park had suggested the infusion of a liter of saline in patients with significant blood loss. This, too, has regained popularity from the work of Shires et al.[131] and of Moyer and his associates,[107] which suggests that the loss of extracellular fluid in shock and burn states is much greater than previously appreciated.

In 1909, Henderson presented an "acapnia" theory of shock.[65] In spite of the misconception of his central theme, he was one of the first to recognize the importance of venous return in shock. He stated: "Venous pressure is, so to speak, the fulcrum of the circulation. Shock, as surgeons use the word, is due to the failure of the fulcrum. Because of diminished venous supply, the heart is not adequately distended in diastole." Judging by their frequent reliance on the central venous pressure as a diagnostic and therapeutic guide to the management of shock states, this statement would be soundly endorsed today by most surgeons.

Physiologists and surgeons combined their efforts in the study of shock during World War I. Measurements of the volume of fluid lost into a crushed limb in the experiments of Cannon and Bayliss suggested that this alone could not account for the degree of shock observed.[25, 26] It was implied that a toxic agent liberated from the crushed tissue might be responsible. The prestige of these investigators did much to advance the "toxic" theory of traumatic shock. Since it had been shown by Dale and Richards only a few years earlier that histamine resulted in profound hypotension when injected into cats, this substance was the principal suspect.[38]

However, the popularity of the toxic theory waned in 1930 when Blalock and Parsons and Phemister, independently repeating Cannon and Bayliss's experiments, showed that if one included in the estimates the volume of fluid lost into tissues just proximal to the level of the crush injury, this volume did correspond to that required to produce an equivalent degree of shock by slow withdrawal from the venous system.[15, 113] Their observations restored the position of inadequate circulating volume as the leading factor in most forms of traumatic shock, a position supported by the extensive clinical experiences of World War II and one that has not been seriously challenged since.

However, interest in toxic humoral substances in shock was soon restored, not only in regard to bacterial endotoxins as the etiologic agents in septic shock, and, as championed by Fine, the final cause of irreversibility in shock of any etiology, but in relation to the contributory roles played by endogenously released vasoactive humoral substances such as histamine, serotonin, bradykinin and other vasoactive peptides, the so-called myocardial-depressant factor, lysosomal enzymes, etc.

Since World War II, experimental studies have continued the development of standard shock preparations, with particular emphasis on a common denominator in irreversible shock. In recent years, the practice of characterizing the events in shock solely in terms of *macrocirculatory* hemodynamics has decreased; the focus is being shifted more and more to changes in regional blood flow, the microcirculation, and the metabolic organ and cellular effects of shock as reflected by changes in organ function, cellular metabolism, intracellular enzyme systems and ultrastructure. Shock literature has reached staggering proportions since World War II; and although many questions have been answered, at least an equal number have been raised.

Classification of Shock

The nomenclature encountered in shock literature can be very confusing. This is exemplified by Table 2–2 which lists some of the forms of clinical and experimental shock commonly mentioned. However, a simpler classification is desirable from both physiologic and therapeutic points of view. The following is a simplified classification of shock similar to that conceived by Blalock in 1934:[16]

TABLE 2–2 FORMS OF SHOCK COMMONLY REFERRED TO IN THE LITERATURE

Allergic Shock	Peptone Shock
Anaphylactic Shock	Septic Shock
Burn Shock	Spinal Shock
Cardiogenic Shock	Surgical Shock
Endotoxin Shock	Tourniquet Shock
Hematogenic Shock	Toxin Shock
Hemorrhagic Shock	Traumatic Shock
Histamine Shock	Tumbling Shock
Neurogenic Shock	Vasogenic Shock
Oligemic Shock	Vasovagal Shock

Hypovolemic Shock. Hemorrhagic shock is the classic example of this type; but in addition to blood loss, any uncompensated loss of extracellular fluid—like that from intestinal obstruction, major burns, crushing injuries, peritonitis or fistulas—can produce it.

Cardiogenic Shock. This implies shock primarily due to ineffective cardiac pumping action. It occurs in instances of myocardial insufficiency (e.g., massive myocardial infarction), with certain cardiac arrhythmias, or when there is mechanical obstruction of the flow of blood into or out of the heart (e.g., cardiac tamponade, massive pulmonary embolism).

Vasogenic Shock. The most common clinical example of this is septic shock, although a number of toxic agents or the sudden release of allergic mediators may produce a similar state (e.g., hymenopterous insect bites, reactions to local anesthetics).

Actually, Blalock included, as a fourth category, "neurogenic shock," but many if not most current treatises of shock disregard this as a separate category and consider it as a "central" form of vasogenic shock. This de-emphasis probably stems in large part from the classic description by Grant and Reeves, in their World War II study of traumatic forms of shock, of a condition called "warm hypotension" in which, despite abnormally low blood pressure, adequate tissue perfusion was maintained as evidenced by skin of normal color and temperature and adequate urinary excretion.[54] This apparent state of reflex vasodilatation with decreased peripheral vascular resistance is not uncommonly briefly seen immediately after significant trauma and cannot truly be considered a form of shock. Otherwise, neurogenic shock is rarely encountered clinically outside of the iatrogenic examples provided by "spinal" anesthesia. Of course, if it were of sudden onset and serious magnitude, neurogenic shock might not be so innocuous, particularly if an arteriosclerotic or otherwise diseased heart was the victim of the sudden loss of venous return it would cause.

Although this classification implies that the cause of the circulatory inadequacy that is called shock can be traced to the function of the pump (heart), the volumes of fluid it circulates (blood and extracellular fluid), or the tone of the conducting vessels (vasomotor activity), it should be emphasized that shock, as it is encountered clinically, frequently represents a combination of more than one of these forms.

Thus, when a patient develops shock following a myocardial infarction, a massive gastrointestinal hemorrhage, or the rigors of ascending cholangitis, there is little question that one is dealing, initially at least, with a simple form of shock—in these instances, cardiogenic, hypovolemic and septic shock respectively—and one can initiate appropriate therapy with some degree of confidence in the diagnosis if not the outcome. However, it is just as common for the etiology to be uncertain, particularly in the postoperative or late post-traumatic periods. Even more perplexing are the frequent instances in which a mixture of contributing elements exists. Next to inadequate volume restoration, failure to recognize later contributions by factors other than the primary etiology factor is probably the most common cause of "refractory shock." MacLean, reviewing an experience in a trauma shock unit, reported that an unrecognized cardiogenic component to shock was the cause of refractoriness and referral to the unit in over 50 per cent of the cases, even though a primary cardiac diagnosis existed in less than 5 per cent.[89] Another common situation is one of hypovolemia associated with septic shock, resulting from a failure to recognize the magnitude of "third space" and insensible fluid losses associated with sepsis. In fact, most cases initially diagnosed as septic shock will turn out to be a combination of hypovolemia in a septic patient, the hypovolemia having been made relatively more significant by the increased circulatory demands imposed by the sepsis. Yet a final example is that of the patient, being treated for cardiogenic shock secondary to myocardial infarction, who develops unrecognized hypovolemia either from rigid fluid restrictions or the shift of extracellular fluid from the intravascular to the extravascular compartment caused by vasopressor therapy. However, as long as one recognizes the limitations of this oversimplified approach to etiologic classification of shock, the atempt to make this categorical distinction clinically is justified by the therapeutic implications, as indicated by the experience of MacLean et al.[89]

Experimental Versus Clinical Shock. Even a casual perusal of shock literature reveals that much disagreement exists in this field. One can find differences of opinion among reputable investigators studying the same problem. One of the most important factors contributing to this is the necessity to study most aspects of the pathophysiology of shock in animals. It is extremely difficult, if not impossible, to conduct truly controlled shock studies on humans. Patients accepted for study in special units have varying medical backgrounds complicated by a variety of intercurrent diseases. Not only do they enter their state of shock by diverse routes, but almost invariably they have undergone a variety of treatments before entering the study unit.

However, in carrying out more detailed, controlled studies of experimental animals, equally formidable barriers are encountered. As Zweifach has indicated, differences in the comparative physiology of laboratory animals present very complex problems in the interpretation of experimental shock studies.[174] Even among animals obtained from a common source, factors such as age, sex, season, nutritional state and intercurrent infection are difficult to control. More important, however, are species differences that limit the extrapolation of findings to human shock.

The animals commonly used in shock experiments differ in the organ system that constitutes their "weak link" in response to shock. For example, the hepatic vein sphincters of the dog are extremely sensitive to changes in pH, adrenergic stimuli and vasoactive substances. The effects of their constriction in shock led many to the impression that severe hepatosplanchnic congestion was a critical factor in determining the lethality of shock. However, these sphincters are not as well developed in most other species and appear to have little significance in primates.[109, 164]

Studies of the hemodynamic response to hypovolemia have often been performed in dogs and cats. However, it has been shown that contraction of the liver and spleen of these animals can add as much as 30 per cent to the active circulating volume. These organs do not have nearly that propensity in man and subhuman primates, in whom the cutaneous circulation appears to act as such a depot.

The intense peripheral vasoconstriction seen in most forms of shock is not uniformly distributed throughout the circulation, and the pattern of distribution varies from species to species. For example, in the shocked rabbit renal cortical ischemia is marked, whereas in the rat or monkey it is mild or absent.

There are also marked species differences in sensitivity to bacterial products, and the relative contents of the vasoactive substances released by certain key organs in response to bacterial toxins are quite variable. The rabbit and cat are extremely sensitive to the lipopolysaccharide extracts of certain bacteria, but the rat and mouse are usually quite resistant to these same endotoxins.

The histological picture of acute endotoxemia varies considerably among species. In the rat, a massive accumulation of leukocytes is seen in the lung; in the rabbit, focal necrosis of the liver and splenitis are encountered; and in the dog, submucosal hemorrhage throughout the intestinal tract appears to be a major pathologic event. In the dog an injection of *E. coli* endotoxin will cause shock characterized by severe vasoconstriction; in the monkey it causes shock with vasodilatation.[172]

Another major problem in experimental shock investigations occurs in experiments that isolate a particular factor for study. The difficulty lies in interpreting the significance of changes in the factor studied in relation to the overall pathogenesis of shock. In focusing on one aspect, overall perspective can be lost as the trail of investigation is followed further and further in that direction. For this phenomenon, Simeone has coined the word "ideolepsis," meaning to be captured by an idea.[137] This has been particularly common in experiments studying the nature of irreversible shock.

The Effects of Shock on Organ Systems

Shock affects every tissue in the body, but because of selective compensatory mechanisms, the tissues of some organs are affected more than others. One of the most controversial issues in medical research has been the relative importance of the functional deterioration of certain vital organ systems in the final capitulation of the body's compensatory and recuperative mechanisms to severe, prolonged shock. The hope that this "irreversibility" is merely a function of our limited state of knowledge has encouraged an intense research interest in this state of shock which, in turn, has greatly extended our knowledge of the effects of shock on the various organ systems. The following discussion summarizes what is known of these effects as well as the conflicting opinions regarding their significance.

The effects of shock on the more important organs systems described below are those resulting from *hypovolemia*, unless otherwise noted. This emphasis is deliberate since hypovolemic shock is the type almost exclusively encountered in the injured patient. However, in discussing the cardiac effects of hypovolemic shock, some comments will also be made regarding the characteristics of cardiogenic shock. The problem of endotoxin or septic shock, as an example of vasogenic shock, will be given separate consideration.

In shock, the endocrine organs are more important for the responses they mediate rather than the effects they suffer. Consequently, they will not be treated separately but dealt with in discussing the organ systems they affect, mainly their circulatory and renal effects.

The Effects of Shock on the Circulatory System. Isolation of the responses of the heart from those of the vessels conducting the blood and lymph and consideration of changes in regional distribution of blood flow separately from changes in the distribution of body fluids are justified only in an attempt to bring some order to the complexities of the circulatory responses to shock. In addition, the coagulation changes attending shock are considered here because of their potential effects on microcirculation.

THE INITIAL CARDIOVASCULAR RESPONSE TO HYPOVOLEMIA. In general, the rate and volume of fluid lost from the effective circulation determine the cardiovascular responses to hypovolemia. At one extreme is a rapid exsanguinating hemorrhage from a large artery, and at the other, an insidious venous ooze or the seeping sequestration of extracellular fluid. In the "open artery" type of bleeding, a profound loss of peripheral vascular resistance occurs in spite of compensating mechanisms. Hypotension is out of proportion to volume loss. Coronary flow, robbed of the driving force of diastole, is greatly impaired, and the rate of deterioration of cardiac function is rapid. The importance of recognizing this form of shock is evident, for prolonging efforts to "catch up" with volume-expanding fluids before surgical intervention in behalf of hemostasis is futile. At the other extreme, the gradual loss of volume, unless quite prolonged, may be entirely compensated for by fluid retention by the kidney and the repartition of body fluids without grossly discernible hemodynamic disturbances.

Between these two extremes lies the more common situation, typified by a combined loss from small arteries, veins and capillaries. Unless the blood loss is arrested, this condition may progress successively to recognizable stages of compensated hypovolemia, impending shock, hypotensive shock and, finally, refractory shock. The volume losses necessary to reach these stages depend on many factors other than the rate of blood loss, among them body position, the stress of other trauma, age and cardiovascular reserve. It has been stated that a 10–15 per cent gradual volume loss usually produces minimal changes, that a 20–30 per cent loss may be compensated for without hypotension, and that a 30–50 per cent loss is required to produce progressive hypotension to a level of 50 mmHg.[99] However, these volume estimates were based largely on studies of the physiologic responses to venesection conducted on healthy young volunteers and were not meant to be applied too literally to patients encountered in the emergency room. Nevertheless, the progression of events demonstrated in these studies can be applied to equivalent stages of circulatory impairment seen clinically.

COMPENSATION. Initial increments of volume loss are compensated by adjustments in venous tone. To some extent this response is an intrinsic one which is not well maintained later in shock.[1] Its mechanism is poorly understood. As hypovolemia progresses, sympathetic neurohumoral activity contributes to the increased venomotor tone. The capacity of the venous system to adjust for volume loss can be appreciated from the fact that fourteen times as much blood normally resides in the systemic veins and venules as in the capillary bed. For this reason venomotor mechanisms are called the "capacitance" system and the "volume effectors," in contrast to arteriolar sphincters that are "pressure effectors" and constitute the "resistance" system.

Even with modest degrees of hypovolemia that can be compensated by adjustments in venous capacity without grossly discernible hemodynamic changes, volume receptors within this system will initiate plasma refilling mechanisms.

When reduction in the capacity of the venous system can no longer compensate for the volume loss, sequential decreases in venous pressure, diastolic filling, stroke volume and arterial pressure result. These effects are short-lived and quickly counterbalanced. They stimulate baroreceptors that respond through the sympathetic neurohumoral axis. These baroreceptors probably exist throughout the circulatory system, but those in the atrium and in the carotid and aortic sinuses are best known. Their relative sensitivity and contribution to vasomotor adjustment are not fully understood. Impulses are relayed first to hypothalamic regulator centers and then to the vasomotor center in the medulla. The efferent arm of this response, the sympathetic nervous system, increases the release of catecholamines at its nerve endings and in the adrenal medulla. The result is an inotropic and chronotropic effect on the heart and a widespread but selective vasoconstriction by which flow is decreased through certain regions of the circulation (e.g., skin, kidney) but not to the heart or brain. Splanchnic, and therefore portal venous, flow is also reduced, but overall hepatic blood flow is partially supported by an increased distribution of cardiac output through the hepatic artery.[76] It has also been shown that the heart is capable of some degree of intrinsic response, that is, independent of nervous and humoral stimuli.

Initially, the combined effect of these compensatory mechanisms is the restoration of arterial pressure, but not without a quickening of the pulse and a narrowing of the pulse pressure.

The skin becomes cool and urinary output decreases. Other expressions of sympathetic overactivity are evident—dry mouth, sweating, pupillary dilation and restlessness. At this stage hypotension may be precipitated by postural elevation or other manipulation of the patient, such as a Valsalva maneuver.

This adrenergic response can counterbalance a considerable degree of acute blood loss (up to 30 per cent) and maintain the integrity of the organism while volume replenishment goes on. If this compensatory capacity is exceeded, generalized circulatory inadequacy (shock) will result. When the blood pressure is used as a reference, the transition into the actual state of shock may seem abrupt; however, most physiologic parameters change gradually throughout the preceding period. In addition to a redistribution of regional blood flow, there is an increased uptake of oxygen from the blood flowing at a reduced rate through the tissues.

DECOMPENSATION. Once a certain stage of inadequate tissue perfusion is reached, a series of vicious cycles is initiated; these progressively interfere with the organism's ability to restore its own integrity. There is a shift to anaerobic metabolism, a depletion of existing energy stores and the development of metabolic acidosis. Acidosis reduces myocardial contractility, depresses the vascular response to catecholamines and promotes intravascular clotting. Reduced flow to the kidney results in a functional shutdown which, in time, will become permanent. This compounds the acidosis and may lead to significant electrolyte disturbances, such as hyperkalemia. Similarly, poor perfusion of the hepatosplanchnic bed may weaken the intestinal mucosa's barrier against bacterial invasion and reduce the reticuloendothelial system's ability to inactivate toxins. These toxins, and tissue ischemia itself cause the release of lysosomal enzymes and other vasoactive humoral substances (histamine, serotonin, bradykinin, myocardial-depressant factor) which in turn profoundly effect vascular tone and integrity, with further volume losses resulting from sequestration and capillary permeability. Initially in shock, there is little arterial hypoxemia unless there is associated trauma. Eventually, however, hypoxemia develops despite a degree of compensatory hyperventilation sufficient to produce hypocarbia, probably because of an elevation of the ventilation perfusion ratio, shunting around the pulmonary vascular bed and an increased arteriovenous difference in the systemic circulation. The continuation of this trend (to hypoxia and hypocarbia) eventually weakens the respiratory drive and may interfere with the autoregulatory capacity of the pulmonary microcirculation. Hypotension decreases coronary flow which in turn further depresses myocardial contractility. The eventual consequences of a weakened heart trying to pump a progressively reduced effective circulating volume requires no further expansion.

THE ROLE OF THE HEART. It is natural and correct to consider the heart an organ of prime importance in shock. However, whether the heart constitutes the weak link in the body's struggle against shock is disputed. Those who contend that cardiac deterioration is *the* factor that determines irreversibility point out that myocardial flow, contractility and oxygen consumption deteriorate progressively as hemorrhagic shock deepens. Cardiac output falls steadily, and terminally there are arrhythmias and a rise in the right atrial pressure. Using serial pressure-output curves, Crowell has demonstrated a progressive weakening of the heart's action.[34] In addition, myocardial structural disintegration has been demonstrated in irreversibly shocked animals.

Nevertheless, the impression has been equally strong that the heart possesses remarkable recuperative powers and responds strongly to an expansion of circulating volume long after a recognizable point of irreversibility has been passed. It has also been shown that cardiac function can be maintained as long as venous return is supported.[166] Indeed, the most impressive evidence of cardiac dysfunction appears only terminally. Even the late elevation of right atrial pressure may be related to pulmonary vasoconstriction.

Thus, experimental evidence to date suggests that although cardiac function deterioration is a striking event late in shock, it occurs when other organs are also showing evidence of terminal decompensation. However, this impression must be tempered by the realization that what may be true for young laboratory animals may not be valid in older human subjects whose cardiac reserve has been lowered by age or disease.

Finally, in resuscitated hemorrhagic shock victims, both experimental and clinical investigations have shown supranormal cardiac outputs despite evidence of inadequate tissue perfusion (e.g., rising blood lactate levels and increasing lactate: pyruvate ratios). Just as an effective circulating blood volume after prolonged hypovolemia may significantly exceed normal limits, so may the circulatory requirements of this post-shock state be excessive. The question that still remains unanswered is whether this refractory state of hyperdynamic circulatory failure represents a failure of the heart, in spite of supranormal effort, to meet the excessive demands placed on it, or whether the cardiac response is appropriate but peripheral factors, such as a-v shunting, abnormal oxygen transport, or widespread cellular dysfunction, are to be blamed.

CARDIOGENIC SHOCK. Shock may, of course, result from primary cardiac lesions, such as myocardial infarction, severe arrhythmias, and acute myocardiopathies, as well as conditions that mechanically interfere with the heart's action, such as cardiac tamponade and pulmonary embolism. Cardiogenic shock can lead to a refractory state by the same series of vicious cycles described in hypovolemic shock. In cardiogenic shock, the pumping action of the heart is not able to maintain a sufficient pressure head for adequate tissue perfusion. There are conflicting opinions regarding the direction in which peripheral vascular resistance changes in response to this so-called forward heart failure. In laboratory preparations of cardiogenic shock, particularly in the dog, peripheral resistance appears to rise and clinically some success has been claimed with vasodilators, particularly in the "low-output" failure encountered after open-heart surgery. Clinical studies, however, report variable changes in peripheral resistance, with many patients staying in the normal range and with the high peripheral resistances characteristic of hemorrhagic shock rarely occurring. The answer may lie in the acuteness with which this failure develops: with slower development some compensation may be afforded by volume expansion and increased tissue extraction of substrates, but in the acutely developing situation, a certain degree of selective vasoconstriction would seem necessary to protect the more vital regional circulations. However, one would not expect the extreme degrees of vasoconstriction and elevated peripheral resistance invoked to compensate for major volume losses.

In earlier years, the direction in which peripheral vascular resistance changed in cardiogenic shock attracted much attention because of its therapeutic significance in regard to the choice of drugs. At that time, a stalemate existed concerning the choice of vasopressor vs. vasodilator drugs. Vasopressors were recommended because they were thought to increase coronary flow and perfusion pressure, but this benefit was offset by increased work of the heart secondary to increased peripheral resistance. Vasodilators on the other hand were felt to decrease cardiac work and increase perfusion through deprived regions of the circulation by decreased resistance to flow; yet a disproportionate reduction in diastolic pressure and therefore coronary flow was feared to further weaken the diseased heart. This conflict has waned with the loss in popularity of both pure vasodilators and vasopressors in favor of drugs which singly or in combination have a positive inotropic effect on the heart with either little effect on the peripheral resistance (glucagon, dopamine) or vasodilatation (isoproterenol), or selective vasoconstriction (mephentermine, epinephrine in small doses).

THE MICROCIRCULATION. Capillary flow is impaired in shock by a combination of factors. As significant hypovolemia occurs, the perfusion pressure is decreased. Sympathetic neurohumoral activity causes a constriction of arteriolar sphincters in most vascular beds. Theoretically, flow into these capillary beds may be further diminished by the passive opening of arteriovenous shunts proximal to the constricted arterioles, but labelled microsphere studies indicate there is no significant degree of anatomic a-v shunting in pure hypovolemic shock.[123] Normally, flow through the capillary circulation is intermittently phased so that only one-third of the channels are open at any one time. This "winking circulation" appears to result from each capillary opening intermittently on demand, probably mediated by locally released vasoactive substances. However, when the perfusion is inadequate, all the capillaries "demand" blood so that the capacitance of the capillary circulation is roughly trebled. The combination of low perfusion pressure and increased precapillary arteriolar resistance allows very little blood into this wide-open capillary bed. The result is a marked degree of stagnation in the microcirculation. This is compounded later in shock by further loss of volume by sequestration and by changes in permeability secondary to ischemia so that fluid shifts into the cell. This offsets the forces contributing to capillary refill and the end result is partial restoration of intravascular volume, an increase in intracellular volume and a contraction in the extracellular, extravascular fluid compartment,[131] as will be discussed more fully under "Changes in Body Fluid Distribution."

Lillehei et al. explain the microcirculation events somewhat differently at this point.[86] They contend that constriction of both the precapillary arteriolar sphincters and the postcapillary venular sphincters is present early in shock. Then the loss of precapillary arteriolar tone occurs while the postcapillary venous sphincters remain constricted so that a "stagnant anoxia" replaces an "ischemic anoxia." The sequestration losses in protracted shock are thus explained by an imbalance between vascular tone on the "resistance" and "capacitance" sides of the capillary bed. This mechanism may apply in the dog and other animals in which the venous sphincters are well developed, but its occurrence in man is highly questionable. Indeed, such an explanation is not necessary. This effect can be just as easily explained by a *relaxation* of tone on the venous side of the circulation. Normally, 25 per cent of the blood volume is present in the heart and pulmonary circulation, 15 per cent in the arterial system and only 4 per cent in the capillary bed. Over 26 per cent of the blood volume resides in the postcapillary venules and 30 per cent in the larger veins. Thus, the venous circulation has the greatest capacity for sequestering blood. The latter contention is supported by the observation that a progressive loss of venous tone occurs in advancing stages of shock. An explanation for this late loss of tone in vascular smooth muscle may be found in the electron microscopic studies of Ashford.[3] He has demonstrated remarkable increases in the intracellular fluid of vascular smooth muscle in advanced stages of shock. It is not hard to understand the inability of the myofibrils to contract when they are separated and disoriented by this abnormal accumulation of cell sap.

Other factors which may be important in these microcirculatory events are the critical closing pressures of arterioles and precapillary sphincters and the increasingly significant effects of changes in viscosity at low-flow situations. Thus, evidence is accumulating which obviates the need to explain the microcirculatory changes in shock entirely on the basis of "sphincters," which has been so popular in the past decade.

COAGULATION CHANGES. The clotting changes associated with shock are considered here because of the implications they have on the microcirculation. There is little doubt that changes in coagulability occur in response to stress, trauma and shock. The state of coagulation represents a dynamic system of checks and balances which act to prevent the development of extremes of hyper- and hypocoagulability. As early as the 1830's Hewson noted that the "blood which was drawn last clotted first in men and animals being venesected."[68] The hypercoagulable state that follows blood loss has a valuable homeostatic function and, in combination with vasoconstriction, helps to stem the loss of blood.

The cause of this increased coagulability has not been fully elucidated but several factors play a role. Locally, damaged tissues and platelets release thromboplastic substances. Platelets also release serotonin, which is thought to contribute to the local vasoconstriction. This probably explains the common observation that a cleanly incised wound bleeds longer than a jagged laceration. However, the clotting response is more than a local one since venesection alone leads to hypercoagulability, particularly if shock supervenes. There is information to suggest that the release of catecholamines and even lysosomal enzymes may contribute to this. The acidosis that accompanies shock appears to be important also. Experimental lowering of the pH by intravenous lactate has been shown to shorten the clotting time.[35] Even heparinized blood can be made *hypercoagulable* if the pH is significantly lowered.[60] Finally, if the acidosis of hemorrhagic shock is prevented by buffering with trishydroxymethanolamine, the severity of the associated clotting changes is greatly ameliorated.[124]

The rate of mobilization of clotting factors is greatly accelerated in response to trauma, although the mechanisms involved are not known.[62] Changes in the electric potential, the release of activators and the factors involved in platelet agglutination and red cell cohesiveness are all under study. An increase in platelet aggregation occurs after stress, trauma or shock, and platelet microthrombi have been demonstrated in movies of the microcirculation by Robb.[119] Similarly, Bjork et al. have shown clumping of red cells[13] and Knisely and his associates, sludging of the blood in postoperative and shock states.[78]

Although the initial response is that of hypercoagulability, this tendency is reversed later if shock is severe and prolonged, and an extreme degree of *hypocoagulability* may result. To some extent this may reflect a loss of clotting factors through hemorrhage and a decrease in production and mobilization of clotting factors secondary to inadequate tissue perfusion. However, the most important factor appears to be the consumption of clotting factors. This is not only a local process at the site of injury, but a disseminated intravascular coagulation as well. Hardaway feels that this results from a combination of capillary stasis and hypercoagulability and that it may contribute greatly to the development of irreversibility as microthrombi block the circulation through vital organs.[60]

In the dog, fibrinolytic activity and circulating anticoagulants do not appear to contribute significantly to this hypocoagulability, which may develop to extreme degrees after two to four hours of hemorrhagic shock.[124] However, clinical observations suggest that these processes may be initiated later when shock is prolonged. One source may be the by-products of coagulation itself. In the proteolytic reaction that produces fibrin from fibrinogen, a fibrin monomer is first released along with two polypeptide fragments. Fibrin is then formed by polymerization of this monomer. These polypeptide byproducts have fibrinolytic activity and one may have vasoconstrictive properties.[80, 101]

Whether these changes in the state of coagulation can lead to significant deleterious effects in clinical shock by a process of disseminated intravascular coagulation is debatable. In histologic studies of human cases of refractory shock, Hardaway et al. have shown that microthrombi and peculiar "globular clots" can be found frequently if looked for.[61] In addition, they presented circumstantial evidence for occlusion of the microcirculation in the form of microinfarcts and petechial hemorrhages. These findings were absent in control patients who died suddenly without passing through a period of protracted shock.

The work of Attar and his associates suggests that there are natural oscillations in coagulability, which, by a system of negative feedbacks, strive to maintain a normal level.[5] In cases of refractory shock they found oscillations that exceeded normal limits in both directions. The magnitude of these oscillations correlated very well with mortality; in nonsurviving patients, they increased progressively to a point of extreme hypocoagulability instead of gradually returning to a normal range.

Simmons et al. recently reported a thorough study of coagulation disorders in Vietnam combat casualties.[139] They studied the acute changes after wounding, after massive transfusion and later in the post-resuscitative period. In the acute phase following wounding and before intravenous therapy, changes in the state of coagulability correlated closely with the degree of hypotension, acidosis and lactacidemia. Those with wounds of mild to moderate severity had normal or shortened prothrombin and partial thromboplastin times. The more severely wounded patients, including those in shock, had normal or prolonged prothrombin and partial thromboplastin times. In general, the severity of the coagulation defects were milder than those seen in experimental canine studies, but showed the same initial phase of hypercoagulability followed by a return to normal or progression into a phase of hypocoagulability. Following the administration of intravenous fluids and blood, a dilutional coagulation picture was produced with the pattern of depression of coagulation factors similar to that of stored bank blood. Platelet levels fell during transfusion to about 100,000/mm.^{3}. Prothrombin times, partial thromboplastin times and fibrinogen levels were less severely affected. Severe operative bleeding was not associated with these relatively mild dilutional changes and the use of fresh blood was rarely warranted. Finally, during early convalescence, coagulation abnormalities were found in approximately one-half of the casualties. These could be correlated with the presence of shock on admission to the hospital, transfusion of *large* quantities of blood and the presence of abnormalities in clotting parameters prior to operation. The prolongation of prothrombin and partial thromboplastin times was much greater than seen earlier. In 20 per cent of the patients, the pattern of recurring cycles of hypocoagulability occurred, and the presence of four or more of these peaks could be correlated with the appearance of life-threatening complications. All the patients who died had clotting abnormalities at some time prior to death. Bleeding episodes requiring reoperation, however, could not be blamed on coagulation abnormalities. Fibrinogen levels were greater than normal in all patients in this third phase. Platelet counts returned to normal over the first week in almost all patients and fibrinolysin values returned toward normal but remained elevated in most patients during the first convalescent week. It was concluded that the coincidence of abnormalities of prothrombin and partial thromboplastin times with thrombocytopenia and fibrinolysis and a relative deficiency of fibrinogen in most seriously wounded patients was consistent with the contention that non-lethal episodes of disseminated intravascular coagulation occurred during recovery from severe trauma and shock.

In summary, there is a hypercoagulable response to hemorrhage that may serve an important homeostatic function. However, when shock is extreme and prolonged, a state of hypocoagulability may ensue as a result of extravasation of clotting factors, decrease in their production and mobilization and, particularly, disseminated intravascular coagulation. This may be aggravated by an increase in fibrinolytic activity and the release of circulating anticoagulants, and by the transfusion of blood deficient in clotting factors. If extreme, this hypocoagulability poses a threat to the bleeding patient and compromises any surgical efforts that may be made on his behalf.

CHANGES IN BODY FLUID DISTRIBUTION. Repartition of body fluids is one of the most important responses to hypovolemia. The translocation of extravascular fluid into the vascular compartment results in a hemodilution which has long been recognized by clinicians in the hematocrit changes that follow hemorrhage.

Volume replenishment can be detected within minutes after a moderate but non-shocking venous hemorrhage (10–20 per cent). After reaching a peak six to ten hours after such a hemorrhage, the rate of refill gradually decreases and is usually completed in 20–40 hours. Electrolyte adjustments take a few days longer and restoration of the red cell mass goes on over approximately a six-week period at rates of 15 to 50 cc. a day.[100]

Only recently have the mechanisms involved in this response finally begun to be uncovered. For years plasma refilling has been explained on the basis of Starling's principle; that is, the lowering of intravascular pressure promotes the ingress of fluid from the extravascular space. Starling suggested that the balance between intravascular and extravascular pressure controlled extracellular fluid movements so that an egress of intravascular fluid occurred with the higher pressure at the arteriolar end of the capillary bed and an ingress of extravascular fluid with the lower pressures at the venular end. This was thought to allow circulation of fluid rich in oxygen and other nutrients out into the extravascular space at the beginning of transit through the capillary bed and its return loaded with carbon dioxide and metabolites at the end. Though attractive, there is growing evidence to suggest that the process is not this simple and that other mechanisms play important roles. This is not to say that the lowering of the intravascular pressure in the capillary bed does not allow fluid to enter from the extravascular space in shock. However, it has been shown that this hemodilution is considerably curtailed by adrenalectomy.[96] In addition, it has been suggested that volume replenishment takes place to a large extent via the lymphatic system. In this regard, Cope and Litwin have shown that the volume and rate of fluid replacement correlated well with increased flow of thoracic duct lymph.[30]

One of the most striking effects of a moderate, non-shocking venous hemorrhage is the decrease in urinary excretion of both water and sodium. Farrell has demonstrated volume receptors in the right atrium which take part in this response.[47] Aldosterone appears to play an important role here and Barter et al. have shown that phlebotomy is a potent stimulus to aldosterone release.[7] Ganong and Mulrow pointed out the importance of the intact kidney in this aldosterone response.[52] The response appears to involve the juxtaglomerular apparatus and macula dense. Renin is released at this site and this proteolytic enzyme acts on a plasma substrate to produce angiotension which, in turn, increases the adrenocortical release of aldosterone.

Aldosterone causes active tubular reabsorption of sodium with obligatory retention of water. It is also thought by some to be necessary for the recruitment of intracellular water in the repartition process. In addition to this aldosterone effect, antidiuretic hormone, release by the hypothalamus-posterior pituitary axis, effects a net retention of sodium-free water, a response which lasts as long as hypovolemia. As the hypovolemia progresses into shock, decreased glomerular filtration further reduces urinary excretion until finally, in deep shock, renal excretion comes to a standstill. The effect of shock on the kidneys will be further elaborated below. How much the blood volume replacement depends on transcapillary refill, increased thoracic duct lymph and retention of salt and water by the renal-adrenal axis has not been established, partly because their relative contributions vary at different stages of shock.

Another aspect of fluid compartment shifts associated with shock that has received intense interest in the last decade is the question of so-called "hidden" extracellular fluid losses. In the 1950's, a number of clinical experiences indicated that intravenous saline infusions could be used to replace lost blood. Experimental investigations indicated that saline infusions were as effective as blood in hemorrhagic shock preparations if three to four times the volume of lost blood was given. Indeed, the survival of shock and burn preparations was often better when crystalloid infusions were given instead of blood. This challenged two time-honored concepts of surgical care: (1) that electrolytes or saline solutions could only incompletely and transiently restore blood volume and (2) that saline solutions were undesirable during or immediately after operation or trauma because of the associated tendency towards salt and water retention. Since, up until the early 1960's, support for this approach was based on equal or better survival rates in animal studies and physiologic tolerance in clinical experiences, it was felt by most that this approach represented something one could get away with, but was not necessarily what was best for the patient. However, in the early sixties, triple isotope studies by Shires indicated that in severe *shocking* degrees of hemorrhage (25 per cent volume loss), there was a much greater reduction in the extracellular fluid space than one would expect from the actual volume lost, a phenomenon that was not observed with lesser, non-shocking degrees of hemorrhage (10 per cent volume loss).[130] There followed a series of reports by other investigators using just about every known isotope technique for measuring extracellular fluid volume, the majority of which refuted Shires' claim. The most common explanation offered for this disagreement was that there was a shift to the right between the control and the post-hemorrhagic radiosulphate equilibration curves so that estimation of the extracellular fluid space from a single 20-minute equilibration sample, as Shires had done, would indicate a reduction, whereas extrapolation from the total curve indicated little change in extracellular fluid volume. However, in fairness, most isotope studies which disputed Shires' conclusions were performed on milder or less prolonged shock preparations.

At the time of this impasse, Borden et al. investigated this problem using an entirely different approach, monitoring interstitial fluid pressure using Guyton's technique.[70] They showed that after prolonged shock, the interstitial fluid pressure was considerably more negative than it was normally, and that restoration of shed blood and even additional colloid solutions did not restore the interstitial fluid pressure to pre-hemorrhage levels, whereas an additional infusion of a crystalloid solution, in an amount equal to 5 per cent of the body weight, did accomplish this end. They contended that whether one could demonstrate it by isotope techniques or not, there was at least a functional ECF deficit following profound hemorrhagic shock as demonstrated by the interstitial fluid pressures. Mathews, using an improved radiosulfate technique and multiple serial samples, was then able to demonstrate two components to the radiosulfate equilibrium curve: an initial fast-equilibrating component, representing the "functional" extracellular fluid volume, and a later more slowly equilibrating component, representing the total extracellular fluid volume.[97] He demonstrated that in moderate shock there was a decrease in the fast-equilibrating or functional compartment and in severe shock, there was a decrease in both the functional and total ECF volume. Restoration of shed blood after severe shock restored total ECF volume. However, only treatment with additional crystalloid solutions restored both slopes to normal. This work appeared to resolve much of the conflict between previous isotope studies.

From the beginning, Shires had claimed that these changes in ECF volume represented a shift of sodium and water into the cells during profound shock, whereas others had claimed that this shift was more apparent than real and actually reflected changes taking place in the interstitium.

It now begins to look like there is justification for both points of view. Cunningham and Shires finally succeeded in showing both a drop in the transmembrane potential of skeletal muscle and an increase in the potassium content of microaspirates of interstitial fluid in severely shocked rats, with the change in membrane potential preceding the rise in potassium in interstitial fluid.[56] This was felt to represent primarily a depression in the activity of the cell membrane sodium pump with the potassium shift occurring secondarily, as a result of a diffusion potential. Hageberg and Haljamäe in Sweden had reached the same conclusion in a series of earlier experiments.[58] They had shown consistent decreases in the transmembrane potential in hemorrhagic shock but had been unable to show significant changes in the sodium and potassium content of skeletal muscle samples. Finally, it became apparent that if diffusion between the interstitium and the vascular compartment was extremely restricted, shifts between the intracellular and extracellular compartments could take place without being reflected in peripheral plasma samples and without being uncovered by analysis of macrotissue samples, which reflect a combination of cellular and interstitial electrolyte composition. They confirmed this suspicion by analysis of washed single cells and showed an average decrease of 26 per cent of intracellular potassium after hemorrhagic shock. Later, directly sampling nanoliter volumes of interstitial fluid, they confirmed the suspected cation shifts. They also showed that skeletal muscle cells taken from severely shocked animals were not able to reaccumulate potassium during prolonged incubation as could cells subjected to milder degrees of shock. Their studies indicated that there was something going on in the interstitial fluid or ground substance that was interfering with the movement of water or at least the diffusion of cations and anions. It is this, it appears, that is responsible for the "functional changes" in extracellular fluid volume.

Some years earlier, Moyer and Butcher, in trying to explain an apparent major expansion in the distribution space of sodium in burns, suggested that connective tissue might trap water in shock and other traumatic states.[106] They pointed out that collagen swelled whenever the pH was altered away from either of its two isoelectric points. Fulton subsequently studied subcutaneously implanted collagen strips and showed that their salt and water content increased after shock, a situation which persisted even after volume restoration.[50] Slonim and Stahl compared the sodium and water contents of cellular tissue (muscle) and connective tissue (tail) in a group of control rats, a group that was severely shocked, and a group that was moderately shocked.[141] In the severely shocked group there was an increase in sodium and water content of both cellular and non-cellular tissue, but in the milder shock group these changes occurred only in the non-cellular or connective tissue. Others have pointed out that the interstitium consists of both a ground substance and a free fluid phase. The ground substance consists of a macromolecular mesh of mucopolysaccharides in which there is "bound" water and the free fluid phase exists between these aggregates. It has been suggested that this sol-gel state can increase its "osmotic activity" in resonse to a number of circulating substances such as acid metabolites, lysosomal hydrolysates and certain hormones, like catecholamines, which are known to be increased in shock. Thus, one currently popular theory is that the "functional" changes in ECF volume can be blamed on changes in the sol-gel state of the interstitial tissues. Drucker's group have made some interesting empiric observations which further support this impression of a functional impairment of extracellular fluid in shock.[51] In their experiments, minute amounts of patent blue dye were injected intradermally through a 25 needle using a constant infusion pump and the size of the dye spots was measured microscopically over extended periods of time. Migration of this dye was resolved in multi-exponential curves with two major phases. The earliest phase of dye spread was solely dependent on available free water in the tissue, that is, interstitial diffusion as opposed to capillary uptake, the latter affecting mainly the later rate of spread and disappearance. They found that both rates were reduced in severe untreated shock subjects, that the administration of blood had little benefit on interstitial diffusion, but improved capillary uptake, whereas administration of salt solutions improved interstitial diffusion but, even when given in three times the volume of shed blood, did not effectively restore capillary uptake and (presumably) flow.

In summary, current thinking favors the existence of deficits in extracellular fluid volume in shock and suggests that there may be a breakdown of the cell membrane ion pump in profound or prolonged shock with a shift to sodium and water to the cells and a diffusion of potassium out of it, but that even in milder degrees of hemorrhage, where this shift does not occur, there are "functional" changes in extracellular fluid volume which may be related to changes in the sol-gel state of the ground substance.

The Effect of Shock on the Kidney. Since 1941 when Bywaters first drew attention to the syndrome of post-traumatic renal shutdown, the effects of shock on the kidney have come under careful scrutiny.[24] The kidney's response to hypovolemia is more complex than originally thought. In addition to previously mentioned aldosterone and antidiuretic effects, Stahl observed a considerable degree of autoregulation.[143] Many of the early investigations measured total renal blood flow. However, it has become apparent that the partitioning of blood between the cortex and medulla plays an important role in regulating renal function. The renal responses to hypovolemia are activated before there is significant hypotension or even generalized vasoconstriction. Initially, the kidney maintains cortical flow by constriction of efferent arterioles, although an intrinsic myogenic mechanism has also been suggested. This is important not only for the maintenance of glomerular filtration but of sodium and water reabsorption. Most of renal oxygen consumption takes place in the cortex where it is utilized largely for the process of sodium resorption in the proximal convoluted tubules. This preferential support of renal cortical flow helps to maintain the osmotic gradients necessary for the countercurrent mechanism of sodium and water reabsorption, a process which has a high energy requirement and which is important in combating hypovolemia.

However, in the face of significant hypotension, there is a disproportionate reduction in renal blood flow. It is reduced from almost 25 per cent of the cardiac output to 7 per cent when the blood pressure is reduced to the 40 to 60 mmHg range, and renal vascular resistance increases as much as sevenfold.[53] Even with non-shocking degrees of hypovolemia, a significant increase in renal vascular resistance and decreased renal blood flow may occur. Once initiated, this renal vasoconstriction may be maintained by intrinsic mechanisms, independent of neural and humoral control, long after hypovolemia is corrected. In studies of regional blood flow in hemorrhagic shock, Rutherford has shown that renal blood flow is the slowest organ flow to return to normal after restoration of blood volume.[123] This supports the earlier observation of Cournand et al. that renal blood flow sometimes did not return to normal in shocked patients for 12 hours after volume restoration.[32]

Although renal cortical flow can be relatively well maintained in the face of moderate degrees of hypovolemia, the compensatory mechanisms do not suffice in profound or prolonged shock. Selkurt's measurements of cortical flow at this stage show that it is severely impaired.[127] Boyland and Ashauer have shown that a washout of the medullary hyperosomotic zone occurs.[20] This event is marked by sodium in the renal venous blood exceeding that of the arterial blood and signals a breakdown of the countercurrent concentrating mechanism. Restoration of blood flow at this stage may result in inability to concentrate urine, which would explain the polyuria that sometimes follows lesser periods of shock. However, as time progresses, ischemic damage to the nephron produces renal shutdown. At one time, the more striking histological changes in the lower part of the nephron led to the impression that the damage was quite selective, hence the long-popular term, "lower nephron nephrosis." Further study, aided by electron microscopic techniques, has established that the entire nephron shares the damaging effect of renal ischemia. Although this damage may be aggravated by the deposition of hemoglobin pigments in transfusion reactions and a proteinaceous material under other circumstances, there is little agreement concerning the extent to which tubular deposits are cause or effect in the renal shutdown that follows hypovolemic shock.

The Effect of Shock on the Lungs. Although a great deal of attention has been given to respiratory impairment at the cellular level, the effects of shock on the organs or respiration received little attention until the late 1960's. Since World War I, descriptions of heavy, wet, congested or hemorrhagic lungs have been described in post mortem examinations of shock victims. Since, to a certain degree, similar findings are present in 80 per cent of all autopsies, particularly in dependent areas, these observations were usually passed off as being due to a combination of prolonged recumbency and terminal congestive failure. After World War II, the term "congestive atelectasis" was used to describe the histologic counterpart of this condition. More recently, many casualties of the Vietnam conflict, resuscitated by rapid transportation and aggressive intravenous therapy from what would have previously been a lethal degree of injury, were observed to develop a progressive and often lethal form of pulmonary insufficiency which did not reach full bloom until 24 to 48 hours after resuscitation. The apparent narrow margin between early death and survival without pulmonary complications may be one of the reasons this pulmonary shock lesion was not fully appreciated before. It is suspected by some that newer approaches to intravenous fluid therapy employing voluminous amounts of crystalloid solutions, particularly in association with loss of pulmonary autoregulatory mechanisms during general anesthesia or hyperventilation, may have converted a relatively innocuous lesion into a serious clinical problem. Nevertheless, there does appear to be a genuine pulmonary shock lesion, the earliest characteristic of which is interstitial edema. Under electron microssopy, dispersion of individual collagen fibers, widening of the thick portions of the alveolar capillary membrane and increased endothelial pinocytosis have been shown by Moss et al.[104] and an inflammatory reaction with erythrocyte aggregation in smaller vessels and layering of leukocytes along the endothelial cell surface has been described by Wilson et al.[170]. Not all these pulmonary changes are pathognomonic of the pulmonary shock lesion since similar findings associated with progressive pulmonary insufficiency have been seen to occur following cardiopulmonary bypass, inhalation burns, fat embolism, etc.; rather the lung appears to show a commonality of response to a wide variety of insults.

A number of etiologic and "treatment" factors have been thought to contribute to this progressive pulmonary insufficiency. These are resuscitational fluid overload,[75] capillary blockage and chemical inflammation from fat embolism,[2] transfusion-induced microembolism from platelet aggregates,[14] microembolism from disseminated intravascular coagulation,[59, 91] capillary lysosomal instability from immunologically active transfused homologous leukocytes,[170, 158] oxygen transport deficits from 2-3 diphosphoglycerate depletion,[60] delayed reductions in surfactant,[66] and hypoxic damage to lining cells between the respiratory bronchiole and the alveoli (which are more dependent upon bronchial than pulmonary flow). In addition, the clinical lesion may be complicated, in an additive cycle, by atelectasis, infection and oxygen toxicity. It is important to point out that although many of the characteristics observed clinically have been produced in experimental shock preparations, no investigator has experimentally reproduced the morphological lesions in association with progressive functional pulmonary insufficiency of *delayed* onset which is so characteristic of the clinical situation. Nor have the pulmonary lesions been prominent in primate experiments unless voluminous crystalloid infusions were administered in resuscitating the subject from shock. The fact that only one of several patients with essentially similar clinical courses will develop the typical picture of shock lung suggests that treatment factors may be to blame. Guyton has produced pulmonary edema in dogs by varying oncotic pressures and pulmonary perfusion pressures according to Starling's hypothesis, supporting the suspicion that the continuation of reduced oncotic pressure following vigorous crystalloid therapy of hemorrhagic shock and intrinsic changes in the pulmonary microcirculation could produce this lesion.[57] However, Moss produced decreased oncotic pressures in resuscitating hemorrhaged baboons with various types of intravenous fluids and did not produce significant pulmonary lesions.[105] The possible loss of autoregulatory capacity of the pulmonary circulation by prolonged hypocarbia and alkalosis may also play a contributory role.

In the typical clinical situation, a day or two after resuscitation from severe trauma with operation and multiple transfusions, the patient begins to hyperventilate and blood gases show a decreased paO_2, $paCO_2$ and increased pH. There is an increased arterial alveolar CO_2 gradient, increased physiologic dead space, and a decreased dynamic complicance (the latter being one of the first indications). Functional pulmonary arteriovenous shunting progressively contributes to the hypoxia even though true anatomic arteriovenous shunts have not been demonstrable by microsphere studies. However, the hypoxia cannot be totally explained by a shunting effect as it appears to be also contributed to by changes in the alveolar capillary membrane, decrease in transit time to the pulmonary capillary bed, decrease in the ventilation-perfusion ratio, etc. Earlier pulmonary shock lesions in the stage of simple interstitial and alveolar edema can be reversed by treatment with concentrated albumin and positive pressure ventilation.

The Effects of Shock on the Liver. The liver ranks high in the chain of vital organs that maintain the organism's integrity. It is the metabolic factory and warehouse of the body. In addition, it is the clearing station for many of the body's endogenous toxins. The importance of its many functions is underscored by the early lethality of hepatectomy. It lies at the estuary of portal flow, the origins of which are that bacterial jungle, the gut. Its well-developed reticuloendothelial system reflects its function in guarding against bacterial assault from within. Finally, it has a unique mixed inflow system. Normally, the arterial inflow supplies only 40–50 per cent of the oxygen consumed by the liver. The portal venous blood, contributing as it does between two-thirds and four-fifths of hepatic blood flow, supplies the remainder. Because the larger portion of the liver's blood and oxygen supply is subject to the physiologic demands of viscera lying upstream from it, the liver should be unusually susceptible to shock and hypoxia. McMichael's observation in cats is pertinent in this regard.[92] When the arterial pressure was dropped from 140 to 180 mm Hg, the oxygen saturation in the portal vein decreased from 68 to 29 volume percentage. It is not surprising then that the liver has been suspected as the body's "Achilles heel" in shock. The pathologic changes observed in the livers of dogs dying after a period of hemorrhagic hypotension tend to re-enforce this suspicion. The livers are heavy and congested, and, microscopically, the sinusoids are packed with red cells. There is central necrosis in the hepatic lobules. Blood drawn from such animals prior to death shows evidence of hepatocellular damage, and levels of blood ammonia are elevated.

As noted, many of these changes can be explained by constriction of hepatic vein sphincters, which in the dog are well developed and very sensitive to acidosis and to certain vasoactive substances released in shock. Anatomic and hemodynamic studies of subhuman primates suggest that these sphincters are not a significant factor in humans.[109, 164] Another species difference which may play a role is the degree of bacterial contamination of the hepatic blood and bile found in the dog. These same factors may be involved in the dog's greater degree of susceptibility to acute occlusion of the hepatic artery or portal vein, as well as to shock. However, regional blood flow studies show that the distribution of cardiac output to the hepatic artery increases as it does to the cerebral and coronary vessels in hemorrhagic shock, and that this greatly offsets the reduction in flow and oxygen to the liver caused by splanchnic vasoconstriction.[76] Furthermore, in the primate, splanchnic vasoconstriction is not as marked as in the dog, and after resuscitation there appears to be a reactive hyperemia in the liver.

Thus, there is reason to believe that the liver may play a more prominent role in the lethality of shock in dogs than it does in humans. This does not mean that hepatic damage does not contribute significantly to the late deterioration that follows protracted shock. It probably does, but convincing evidence of the significance of hepatic dysfunction in clinical shock has not been developed.

The Effect of Shock on the Gastrointestinal Tract. Striking changes in the gastrointestinal tract occur in dogs subjected to lethal degrees of hemorrhagic or endotoxin shock. There is a marked increase in the weight of the splanchnic viscera and both gross and microscopic evidence of congestion, edema and focal hemorrhage. Most impressive are the widespread foci of hemorrhagic necrosis in the intestinal mucosa. These changes have suggested that the effects of shock on the gastrointestinal tract might be a major lethal factor. Originally, hepatosplanchnic congestion was held responsible for the mucosal lesions. However, when provision was made for decompression of the portal system by the prior construction of a portacaval shunt, little if any measurement was noted in the dog's response to shock. In particular, the hemorrhagic mucosal lesions still occurred.[49] On the other hand, Lillehei found that these lesions did not occur and that survival was improved if the superior mesenteric artery was selectively perfused during the shock period with oxygenated blood at normal pressures.[85] This implies that these lesions were the result of poor inflow into the splanchnic bed rather than obstructed outflow. Since similar lesions were observed after toxic doses of epinephrine, it was surmised that prolonged vasoconstriction in the splanchnic bed was responsible.

Subsequently, Bounous et al. have shown that these mucosal lesions could be prevented by giving a trypsin inhibitor or by prior ligation of the pancreatic duct.[18] They demonstrated that the mucous covering of the intestinal villi disappeared and that biosynthesis of mucin in the mucosal cells ceased during the course of hemorrhagic shock.[19] These findings suggest the possibility that, in protracted shock, either because of focal ischemia or because the high energy requirements of mucin production cannot be met, there is a loss of the protective mucous covering and the intestinal villi have no defense against intraluminal trypsin. The result is widespread hemorrhagic necrosis of the mucosa.

Darin et al. have been able to prevent these lesions in an endotoxin shock preparation by exclusion of the small intestine from the gastrointestinal stream.[45] However, pursuing this further, they found that neither diversion of pancreatic nor biliary drainage was as effective in preventing the mucosal lesions as total gastrectomy or subtotal gastrectomy with vagotomy. They also point out that all animals died regardless of the presence or absence of the intestinal lesion. Unfortunately, they used a dose of endotoxin that produced 100 per cent mortality in the controls so that a "supralethal" dose may have obscured some degree of benefit from the prevention of hemorrhagic necrosis. Gurd et al. have also been able to prevent this lesion by hypertonic glucose instilled intraluminally.[27] This is thought to provide an available energy substrate in the face of shock.

In considering the significance of these intestinal lesions, it must be kept in mind that they are not an outstanding characteristic of primate shock. However, in spite of this reservation, one cannot dismiss the possible importance of the gastrointestinal effects of shock in the human. It is still possible that a breakdown in the gastrointestinal barrier against bacteria and exogenous toxins could occur in humans without the association of the striking hemorrhagic mucosal lesions seen in dogs. This point has been made convincingly by recent studies of the back diffusion of hydrogen ion through the gastric mucosa following the ingestion of alcohol and certain drugs (e.g., aspirin, indomethicin) and following shock. As pointed out by Silen, this invisible but striking breakdown in the gastric mucosal barrier to back diffusion of hydrogen ion, combined with a concomitant release of pepsin, may be the common mechanism for the erosive gastritis and stress ulcers which occur under these circumstances and which, unlike the hemorrhagic enteritis of canine shock, has a very real and serious clinical counterpart.[136]

Endotoxin and Septic Shock

For some years investigators have studied experimental preparations in which shock was produced by injections of a high molecular weight phospholipid-polysaccharide-protein complex derived from the cell wall of certain gram-negative bacteria, particularly *E. coli*. This substance, called endotoxin, is generally thought to be responsible for the state of shock occasionally seen with certain clinical infections. The basis for endotoxin shock is still thought to be a hypersensitivity reaction or an accelerated Schwartzman's phenomenon. For example, the California hagfish shows no tissue response to injected antigen and is completely resistant to the lethal effects of endotoxin. The same bacteria that possess this endotoxin are commonly responsible for these infections, and the injection of this endotoxin mimics many of the changes seen clinically. Some have taken exception to this conclusion, pointing out that human septic shock is nearly always associated with a bacteremia and that certain hemodynamic parameters, particularly peripheral vascular resistance, do not consistently follow the pattern observed after endotoxin injection. However, these differences may be explained by species differences in response to endotoxin, superimposition of endotoxemia on the dynamic picture of a systemic infection rather than the normal baseline of experimental studies and, finally, the variable release pattern of endotoxin in clinical infections compared with the single lethal dose usually used experimentally.

The Effects of Shock on Bacterial Defense Mechanisms. There seems to be little doubt that the body's bacterial defense mechanisms are profoundly impaired in shock. Impressive laboratory evidence of this has nurtured the idea that an overwhelming endotoxemia is the essence of irreversible shock regardless of the participating cause. However, until recently, the mechanisms themselves have not been studied in detail.

Olledart and Mansberger have presented evidence indicating that this impairment is due to a combination of reduced opsonization, decreased contact time between the bacterium and the phagocyte and reduced phagocytic ability.[111]

Complement, which is a complex system of at least six components, sensitizes the bacterium and facilitates contact between it and the natural antibody. This process, called opsonization, appears to injure the bacterium and render it less resistant to phagocytosis. Contact between the sensitized bacteria and phagocytes takes place largely in the reticuloendothelial system, the greater portion of which lies in hepatosplanchnic viscera which, in turn, are particularly poorly perfused in shock. This circulatory impairment not only affords less opportunity for the reticuloendothelial system to make contact with bacteria, but the phagocytic cells themselves are damaged. These authors also noted that all three phases of antibacterial activity were even further impaired by transfusions of homologous (ACD) bank blood.

Pagano and Mersheimer have studied the immunological response to shock.[112] They found a fall in complement, an elevation of lysosome enzymes in the serum, the formation of substances that increase capillary permeability and the appearance of an abnormal toxic immunoprotein which suggested that an autologous immunotoxic reaction occurs. They point out that soluble antigen antibody complexes, which utilize complement in forming this abnormal immunoprotein, are found in old nonfrozen serum, which may explain Olledart's observation on the effects of blood transfusion.

Rutenburg et al. have isolated a splenic fraction capable of rapidly degrading endotoxin.[122] This fraction contains a protein with esterase-like activity. Indirect biologic assays indicate its activity is reduced in hemorrhagic shock. This has been presented as additional support of endotoxemia as the cause of irreversible shock. Conceding that the antibacterial defense mechanisms are significantly impaired in these experimental shock models, one cannot freely extrapolate these observations to the clinical counterpart since, as Zweifach has pointed out, marked species differences exist in bacterial flora, sensitivity to bacterial products, the target organ in endotoxemia, functional capacities of the reticuloendothelial system, opsonizing ability and the ability to develop tolerance.[174]

Hemodynamic Changes in Endotoxin and Septic Shock. After the injection of endotoxin there is a sudden fall in blood pressure. In a dog there is a moderate drop in plasma volume with a marked decrease in venous return. Although the heart is not immune to the effects of endotoxin, most of the circulatory changes appear to be related to peripheral effects. The decrease in venous return is due primarily to pooling in the hepatosplanchnic bed. This is caused by constriction of hepatic vein sphincters from histamine released by endotoxin. Wide species variations in the regional distribution of histamine and in the development of hepatic vein sphincters partly explain species variations in the hemodynamic responses to the injection of endotoxin. However, most of the other species differences appear to be quantitative rather than qualitative. Thomas et al. have shown that injections of viable washed *E. coli* and injections of *E. coli* endotoxin each produce similar hemodynamic responses (to each other) in dogs and in monkeys.[157]

After the initial hypotensive response to endotoxin injection, the blood pressure is returned toward normal by the pressor effect of released catecholamines. Then, depending on the lethality of the dose given, it will either be maintained or gradually decline again as the animal sinks into a state of profound and lethal shock, which is virtually indistinguishable from the refractory stages of shock from hemorrhage or other causes. The intense vasoconstriction wanes as catecholamine activity is overshadowed by the effects of histamine and vasoactive polypeptides.[156] Vasomotor tone collapses with peripheral pooling, loss of effective circulating blood volume and increased capillary permeability and loss of fluid into the extravascular space. That some of this vasomotor collapse may be intrinsic, secondary to damage to vascular smooth muscle, is suggested by the electron microscopic studies of Ashford.[3]

It has previously been mentioned that the hepatosplanchnic pooling that characterizes the canine response to endotoxin is comparatively insignificant in the monkey.[164] In addition, the marked increase in peripheral resistance observed in the dog is not found in the cat or monkey. These species differences have been used to explain dissimilarities between experimental endotoxin shock preparations and the clinical picture of septic shock. However, there is even a disagreement about what hemodynamic changes are characteristic of septic shock in the human. Originally, clinical septic shock was thought to be a problem of vasomotor collapse with peripheral pooling of blood. Udhoji and Weil in a careful hemodynamic study of six patients, suggested that this was due not to arteriolar dilatation but to failure of venous return secondary to changes in the venous or capacitance sphincters.[161] On the other hand, most of the patients studied by Thal and Wilson showed a normal blood volume, decreased peripheral resistance, but an increased cardiac index.[155] It is apparent that the hemodynamic picture is quite variable. This may be the result of differences in the state of the circulation imposed by the underlying infection prior to the onset of septic shock. Siegel and Del Guercio's study has documented the correlation of this variability with cardiac output and the degree of pulmonary and systemic arteriovenous "shunting" with many patients exhibiting a syndrome of high output circulatory failure.[135]

MacLean et al. described four different groups of septic shock patients by arbitrarily separating 56 consecutive cases according to whether they had a high or low central venous pressure (CVP) and whether they were alkalotic or acidotic.[90] Half the patients fell into Group 1 with a high CVP and a normal or high pH. Twenty-four of these survived their shock episode. This group was thought to represent the typical early septic shock picture, characterized by hyperventilation and respiratory alkalosis and a high CVP, high cardiac index, low peripheral resistance with warm, dry skin in the face of hypotension, oliguria and lactacidemia. In the second group of 11 patients with a high CVP and acidosis, only one survived. These patients showed the same hyperdynamic circulatory state but were thought to have become acidotic, because even their increased cardiac output was insufficient to meet the increased circulatory demands of their septic state. Pulmonary edema was a prominent additional feature in this group and it did not respond to conventional therapy. In Group 3, there were 10 patients with a low CVP and a normal or high pH. Nine of these were resuscitated from shock. These patients were relatively hypovolemic and responded to intravenous fluids. The fourth group were acidotic with a low CVP and all seven died. The authors suggested that the variable patterns described in previous studies of septic shock were related to two factors, the relative ability of the heart to meet the increased circulatory demands placed on it and the patient's state of hydration or blood volume. Half of the patients who died were unable to raise their cardiac outputs. The authors suggested that the other half who died in spite of a supranormal cardiac output must have succumbed for one of three reasons: (1) their cardiac output was still not sufficient to meet the increased needs of the body, (2) enough oxygen and metabolites were not reaching the vital tissues because of arteriovenous shunting or (3) there was a failure of tissue utilization of the oxygen and nutrients delivered to it because of deteriorization or death of the cells.

Siegel et al. reported similar findings in comparing a series of septic shock patients with those suffering from other forms of shock.[134] They pointed out that all patients in septic shock, regardless of cause or bacterial etiology, have a significantly decreased vascular tone as compared to non-septic shock patients. That is, at a given systemic flow, the vascular resistance is less in septic shock than in other forms of shock, a relationship which holds true over the entire range of cardiac outputs. They also noted signs of anaerobic metabolism in spite of high cardiac outputs. Patients with septic shock showed a different pattern with regard to the effectiveness of their oxygen transport mechanisms in that oxygen consumptions vary independently of cardiac index. The hyperdynamic or high output failure patients with septic shock exhibited very inefficient oxygen extraction. To achieve a normal oxygen consumption, they required two to four times the cardiac output needed by normal patients. Those patients with septic shock and a little cardiac output had similar oxygen transport patterns to the non-septic shock patients. Finally, every patient they studied with septic shock had a diminished ventricular function relationship, in that the relationship between stroke work and the venous pressure was decreased. The high cardiac output cases obviously had a better ventricular function than those with low cardiac output, but the eventual incidence of myocardial failure was equal in both groups.

The Endotoxin Theory of Irreversible Shock. The possibility that overwhelming endotoxemia might be the final common denominator in irreversible shock, regardless of the precipitating factor, has been suggested by Fine.[116] Attention was initially attracted to this possibility by the strikingly similar pathologic changes in the hepatosplanchnic bed in dogs subjected to hemorrhagic shock and lethal injections of endotoxin. Since the splanchnic viscera represent a major interface of bacterial growth with the body's defense mechanisms, it was suggested that, in severe shock of any origin, the reticuloendothelial system—which normally detoxifies any endotoxin which might be absorbed from bacteria in the gut—may be rendered ineffective, resulting in an overwhelming endotoxemia. Evidence was presented in support of this contention. The toxicity of blood taken from animals suffering from irreversible hemorrhagic shock suggested a transferable factor. It was shown that there was a decreased tolerance to hemorrhage after blockade of the reticuloendothelial system, and increased tolerance could be achieved by multiple sublethal doses of endotoxin. Experiments in the same laboratory showed that sterilization of the gut gave a significant degree of protection against the lethality of hemorrhagic shock. More recently, Rutenburg et al.[122] have shown by indirect assay that the spleen's ability to detoxify endotoxin was impaired by hemorrhage. Finally, support can be drawn from the growing evidence that the body's antibacterial defense mechanisms are greatly impaired in hemorrhagic shock[111] and from the demonstration of Bounous and associates of the breakdown of the integrity of the mucosal barrier of the gut in shock.[18, 19]

Nevertheless, formidable barriers were raised against the acceptance of this theory. First, both Lillehei and Simeone failed to confirm a protective effect of gut sterilization against the lethality of hemorrhagic shock.[85, 137] Secondly, McNulty and Linares showed that germ-free rats were no more tolerant of hemorrhagic shock than littermates reared in a contaminated environment.[93] In addition, Sanford and Noyes were unable to detect the absorption of isotope-tagged endotoxin instilled into the gut of dogs in hemorrhagic shock in quantities 1000 times greater than detectable after intravenous infusion.[125] In rebuttal, Fine has dismissed the failure of others to confirm his observations on the benefit of gut sterilization as the result of technical differences. He points out that even germ-free animals eat food that has ample quantities of dead bacteria in it. Furthermore, workers in his laboratory feel they have been able to detect circulating endotoxin in hemorrhagic shock by indirect assay.

As this controversy continues without clear-cut victory for either side, much valuable information is being gained about the effects of endotoxin. Evidence has been presented that many of the effects of endotoxin may be mediated through the nervous system. Penner and Bernheim found that one-twentieth of the intravenous lethal dose would be fatal if injected into the third ventricle.[114] Fine and his coworkers found denervation procedures to be more effective than adrenergic blocking agents and feel it produces a more selective benefit.[173] In one experiment they denervated one-half of the spleen and three weeks later subjected the animals to hemorrhagic shock. They observed that the nondenervated half of the spleen lost two-thirds of its norepinephrine content and its ability to detoxify endotoxin, while the denervated half did not lose its endotoxin detoxifying ability or its norepinephrine content and did not change in size, shape or color.

There is also evidence that the lethal effect of endotoxin is largely due to a direct action on the cell. Simeone feels that, in endotoxin shock, tissue damage occurs at the outset, in contradistinction to other types of shock in which it occurs as the late effect of inadequate tissue perfusion.[138] Thal et al. feel that endotoxin might interfere directly with the intracellular enzyme systems involved in aerobic metabolism.[154] Bell and Schloerb have shown a relatively greater fall in intracellular pH in endotoxin shock than in hemorrhagic shock.[11] Rush has even noted acidosis following doses of endotoxin so small that hypotension was not provoked.[121] More will be said of the effects of endotoxin on the cell later in this chapter.

Vasoactive Substances in Shock

The control of flow through the peripheral circulation in shock is a complex process. Peripheral resistance reflects the summation of intrinsic, neural and humoral vasomotor adjustment to changes in cardiac output and blood volume. It is difficult, if not impossible, to isolate their relative contributions. This difficulty is exemplified by attempts to separate the effects of the sympathetic neurohumoral axis that are mediated by catecholamines released from the adrenal medulla from those of the sympathetic nerve endings. If a sympathectomy is done, the sensitivity of effector sites to centrally released catecholamines is heightened. If the adrenals are removed, cortical as well as medullary function is eliminated.

Equally difficult is the attempt to estimate the relative contributions of vasoactive humoral agents in shock. This is compounded by species variations in both sensitivity to these substances and the pattern of end organ response. Understandably, the study of vasoactive substances in human shock has been limited.

Peripheral blood levels of these substances do not necessarily reflect their activity. A substance may be released, exert its effects locally and be quickly degraded without its peripheral level becoming significantly elevated. On the other hand, the action of one of these substances may be blocked by drugs or other agents so that their effect may be minimal in spite of high circulating levels.

Some vasoactive substances, such as adrenaline and serotonin, can produce different, even opposite, effects at different dosage levels or in the face of differences in existing vasomotor tone. Furthermore, many of these agents act on the same receptor site. Finally, one must also consider the influence of background factors, such as pH, the concentration of certain electrolytes and the sensitivity of the end organ.

These limitations should be kept in mind during the following discussion of the effects of these vasoactive agents in shock.

Catecholamines. Properly defined, catecholamines are any low molecular weight substances combining a catechol nucleus and an amine group, but the term is usually reserved for dopamine and its metabolic end products, norepinephrine and epinephrine. They are synthesized in the brain, in the chromaffin cells of the adrenal medulla and at sympathetic nerve endings from tyrosine. In addition to tissues which can synthesize catecholamine, many other tissues are capable of removing it from the circulation and storing it. The synthesis, release, breakdown and degradation of catecholamines as well as other pertinent details of their metabolism have been fully reviewed by Wurtman.[171]

The actions of the catecholamines are variable. Attempts have been made to organize their effects in terms of alpha and beta receptors. These may not be receptors in the usual physiologic sense, but rather key enzymatic processes. Sutherland and Rall have presented evidence suggesting that the beta receptor may be the cyclizing enzyme that catalyzes the conversion of ATP to cyclic 3,5 adenosine monophosphate (3,5 AMP), a key reaction in the hormonal control of certain energy systems.[150]

Epinephrine appears to act predominantly on the beta receptor when given in small doses, whereas at higher doses, its alpha effect predominates. Norepinephrine also has both alpha and beta effects, although the alpha effects predominate at all doses. The most important expression of alpha activity is the excitation of smooth muscle, particularly vascular smooth muscle. Beta stimulation, on the other hand, produces an inotropic and chronotropic effect on the heart, a mobilization of glucose from glycogen stores and free fatty acid from adipose tissue, a release of ACTH and relaxation of smooth muscle. Thus, the overall hemodynamic effects of catecholamine release depend on the relative levels of epinephrine and norepinephrine. When the alphamimetic effects predominate , there is an increased arteriolar tone, venous pooling and bradycardia, whereas the betamimetic effects lead to decreased arteriolar constriction and an increase in heart rate and stroke volume. These usually act in combination, and the differences in end organ sensitivity to each provide a selective hemodynamic response.

Thus, the usual effects of combined catecholamine activity are an increase in blood flow to the heart, brain and striated muscle and a decrease in the flow to the skin, hepatosplanchnic area and kidney, just what one would expect from the "flight or fight" function of the sympathetic nervous system. In hemorrhagic shock, the regional blood flow pattern is thought to be influenced by catecholamine release, but it differs slightly from that above in that flow to striated muscle is diminished and splanchnic vasoconstriction is partly compensated for by an increased distribution of cardiac output through the hepatic artery.

In experimental shock preparations, high catecholamine levels are found in the blood. Since high doses of norepinephrine can produce pathologic changes identical to those seen with lethal degrees of endotoxin or hemorrhagic shock, some have contended that it is the excessive and prolonged catecholamine activity that causes the irreversible effects of shock. Although the deleterious effects of excessive catecholamine activity are not challenged, most feel that inadequate tissue perfusion of any cause will lead to the same end result. Furthermore, alpha blocking agents given in the refractory stages of shock are not protective. Indeed, late in shock there appears to be a profound loss of vasomotor tone and, in endotoxin shock at least, 80 per cent of the vasoactivity at the stage appears to be derived from histamine and vasoactive polypeptides.[79] The central point in this debate is whether catecholamine activity is physiologic and reversible or excessive and self-perpetuating. On this there is no general agreement.

Histamine. In 1912 Dale and Richards discovered that histamine was a vasodilator that increased tissue permeability and, when given to cats in large doses, produced severe hypotension.[38] When the experiments of Cannon and Bayliss shortly after this suggested a toxemic basis for traumatic shock, histamine became a prime suspect.[26] The initial hypotensive episode that follows the injection of endotoxin in dogs has been shown to be due to hepatosplanchnic pooling secondary to the effect of histamine on hepatic vein sphincters. It can be mimicked by histamine injection, prevented by prior histamine depletion using 48/80, and blocked by dibenzyline.[69]

Thal and his associates have studied the pattern of histamine activity after both endotoxin and exotoxin injection.[79] After the initial peak there is a secondary rise late in the course of the shock at which time histamine and vasoactive polypeptides contribute most of the total vasoactivity. Thal has also shown that endotoxin releases histamine in vivo and, if first incubated with blood or tissue homogenates, releases it in vitro as well. He found the tissues that liberate the largest amount of histamine are the liver, pancreas and upper small intestine and that greater amounts of histamine are released after portal than systemic injection of endotoxin. Hepatectomy and evisceration experiments suggest that the initial peak of histamine is released mainly from the hepatosplanchnic bed, whereas the terminal rise results from slower biosynthesis in other tissues. Schayer's experiments have suggested to him that the local synthesis of histamine by histidine decarboxylase may, in balance with the catecholamines, exert a controlling influence on the microcirculation.[126]

The loss of arteriolar resistance, increased capillary permeability and persistent venous sphincter tone, which are thought to be characteristic of the late stages of shock in the dog, have been explained by some as indicating a predominance of histamine over catecholamines at this point. Thal's assays of histamine and catecholamine activity injection are compatible with this contention. The work of Visscher and associates suggests that the increased capillary permeability from histamine may be the result of postcapillary venular spasm alone.[163] However, it must be remembered that this impression of histamine's effect on the venous outflow sphincters has been derived mainly from canine experiments. As shown by Brockman and Vasko and Waldhausen et al., these changes are much less marked in subhuman primates.[21, 164] Histamine stores in primates also differ in amount (less) and pattern of distribution from dogs. Thus, while the role of histamine in human shock is still unsettled, its importance appears to be waning.

Serotonin. 5-Hydroxytryptamine, or serotonin, is widely distributed throughout the body and is particularly abundant in the brain, upper small intestine, platelets and mast cells. Elevations in circulating serotonin levels have been demonstrated in both experimental and clinical shock studies. Serotonin is capable of amphibaric effects. It may raise or lower the blood pressure under different circumstances, usually acting in opposition to the existing direction of change. Its contribution to total vasoactivity in the canine endotoxin shock studies of Thal was definitely less than histamine. One of the areas in which serotonin has been suspected of contributing most to the pathogenesis of shock is the pulmonary circulation. Serotonin greatly increases pulmonary vascular resistance and, unlike a similar response to histamine, this is independent of any bronchoconstrictive effects.[102] It has been suggested that the *drop* in peripheral resistance and the narrowing of a-v oxygen differences seen late in shock may represent the opening of a-v shunts secondary to serotonin release, similar to the effect described in the carcinoid flush.[40]

However, the evidence that serotonin exerts a significant systemic hemodynamic effect in shock is not substantial. Nevertheless, at a local level, the release of serotonin from injured platelets may play an important role in the clotting and constriction of injured vessels. In addition, the tendency for platelet aggregation after trauma may be the result of serotonin release.[151]

Vasoactive Polypeptides. Recent years have witnessed a growing interest in certain plasma polypeptides possessing powerful vasoactive properties. This began with Werle's work on a hypotensive proteolytic substance derived from the pancreas[168]. This substance, called kallikrein, was first thought to exert its effect directly, but further research has established that it activated polypeptides from their precursors in the plasma or the pancreas, probably through another enzyme system, the kinases. Trypsin and other proteolytic enzymes also appear capable of activating these kinin peptides and, in turn, along with kallikrein, these proteases may be activated by Hageman factor, plasmin and possibly endotoxin. With the uncovering of this complex system of interacting enzymes, there has been a renewed interest in the pathogenesis of shock resulting from pancreatitis and endotoxemia.

The best known of the kinin peptides is bradykinin, a nonapeptide whose amino acid sequence has been determined. It is known to produce vasodilation, smooth muscle relaxation, increased capillary permeability, leukocytic infiltration and pain, all of which are interrelated, suggesting that bradykinin may be the mediator of the local inflammatory response and an important factor in local microcirculatory control in other situations. In comparative tests it is a more potent universal vasodilator than histamine.

Bradykinin release has been detected in both experimental and clinical shock studies.[77, 80] In hemorrhagic shock, bradykininogen levels rose initially then fell below control levels.[41] Kobold, Thal and associates have compared the relative contributions of vasoactive polypeptides and catecholamines, histamine and serotonin to total vasoactivity at different stages of endotoxin shock using a strip of ox carotid.[80] Their studies suggest that these vasoactive polypeptides, along with histamine, contribute heavily late in shock.

The hyperdynamic circulatory state seen in early septic shock and in the late refractory stages of shock of other etiologies is compatible with and suggestive of the systemic effects of kinins on the circulation. However, the role of these peptides in the pathogenesis of these shock states has been generally downgraded because their supposed short half-life had relegated them, in the thinking of most investigators, to playing only a local humoral role. And yet, the demonstration that the hypotensive response to intravenous bradykinin in the rat was only one-fiftieth that of an aortic injection[48] led to the realization that the apparent minor systemic effect of intravenous bradykinin and its presumed short half-life are due to its extremely effective (90–98 per cent) breakdown during passage through the lungs by a system of pulmonary kininases suspected of being located in the pinocytotic vesicles directly under the pulmonary capillary endothelium.[115]

Work by Wilson suggests that the enzymes in these vesicles are depleted in the lungs of animals subjected to shock.[170] It is further known that the pulmonary kininase system is subject to tachyphylaxis and can be overwhelmed by larger doses of bradykinin.[12] Acute pulmonary edema has been produced in normal rats by this means.[66] Furthermore the electron microscopic appearance of tissues perfused with kinins is not unlike that demonstrated for shock lung, with opening up of the septa between endothelial cells, pouring out of plasma and large protein molecules into the interstitial space, etc.[153] Bradykinin is more powerful than either histamine or serotonin in producing these tissue changes. Finally, the demonstrated protection from "shock lung" by hilar cross-clamping during shock[169] and the sparing of the downstream lung of two lungs perfused in series from a similar pulmonary lesion produced by extracorporeal perfusion with autologous blood[142] could be equally well blamed on circulating humoral substances as on microemboli or fat emboli.

It has been demonstrated in experimental shock that lysosomal disruption occurs and lysosomal products have been revealed in the peripheral circulation in both experimental and clinical shock.[117, 88] Kinin-forming enzymes in the tissues are lysosomal in origin with optional activity in the lower pH range seen in shock, whereas kinin inhibitors or kininases are less efficient at these pH's. These factors suggest the possibility that significant amounts of vasoactive polypeptides may be released during shock and eventually might not only contribute significantly to the pathogenesis of shock lung but, having overwhelmed or bypassed the pulmonary kininase system, may reach the systemic arterial circulation in increasing amounts and contribute to the hyperdynamic circulatory failure which characterizes refractory stages of some types of clinical shock. At the moment this is merely conjecture or at best circumstantial evidence which awaits proper clinical investigation.

Another vasoactive polypeptide, apparently unrelated to the kinins, has recently been brought to the forefront of shock research. It is called MDF, or myocardial depressant factor. Although a similar substance was identified earlier by Brandt et al. as a vasodepressor factor following declamping shock, its role in the pathogenesis of shock has been mainly elaborated by the work of Lefer and his associates.[82] Brand and Lefer originally identified this substance in the plasma of cats after severe hemorrhagic shock. Plasma samples were shown to decrease the developed tension of isolated cat papillary muscles, which has remained the basis for its bioassay. High activities of plasma cathepsin-like substances appearing in the blood prior to increased levels of MDF suggested that the appearance of MDF may be related to enzymatic cleavage of plasma proteins by proteases. MDF has since been found in the plasma of animals subjected to hemorrhagic shock, pancreatitis, endotoxin shock, splanchnic ischemia and cardiogenic shock. Lovett et al. studied the plasma of 24 patients for the myocardial depressant factor; 14 of the patients were in severe shock and 10 were controls.[88] A significantly higher plasma MDF level and lysosomal enzyme activities were present in the plasma of patients with circulatory shock. In 10 of 14 there was evidence of impaired myocardial function at the time the specimen was obtained.

In spite of this suggested information, the relative importance of MDF in the pathogenesis of irreversible shock has not been established, particularly since in many other similar shock preparations in other laboratories, alterations in myocardial contractility have not been considered a significant finding. Greenfield et al. performed cross-circulation experiments between normal isolated hearts in dogs in terminal shock, 18–21 hours after administration of endotoxin.[55] The cross-circulation was carried out for a period of three hours and compared to control animals studied similarly but without endotoxin administration. Isometric cardiac performance (measured by intraventricular balloon distention) was *not* impaired in the endotoxin group, which actually showed consistently better time-tension curves and pressure work than control animals. No alteration in force-velocity curves was noted in either group. Increases in both oxygen uptake and pressure work in the endotoxin group indicated no changes in calculated myocardial efficiency. The conclusion of these investigators was that no deleterious effect on the normal heart perfused with blood from a dog in terminal endotoxin shock could be demonstrated to substantiate the primary role suggested for the myocardial depressant factor.

More damning has been the report by one of Lefer's former coworkers that plasma MDF has been identified as salt and represents an artifact of the bioassay system, and that its depressant activity plays no significant role in shock.[165] Following this, however, Lefer's laboratory claims to have not only identified but synthesized MDF.

Angiotensin. Angiotensin is a potent vasoactive octapeptide formed by the action of the renal protease renin on the plasma precursor angiotensinogen. Its hemodynamic effects are essentially the reverse of bradykinin. It is a more potent and universal vasoconstrictor than norepinephrine. Evidence from human and animal studies suggests that angiotensin increases vascular resistance by constricting arteriolar sphincters, without the degree of postcapillary resistance seen with norepinephrine.[87] Thus, it has been suggested that angiotensin reduces capillary hydrostatic pressure and allows rather than retards transcapillary plasma refilling. This impression that angiotensin may support the blood pressure more physiologically has led to its evaluation as a therapeutic agent for hypotensive states with conflicting conclusions that may eventually be resolved by establishment of proper dosage levels.

At present, there is not enough information to allow firm conclusions to be drawn about the natural or therapeutic role angiotensin plays in various shock states. Its relationship to aldosterone production has been discussed earlier in this chapter.

Prostaglandins. Prostaglandins are a family of structurally related, hormone-like substances with extremely powerful activity effecting a wide range of physiologic processes. Many of the prostaglandins have marked hemodynamic effects and it is understandable that they are suspected of playing a role in the pathogenesis of refractory shock. However, at the moment, there is no evidence that their action is anything other than physiologic in facilitating the actions of hormones and nerves at the common interface of the cell membrane.

The Effects of Shock on the Cell and on Metabolism

As stated earlier, the decreased arteriovenous oxygen differences which characterize the hyperdynamic circulatory failure of late shock could be due to a circulatory system driven beyond the perfusion demands of the tissues, opening of arteriovenous shunts, abnormalities in oxygen transport, or the inability of dead, dying or deranged cells to utilize oxygen. There is a growing conviction that the latter is the case, and in the final analysis, mortality is determined at a cellular level. More is implied by this than simply an equation of cellular death with its summation or the death of the whole organism. Rather it is felt that some discrete form of cellular damage of dysfunction is *primarily* responsible for the refractory state that develops in protracted shock. This view is most plausible for endotoxin shock, in which, as outlined in the preceding section, there is evidence for a direct, early toxic effect on the cell. Even those who do not share this conviction can, for therapeutic reasons, share the hope that some discrete and correctable metabolic change in the cell can be faulted in irreversible shock.

The work of Bryant et al. suggests that further investigation in this direction may be rewarding.[22] They studied three groups of dogs which had been bled to 40 mmHg and maintained at this level until they had reached a recognizable stage of irreversibility (25 per cent uptake from the bleeding reservoir). After reinfusion of the remainder of the shed blood, they assisted the circulation of one group with a two-hour partial venoarterial bypass, synchronized to deliver blood during diastole. None of this group survived. In a second group, cross circulation through a donor dog but without mechanical circulatory support provided only a 10 per cent survival. However, in the third group in which they continuously cross-circulated the blood through a donor dog as well as applied synchronized circulatory assistance with a partial venoarterial bypass, there was an 80 per cent survival. They concluded that "the addition of the metabolic reservoir of a donor dog to an animal in irreversible hemorrhagic shock can lead to successful resuscitation when combined with synchronous pumping for the failing circulation."

The hope that irreversible shock merely represents a limitation in our present state of knowledge has stimulated many investigations into the cellular changes in shock and their metabolic effects. Just as the focus of attention on the circulatory changes in shock has been carried to the level of the microcirculation, so have the studies of metabolic responses gone beyond the measurement of blood levels of glucose, oxygen, carbon dioxide, pH and electrolytes. However, complex technical problems associated with study at the cellular level still greatly limit the information that can be gained by such endeavors.

If the functional and structural integrity of the cell is to be maintained, it must be able to generate energy. This requires access to an adequate supply of oxygen and nutrients. Most of the energy generated by the cell is captured in the terminal phosphate bond (~p) of adenosine triphosphate (ATP), although considerable storage capacity is provided by the transfer of this terminal phosphate bond to creatinine. Ninety per cent of the ~p is generated aerobically and captured by a most efficient energy trapping system, a chain of flavoproteins and cytochrome oxidases called the respiratory enzymes. This chain carries the two hydrogen atoms generated by oxidative reduction through a graded series of energy levels, with lipoproteins assisting in each transfer. At each level ~ p's are generated until the two hydrogen atoms are finally united with oxygen to form water. Essentially, all the energy captured by this system is derived from the reactions of the Krebs cycle into which acetyl CoA (the two-carbon unit of carbohydrate), fat and protein breakdown are fed. This highly organized process operates wholly within the mitochondria and in the presence of oxygen.

The cell performs many functions on its own behalf that require this energy. The sodium ion pump that maintains membrane potential and permeability and the active transport of certain substances across the cell membrane and between the cytoplasm and the mitochondria and other components of cell ultra structure are prime examples of this. In addition, the survival of the organism as a whole depends on such specialized, energy-dependent, cellular functions as the contraction of cardiac, smooth and striated muscle, the transmission of nerve impulses, the metabolic activity of hepatic cells, the refining of urine by the kidney's countercurrent multiplier sodium pump system and the production of mucin, surfactant and various exocrine and endocrine substances.

The importance of continued energy production by the cell seems obvious. This does not necessarily mean that energy depletion is *the* critical factor in the outcome of shock. Nor has a discrete cause for the breakdown in cellular metabolism been identified, although several possibilities have been entertained.

The natural suspect, of course, is inadequate oxygen supply to the cell. If oxygen is no longer available to accept the hydrogen atoms at the end of the respiratory enzyme chain, this system will grind to a halt, forcing the cell to utilize anaerobic pathways, which are a rather limited source of energy. Although a switch to anaerobic metabolism is characteristic of shock states, the explanation seems to be more complex than the unavailability of oxygen. Oxygen consumption appears to be normal until the terminal phase of shock. Triner et al. have shown that it is even increased during compensated (normotensive) hypovolemia, probably as a result of sympathetic activity.[159] Also, although oxygen availability may be reduced, some oxygen must be available to the tissues and, even when tissue perfusion is reduced, increased arteriovenous oxygen differences suggest that this is at least partially compensated for by increased oxygen uptake, facilitated by the characteristics of the hemoglobin-oxygen dissociation curve.

Nevertheless, a switch to anaerobic glycolysis does occur relatively early in shock. Shumer has shown by studying the relative amounts of C^{14} labelled glucose that appeared downstream in metabolic intermediates, that a metabolic block appeared in shocked animals in the metabolic pathway between pyruvate and acetyl CoA.[132] Furthermore, later in shock there are *decreases* in arteriovenous oxygen differences and oxygen consumptions. Although the latter have been explained by the opening of arteriovenous shunts and the bypassing of the capillary circulation or defects in oxygen transport, such as the change in oxygen-hemoglobin affinity brought about by decreased levels of 2-3 diphosphoglycerate, it is more likely that they are the result of the lack of utilization by damaged cells. Bounous and his associates have shown that the decreases in oxygen consumption by the splanchnic bed correlate well with mortality.[17] The failure of hyperbaric oxygen therapy at this point in shock would also suggest that cellular dysfunction has occurred that prevents utilization of oxygen.[73]

It has been suggested that the *acidosis* that develops during shock has an adverse effect on cell function. As shock deepens and the cell turns more and more to anaerobic glycolysis, pyruvate is converted to lactate rather than being processed through the Krebs cycle. Huckabee has shown that the excess accumulation of lactate is a fairly sensitive index of cellular hypoxia, a phenomenon long known by the name of "oxygen debt."[72] This metabolic acidosis, from the accumulation of lactate, carbon dioxide and other acidic metabolites, is at first compensated for by hyperventilation so that the pH of *peripheral arterial blood* may even suggest an alkalosis. In fact, studies of combat casualties in Vietnam[28, 29] and civilian clinical investigations[8] have indicated that in healthy young subjects (and when hemorrhage is not too rapid or hypotension too prolonged) acidosis is *not* a regular accompaniment of shock. In fact, hyperventilation will usually have caused some degree of alkalosis. Unlike canine studies of the past, recent primate shock studies[123] have shown that periods of hemorrhagic hypotension, sufficiently profound and prolonged to be lethal, may not be associated with acidosis until the terminal phase. Nevertheless, even in these situations the venous pH is usually relatively low, suggesting a masked, concomitant metabolic acidosis. If this situation persists long enough, especially in older patients or those with multiple injuries or intercurrent disease such as diabetes, the respiratory compensation will fail and metabolic acidosis will predominate. Until that time, the routine use of buffering agents or infusions of lactated Ringer's solution rather than saline in resuscitation will not only have been unnecessary but may have been deleterious.

To a degree, acidosis has a homeostatic value. It facilitates the release of oxygen and the uptake of carbon dioxide in the tissues, increases the coagulability of blood, and results in increases in respiratory rate, cerebral circulation and arterial pressure.

However, *profound* degrees of acidosis have been shown to decrease myocardial contractility, to decrease the vasomotor response to humoral agents, and, in dogs, to produce a constriction of venous (capacitance) sphincters. More telling may be its effects inside the cell. It may interfere with cellular metabolism if the pH is lowered beyond the optimum range of key intracellular enzymes, or it may result in the rupture of lysosomal membranes, releasing harmful proteolytic enzymes within the cell. Neither of the latter suggestions can be considered more than conjectural at present.

Some experiments have shown beneficial effects in shock from buffering therapy, using $NaHCO_3$ or the buffer amine, trishydroxymethanolamine. Like almost all therapeutic measures claiming success in the treatment of experimental shock, this benefit is not significant once a stage of recognizable "irreversibility" has been reached. However, these measures do seem to result in improved urinary output[110] and an amelioration of clotting abnormalities in in shocked animals[124] and, in combination with increased oxygen delivery, to provide a significant increase in survival.[95]

It has been known since Claude Bernard's experimental observations in 1877 that the blood sugar became elevated in shock. This was eventually attributed to the hepatic glycogen mobilization effect of catecholamine release, although Carey's recent work suggests that the initial hyperglycemia is not simply an epinephrine effect.[37] After an initial increase, probably from the release of preformed insulin, the insulin response to this hyperglycemia appears to be depressed, probably as a result of severely reduced pancreatic blood flow. Coran's studies suggest that the hypotensive baboon is both physiologically and immunochemically insulin-deficient.[31] On the other hand, in milder degrees of shock, as in volunteers to hemorrhage by Skillman, insulin production may be increased.[140] In any event, in late shock hypoglycemia intervenes and is characteristic of the terminal state. Since severe hypoglycemia can produce hypotension, its role in terminal shock has been considered. However, infusions of hypertonic glucose at this stage of shock have no effect on the outcome or even the hemodynamic picture.

Glucose makes a relatively greater contribution to total body energy in shock and trauma, but, as in the normotensive state, fatty acids still constitute the main circulating energy source. Like glucose, fatty acids are mobilized and released in response to epinephrine. It would appear from Drucker's work that the changes in the peripheral levels of glucose and fatty acids in response to hemorrhagic shock depend on the rapidity and depth of the hemorrhage.[46] With slow hemorrhage, plasma-free fatty acids increased initially and then decreased later as hyperglycemia developed. However, if the volume lost was rapid enough, hyperglycemia occurred early and free fatty acids decreased. As pointed out by Cahill, a labile protein pool exists and provides the body requirements for glucose when glycogen stores are depleted.[43] But all protein, in contrast to fats, exists in the body for a purpose, so there is no expendable depot of nitrogen.

Once the essential nutrients become unavailable and the cell's energy stores are depleted, the cell is forced, in a sense, to turn on itself for other sources of energy. Steinberg has shown that cells may survive for up to two hours with no external source of nutrients.[144] However, in doing so, they penalize themselves since *structural phospholipids* are one of the major components depleted by this effort.

Loss of the structural integrity of the cell membrane and ultrastructure has important consequences beyond those of increased permeability. The mitochondrial apparatus may not be able to function if the intricate structural and spatial arrangements of its enzyme network are disrupted, preventing enzymes involved in a chain of related biochemical reactions from "getting together." Structural changes in the mitochondria have been demonstrated by electron microscopic techniques in the tissues of animals subjected to shock or hypoxia[4, 149] Others have only reported mitochondrial swelling, but even this may interfere with function. Thus, it is possible that the configurational templates that are felt to be so vital for molecular synthesis might be disrupted and the maintenance of ion gradients and the active transport of substances vital to cell life no longer possible.

Disruption of the limiting membranes of the lysosomes inside the cell is one of the more interesting recent proposals. These subcellular structures are thought to play a protective role by isolating the cell from essential but potentially destructive enzymes such as proteases, esterases, hydrolases and phosphatases. The works of DeDuve have drawn attention to this possibility and indeed the lysosomal apparatus has been considered the cell's "suicide sac."[39] Lysosomes appear to be disrupted when the cell is subjected to anoxic injury, and the appearance of proteolytic enzymes in the peripheral circulation in certain shock states may be a reflection of this. Their release may in turn activate the kinase system, with the release of vasoactive polypeptides and the initiation of intravascular clotting.

Mela et al. have shown that lysosommal derangements observed following endotoxin injection.[98] Lefer et al. have shown increased cathepsin-like activity in association with increased myocardial depressant factor in shock.[82] On the other hand, Shumer could not show lysosomal enzymes in circulating blood after hemorrhagic shock.[133]

Janoff et al. have shown that graded injury (drum shock), and Weissmann and Thomas that steroids, may increase the resistance of lysosomes to rupture.[74, 167] The acquired tolerance to shock and the beneficial effects of steroids may have some foundation in these observations.

The question has been raised whether, in shock, there is a weak link in the chain of intracellular enzymes that support cell life or whether the abnormal metabolism simply reflects a summation of effects. At the moment, there is no answer to this question. Some have even suggested that cellular metabolism is not intrinsically abnormal but reflects only inadequate tissue perfusion. McShan et al. in 1945 and LePage found decreases in tissue levels of high energy phosphate compounds and energy-yielding substrates in rats subjected to drum shock and to hemorrhagic shock.[94, 83, 84] However, Rosenbaum et al. found that the decreases in high energy phosphate compounds in the liver of bled dogs did not correlate with their response to reinfusion.[120] Stoner and Threlfall, using a tourniquet shock model, found that these compounds were not significantly depleted in muscle outside the injured limb.[147] They found a decrease in body temperature and heat production that correlated well with lethality. Subsequent studies suggest that this is not related to decreased energy production, although Stoner now admits that the latter occurs terminally.[146] Kovach and Fonyo found, in rats shocked by freezing their hind limbs, that cerebral energy-rich compound were unaltered even in terminal stages.[81] However, it should be pointed out that the cerebral circulation, like that of the heart, is selectively spared in shock.

Strawitz and Hift subjected dogs to three to five hours of hemorrhagic shock then sacrificed the animals without reinfusing the shed blood.[148] They found mitochondrial abnormalities in the heart, liver and kidney. Although myocardial mitochondria retained their capacity for oxidative phosphorylation in vitro, their phosphate-oxygen ratios suggest that this process may have been impaired. In vitro studies, such as these, must be interpreted with caution because the mitochondrial preparation may not reflect in vivo function. This is because these organelles are again placed in an optimum environment during such studies, and significant distortions in spatial relationships of related enzymes may be masked by the preparation process that breaks up the mitochondria so that that function possible through random association is measured.

Recent investigations by Baue et al. have demonstrated a partial uncoupling of ATP-dependent and ATP-yielding reactions.[9] Liver mitochondria of shocked animals had a decreased ability to resynthesize ATP from ADP, particularly with DPN-linked substrates, such as alphaketoglutarate. These changes were revised by volume restoration and appeared to correlate with changes in the cation content (increased sodium and decreased potassium and bound magnesium) of the mitochondrial. Increased activity of the transport enzyme sodium and potassium ATP-ase was also found. This finding fit well with changes in cell membrane potential in shock reported by others and was thought to indicate that the cell membrane might be the initial weak point in the functional disintegration of the cell.

Empirical evidence that these ATP-generating reactions or the enzymes responsible for them may be impaired in shock has been presented by the observations of Talaat et al. and Sharma and Eiseman, who showed beneficial effects from infusions of ATP in shock preparation.[152, 128] Similarly, Hashimoto and Cowley have noted a protective effect from mitochondrial suspensions.[64] It must be pointed out that these therapeutic measures were effective only when given at a time when infusion of shed blood would still have resulted in survival. It has been noted that ATP has vasodilatory properties. However, in Sharma and Eiseman's experiment, this effect of ATP was apparently ruled out by the fact that control groups, given doses of AMP and dibenzyline which produced an equivalent vasodilation, did not show the same protection.

Recently, there has been a great deal of interest in cyclic 3,5 AMP, a substance produced from ATP by the cyclizing enzyme located on the cell membrane. This molecule is thought to be an important intracellular mediator of certain hormone-controlled, energy-requiring organ functions such as the phosphorylation of glucose in the liver, steroid synthesis by the adrenals and sex hormone production by the ovaries. Sutherland and Rall, who showed that this cyclase system is responsible for the activation of phosphorylase, have suggested that his process may be the key to ATP's role in the sodium ion pump, inotropic effects on the heart, smooth muscle relaxation and the mobilization of free fatty acids from adipose tissue.[150] The fact that many substances acting on the beta receptor, such as catecholamines, isoprenaline, glucagon, serotonin and acetycholine, have similar effects on this cyclizing reaction suggests that this enzyme, and not a receptor site in the usual physiologic sense, may be the beta receptor.

Although many of the statements in this section are obviously conjectural, investigations should greatly increase our understanding of the cellular responses to shock.

Finally, although this resume of the physiologic and metabolic responses to shock reflects serious limitations of our state of knowledge, it should also be evident that much progress has been made and that much more can be expected in the future.

REFERENCES

1. Alexander, R. S.: Venomotor tone in hemorrhage and shock. Circ. Res. *3*:181, 1955.
2. Ashbaugh, D. and Uzawa, I.: Respiratory and hemodynamic changes after injection of free fatty acids. J. Surg. Res. *8*:417, 1968.
3. Ashford, T.: A lesion in vascular smooth muscle in shock and its response to corticosteroid: Electron microscopic study. (Paper presented before the American Surgical Association, March, 1966.) Ann. Surg. *164*:575, 1966.
4. Ashford, T. P., and Burdette, W. J.: Response of the isolated perfused hepatic parenchyma to hypoxia. Ann. Surg. *162*:191, 1965.
5. Attar, S., Kirby, W. H., Jr., Masaitis, C., Mansberger, A. R., Jr., and Crowley, R. A., Coagulation changes in clinical shock: I. Effect of hemorrhagic shock on clotting time in humans. Ann. Surg. *164*:34, 1966.
6. Bains, J. W., Crawford, D. T., and Ketchman, A. S.: Effect of chronic anemia on wound tensile strength: Correlation with blood volume, total red blood cell volume and proteins. Ann. Surg. *164*:243, 1966.
7. Bartter, F. C., Biglieri, E. G., Pronove, P., and Delea, C. S., Effect of changes in intravascular volume on aldosterone secretion in man. *In* Muller, A. F., and O'Connor, C. M. (eds.): International Symposium on Aldosterone. Boston, Little, Brown and Co., 1958, p. 100.

8. Bassin, R., Vladek, B. C., Kark, A. E., and Shoemaker, W. C.: Rapid and slow hemorrhage in man. Ann. Surg. *173*:325, 1970.
9. Baue, A. E., and Sayeed, M. M.: Alterations in the functional capacity of mitochondria in hemorrhagic shock. Surgery *68*:40, 1970.
10. Baue, A. E., Wurth, M. A., and Sayeed, M. M.: The dynamics of altered ATP-dependent and ATP-yielding cell processes in shock. Surgery *72*:94, 1972.
11. Bell, D. J., and Schloerb, R. R.: Cellular response to endotoxin and hemorrhagic shock. Surgery *60*:69, 1966.
12. Biron, P.: Pulmonary extraction of bradykinin and eledoisin. Rev. Can. Biol. *27*:75, 1968.
13. Bjork, V. I., Intouti, F., and Norlung, S.: Correlation between sludge in the conjunctiva and the mesentery. Ann. Surg. *159*:428, 1964.
14. Blaisdell, F. W., and Stallone, R. J.: The mechanism of pulmonary damage following traumatic shock. Surg. Gyn. Obst. *130*:15, 1970.
15. Blalock, A.: Experimental shock: The cause of the low blood pressure produced by muscle injury. Arch. Surg. *20*:959, 1930.
16. Blalock, A., Acute circulatory failure as exemplified by shock and hemorrhage. Surg. Gynec. Obst. *58*:551, 1934.
17. Bounous, G., Hampson, L. G., and Gurd, F. N.: Regional blood flow and oxygen consumption in experimental hemorrhagic shock. Arch. Surg. *87*:340, 1963.
18. Bounous, G., McArdle, A. H., Hampson, L. G., and Gurd, F. N.: The cessation of intestinal mucus production as a pathogenic factor in irreversible shock. Surg. Forum *16*:11, 1965.
19. Bounous, G., McArdle, A. H., Hodges, D. M., Hampson, L. G., and Gurd, F. N.: Biosynthesis of intestinal mucin in shock: Relationship to tryptic hemorrhagic enteritis and permeability to curare. Ann. Surg. *164*:13, 1966.
20. Boyland, J. W., and Asheur, E.: Depletion and restoration of medullary osmotic gradient in dog kidney. Arch. Ges. Physiol. *276*:99, 1962.
21. Brockman, S. K., and Vasko, J. S.: Hemodynamics in endotoxin shock. Surg. Forum *17*:17, 1966.
22. Bryant, L. R., Rush, B. F., Jr., Houck, G. R., and Sexton, R.: Parabiotic resuscitation in irreversible hemorrhagic shock. Surg. Forum *17*:17, 1966.
23. Burke, J. F.: Identification of the sources of staphyloccocus contaminating the surgical wound during operation. Ann. Surg. *158*:898, 1963.
24. Bywaters, E. G. L.: ischemic muscle necrosis. J.A.M.A. *124*:1103, 1944.
25. Cannon, W. B.: Traumatic Shock, New York, D. Appleton and Co., 1923.
26. Cannon, W. B., and Bayliss, W. M.: Muscle injury in relation to shock. Report of Shock Committee, March, 1919. No. 26, 19–23, cited by Blalock (reference 9).
27. Chiu, C. J., Scott, H. J., Gurd, F. N.: Intestinal mucosal lesion in low-flow states: II. The protective effect of intraluminal glucosa as energy substrate. Arch. Surg. *101*:484, 1970.
28. Cloutier, C. T., Lowery, B. D., and Carey, L. C.: Acid-base disturbances in hemorrhagic shock. Arch. Surg. *98*: 551, 1969.
29. Collins, J. A., Simmons, R. L., James, R. M., Bredenberg, C. E., Anderson, R. W., and Heistercamp, C. A.: Acid-base status of seriously wounded combat casualties: I. Before treatment. Ann. Surg. *171*:595, 1970.
30. Cope, O., and Litwin, S. B.: Contribution of lymphatic system to replenishment of plasma volume following hemorrhage. Ann. Surg. *156*:655, 1962.
31. Coran, A. G., Cryer, P. E., Horwitz, D. L., and Herman, C. M.: Fat and carbohydrate metabolism during hemorrhagic shock in the unanesthetized baboon. Surg. Forum *22*:9, 1971.
32. Cournand, A., Riley, A. R., Bradley, S. E., Breed, E. S., Noble, R. P., Lawson, H. D., Griegersen, M. I., and Richards, D. W.: Studies of the circulation in clinical shock. Surgery *13*:964, 1943.
33. Crile, G. W., and Lower, W. E.: Anoci-Association, Philadelphia, W. B. Saunders Co., 1914.
34. Crowell, J. W.: Cardiac deterioration as the cause of irreversibility in shock. *In* Mills, L. C., and Moyer, J. H. (eds.): Shock and Hypotension. The Twelfth Hahnemann Symposium. New York, Grune and Stratton, 1965.
35. Crowell, J. W., and Houston, B.: The effect of acidity on blood coagulation. Am. J. Physiol. *201*:379, 1961.
36. Cunningham, J. N., Jr., Shires, G. T., and Wagner, Y.: Cellular transplant defects in hemorrhagic shock. Surg. *70*: 215, 1971.
37. Curtin, R. A., Sapira, J. D., Danon, A., and Carey, L. C.: Comparison of exogenous and endogenous epinephrine on hyperglycemia in unanesthetized pigs. Surg. Forum *22*:85, 1971.
38. Dale, H. H., and Richards, A. N.: Vasodila-

tory actions of histamine and other substances. J. Physiol. 52:110, 1918.
39. DeDuve, C.: Lysosomes: A New Group of Cytoplasmic Particles. Subcellular Particles, New York, The Ronald Press Co., 1959.
40. Dillinger, M. R., and Gardner, B.: Newer aspects of the carcinoid spectrum. Surg. Gyn. Obst. *123*:1335, 1966.
41. Diniz, C. R., and Carvalho, I. F.: Micromethod for determination of bradykinogen under several conditions. Ann. N. Y. Acad. Sci. *104*:77, 1963.
42. Douglas, D. M.: The healing of aponeurotic incisions, Br. J. Surg. *40*:79, 1952.
43. Drucker, W. R.: What's new in shock and metabolism. Surg. Gyn. Obst., *132*: 234, 1971.
44. Dunphy, J. E., and Jackson, D. S.: Practical aspects of experimental studies in the care of the primary closed wound. Am. J. Surg. 104:273, 1962.
45. Evans, W. E., Shore, R., and Darin, J. C.: Studies in Endotoxin Shock. II. Relationship of the Pancreas and Gastric Secretion. Paper presented before the 27th Annual Meeting of the Society of University Surgeons, February, 10, 1966.
46. Farago, G., Levene, R. A., Lau, T. S., and Drucker, W. R.: Availability of lipid for energy metabolism during hypovolemia. Surg. Forum *22*:7, 1971.
47. Farrell, G. L.: Physiological factors which influence secretion of aldosterone. Recent Progr. Hormone Res. *15*:275, 1959.
48. Ferreira, S. H., and Vane, J. R.: The disappearance of bradykinin and eledoisin in the circulation and vascular beds of cats. Br. J. Pharm. *30*:417, 1967.
49. Frank, H. A., Glotzer, P., Jacob, S. W., and Fine, J.: Hemorrhagic shock in Eck fistula dogs. Am. J. Physiol. *167*:508, 1951.
50. Fulton, R. L.: Adsorption of sodium and water by collagen during hemorrhagic shock. Ann. Surg. *172*:861, 1970.
51. Gallie, B. L., Koven, I. H., Lo, S. F., Taubenfligel, V., and Drucker, W. R.: Correction of the interstitial diffusion defect in hemorrhagic shock by balanced salt solution. Surg. Forum, *22*:21, 1971.
52. Ganong, W. F., and Mulrow, P. J.: Role of kidney in adrenocortical response to hemorrhage in hypophysectomized dogs. Endocrinology *70*:182, 1962.
53. Goetz, R. H., Selmonosky, C. A., and State, D.: Effect of amine buffer tris (hydroxylmethyl) amino methane (THAM) on renal blood flow during hemorrhagic shock. Surg. Gyn Obst. *117*:715, 1963.
54. Grant, R. T., and Reeves, E. B.: Observations on the general effects of injury in man. Med. Res. Council, Spec. Rep. Ser. No. 277. London, His Majesty's Stationery Office, 1941.
55. Greenfield, L. J., McCardy, J. R., Hinshaw, L. B., and Elkins, R. C.: Preservation of myocardial function during cross-circulation in terminal endotoxin shock. Surg *72*:111, 1972.
56. Gross, S. D.: System of Surgery, 1850. Cited by Mann, F. C.: Bull. Hopkins Hosp. *25*:205, 1914.
57. Guyton, A. C., and Lindsay, A. W.: Effect of elevated left arterial pressure and decreased plasma protein concentration on the development of pulmonary edema. Circ. Res. *7*:649, 1959.
58. Haljamäe, H.: "Hidden" cellular electrolyte responses to hemorrhagic shock and their significance. Rev. Surg. *27*:315, 1970.
59. Hardaway, R. M.: Disseminated intravascular coagulation in experimental shock. Am. J. Cardiol. *20*:161, 1967.
60. Hardaway, R. M.: Intravascular coagulation in irreversible shock. *In* Mills, L. C., and Moyer, J. H. (eds.): Shock and Hypotension. The Twelfth Hahnemann Symposium, New York, Grune and Stratton, 1965.
61. Hardaway, R. M., Chun, B., and Rutherford, R. B.: Histologic evidence of disseminated intravascular coagulation in clinical shock, Vasc. Dis. *2*:254. 1965.
62. Hardaway, R. M., Johnson, D. G., Elovitz, M. J., Houcin, D. N., Jenkins, E. B., Burns, J. W., and Jackson, D. R.: Studies on the fibrinogen replacement rate in dogs. Ann. Surg. *160*: 835, 1964.
63. Harkins, H. M.: Wound healing. *In* Allen, J. G., Harkins, H. M., Moyer, J. H., and Rhoads, J. E. (eds.): Surgery Principles and Practice. Philadelphia, J. B. Lippincott Co., 1957.
64. Hashimoto, S., and Cowley, R. A.: Treatment of experimental shock in dogs with mitochondria. Surg. Forum *15*: 10, 1964.
65. Henderson, Y.: Acapnia and shock. Am. J. Physiol. *24*:66, 1909.
66. Henry, J. N., McArdle, A. H., Bounous, G., Hampson, L. G., Scorr, H. J., and Gurd, F.: The Effect of Experimental Hemorrhagic Shock on Pulmonary Alveolar Surfactant. (Paper presented at 26th Annual Session

of the American Association for the Surgery of Trauma, October 9, 1966.)
67. Henry, J. N., McArdle, A. H., and Bounous, G. et al.: The effect of experimental hemorrhagic shock on pulmonary alveolar surfactant. J. Trauma 7:691, 1967.
68. Hewson, W.: *In* Gulliver, G. (ed.): The Work of William Hewson, F.R.S. London, Sydenham Society, 1846, p. 46.
69. Hinshaw, L. B., Brake, C. M., and Emerson, T. E.: Biochemical and pathologic alterations in endotoxin shock. *In* Mills, L. C., and Moyer, J. H., (eds.): Shock and Hypotension. The Twelfth Hahnemann Symposium. New York, Grune and Stratton.
70. Hopkinson, B. R., Borden, J. R., Heyden, W. C., and Schenk, W. G.: Interstitial fluid pressure changes during hemorrhage and blood replacement with and without hypotension. Surgery *64*:68, 1968.
71. Howard, J. E. (ed.): Battle Casualties in Korea. Washington, D.C., Government Printing Office, 1955.
72. Huckabee, N. E.: The relationship of pyruvate and lactate during anaerobic metabolism. J. Clin. Invest. *37*:264, 1958.
73. Jacobson, Y. G., DeFalco, A. J., Mundth, E. D., and Keller, M. A.: Hyperbaric oxygen in the therapy of experimental shock. Surg. Forum. *16*: 15, 1965.
74. Janoff, A., Weismann, G., Zweifach, B. W., and Thomas, L.: Pathogenesis of experimental shock: IV. Studies on lysosomes in normal and tolerant animals subjected to lethal trauma and endotoxemia. J. Exp. Med. *116*:451, 1962.
75. Jenkins, M. T., Jones, R. F., Wilson, B., and Moyer, C.: Congestion atelectasis; complications of intravenous infusions of fluids. Ann. Surg. *132*: 327, 1950.
76. Kaihara, S., Rutherford, R. B., Schwentker, E. P., et al.: The distribution of cardiac output of experimental hemorrhagic shock in dogs. J. Appl. Physiol. *27*:218–222, 1969.
77. Kalfus, L., and Thal, A. P.: Plasma kinin and kininase in various forms of shock. Fed. Proc. (Part I) *23*:539, 1964.
78. Knisely, M. H., Eliot, T. S., and Bloch, E. H.: Sludged blood in traumatic shock. Arch. Surg. *51*:220, 1945.
79. Kobald, E. E., Lobell, R., Katz, W., and Thal, A. P.: Chemical mediators released by endotoxin. Surg. Gyn. Obst. *118*:807, 1964.
80. Kobald, E. E., Lucas, R., and Thal, A. P.: Chemical mediators in clinical septic shock. Surg. Forum *14*:16, 1964.
81. Kovach, A. G. B., and Fonyo, A.: Metabolic response to injury in cerebral tissue. *In* Stoner, H. B., and Threlfall, C. J. (eds.): The Biochemical Response to Injury. Philadelphia, F. A. Davis Co., 1960, pp. 129–160.
82. Lefer, A. M., and Martin, J.: Relationship of plasma peptides to the depressant factor in hemorrhagic shock. Circ. Res. *26*:59, 1970.
83. LePage, G. A.: Biological energy transformations during shock as shown by their tissue analyses. Am. J. Physiol. *146*:267, 1946.
84. LePage, G. .A.: The effects of hemorrhage on tissue metabolites. Am. J. Physiol. *147*:446, 1946.
85. Lillehei, R. C.: The intestinal factor in irreversible hemorrhagic shock. Surgery *42*:1043, 1957.
86. Lillehei, R. C., Longerbeam, J. K., Block, J. H., and Manax, W. G.: The nature of irreversible shock. Experimental and clinical observations. Ann. Surg. *160*:682, 1964.
87. Lister, J., McNeil, L. F., Marshal , V. C., Pizak, L. F., Dagher, F. J., and Moore, F. D.: Transcapillary refilling after hemorrhage in normal man: Basal rates and volumes; effect of norepinephrine. Ann. Surg. *158*:698, 1963.
88. Lovett, W. L., Wangensteen, S. L., Glenn, T. M., and Lefer, A. M.: Presence of a myocardial depressant factor in patients in circulatory shock. Surgery *70*:223, 1971.
89. MacLean, L. D., Duff, J. H., Scott, H. M., and Derftz, D. J.: Treatment of shock in man based on hemodynamic diagnosis. Surg. Gyn. Obst. *120*:1, 1965
90. MacLean, L. D., Mulligan, W. G., McLean, A.P.H., and Duff, J. H.: Patterns of septic shock in man—A detailed study of 56 patients. Ann. Surg. *166*: 543, 1967.
91. McKay, D. G.: Trauma and disseminated intravascular coagulation. J. Trauma 9:646, 1969.
92. McMichael, J.: The oxygen supply of the liver. Quart. J. Exper. Physiol. *27*: 73, 1937.
93. McNulty, W. P., Jr., and Linares, R.: Hemorrhagic shock of germfree rats. Am. J. Physiol. *198*:141, 1960.
94. McShan, W. H., Potter, V. R., Goldman, A., Shipley, E. G., and Meyer, R. K.: Biologic energy transformation during shock as shown by blood chemistry. Am. J. Physiol. *145*:93, 1945.
95. Manger, W. M., Nahas, G. G., Hassam, D., Habif, D. V., and Papper, E. M.: Effect of pH control and increased O_2 delivery on the course of hemor-

rhagic shock. Ann. Surg. *156*:503, 1962.

96. Marks, L. J., King, D. W., Kingsbury, P. F., Boyett, J. E., and Dell, E. S.: Physiologic role of the adrenal cortex in the maintenance of plasma volume following hemorrhage of surgical operation. Surgery *58*:510, 1965.
97. Mathews, R. E., and Douglas, G. J.: Sulphur-35 measurements of functional and total extracellular fluid in dogs with hemorrhagic shock. Surg. Forum *20*:3, 1969.
98. Mela, L. M., Miller, L. D., and Nicholas, G. G.: Influences of cellidas andosis and activated cation concentrations on shock-induced mitochondrial damage. Surgery *72*:102, 1972.
99. Moore, F. D.: Metabolic Care of the Surgical Patient. Philadelphia, W. B. Saunders Co., 1960.
100. Moore, F. D.: The effects of hemorrhage on body composition. New Eng. J. Med. *273*:567, 1965.
101. Moore, F. D., and Ball, M. R.: The Metabolic Response to Surgery. No. 132 in American Lecture Series. Springfield, Ill., Charles C Thomas, 1952.
102. Moore, T. C., Normel, L., and Eiseman, B.: Effect of histamine and serotonin on blood flow and tracheal resistance in the isolated perfused lung. Surgery *57*:730, 1965.
103. Morris, R.: Personal communication.
104. Moss, G. S., Das Gupta, T. K., Newsom, B., and Nyhus, L. M.: Morphologic changes in the primate lung after hemorrhagic shock. Surg. Gyn. Obst. *134*:3, 1972.
105. Moss, G. S., Proctor, H. J., Herman, C., Homer, L. D., and Litt, B. O.: Hemorrhagic shock in the baboon: I. Circulatory and metabolic changes. J. Trauma *8*:837, 1968.
106. Moyer, C. A., and Butcher, H. R.: Burns, Shock and Plasma Volume Regulation. St. Louis, C. V. Mosby, 1967.
107. Moyer, C. A., Margraf, H. W., and Monafo, W. W.: Burn shock and extravascular sodium deficiency. Treatment with Ringer's solution with lactate. Arch. Surg. *90*:799, 1965.
108. Nayman, J.: Effect of renal failure on wound healing in dog's response to hemodialysis following uremia induced by uranium nitrate. Ann. Surg. *164*:227, 1966.
109. Neill, S. A., Gaisford, W. D., and Zuidema, G. D.: A comparative anatomic study of the hepatic veins in the dog, monkey and human. Surg. Gyn. Obst. *116*:451, 1963.
110. Nelson, R. M., Poulson, A. M., Lyman, J. H., and Henry, J. W.: Evaluation of tris (hydroxymethyl) aminomethane: (THAM) in experimental hemorrhagic shock. Surgery *54*:86, 1963.
111. Olledart, R., and Mansberger, A. R.: The effect of hypovolemic shock on bacterial defense. Am. J. Surg. *110*: 302, 1965.
112. Pagano, V. P., and Mersheimer, W. L.; Immuno-chemical changes observed with shock. Surg. Forum *16*: 45, 1965.
113. Parsons, E., and Phemister, D. B.: Hemorrhage and "shock" in traumatized limbs: Experimental study. Surg. Gyn. Obst. *51*:196, 1930.
114. Penner, A., and Bernheim, A. I.: Studies in the pathogenesis of experimental dysentery intoxication. J. Exp. Med. *111*:145, 1960.
115. Piper, P. J., and Vane, J. R.: Release of additional factors in anaphylaxis and its antagonism by anti-inflammatory drugs. Nature *223*:29, 1969.
116. Ravin, H. A., and Fine, J.: Current concepts and controversies on traumatic shock. Progr. Surg. *3*:102, 1963.
117. Reich, T., Dierolf, B. M., and Reynolds, B. M.: Plasma cathepsin-like acid proteinase activity during hemorrhagic shock. J. Surg. Res. *5*:116, 1965.
118. Rhoads, J. E., and Howard, J. M.: The chemistry of trauma. Springfield, Ill., Charles C Thomas, 1963.
119. Robb, H. J.: The role of micro-embolism in the production of irreversible shock. Ann. Surg. *158*:685, 1963.
120. Rosenbaum, D. K., Frank, E. D., Rutenburg, A. M., and Frank, H. A.: High energy phosphate content of liver tissue in experimental hemorrhagic shock. Am. J. Physiol. *188*:86, 1957.
121. Rush, B. J.: Discussion of Bell, D. J., and Schloerb, P. R.: Cellular response to endotoxin and hemorrhagic shock. Surgery *60*:69, 1966.
122. Rutenburg, S. H., Rutenburg, A. M., Smith, E. E., and Fine, J.: On the nature of tolerance to endotoxin. Proc. Soc. Exp. Biol. Med. *118*:620, 1965.
123. Rutherford, R. B., and Trow, R. S.: The pathophysiology of irreversible hemorrhagic shock in monkeys. J. Surg. Res. (accepted for publication).
124. Rutherford, R. B., West, R. L., and Hardaway, R. M.: Coagulation changes during experimental hemorrhagic shock. Ann. Surg. *164*:203, 1966.
125. Sanford, J. P., and Noyes, H. E.: Studies on the absorption of Escherichia coli endotoxin from the gastrointestinal tract of dogs in the patho-

genesis of "irreversible" hemorrhagic shock. J. Clin. Invest. *37*: 1425, 1958.

126. Schayer, R. W.: Relationship of stress-induced histidine decarboxylase activity in histamine synthesis to circulatory homeostasis and shock. Science *131*:226, 1960.
127. Selkurt, E. E.: Renal blood flow and renal clearances during hemorrhage and shock. *In* Block, K. D.: Shock Pathogenesis and Therapy. Berlin, Springer-Verlag, 1962, p. 445.
128. Sharma, G. P., and Eiseman, B.: Protective effects of adenosine triphosphate in experimental hemorrhagic shock. Surg. Forum *15*:27, 1964.
129. Sherry, S.: Homeostatic mechanisms and proteolysis in shock. Fed. Proc. (Suppl.): *9*:209, 1961.
130. Shires, G. T., Brown, F. T., Canizaro, P. C., and Somerville, N.: Distributional changes in extracellular fluid hemorrhagic shock. Surg. Forum *11*:115, 1960.
131. Shires, G. T., Carrico, C. J., and Cohn, D.: The role of the extracellular fluid in shock. *In* Hershey, S. (ed.): Shock, Boston, Little, Brown and Co., 1964.
132. Shumer, W.: Localization of the energy pathway block in shock. Surgery *64*:55, 1968.
133. Shumer, W., Kapica, S. K., Teng, Ta-Lee: Validity of the hysosomal therapy of oligemic shock. Arch. Surg. *99*: 325, 1969.
134. Siegel, J. H., Goldwyn, R. M., and Friedman, H. P.: Pattern and process in the evolution of human septic shock. Surgery *70*:232, 1971.
135. Siegel, J. J., and Del Guercio, L. R. M.: The High Cardiac Output Syndrome and Ventricular Failure—A Problem in Surgical Management. (Paper presented before the Halsted Society, Baltimore, Maryland, September 16, 1966.)
136. Silen, W.: Horizons in gastrointestinal research. Surgery *72*:91, 1972.
137. Simeone, F. A.: Shock, trauma and the surgeon. Ann. Surg. *158*:759, 1963.
138. Simeone, F.: Discussion of Rosenberg, J. C., and Rush, B. J.: Basic biochemical difference in endotoxin and hemorrhagic shock. Surg. Forum *16*:23, 1965.
139. Simmons, R. L., Collins, J. A., Heistercamp, C. A., et al.: Coagulation disorders in combat casualties. Ann. Surg. *169*:455, 1969.
140. Skillman, J. J., and Moore, F. O.: Volume regulatory and endocrine relationships after blood loss in man. Ann. N. Y. Acad. Sci. *150*:639, 1968.
141. Slonim, M., and Stahl, W. M.: Sodium and water content of connective versus cellular tissue following hemorrhage. Surg. Forum *19*:53, 1968.
142. Spencer, F. C.: Personal communication.
143. Stahl, T. H.: Pressure-flow factors in the renal excretory response to hemorrhage. Surg. Forum *16*:23, 1965.
144. Steinberg, D.: Paper presented at The Conferences on Energy Metabolism and Body Fuel Utilization, Boston, Massachusetts, July 13, 1966.
145. Steward, J. M.: Peptide Hormones. Annual Reports in Medicinal Chemistry, 1969, C. K. Cain (ed.).
146. Stoner, H. B.: Paper presented at The Conferences on Energy Metabolism and Body Fuel Utilization, Boston, Massachusetts, July 13, 1966.
147. Stoner, H. B., and Threlfall, C. J.: The effects of nucleotide and ischemic shock on the level of energy-rich phosphates in the tissues. Biochem. J. *58*:115, 1954.
148. Strawitz, J. G., and Hift, H. L.: The structure and function of mitochondria in irreversible hemorrhagic shock. Proc. Soc. Exper. Biol. Med. *91*:641, 1956.
149. Strawitz, J. G., and Hift, H.: Subcellular changes in hemorrhagic shock. *In* Mills, L. C. and Moyer, J. H. (eds.): Shock and Hypotension. The Twelfth Hahnemann Symposium. New York, Grune and Stratton, 1965.
150. Sutherland, E. W., and Rall, T. W.: The relationship of adenosine 3-5 phosphate and phosphorylase to the action of catecholamines and other hormones. Pharmacol. Rev. *12*:265, 1960.
151. Swank, R. L., Hissen, W., and Bergentz, S. E.: 5-Hydroxytryptamine and aggregation of blood elements after trauma. Surg. Gyn. Obst. *119*:779, 1964.
152. Talaat, S. M., Massion, W. H., and Schilling, J. A.: Effects of adenosine triphosphate administration in irreversible hemorrhagic shock. Surgery 55:813, 1964.
153. Teplitz, C.: The ultrastructural basis for pulmonary pathophysiology following trauma. Pathogenesis of pulmonary edema. J. Trauma *8*:700, 1968.
154. Thal, A. P.: Discussion of Rosenberg, J. C., and Rush, B. J.: Basic biochemical difference in endotoxin and hemorrhagic shock. Surg. Forum *16*:23, 1965.
155. Thal, A. P., and Wilson, R. F.: *In* Current Problems in Surgery. (A series of monthly clinical monographs.) Chicago, Year Book Medical Publishers, Inc., September, 1965.
156. Thal, A. P., Wilson, R. F., Kalfuss, L., and

Andre, J.: The role of metabolic and humoral factors in irreversible shock. *In* Mills, L. C., Moyer, J. H., (eds.): Shock and Hypotension. The Twelfth Hahnemann Symposium, New York, Grune and Stratton, 1965.

157. Thomas, C. S., Jr., Melly, M. A., Koenig, M. G. et al.: The hemodynamic effects of viable gram-negative organisms. Surg. Gyn. Obst. *128*:753, 1969.
158. Thompson, J. S., Severson, C. D., Parmely, M. J., et al.: Pulmonary "sensitivity" reactions induced by transfusion of non H-L-A leukoagglutinins. New Eng. J. Med. *284*:1120, 1971.
159. Triner, L., Nahas, G. G., Small, H. S., Lee, A. St. J., and Habif, D. V.: Increase of O_2 uptake during hemorrhage and after transfusion. Surg. Forum *16*: 21, 1965.
160. Udenfriend, S.: Formation of hydroxyproline in collagen, Science *152*:1335, 1966.
161. Udhoji, V. N., and Weil, M. H.: Hemodynamic and metabolic studies on shock associated with bacteremia. Ann. Intern. Med. *62*:966, 1965.
162. Valeri, C. R.: Viability and function of preserved red cells. New Eng. J. Med. *284*:81, 1971.
163. Visscher, M. D., Haddy, F. J., and Stephen, G.: Physiology and pharmacology of lung edema. Pharmacol. Rev. *8*:389, 1956.
164. Waldhausen, J. A., Abel, F. L., and Selkurt, E. E.: Splanchnic blood flow in the monkey during hemorrhagic shock. Surg. Forum *15*:7, 1964.
165. Wangensteen, S. L., Ramey, W. G., Ferguson, W. W., and Starling, J. R.: Plasma myocardial depressant activity (shock factor) identified as salt in the cat papillary muscle bioassay system. J. Trauma *13*:181, 1973.
166. Weidner, M. G., Albrecht, M., and Clowes, G. H.: Relationship of myocardial function to survival after oligemic hypotension. Surgery *55*:73, 1964.
167. Weissman, G., and Thomas, L.: Studies on lysosomes: I. Effects of endotoxin, exotoxin tolerance, and cortisone on release of enzymes from granular fraction of rabbit fever. J. Exp. Med. *116*:433, 1962.
168. Werle, E.: Kallikrein, Kallidin and Related Substances, Polypeptides Which Affect Smooth Muscles and Blood Vessels. New York, Pergamon Press, 1960.
169. Willwerth, B. M., Crawford, F. A., Young, W. G., Jr., et al.: The role of functional demand on the development of pulmonary lesions during hemorrhagic shock. J. Thorac. Cardiovasc. Surg. *54*:658, 1967.
170. Wilson, J. W., Ratliff, N. B., and Hackel, D. B.: The lung in hemorrhagic shock. Am. J. Pathol. *58*:337, 1970.
171. Wurtman, R. J.: Catecholamines. New Eng. J. Med. Medical Progress Series, Boston, Little, Brown and Co., 1966.
172. Wyler, F., Forsyth, R. P., Nies, A. S., Neutze, J. M., and Melmon, K. L.: Endotoxin induced regional circulatory changes in the unanesthetized monkey. Circ. Res. *24*:777, 1969.
173. Zetterstrom, B. E. M., Palmerio, C., and Fine, J.: Protection of functional and vascular integrity of the spleen in traumatic shock by denervation. Proc. Soc. Exp. Biol. Med. *117*:373, 1964.
174. Zweifach, B. W.: Aspects of comparative physiology of laboratory animals relative to the problems of experimental shock. Fed. Proc. (Suppl.) 9:18, 1961.

chapter

3

THE TREATMENT OF SHOCK

John A. Collins, M. D., and Walter F. Ballinger, M.D.

INTRODUCTION

Shock in the injured patient represents one of the most trying challenges for the clinicians caring for these patients, to the investigators searching for the causes and mechanisms of failure of treatment, and to those concerned with the organization of systems designed to improve the care of these patients from the time of injury. The clinician is truly "under the gun"—his decisions and interventions must be rapid and correct. His immediate field of concern involves all the vital organs and systems and a host of rapidly life-threatening specific injury patterns. His view must be broad yet detailed, and the most important decisions are usually made on the basis of his examination of the patient, often without time for the luxury and comfort of laboratory or radiologic confirmation of his findings. There are very few parallel situations in modern medicine.

Those who seek answers to clinical problems in the laboratory have abundant material centered on basic physiology and ranging from complex integrated systems to subcellular particles. Most patients who now die of injuries after reaching a hospital alive are theoretically salvageable. They die of what appear to be preventible complications, most of which are sequelae of shock. Reducing this fraction is the scientific challenge.

Perhaps more than with any other disease entity, the results obtained in caring for the seriously injured reflect the excellence of health care as a broadly conceived system. It is likely that the greatest number of preventable deaths occur before the patient ever gets to a treatment facility, and many of these are from untreated shock. It is no longer tenable to state that medical care and concern begin at the hospital door—they begin at, when, and where the patient is injured. The system used for treating combat casualties in Vietnam probably will not be duplicated in the United States, but there are obvious elements of communication, transportation, and regionalization which can and should be developed. It is particularly distressing to think of the enormous national commitment in money, equipment, training and personnel that has gone into this magnificently effective system of caring for the injured, which apparently will now be allowed to disband, run down, and rust, while disorganized, inefficient, sporadic, misdirected and generally wasteful efforts to duplicate it will be made in the civilian sector, with the bill paid by the same nation and the same taxpayers. The military have always needed a mission while waiting for wars to happen. They have in hand now a system which can perfectly match an urgent national need. Never before in our history have they so urgently needed a reaffirmation of their social value, both for themselves as individuals and for the society which supports them. The opportunity is passing; the decision will be made by political leaders, but not without impetus from the military.

This chapter will emphasize the treatment of shock as it occurs in the acutely injured patient. The main focus will be on clinical data, when available, concerning shock due to hemorrhage. This is not meant to imply that shock due to sepsis or myocardial infarction does not occur following trauma. It is rather an effort to make the best use of available space in a work dealing with the injured patient. Some overlapping with other chapters is unavoidable, but this has been kept to a minimum. Several points of current interest or controversy have been developed in some detail, but it is obviously impossible to be comprehensive in depth within these space limitations. We have emphasized clinical, scientific, and organizational considerations.

CAUSES OF SHOCK IN ACUTELY INJURED PATIENTS

Far and away the commonest cause of circulatory collapse in injured patients is blood loss. Often this is evident from examination of the patient, but appearances are too often deceiving. The patient who arrives with a face and shirt covered with blood from a scalp laceration may be accompanied by a distraught or hysterical family and attract the attention of the entire waiting room. Most of the time he has lost less than one-tenth the amount of blood lost by the patient with a fractured femur who arrives quietly in a stretcher without a drop of blood on him.

Many guidelines and rules of thumb have been devised for estimating the blood lost with "typical" injuries, but the variations are too great in individual patients to make them of much use.[13, 29, 60, 73] An awareness of the potential magnitude of hidden blood loss can be gained from simple arithmetic (Fig. 3–1). If a thigh of average dimensions is considered to be a cylinder for computational purposes, an

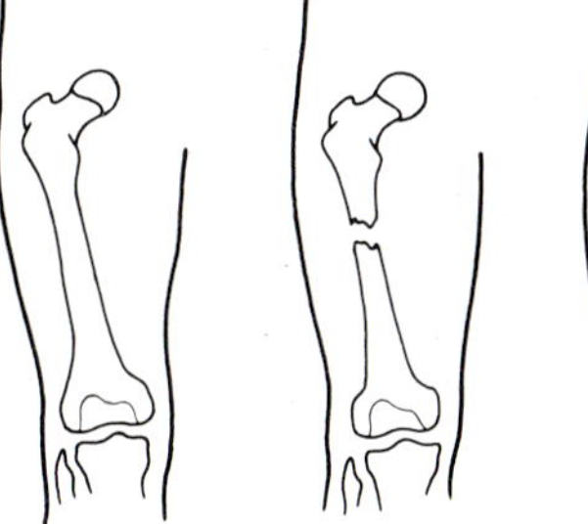

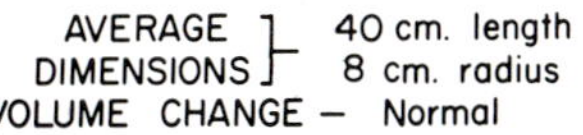

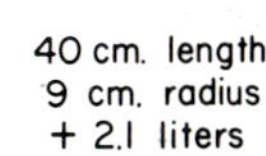

Figure 3–1 Injured thigh considered as a cylinder for computational purposes: change in volume (=blood loss) corresponding to changes in radius.

increase of only 1 cm. in the average radius of that thigh represents a net gain of 2 L. in volume. If the increase in radius is 2 cm., the volume gain is 4.5 L. over normal. In the acutely injured patient, such acute changes in dimensions are largely due to bleeding into injured tissues. Even the relatively small upper arm can contain a significant amount of shed blood.

With the abdomen, the situation is particularly misleading because the length of the abdominal cavity can and does change in a totally inapparent manner by raising the diaphragms. This may in fact be the dominant dimensional change early after abdominal injury. If we consider concurrent and equal changes in the dimensions of radius and length of our typical abdominal "cylinder" (Fig. 3–2), a gain of 1 cm. represents a volume of change of 2.9 L. A gain of 2 cm. represents a volume change of 6.1 L. Changes of this magnitude are not very evident externally. Abdominal swelling in an injured patient may be due to accumulation of air in the intestinal tract, especially the stomach, and to the sequestration of predominantly extracellular-type fluid in the enteric canal, and/or the peritoneal cavity. Nevertheless, a briskly bleeding vessel or viscus within the peritoneal cavity can pour essentially whole blood into that cylinder before these other materials add to the dimensional changes. *A patient can exsanguinate into the peritoneal cavity without any dramatic external change in abdominal dimensions or appearance.* It can be a tragic blunder to assume that because the abdomen is not distended, hypotension is not due to intra-abdominal bleeding.

Any sizable area can, of course, "hide" blood loss, including the retroperitoneal areas, the buttocks, and the shoulder girdle. In dealing with nonblood losses, one must consider the potential for sequestration in any tissue where fluid can accumulate (e.g., the enormous fluid losses into skin and subcutaneous tissues in extensively burned patients). The problems of estimating blood loss in the injured patient are further complicated by the non-linear relationship between the signs and symptoms of hypovolemia and the volume of blood lost, which will be considered later.

Specific types of injuries may result in losses of fluids other than blood. Burns are the best example, in which extracellular-type fluid and plasma are lost in very large amounts, producing profound shock in the extensively burned individual. Crushing types of injury can produce losses of all three types of fluid. In a situation that has become fortunately rare, tourniquets left on limbs tightly enough and long enough can result in rapid sequestration of plasma and extracellular fluid in the ischemic limb after release. It is also rare to see venous return so extensively interrupted at the time of injury as to pro-

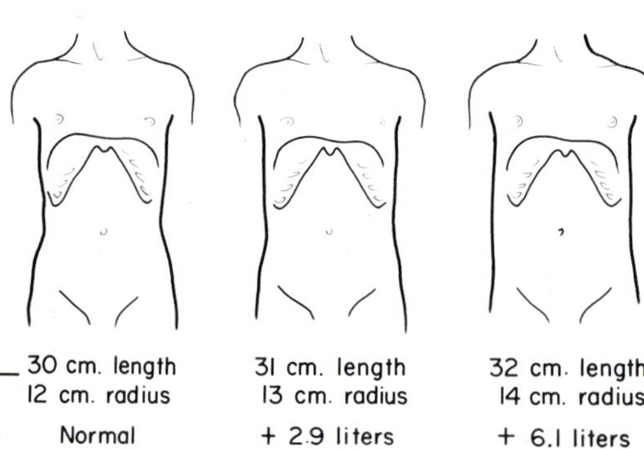

Figure 3–2 Injured abdomen considered as a cylinder for computational purposes: change in volume corresponding to changes in length and radius. Change in length occurs as raising of the diaphragms and thus remains inapparent to external examination. Exsanguination can occur with minimal change in external appearance.

duce massive fluid sequestration in the hind-quarter, but this can be a life-threatening complication of acute iliofemoral thrombosis whenever it occurs. Whatever the mechanism of injury, the presence of shed blood in body cavities or in soft tissues evokes an inflammatory response which is accompanied by the sequestration of extracellular-type fluid in varying amounts. With time, then, blood which is "shed internally" and the responses to the injuring force cause the additional loss of extracellular fluid which may exceed the volume of blood lost.

The acutely injured patient may be hypotensive for reasons other than blood loss. Pericardial tamponade is one of the most important because it can be so rapidly lethal, yet sometimes can be rapidly relieved in the emergency room. The usual signs of distant heart sounds, paradoxical pulse, narrow pulse pressure, distended neck veins, large globular heart shadow on x-ray are all of very limited value in the acutely injured patient. Concomitant blood loss may mask some of the circulatory signs, heart sounds can be hard to evaluate with associated injuries and blood loss, and the previously normal pericardium does not stretch easily when acutely distended. The absence of any or all of these signs does not rule out tamponade. It must be considered in the differential diagnosis of all hypotensive patients who are known or are likely to have sustained a significant injury to the chest. It must be looked for in all patients with known chest injury. The key to detection in the seriously injured patient is accurate monitoring of the central venous pressure. By definition, if tamponade is occurring, an accurately measured central venous pressure will be elevated. The concurrence of an elevated central venous pressure and systemic hypotension in an acutely injured patient means that pericardial tamponade must be seriously considered. Occasionally, tension pneumothorax will produce this picture, but other signs usually point to this diagnosis. Injury rarely produces an acute true superior vena caval syndrome. Heart failure from any cause and pulmonary embolism must, of course, also be considered if appropriate to the clinical circumstances.

Advanced ventilatory disorders may produce hypotension in the injured patient. Tension pneumothorax will do this as it develops. Airway obstruction, large sucking chest wounds, bilateral pneumothorax, massive aspiration, to name a few, can result in hypotension when hypoxemia becomes preterminal. It should be remembered, however, that hypertension is the usual response to acute CO_2 retention, but this may not occur in a hypovolemic patient.

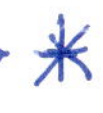

An acute spinal cord injury can cause hypotension in the same manner that spinal anesthesia can, by acute removal of the neural control of arteriolar constriction in much of the vascular system. This is usually well tolerated unless central aortic pressure drops markedly or there has been significant blood loss. It is surprising how easy it is to temporarily overlook a cord level when more attention-getting injuries are present. Needless to say, intact motion and sensation even in injured legs can be determined in a very few seconds. Detecting an acute spinal level is more important for the correct handling of the patient during resuscitation and evaluation than for the few times it acts as the cause of hypotension.

Although spinal injuries can cause hypotension, it is a good policy *never to consider a head injury as the cause of hypotension or shock.* It is true that the head, scalp and face have a large blood supply and that blood loss from soft tissue damage can be severe, but this should be evident. Intracranial bleeding and brain injury do not often cause hypotension except with terminal decompensation or compression of the medullary centers. The standard response to increased intracranial pressure is peripheral vasoconstriction and a *rising* blood pressure. Hemorrhage

may, of course, mask this response. The occurrence of hypotension in a patient with a serious head injury necessitates a careful search for its cause. If the central venous pressure is low and other evidence indicates hypovolemia, blood loss must be assumed and accounted for. The abdomen is very hard to evaluate in these patients. If no other site of blood loss is found, firm objective evidence must be obtained that rules out intra-abdominal bleeding. (See chapter on abdominal injuries.)

It is always possible that the patient became hypotensive for a reason not related to his injury. Some patients have accidents because of myocardial infarctions, pulmonary emboli, drug reactions, or hypoglycemia. These are rare occurrences. More often, a patient will have a myocardial infarction as a result of hypotension and hypovolemia, and this may then become the dominant circulatory factor. Tunnel vision in any field of medicine is usually rewarded with avoidable failure. This is no less true when taking care of injured patients.

THE CIRCULATORY, METABOLIC, AND ENDOCRINE RESPONSE TO HEMORRHAGE IN MAN

A great deal of experimental work has been done on the responses to hemorrhage. Much of the work in animals is of limited value because of species differences and the use of anesthesia. There have been several studies directly in man, in both injured patients and normal volunteers.[8, 13, 19, 19, 22, 27, 29, 41, 45, 48, 51, 54, 56, 60, 65, 67, 69, 73, 77, 81, 91, 98, 100, 102, 106, 108, 115, 116, 120, 122, 124, 126, 127, 137, 142] This brief and oversimplified version of the sequence of events that follows blood loss is based whenever possible on studies in man in which blood volume and/or blood loss has been measured as well as the pertinent variable (Table 3–1, Fig. 3–3).

The first response to blood loss is contraction of the great veins, the "capacitance" system. This is probably under neural control and results in a smaller vascular space in which the resulting blood volume can function with little change elsewhere in the system.

TABLE 3–1 COMPOSITE OF REPORTED RESPONSES TO HEMORRHAGE IN MAN*

BLOOD LOSS	VASCULAR RESPONSE	ENDOCRINE RESPONSE	METABOLIC RESPONSE	SIGNS AND SYMPTOMS
Minimal (15%)	Contraction of great veins; recruitment of ECF	Slight	Slight	Usually transient
Moderate (30%)	All of above. Arteriolar constriction with reduced flow to skin and muscle. Decreased cardiac output; narrow pulse pressure; tachycardia.	Increase in aldosterone, ADH, growth hormone. Variable increase in cortisol, catecholamines. No increase in insulin.	Increased glycolysis and mild hyperglycemia. Increased lipolysis and free fatty acid levels. Small increase in lactate levels. Hyperventilation with alkalemia. Oxygen consumption may be increased. Decreased urinary sodium and volume.	Thirst, orthostatic hypotension, apprehension, weakness, pallor, cool skin.
Severe (45%)	All of above. Cardiac output less than 50% normal. Hypotension. Most of remaining cardiac output to heart and brain.	All of above. Marked increase in catecholomines.	Severe lactic acidosis. Severe oliguria. Mixed venous P_{O_2} approaching 20 mm. Hg or less.	Air hunger. Deteriorating state of consciousness.

*Note: individual variation is most marked at the 15 per cent hemorrhage level.

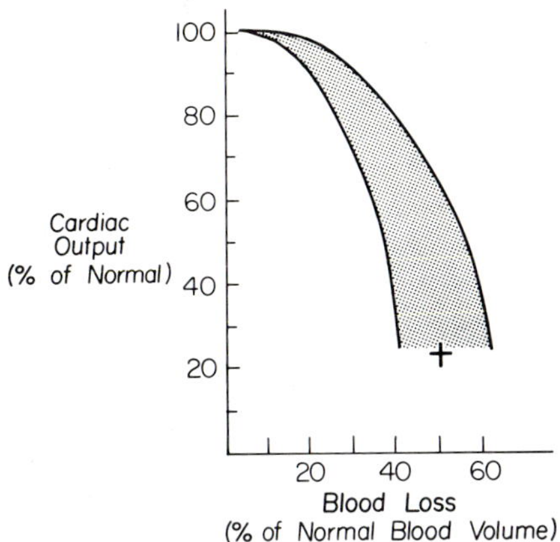

Figure 3–3 A schematic representation of reported changes in cardiac output corresponding to acute changes in blood volume. A considerable range of response is indicated. Data is least complete at the largest volume losses. Sources are cited in the text.

It is therefore a very efficient response, similar to an endogenous blood bank. However, it can buffer the loss of only about 10 per cent of the normal blood volume. At the same time, some net inflow of extracellular fluid to the vascular space begins. Cardiac output and oxygen consumption do not change and the endocrine and metabolic changes are minimal.

At about 15 to 20 per cent blood volume loss, more extensive changes occur. The compensatory ability of the capacitance response has been exceeded. The ability of the extracellular space to replenish plasma volume is still intact in a normally nourished and hydrated individual, but this will take hours to occur. Tachycardia results from sympathetic stimulation of the heart which moves it to a new work-pressure relationship in which a higher output is achieved for a given filling pressure. This involves more biologic work by the heart muscle, requiring coronary dilatation and an increased fraction of the cardiac output diverted to the heart itself. Blood flow to skin and muscle may be reduced by arteriolar construction. Endocrine responses are more evident now, with increased aldosterone and antidiuretic hormone levels, resulting in salt and water retention and a lower urinary output. Growth hormone and epinephrine and norepinephrine levels may increase; cortisol levels may or may not increase. Blood sugar and free fatty acid levels will rise, oxygen consumption will *increase* and lactate levels may rise slightly. Hyperventilation will begin with a resulting alkalemia. It is this range of blood loss at which cardiac output begins to decrease, and systolic blood pressure and central venous pressure fall somewhat. The patient may experience thirst, weakness and some apprehension. He will begin to look pale and his skin will get cool. He may well exhibit orthostatic hypotension and become light-headed, nauseated or even lose consciousness on sitting up. This is the range of blood loss (15–20 per cent) with the greatest individual variability of response, varying from partial decompensation and a clinical picture of severe shock in some patients to a deceptively intact appearance in others. This intact appearance is dangerous because decompensation may occur suddenly with relatively small further losses and will almost certainly occur if the patient is given general anesthesia without some form of effective replacement.

At a 30 per cent loss of blood volume, practically all patients will exhibit at least some of the signs and symptoms of the shock syndrome: thirst, pallor, cool skin, severe orthostatic hypotension, tachycardia, oliguria and a systolic blood pressure below 100, even when supine. Cardiac output is now significantly reduced despite the institution of perfusion priorities by arteriolar constriction. Blood flow to the viscera is maintained at the expense of the carcass, and even visceral flow is now becoming altered in distribution to protect the heart and brain. Renal blood flow decreases as renal vascular resistance increases. The endocrine responses are now more marked. Lactic acid levels are significantly elevated.

If blood loss continues, all of the compensatory responses are exceeded and blood flow to the heart and brain decreases. Air hunger is marked and the patient will lose consciousness. Metabolic acidosis becomes profound as blood flow to the liver falls below a critical level. A blood volume 50 per cent of normal cannot be tolerated for long. Even with a loss of 50 per cent which has been stopped, expansion of plasma volume from endogenous sources alone may not occur in time. When central aortic pressure falls below the level at which coronary perfusion can be maintained, cardiac output falls with a further fall in central aortic pressure (the adrenergic neural and humoral responses already at maximum levels so that vascular resistance cannot increase further to maintain pressure), which in turn causes a further fall in coronary perfusion. Once this vicious circle is entered, death rapidly ensues.

This "classical" pathophysiologic interpretation of hemorrhagic shock as a circulatory phenomenon is incomplete. A prolonged, severe reduction of peripheral and visceral blood flow will lead to one of a number of possible breakdowns in various organs and systems, distinct from the circulatory system, described in a later section. The initiating mechanism for all of these events may occur at the cellular level. One school of thought holds that lysosomal membrane disruption can occur in ischemic cells, leading to self-destruction and more widespread harm.[4, 14, 71] The evidence for this is very incomplete at best, with some evidence against it. Perhaps more pertinent are the studies on mitochondrial changes that occur after prolonged hypoperfusion, with the demonstration of decreased efficiency of oxidative phosphorylation and some failure to maintain normal electrolyte gradients.[10, 86]

TREATMENT

Successful treatment of the injured patient in shock requires rapid and correct assessment of the entire clinical situation, the establishment of appropriate priorities (both therapeutic and diagnostic) and rapid correction of the important disorders. Shock is an immediately life-threatening disorder and will be one of the highest priorities for management in any injured patient.

Evaluation

Evaluation of the hypotensive injured patient will require, in addition to the essential history and rapid physical examination, the measurement of central venous pressure (CVP). This will aid in diagnosis, provide a large-bore catheter for rapid infusion and help in determining the volume of fluid required. Common sense dictates that if blood loss is an obvious cause and there is little question of tamponade, time should not be wasted in inserting a central catheter if it cannot be done quickly and safely. If there is no one present who is experienced in the insertion of central catheters, it is better to secure a portal through a peripheral vein until such help arrives. The acutely injured patient is not a good subject on which to gain initial experience in the insertion of central venous catheters. The situation is urgent so that insertion will be hurried, the commonly used veins will be smaller than usual because of blood loss, the patient may be restless and uncooperative, and the common complications of insertion will be poorly tolerated if they occur.

If a central venous catheter is inserted, it is mandatory that its position be confirmed by x-ray before important decisions are based on the pressure readings obtained. In perhaps 10 per cent of the cases, even a well-inserted catheter will lodge in an aberrant (non-superior caval) position, usually the internal jugular vein. This position can yield falsely high CVP values if the catheter becomes wedged. We have seen a patient with a bisected liver and massive blood loss in whom blood was withheld and a pericardiocentesis almost undertaken because of a "CVP" of 16 cm. of water, profound hypotension, and a crushing chest injury. The chest x-ray arrived in time to indicate a jugular position of the catheter. The true CVP was 0 and the patient urgently needed rapid transfusion through multiple portals and a laparotomy.

A post-insertion x-ray will also reveal many of the other complications of central venous catheter insertion: pneumothorax, severed catheter, intracardiac position and sometimes an extravascular location. Pneumothorax especially should be detected before anesthesia is given with positive pressure ventilation, because a small tear in the lung can become the source for a tension pneumothorax in a patient who is unconscious and whose chest is draped out of sight. An intracardiac position of the tip of a polyethylene catheter has resulted in 12 reported deaths from perforation of the heart with resulting tamponade.[16] Many more have undoubtedly gone unreported. An intracardiac position should not be allowed to persist.

The two conditions besides hemorrhage which most commonly produce severe hypotension in injured patients are pericardial tamponade and tension pneumothorax. The signs of tension pneumothorax are well known and the condition is not usually subtle, provided it is considered. On the other hand, an unexpectedly elevated CVP may be the only clue to tamponade, and CVP therefore should be measured in all hypotensive patients with known or suspected chest injuries. Both tension pneumothorax and pericardial tamponade should be treated when diagnosed. Both may have to be treated before x-ray confirmation can be obtained.

If the extent of injury and blood loss is evidently limited and if the hypotension is rapidly reversed with fluid administration, catheterization of the urinary bladder can often be avoided. If shock has been severe, blood loss apparently great, the response to treatment slow, the anticipated operation long, if there is injury to the pelvis, if there is blood in a voided specimen or the patient cannot void, or if one is dealing with a known diabetic, it will almost always be advisable to catheterize the bladder and monitor urinary output.

Arterial blood gas analysis may reveal unsuspected hypoxemia, which if uncorrected will worsen the impairment of oxygen delivery that is the central event in hemorrhagic shock. An appreciable degree of metabolic acidosis (base deficit) indicates a long duration or profound degree of shock or the presence of some other factor, such as diabetic ketoacidosis. The absence of a marked metabolic acidosis does not mean that significant blood loss or circulatory deterioration has not occurred. It is clear that metabolic acidosis is a relatively late development in injured patients and that the state of acid-base balance does not correlate well with the clinical situation soon after injury.[31, 39] Sampling the central venous P_{O_2} can provide a valuable indicator of circulatory status. A mixed venous P_{O_2} near 20 mmHg indicates a severely stressed circulatory system which is barely supplying enough oxygen to maintain life. A mixed venous P_{O_2} of 40 mmHg generally indicates that the circulatory system is easily meeting the demands placed upon it. A rising mixed venous P_{O_2} is usually a sign of improving circulatory status, while a falling mixed venous P_{O_2} is cause for concern. The central venous catheter usually yields superior caval blood, which under conditions of stress has a somewhat higher P_{O_2} than true mixed venous blood, but the general relationships remain the same.[68]

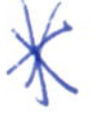

Hemorrhage

When hemorrhage is occurring, every expedient method to stop the loss of blood must be taken. Pressure on an external bleeding site will usually suffice. Splinting of major fractures is very important; a one-liter hemorrhage can be prevented by early use of a Thomas splint. In some instances, early laparotomy becomes a resuscitative measure. If the rate of loss is rapid enough, anesthesia and operation may be necessary before blood pressure and urine flow have been restored. In such conditions of massive internal hemorrhage, the earlier the operation the better.

When shock is judged to be due to blood loss, as it usually will be in the injured patient, one is faced with two decisions: how much fluid to give and what kind to use. The simplest guides for the optimum volume are those that indicate a reversal of the shock state: improved color and warmth, loss of apprehension or improvement in state of consciousness, slowing pulse, rising blood pressure, increasing urinary output, slowing respiratory rate, ability to sit up without faintness or hypotension. The central venous P_{O_2}, described above, appears to be a valuable objective indicator of circulatory status and deserves wider application. The CVP must be used cautiously. There is a wide variation in normal CVP within any population and even in the same individual at different times.[56, 98] The relationship between CVP and blood volume has been thoroughly demonstrated to be a very imprecise one with considerable variability.[54, 56, 80, 98, 138, 142] The absolute value of the CVP also depends on an imprecise anatomic landmark, the level of the middle of the right atrium as judged externally. The change in the CVP is more valuable than the absolute value (unless this is elevated). A CVP that rises appreciably with the infusion of a few hundred milliliters of crystalloid solution usually indicates a full blood volume. A CVP that does not change with the rapid infusion of blood indicates hypovolemia or an erroneous reading.

Three errors are commonly made in the use of CVP monitoring in injured patients. The position of the catheter is sometimes not confirmed before treatment decisions are made. The absolute value of the CVP is too often taken as an indication of the presence or absence of normovolemia or hypovolemia. Finally, perhaps most commonly, the CVP is relied upon to detect fluid overload when administering crystalloid solutions. Gross overloading with simple salt solutions can occur with a normal central venous pressure. The study in dogs by Johnson and Lambert is a dramatic demonstration of this principle.[72] We have seen far too many typical clinical examples. The central venous pressure measures a result of the interaction of blood volume, venous tone, and the efficiency of the right heart as a pump. Crystalloid solutions expand the extracellular volume primarily, and relatively small fractions remain in the plasma space if blood loss has been extensive or if plasma-specific osmotic activity is low. The central venous pressure does not measure changes in the interstitial fluid space, which is where flooding occurs with the use of saline solution. The pulmonary interstitial space is part of this compartment. In addition, whatever saline stays in the plasma space dilutes the plasma-specific osmotic activity and changes the Starling relationships to favor edema formation at lower pressures.[55, 76] After alveolar flooding occurs, the central venous pressure may rise as a result of increased pulmonary vascular resistance and myocardial hypoxia.

On theoretical grounds one would expect that patients who have been severely hypotensive from blood loss would require a greater than normal blood volume for optimal resuscitation, due to the requirements for higher cardiac output during recovery and the presumed diffuse vasodilatation following the previous vasoconstriction. Certainly, animals who are resuscitated with something in addition to the volume of blood shed seem to do better.[44, 116] MacLean and associates presented evidence confirming this point, but it appears from their presentation that at least some of these patients were septic.[81] Studies on blood volumes in resuscitated combat casualties in South Vietnam by the United States Army Surgical Research Team have, however, raised some interesting questions. Simmons and associates found that the most severely injured patients, requiring the largest amounts of blood replacement, were consistently "undertransfused", that is, their total blood volumes were less than the predicted normal and less than casualties who were also transfused but who had been less severely injured.[119] The differences were greater than could be accounted for by the expected loss of up to 25 per cent of the transfused red cells in the 24 hours after transfusion. The delay in plasma refilling noted in a later study could have been due to continuing third-space losses.[45] Blood volumes returned to normal on the second or third postoperative day, with some "overshoot." These patients were transfused according to the usual criteria of blood pressure, pulse rate, urinary output and central venous pressure. The central venous pressure was slightly lower on average in the heavily transfused group, but there was no impressive difference in any of these criteria. The implication is that severely injured patients tend to manifest satisfactory clinical signs of recovery at a lower than "normal" blood volume, contrary to theoretical expectations. Cleland and associates found a lower than normal plasma volume with an increased extracellular fluid volume following cardiopulmonary bypass, despite equal or higher right atrial pressures and normal protein concentrations.[30] They postulated a persistent contraction of the capacitance vessels. Friedman et al. also reported a lower blood volume to CVP ratio in a mixed group of ill patients.[54] Northfield and Smith reported that transfusing patients with gastrointestinal hemorrhage to a normal CVP (5 cm. water) restored a normal blood volume, but their illustration indicates that the average post-transfusion blood volume was less than normal.[98] Wilson et al. found almost no relationship between blood volume and CVP, but unfortunately did not distinguish patients with hemorrhage and trauma from those with known heart failure and sepsis.[142] If there is persistent contraction of the capacitance system following blood loss and transfusion, one can easily visualize another mechanism predisposing to the development of pulmonary congestion after resuscitation in seriously injured patients. Four of the 29 casualties in Simmons' study developed postoperative pulmonary edema. None had a larger than predicted blood volume; two, in fact, were in the "undertransfused" group. One wonders what would have happened had resuscitative fluids been pushed to achieve a higher central venous pressure. Further investigation along these lines is clearly needed.

Blood

Of the fluids available for resuscitation, only whole blood or red cell preparations have the ability to restore oxygen-delivering capacity. This means that very large single hemorrhages or extensive continuous or repeated blood loss must be treated with whole blood at least in part. These preparations, then, constitute the basis for fluid replacement in the seriously hemorrhaged patient. Besides oxygen-delivering capacity, whole blood supplies, for the most part, a fairly normal spectrum of plasma proteins for osmotic, immunologic and clotting effects. The volume of fluid transfused is largely the volume of fluid that remains in a normal circulation and persists there for a significant period of time. The anticoagulant solution (NIH-A) supplies an extra 15 mEq. of sodium and 67.5 ml. of water per unit of blood. Because citrate is so rapidly metabolized, this sodium has an effect like that of sodium bicarbonate. Thus, even before the measurements of extracellular fluid spaces and their real or imagined shifts, blood for replacement was supplied with a built-in excess of 10–15 per cent as a sodium solution in a slightly hypertonic form (222 mEq./L.).

The disadvantages of whole blood transfusion are well known and very significant. Most serious is the fact that blood transmits disease, and a definite mortality rate results, sometimes estimated at one death per thousand transfusions. Screening for Australia antigen will not remove all the hepatitis carriers—perhaps less than half. Prophylactic use of pooled gamma globulin may not be protective.[59] The problem thus remains a serious one that will not be eliminated even if present plans to eliminate high-risk "commercial" blood are successful. Blood is immunologically active and can cause serious reactions during administration, as well as immunization against future administration. It should not be given without determining immunologic compatibility, which causes a significant delay. Procurement of blood is difficult and sporadic, and the proper type may not be available when it is needed. Blood must be carefully refrigerated and protected from repeated handling and agitation, and it has a relatively short shelf life. It is very expensive and is becoming more so.

When blood must be given rapidly and in large quantities, a number of other toxicities become possible.[20, 36] Ironically, the classic problems of massive transfusion, excess citrate and potassium, and clotting factor depletions are usually of lesser practical importance. Citrate toxicity is probably rare and certainly unpredictable.[21, 97] Available evidence indicates that it is not to be expected at transfusion rates below one unit of blood every five minutes to an average adult with a reasonably intact circulation and a functioning liver.[20, 115] Hyperkalemia has not been characteristic of heavily transfused patients unless severe acidosis occurs, in which case the hyperkalemia may be related more to the acidosis.[20, 23, 141] Clotting factor depletion is a more complex problem. The clotting factors in which blood is seriously deficient are platelets and factors V and VIII, but even these latter two are present in detectable amounts. Studies on clotting changes during massive transfusion have been rare. In both the Korean and Vietnam wars and in one well-documented civilian series, heavily transfused patients rarely exhibited platelet counts below 75,000/mm.[58, 113, 118, 141] The Naval Research Team, however, found more severe thrombocytopenia in their studies on heavily transfused combat casualties.[89] More sophisticated studies of clotting function indicated that shock itself was the probable cause of serious clotting defects, which, in fact, could be partially corrected by the use of 2- to 3-week-old blood.[118] A large number of surgeons can personally attest to the ability to safely and uneventfully perform massive soft-tissue debridements in combat casualties who have received liters of stored bank blood immediately before operation.

Acidosis has received some attention as a logical consequence of massive transfusion, since stored blood contains a high acid load and the severely hemorrhaged patient is usually tending in that direction. Both the endogenous (shock) and the exogenous (transfused) acid loads, however, are organic acids that are very rapidly metabolized when circulation is restored. The sodium citrate of the anticoagulant acts as an alkalinizing agent, and further alkalinization seems necessary only with apparent failure of resuscitation.[40] In those circumstances, citrate excess is as likely and calcium should also be given.

The low temperature of stored blood can induce hypothermia in the recipient, which in turn can impair the ability to metabolize organic acids and various drugs and can create increased oxygen requirements to maintain body temperature.[17] If cold blood is given under pressure through a central venous catheter, it could conceivably emerge as a jet and differentially cool one area of the heart, setting up an arrhythmogenic zone. Visual inspection of the filter after clinical transfusion often reveals gross blood clots. If numerous transfusions are given under pressure through the same filter, some of this material must reach the patient. Microscopic aggregates of cells and cellular debris are demonstrable in stored blood. A series of studies from the United States Army Surgical Research Team in South Vietnam has dealt with the problem of microembolism resulting from extensive transfusion.[85, 94] Screen filtration pressures were used in some of these studies, and an exact interpretation of the significance of such changes is not possible, but the possibility and even likelihood cannot be denied. It was difficult to relate changes in pulmonary function to transfusion alone because the most heavily transfused were the most extensively injured,[35, 78] but it is likely that the basically healthy young adults studied in South Vietnam were better able to withstand pulmonary embolization than the usual civilian casualty would be.

Protein denaturation occurs with exposure to foreign surfaces, gas interfaces, and perhaps the temperature of storage and initial severe acidity as the first fractions of collected blood enter the undiluted anticoagulant. Such denaturation has been proposed as a cause of morbidity with the pump-oxygenator. The effect of the nature of blood surface contact on the subsequent mortality of shocked, transfused dogs is impressive,[66, 111] and it is interesting to note that the occasional study in which untreated animals or those treated with asanguineous fluids do better than those reinfused with shed blood often involves extensive handline, glass contact or gas bubbling of the shed blood.[18, 46]

Serotonin and perhaps other vasoconstrictive amines are released from the breakdown of platelets and leukocytes during storage. Some of the intermediate clotting factors are activated during storage and perhaps can facilitate the occurrence or progression of intravascular clotting. Stored homologous blood may worsen the impairment of antibacterial defenses after shock.[99] Increased pulmonary vascular resistance and periarterial hemorrhages were found in dogs given "compatible" homologous but not autologous blood.[136] A graft-against-host reaction (transfused lymphocytes attacking the recipient) has been postulated when fresh blood is used, but its occurrence remains highly speculative.[87]

One can expect a loss of up to 25 per cent of the transfused red cells in the day following transfusion, the exact percentage depending on the age of the blood. This results in a significant loss of oxygen-carrying capacity and perhaps of blood volume in the early recovery period.

Perhaps the most serious detrimental effect of massive transfusions of stored blood has only recently come to light. A potentially harmful shift of the oxygen-hemoglobin dissociation curve in stored blood was documented in 1954, but little attention was paid to it.[135] The recent elucidation of the role of 2,3-diphosphoglyceric acid (2,3-DPG) in regulating oxygen dissociation and its evident physiologic importance led to a reinvestigation of stored blood and the discovery that it is severely depleted of 2,3-DPG.[133] This depletion takes hours to be corrected after transfusion. Levels of 2,3-DPG have been very low and hemoglobin-oxygen affinity abnormally high in massively transfused patients.[83, 130, 134, 135] A detrimental effect of such increased oxygen affinity has not been easy to demonstrate at normal hematocrits, however, and many more studies are necessary to establish the clinical importance of these changes. The coming change to CPD as the standard anticoagulant will result in a significant improvement in the oxygen affinity of stored blood, although it will still be significantly abnormal.

The accumulated clinical experience with massive transfusion indicates that this impressive list of problems has not prevented clinical success in resuscitation. Much more data is needed in many of these areas, but the remarkable resiliency of the human system is often able to overcome these insults even after severe injury and hemorrhage. Clearly, however, improvements are badly needed in the safety, effectiveness and availability of blood transfusion. It remains the keystone of resuscitation.

Crystalloid Solutions

The currently most popular alternatives to the use of whole blood in injured patients in the United States are the "crystalloid" solutions. Crystalloid solutions are simple electrolyte solutions that mimic interstitial fluid. They are basically isotonic sodium chloride with variations which are generally of little importance except when very large volumes are infused rapidly or when renal function is poor. The United States Navy Surgical Research Team compared acid-base and electrolyte changes in combat casualties resuscitated with large amounts of saline solution and with lactated Ringer's solution.[23] There was little difference in the average blood electrolyte and acid-base values for the two groups. When patients with cholera were resuscitated with saline solution, however, the metabolic acidosis persisted.[24] These patients are unusual in that they have a severe subtraction metabolic acidosis (loss of alkaline gastrointestinal secretions), a situation very different from the usual injured and hemorrhaging patient whose acidosis is due to an accumulation of organic acids that are rapidly "burned off" when circulation is restored.[40]

The crystalloid solutions have a number of important advantages as resuscitative fluids. They are cheap, plentiful, easily stored and readily available, and they can be administered instantly; they do not transmit communicable diseases, they are nonimmunogenic and they are essentially nontoxic except for total fluid load. A broad clinical experience indicates that simple saline solutions are effective plasma volume expanders in many clinical situations. Careful studies on blood volume changes in volunteers with moderate hemorrhages indicate a somewhat preferential retention of infused saline solution in the plasma space, approaching 35 to 40 per cent of the initially infused fluid.[91, 102] The long-term effects on plasma volume are less clear and may be strongly influenced by individual renal function, prehemorrhage protein stores and associated abnormalities.[57] The effectiveness of crystalloid replacement for very large hemorrhages is much less certain.[131] Judicious use of saline solutions has reduced the amount of blood used in resuscitation and in the operating room with little apparent loss of effectiveness.[110] The United States Navy Surgical Research Team favored a blood-plus-saline regimen over a blood-plus-colloid approach after a direct clinical comparison of the two in South Vietnam.[23] Less objectively analyzed experience throughout the combat zone agreed with this practice.

The disadvantages of simple saline solutions are those of all nonoxygen-carrying plasma expanders, plus the important feature of lack of plasma-specific osmotic activity. These fluids expand the extracellular fluid space, with plasma volume expansion resulting as a compartment of this extracellular space. To the extent that the plasma volume is expanded, its specific osmotic activity relative to the interstitial space is reduced. The specific disadvantages of these fluids are flooding of the extracellular space and reduction in plasma-specific osmotic activity, which promote the development of interstitial edema which can be damaging in the lungs.

Several factors increase the chance of inadvertent flooding unless great care is taken in the use of these fluids. First, the more blood that is lost, the greater is the relative requirement for crystalloid solution needed to restore the circulation.[95] This is at least partly due to the loss of plasma-specific osmotic activity. The relationship is not a constant one, nor does it run in a straight line. Rather, it is a sharply rising curve, with ever-increasing amounts of saline solution required to replace succeeding increments of blood loss. In a situation of continuing hemorrhage in which saline solution is being given to maintain blood pressure, gross flooding can easily occur unless one keeps track of the amount of blood lost and the amount of crystalloid solution given. Second, the central venous pressure may not indicate gross overloading with crystalloid infusions, as has been discussed already. Third, seriously injured patients will retain infused salt and water to an abnormal degree, perhaps even greater than is evident from input and output data.[57, 62, 70] The kidneys cannot be relied on to make up for the therapeutic excesses.

One of the reasons for the growth in popularity of the crystalloid solutions was the demonstration by Shires and coworkers of a sizable loss of extracellular fluid in hemorrhagic shock, apparently through internal shifts into the intracellular space.[116] It was found by others that much of the apparent loss was due not to true shifts of fluid but rather to a delay in equilibration of the markers used for measurement.[8, 30, 91, 108, 114] Most researchers now agree that such shifts, if they occur, are found only rather late in profound hypotension, and the magnitude of the shift is relatively modest—10 to 15 per cent of the extracellular fluid space, or 1 to 2 L. of saline solution for an adult. The term "functioning extracellular space" has been devised to emphasize the delay in equilibration that occurs after shock,[88] but there is no clear evidence as yet of the physiologic significance, if any, of this phenomenon.

There are, however, other cogent reasons to add an extracellular-like fluid to the resuscitative regimen. Injured patients will sequester significant amounts of fluid in areas of injury during the following one or two days. The size of this space will be proportional to the size and seriousness of the physical damage to tissues and will be increased by such complications as paralytic ileus or peritonitis. It could eventually equal a large fraction of the normal extracellular fluid volume. Perhaps more important are the considerations of preventing renal failure in the seriously injured patient. Most evidence points in the same direction. The earlier that normal blood flow is reestablished, the lower will be the incidence of renal failure after injury. In addition, the early institution of a saline diuresis will protect experimental animals from a number of combined insults that would otherwise produce renal failure.[47, 96, 128] There may be at least two protective mechanisms. One appears to be prevention of the intratubular precipitation of certain products of tissue destruction by preventing the persistence of a slow flow of concentrated, acidic urine in the tubules. Another may be related to a reduction in oxygen requirements by the tubules during diuresis. Whether or not there is any specific redistribution of blood flow in the kidneys as the result of diuresis is not certain. All these considerations favor the use of large volumes of both blood and saline solutions early in resuscitation when renal function alone is considered. The incidence of post-traumatic renal insufficiency has been much lower in the Vietnam war than it was in the war in Korea. Many casualties have been resuscitated earlier, which certainly is a contributing factor, but additional saline solutions and osmotic diuretics, especially mannitol, have been used liberally. High urine outputs have been achieved early in the course of resuscitation. Civilian centers using liberal amounts of saline solutions also claim a lower incidence of acute tubular necrosis.[11]

Plasma and Artificial Colloids

Plasma has been remarkably inefficient as the sole resuscitative fluid for the treatment of hemorrhage in many experiments. There was widespread dissatisfaction with its use in World War II, and the switch to whole blood as the prime resuscitative fluid seemed to yield much better results.[74] The reasons for this poor performance are not clear but may relate to denaturation of proteins during processing. The major role for these fluids today is to restore some plasma-specific osmotic activity in patients receiving crystalloid solutions and occasionally in small volumes as temporary blood substitutes. Pooled plasma and even single donor units of plasma should not be used except for very specific indications; the risk of hepatitis is too great. Certain processed fractions, such as albumin, provide the osmotic activity at a very much smaller risk of hepatitis.

The artificial colloids in the United States are mainly the dextrans and hydroxyethyl starch. All of these materials interfere with clotting and should not be given to a total dose exceeding 1 to 1.5 liters in 24 hours. This seriously limits their usefulness. In addition, there are serious questions about the renal toxicity of low molecular weight dextran.[26, 36 82] This material has been pushed aggressively for its flow-improving properties, which in fact may not exist at the blood levels that can be safely achieved clinically.[25, 33, 75] At this stage of uncertainty, we do not consider it an acceptable fluid for use in acutely injured patients.

Hemodilution

The success of hemodilutional methods in cardiopulmonary bypass and of extensive use of crystalloid solutions in treating injured patients has led to much current discussion of the advantages of deliberate hemodilution in resuscitation. It is clear that a previously normal mammal can tolerate acute lowering of hematocrit to at least half normal levels provided total blood volume is maintained. These studies have helped establish a basic principle of resuscitation from severe hemorrhage, that flow is more important than hematocrit until very low levels of hematocrit are reached. As the viscosity of blood is directly related to the hematocrit, some have extrapolated these observations to conclude that a low hematocrit is *desirable* during resuscitation. What pertinent experiments have been done indicate that the normal ratios are "optimal": the studies of Crowell and co-workers[42] on hemorrhagic hypotension (optimal hematocrit, 42 per cent) and of Smith and Crowell[125] on induced severe hypoxemia (optimal hematocrit, 40–41 per cent) in dogs, and indirect measurements of tissue oxygen tensions[9] (steady decrease below hematocrit, 45 per cent) or of oxygen consumption and lactate production[61] (best above 34 per cent), as well as other, less elegant studies measuring "oxygen transport" (arterial oxygen content times cardiac output), support the 40 per cent range as one of optimal circulatory efficiency. Crowell and Smith have attempted to formulate mathematical expressions that can be solved for the optimal hematocrit under changing conditions.[43] Clinically available data support the more normal hematocrits in that congestive heart failure or angina can be relieved in some chronically anemic patients and exercise tolerance improved in most when hematocrits are raised, indicating a beneficial effect on the cardiac work/oxygen delivery relationship. Even more relevant to resuscitation of the injured patient are recent studies on the interrelationships between hematocrit, oxygen affinity, and survival from hemorrhage.[38] Rats treated for hemorrhage with stored blood with high oxygen affinity did just as well as those treated with fresh blood when the hematocrit was normal, but when the hematocrit was reduced to half normal there was a marked increase in the mortality of those receiving the stored blood. The combination of hemodilution and increased oxygen affinity (which occurs during storage of blood) was clearly detrimental. Naturally occurring hemoglobin variants with altered oxygen affinity are being identified; the clinical features of "normal" hematocrit, exercise tolerance, etc. indicate how closely the oxygen-binding properties of hemoglobin are related to the optimal hematocrit ratio.[103] The "normal" hematocrit seems to vary directly with affinity of hemoglobin for oxygen, indicating that as yet unidentified regulatory mechanisms will choose the lowest hematocrit compatible with a certain level of oxygen delivery (tissue P_{O_2}?) at a certain resting cardiac output. The regulatory system must be a fairly complex yet very basic one, as is the entire question of what is the optimal hematocrit.

Summary

Red cells will be required for resuscitation when blood loss approaches half the normal blood volume (less blood loss will be tolerated by patients with vascular or cardiopulmonary disease). In seriously injured patients, blood then remains the key resuscitative fluid. Non-red cell–containing fluids have useful roles in limiting or eliminating the need for blood with limited hemorrhages, in keeping the patient alive until blood can be obtained, in replacing hidden losses of extracellular fluid and in promoting an early and sustained output of urine to minimize post-traumatic renal failure. All of the non-blood fluids have serious disadvantages, but the crystalloid solutions appear to be the most useful. Stored blood itself has very serious disadvantages which may be lessened by investigative and organizational work now in progress.

WHY DOES RESUSCITATION FAIL?

Resuscitation can fail if the injuries sustained are incompatible with survival. This is not really a failure of resuscitation, but rather a reflection of our limitations in other fields. Brain injury is the usual culprit in this situation, but extensive destruction of any of the "vital" organs can be the cause. Certain developments could improve these results; temporary replacement of pulmonary function for several days while the injured lungs recover is perhaps the nearest to realization. Transplantation is not likely to be a useful approach in the acutely injured patient until a radically different method is devised that does not require generalized immunosuppression.

Certain associated diseases carry a higher risk of failure and are really a variation of the above theme. Patients with myocardial or coronary insufficiency do very poorly because the ability of the heart to increase its work is one of the key elements in maintaining an intact circulation during loss of blood. The ability of the coronary vessels to dilate is essential because of the peculiar situation in which the heart extracts nearly all the usable oxygen from its blood supply, leaving very little reserve. Preexisting renal and pulmonary disease make subsequent organ failure more likely. Hepatic insufficiency is associated with a high mortality in shock of all forms because of the essential role of the liver in intermediary metabolism. The higher risk in diabetics probably reflects arterial insufficiency and perhaps the impairment in energy metabolism.

All experimental studies clearly show the critical importance of the duration of shock in determining the outcome. This has been hard to document in clinical material because of the element of selection—the seriously injured die before reaching treatment if the delay is long and therefore are eliminated from the statistics. In Vietnam, for instance, no one who has been there can possibly doubt that very rapid helicopter evacuation and the organization of medical care has saved many lives that would have been lost in other wars or even today in the middle of most American cities. The same system has also rescued irretrievably injured casualties who previously would have died in the field. The statistics as a result are paradoxically not quite as good as they were in the Korean War. We can hope that major advances in the care of injured patients in the United States in the coming years will occur in the areas of transportation and organization, because so much can be gained here. Reducing the time from injury to informed treatment will greatly improve the survival rate among potentially salvageable casualties.

In considering the various specific organs and systems in an analysis of resuscitation failures, one must be cautious in interpreting published statistics which are often devised to prove a point, follow a fad, or justify requests for further funding. Patients who die of organ or system failure following injury and resuscitation usually die of multisystem failure. In some patients a single event or failure clearly led to the others, but this analysis is usually missing from statistics relating predominantly to one or another system.

Circulatory failure has received by far the most attention in experimental work on hemorrhagic shock using laboratory animals. The concept of "irreversible shock" arose from work in which animals died in shock long after all their shed blood had been restored.[139] Patients have rarely exhibited this phenomenon, however, at least in its pure form. Several groups of clinical investigators have tried to abolish the concept as being potentially harmful in the clinical context.[13, 69, 127] This question is closely linked to that of the role of the heart in persistent circulatory failure. The heart is potentially vulnerable because of a number of peculiarities in its oxygen supply. The heart normally extracts almost all of the available oxygen from its blood supply, leaving very little reserve. Increased demands must be met by increases in coronary blood flow. Coronary blood flow is dependent on central aortic diastolic pressure and on the ability of the coronary vessels to dilate. Most of coronary flow occurs during diastole, so that the total fraction of time that the heart spends in diastole also influences flow. Everything that happens during severe hemorrhage challenges this system: diastolic pressure falls, the work demands on the heart increase and a higher fraction of time is spent in systole. These events place a very critical demand on the coronary vessels to dilate, and this certainly forms one of the weak links in the patient's defenses against hemorrhage.

In the animal models, although there is evidence on both sides, it seems clear that the heart retains enough functioning reserve to prevent death and that impaired venous return and decreased coronary flow are the prime causes of the low cardiac output.[63, 90, 104, 109, 117] Most of what we have seen as persistent, volume-resistant circulatory failure has occurred in patients with arteriosclerotic coronary disease following prolonged or very severe hypotension. These patients died in a setting compatible with acute heart failure. Ability to measure left atrial pressures would have provided valuable information. This situation does occur, albeit rarely, in younger patients but is almost always accompanied by clotting abnormalities and renal and pulmonary failure.

The clotting system can deteriorate to the point of diffuse uncontrollable bleeding. This usually occurs after very severe blood loss and almost never with losses less than 30 per cent unless a mismatched blood transfusion is involved. Disseminated intravascular coagulation is a well-documented sequel of hemorrhage in animals.[64, 84] In man the situation is complicated by the effects of injury with the probable release of tissue thromboplastins and local platelet sequestration, but well-documented cases have occurred after hemorrhage alone. When truly pathological bleeding develops, the prognosis is poor. Heparin and clotting factor replacement may improve clotting factor levels in the circulation, but renal, pulmonary and persistent circulatory failure are the usual concurrences with death within 24 hours. As several semi-detached and wise observers have commented, the most common significant clotting deficit in injured patients is silk, a principle which should always be kept in mind, but when this kind of pathological bleeding occurs it is obvious even to the skeptics.

Renal failure is one of the classical causes of resuscitative failure in injured patients. It became recognized as an entity in its own right during World War II, was further elucidated during the Korean War and has since then been refined by the recognition of a spectrum of forms and degrees and by the impact of hemodialysis. Unfortunately, hemodialysis is far more successful in treating renal failure in medical patients. Renal failure after major injury still carries a very high mortality.[15, 96, 107, 143] The causes and mechanisms are debated. Tubular precipitation with mechanical blockage, uncontrolled back diffusion of urine, renal tubular toxins, ischemic damage due to prolonged vasoconstriction or shunting of blood away from the cortex, interstitial edema sufficient to cause mechanical obstruction, disseminated intravascular coagulation and other factors have been advanced as causes for acute renal failure following injury.[47, 96] No single animal model duplicates the antecedent clinical setting and the pathological and physiological picture found in patients. Renal failure sometimes follows apparently moderate degrees of hemorrhage and injury, and its cause then is particularly puzzling. Experimental and uncontrolled clinical experience indicates that the early institution of a diuresis may lower the incidence of post-traumatic renal failure. The incidence of post-traumatic renal failure in Vietnam was much lower than had been expected. How much of this reduction was due to the aggressive use of crystalloid solutions and diuretics and how much to the reduction in the delay between wounding and treatment cannot be determined.

Pulmonary failure in seriously injured patients is a topic of considerable recent interest and concern. It is probably more than coincidence that the incidence of pulmonary problems seemed to rise at the time when fluids for resuscitation were being used more and more aggressively. In addition to this, recognition of ventilatory failure is now much better because of the widespread use of blood gas analysis. Unexpected deaths and "cardiac arrests" in former days were often undoubtedly the result of unrecognized and hence untreated ventilatory failure. One of the valuable medical lessons of the war in Vietnam has been the awareness of the difficulty in detecting significant hypoxemia clinically and an awareness of how commonly patients with multiple system injury become hypoxemic.

The important principle that follows from these observations is that routine arterial blood gas analysis is advisable in the seriously injured patient. The frequency of sampling should be determined by the status of the patient and should be more frequent in the more seriously ill and in those with conditions that carry an extra risk of pulmonary impairment. Use of oxygen therapy should not be indiscriminate, however. Oxygen is itself potentially damaging to alveoli, and the inspired oxygen tension should be no higher than is necessary to nearly completely saturate hemoglobin with oxygen. Since an arterial P_{O_2} of 70 mmHg usually signifies 90 per cent saturation or better, there is little to be gained by increasing the inspired oxygen concentration to raise Pa_{O_2} above this level. In addition, oxygen that is delivered without adequate humidification can create a serious impairment to the clearing of bronchial secretions. Once hypoxemia is detected, however, it should be treated promptly and to the extent necessary. There is probably more damage done by delaying the use of ventilatory assistance than by over-agressive intervention. Indirect evidence indicates that early and correct ventilatory assistance can prevent much more serious pulmonary insufficiency a day or two later. This complex of problems appears to be much more easily halted and reversed in its early stages.

There are many well documented causes of hypoxemia in injured patients; these have been reviewed elsewhere.[35, 49, 92] The effects of severe hemorrhage on pulmonary function are also rather well documented.[37] Gas exchange is well maintained during hemorrhage. The ratio of dead space to tidal ventilation increases as reduced pulmonary blood flow occurs mainly through dependent parts of the lungs under the influence of gravity while ventilation of the upper parts continues. After reinfusion of shed blood, there is a variable amount of congestion, interstitial edema, leucocyte and platelet aggregation, and loss of compliance, but gas exchange remains intact in most experiments. These changes do not progress, but rather improve during the days following resuscitation. The degree of change may be related to the type of fluid used for resuscitation. Severe hemorrhage and resuscitation, then, do effect the lungs in a detrimental way, but a progressive or late-appearing syndrome has not been produced in animals. It is likely that ventilatory failure in patients after resuscitation is due at least in part to other causes. Ventilatory failure forms a broad spectrum of severity in the post-traumatic patient. The requirement for mechanical ventilatory support does not imply a poor prognosis, although specific mortality rates are hard to derive because of the heterogeneity of the population.

Sepsis continues to be one of the main causes of eventual failure in the treatment of seriously injured patients. This tends to be obscured by the interest devoted to pulmonary and renal failure. Many instances of pulmonary and renal failure following injury are in fact consequences of uncontrolled infection. It has been estimated that sepsis was the leading primary cause of death among potentially salvageable American combat casualties in Vietnam who lived to receive resuscitative measures. The impairment of antimicrobial defenses that results from serious injury and shock is poorly characterized and poorly understood. Reticuloendothelial system function is demonstrably impaired in proportion to the degree of shock.[7, 112] Leucocyte function is less easily studied,[1, 140] as are the specific and non-specific humoral defense mechanisms.[3, 32] Clinical evidence is quite clear, however. The state of antimicrobial defenses after severe injury is one of the relatively neglected scientific areas of investigation in trauma. Newer methods are sorely needed.[2, 5]

Because of the relative paucity of knowledge in this area, a number of clinically important questions remain unanswered. The role of antibiotic therapy in the seriously injured patient has not been defined precisely. In contaminating wounds of the peritoneal cavity, early prophylactic use of appropriate antibiotics appears to decrease later morbidity from sepsis.[5] At the other end of the spectrum, it is doubtful that prophylactic antibiotic therapy improves results in patients with "clean" injuries (ruptured spleens, pelvic fractures, etc.). In between are patients with contaminated wounds involving soft tissues only. These are currently handled either with or without antibiotic coverage depending on the size of the wound, completeness of debridement, interval from injury to debridement, and the habits of the surgeon. Whether the occurrence of significant hypotension in an injured patient is itself an indication for the use of antibiotics remains open to question. We currently think it is not.

Stress ulceration is a cause of resuscitative failure that usually follows other complications.[6, 50, 79, 101] It is not often seen in an uncomplicated convalescence but is more often a complication of complications, especially sepsis, and often fulfills the role of delivering the coup de grace. Recent investigations indicate that the mucosal barrier function of the stomach may be impaired after serious injury, thereby explaining the paradoxically lower free acid content in the stomachs of patients at higher risk of acute ulcerative complications and the somewhat peculiar pattern of distribution of these ulcers.[105, 121, 129]

A number of hemodynamically active drugs have been proposed for use in resuscitation from shock, especially isoproterenol and steroids. These agents are usually discussed in the context of treatment-resistant septic shock or cardiogenic shock, but proposals have been made for use in hypovolemia. This appears to be generally unnecessary, and routine use of such drugs is therapeutically meddlesome and potentially dangerous. Volume replacement is clearly the first priority and is usually all that is necessary. Even established metabolic acidosis in hypovolemic patients will usually respond to volume replacement without alkalinizing agents.[40] Steroids can potentiate the susceptibility to infection and to stress ulceration and isoproterenol is potentially arrhymogenic and requires a large increase in coronary flow to accomplish an increase in cardiac output. There is little or no clinical evidence favoring the use of these agents in uncomplicated hypovolemia; the experimental evidence relating to their use is inconsistent or contradictory. Even liberal use of sodium bicarbonate, which is relatively benign and has more to recommend its use, can quickly add up to a large sodium load which may not be easily handled after resuscitation is complete.

Ironically, the laboratory models for hemorrhagic shock are best suited for a condition we rarely see: unexplained, post-resuscitative, volume-resistant circulatory failure. They fail to produce the problems more commonly seen in patients: renal failure, pulmonary insufficiency and stress ulcer. This illustrates the very great importance of maintaining research into shock in the clinical context.

One patient we recently encountered illustrates a number of points. A 74-year-old man was struck by an automobile while crossing the street, sustaining an injury to his thigh and a bump on the head. He was taken to a local hospital where a scalp laceration was sutured. X-rays revealed a skull fracture and a supracondylar fracture of the femur. A Thomas splint was applied and arrangements made to transfer the patient to a university center because of the skull fracture. The patient became hypotensive and restless. Intravenous fluids were given in the form of dextrose in water, and the patient was given a narcotic and a phenothiazine for his restlessness. He arrived in transfer three hours after his injury profoundly hypotensive, barely arousable and almost anuric. The fractured thigh was grossly swollen and tense and the limb distally was cool and pulseless. The central venous pressure was 0 and there was S-T segment depression on EKG. The accompanying x-rays revealed that the skull "fracture" was an anatomic variant. The patient was given lactated Ringer's solution and levarterenol to maintain a systolic pressure of 90 mmHg until crossmatched blood was available. Five units of blood administered rapidly through multiple portals failed to sustain a systolic pressure of 100 mmHg. An arteriogram revealed a transected popliteal artery. The patient was anesthetized, the limb explored and the artery repaired, and a pin inserted in the tibial tubercle and skeletal traction begun. Bleeding was diffuse and became uncontrollable and generalized, involving all known venepuncture sites and the respiratory and gastrointestinal tracts. Pressure was applied where possible. Laboratory studies revealed a marked thrombocytopenia, hypofibrinogenemia, marked decrease in factor V and factor VIII, and a high titer of fibrin split products. Continuous intravenous heparin was given as well as fresh blood and fresh-frozen plasma. The clotting studies all improved but the patient continued bleeding. He went through an episode of pulmonary edema requiring continuous positive pressure ventilation for control, remained severely oliguric, never regained consciousness, never sustained an acceptable blood pressure despite raising his CVP to 15 cm. water, and died 15 hours after admission.

The mistakes made at the first hospital are obvious and fundamental. The true nature of his disorder, blood loss, was not recognized because it was hidden. When he was given fluids, it was the wrong kind. He was treated for the restlessness that represented cerebral hypoxia with central nervous system depressants. He was transferred to another hospital for the wrong reason. Obviously, he had been taken for emergency care to a facility that was not capable of the job, at least at that time. The mistakes did not end with his arrival at the university center. It is very poor practice to treat blood loss with vasoconstrictors. If the degree of hypotension was thought to be so life-threatening, as it may indeed have been in a man of this age, type-specific but uncrossmatched blood would have been available in ten minutes and would have been a better choice. In most hospitals at least 45 minutes will elapse before crossmatched blood is available. Some patients must receive blood sooner, and type-specific blood with a fast-slide crossmatch is usually the best alternative. Finally, in someone in this desperate condition an amputation may have been a better choice than a vascular reconstruction. Even better would have been no operation at all if the bleeding into the thigh could have been controlled by pressure, but this is a very difficult decision to make without the benefit of hindsight. His course illustrates the principle of multisystem failure, the occurrence of disseminated intravascular coagulation in patients with prolonged and volume-resistant circulatory failure, and the occurrence of renal and pulmonary failure in this setting.

In summary, seriously injured patients who reach a hospital alive but do not survive die for a variety of reasons. Some have injuries incompatible with life and little can be done. Some have associated diseases that seriously impair the reserve necessary in certain systems to withstand the stress of hemorrhage and injury. Most will have identifiable failures in various systems, usually several: renal, pulmonary, clotting, antibacterial defense or upper gastrointestinal. Circulatory failure usually occurs because vascular disease will not allow adequate coronary perfusion at low pressures and high work demands. In all of these considerations, reducing the delay between injury and treatment and insuring satisfactory initial management will do more to improve results than any immediately foreseeable scientific development.

REFERENCES

1. Alexander, J. W., Dionigi, R., and Meakins, J. L.: Periodic variation in the antibacterial function of human neutrophils and its relationship to sepsis. Ann. Surg. *173*: 206, 1971.
2. Alexander, J. W., and Meakins, J. L.: Natural defense mechanisms in clinical sepsis. J. Surg. Res. *11*:148, 1971.
3. Alexander, J. W., and Moncrief, J. A.: Alterations of the immune response following severe thermal injury. Arch. Surg. *93*:75, 1966.
4. Alho, A.: Lysosomal functions in circulatory shock. Ann. Clin. Gyn. Fenn. *60*:159, 1971.
5. Altemeier, W. A.: The significance of infection in trauma. Bull. Am. Coll. Surg. *57*(1 Feb.):7, 1972.
6. Altemeier, W. A., Fullen, W. D., and

McDonough, J. J.: Sepsis and gastrointestinal bleeding. Ann. Surg. *175*:759, 1972.
7. Altura, B. M., and Hershey, S. G.: Sequential changes in reticuloendothelial system function after acute hemorrhage. Proc. Soc. Exper. Biol. Med. *139*:935, 1972.
8. Anderson, R. W., Simmons, R. L., Collins, J. A., Bredenberg, C. E., James, P. M., and Levitsky, S.: Plasma volume and sulfate spaces in acute combat casualties. Surg. Gynec. Obstet. *128*:719, 1969.
9. Bartlett, D., and Tenney, S. M.: Tissue gas tensions in experimental anemia. J. Appl. Physiol. *18*:734, 1963.
10. Baue, A., and Sayeed, M. M.: Alterations in the functional capacity of mitochondria in hemorrhagic shock. Surgery *68*:40, 1970.
11. Baxter, C. R., Canizaro, P. C., Carrico, C. J., and Shires, G. T.: Fluid resuscitation of hemorrhagic shock. Postgrad. Med. *48*:95, 1970.
12. Bayliss, W. M.: Intravenous Injection in Wound Shock. London, Longman, Green and Co., 1918.
13. Beecher, H. K., Burnett, C. H., Shapiro, S. L., Sunione, F. A., Smith, L. D., Sullivan, E. R., and Mallory, T. B.: The physiologic effects of wounds. Medical Dept., U.S. Army: Surgery in World War II. Off. Surg. Gen., Dept. Army, Wash., D.C., 1952.
14. Bell, M. L., Herman, A. H., Smith, E. E., Egdahl, R. H., and Rutenberg, A. M.: Role of lysosomal instability in the development of refractory shock. Surgery *70*:341, 1971.
15. Berne, T. V., and Barbour, B. H.: Acute renal failure in general surgical patients. Arch. Surg. *102*:594, 1971.
16. Bone, D. K., Maddrey, W. C., Eagen, J., and Cameron, J. L.: Cardiac tamponade: a fatal complication of central venous catheterization. Submitted for publication.
17. Boyan, C. P., and Howland, W. S.: Blood temperature: a critical factor in massive transfusion. Anesthesiol. *22*: 559, 1961.
18. Brand, E. D., Suh, T. K., and Avery, M. C.: Reversal of postoligemic shock in the cat by hypervenolaric massive fluid therapy. Am. J. Physiol. *211*: 1232, 1966.
19. Bull, J. P.: Circulatory responses to blood loss and injury. Progr. Surg. *4*:35, 1964.
20. Bunker, J. P.: Metabolic effects of blood transfusion. Anesthesiol. *27*:446, 1966.
21. Bunker, J. P., Stetson, J. B., Coe, R. C., Grillo, H. C., and Murphy, A. J.: Citric acid intoxication. J.A.M.A. *157*:1361, 1955.
22. Cannon, W. B.: Traumatic Shock, New York, Appleton, 1923.
23. Carey, L. C., Cloutier, C. T., and Lowery, B. D.: The use of balanced electrolyte solution for resuscitation. *In* Fox, C. L., Jr., and Nahas, G. G., eds.: Body fluid replacement in the surgical patient. New York, Grune & Stratton, 1970, p. 200.
24. Carpenter, C. C. J., Biern, R. O., Mitra, P. P., Sack, R. B., Dons, P. E., Wells, S. A., and Khaura, S. S.: Electrocardiogram in Asiatic cholera; separate studies of effects of hypovolemia, acidosis, and potassium loss. Brit. Heart J. *29*:103, 1967.
25. Chien, S., Usami, S., and Gregersen, M. I.: Effects of plasma expanders on blood viscosity. *In* Fox, C. L., Jr., and Nahas, G. G., eds.: Body fluid replacement in the surgical patient. New York, Grune & Stratton, 1970.
26. Chinitz, J. L., Kim, K. E., Onesti, G., and Swartz, C.: Pathophysiology and prevention of dextran-40-induced anuria. J. Lab. Clin. Med. *77*:76, 1971.
27. Chute, A. L., Cleghorn, R. A., and Lathe, G. A.: Reports of no. 1 research unit. Ottawa, Proc. 8th Meeting Assoc. Canad. Army Med. Res. *2*:(1945).
28. Clarke, R., Fisher, M. R., Topley, E., and Davies, J. W. L.: Extent and time of blood loss after civilian injury. Lancet *11*:381 (1961).
29. Clarke, R., Topley, E., and Flear, C. T. G.: Assessment of blood loss in civilian trauma. Lancet *1*:629, 1955.
30. Cleland, J., Pluth, J. R., Tauxe, W. N., and Kirklin, J. W.: Blood volumes and body fluid compartment changes soon after closed and open intracardiac surgery. J. Thorac. Cardiovasc. Surg. *52*:698, 1966.
31. Cloutier, C. T., Lowery, B. D., and Carey, L. C.: Acid-base disturbances in hemorrhagic shock. Arch. Surg. *98*: 551, 1969.
32. Cohnen, G.: Changes in immunoglobulin levels after surgical trauma. J. Trauma *12*:249, 1972.
33. Collins, G. M., and Ludbrook, J.: The rheologic properties of low molecular weight dextrans: fact or fancy? Amer. Heart J. *72*:741, 1966.
34. Collins, J. A.: First six months' activities, Walter Reed Army Institute of Research, Surgical Research Team, Vietnam. Off. Surg. Gen., Dept. Army, Wash., D.C., 1967.
35. Collins, J. A.: The causes of progressive pulmonary insufficiency in surgical patients. J. Surg. Res. *9*:685, 1969.
36. Collins, J. A.: Fluid replacement in trauma. *In* Practice of Surgery: Current Review. Ballinger, W. F., and

Drapanas, T., eds. St. Louis, C. V. Mosby Co., 1972.
37. Collins, J. A., Braitberg, A., and Butcher, H. R.: Changes in lung and body weight and lung water content in rats treated for hemorrhage with various fluids. Surgery *73*:401, 1973.
38. Collins, J. A., Braitberg, A., and Strechenberg, L.: Interaction between hematocrit and hemoglobin-oxygen affinity on survival of rats following hemorrhage shock. Submitted for Publication.
39. Collins, J. A., Simmons, R. L., James, P. M., Bredenberg, C. E., Anderson, R. W., and Heisterkamp, C. A.: The acid-base status of seriously wounded combat casualties: I. Before treatment. Ann. Surg. *171*: 595, 1970.
40. Collins, J. A., Simmons, R. L., James, P. M., Bredenberg, C. E., Anderson, R. W., and Heisterkamp, C. A.: Acid-base status of seriously wounded combat casualties: II. Resuscitation with stored blood. Ann. Surg. *173*: 6, 1971.
41. Cournand, A., Riley, R. L., Bradley, S. E., Breed, E. S., Noble, R. P., Lausen, H. D., Gregersen, M. I., and Richards, D. W.: Studies of the circulation in clinical shock. Surgery *13*:964, 1963.
42. Crowell, J. W., Ford, R. G., and Lewis, V. M.: Oxygen transport in hemorrhagic shock as a function of the hematocrit ratio. Amer. J. Physiol. *196*:1033, 1959.
43. Crowell, J. W., and Smith, E. E.: Determinant of the optimal hematocrit. J. Appl. Physiol. *22*:501, 1967.
44. Dillon, J., Lynch, L. J., Myers, R., and Butcher, H. R.: The treatment of hemorrhagic shock. Surg. Gynec. Obstet. *122*:967, 1966.
45. Doty, D. B., Moseley, R. V., and Simmons, R. L.: Sequential changes in blood volume after injury and transfusion. Surg. Gynec. Obstet. *130*:801, 1970.
46. Drucker, W. R., Holden, W. D., Kingsbury, B., Hofmann, N., and Graham, L.: Metabolic aspects of hemorrhagic shock. II. Metabolic studies on the need for erythrocytes in the treatment of hypovolemia due to hemorrhage. J. Trauma *2*:567, 1962.
47. Earley, L. E.: Pathogenesis of oliguric acute renal failure. New Eng. J. Med. *282*:1370, 1970.
48. Ebert, R. V., Stead, E. A., Jr., and Gibson, J. G.: Response of normal subjects to acute blood loss with special reference to the mechanism of restoration of blood volume. Arch. Intern. Med. *68*:578, 1941.
49. Eiseman, B., and Ashbaugh, D. G.: Pulmonary effects of nonthoracic trauma. J. Trauma *8*:625, 1968.
50. Eiseman, B., and Heyman, R. L.: Stress ulcers—a continuing challenge. New Engl. J. Med. *282*:372, 1970.
51. Emerson, C. P., and Ebert, R. V.: A Study of shock in battle casualties. Ann. Surg. *122*:745, 1945.
52. Evans, E. I., Hoover, M. J., James, G. W., and Alm, T.: Studies on traumatic shock. I. Blood volume changes in traumatic shock. Ann. Surg. *119*:64, 1944.
53. Fisher, M. R.: Clinical signs following injury in relation to red cell and total blood volume. Clin. Sci. *17*:181, 1958.
54. Friedman, E., Grable, E., and Fine, J.: Central venous pressure and direct serial measurements as guides in blood volume replacement. Lancet *2*:609, 1966.
55. Gaar, K. A., Jr., Taylor, A. E., Owens, L. J., and Guyton, A. C.: Effect of capillary pressure and plasma protein on development of pulmonary edema. Am. J. Physiol. *213*:79, 1967.
56. Gauer, O. H., Henry, J. P., and Sieker, H. O.: Changes in central venous pressure after moderate hemorrhage and transfusion in man. Circ. Res. *4*:79, 1956.
57. Gollub, S., Schechter, D. C., Schaefer, C., Svigals, R., and Bailey, C. P.: Absolute hemodilution cardiopulmonary bypass: free water distribution and protein mobilization in body compartments. Amer. Heart J. *78*: 626, 1969.
58. Gollub, S., Ulin, A. W., Winchell, H. S., Ehrlich, E., and Weiss, W.: Hemorrhagic diathesis associated with massive transfusion. Surgery *45*:204, 1959.
59. Grady, G. F., Bennett, A. J. E. et al.: Risk of post-transfusion hepatitis in the United States: A prospective cooperative study. J.A.M.A. *220*:692, 1972.
60. Grant, R. T., and Reeve, E. B.: Observations on the general effects of injury in man. Spec. Rep. Ser. Med. Res. Coun. (London) No. 277, 1951.
61. Gump, F. E., Butler, H., and Kinney, J. M.: Oxygen transport and consumption during acute hemorrhage. Ann. Surg. *168*:54, 1968.
62. Gump, F. E., Kinney, J. M., Iles, M., and Long, C. C.: Duration and significance of large fluid loads administered for circulatory support, J. Trauma *10*:431, 1970.
63. Guyton, A. C., and Crowell, J. W.: Dynamics of the heart in shock. Fed. Proc. *20*:51, 1961.
64. Hardaway, R. M.: Syndromes of Disseminated Intravascular Coagulation.

Springfield, Ill., Charles C Thomas, 1966.
65. Hardaway, R. M., James, P. M., Anderson, R. W., Bredenberg, C. E., and West, R. L.: Intensive study and treatment of shock in man. J.A.M.A. *13*: 199, 1967.
66. Hardaway, R. M., Johnson, D. G., Houchin, D. N., Jenkins, E. B., Burnes, J. W., and Jackson, D. R.: The influence of extracorporeal handling of blood on hemorrhagic shock in dogs. Exp. Med. Surg. *23*:28, 1965.
67. Hopkins, R. W., Sabga, G., Penn, I., and Simeone, F. A.: Hemodynamic aspects of hemorrhagic and septic shock. J.A.M.A. *191*:127, 1965.
68. Horovitz, J. H., Carrico, C. J., and Shires, G. T.: Venous sampling sites for pulmonary shunt determinations in the injured patient. J. Trauma *11*: 911, 1971.
69. Howard, J. M., ed.: Battle Casualties in Korea: Studies of the Surgical Research Team. Army Med. Service School, Walter Reed Army Med. Center, Wash. D.C.
70. Hutchin, P., Terzi, R. G., Hollandsworth, L. C., Johnson, G., and Peters, R. M.: The influence of intravenous fluid administration on postoperative urinary water and electrolyte excretion in thoracic surgical patients. Ann. Surg. *170*:813, 1969.
71. Jannoff, A., Weissmann, G., Zweifach, B. W., and Thomas, L.: Pathogenesis of experimental shock. IV. Studies on lysosomes in normal and tolerant animals subjected to lethal trauma and endotoxemia. J. Exp. Med. *116*:451, 1962.
72. Johnson, G., Jr., and Lambert, J.: Responses to the rapid intravenous administration of an overload of fluid and electrolytes in dogs. Ann. Surg. *167*:561, 1968.
73. Keith, N. M.: Blood volume changes in wound shock and primary hemorrhage. Report No. IX, Spec. Rep. Series No. 27. Great Britain Medical Res. Council, London, March, 1919, p. 5.
74. Kendrick, D. B.: Medical Department, United States Army. Blood Program in World War II. Off. Surg. Gen., Dept. Army, Washington, D.C., 1964.
75. Kilman, J. W., Waldhausen, J. A., and Schumacker, H. B.: Effects of low molecular weight dextran on peripheral blood flow with controlled cardiac output. Ann. Surg. *166*:190, 1967.
76. Levine, O. R., Mellins, R. B., Senior, R. M., and Fishman, A. P.: The application of Starling's law of capillary exchange to the lungs. J. Clin. Invest. *46*:934, 1969.
77. Lister, J., McNeill, I. F., Marshall, V. C., Plzak, L. F., Jr., Dagher, F. J. and Moore, F. D.: Transcapillary refilling after hemorrhage in normal man: basal rates and volumes; effect of norepinephrine. Ann. Surg. *158*:698, 1963.
78. Lowery, B. D., Cloutier, C. T., and Carey, L. C.: Blood gas determinations in the severely wounded in hemorrhagic shock. Arch. Surg. *99*:330, 1969.
79. Lucas, C. E., Sugawa, C., Riddle, J., Rector, F., Rosenberg, B., and Walt, A. J.: Natural history and surgical dilemma of "stress" gastric bleeding. Arch. Surg. *102*:266, 1971.
80. MacLean, L. D.: Blood volume versus central venous pressure in shock. Surg. Gynec. Obstet. *118*:594, 1964.
81. MacLean, L. D., Duff, J. H., Scott, H. M., and Peretz, D. I.: Treatment of shock in man based on hemodynamic diagnosis. Surg. Gynec. Obstet. *120*:1, 1965.
82. Mailloux, L., Swartz, C. D., Capizzi, R., Kim, K. E., Onesti, G., Ramirez, O., and Brest, A. N.: Acute renal failure after administration of low-molecular-weight dextran. New Eng. J. Med. *277*:1113, 1967.
83. McConn, R., and Derrick, J. B.: The respiratory function of blood: transfusion and blood storage. Anesthesiol. *36*:119, 1972.
84. McKay, D. G.: Disseminated Intravascular Coagulation. New York, 1965.
85. McNamara, J. J., Molot, M. D., and Stremple, J. F.: Screen filtration pressure in combat casualties. Ann. Surg. *172*:334, 1970.
86. Mela, L. M., Miller, L. D., and Nicholas, G. G.: Influence of cellular acidosis and altered cation concentrations on shock-induced mitochondrial damage. Surgery *72*:102, 1972.
87. Melrose, D. G., Nahas, R., Alvarez, D., Todd, I. A. D., and Dempster, W. J.: Postoperative hypoxia after extracorporeal circulation: a possible graft against host reaction (preliminary communication). Experientia *21*:47, 1965.
88. Middleton, E. S., Mathews, R., and Shires, G. T.: Radiosulphate as a measure of the extracellular fluid in acute hemorrhagic shock. Ann. Surg. *170*:174, 1969.
89. Miller, R. P., Robbins, T. O., Tong, M. J. et al.: Coagulation defects associated with massive blood transfusions. Ann. Surg. *174*:794, 1971.
90. Monroe, R. G., Gamble, W. J., LaFarge, C. G., Aquilar, S. R., and Goldblatt, A.: A comparison of the effect of hemorrhage and infused catecholamines on ventricular performance, coronary flow, and myocardial oxy-

gen consumption. J. Pharmacol. Exper. Therap. *153*:455, 1966.

91. Moore, F. D., Dagher, F. J., Boyden, C. M., Lee, C. J. and Lyons, J. H.: Hemorrhage in normal man: I. Distribution and dispersal of saline infusions following acute blood loss—clinical kinetics of blood volume support. Ann. Surg. *163*:485, 1966.
92. Moore, F. D., Lyons, J. H., Pierce, E. C., Morgan, A. P., Drinker, P. A., MacArthur, J. D., and Dammin, G. J.: Post-traumatic Pulmonary Insufficiency. Philadelphia, W. B. Saunders Co., 1969.
93. Morgan, I. O., Little, J. M., and Evans, W. A.: Renal failure associated with low molecular weight dextran infusion. Brit. Med. J. *2*:737, 1966.
94. Moseley, R. V., and Doty, D. B.: Changes in the filtration characteristics of stored blood. Ann. Surg. *171*:329, 1970.
95. Moss, G.: Fluid distribution in prevention of hypovolemic shock. Arch. Surg. *98*:281, 1969.
96. Muehrcke, R. C.: Acute Renal Failure: Diagnosis and Management, St. Louis, C. V. Mosby Co., 1969.
97. Nakasone, N., Watkins, E., Janeway, C. A., and Gross, R. E.: Experimental studies of circulatory derangement following the massive transfusion of citrated blood. J. Lab. Clin. Med. *43*:184, 1954.
98. Northfield, T. C., and Smith, T.: Physiologic significance of central venous pressure in patients with hemorrhage. Surg. Gynec. Obstet. *135*:267, 1972.
99. Ollodart, R., and Mansberger, A. R.: The effect of hypovolemic shock on bacterial defense. Am. J. Surg. *110*:302, 1965.
100. Prentice, T. C., Olney, J. M., Artz, C. P., and Howard, J. M.: Studies of blood volume and transfusion therapy in the Korean battle casualty. Surg. Gynec. Obstet. *99*:542, 1954.
101. Pruitt, B. A., Foley, F. D., and Moncrief, J. A.: Curling's ulcer: a clinical-pathology study of 323 cases. Ann. Surg. *172*:523, 1970.
102. Pruitt, B. A., Moncrief, J. A., and Mason, A. D.: Efficacy of buffered saline as the sole replacement fluid following acute measured hemorrhage in man. J. Trauma *7*:767, 1967.
103. Ranney, H. M.: Clinically important variants of human hemoglobin. New Eng. J. Med. *282*:144, 1970.
104. Regan, T. J., LaForce, F. M., Teres, D., Block, J., and Hellems, H. K.: Contribution of left ventricle and small bowel in irreversible hemorrhagic shock. Am. J. Physiol. *208*:938, 1965.
105. Robbins, R., Idjadi, F., Stahl, W. M., and Essiet, G.: Studies of gastric secretion in stressed patients. Ann. Surg. *175*:555, 1972.
106. Robertson, O. H., and Bock, A. V.: Memorandum on blood volume after hemorrhage. Report No. VI, Spec. Rep. Series No. 25, Great Britain Med. Res. Council, London, Aug. 1918, p. 226.
107. Rosenberg, I. K., Gupta, S. L., Lucas, C. E., Khan, A. A., and Rosenberg, B. F.: Renal insufficiency after trauma and sepsis. Arch. Surg. *103*:175, 1971.
108. Roth, E., Lax, L. C., and Maloney, J. V.: Ringer's lactate solution and extracellular fluid volume in the surgical patient: a critical analysis. Ann. Surg. *169*:149, 1969.
109. Rothe, C. F.: Heart failure and fluid loss in hemorrhagic shock. Fed. Proc. *29*: 1854, 1970.
110. Rush, B. F., and Stewart, R. A.: More liberal use of a plasma expander: impact on a hospital blood bank. New Eng. J. Med. *280*:1202, 1969.
111. Rush, B. F., and Wilder, R. J.: Mortality and renal tubular necrosis in hemorrhagic shock in dogs: the effect of blood handling. Surg. Forum *14*:1, 1963.
112. Schildt, B. E., and Low, H.: Relationship between trauma, plasma corticosterone and reticuloendothelial function in anaesthetized mice. Acta Endocrinol. *67*:141, 1971.
113. Scott, R., and Crosby, W. H.: Changes in coagulation mechanism following wounding and resuscitation with stored blood; a study of battle casualties in Korea. Blood *9*:609, 1954.
114. Serkes, K. D., and Long, S.: Changes in extracellular fluid volume after hemorrhage and tourniquet trauma. Surg. Forum *17*:58, 1966.
115. Shenkin, R. A., Cheney, R. H., Govons, S. R., Hardy, J. D., Fletcher, A. G., Jr., and Starr, I.: On the diagnosis of hemorrhage in man: a study of volunteers bled large amounts. Amer. J. Med. Sci. *208*:421, 1944.
115a. Shields, C. E., Dennis, L. H., Eichelberger, J. W., and Conrad, M. E.: The rapid infusion of large quantities of ACD adenine solution into humans. Transfusion *7*:133, 1967.
116. Shires, T., Cohn, D., Carrico, J., and Lightfoot, S.: Fluid therapy in hemorrhagic shock. Arch. Surg. *88*:688, 1964.
117. Siegel, H. W., and Downing, S. E.: Contributions of coronary perfusion pressure, metabolic acidosis and adrenergic factors to the reduction of myocardial contractility during hemorrhagic shock in the cat. Circ. Res. *27*:875, 1970.

118. Simmons, R. L., Collins, J. A., Heisterkamp, C. A., Mills, D. E., Anderson, R., and Phillips, L. L.: Coagulation disorders in combat casualties. II. Effects of massive transfusion. Ann. Surg. *169*:462, 1969.
119. Simmons, R. L., Heisterkamp, C. A., Moseley, R. V., and Doty, D. B.: Post-resuscitative blood volumes in combat casualties. Surg. Gynec. Obstet. *128*:1193, 1969.
120. Skillman, J. J., Awwad, H. K., and Moore, F. D.: Plasma protein kinetics of the early transcapillary refill after hemorrhage in man. Surg. Gynec. Obstet. *125*:983, 1967.
121. Skillman, J. J., Gould, S. A., Chung, R. S., and Silen, W.: The gastric mucosal barrier: clinical and experimental studies in critically ill and normal man, and in the rabbit. Ann. Surg. *174*:911, 1971.
122. Skillman, J. J., Hedley-White, J., and Pallotta, J. A.: Cardiorespiratory, metabolic and endocrine changes after hemorrhage in man. Ann. Surg. *174*:911, 1971.
123. Skillman, J. J., Lauler, D. P., Hickler, R. B., Lyons, J. H., Olsen, J. E., Ball, M. R., and Moore, F. D.: Hemorrhage in normal man—effect on renin, cortisol, aldosterone and urine composition. Ann. Surg. *166*:865, 1967.
124. Skillman, J. J., Olson, J. E., Lyons, J. H. and Moore, F. D.: The Hemodynamic effect of acute blood loss in normal man, with observations on the effect of the Valsalva maneuver and breath holding. Ann. Surg. *166*:713, 1967.
125. Smith, E. E., and Crowell, J. W.: Influence of hematocrit ratio on survival of unacclimatized dogs at simulated high altitude. Amer. J. Physiol. *205*:1172, 1963.
126. Smith, L. L., Hamlin, J. T., Walker, W. F., and Morre, F. D.: Metabolic and endocrinologic changes in acute and chronic hypotension in man. Metab. *8*:862, 1959.
127. Smith, L. L., and Moore, F. D.: Refractory hypotension in man—is this irreversible shock? New Eng. J. Med. *267*:734, 1962.
128. Stahl, W. M., and Stone, A. M.: Prophylactic diuresis with ethacrynic acid for prevention of postoperative renal failure. Ann. Surg. *172*:361, 1970.
129. Stremple, J. F., Molot, M. D., McNamara, J. J., Mori, H., and Glass, G. B.: Posttraumatic gastric bleeding. Arch. Surg. *105*:177, 1972.
130. Sugerman, H. J., Davidson, D. T., Vibul, S. et al.: The basis of defective oxygen delivery from stored blood. Surg. Gynec. Obstet. *131*:733, 1970.
131. Takaori, M., and Safar, P.: Treatment of massive hemorrhage with colloid and crystalloid solutions. J.A.M.A. *199*:297, 1967.
132. Thal, A. P., Brown, E. B., Hermreck, A. S., and Bell, H. H.: Shock: A Physiologic Basis for Treatment. Chicago, Year Book Medical Publishers, 1971.
133. Valeri, C. R.: Viability and function of preserved red cells. New Eng. J. Med. *284*:81, 1971.
134. Valeri, C. R., and Collins, F. B.: The physiologic effect of transfusing preserved red cells with low 2,3-diphosphoglycerate and high affinity for oxygen. Vox. Sang. *20*:397, 1971.
135. Valtis, D. J., and Kennedy, A. C.: Defective gas transport function of stored red blood cells. Lancet *1*:119, 1954.
136. Veith, F. J., Hagstrom, J. W. C., Panossian, A., Nehlsen, S. L., and Wilson, J. W.: Pulmonary microcirculatory response to shock, transfusion, and pump-oxygenator procedures: a unified mechanism underlying pulmonary damage. Surgery *64*:95, 1968.
137. Warren, J. V., Brannon, E. S., Stead, E. A., Jr., and Merrill, A. J.: The effect of venesection and the pooling of blood in the extremities on the atrial pressure and cardiac output in normal subjects with observations on acute circulatory collapse in three instances. J. Clin. Invest. *24*:337, 1945.
138. Weil, M. H., Shubin, H., and Rosoff, L.: Fluid repletion in circulatory shock: central venous pressure and other practical guides. J.A.M.A. *192*:668, 1965.
139. Wiggers, C. J.: Physiology of Shock, New York, Commonwealth Fund, 1950.
140. Williams, A. D., Mandell, G. L., and Lefer, A. M.: Phagocytosis and bactericidal activity of leucocytes in hemorrhagic shock. Infection and Immunity *2*:345, 1970.
141. Wilson, R. F., Mammen, E., and Walt, A. J.: Eight years of experience with massive blood transfusions. J. Trauma *11*:275, 1971.
142. Wilson, R. F., Sarver, E., and Birks, R.: Central venous pressure and blood volume determinations in clinical shock. Surg. Gynec. Obstet. *132*:631, 1971.
143. Zimmerman, J. E.: Respiratory failure complicating post-traumatic acute renal failure: etiology, clinical features and management. Ann. Surg. *174*:12, 1971.

chapter

4

CARDIOPULMONARY RESUSCITATION AND ANESTHESIA IN TRAUMA

Donald W. Benson, M. D.

CARDIOPULMONARY RESUSCITATION

In the context of trauma therapy there can be no clear-cut definition of cardiopulmonary resuscitation. It could be said that the initial phase of therapy in trauma is frequently resuscitative in scope, if not in actual fact. There are many degrees of the resuscitative effort, and it is obviously difficult to delineate specific therapy in resuscitation for all the various kinds of trauma.

As the title implies, the resuscitation effort is concerned with the cardiovascular system and the respiratory system. In clinical experience, they cannot be separated. For the sake of clarity, however, respiratory resuscitation will be considered first, separately from cardiac resuscitation. This is done with some purpose. In working with those who are learning resuscitative techniques, it soon becomes apparent that comprehension and management of inadequacies of the cardiovascular system are easier. For this reason, the novice will often seriously neglect the respiratory system in resuscitation. Adequate oxygenation and removal of carbon dioxide from circulating blood is a primary purpose of the circulation; to neglect its ventilation is to defeat the over-all effort. Obviously there is the other extreme of neglecting the circulatory aspect. Empirically, however, this is rarely done even though the respiratory resuscitation may be quite inadequate.

Inadequacies of the Respiratory Effort

Normal respiration is maintained by a well balanced mechanism involving a carbon dioxide stimulus acting on the central nervous system, which in turn activates the respiratory musculature to provide pulmonary ventilation. Breakdowns in this mechanism can occur readily in trauma and are common causes of death, for example, in serious head trauma or high spinal cord injury. With neurological damage there may be no impairment of the respiratory system itself. Early recognition of inadequate ventilation caused by neural involvement and prompt initiation of artificial ventilation are extremely important.

Events similar to those which occur with head trauma are often seen with severe shock from hemorrhage. Undoubtedly the mechanism is closely related, since the central nervous system is made moderately ischemic by hypotension or inadequate cardiac output, and the neuro-activating centers fail to respond to normal carbon dioxide or hypoxic stimuli. Adequate ventilation, hopefully with a high oxygen concentration, and resuscitation of the cardiovascular system may make salvage possible.

Inadequacies of the ventilation effort can, of course, arise as a part of multiple trauma. Fractures of many ribs may reduce the efficiency of respiration and allow carbon dioxide retention and inadequate oxygenation. This is often an insidious process and results in many of the signs and symptoms of hemorrhagic shock, even though shock is not present. Pneumothorax, tension pneumothorax, hemothorax and hemopneumothorax can all present with varying degrees of respiratory insufficiency. These factors must be considered in the differential diagnosis whenever trauma has occurred to the chest wall, especially if the patient appears cyanotic or manifests sweating, a rapid pulse and the agitation of carbon dioxide retention and hypoxia.

With the advent of high speed travel in automobiles, there has been an increase in the number of chest wall and lung injuries and a further increase may be expected. The treatment of these chest injuries, which in themselves provoke respiratory inadequacy, is considered in detail elsewhere. However, the recognition and the early treatment of such situations is vital to the stabilization and maintenance of these victims. For example, the patient with a severely crushed chest who may not have a pneumothorax may nevertheless die unless he is supported, at least temporarily, by positive pressure ventilation.[1] This, of course, can be done by various methods, described in some detail later. What is most important is that these factors be recognized and immediately treated.

Airway Obstruction

Even without trauma, unconsciousness can produce organic obstruction to the upper airway by the simple apposition of the base of the tongue with the posterior wall of the pharynx. This is undoubtedly the most common form of respiratory obstruction; in fact, it is nothing more than a variant of snoring. The patient who has been knocked unconscious by a severe blow to the head may have some ability to breathe; that is, his response to carbon dioxide and hypoxia may still be present, though inadequate. Under this circumstance, such a minimal form of respiratory obstruction may cause him to stop breathing. The obstruction may be simply and quickly cleared by manipulation of the mandible to elevate the base of the tongue from the posterior wall of the pharynx or to insert some device that will clear the airway (Fig. 4–1).

INJURIES TO HEAD. Severe facial fractures involving the maxillae and the mandible, plus the associated contusion of soft tissues, may distort the airway in the head to such a degree that it will be obstructed. For example, large hematomas in the posterior wall of the pharynx which have totally obstructed the airway have been unrecognized and the patients have died. If simple manipulation

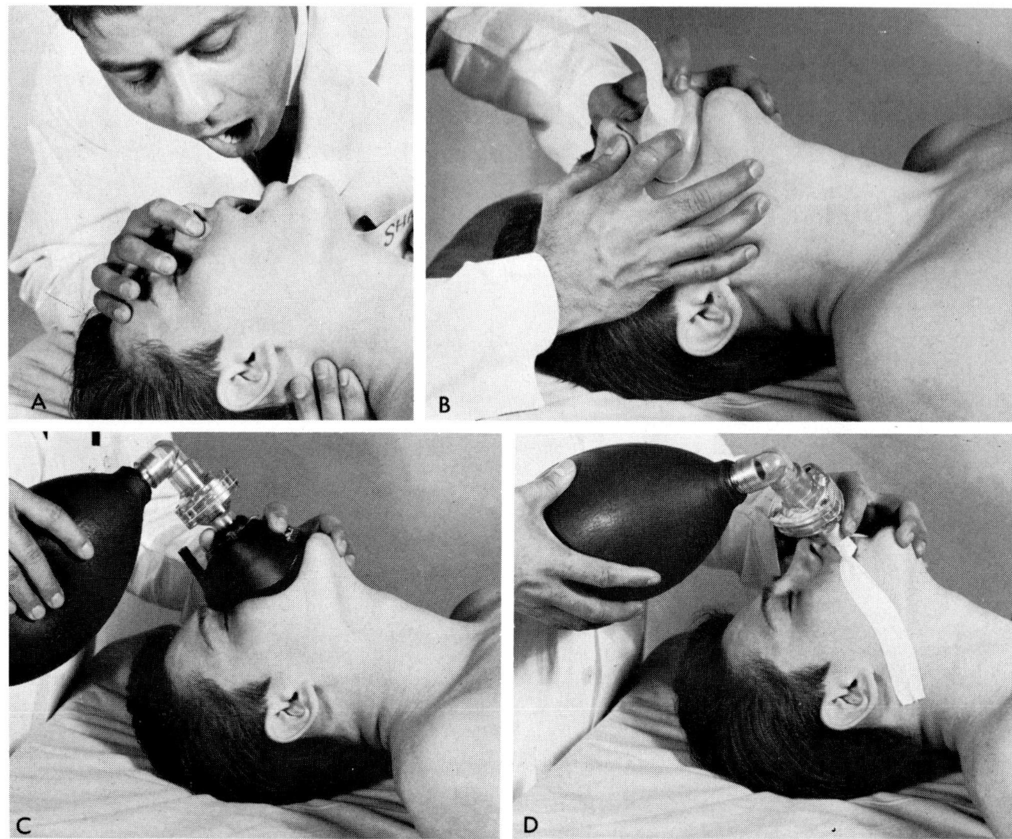

Figure 4–1 Essentials of respiratory resuscitation technique. *A*, Mouth-to-mouth respiration. Note neck extension. *B*, Mouth-to-airway. Note neck extension and seal around lips. *C*, Bag and mask with non-rebreathing valve. *D*, Bag with non-rebreathing valve on endotracheal tube.

does not relieve obstruction in the severely injured upper airway, a diagnosis of obstruction caused by fractures or swelling should be considered and a means of bypassing this obstruction undertaken. These could include the insertion of an endotracheal tube, bronchoscope or an oropharyngeal airway or, if these are impossible, a tracheostomy should be done.

At the same time that multiple trauma may occur around the face in the upper part of the airway, there may be obstruction because of bleeding, salivation or regurgitation. Especially in the partially unconscious patient this may result in obstruction of the larynx and laryngospasm or aspiration into the tracheobronchial tree with resultant peripheral obstruction. This may produce severe atelectasis and pneumonia. Such foreign material should be removed as soon as possible. High speed impacts may, for example, push stomach contents into the upper airway where they may cause obstruction or may be aspirated into the entire tracheobronchial tree.

INJURIES TO NECK. Severe trauma to the larynx and trachea has become more commonplace, in spite of the fact that this part of the airway is relatively well protected by the thoracic cage. There are reported incidents of fractures and even separation of the trachea without a fractured sternum.[18] The author recalls one such case in which the trachea was fractured approximately two rings above the carina and did not manifest itself for 48 hours, when it finally began to close. Obstruction somewhere in the respiratory tree was recognized. A tracheostomy was done, which did not suffice since it did not bypass the obstruction at the lower part of the trachea. At length this problem was recognized and a very small endotracheal catheter was passed through the obstruction; this maintained the patient until surgical intervention could be carried out.

A fractured larynx is no longer an uncommon accident. Sandlot baseball, for example, contributes a number of these injuries. Hematoma formation can result in complete obstruction of the airway which, if not relieved, is fatal. Both these conditions can be remedied by bypassing the obstruction. The treatment is obvious and often simple; actual recognition may be delayed and a high degree of suspicion must be maintained.

At first some of these obstructions seem technically almost impossible to bypass, and success depends upon personal ingenuity and availability of equipment and assistance. In fact, some resuscitations depend on immediate thoracotomy, which may not be feasible under all emergency circumstances. However, in many salvageable patients of the type described previously, trouble from respiratory obstruction develops relatively slowly. In fact, this may occur after the patient is in the hospital accident room or has been placed on the ward. This is when vigilance sometimes drops and the insidious effects of respiratory obstruction go unrecognized.

Technique of Respiratory Resuscitation

Stated most simply, respiratory resuscitation is the provision of a means for the movement of air in and out of the alveoli of the lung to provide adequate ventilation of the circulating blood. As suggested by the foregoing discussion, the problem involves two major categories: (1) creating and maintaining an airway to the alveoli, and (2) supplying the necessary means of pushing air into the alveoli and getting it out. These categories include both emergency and definitive measures.

Obstruction by Tongue. Establishing a patent airway in a patient whose airway has not been deranged by trauma is now a routine technique. As stated, the most common form of obstruction is pressure of the base of the tongue against the posterior wall of the pharynx, which occludes the airway. Various techniques have been established to relieve this. The first and probably the simplest is hyperextension of the head on the shoulders.[7] The hand is placed on the vertex of the head and the back of the head is pushed downward toward the shoulders to hyperextend the neck. At the same time a hand may be placed on the tip of the chin to further hyperextend. This maneuver elevates the entire contents of the neck away from the spinal column and at the same time tends to clear the airway. Blowing through the mouth to produce positive pressure is somewhat more difficult with this maneuver and consequently the nose is usually used. The rescuer's mouth is placed over the victim's nose and the victim's mouth is closed. With a good expiratory effort, air is blown into the patient's lungs.

Another variant of this technique is to place one hand under the neck of the victim and elevate it slightly from the flat surface on which he is lying so that the head tends to fall back. The thumb and forefinger of the other hand close the nose and the heel of the hand pushes down the forehead to hyperextend the neck. These maneuvers cause the mouth to open and the rescuer can then place his mouth over that of the patient and exhale air into the victim's lungs. The pressure created in the upper airway helps to open it up and make it more patent. The maintenance of a small amount of positive pressure tends to push the tongue and the soft tissue of the pharynx aside and to make the passage clear (Fig. 4–1).

One of the first techniques developed was the mouth-to-mouth method, in which the mandible is elevated by thumb and forefinger and the mouth is held open while the other hand is used to hyperextend the head and close the nostrils.[19] The rescuer then places his mouth over this thumb and the victim's mouth and blows air into the lungs.

For the resuscitator who is a professional (that is, a physician or paramedical person) the use of an oral airway is probably the most convenient method (Fig. 4–1). There are a number of these commercially available at the present time. They usually assume an S shape, which makes it possible to get behind the base of the tongue of the victim and at the same time provide an accessible tip for blowing into the patient's lungs. The obvious advantage is that a good clear airway is secured by the careful placement of the device. This is achieved with the risk of possible regurgitation or even laryngospasm. Furthermore, it is frequently difficult to get a good seal around the mouth so that enough pressure can be put into the airway to make ventilation possible.

Obstruction by Foreign Bodies. One must remember that while these efforts are going on, there may be foreign material in the airway which needs to be cleaned out. Even before the placement of an airway, or before mouth-to-mouth breathing, one should look for such things as broken dentures, chewing gum, cuds of tobacco, regurgitated debris, blood and secretions. Any of these should be removed before any respiratory effort is carried out. This is best done with some suction device; but under emergency situations such may not be available, and it can be accomplished by turning the victim on his side and cleaning out the mouth and the pharynx with a handkerchief or even a finger.

Endotracheal Intubation. More definitive means of making a patent airway are endotracheal intubation by direct laryngoscopy, by a blind technique or by tracheostomy. Unfortunately, the novice rescuer frequently equates endotracheal intubation with respiratory resuscitation. The consequence is that much time and effort is expended in establishing an airway by endotracheal intubation, while the patient suffers greater and greater hypoxia.

For the good of the patient, ventilation by one of the emergency techniques, such as mouth-to-mouth, is extremely important prior to the attempt to place an endotracheal tube. It permits a few seconds or even minutes of effort to be expended during intubation while the lung is reasonably full of oxygen. At times it is absolutely essential to place an endotracheal tube in order to effect respirations. Without question, there are many instances when even the most able rescuer cannot make a patent airway and has to resort to an endotracheal tube. However, under most circumstances, emergency measures should be utilized preparatory to intubation.

Tracheostomy. Tracheostomy, although appearing dramatic and simple, can be excessively prolonged in the presence of inadequate ventilation. The patient may die or suffer brain damage because of the hypoxia occurring during the operation. When the need for a tracheostomy is apparent and there is difficulty in maintaining an airway, it is much safer for an endotracheal tube or a bronchoscope to be inserted and for the tracheostomy to be done over such a device. There is then constant assurance of an adequate airway during a procedure which, in itself, can cause temporary airway obstruction.

Circumventing Obstruction. Considerable ingenuity must be exerted by the would-be rescuer to circumvent some obstructions resulting from severe upper airway trauma. Finding the larynx with the laryngoscope in the presence of much blood and secretions may be actually impossible in a patient with a badly mangled face. Another example is the patient with a fractured trachea, described previously. In such instances, use of an excessively long endotracheal tube is indicated, despite the fact that it may pass into the right main bronchus and temporarily, at least, produce unilateral obstruction. However, if it gets past the tracheal obstruction, it may be lifesaving. Such a clinical example also emphasizes that in emergency situations it is wiser to depend on a small endotracheal tube than a larger one, primarily because the smaller tube is easier to insert and is of itself less likely to cause trauma.

Methods of Alveolar Ventilation. There are several available methods for moving air into the respiratory tree for alveolar ventilation. The first is expired air ventilation from the mouth of the rescuer. The oxygen and carbon dioxide tensions of the expired air of the rescuer are such that they can maintain good alveolar tensions in the victim for extended periods of time.[6]

It is even possible to enrich the oxygen concentration by having the rescuer breathe oxygen whenever possible by placing a catheter in the corner of his mouth or by inspiring oxygen from a mask during his own inspiration. Positive pressure by expired air can be applied over the nose or mouth or into the endotracheal tube or airway. The main difficulty is overcoming of the natural revulsion of placing one's mouth over the soilage that may be present around the mouth or a bleeding tracheostomy site.

It is also not well appreciated that higher pressures and larger volumes than normal must be blown by the rescuer to achieve ventilation. With the leaks that are inherently present it is usually necessary to apply large volumes and considerable pressure, especially in ventilating an adult. This may cause hyperventilation on the part of the rescuer and he may become dizzy and be unable to continue.

Bag and Mask Ventilation. The most common approach by physicians is the use of a bag and mask. There are many varieties of these devices available in hospital wards, emergency rooms and ambulances. The simplest is the bag and mask that is fed oxygen from an accompanying tank. Since a device such as this is not valved or constructed in such a way to fill itself with room air, a flow of at least six to eight liters of oxygen is essential to keep the concentration of carbon dioxide diluted to a level that will not be toxic. A further complication is that unless one is experienced it is quite difficult to achieve a good fit with a face mask and not have leaks around the edge of the mask. These bag and mask arrangements can usually be adapted to fit endotracheal tube connectors or tracheostomy tubes.

The so-called nonrebreathing bags and masks are a real boon for respiratory resuscitation. These devices usually consist of a respiratory bag that is self-expanding and valves that are so arranged that when the bag is squeezed, air is forced into the patient; when the bag is allowed to relax and fill, the patient can expire passively to the outside atmosphere. The air in the bag can also be enriched by oxygen introduced through a port available on the apparatus. Many of these devices are distributed commercially and they are suitable for practically any application in respiratory resuscitation. All have the so-called standard fittings for face masks as well as for endotracheal connectors. As indicated, the problem of getting a good tight fit around the mask still exists; in the event that this cannot be achieved, mouth-to-mouth breathing may be a better answer than to persist in an effort to achieve ventilation with the device.

VENTILATION BY ANESTHESIA MACHINE. Anesthesia machines will, of course, function as well as any of the devices mentioned. In most emergency rooms, gas machines are kept on hand for the administration of anesthesia and should be available for resuscitation as well. These can be equipped to fit either face masks or endotracheal tubes. Those individuals concerned with resuscitation of patients, whether they be anesthetists or not, must be thoroughly acquainted with gas machines so that they can respond readily in emergencies by proper application of the equipment. Only oxygen should be used in the resuscitation effort, and the machine must be checked to be certain that all anesthetic agents are turned off.

MECHANICAL VENTILATORS. For prolonged respiratory resuscitation, the use of a dependable mechanical ventilator is helpful. The many considerations concerning these devices cannot be detailed here, but it should be emphasized that it is absolutely essential that the user understand precisely how the mechanical ventilator works. Respirators function on various principles and any given respirator will provide adequate ventilation if operated by someone who truly knows how to use it. One must be absolutely certain, for example, that the volume given to the patient is providing adequate alveolar ventilation and is not allowing progressive atelectasis to ensue. This can be a certainty only when the user knows the respirator's capabilities and how to accomplish this end.

There are a number of pressure activated respirators available in emergency rooms, operating rooms, ambulances and elsewhere, which, in the hands of trained rescuers, function well in providing adequate ventilation. It is not commonly understood, however, that these devices cannot be used when applying external cardiac massage. When the chest wall is depressed, there is a rapid rise in pressure within the tracheobronchial tree. This transmits itself to the respirator and the respirator then cycles automatically into a reverse or expiratory phase. Obviously, if the cardiac resuscitation is being done at 60 to 70 compressions a minute, the respirator will cycle that frequently. This does not allow time for adequate inspiration to provide alveolar ventilation. It follows then that the use of such a respirator is contraindicated in combined cardiopulmonary resuscitation. Physicians in charge of resuscitation in hospital emergency rooms or acting as advisers to ambulance crews should be aware of this danger and stress its importance to those in their charge. Several deaths have resulted from a misunderstanding of this principle.

The use of a mechanical ventilator during resuscitation is usually unnecessary because of the number of individuals around who can breathe for the patient with a bag. If a mechanical ventilator is necessary the pressure limiting devices can be used with the clear understanding that they must be given time to inflate the lung ten to twelve times a minute, thus requiring the compression of the chest to be stopped for a beat or two. This inherently results in a decreased minute output and should be avoided if possible. It is more appropriate to use a volume-limited ventilator which does not respond to the pressures created by chest compression. A setting on the ventilator of a respiratory frequency and a tidal volume which would result in normal ventilation should be adequate for ventilation during the resuscitation period.

Timing of Tracheostomy. Another important error in many resuscitation efforts is that a tracheostomy is often done far too early in the course of therapy. There are many reasons for performing an early tracheostomy, but if other maneuvers are to be carried out under general anesthesia, such as the removal of a ruptured spleen, or the repair of a fractured long bone of the leg, the tracheostomy may be left until last. Resuscitative and anesthetic management of an acute emergency is far better managed through an endotracheal tube than through a fresh tracheostomy. This is true for several reasons. First, the tracheostomy often bleeds excessively. Second, frequently there is not adequate equipment available for making proper connections to the tracheostomy so that a good tight fit can be achieved. Third, all too often the anesthetist finds himself virtually in the operative field, creating unnecessary difficulties for the surgeon.

Thought should be given to whether a tracheostomy should be done early in the total resuscitative effort or whether an endotracheal tube would suffice until definitive therapy can be carried out. At this time, a tracheostomy can be performed under ideal circumstances and the patient then placed on a respirator, if necessary. Early tracheostomy should be done when obvious circumstances require it; nevertheless, there are many times when tracheostomy is advisably delayed because there are better means for giving adequate ventilation and controlling the patient under these situations.

Cardiac Resuscitation

As stated, one cannot truly make a dichotomy between cardiac and pulmonary resuscitation; they must be considered together. However, too much emphasis cannot be given to the fact that adequate ventilation must be assured before cardiac resuscitation will work.

Diagnosis of Cardiac Arrest. Recognition of cardiac arrest or of a totally inadequate cardiac output is more difficult in injured patients than in the usual situation in patients in the operating room or in the hospital ward. The presence of severe shock frequently complicates the picture. Nevertheless, the rescuer must make some immediate evaluations concerning the adequacy of circulation. The first and most frequently utilized measure is the pulse. In the severe shock of hypovolemia, pulses may be undetectable in the more peripheral arteries such as the radial, but they may be felt in central arteries such as the femoral or the carotid. However, even these pulses may be absent in some instances, and heart sounds may be very difficult to hear.

Another sign of circulatory inadequacy that is quite reliable is the degree of dilatation of the pupil of the eye. This is fairly sensitive since it usually dilates rapidly when cardiac arrest occurs. Patients with severe head trauma may have dilatation of one or both pupils in the presence of adequate cardiac and circulatory activity. However, in the absence of peripheral arterial pulses or other similar indications of shock, the presence of a dilated pupil strongly suggests an inadequate circulation that must be supported promptly. A third sensitive measure of the adequacy of circulation is respiration. If cardiac arrest is present or if cardiac output is so low that the brain is moderately deprived of oxygenated blood, respiration will usually cease. Thus, if a patient is breathing on his own and pulses cannot be felt, there must then be some circulatory activity which is at least partially adequate. Again it must be remembered that trauma complicates the picture since many forms of trauma may in themselves cause cessation of respiration.

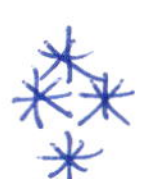

The absence of electrical activity of the heart during electrocardiography certainly is indicative of cardiac arrest. Delay in obtaining an electrocardiogram may be unduly prolonged. Furthermore, it does not by any measure indicate adequacy of cardiac output. A seemingly normal electrocardiogram can exist in the presence of an extremely low cardiac output which is inadequate for cerebral or coronary perfusion. Often cardiac massage may be necessary in a patient with an apparently normal electrocardiogram.

Cardiac Massage

When it has been ascertained that cardiac arrest is present or that cardiac output is of such low level that it cannot maintain adequate tissue perfusion, some form of cardiac massage must be instituted. One of the requisites of successful resuscitation is reduction of the period of inadequate circulation to an absolute minimum.

An aggressive attitude must be taken at all times toward the reinstitution of a normal or near normal cardiac beat and output. The function of either external or internal cardiac massage is to maintain some circulation of the brain, heart and other vital organs of the body to prevent biological death. This term is used to designate death of cells in contradistinction to the term clinical death, which implies cessation of respiration and circulation. If clinical death occurs abruptly in near normal circumstances, biological death may take as long as six minutes to ensue. It has been demonstrated repeatedly that it is possible to provide a marginal circulation to the various vital organs of the body for significant periods of time, supporting life in the face of cardiac arrest and clinical death. Thus, the function of the cardiac portion of cardiopulmonary resuscitation is to maintain a modicum of circulation until such time as the heart can be brought back to function in its normal manner with a cardiac output that is adequate to perfuse the vital organs of the body.

An adequate cardiac output, of course, depends upon a venous return which is commensurate with the desired output. It follows, therefore, that total blood volume may be inadequate to provide an adequate cardiac output, especially in trauma in which hemorrhage is frequent. Thus at the same time that cardiac massage is being carried out, it is essential to replace deficits in the blood volume. This should be done at the same time as the resuscitation effort.

It is emphasized again that the first resuscitative effort must be to provide a lung full of fresh air. The blood pumped through the lung will then be adequately ventilated and will provide oxygen to the myocardium. Three or four good respiratory excursions of the lung by the mouth-to-mouth technique or by bag and mask, or by other mechanical means previously detailed, will usually do this. The rescuer then should commence external or internal cardiac massage.

The question of whether external or internal cardiac massage is more efficient is frequently raised. From the point of view of this author, there are few instances indeed where internal massage is necessary. The cardiac output obtainable by external massage is, in almost all instances, as good as that obtained with internal massage. There is abundant clinical documentation of this.[10] There are, however, certain indications for internal cardiac massage. These are: (1) the presence of a tension pneumothorax or a pneumothorax of such severity that excessive arteriovenous shunting of blood is occurring within the lung; (2) indications of rather marked bleeding within the chest which might be the inciting cause of the arrest; and (3) a severely crushed or injured chest on which placement of hands and the compression of the heart may be dangerous.

Another good reason to perform internal cardiac massage is experience in its use and lack of experience with external massage. It must be understood, however, that internal massage inherently causes delay in the reestablishment of a cardiac output. This is partly due to an unavoidable delay as the rescuer decides whether the drastic step of emergency thoracotomy should be undertaken. Furthermore, it takes most individuals at least one minute to get inside the chest and to open the pericardium so that adequate massage can be carried out. In external massage, output can be achieved immediately by the proper placement of hands and compression of the sternum. The delay of preparation for internal massage may be fatal for the patient if the heart has been arrested for a preceding minute or two; this delay is not necessary in external cardiac massage, which can be begun at once. External massage can be done and then, if it is felt necessary, internal massage can be carried out.

Another possible indication for internal cardiac massage is the lack of a suitable external defibrillator. Although most hospitals are now set up to handle cardiopulmonary resuscitation, they may be prepared only for internal defibrillation. Whereas the external defibrillator can be used in open chest resuscitation by simply placing the electrodes on the chest wall, the internal defibrillator does not provide enough energy to penetrate the chest.

Technique of External Cardiac Massage. Although the various techniques of cardiac massage have been published many times elsewhere, it is worthwhile to repeat them in the context of a book on trauma.[12] Responsibility for the care of injured patients certainly requires familiarity with this modality for circulatory support, especially since the group of patients involved is apt to be younger than the general hospital population and the opportunity for cardiac salvage greater. For this reason, if for no other, cardiopulmonary resuscitation efforts carried out by a trauma team should always be adequate and well done.

With the patient supine and on a firm surface, external cardiac massage is carried out simply by placing the hands on the sternum in such a position that they produce compression through a narrow line of the heel of the hand pressing upon the lower third of the sternum (Fig. 4–2). The force is conducted to the heart, which is squeezed against the spine. The force necessary to do this is approximately 60 to 70 pounds in the average individual. It may be somewhat greater in the more muscular or emphysematous person but, by and large, it need not exceed this amount. The sternum should be depressed approximately 2.5 in. or to such a degree that a pulse wave can be felt by a second observer with a hand on the femoral pulse. It must be re-emphasized that an adequate blood volume and an oxygenated lung are necessary companions to effective cardiac massage.

The rescuer should compress the heart approximately 60 to 70 times per minute in an adult. In children, the chest is usually more flexible and smaller and will rise more rapidly and thereby allow more frequent compressions. A rate of 90 to 100 times a minute is preferable in younger adults and children. The pressures needed are proportionately less.

If a rescuer is working alone it is necessary that he compromise the rate of external cardiac massage to some degree to provide ventilation at the same or nearly the same time. It is recommended that the rescuer give approximately 12 to 15 squeezes on the heart and then breathe for the patient three to four times. Under the circumstances, this will allow both parts of the total resuscitation effort to be carried out at the same time.

Once a second rescuer arrives both efforts can be carried out simultaneously. It is much better if the respiratory resuscitation can be rhythmically coordinated with that of external cardiac massage. This may be quite difficult in actual practice, but if a good airway is obtained and as long as the respiratory exchange is being carried out well by one of the rescuers, cardiac massage can be continued right on through each breath. If, however,

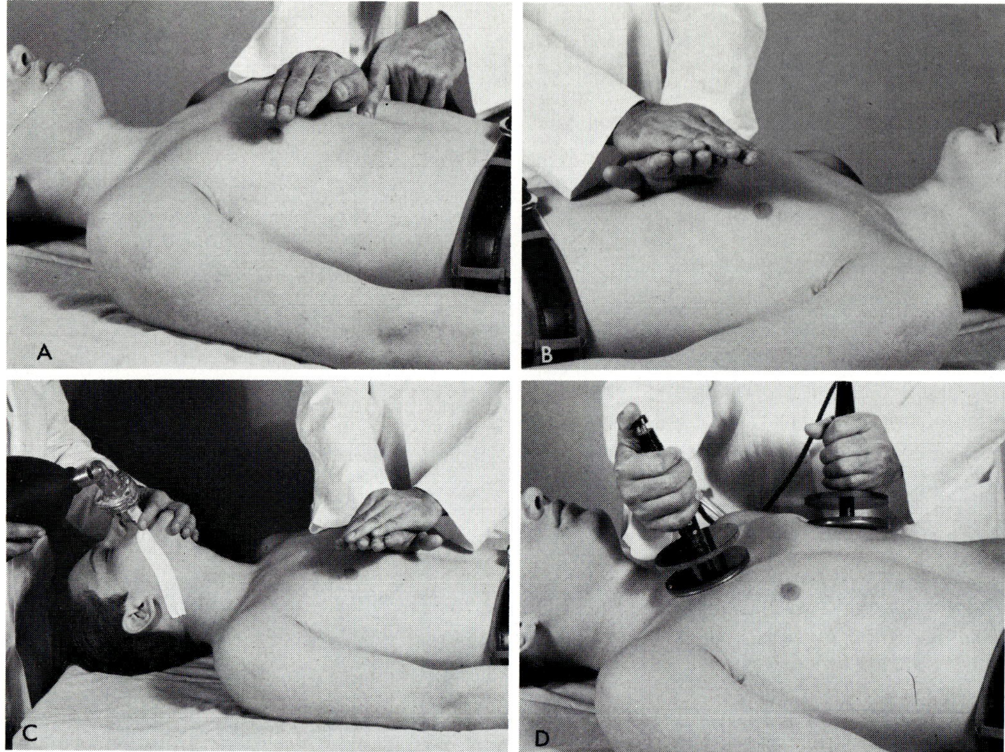

Figure 4–2 Essentials of cardiac resuscitation technique. *A*, Locating tip of sternum and placement of heel of one hand over lower third of sternum. *B*, Both hands in place. Elevation of fingers is accentuated to emphasize point pressure through heel of hand. *C*, Position of two rescuers carrying out cardiopulmonary resuscitation. *D*, Placement of electrodes for defibrillation.

there is any doubt about the airway, as occurs frequently in trauma, the respiratory resuscitator should ask his cardiac colleague to stop momentarily while he ascertains whether the lungs are being filled. After a breath or two, chest massage may be started again. Some have suggested that a rhythm be set up, such as 10 or 12 squeezes on the chest followed by one or two breaths and so on. This does represent a compromise to an already decreased cardiac output and, if possible, ventilation should be carried out directly through the external cardiac massage effort.

Adjuvant Drug Therapy. It should be kept in mind that drug therapy is no substitute for adequate cardiac output by compression and ventilation. In fact no drug will work adequately if there is not a modicum of oxygenated blood being circulated. Drug therapy should be kept simple and appropriate. During the initial resuscitation period of the heart very few drugs are required.

If after one or two minutes there is no obvious return of cardiac output as evidenced by return of carotid or femoral pulsation, the resuscitator should resort to the aggressive use of drugs beginning with epinephrine.[17] A positive inotropic and chronotropic effect is produced on the heart and peripheral vasoconstriction occurs, providing an increase in peripheral resistance. The suggested dosage is 0.5 mg. or 5 ml. of a 1:10,000 solution of epinephrine given intravenously if there is an adequate I.V. at this time or injected directly into the heart. The cardiac injection is accomplished by passing the needle directly along the left side of the sternum between the fourth and fifth ribs. Because of the complications of bleeding from a perforated coronary or a pneumothorax, the intravenous route is more desirable than the direct cardiac.

The second drug which is of great importance is a buffering agent to combat acidosis. Most commonly this is sodium bicarbonate solution. The drug is packaged in 40 ml. screw-top bottles containing 40 mEq. of sodium bicarbonate in a sterile solution. In the average adult the entire 40 ml. should be injected intravenously after the first two or three minutes of cardiac arrest. The reason for this has been demonstrated many times.[21] At the time of cardiac arrest, severe oxygen deprivation of peripheral tissues occurs. Immediately, production of lactic acid and probably fatty acids ensues. The circulatory system rapidly manifests acidosis and under these circumstances the heart has little chance of recovery. It has been further suggested that neither endogenous nor exogenous epinephrine functions well in an acid medium. Sodium bicarbonate should be given in the same quantity roughly every 5 to 10 minutes throughout the resuscitation effort.

Sodium bicarbonate is now available in a 500 ml. bottle at a 5 per cent concentration in sterile water. This can be administered at a rate of 25 to 50 ml. per minute. Overdosage must be guarded against since severe hypernatremia can result from giving large quantities of sodium bicarbonate.

Tris-buffer, commonly known as THAM, has been used to combat metabolic acidosis. This drug, previously available only as a powder and consequently not well adapted for quick resuscitation efforts, is now available in a 0.3 M solution which is stable. This can be administered at a rate of 40 ml. per minute to a total dose of 300 ml. After this initial dose the arterial pH should be monitored prior to giving subsequent doses.

A third drug which is frequently useful is calcium chloride in a 10 per cent solution. This drug has been used by many to provide an increased tone to the heart, although its effectiveness has been questioned. When a beat is felt that is probably too weak to reflect sufficient cardiac output, calcium chloride will frequently improve the force of contraction to such a degree that the cardiac output becomes nearly normal.[11]

A fourth drug of demonstrated value is one of a group of agents best termed chronic vasoconstrictors. The drugs commonly used in this situation are levarterenol (32 mg. in 500 ml. of fluid) or metaraminol (100 mg. in 500 ml. of fluid). By producing strong vasoconstriction in the peripheral portions of the circulation, major quantities of blood are diverted into the coronary and cerebral circulation and a high arterial pressure can be maintained. As soon as possible the use of either of these drugs should be curtailed or stopped to prevent the secondary effects inherent in prolonged vasoconstriction.

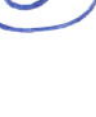

An electrocardiogram is of great assistance in planning further therapy of the arrested heart. It is not necessary, however, to wait until an electrocardiogram is seen before aggressively utilizing the drugs mentioned and even proceeding to defibrillate the heart. The importance of aggressiveness and speed cannot be overemphasized. Most patients who survive cardiac arrest have been resuscitated within the first eight to 10 minutes. Often an electrocardiogram cannot be obtained in that length of time. If the heart does not return to a palpable beat within five to 10 minutes the operator may assume that the heart is fibrillating and proceed to give it a defibrillating shock. If the heart is beating poorly or in asystole, such a shock will not harm it and if the heart is fibrillating it may well return it to a normal rhythm.

Defibrillators

The technical aspects of electrical defibrillation of the heart are too extensive to be detailed here.[13,14,22] There are both external and internal defibrillators, as well as alternating current and direct current types. These are so constructed that when used properly they will impart electrical energy into the fibrillating heart to depolarize the myocardium and thus allow it to restart in a synchronized fashion. The energy levels from the internal defibrillators are not adequate to go through the chest wall and give a sufficient shock to the heart. On the other hand, the external defibrillators provide an energy level which may actually burn the heart if applied directly to it.

External Defibrillation. These devices must be used appropriately. The placement of the paddle electrodes is important, as is a good skin or heart contact. In external defibrillation, the electrodes are rubbed with an electrode paste and their surfaces are then rubbed directly into the skin at the appropriate sites to reduce the skin resistance. Firm pressure is placed on the electrodes to give as strong a contact as possible. Loose contacts cause increased resistance and will result in burning of the skin. The electrodes should be placed on the long axis of the heart. One is placed just below the clavicle and to the right of the sternum, while the other is placed over the presumed position of the apex of the heart. Usually this is at the midclavicular line at about the 5th or 6th left interspace. There are now paddles available that can be placed in the back and the front of the patient so that the current goes directly through the heart rather than following a curving path from the front through the heart and then back to the front again, as it does with the two anterior placements (Fig. 4–2).

Internal Defibrillation. For internal defibrillation, the electrodes are usually provided with suitable pads that can be soaked in saline to provide good contact with the heart. One is placed at the apex of the heart and the other at the base of the heart or wherever the ventricles are accessible. Every effort should be made to make as much of the current as possible go through the heart.

The commercially available defibrillators are all based on similar general principles. They tend to vary only in minor characteristics which represent more the current attitudes of the developers or consultant physicians. Physicians concerned with the use of defibrillators should study them well and recognize them as potent energy sources. This means learning the settings such as voltages and times for internal and external defibrillation in adults and children for their particular instrument. Table 4–1 may be used as a rough guide if these settings are not known.

Adjuvant Drugs. The electrocardiogram can demonstrate the degree of activity of fibrillation, and if it is of poor quality, epinephrine should be introduced into the circulation either intravenously, if a good vein is open, or directly into the heart to enhance the fibrillatory activity. This may seem contrary to logical judgment, but it is now clinically accepted that epinephrine-enhanced fibrillation is easier to shock to a normal rhythm than the weak fibrillation that is often present after cardiac arrest.

When the heart is restored to a rhythm that produces ventricular contractions it frequently needs further massage until it is adequately oxygenated to the point at which it is beating well on its own. Massage should be continued until it is felt that the cardiac output is suitable to maintain the myocardial contraction and to supply body tissues as well. At the same time, the patient may resume breathing on his own, but if the respirations are inadequate they should also be assisted or controlled until such time as ventilation becomes completely adequate.

In the event that the heart cannot be defibrillated, the use of one of the cardiac depressants is indicated. The most commonly used drug at the present time is lidocaine. The first

TABLE 4–1 USE OF DEFIBRILLATORS

	OPEN CHEST DEFIBRILLATION	
A.C.	110 to 180 volts	0.1 to 0.2 second
	Shock may be prolonged to 0.5 to 1.0 second at the risk of burning. Serial shocks may be given approximately 1 second apart.	
D.C.	20 to 60 watt-seconds	Duration fixed
	CLOSED CHEST DEFIBRILLATION	
A.C.	440 to 880 volts	0.25 second (Serial shocks may be given)
D.C.	80 to 400 watt-seconds	Duration fixed
	The lower energy levels are meant for children, the higher for adults. The higher levels may be needed in children with large hearts.	

dose is administered as 10 ml. of a 1 per cent solution or 100 mg. in an intravenous push. Subsequent doses can be given in the same or smaller increments, depending upon the clinical indications. It is probably best to slowly drip in a 0.1 per cent solution if cardiac irritability persists. The total amount given over a 20–30 minute period should not exceed 400–500 mg. if possible. Too rapid administration may result in severe central nervous system depression or a convulsion.

Until some beat is established the above mentioned drugs are quite adequate. Subsequent therapy will depend on the status of the heart. A favorite drug for a poorly beating heart with very little cardiac output is isoproterenol. This is given carefully in an intravenous drip at a rate of 4 micrograms per minute in a concentration of 1 mg. per 100 cc. Great care must be exercised utilizing this drug because it easily provokes a severe tachycardia which may revert to fibrillation. The place of atropine is open to question. However, in the instance of a very slow rate or a heart block with a good pulse it is probably appropriate to give .5 mg. of atropine intravenously.

The administration of drugs must be accompanied by good ventilation and external cardiac massage. If the drugs are given through an intravenous route they must be massaged into the heart and out into the arterial side before they can be effective.

Cessation of Treatment. It is difficult to decide when to stop cardiopulmonary resuscitation after apparent failure. It is presumed that physicians who will be handling cases of trauma will have considerable insight into some aspects of the status of the patient, including the possibility of salvage from other injuries and the probable length of time of cardiac arrest. Most of those involved with resuscitation consider that efforts at continued resuscitation should cease when there are signs of central nervous system death. Diminution of previous activity of the central nervous system as manifested by lack of breathing or failure of the pupils to constrict are among such signs. If the electrocardiogram shows a low voltage QRS complex, a continued asystole which cannot be corrected, or a ventricular fibrillation pattern which cannot be broken, there is little or no hope of restoring such a failing heart. It is wrong to indicate specific time duration for a resuscitative effort or signs or symptoms which should be relied upon. Each physician should make up his own mind, depending upon the circumstances, when he should stop. Young children with signs of central nervous system death have been brought back to a normal or near normal status, but adults with the same degree of symptomatology will usually die. If the rescuer has provided adequate external cardiac massage and expired air ventilation, has been aggressive with the use of drugs and has taken care of whatever inciting factors he can, he should feel he has done everything possible under the circumstances and desist from further efforts.

Postresuscitative Care

Postresuscitative care deserves an entire chapter, but a few general principles should be noted here. Central nervous system damage in some measure nearly always occurs if cardiac arrest lasts longer than three to four minutes.[3] Cerebral edema secondary to the ischemia and hypoxia must be minimized if possible. Hypothermia of the patient by surface cooling to 30 to 32° C. should be instituted as soon as there is an indication of brain damage and should be maintained for 48 to 72 hours.

Mannitol in a 20 per cent solution, 1 to 1.5 gram per kilogram, may be used to further aid in minimizing cerebral edema. This dose can be repeated once or twice a day as indicated. Good urine output, however, is essential for the osmotic diuresis to reduce the brain water.

Corticoids have been in and out of favor for reducing brain edema. Most neurosurgeons at the present time feel that dexamethasone 4 mg. intramuscularly every six hours for the average adult is of some help.

The maintenance of an airway and also adequate respirations in the comatose patient may also be a part of postcardiac arrest therapy. A tracheostomy may be necessary to handle the secretion problems and to provide a port for a respirator. The adequacy of ventilation must be checked with blood gas measurements. The need for unusually vigilant and massive nursing care during this time cannot be overemphasized. This, plus the removal of the inciting factors of the cardiac arrest and the careful monitoring and restabilizing of a severely insulted cardiovascular system, may result in the salvage of an otherwise dead patient.

BASIC STEPS IN CARDIOPULMONARY RESUSCITATION IN TRAUMA

I. Recognize the problem
   A. Check pulse and respiration
   B. Check EKG if patient is being monitored
   C. Check pupils
II. Commence resuscitative measures
   A. Make an airway and ventilate
   B. External cardiac massage
   C. Check for and remove or bypass inciting factors if possible
      1. Airway obstruction
      2. Pneumothorax
      3. Hemothorax
      4. Pericardial tamponade
      5. Hemorrhage
III. Definitive therapy
   A. Establish a good intravenous route (i.e., cut down)
   B. Administer epinephrine 0.5 mg. or 5 ml. of a 1:10,000 solution intravenously or intracardiac every 5 minutes
   C. Give sodium bicarbonate (40 mEq. in 40 ml.) through cut down
   D. Maintain a high perfusion pressure with levarterenol solution (32 mg. in 500 ml.) or metaraminol solution (200 mg. in 500 ml.)
   E. Ventilate and circulate
   F. Get EKG machine and defibrillator and attach patient to EKG. Determine type of arrest
   G. If profound cardiovascular collapse is present give 0.5 gm. of calcium chloride (5 ml. of 10 per cent solution)
   H. If asystole is present give cardiotonic drug such as epinephrine. Continue ventilation and massage
   I. If ventricular fibrillation is present establish strong fibrillation by administering epinephrine and giving good ventilation and massage

1. Countershock with appropriate defibrillator
2. If fibrillation persists or if rhythm keeps reverting to fibrillation give a depressant before shocking.
   a. Lidocaine 100 mg. (10 cc. 1 per cent) as an I.V. push
   b. Lidocaine 0.1 per cent slow I. V. drip

J. At any time interrupt the foregoing proceedings to insert an endotracheal tube rapidly and/or switch to a technique to provide an oxygen-enriched atmosphere for ventilation (preferably 100 per cent)

K. Under special circumstances consider internal cardiac massage
1. Pneumothorax *
2. Intrathoracic bleeding *
3. Pericardial tamponade *

IV. After return of functional circulation and respiration provide suitable support and observation

A. May require respirator

B. Monitor EKG

C. Consider measures to minimize cerebral edema
1. Hypothermia
2. Osmotic diuretics
3. Steroids

ANESTHESIA IN TRAUMA

There is no distinct transition from the resuscitation of the injured patient to the anesthesia care necessary during emergency surgery. The anesthetist must vigorously continue the resuscitative procedures started in the emergency room such as assuring adequacy of ventilation and continuing venous transfusion. At the same time, he must superimpose upon them an anesthetic state suitable for the performance of surgery.

The most important consideration for the anesthetist is to insure adequate ventilation. This may require placement of an endotracheal tube and assisted or controlled ventilation or continuous observation of spontaneous ventilation. The second consideration is maintenance of circulation. This usually involves continuous infusion of blood, plasma or crystalloids in quantities adequate to balance losses, past and continuing.

Choice of Anesthetic Drug and Technique

The choice of an anesthetic drug and technique is based upon the need to provide optimal conditions for surgical intervention. It depends upon whether a qualified anesthetist is present to administer anesthesia or whether the patient can be better handled by a local or regional anesthetic administered by the surgeon. Either the anesthetist or the surgeon must decide the technique and agents to be used.

In most instances it can be stated unequivocally that general anesthesia with proper control of the airway provides the optimal situation for surgery immediately after trauma. The development of new drugs and techniques has made this more feasible. Formerly, in World War II for example, trained anesthetists were few, and surgeons themselves had to administer the anesthesia. General anesthesia is particularly indicated by multiple injuries involving many parts of the body and inability of the patient to cooperate because of pain, confusion from central nervous system damage, or intoxication. In some cases, fear of a full stomach, the involvement of limbs such as hand injuries or foot injuries or the necessity for a single anesthetist to manage several patients may make the use of local or regional anesthesia mandatory or preferable.

GENERAL ANESTHESIA

Safe general anesthesia can be administered for nearly every type of trauma. The primary requisite is a secure airway that will obviate the possibility of aspiration of stomach contents. An endotracheal tube can be placed in the semiconscious or unconscious patient directly without the need for any local anesthesia or narcotic depressant. If the patient is awake it can be done under local anesthesia.

The most common method used at present is the so-called crash technique. The lungs are purged of nitrogen by the nonrebreathing of oxygen or by the use of high flows of oxygen (10 to 12 liters per minute) in a gas machine. This can be achieved in six to eight minutes of breathing. The patient is placed in a head-up position of reverse Trendelenburg (10 to 15 degrees) to minimize the possibility of spill from the esophagus during the relaxation phase. Approximately 150 to 200 mg. of thiopental sodium or a similar fast acting barbiturate is injected intravenously to cause the patient to lose consciousness. This is followed immediately with 80 to 100 mg. of succinylcholine. This produces complete relaxation. An endotracheal tube is then directly installed without ventilating, which might of itself push stomach contents up into the pharynx. Once the tube is in place the cuff is inflated and ventilation can be carried out with minimal danger of aspiration.

This securing of the airway is of vital importance and primary to all further anesthetic procedures. It should be considered vital in all types of trauma, even those of a minimal nature, since aspiration is probably the most serious threat to the patient.

Nitrous Oxide. Once the airway is secured general anesthesia can be carried on in a number of ways. By far the simplest and most easily managed is the use of nitrous oxide and oxygen mixtures plus succinylcholine for relaxation. The use of these two drugs results in a minimal change in cardiovascular reflex response, allowing the patient to reflect in his usual way the effects of blood loss. The concentration of nitrous oxide should be sufficient to provide adequate hypnosis and analgesia but not of such degree that hypoxia might result. This usually amounts to 60 to 70 per cent nitrous oxide. The succinylcholine is used for relaxation but also, of course, provides total paralysis so that the patient cannot move or make a sign reflecting a painful stimulus.

It must be borne in mind that adequate concentrations of nitrous oxide to remove the possibility of pain and the subsequent memory of it must be maintained at all times. This technique is probably the choice of most anesthetists since there is little or no cardiovascular depression inherent in the technique other than that which might be produced by artificial ventilation.

Cyclopropane. Cyclopropane has long been the choice of anesthetists administering anesthesia to patients in shock or with low blood volumes. The drug is able to maintain considerable peripheral vascular tone, which makes maintenance of blood pressure possible and at the same time allows a high concentration of oxygen. Diethyl ether, although of not quite the capabilities of cyclopropane, has been utilized in much the same way. However, in most operating rooms where massive trauma is treated, the use of cautery makes it practically impossible to utilize these explosive gases any longer. The use of cyclopropane in The Johns Hopkins Hospital has dropped from a high of about 30 per cent of all anesthesias given 10 years ago to less than 1 per cent at the present time.

Halothane. Halothane has been highly publicized for use in the shocked patient because of its ability to produce some peripheral vasodilation and provide more adequate flows to body tissues.[5] When there is good volume replacement this has been shown to be true. Often, however, there has been inadequate volume replacement or there is continuing hemorrhage, and blood pressures fall far too low to be adequate. Once the intravascular volume has been reestablished, halothane is an excellent drug and probably the one of choice to provide a comfortable anesthesia level with the accompanying attributes of high oxygen content plus good peripheral vasodilation.

The question of the use of halothane

when there has been trauma to the liver is certain to arise. Our present understanding of halothane toxicity strongly suggests that it in no way harms the liver in this context. A preexisting sensitivity of some sort must be present before the typical lesions of halothane hepatitis occur. It would seem, therefore, that in view of the already mentioned attributes halothane is a good choice of an anesthesia in the traumatized patient.

The selection of curare as the relaxant with any of the other anesthetic drugs is open to question because of its long lasting qualities and its penchant for producing drops in blood pressure. Nevertheless, when blood volume has been adequately re-established curare can be used as in elective surgery.

Some Contraindications. There is a common feeling among anesthetists that some anesthesia must be given under all circumstances. In many situations of trauma, however, the patient is totally unresponsive because of central nervous system damage or shock and really needs no anesthetic drug. His interests are better served by good ventilation with oxygen and relaxation with succinylcholine. It should be further pointed out that most patients who have undergone serious trauma are amnesic from sometime just prior to the event and often for several days after seeming to return to consciousness. The use of any anesthetic drug in such circumstances is open to question. When the circulatory system is unstable, even nitrous oxide can produce a mild depression resulting in serious cardiac arrhythmia which may deteriorate to asystole or ventricular fibrillation.

The use of specific agents for producing peripheral vasodilation is a moot question at the present time. Such drugs as promethazine, chlorpromazine and Dibenzyline have been shown experimentally to produce good peripheral vasodilation under conditions of shock and to enhance the flow of blood into peripheral areas. It must be pointed out that these drugs are protective only under optimal conditions, and in general such conditions do not prevail at the time of surgery on the injured patient. At present it seems best to omit these drugs from the usual routine care of such patients.

LOCAL OR REGIONAL ANESTHESIA

In his book *Resuscitation and Anesthesia for Wounded Men* Beecher points out that in a survey made in September, 1943, the use of spinal anesthesia in advanced hospitals was approximately 20 per cent.[2] A year later it had fallen to 3 per cent. He pointed out that the circulatory condition of such patients was already so precarious that spinal anesthesia often caused a rapid deterioration. This is the consensus of most anesthetists at the present. The removal of protective reflexes, which is inherent in spinal or epidural anesthesia, reduces their value in the care of injured patients.

Spinal anesthesia should be relegated to use in those patients whose circulating volumes have been well re-established and in whom the injury is sharply circumscribed to the lower limbs. Here a spinal or epidural anesthesia can be kept below the twelfth dermatone, diminishing the possibility of interruption of the sympathetics and rapid fall in blood pressure. If active bleeding is taking place or if excessive bleeding is likely to occur, the use of this type of regional anesthesia is open to question. In the event that there is a special indication, such as severe respiratory disease, emphysema or asthma, such a choice may be necessary. Also, where personnel competent to handle general anesthesia care is not available, spinal or epidural may be a necessary choice. However, the patient must be properly prepared prior to this anesthesia and carefully guarded against the usual difficulties involved in marked peripheral vasodilation, which may occur.

Another complicating factor which

negates the use of these regional techniques is the somewhat unknown quality of the surgery being undertaken. Not infrequently the site of surgical intervention must be extended above and beyond the portions of the body anesthetized. Furthermore, if the single shot spinal or epidural is used and the surgery takes much longer than had been supposed, a general anesthesia must be begun under less than desirable circumstances. It is not prudent to use spinal or epidural anesthesia for lower abdominal intervention unless the patient has been well prepared and the resuscitative techniques such as endotracheal intubation equipment, anesthesia machine and capable personnel are available.

Nerve Block. Nerve blocks and local infiltration can be of great value to the trauma surgeon. It should be pointed out, however, that these techniques are too often utilized in emergency rooms in situations which ask far too much of these methods and run the risk of local anesthetic intoxication and reaction. The more complicated nerve blocks, such as sciatic and femoral blocks and supraclavicular brachial plexus blocks, should be done by qualified personnel. Trauma surgeons who find that they often have to work without the services of an anesthesiologist should learn to do such blocks as these under the tutelage of a competent anesthesiologist prior to trying them in the acute trauma situation. A definitive text such as Moore's *Regional Block* should be available in the accident room and operating rooms where care of injured patients is undertaken.[15]

ANESTHESIA FOR ARM. The hand and forearm are probably more involved in trauma than any other extremity. This is frequently a circumscribed injury requiring early surgical intervention. If a competent anesthesiologist is available, a brachial plexus block can be given by the supraclavicular technique. The hazards of intravascular injection and pneumothorax are too frequent in this block for it to be done by a neophyte.

A better approach is to utilize the currently popular perivascular axillary technique. Here the cords of the brachial plexus are infiltrated by depositing a large volume of anesthetic solution around the axillary artery as it appears just beneath the pectoralis major. The vessel can be readily felt and a solution of 1 per cent lidocaine containing 1:100,000 adrenaline can be deposited easily around the artery. It will diffuse readily upwards toward the major part of the brachial plexus and provide essentially as good anesthesia as can be achieved by the supraclavicular approach. A volume of 30 to 40 ml. is usually necessary to accomplish this. This block facilitates surgery on the forearm and hand immensely and can be done with a little practice by the trauma surgeon.

Nerve blocking further down the arm, at the antecubital space for the ulnar, median and radial nerves for instance, is easily accomplished if the anatomy is known. The same is true of the wrist. It should be pointed out, however, that for most procedures in the hand simple wrist blocks are not adequate. The axillary block again will suffice for what these blocks are capable of doing and will also allow the use of a tourniquet to aid in control of bleeding.

ANESTHESIA FOR LOWER LIMBS. In the lower limbs the situation is not quite so favorable: for example, for procedures on the foot, the sciatic and the femoral nerves must be blocked. To consistently do this well requires considerable experience. Furthermore, the quantity of drug necessary for this block is often very close to the toxic level and may result in marginal or actual local anesthetic toxicity.

Blocks of the lower limbs are difficult and give adequate anesthesia only when administered by an expert. Blocking of the sciatic and femoral nerves will generally suffice for operations or manipulations below the knee. If the operation needs to be extended, it is frequently necessary to block the obturator and the lateral femoral cutaneous nerves. By the time this has been done the quantity of local anesthetic drug is frequently near the toxic level or has exceeded it. If a regional technique is the one of choice it seems more appropriate to use a low spinal or epidural anesthesia in this instance.

The advantage of the nerve blocking techniques over spinal anesthesia, especially in the lower limbs, is that they do not involve the sympathetic nervous system to as great a degree as the spinal anesthetic. The peripheral vasodilation is not nearly so severe and the accompanying cardiovascular effects are not so noticeable.

LOCAL INFILTRATION. Except for minor lacerations involving the skin and subcutaneous tissue, local infiltration is not the best choice for anesthesia. It frequently involves many passes of needles through contaminated areas, increasing the possibility of infection. Also, there is a tendency to disregard the quantity of anesthetic drug used and frequently much is required. This can result in a catastrophic systemic reaction to the local anesthetic. If simple infiltration is decided upon, the lowest concentration of the drug and the least amount possible to perform the surgery should be used. With lidocaine, for example, a concentration of 0.5 per cent is adequate and will allow approximately 100 ml. of solution to be injected with reasonable safety. The toxic total dose of lidocaine for the average adult is 500 mg. To further reduce the toxicity the solution should contain epinephrine in a 1:200,000 dilution.

INTRAVENOUS REGIONAL ANESTHESIA

The intravenous regional technique is applicable to the surgical repair of trauma to the lower arm and hand and to the foot and lower leg to slightly above the ankle level. In this technique the limb is held well above the level of the heart for 2 to 3 minutes to reduce the blood volume in the limb and then the circulation is occluded by tourniquet and the venous system is infused with a dilute solution of a local anesthetic agent. The tourniquet must be maintained in the inflated position for at least 15–20 minutes to reduce the possibility of a rapid influx of local anesthetic agent into the general circulation.

The usual technique is as follows. Two tourniquets are placed around the limb. When the lesion is in the hand, the tourniquets are generally placed on the forearm well above the site of surgery. When the lesion is in the forearm, the tourniquets are placed on the upper arm. In the lower limb best results are achieved when the tourniquets are placed about midway on the lower leg. Tourniquets can be used on the upper portion of the leg and surgery can be performed higher up on the limb than is indicated above. However, the quantity of drug necessary to perform procedures in this instance is toxic if it escapes and it is therefore not recommended. The limb is then prepared and draped and a small sterile intravenous needle, such as a butterfly type needle with a small catheter attached, is inserted into a vein. The limb is then elevated for 3 minutes to drain some of the blood and the most proximal cuff is inflated. If the cuff is on the lower arm 30 ml. of 0.5 per cent Xylocaine is injected through the I.V. needle. If the cuff is on the upper arm 40 ml. of this solution is utilized and in the leg 60 ml. The onset of anesthesia is within 3–5 minutes. At this time the distal cuff is inflated over the area which has now been anesthetized and serially the proximal cuff deflated.

As was stated above, if the surgery lasts only a matter of a minute or two the cuff should be left up for 15 to 20 minutes to allow some detoxification of the drug. After this time the cuff can be deflated with impunity. The duration of surgery is usually based on how long the tourniquet can be left up safely. In general, it may be said that 90 minutes is a reasonable limit for this type of anesthesia.

Toxicity of General and Local Anesthesia

No matter what drug or technique for anesthesia is used, it must be remembered that the circulating blood volume in an injured patient is nearly always reduced. As a result, the usual dose of any given drug will achieve a higher level in the circulation than under normal circumstance and, consequently, be more toxic. For example, in some forms of trauma the blood volume may be reduced as much as 30 to 40 per cent with reasonable compensation of blood pressure by peripheral vasoconstriction. The injection of a usual dose of thiopental sodium will provide a much higher concentration than if the blood volume were normal. This same general approach holds for local anesthesia as well. Here the absorption of the drug from the site of injection may produce a far higher level than would usually be achieved; this may result in systemic toxicity and central nervous system excitation proceeding to convulsions and severe cardiovascular depression. For the most part lower concentrations and smaller quantities of drugs are necessary in injured patients than in normal elective surgical patients.

Aspiration

The lack of preparation of an injured patient always makes the specter of inadvertent regurgitation and aspiration one of the most serious aspects of anesthesia. As stated earlier, one appoach to this problem is to utilize some form of awake intubation or crash induction with rapid placement of the endotracheal tube. The question is often asked whether waiting four to six hours will provide protection against aspiration. The safest answer is that when trauma occurs, gastric emptying ceases. If anything, there is a gradual collection of gastric secretions with the food that has been in the stomach and which remains for a long period of time. There is no certain time period beyond which one can say that the patient is safe from the possibility of aspiration. It is far better always to assume that aspiration is a potential hazard and treat the patient with this in mind.

Aspiration may have occurred at the time of injury and, under this circumstance, it must be treated as soon as possible. Bronchoscopy has questionable value in the acutely injured patient because of the difficulty of maintaining adequate ventilation during the procedure. The removal of aspirated matter through a wide-bore endotracheal tube will usually accomplish just as much. If aspiration is suspected tracheobronchial toilet should be instituted as soon as possible. As large a suctioning catheter as can be safely fitted through the endotracheal tube should be used, with the suction turned off during the passage of the catheter into the trachea. Vigorous ventilation with oxygen should precede this maneuver and also follow it as soon as possible.

When no more aspirate can be pulled out it is the author's practice to lavage the tracheobronchial tree with small quantities of normal saline. In the average adult this would be 40 to 50 ml. and in the child six to eight years of age approximately 5 to 10 ml. As soon as the saline is instilled it is removed with the suction catheter. Extensive lavage is of questionable value, as is the use of sodium bicarbonate solutions and solutions containing corticoids.

The consequences of aspiration are extremely serious and difficult to combat. At the present time the best treatment is continuous positive pressure ventilation. Coupled with antibiotic therapy and careful tracheobronchial toilet, this is the only hope of salvage in these patients.

Cardiovascular Stability

The maintenance of circulating volume or building the volume to a normal level during the course of anesthesia is a primary responsibility of the anesthetist. Several intravenous routes should be insured prior to the beginning of anesthesia and surgery. A venous pressure manometer should be attached to one of the intravenous catheters and, if the degree of trauma and blood loss warrant it, a urinary catheter should be inserted into the bladder. These latter two, plus the usual blood pressure cuff, are the best available methods for monitoring the adequacy of circulation on a minute-to-minute basis.

Blood pressure and pulse rate can be modified somewhat by anesthetic drugs, but if these are kept at a minimum as was suggested earlier, a falling blood pressure and a rising pulse rate will reflect inadequate intravascular volume. On the other hand, a catheter for measuring central venous pressure will give a general reflection of the state of the circulatory bed. Central venous pressure should not be construed to give a precise indication of the status of the circulation; more emphasis should be placed on interpreting changes of central venous pressure.

Many remarkable attributes have been ascribed to venous pressure, but in truth this measurement reflects primarily the status of the right ventricle and the filling pressure on the right side of the heart. A rapidly rising venous pressure may suggest a full circulation or a failing right heart. Clinical acumen must be utilized to determine which of these is the case. Urinary flow is a sensitive sign of adequacy of organ perfusion. If urine output diminishes, it suggests either inadequate volume or inadequate extracellular fluid.

The level at which arterial blood pressure should be maintained is dependent upon the status of the circulatory bed of the patient, i.e., whether arteriosclerotic disease, a previous hypertensive state, and so forth, are present. In the normal healthy adult, for example, blood pressure can be allowed to remain at the level of 80 mm. of mercury systolic for rather long periods of time without harm. However, if the patient has coronary arteriosclerosis, 80 mm. of mercury may be an inadequate pressure head to provide coronary circulation. The adequacy of peripheral circulation will usually manifest itself in maintenance of warm skin temperature and dryness. A cold, clammy, blanched skin suggests pronounced vasoconstriction, probably on the basis of an inadequate volume.

Transfusions

The administration of blood in large amounts in a short period of time can cause considerable distortion of the body's hemostatic mechanisms. Bank blood is usually low in pH because of considerable acid produced by glycolysis, and the blood itself is cold relative to body temperature. Howland and his associates suggest the administration of 44.7 mEq. of sodium bicarbonate with every four to five 500 ml. transfusions to minimize the acidotic effects of bank blood.[9] They further suggest that in rapid and large transfusions the blood be warmed to near body temperature.[4] To facilitate this there are available, at the present time, a number of types of water baths through which blood can be passed to bring it up to body temperature as it is infused into the body. Results suggest that this is a much more physiological approach to rapid infusion of large quantities of blood than has previously been utilized.

The use of the calcium ion for counteracting the effect of the citrate used in bank blood is open to serious question. Again Howland et al. have pointed out that in the average adult citrate intoxication is no serious problem.[8] They suggest that the calcium ion need not be given to improve the coagulability of blood once it is in the body. They further suggest that the calcium ion may account for a number of ventricular fibrillations which occur during rapid transfusions. In adults this may certainly be true. However, in children, in whom the infusion of blood may be relatively much more rapid and in comparably larger quantities than in the adult, the calcium ion may be of considerable import and small quantities such as 2 ml. of a 10 per cent calcium gluconate solution given after each 200 to 300 ml. of blood may remarkably improve the contractility of the heart and improve its output. At any rate it seems apparent that the warming of blood and the use of antiacidosis substances such as sodium bicarbonate are of real value in rapid transfusion.

It should also be kept in mind that bank blood characteristically has a higher serum concentration of potassium than circulating blood. This can be exceptionally high and may result in symptoms of hyperkalemia. This is more likely to occur during the postoperative period than the intraoperative period. If urine output is kept up the possibility is also minimized.

When large volumes of blood are transfused, there is always the possibility of a transfusion reaction. This, of course, can happen with small transfusions as well. When the patient is under anesthesia, reactions are difficult to recognize. Characteristically, they produce drops in blood pressure and oozing from the wound margins and, in allergic reactions, a rash is sometimes present. Especially when blood is obtained on emergency cross-match, a high degree of suspicion must be continuously entertained for this possibility. The treatment is antihistaminics for the allergic reactions and, for the more serious hemolytic reactions, maintenance of urine flow with alkalinization if this is possible at the time.

Infusions

The loss or unavailability of third space fluids or extracellular fluids is a very real problem during severe shock and trauma. Shires and co-workers have pointed out the advisability of supplementing blood transfusion with an equal quantity of lactated Ringer's solution to minimize this effect.[20] They suggest giving volume for volume of blood and Ringer's lactate during rapid transfusion besides supplementing the infusion with approximately 7 ml. per kg. per hour of Ringer's lactate during the course of surgery. This work has been seriously disputed because of errors made in measurement of the magnitude of the third space. Be that as it may, these workers pointed out a situation which frequently does exist, i.e., there is a relative loss of fluid because of the inability of the circulation during shock to keep all fluid spaces in dynamic equilibrium. In the author's experience, the suggestions that Shires makes will frequently result in an overload of the circulation. It is more appropriate to rely upon general clinical evaluation, central venous pressure and urine output as indicators for the need for crystalloids. Providing that there is adequate cardiac output and the kidneys have not shut down, the urine flow is a sensitive indicator of the adequacy of extracellular fluid volume. The nature of the fluids utilized should depend on patient needs. In the absence of definite criteria, a balanced salt solution such as Ringer's lactate is considered best.

Vasopressors

Vasopressors, which had been used extensively, have fallen under a cloud in the past few years. They have been shown to cause moderate degrees of metabolic acidosis, probably on the basis of their ability to close off peripheral areas and cause ischemia.[16] However, when severe drops in blood pressure occur that may threaten life and when adequate fluids, mainly blood, for reconstituting the circulation are lacking, these drugs may be lifesaving. They should be saved for such situations, however, and not used as a routine method for maintaining a blood pressure which of itself can hide the true status of the circulation. It has been the author's habit when such drugs were needed to utilize a drug such as ephedrine, which has a vasoconstricting effect and an inotropic effect on the heart, to minimize the possibility of precipitating heart failure. The dose of ephedrine is usually 25 mg. intravenously. A mixture of 1 mg. phenylephrine and 15 mg. of mephentermine will accomplish the same result with probably somewhat better cardiac output. It is certainly wrong to say that one should never use vasopressors, but their use in a continuous infusion to maintain blood pressure in the usual situations in trauma is unwise.

The Failing Heart

After prolonged shock the heart may begin to manifest signs of impending failure, especially during anesthesia. This is usually reflected in an elevated central venous pressure; sometimes rales in the lungs can be heard. This can occur in children without disease as well as in elderly people who have cardiovascular disease. Not infrequently one's clinical judgment may indicate that a patient has been adequately transfused and the central venous pressure may have become elevated, yet the arterial blood pressure may not rise. Digitalization is warranted in these situations; if done carefully no harm can result even though it may have been unnecessary. The author's preference is for digoxin since it is a rapidly acting drug, manifesting its first activity within about 30 minutes, and it can be used easily for long term digitalization. The digitalizing dose of this drug is approximately 30 μg. per kg. in the average adult, increasing to 50 μg. per kg. in small children. Half the digitalizing dose is given intravenously, with a quarter of the dose following in 6 hours and a second quarter in another 6 hours. Electrocardiograms should be taken serially after operation to pick up any possible digitalis intoxication.

Another drug of great value after the heart has been insulted by hypoxia and shock is isoproterenol. It is used in a manner similar to that suggested for cardiac resuscitation. It provides a pronounced inotropic effect as well as a chronotropic effect and can be of great value to support the heart until it can detoxify itself by good coronary perfusion and the effects of previously administered digitalis are achieved. It must be administered very carefully to provide an optimal heart rate and cardiac output. This is generally done by utilizing some sort of intravenous pump or a microdrip intravenous set. A solution containing 1 mg. per 100 ml. is administered at approximately 4 micrograms (0.4 ml.) per minute and adjusted for the desired result.

Mechanical and Anatomical Derangements of the Lung

Severe contusions of the lung can occur without fracture of ribs and early obvious changes in the respiration. These may gradually manifest themselves during surgery when there may be a notable change in the compliance of the lung noticed by the anesthetist as he ventilates the patient. This may be the result of interstitial hemorrhage which produces a very stiff lung and can also result in an abnormality of the ventilation perfusion ratio. The patient may gradually manifest hypoxia, requiring higher and higher concentrations of oxygen in the inspired gas mixture.

A second cause for a change in compliance is aspiration which is undetected. Gastric juice can produce severe bronchospasm and atelectasis which is continually progressive and produces a picture not unlike that seen in the contused lung. Both of these call for continuous positive pressure ventilation to limit the encroachment of the process on more of the normal lung. There is little more that the anesthetist can do except to be continuously aware of this possibility and to treat it with higher and higher concentrations of oxygen plus higher ventilation pressures. The ventilation pressures, of course, can reach the point of diminishing the venous return and some compromise will usually have to be reached.

There are other causes of stiff lungs and these are usually related to congestion of the circulatory bed of the lung. Heart failure can produce this situation and must be remedied by digitalization. Circulatory overload can give the appearance of heart failure and again will produce stiff lungs. A third but less common entity is cardiac tamponade, with multiple trauma. This may occur and be undetected until it produces a high pressure in the pulmonary bed, which will necessitate high ventilation pressures.

A complication of trauma, which may not make itself manifest until the patient is anesthetized, is pneumothorax. There may be actual perforation of the lung or contusion which weakens the integrity of the lung, and during positive pressure ventilation gas may escape into the pleural space. Sudden changes in lung compliance and evidence of hypoxia should suggest this. Rapid placement of intrapleural catheters is the treatment. If severe contusion or a flail chest is already present, catheter drainage should be instituted prior to the administration of anesthesia. Even minimal amounts of pneumothorax with the accompanying shunting may be fatal to these patients.

Special Monitoring

When special monitoring devices are available the anesthetist should utilize them if they can provide information that will be helpful in the over-all care of the patient. Certainly an electrocardiograph monitoring oscilloscope can be of great value. This is especially true when the anesthetist is extremely busy with ventilation and transfusion problems and can only give a quick glance to an oscilloscope to ascertain the status of the heart. The oscilloscope can be helpful as well in the treatment of cardiac arrhythmias which might occur during digitalization and in cardiac resuscitation if it becomes a part of the procedure.

The measurement of blood pressure by an intra-arterial needle is a nicety which is worth having if it is available and can easily be applied. In general, however, this is rarely the case. The same holds for the electroencephalograph. Its value in the care of the trauma patient lies more in the determination of the integrity of the central nervous system than as a guideline for treatment.

Metabolic acidosis, respiratory acidosis and arterial hypoxia produced by intrapulmonic shunts and ischemia are all possibilities in an injured patient undergoing surgery and being observed in the post-surgical period. Clinical evaluation of any or all of these entities is extremely difficult by simple observation. Arterial sampling of blood for measurement of pCO_2, pO_2 and pH and the calculation of the buffering qualities of the blood have now become commonplace. It is essential that these measurements be utilized frequently for proper therapy. The adequacy of ventilation, for example, can be best judged by evaluation of the arterial pCO_2. pCO_2 above 40 mmHg generally means carbon dioxide retention. pO_2 below 60 with the patient breathing room air suggests intrapulmonic shunts such as those caused by atelectasis or pneumonia. The blood pH reflects the changes produced both by ventilation and ventilation/perfusion abnormalities and those produced by hypoxia as the result of tissue ischemia and/or ventilatory hypoxia. In all events these must be corrected toward normal. This therapy is beyond the scope of this chapter, but the importance of the utilization of these parameters in therapy cannot be overstressed.

POSTOPERATIVE CARE

The role of the anesthetist in the postoperative period is that of a member of a team of physicians interested in the well-being of the patient. His special training is usually helpful in evaluating and maintaining respiration and aiding in the maintenance of circulatory homeostasis.

Postoperative support of ventilation may be part of anesthesia or it may be a part of the over-all therapy. In some instances the anesthetic drugs and the relaxants may have a hang-over effect that can result in an insidious decrease in ventilation to the point at which respiratory arrest and subsequent cardiac arrest ensue. It is the author's opinion that when relaxants have been used in large amounts, the patient should be respired postoperatively until there is absolute certainty that the drugs have been detoxified. The use of the nitrous oxide, oxygen and succinylcholine technique may well result in a prolonged diminished ability of the patient to ventilate.

A further indication for postoperative ventilation is compensation for the metabolic acidosis that may result from a period of shock. The patient may be too fatigued or splinting too much to handle this on his own. Mild hyperventilation will solve this problem and at the same time prevent early postoperative atelectasis which may result from reduced tidal volumes.

Endotracheal tubes can be left in place with impunity for 24 to 48 hours. This is often a more conservative approach than performing a tracheostomy which might result in wound infection and/or intrapulmonary infection. When endotracheal tubes are left in place for the support of ventilation, they should be carefully secured and supported. Three to 5 mg. of morphine given intravenously will usually keep the patient from coughing and bucking and will also help to control his pain. Another indication for postoperative ventilation is the necessary use of certain antibiotics in the peritoneal cavity. When peritoneal soilage is severe because of trauma, some surgeons feel that irrigation of the cavity with an antibiotic solution such as neomycin in normal saline helps to reduce postoperative infection. It must be borne in mind that there are a number of antibiotics which have a synergistic effect with relaxants and can of themselves produce a curare-like effect on the myoneural junction. This can result in prolonged respiratory paralysis, necessitating the use of postoperative ventilation.

When the thorax has been injured or when aspiration or injury to the lungs has occurred, continuous postoperative ventilation is usually an important part of the over-all therapy. When this is expected it is, of course, advisable to do a tracheostomy at the end of the surgical procedure and to insert a tracheostomy tube suitable for the respirator that will be utilized. In general, this is some form of a cuffed tracheostomy tube; many are available commercially at the present time. Such patients are a special problem and their care is most difficult. They require intensive observation by physicians and nurses. The insistence on aseptic technique to eliminate the possibility of introducing infection is paramount.

Continuous Positive Pressure Breathing

In trauma to the lungs produced directly or that caused indirectly by shock there is a strong tendency toward alveolar collapse and a marked increase in intrapulmonic shunting. This can be best treated by utilizing a continuous end-positive expiratory pressure of 5 to 10 cm./H_2O with a patient on a ventilator, thus keeping the alveoli expanded. To accomplish this most simply the expired gases from the patient are allowed to escape under water much as in a chest drainage bottle with the height of the column adjusted to the desired pressure. For example, if an end-positive pressure of 5 centimeters is desired, the end of the tube for the escaping gases is submerged 5 centimeters. This technique is extremely helpful after severe lung contusion and with the development of atelectasis or other changes which occur after severe trauma. It must be kept in mind, however, that this technique also can compromise venous return to the heart and thus cause a drop in blood pressure. Frequently, the peripheral venous pressure must then be raised by additional volume expansion to compensate for this.

REFERENCES

1. Avery, E. E., Mörch, E. T., and Benson, D. W.: Critically crushed chest. J. Thoracic Surg. *32*:291, 1956.
2. Beecher, H. K.: Resuscitation and Anesthesia for Wounded Men. Springfield, Ill., Charles C Thomas, 1949, p. 146.
3. Benson, D. W., Williams, G. R., Jr., Spencer, F. R., and Yates, A. J.: The use of hypothermia after cardiac arrest. Anesth. Analg. *38*:423, 1959.
4. Boyman, C. P., and Howland, W. S.: Cardiac arrest and temperature of bank blood. J.A.M.A. 183:58, 1963.
5. Collins, W. L., and Fabian, L. W.: Halothane anesthesia during hypovolemic hypotension. *In* Clinical Management of the Patient in Shock. Philadelphia, F. A. Davis Co., 1965, pp. 119—135.
6. Elam, J. O., Brown, E. S., and Elder, J. D., Jr.: Artificial respiration by mouth-to-mask method; study of respiratory gas exchange of paralyzed patients ventilated by operators' expired air. New Eng. J. Med. *250*:749, 1954.
7. Elam, J. O., Greene, D. G., Schneider, M. A., Ruben, H. M., Gordon, A. S., Husted, R. F., Benson, D. W., Clements, J. A., and Ruben, A.: Head-tilt method of oral resuscitation. J.A.M.A. *172*:812, 1960.
8. Howland, W. S., Schweizer, O., and Boyan, C. P.: Massive blood replacement without calcium administration. Surg. Gynec. Obstet. *118*:814, 1964.
9. Howland, W. S., Schweizer, O., and Boyan, C. P.: The effect of buffering on the mortality of massive blood replacement. Surg. Gynec. Obstet. *121*:777, 1965.
10. Jude, J. R., Kouwenhoven, W. B., and Knickerbocker, G. G.: External cardiac resuscitation. Monographs in the Surgical Sciences *1*:59, 1964.
11. Kay, J. H., and Blalock, A.: The use of calcium chloride in the treatment of cardiac arrest in patients. Surg. Gynec. Obstet. *93*:97, 1951.
12. Kouwenhoven, W. B., Jude, J. R., and Knickerbocker, G. G.: Closed chest cardiac massage. J.A.M.A. *123*:1064, 1960.
13. Kouwenhoven, W. B., and Kay, J. H.: A simple electrical apparatus for the clinical treatment of ventricular fibrillation. Surgery 30:781, 1951.
14. Lown, B.: Comparison of AC and DC electroshock across the closed chest. Am. J. Cardiol. *10*:223, 1962.
15. Moore, D. C.: Regional Block. Springfield, Ill., Charles C Thomas, 1965.
16. Morris, R. E., Jr., Graff, T. D., and Robinson, P.: Metabolic effects of vasopressor agents. Bull. N. Y. Acad. Med. *42*:1007, 1966.
17. Pearson, J. W., and Redding, J. S.: The role of epinephrine in cardiac resuscitation. Anesth. Analg. *42*:599, 1963.
18. Quattlebaum, J. K., Jr.: Stricture of the trachea following traumatic fracture; successful excision and anastomosis. A.M.A. Arch. Surg. 76:417, 1958.
19. Safar, P.: Ventilatory efficacy of mouth-to-mouth artificial respiration. Airway obstruction during manual and mouth-to-mouth artificial respiration. J.A.M.A. 166:335, 1958.
20. Shires, T., Coln, D., Carrica, J., and Lightfoot, S.: Fluid therapy in hemorrhagic shock. Arch. Surg. *88*:688, 1964.
21. Stewart, J. S., Stewart, W. K., and Gillies, H. G.: Cardiac arrest and acidosis. Lancet *2*:964, 1962.
22. Zoll, P. M., Linenthal, A. J., Gibson, W., Paul, M. H., and Norman, L. R.: Termination of ventricular fibrillation in man by externally applied electric countershock. New Eng. J. Med. *254*: 27, 1956.

chapter

5

ACUTE RENAL FAILURE FOLLOWING TRAUMA

Charles B. Manley, M.D.
and Alan M. Robson, M.D.

INTRODUCTION

The clinical syndrome of acute renal failure was first well defined by Bywaters after observing many cases associated with crush injury during the London blitz in World War II. The conservative dietary regimens developed by Borst in the Netherlands and by Bull in England, following the war, increased the survival rate of patients with acute renal failure. In recent years, the development of renal dialysis and transplantation has markedly transformed the management of this problem.

Trauma victims are especially liable to develop acute renal failure. Since recognition and correct management in the early phases of the condition can significantly reduce complications and improve prognosis, it is important that surgeons attending these trauma patients should have a thorough understanding of the principles of diagnosis and management.

ETIOLOGY

Acute renal failure can be defined as progressive azotemia in a patient who previously had normal renal function. It is usually associated with oliguria—a urine output of less than 400 ml. per day—although on occasions a polyuric form of the syndrome with daily urine volumes in excess of 1500 ml. may be seen. While the latter condition portends a better prognosis, it is probably not a separate entity but only represents a later stage of the disease process after a transient or unrecognized oliguric phase.

There are many causes of acute renal failure. The more common ones are listed in Table 5–1. A time-honored approach to etiology that continues to be worthwhile provides a subdivision of acute renal failure into three distinct clinical groups: prerenal, renal and post-renal. This differentiation is important, since the management in each of these groups differs.

TABLE 5–1 MAJOR CAUSES OF ACUTE RENAL FAILURE*

A. Pre-renal (circulatory inadequacy)
   1. Fluid and electrolyte depletion
   2. Hemorrhage
   3. Myocardial infarction
   4. Septicemia
B. Post-renal (obstruction)
   1. Prostatism
   2. Bladder or other pelvic or retroperitoneal tumors
   3. Renal calculi
   4. Ureteral blockage after surgery or instrumentation
C. Primary renal injury
   1. Acute tubular necrosis and cortical necrosis due to direct renal injury
      a. "Ischemic" (consequent to circulatory inadequacy, post-surgical, obstetric [septic abortion, premature placental separation], etc.)
      b. Toxins (carbon tetrachloride, heavy metals [mercury etc.], methanol, ethylene glycol and many others)
      c. Hemolysis (mismatched transfusion, etc.)
      d. Crush injuries
      e. Burns
   2. Acute glomerulitis (post-streptococcal glomerulonephritis, nephritis in vasculitis, periarteritis, lupus nephritis, etc.)
   3. Arterial or venous obstruction (embolus, thrombosis, aneurysm)
   4. Acute pyelonephritis, papillary necrosis
   5. Severe hypercalcemia
   6. Intrarenal precipitation (sulfonamides, urates after toxic drug therapy, myeloma protein after pyelogram, etc.)

*From Levinsky, N. G.: Acute Renal Failure. *In* The Management of Emergencies, New Eng. J. Med. [Suppl.], 1966.

Pre-Renal

Pre-renal failure is characterized by the occurrence of azotemia and oliguria in the absence of demonstrable structural changes in the kidney. It is seen with hypovolemia, with a decreased cardiac output or with shock. Of these factors, hypovolemia is the most common. It may result from fluid loss due to severe burns, peritonitis or ileus with third-space sequestration of fluid, excessive vomiting or diarrhea, enteric fistulae, prolonged gastric suction and, of course, hemorrhage. Decreased cardiac output might follow hypovolemia, but other causes such as the coincident development of a myocardial infarction or an arrhythmia with left ventricular failure should be considered. Shock may result from hypovolemia but can also occur with septicemia or sensitivity reactions in the absence of significant volume contraction.

The consequence of these pre-renal factors, regardless of cause, is hypotension and marked diminution of renal blood flow. A concomitant decrease in glomerular filtration rate results in progressive azotemia. An increase in fractional reabsorption of the glomerular filtration by the renal tubules potentiates the decreased filtration rate in the production of marked oliguria. If the pre-renal failure is recognized and adequate corrective measures are undertaken, the changes can be reversed without ensuing renal damage. Conversely, if the situation is not recognized promptly, acute tubular necrosis may develop.

Renal

While acute renal failure may occur in association with many forms of intrinsic renal disease, such as acute glomerulonephritis, the most common renal pathologies resulting from trauma are acute tubular necrosis, renal artery or vein occlusion and renal cortical necrosis. Acute tubular necrosis due to toxic or ischemic factors may involve any portion of the proximal nephron, thus explaining the abandonment of the former term for this condition, "lower nephron nephrosis". Precipitating factors are numerous and include nephrotoxins, hemolytic reactions and, as mentioned above, uncorrected pre-renal failure of whatever cause. Traumatic renal artery thrombosis requires early diagnosis and prompt treatment if infarction is to be averted. Similarly, the prognosis for renal vein thrombosis is improved if the lesion is diagnosed early and treated without delay. Fulminant, ischemic necrosis of the cortex is clearly distinguishable pathologically but often not clinically from acute tubular necrosis, so that renal biopsy is usually necessary for differentiation. Cortical necrosis most often follows obstetrical complications but may be seen with severe hemorrhage, infarction or trauma.

Post-Renal

Blunt or penetrating trauma to any portion of the urinary tract from the kidney to the urethra may result in acute renal failure either by direct injury to the renal parenchyma or by inducing pre-renal factors (see Chapter 12). In addition, post-renal failure may occur due to obstruction of the urinary passages by extrinsic compression from hematomas and displaced bony fragments, or intrinsically by massive blood clots or sloughed renal papillae. Disruption of urinary conduits with extravasation and reabsorption of urine, as with intraperitoneal rupture of the bladder, may produce an acute renal failure syndrome despite normally functioning kidneys. Surgical trauma most often involves inappropriate ligation or resection of the ureter. Finally, it should not be forgotten that pre-existing obstructive abnormalities such as anomalies, calculi or neoplasms may be present, rendering these organs more susceptible to trauma.

Other Causes

Surgical patients may develop acute renal failure associated with such conditions as acute peritonitis, acute pancreatitis, gastrointestinal obstruction or with any major or prolonged operative procedure without any obvious precipitating cause. In approximately 30 per cent of patients, no etiology may be apparent.

CLINICAL FEATURES

The insidious onset of acute renal failure in the emergency or recovery room setting is often overlooked by physicians not anticipating its possibility. Urine output provides the key to early recognition. At this time, an indwelling catheter serves a dual purpose in assessing the possibility of injury to the bladder or urethra and in monitoring urine output (see Chapter 12). An hourly urine volume of 20 ml. or less is compelling evidence for acute renal failure and a tentative diagnosis should be made. If the oliguria is not recognized promptly the syndrome presents as a rapidly rising BUN or as a manifestation of intravenous fluid overload with water intoxication, congestive heart failure or pulmonary edema.

While the course of acute renal failure associated with increased catabolic states such as infection, surgery or accidental trauma may be quite variable, that of uncomplicated acute tubular necrosis is quite predictable and serves as a guide for management. Five distinct clinical stages are recognized: onset, oliguric-anuric, diuretic, recovery and convalescent.

The onset stage is that short period between the acute precipitating event and the onset of oliguria. This may

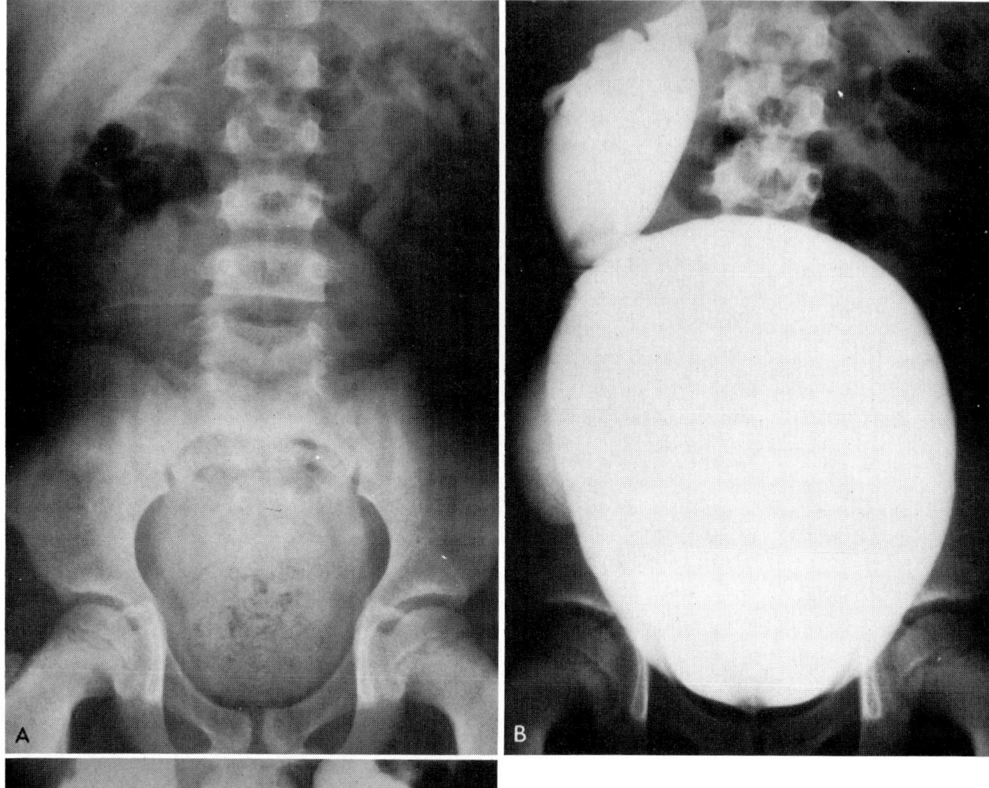

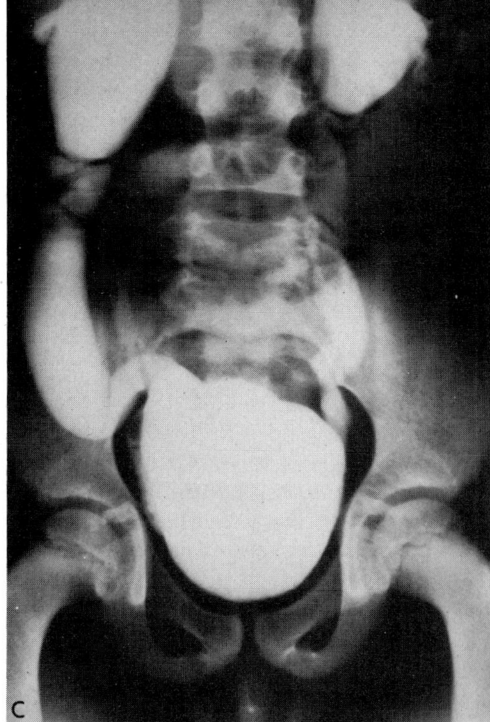

Figure 5–1 Renal failure with unsuspected obstructive uropathy. This azotemic 9-year-old boy, with a familial history of nephritis, was hospitalized for renal biopsy. There was no history of voiding difficulty, urinary infection or other GU problems. Physical examination was unremarkable, including a flat, soft abdomen. Neurological examination was negative. The kidneys failed to visualize on IVP; however, a plain film of the abdomen 24 hours later unexpectedly revealed a faintly visualized mass filling the the abdomen (A). Catheterization and cystogram confirmed this to be a markedly enlarged, thin and atonic bladder which was devoid of sensation (B). A post-void film (C) demonstrated severe bilateral reflux with residual urines measured at 500–700 ml. After a voiding cystourethrogram showed no urethral outlet obstruction, a diagnosis of Megacystitis syndrome was made.

be as long as a week for carbon tetrachloride-induced ATN but is generally very brief with shock or trauma.

The oliguric-anuric stage usually lasts 8 to 15 days but occasionally may persist for much shorter or longer periods. Anuria is rare with uncomplicated ATN and persistence beyond two weeks carries a poor prognosis. As mentioned above, recognition of the condition is usually made at this time, either by noting the decreased urine output or by progressive symptoms of uremia such as hiccups, nausea and vomiting, confusion and somnolence. Signs of pericarditis or congestive heart failure may be prominent. The daily rise in BUN is approximately 20–30 mg. per cent in uncomplicated cases but may be much greater with trauma, burns and infection. The postoperative patient is more prone to infection and dehiscence of wounds occurs about 50 per cent of the time. Hyperkalemia, metabolic acidosis and overhydration are common factors of this stage.

The diuretic stage begins when the urine volume first exceeds 400 ml./day and extends until the daily rise in BUN has ceased. While giving the first indication of recovery, the diuresis should not prompt undue sense of relief, as 25 to 50 per cent of deaths occur during this stage of the disease. The degree of overhydration determines the magnitude of diuresis and careful monitoring of body weight, central venous pressure, blood and urine electrolytes and intake and output is necessary during this labile period of 4 to 8 days.

The recovery stage corresponds to the beginning drop in BUN until it has stabilized or returned to normal range. In some patients the BUN remains permanently elevated, reflecting irreversible damage. Creatinine or inulin clearances may require additional months before reaching maximal values.

The convalescent stage follows and a period of several months is needed for full recovery from anemia, nutritional depletion and metabolic exhaustion.

DIAGNOSIS

Before a diagnosis of acute renal failure is established, it is important to consider other causes of uremia and oliguria and to exclude the presence of pre-existing chronic renal disease.

Neither azotemia nor aliguria alone is sufficient to make the diagnosis. Blood urea nitrogen (BUN) levels above "normal" values may result from high dietary protein intake or from excessively elevated urea production rates. The latter may follow extensive trauma with reabsorption of large areas of necrotic tissue, with gastrointestinal hemorrhage or with hypercatabolic states such as those associated with burns or infection. An elevated BUN may also occur with urine reabsorption following ureterointestinal urinary diversion or with intraperitoneal extravasation from a ruptured bladder.

Similarly, a reduction in urine flow rate does not necessarily indicate renal failure. A normal person can excrete the necessary daily solute load in a urine volume of 400 to 500 ml. This low urine flow rate may result from either the appropriate or inappropriate release of antidiuretic hormone in response to injury, anesthetics or surgery or from a fluid regimen that is inadequate to match losses.

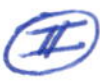

Catheterization may be necessary to exclude urinary retention of the bladder, a condition that cannot be accurately assessed by physical examination. Many a reputation has been tarnished by this simple oversight.

If not necessary for the treatment of lower urinary tract injury or obstruction, and as soon as the status of renal function is determined, the catheter should be removed to avoid introduction of infection. If the catheter is

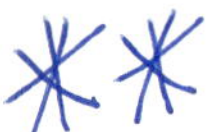

TABLE 5–2 A SUMMARY OF DIAGNOSTIC CONSIDERATIONS IN ACUTE RENAL FAILURE

A. Does the patient have renal failure?
   1. Is there oliguria (urine volume 20 ml./hr. or less)?
      a. Is there bladder retention?
      b. Could this be due to dehydration or blood volume contraction?
      c. Is there another stimulus for ADH release?
      d. Could he have inappropriate ADH release?
      e. Could he have a polyuric form of acute renal failure?
   2. Is he uremic?
      a. Could this be due to increased urea production, e.g., from G.I. hemorrhage or tissue necrosis?
      b. Was there pre-existing renal disease?
B. Is the renal failure acute or chronic?
   1. Is there a history suggestive of previous renal disease?
   2. Has the patient had previous hospitalizations, visits to a physician, life insurance or army medical examinations?
   3. If the patient is female, does she have an obstetric history of toxemia of pregnancy?
C. Tentative diagnosis of acute renal failure: is it post-renal, renal or pre-renal?
D. Rule out post-renal factors
   1. Radiography
      a. K.U.B.
      b. Intravenous urography?
      c. Cystoscopy with retrograde ureterograms
      d. Renal arteriogram?
   2. Radioisotope renograms
E. Renal or pre-renal?
   1. Urinalysis
   2. Urine sodium
   3. U/P creatinine ratio
   4. Therapeutic trial volume expansion or diuretics
      a. Could the patient have fluid overload?
      b. Is central venous pressure being monitored?
      c. Is it safe to catheterize bladder to monitor rate of urine flow?

introduced aseptically and with careful closed-system management, it should be possible, if needed, to leave indwelling for 24 to 48 hours without development of infection. On the other hand, many do not understand that once bacteriuria has occurred, the catheter should not be removed until appropriate antibiotic therapy has been instituted.

In regard to the possibility of pre-existing chronic renal disease, the history is only of occasional benefit. Unfortunately, chronic renal failure often develops so insidiously that the person is unaware of any problems until he presents to a physician with renal function below 10 per cent of normal. Information from past hospitalizations, insurance examinations, military physicals and obstetrical records may be helpful. Other historical clues include hematuria, proteinuria, high blood pressure, recurrent urinary infections or complaints of malaise, unexplained nausea, vomiting, anorexia or nocturia.

Physical examination is also of limited value but might reveal impaired growth or deficient secondary sex characteristics, opaque white fingernails, skin pallor or discoloration, hypertension, fundoscopic abnormalities or pericardial friction rub, all of which may be associated with chronic uremia.

Small, symmetrical renal outlines on a plain film of the abdomen suggest chronic renal disease although normal size does not exclude it. An unexplained normocytic, normochromic anemia is also supportive evidence of this diagnosis. Secondary hyperparathyroidism is an important indication of chronic renal disease. Subperiosteal bone reabsorption in the phalanges of the hand is seen radiographically. Other evidence includes elevation of the serum alkaline phosphate and a relatively well-maintained serum calcium in the presence of hyperphosphatemia.

Once it has been established that oliguria and azotemia result from acute renal failure, it is necessary to determine whether this is on the basis of a pre-renal, renal or post-renal lesion.

DETERMINATION OF CAUSE OF ACUTE RENAL FAILURE

Post-Renal

It is rare for a pre-renal or renal lesion to result in complete anuria, and any patient who presents with anuria or severe oliguria should be considered to have a post-renal etiology until this diagnosis has been eliminated by the appropriate investigations. This is best accomplished by radiography which may also give information about pre-existing renal disease and may, at the same time, reveal lower urinary tract injury requiring surgical correction (see Chapter 12). The importance of excluding a post-renal lesion relates to the considerable prompt improvement that usually follows relief of obstruction.

RADIOGRAPHY

Plain films of the abdomen and high-dose intravenous urograms are usually of limited value. Radio-opaque calculi and nephrocalcinosis may be noted on a plain film. Bilateral, small, symmetrical renal outlines usually indicate chronic end-stage renal disease. Intravenous urograms may reveal obstructive uropathy; however, visualization of contrast media is unlikely to occur with a BUN of 80 mg. per cent or greater. The hypertonic solution used in these studies may further expand an already overloaded plasma fluid volume so that this procedure should not be considered a routine investigation for patients with acute renal failure.

In most instances, cystoscopy with retrograde urography is necessary to rule out post-renal failure due to obstructive lesions. An increased awareness of the potential hazards of introducing infection has led to improved techniques so that minimal risk is incurred. Aseptic technique is mandatory. An antibiotic such as neomycin is often added to the contrast media. A retrograde ureterogram is now generally preferred rather than introduction of a ureteral catheter to the renal pelvis. A ureteral catheter with a bulb or acorn-shaped tip is introduced under cystoscopic vision just into the ureteral orifice which momentarily occludes the ureter while 5 to 7 ml. of contrast media is introduced. Care must be taken not to overfill the collecting system. The catheter is withdrawn immediately after the film is taken, allowing release of the contrast. Delayed films after several minutes help confirm impaired drainage of obstructed systems.

Some difference of opinion concerns the necessity of demonstrating the appearance of only one or both upper urinary tracts. The unilateral advocates worry about increased morbidity; the bilateral advocates worry about the occasional unilateral obstruction opposite a kidney with vascular impairment, the latter chosen by chance for the retrograde. Both concerns are of little moment but if there is any reasonable doubt, both ureters should be injected.

RADIOISOTOPE RENOGRAM

Extensive pelvic trauma, such as pelvic fracture with rupture of the urethra or bladder, may prevent the use of retrograde ureterograms to rule out upper tract obstruction. In these instances, radioisotope renography using I^{131} labeled sodium orthoiodo-

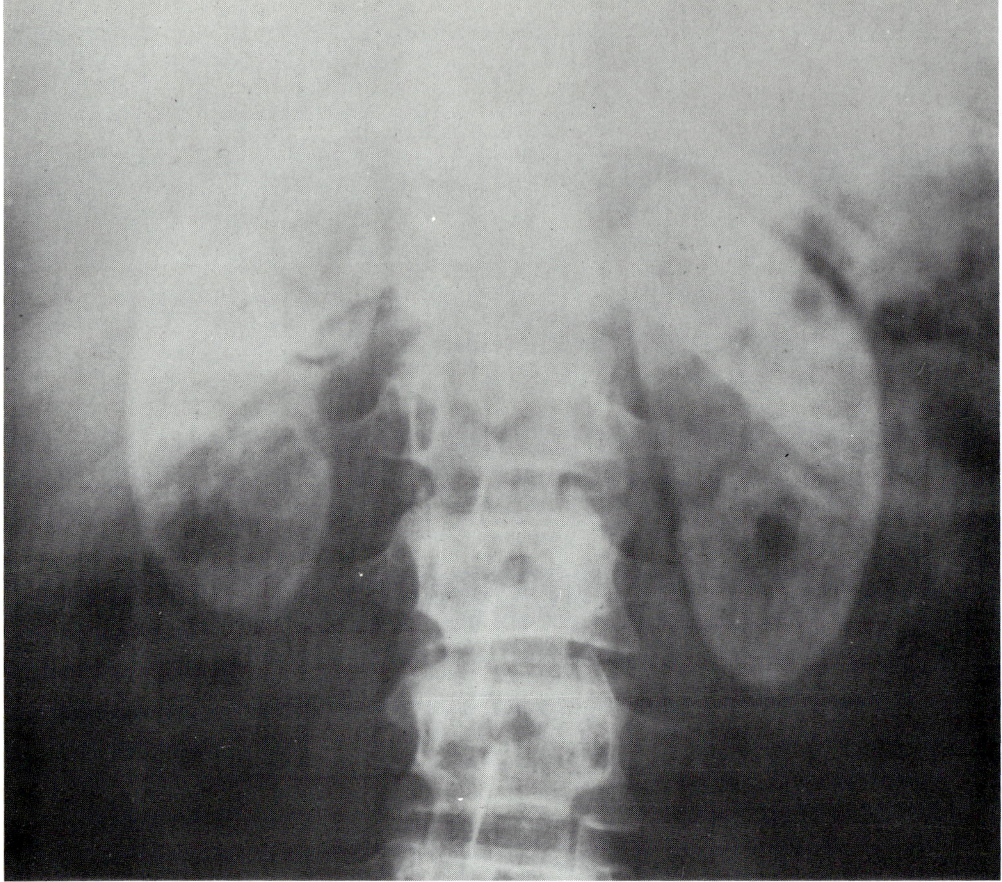

Figure 5–2 Renal cortical calcification. A plain film of the abdomen demonstrating bilateral, diffuse, renal calcifications with an unusual survival several years following acute cortical necrosis.

hippurate (Hippuran) provides an alternative but less certain means of investigation. It is a relatively safe and simple test not requiring instrumentation and can be completed within 10 to 12 minutes. A renogram showing a continuing, rising excretory phase would suggest obstructive uropathy in contrast to a flat curve with acute tubular necrosis. Lack of a vascular phase would be suggestive of renal artery occlusion.

Renal or Pre-Renal

Post-renal lesions account for a relatively small percentage of patients with acute renal failure and after exclusion of these etiologies attention must be directed toward differentiating between pre-renal and renal causes. The importance of this relates to the difference in management of these two pathophysiologically distinct entities. The former usually requires replacement therapy with the administration of large volumes of fluid and electrolytes, the latter usually requires restriction of intake of these agents. The administration of injudicious amounts of fluids and electrolytes to a patient with acute tubular necrosis may well result in edema, circulatory overload, hypertension and heart failure.

Evidence for pre-renal failure can often be obtained from a detailed review of the patient's fluid and electrolyte balance, from review of the blood pressure chart and from a careful examination. When calculating fluid balance it is important to include insensible fluid loss and to try to determine whether there is pooling of fluid in a third-space compartment such as the gastrointestinal tract. If this occurs, total fluid balance may be well maintained but volume contraction may be present. Similarly, a blood pressure which appears normal may represent hypotension if the patient was previously hypertensive. Physical examination in a patient with acute renal failure should also concentrate on determining the patient's current status of fluid balance, whether there is circulatory overload or depletion and whether there may be pooling of fluid in compartments, such as the gastrointestinal tract, or as either ascites or edema. Dry mucous membranes may indicate that a patient is dehydrated, but it is important to remember that the patient with acute renal failure usually is acidotic and frequently breathes through his mouth. Thus, a dry mouth may be found even in the presence of edema or circulatory overload. Central venous pressure measurements may also be helpful.

History and physical examination usually do not provide sufficient information to establish the cause of renal failure and additional tests are necessary.

URINALYSIS

A urinalysis should be performed in all patients with acute renal failure. Unfortunately, it is not always diagnostic in separating intrinsic renal failure from extrinsic lesions, nor will it necessarily indicate the nature of an underlying renal lesion.

The gross appearance of the urine may indicate the presence of hematuria, hemoglobinuria, myoglobinuria or bilirubinuria. With fresh bleeding into the genitourinary tract the urine appears red, but if the blood is in contact with an acid urine for any length of time, hemoglobin is converted to acid hematin, giving the urine a characteristic brown or coffee color. Hematuria should be distinguished from hemoglobinuria, the former occurring with trauma to the kidney, the latter indicating intravascular hemolysis. This can usually be achieved using one of the dipsticks which detects hemoglobin in urine and microscopy, which will indicate the presence of red cells in the urine. Even though red cells will lyse in hypotonic urine, microscopic examination of a fresh urine sample will usually indicate whether bleeding has occurred into the genitourinary tract.

The measurement of urine specific gravity is sometimes helpful in distinguishing the cause of oliguria. Even in patients with low urine output this measurement can be obtained on a very small sample of urine using the refractometer. In chronic renal disease there is usually isosthenuria with specific gravity varying little and being close to 1.010. In pre-renal failure or with acute glomerular disease the urine specific gravity is usually high, often being 1.025 or greater. In acute tubular necrosis the value is usually around 1.010.

Proteinuria is a non-specific finding. Red cell, white cell, hemoglobin or myoglobin casts as well as renal tubular cells may be seen either in acute tubular necrosis or in glomerulonephritis. Evidence of infection such as pyuria and bacteriuria suggests the possibility of obstructive uropathy but could also relate to a prior catheterization.

URINE CHEMISTRIES

Measurement of the urine sodium concentration can be of considerable help in differential diagnosis, providing this determination is made on urine obtained during oliguria. In pre-renal failure, renal perfusion is decreased, there is a decrease in glomerular filtration rate per nephron

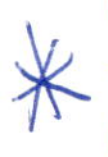

and there is a high fractional reabsorption of the filtered sodium by the renal tubule. As a result, urine sodium levels are low, usually below 20 mEq./L. and often as low as 5 mEq./L. Conversely, in renal failure with extensive renal tubular damage, the urine has a much higher sodium concentration characteristically around 60 mEq./L. or greater.

The presence of pre-existing chronic renal disease may make interpretation of urinary sodium levels difficult. For example, urine sodium in a dehydrated patient with chronic renal disease is usually higher than that seen in a dehydrated patient with previously normal kidneys. Also, the decrease in GFR per nephron seen in patients with acute glomerulonephritis usually results in a low urine sodium during the oliguric phase and may be confused with the similar finding in volume contraction (see Table 5–3).

Measurement of urine osmolality is of relatively little help in determining the cause of acute renal failure. Urine osmolality results principally from the urea, sodium and chloride concentrations in the urine. In renal hypoperfusion, urine sodium and chloride levels are low but urea concentrations are high. In acute tubular necrosis, urine sodium and chloride levels are higher but urea concentrations are lower so that urine osmolalities may be similar in the two situations.

U/P CREATININE RATIOS

For this test, specimens of urine and plasma are obtained simultaneously during oliguria and submitted for creatinine determination. The ratio of urine to plasma creatinine concentration gives an approximate estimate of fractional water reabsorption by the renal tubule. In dehydration and pre-renal failure, renal tubular fluid reabsorption is great and the U/P creatinine ratio is above 20, usually being 50 or greater. In acute tubular necrosis, tubular fluid reabsorption is reduced with the U/P creatinine ratio characteristically being below 20 and frequently 10 or less.

The urine to plasma urea ratio has been used for the same purpose but is less satisfactory because urea diffuses more readily across the renal tubule than does creatinine.

BLOOD CHEMISTRIES

Serum electrolytes, blood urea nitrogen and creatinine levels do not help to distinguish the type of renal

TABLE 5–3 CHEMISTRIES IN ACUTE RENAL FAILURE*

CONDITIONS	U/P CREATININE RATIO	URINE SODIUM CONCENTRATION
PRE-RENAL	Usually > 20; often > 50	Usually <20 mEq./L.; often <10 mEq./L.
PRIMARY RENAL		
Oliguric	Usually < 20; often < 15	Usually > 30–40 mEq./L.
Nonoliguric	Usually < 20; often < 15	Usually < 20; often < 15
POST-RENAL	Variable; often high in short-term obstruction and low after prolonged obstruction	Variable; may be low in short-term partial obstruction

*From Smith, J. W., ed.: Manual of Medical Therapeutics (19th Ed.) Boston, Little, Brown & Co., 1969.

failure but should be obtained as part of the initial evaluation since these values are needed to plan therapy on a rational basis.

In acute renal failure when there is little tissue trauma, no major bleeding and no cause for increased tissue catabolism, blood urea nitrogen may increase as little as 15 mg./100 ml./day but when any of these complications exists, the increase in blood urea nitrogen may be 50 mg./100 ml./day or greater. Similarly, with increase in catabolic rate the serum potassium in a patient with acute renal failure may increase by 2 mEq./L./day and the serum bicarbonate may fall by 5 or more mEq./L./day, indicating the need for frequent monitoring of these parameters.

MANNITOL ADMINISTRATION

The administration of mannitol has been used both as a diagnostic test and as therapy in oliguric patients. Since mannitol is not effective after acute tubular necrosis has developed, there is little value in its administration if the insult resulting in the oliguria occurred more than 48 hours previously. The bladder should be emptied by urethral catheterization and up to 25 gm. of 20 per cent mannitol is given intravenously over a 20-minute period. The subsequent urine flow rate should be carefully monitored. If there is no resultant diuresis it can be concluded that intrinsic renal damage has already occurred. If a diuresis ensues, usually within 30 minutes, there is some evidence to suggest that this therapy may prevent progression to acute tubular necrosis, possibly by increasing renal blood flow. Under these circumstances mannitol can be infused to maintain a urine flow rate of 60–100 ml./hr. Mannitol administration may result in significant expansion of the blood volume and should be given with caution if there is evidence of circulatory overload.

FUROSEMIDE OR ETHACRYNIC ACID ADMINISTRATION

Many centers prefer the use of either intravenous furosemide (Lasix) or ethacrynic acid (Edecrin) over mannitol administration as a diagnostic test since neither of these diuretic agents result in expansion of blood volume and either may be effective in patients resistant to mannitol. The test is performed in a similar manner to that outlined for mannitol, the dose of Lasix being 80 mg. and that of Edecrin 50 mg. If a diuresis occurs following this therapy, the drug can be repeated after 2 to 4 hours using the same dosage. The efficacy of larger doses has yet to be proven.

RENAL BIOPSY

Renal biopsy may clarify the diagnosis in selected instances of acute renal failure. Although acute tubular necrosis is frequently associated with typical pathologic changes (see Fig. 5–3), the biopsy is not always diagnostic and patients with clinical acute tubular necrosis may not show any histologic abnormalities. Similarly, biopsies from patients with cortical necrosis may show normal tissue since this lesion is frequently patchy and the tissue may have been obtained from relatively unaffected cortex.

It should be emphasized that renal biopsy carries a higher morbidity in patients with renal failure than in healthy subjects and should only be performed when there are good indications. If possible, the procedure should be postponed until anemia, uremia and hypertension have been controlled.

MANAGEMENT

In the preceding section emphasis has been placed on determining the underlying cause for acute renal fail-

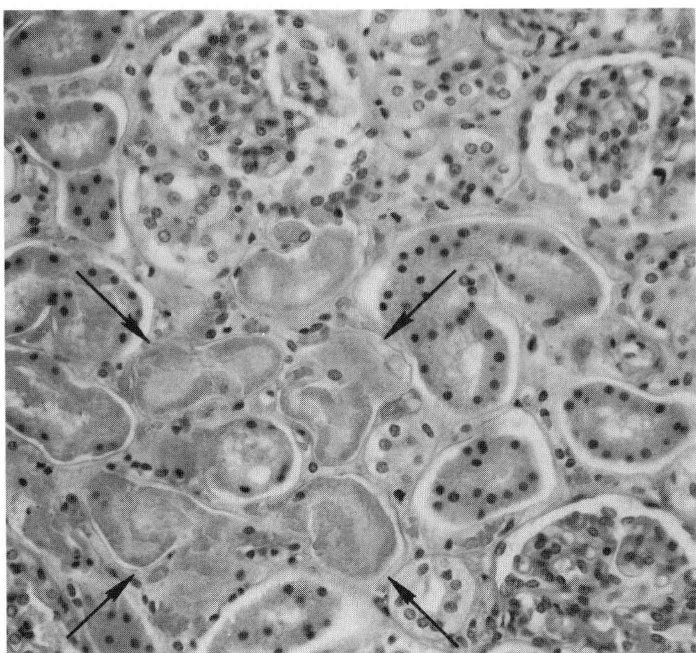

Figure 5–3 Acute tubular necrosis. The arrows indicate characteristic tubular profiles with coarsely granular cytoplasm and absent or greatly diminished numbers of nuclei. (H&E × 250. Photomicrograph courtesy of Dr. J. M. Kissane.)

ure. This is imperative since management of the patient with a post-renal or a pre-renal etiology differs from that of the patient with acute tubular necrosis. In the former, relief of obstruction or correction of damage to the lower urinary tract is of paramount importance. In pre-renal failure, supportive measures such as extracellular fluid volume expansion designed to improve renal perfusion are required. In renal lesions therapy depends on the state of hydration of the patient and the degree of electrolyte imbalance but usually consists of restriction of the amount of fluid and electrolytes administered, correction of electrolyte abnormalities and modification of drug dosages. These areas are discussed in greater detail below.

Post-Renal Failure

Relief of upper urinary tract obstruction essentially involves either retrograde ureteral catheterization or nephrostomy. Ureteral catheterization can be performed in a few minutes under local anesthesia and may be life-saving in acute fluid-overload situations. However, the catheter is difficult to maintain for more than a few days. Nephrostomy requires a patient of reasonable risk for open surgery but can be used as a means of diversion for weeks or months. Accordingly, ureteral catheterization is often used initially to be replaced by nephrostomy as the patient's improved condition allows.

Patients with persisting partial obstruction of the urinary tract frequently are polyuric. However, a life-threatening diuresis and natriuresis may occur when the obstruction is relieved. Urine volumes up to 15 liters per day may be seen with sodium excretion rates being increased up to 1900 mEq./day. The precise mechanisms responsible for these changes have yet to be delineated but it is inappropriate for the patient's state of hydration and may result in depletion of the extracellular fluid volume, vascular collapse and death. This phenomenon should be watched for in any patient who has had obstruction relieved and is treated by the replacement of appropriate amounts of fluids and electrolytes. Urine volumes and electrolyte concentrations should be carefully monitored during this phase to enable the correct replacement therapy to be calculated.

Pre-Renal Failure

The declining incidence of acute renal failure associated with surgery or trauma is believed due to many factors, one of which is the early recognition and correction of pre-renal factors. The aim of therapy is to restore renal perfusion by correcting the underlying cause. This may necessitate the administration of one of the digitalis preparations to improve cardiac output, the administration of blood to replace blood loss, the administration of extracellular fluid and electrolytes to correct deficits or the administration of pressor agents to correct hypotension due to causes other than volume depletion. Levophed (norepinephrine) and other pressor substances should be used sparingly since a decreased renal perfusion may result even when blood pressure has been increased.

Volume depletion should be treated by the intravenous administration of fluid that has a composition similar to that of extracellular fluid. Commercial solutions with this composition are available but a suitable solution can be constituted by mixing 750 ml. isotonic saline, 225 ml. 5 per cent dextrose in water and 25 ml. sodium bicarbonate (3.75 gm. in 50 ml.). Each liter of this solution provides 137 mEq. sodium, 115 mEq. chloride and 22.5 mEq. bicarbonate. Occasionally, potassium chloride may be added to the solution in a concentration of up to 4 mEq./L. Two or more liters of this synthetic ECF solution may be needed to correct volume contraction; however, the patient's response to therapy must be closely watched and central venous pressure should be monitored. At any sign of the development of circulatory overload the fluid administration should be discontinued. At this stage if there is no evidence of reversal of the renal failure, the diagnosis of dehydration as a cause of the renal failure should be reconsidered. It is preferable to have dialysis facilities available if a therapeutic trial of volume expansion is to be undertaken, since forcing fluids will not induce a diuresis in a patient with primary renal failure and may precipitate heart failure if the initial diagnosis of volume depletion was incorrect. Under such circumstances dialysis may be required to remove the excess fluid administered.

As mentioned previously, it may be difficult in some patients to determine whether renal failure is due to a pre-renal or a renal lesion and a trial of furosemide, ethacrynic acid or mannitol, using the regimens already outlined, may help to establish the diagnosis and may be of therapeutic merit.

Primary Renal Failure

As outlined earlier, the oliguric phase of acute tubular necrosis may last for as short a time as two days or up to 35 days and is followed by a diuretic phase. Treatment of the oliguric phase is exacting. It is summarized in Table 5–4 and is described in some detail on the following page.

OLIGURIC PHASE

Fluid and Electrolyte Balance. The prevention of fluid overload in the oliguric phase is one of the main reasons for improvement in the prognosis for patients with acute renal failure. Fluid requirements are calculated from the patient's fluid losses. This includes insensible loss plus

TABLE 5–4 SUMMARY OF THERAPEUTIC CONSIDERATIONS IN THE OLIGURIC PHASE OF ACUTE RENAL FAILURE

A. Fluid restriction.
   Depends on patient's status of fluid balance. Remember insensible fluid loss and ongoing abnormal losses.
B. Sodium restriction.
   If patient not volume contracted, sodium intake usually restricted to 17 mEq./day (1 gm. salt). Monitor patient's fluid sodium balance carefully.
C. Potassium restriction.
   Always watch for hyperkalemia even when intake of potassium is reduced.
D. Modification of drug dosages.
E. Maintenance of nutrition.
   Dietary protein restriction not always required. Try to provide patient with adequate caloric intake if possible.
F. Correction of acidosis.
   Not necessary to obtain a normal plasma bicarbonate.
G. Anemia.
   Consider use of packed cells. Whole blood may produce volume overload.
H. Hypertension.
   Drugs may be ineffective if significant volume overload present and dialysis may be required.
I. Anabolic steroids.
J. Infections.
   Treat existing infections—prophylactic treatment not indicated.
K. Mouth hygiene.
L. Nursing care to prevent bed sores.

fluid lost by other routes such as urine, gastric drainage or wound drainage. Insensible loss for an average adult is calculated as 300–400 ml./day with this figure increasing by 10 per cent for each degree rise in body temperature above normal. If the patient's degree of hydration is satisfactory, fluid intake should equal fluid loss. If the patient is overhydrated the amount of fluid allowed is decreased to less than that lost. Fluid intake is usually not restricted to less than 400 ml./day. If the patient is able to eat it is impossible to provide a palatable diet providing less than this amount of fluid. When calculating fluid intake it is important to remember the fluid contained in the diet and to subtract this from the total allowance.

Most patients with acute renal failure require restriction of their sodium intake. Sodium balance is calculated in a similar manner to that for water. Usually a one-gram salt (17 mEq./Na) diet is instituted. This may result in a small positive sodium balance but in the interests of palatability greater dietary restriction of sodium is not desirable. If a patient has a significant sodium loss from any source and if he is in good electrolyte balance the loss of sodium should be measured and replaced in equimolar amounts. If the patient is catabolic and requires frequent dialysis (e.g., daily), sodium restriction may be relaxed since electrolyte balance can be maintained by dialysis.

Potassium. Hyperkalemia is frequently seen in renal failure, especially if the patient has been subjected to trauma or has significant tissue necrosis. Hemolysis of the blood specimen will result in an inaccurate potassium determination. The sample should be obtained without tourniquet, without the use of excess suction and should be transferred into a dry tube after the needle has been removed from the syringe. It is preferable to use plasma for the determination; if serum is used it should be withdrawn without disturbing the clot. In addition to measuring serum potassium, an EKG should be obtained from any patient suspected of being hyperkalemic. The characteristic electrocardiographic changes of hyperkalemia are shown in Figure

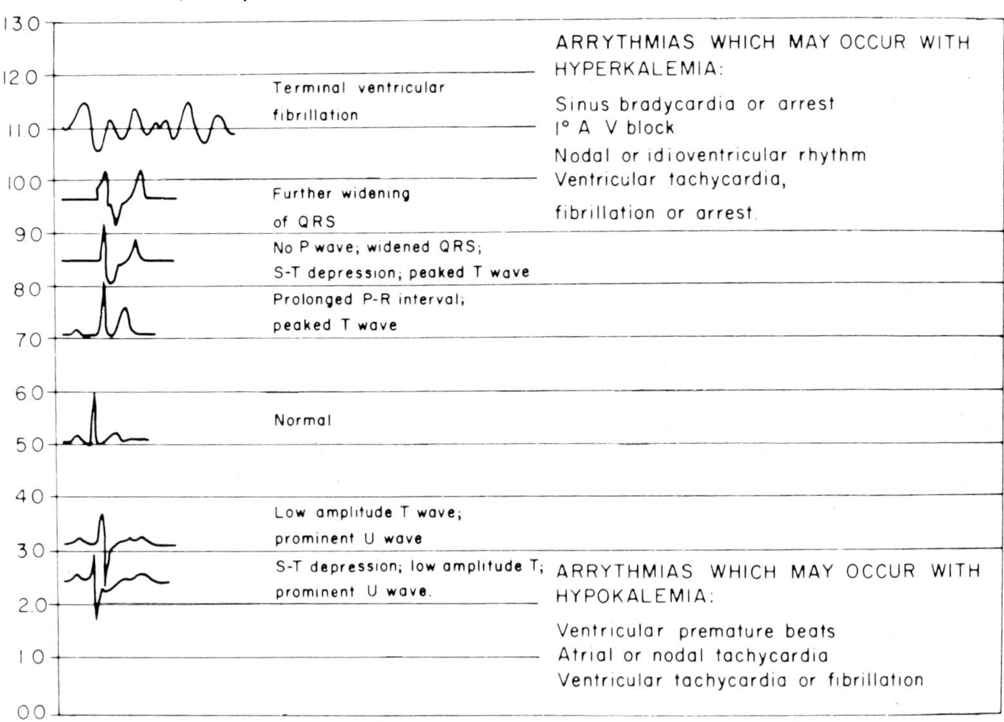

Figure 5–4 Electrocardiographic changes of hyperkalemia. (From "Principles of Pediatric Fluid Therapy," *Health Care World-Wide*, Abbott Laboratories.)

5–4. If the EKG shows hyperkalemic changes or if serum potassium levels are above 6.5 mEq./L., the patient should be treated as a medical emergency. Elevated serum potassium levels below this level require treatment but usually need not be treated as urgently. Serum potassium levels above 8 mEq./L. not only require emergency therapy but also dialysis to induce negative potassium balance.

The emergency treatment of hyperkalemia consists of administering calcium gluconate intravenously in a dose of 5 to 10 ml. of a 10 per cent solution given over a two-minute period to counteract the toxic effect of an elevated serum potassium on the heart. The EKG should be monitored continuously during this therapy. The onset of action requires one to five minutes and its effects may last for 30 minutes to two hours. Calcium should not be administered if the patient is receiving digitalis preparations.

Serum potassium can be lowered by the intravenous administration of 45 mEq. of sodium bicarbonate over a five-minute period. Effects occur within five to 10 minutes and last for about two hours. The dose may be repeated 10 to 15 minutes later if EKG abnormalities persist. Sodium bicarbonate causes an intracellular shift of potassium and does not result in negative potassium balance.

A similar effect to that seen with bicarbonate may be obtained by giving 10 units of regular insulin in 200 to 500 ml. of 10 per cent glucose intravenously over a 30-minute period. This will lower the serum potassium within one hour and will remain effective for up to 24 hours. Glucose and insulin administration is preferable to sodium bicarbonate in fluid-overload situations.

After emergency treatment, negative potassium balance should be induced by the use of either Kayexelate or dialysis. With less severe hyperkalemia the use of the ion exchange resin Kayexelate is satisfactory. Fifty grams of the resin and 50 grams of sorbitol are mixed in 200 ml. of water and given as a retention enema using an inflatable catheter, if needed, to help retention. Alternately, the resin can be given orally in a dose of 20 to 50 grams of Kayexelate in 15 ml. of sorbitol solution four times a day.

The resin requires two or more hours to be effective but has the advantage of removing approximately 1 mEq. of potassium from the patient per gram of Kayexelate administered. It should be noted that there is an equivalent exchange of sodium so that the patient gains sodium with this therapy.

With more severe levels of hyperkalemia, control can be achieved using the emergency methods outlined while preparing for dialysis. Both hemodialysis and peritoneal dialysis are effective in removing potassium. However, it may require two hours from the onset of preparation until the serum potassium begins to decrease when using either method.

Nutrition. The use of a 20-gm. protein diet may limit the rate at which azotemia develops but is of little therapeutic value if the patient has markedly increased catabolism or has significant tissue breakdown from trauma. Dietary protein restriction limits the calorie intake of the patient. It is probably more important to design a diet which allows the patient a minimum of 1500 to 2000 calories and to restrict dietary protein to this level of diet. In hypercatabolic patients survival is improved if the diet is liberalized and the patient is dialysed more frequently—often on a daily basis. This regimen usually increases the patient's feeling of well-being as well as improving prognosis.

The protein-restricted diet may be of significant advantage in minimizing hyperkalemia or acidosis in patients who are not hypercatabolic. The diet should be designed to use proteins of high biologic value whenever possible. The use of large amounts of oral fats or carbohydrates in an attempt to provide adequate calories is usually associated with nausea and vomiting and is not advocated.

Even with the best-designed dietary regimen acute renal failure patients lose approximately one pound of body weight per day. This progressive weight loss should not be interpreted to indicate volume depletion.

Other Factors. Acidosis is frequently seen in acute renal failure and is difficult to treat because the administration of bicarbonate requires the administration of sodium. A moderate reduction of serum bicarbonate to between 12 and 20 mEq./L. is usually well tolerated by the patient and rarely requires treatment. More severe or symptomatic acidosis usually requires dialysis.

Anemia should be treated with packed cells given in the smallest volume possible to maintain the hematocrit at about 25 per cent. Cardiac output is little affected until the hematocrit falls below this level. Attempts to achieve higher hematocrit values may well result in circulatory overload.

Symptomatic hypocalcemia may be very difficult to control because serum phosphorus levels are usually markedly elevated. The use of oral aluminum hydroxide gels may lower the serum phosphorus but persistent problems are best treated by dialysis.

Hemorrhage is a common problem in acute renal failure. Many defects in the coagulation system have been described and it is rare for only a single factor to be abnormal. Unnecessary trauma such as excessive venipunctures, intramuscular injections or the prolonged use of nasogastric tubes should be avoided. Hemostasis can usually be accomplished by local pressure or the use of topical thrombin with gel foam. Occasionally, the level of a coagulation factor is deficient, requiring replacement with fresh blood or the appropriate factor.

Hypertension is frequently difficult

to control. Methyldopa (Aldomet) is usually the drug of choice but may be ineffective if there is considerable circulatory overload, necessitating dialysis.

Infection is a frequent complication of acute renal failure and one of the more common causes of death. The physician should be alert for any evidence of infection, should identify the causative organism and treat appropriately. The prophylactic use of antibiotics usually results in infection with a resistant organism and should not be employed.

Anabolic steroids may reduce negative nitrogen balance during the oliguric phase of renal failure and are frequently used. These drugs may produce virilism in women if used for prolonged periods and should not be given if there is evidence of liver dysfunction. Suitable agents include methandrostenolone (Dianabol 5–10 mg. daily by mouth) and nandrolone phenpropionate (Durabolin 25–50 mg. I.M. weekly). A longer-acting agent, nandrolone decanoate (Deca-Durabolin), can be given I.M. in a dose of 50 to 100 mg. every three or four weeks.

Convulsions in patients with acute renal failure should be controlled with short-acting barbiturates given either I.M. or I.V. These drugs are excreted through the liver and therefore are more suitable in renal failure than long-acting barbiturates which are excreted in part by the kidney.

Nausea, pruritus and hiccups can be distressing features in this syndrome and are best treated with either prochlorperazine (Compazine) or chlorpromazine (Thorazine), initially given in a dose of 5 to 10 mg. every 4 hours.

Renal failure is frequently complicated by drying and cracking of the lips, gingivitis and parotitis. The administration of fluids and nutrition by mouth often helps to stimulate salivary flow and to postpone the onset of these complications which are extremely distressing for the patient. In addition, a meticulous program of mouth care including the chewing of gum may prevent the onset of parotitis.

Modification of Drug Dosage. Since many drugs are excreted by the kidney it is important to review a patient's therapy to determine whether modification of dosage is required when renal failure ensues. Some drugs such as penicillin are excreted primarily by the kidney but the difference between therapeutic and toxic levels is great and failure to modify the dose of this drug rarely results in any problems. Conversely, administration of the conventional maintenance dosage of digitalis preparations to a patient with renal shutdown will result in accumulation and toxicity. The dose of digitalis preparations required for digitalization in such patients is usually normal (we calculate it as 75 per cent of the usual dose, working on the principle that it is always easier to give the remaining 25 per cent if needed than it is to remove any excess administered drug). The maintenance dose must be reduced in proportion to the loss of renal function, giving half as much with 50 per cent loss of glomerular filtration rate and so forth until virtually no maintenance dose is given for patients with complete renal shutdown. The reduction in dosage can be accomplished either by reducing individual doses or by giving the usual maintenance dose but at appropriately increased intervals. Similar dosage schedules should be calculated for potentially toxic antibiotics such as kanamycin (Kantrex) or gentamicin (Garamycin).

A useful rule of thumb has been developed for kanamycin (Kantrex). The usual initial dose of the drug is given. Maintenance doses are given at intervals of nine hours times the serum creatinine level. Thus, in a patient with a serum creatinine of 3 mg./100 ml. the maintenance dose would be given every 27 hours.

Much has been written regarding reduced drug dosages in patients with renal failure (see Table 5–5 and References). If such information is not

TABLE 5–5 INFLUENCE OF RENAL FAILURE ON DOSAGES OF SELECTED COMMON DRUGS*

DRUG	MAINTENANCE DOSE INTERVALS				SIGNIFICANT DIALYSIS OF DRUG (H. HEMODIALYSIS; P. PERITONEAL DIALYSIS)	ROUTE OF EXCRETION NORMAL HALF-LIFE	TOXIC EFFECTS †REMARKS
		RENAL FAILURE					
	NORMAL	MILD	MODERATE	SEVERE			
Antibiotics							
Ampicillin	Q6h	Q6h	Q6h	Q8–12h†	Yes (H)	Renal Hepatic 1.5 h	†If high urine level desired, normal dosage intervals needed
Carbenicillin	Q6h	Q6h	Q6h	Q8–12h (×1.5–2)	Yes (HP)†	Renal Hepatic 1.5 h	†May add to peritoneal dialysate at desired serum level (e.g., 100 μg./ml.)
Cephalothin	Q6h	Q6h	Q6h	Q8–12h (×1.5–2)	Yes (HP)†	Renal Hepatic 0.5–0.85h	†Only moderate dialysis; if high therapeutic level needed, add one maintenance dose after H, or add drug to P dialysate at desired serum level (e.g., at 20 μg./ml.)
Chloramphenicol	Q6h	unchanged	unchanged	unchanged	No (HP)	Hepatic (Renal) 2.5h	Bone marrow toxicity adds to uremic marrow suppression
Colistimethate (Colistin)	Q12h	Q24h (×2)	Q36–60h (×3–5)	Q60–90h (×5–8)	Yes (P) No (H)	Renal 2h	Nephrotoxic; peripheral neuropathy; respiratory paralysis
Gentamicin	Q8h	Q8–12h (×1.5)	Q12–24h (×1.5–3)	Q48h (×6)	Yes (H)	Renal 2.5h	Ototoxic; nephrotoxic: incidence less than colistin or kanamycin
Kanamycin	Q8h	Q24h (×3)	Q24–72h (×3–9)	Q72–96h (×9–12)	Yes (HP)‡	Renal 3–4h	Nephrotoxic; ototoxic †Specific formula is available ‡May add to P dialysate at desired serum level (e.g., 20 μg./ml.)

Penicillin G	Q8h	Q8h	Q8h	Q12h (×1.5)	No (HP)	Renal Hepatic 0.5h	Convulsions with very high levels (hyperkalemia; penicillin G potassium has 1.7 mEq. K+ per 1 million units)
Sulfasoxisole†	Q6h	Q6h	Q8–12h (×1.5–2)	Q12–24h‡ (×2–4)	Yes (P)	Renal 3–4h	Rare crystalluria †Sulfadimidine provides adequate urine levels without greatly increased blood levels in renal failure ‡If high urine level desired, normal dosage intervals needed
Tetracycline	Q6h	Q12h (×1.5–2)	Q24–48h (×6–8)	Q72h (×12)	No (HP)	Renal Hepatic 6–8h	May potentiate acidosis; catabolic; increases BUN
Antihypertensive Agents							
Methyldopa	Q6h	Q6h	Q8–12h† (×1.5–2)	Q12–18h† (×2–3)	Yes (H)	Renal Hepatic	Prolonged hypotension †Blood pressure best guide to dose intervals
Cardiac Glycosides							
Digoxin	Q12h	Q24h† (×2)	Q24h–36h† (×2–3)	Q36–48† (×3–4)	No (HP)	Renal (Nonrenal: 15%) 36h	Adds to uremic GI symptoms arrhythmias †Common clinical practice dictates cutting size as well as interval of maintenance dose; blood level best guide

*From Bennett, W. M., Singer, I., and Coggins, C. H.: J.A.M.A. *214*:1468, 1970.

readily available, a telephone call to the drug manufacturer can be very helpful.

Dialysis. Dialysis facilities should always be available for the patient with acute renal failure. In the early days of dialysis, this procedure was rarely performed until the blood urea nitrogen rose to 200 mg. per cent or greater. It is now apparent that better results are obtained by dialysing patients at an earlier stage of their disease, especially if they present with symptoms of uremia. Other indications for dialysis include hyperkalemia, severe acidosis, hypocalcemia with hyperphosphatemia, circulatory overload, anemia (especially in the face of an increased blood volume) and intractable hypertension.

The decision whether to employ hemodialysis or peritoneal dialysis is influenced by many factors. Hemodialysis corrects biochemical abnormalities more rapidly than peritoneal dialysis but these rapid changes in the milieu may result in the well-described "disequilibrium syndrome." Moreover, hemodialysis requires cannulation of an artery and vein and heparin must be administered to prevent coagulation of the blood in the artificial kidney. Preparation of the patient for hemodialysis may take a considerable period of time and an artificial kidney may not be available when needed.

Many surgical units use peritoneal dialysis as the method of choice. This method is often more readily available than is hemodialysis but it, too, has disadvantages. With a recent abdominal operation, dialysis fluid may leak through the wound or cause dehiscence. Introduction of the peritoneal dialysis catheter may perforate the bowel if adhesions are present. Ileus impairs the effectiveness of exchange across the peritoneum. Peritoneal dialysis is also associated with marked protein loss which may be a significant factor in a debilitated patient.

Under ideal circumstances with adequate facilities and staff, the optimum results are probably obtained by maintaining the blood urea nitrogen below 100 mg. per cent at all times. In patients with severe trauma, this may necessitate daily hemodialysis but has the advantage of allowing a more liberal dietary regimen.

EARLY DIURETIC PHASE

As mentioned earlier, the onset of diuresis in a patient with acute renal failure is an encouraging sign, but the physician must not relax his vigilance since 25 to 50 per cent of deaths from acute renal failure occur during this phase of the disease. The most common complications at this stage are infection and electrolyte depletion.

During the early diuretic phase both glomerular and tubular functions are depressed and the urine usually contains high levels of sodium and potassium. This may represent the loss of edema fluid accumulated during the period of oliguria, however, in some patients the natriuresis and kaliuresis are inappropriate and can threaten the patient's survival. If there is no contraindication, free access to salt and water should be allowed during the first few days of the diuretic phase. Frequently, this provides adequate replacement of urinary losses of electrolytes and water. If oral intake is insufficient, replacement of electrolytes and fluid must be given by intravenous infusion. The great importance of carefully monitoring the patient during this phase of the disease must be emphasized. As the diuretic phase of ATN continues, renal function progressively improves and the kidney is better able to regulate body composition.

PROGNOSIS

Prior to the advent of the artificial kidney and other modern forms of therapy, the death rate in patients with acute renal failure was greater than 90 per cent. Although present figures show a marked improvement in survival, the death rate is still high. In reports recently published from several large referral centers, 53 per cent of patients died despite intensive dialysis. This figure was obviously influenced by the type of patient being treated at these centers, often older patients and those with prolonged oliguria and severe complicated illnesses being seen. Milder forms of the syndrome were not usually referred. However, this experience illustrates that acute renal failure is still a serious medical problem.

The etiology of renal failure affects survival rate. In the patients cited above, 88 per cent with obstetrical causes for renal failure survived in contrast to 40 per cent with a post-surgical or traumatic etiology. Survival from acute renal failure in older patients undergoing surgery is uncommon.

Mortality factors are numerous but infection is probably the most common, accounting for approximately one-third of all deaths. Gram-negative organisms are often responsible with pneumococci, clostridia and fungal infections also being seen. Fungal infections due to Candida are occurring with increasing frequency. A high percentage of patients die from their primary disease even though the renal failure may have been reversed. Hemorrhage, hyperkalemia and other electrolyte abnormalities, unexplained shock, digitalis intoxication and uremia are other causes of death commonly seen.

CONCLUSIONS

The patient with acute renal failure has the greatest chance of survival if referred to a medical center equipped with dialysis facilities, to be treated by a medical team experienced in dealing with these problems. However, early recognition, appropriate diagnosis and prompt conservative management will also result in markedly improved survival.

Physicians dealing with trauma should always be alert for the development of acute renal failure and should be familiar with the principles of management of this syndrome. It is these areas which have been stressed in the foregoing discussion.

REFERENCES

Reviews

Muehrcke, R. C.: Acute Renal Failure: Diagnosis and Management. C. V. Mosby Company, St. Louis, 1969.

Dossetor, J. R., and Gault, M. H.: Nephron Failure. Charles C Thomas, Springfield, Ill., 1971.

Schreiner, G. E.: Acute renal failure. *In* Renal Disease. (2nd Ed.) D. A. K. Black, ed. F. A. Davis Co., Philadelphia, 1967, p. 309.

Merrill, J. P.: Acute renal failure. *In* Diseases of the Kidney. (2nd Ed.) M. B. Strauss, and L. G. Welt, eds. Little, Brown and Company, Boston, 1971, p. 637.

Diagnostic Tests

Blaufox, M. D., ed.: Evaluation of renal function and disease with radionuclides. University Park Press, Baltimore, 1972.

Management

Anderson, E. E.: Surgery of dialysis. *In* Urologic Surgery. (1st Ed.) J. F. Glenn and W. H. Boyce, eds. Hoeber Medical Division, Harper & Row, New York, 1969, p. 746.

Bennett, W. M., Singer, I. and Coggins, C. H.: A practical guide to drug usage in adult patients with impaired renal function. J.A.M.A. *214*:1469, 1970.

Levinsky, N. G.: Acute renal failure. *In* Management of Emergencies. New Eng. J. Med. *274*:1016, 1966.

Lewis, E. J., and Magill, J. W., eds.: Nutritional aspects of uremia. Amer. J. Clin. Nutr. *21*: 349–643, 1968.

Milne, M. D., ed.: Management of renal failure. Brit. Med. Bull. *27*:95–185, 1971.

Smith, D. R., Schulte, J. W. and Smart, W. R.: Surgery of the kidney. *In* Urology. (3rd Ed.) M. R. Campbell and J. H. Harrison, eds. W. B. Saunders Co., Philadelphia, 1970, p. 2186.

Prognosis

Stott, R. B., Cameron, J. S., Ogg, C. S. K., and Bewick, M.: Why the persistently high mortality in acute renal failure? Lancet *2*:75, 1972.

Lordon, R. E., and Burton, J. R.: Post-traumatic renal failure in military personnel in Southeast Asia. Amer. J. Med. *53*:137, 1972.

chapter

6

INJURIES OF THE HEAD AND SPINAL CORD

A. Earl Walker, M.D.
George B. Udvarhelyi, M.D.
J. Donald McQueen, M.D.
Charles D. Ray, M.D.
Edward R. Laws, Jr., M.D.
and
Perry Black, M.D., C.M.

INTRODUCTION

A. Earl Walker, M.D.

When hand to hand combat was common, the head apparently was recognized as a vulnerable target. Helmets—often bulky, heavy and obviously uncomfortable—are depicted in the graphic records of early ages. Although the uniform of the warrior has changed greatly, the use of protective head gear has remained a symbol of the profession. When gunpowder was introduced, the larger parts of the body became easy targets for balls and bullets, but the head still required a helmet of some type.

The importance of head injuries in early times is further documented by the emphasis placed upon it in ancient medical and surgical manuscripts. Breasted's papyrus devoted a section to head wounds. Hippocrates likewise has a book *Of Injuries of the Head.* In Roman and Byzantine manuscripts a prominent place is given to discussion of these wounds. In the Middle

Ages the surgical treatment of head injuries apparently fell into disrepute, perhaps because treatment by trephination of such injuries increased rather than decreased their morbidity and mortality.

In later centuries, as modern warfare developed high velocity arms that could mortally wound an individual with an injury of the chest or of the abdomen, the head was no longer the prime target of the soldier. However, in recent years the frequency and seriousness of head injuries have again come to the fore. Not open warfare but accidents, especially automobile, have subjected the head to trauma.

In most countries of the world, accidents are the number one cause of death in young people. In Canada they kill more people between infancy and middle age than any other condition. These injuries do not all involve the central nervous system. However, 60 per cent of all traffic accidents involve the head and in the category of fatal accidents the percentage rises to 70. In two-thirds of these cases, the injuries to the head are the cause of death. This figure is about the same in all populous countries of the world, although in underprivileged lands where car traffic is minimal, falls or assaults are more common causes of head injury.

The tremendous increase in traffic accidents is attributable to the increase in the number of cars on the road and to the speed of travel. Safety measures in the design of cars and the construction of roads have advanced, but not to the extent that they have in industry. Because of the vested interest of industrial firms in their workers, preventive measures for the protection of the employees have been adopted. On the other hand, although a great number of safety measures have been suggested for the regulation of automobiles and their use, relatively few have been put into practice.

The magnitude of the accident problem is difficult to define accurately because of the lack of precise figures. Automobile collisions causing a certain amount of damage must be reported, but many car accidents do not involve a second party. Falls and injuries in the home are rarely brought to the attention of the accident prevention bureaus, yet they constitute about one-third of all accidents. It has been estimated that each year one person in 200 will require medical care for a head injury. At the present time, approximately 1 per cent of the entire working community is disabled on any one day as the result of a head injury.

The problem concerns not only the safety divisions of the bureaus of traffic and roads but is of serious moment to the medical profession since trauma constitutes one of the major conditions with which physicians must contend. This problem is of particular interest to the general practitioner because he is usually the first to see the person with a head injury; and what he does in the first few hours may be the difference between life and death or permanent disability. Accordingly, it is imperative that general practitioners and house officers serving in emergency treatment rooms be well informed about the emergency treatment of head injuries. Unfortunately, many medical school courses emphasize long-term treatment of head injuries to the neglect of emergency treatment. House officers are too often more prone to rush the patient from the accident room to the x-ray department to check for skull fracture than to determine that the airway is patent and that shock is adequately treated. The best methods of maintaining pulmonary ventilation should be clearly understood. In such cases intratracheal intubation is of great importance. The administration of oxygen to such patients may be life-saving, or at least "brain saving."

The role of the general surgeon and the emergency room surgeon in such cases is of extreme importance. By the time a specialist in neurological surgery is called and sees the patient, the patient's fate is often decided. Bleeding into the intracranial cavity, an important factor in acute head injuries, is an extremely common cause of death and is thought to occur in almost 50 per cent of individuals who have prolonged periods of unconsciousness following a head injury. Studies by medical examiners in a number of different countries have indicated that intracranial hemorrhage is a cause of death in approximately 35 to 50 per cent of patients who come to autopsy following head injury. Sano[57] reported that 34.2 per cent of *500 medical examiner's cases* in Tokyo had had intracranial hemorrhage.

If an individual is comatose an hour after an accident, there is an estimated 50 per cent chance of a massive hemorrhage, with or without brain damage. Because the general practitioner or surgeon often hesitates to call a specialist so early, many people die from such hemorrhages without having received adequate treatment. Frohwein, in Germany, estimated that 30 per cent of patients with head injury had unrecognized hematomas in spite of improved techniques for their diagnosis.

As knowledge of a subject develops, concepts are denoted by terms incorporated into the common usage. By the time a term is generally accepted in a subject that is not well understood or that is in a state of flux the connotation of that term may no longer be valid. Thus, words in common usage may denote outmoded scientific concepts. Many such examples might be cited in the field of head injuries. Concussion, contusion and compression are time-honored terms that are used differently by the laity and the medical profession. Even more recently introduced terms such as acceleration-deceleration and compression concussion are often misused, for the former was once considered unassociated with a rise in intracranial pressure, and the latter to be due to intracranial hypertension. It is now known that both are related to intracranial stresses, one of which is hypertension. In an attempt to lessen the confusion concerning nomenclature, the terms used in this section will follow the glossary recently formulated by the Nomenclature Committee of the Congress of Neurological Surgeons. A few of the more common terms are given here.

Consciousness. A state of general wakefulness and responsiveness to environment. Impairment of consciousness may be of any degree of severity. Terms such as lethargy, drowsiness, stupor, semicoma and coma are commonly used, with varying connotations. There is no unanimity of opinion on the precise meaning of these terms.

Brain Concussion. A clinical syndrome characterized by immediate and transient impairment of neural function, such as alteration of consciousness, and disturbance of vision and equilibrium, due to mechanical forces.

Brain Contusion (Bruise). A structural alteration of the brain, usually involving the surface, characterized by extravasation of blood cells and death of tissue, with or without edema. Clinical manifestations of the contusion depend on the area and the extent of the injured tissue.

Closed Head Injury. A head injury in which continuity of the scalp and mucous membranes is maintained.

Open Head Injury. A head injury in which there is loss of continuity of scalp or mucous membranes. The term is sometimes used to indicate a communication between the exterior and the intracranial cavity. (See Penetrating Wound.)

Penetrating Wound. An open wound in which the dura mater is pierced.

The following sections dealing with more specific aspects of head and spinal cord injury are, for the reasons mentioned, written for the general surgeon and house officer rather than for the neurosurgical specialist.

THE DIAGNOSIS OF CRANIOCEREBRAL INJURIES

George B. Udvarhelyi, M.D.

In civilian practice a majority of the patients brought into the emergency rooms of hospitals with craniocerebral trauma have injuries of the closed type. By definition, in closed head injuries the brain and its coverings have not been penetrated by any missile and there is no evidence of compound fracture of the skull with subsequent exteriorization of the brain. In cases of compound fractures of the skull, the injury is usually apparent to the layman who may be present at the time of the injury and to the physician who receives the injured patient. The real diagnostic difficulty in closed head injuries lies in the correct and timely recognition of intracranial damage.[5]

THE IMPORTANCE OF A CAREFUL HISTORY

Even in cases that represent an extreme surgical emergency, clear-cut information about the type and mode of injury has great practical value. Eyewitness descriptions of the accident should be carefully evaluated. If the patient has already been seen by a physician before arriving at the emergency treatment room of the hospital, the doctor's findings, if known, should be meticulously recorded.

Injuries to the central nervous system may be manifest in various ways. In general, any moderately severe head injury will cause some interruption of the normal function of the central nervous system. In most instances this is not specific; von Monakow[43] called the effect of any sudden impact on the structure of the brain "diaschisis." In moderate-to-severe head injuries, loss of consciousness at the outset is the rule. Since the subsequent prognosis for recovery depends partly on the length of the period of unconsciousness, reliable information on this is very helpful.

In addition to the immediate derangement of the function of the brain as a whole, local damage to various parts of the brain or its coverings may occur at the time of the head injury. Such local damage may be masked in the beginning by the immediate generalized effect of the injury. However, quite often it is possible to detect symptoms that indicate motor weakness of one side of the body or of individual limbs, brainstem involvement, pupillary disturbances and faulty coordination of the eye movements, and so forth. Changes in vital signs (pulse rate, blood pressure, respiration and temperature) also occur. Slowing of pulse and respiration coupled with elevation of blood pressure and temperature indicates increasing severity of head injury.[77] It should be emphasized, however, that concomitant injuries to other systems often complicate the clinical picture. Their recognition at the time of the injury is important in choosing an intelligent plan for step-by-step management of the patient.

Although the causal relationship between the injury and subsequent brain damage can usually be established, the examiner must also consider the possibility of pre-existing disease processes, such as diabetes, hypertension, renal insufficiency or a severe heart condition, since these may worsen as a result of the head injury. Occasionally, head injuries produce bleeding from a congenital vascular malformation, aneurysm or tumor; therefore, relevant data about the patient's status prior to the injury may be of great help in arriving at the right diagnosis. It is also important to investigate the possibility of concomitant injury to the cervical spine, a not uncommon occurrence when there are severe head injuries (Fig. 6–1).

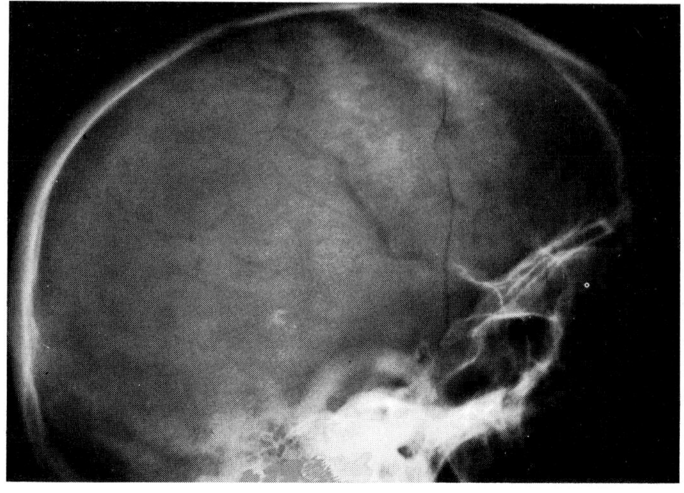

A

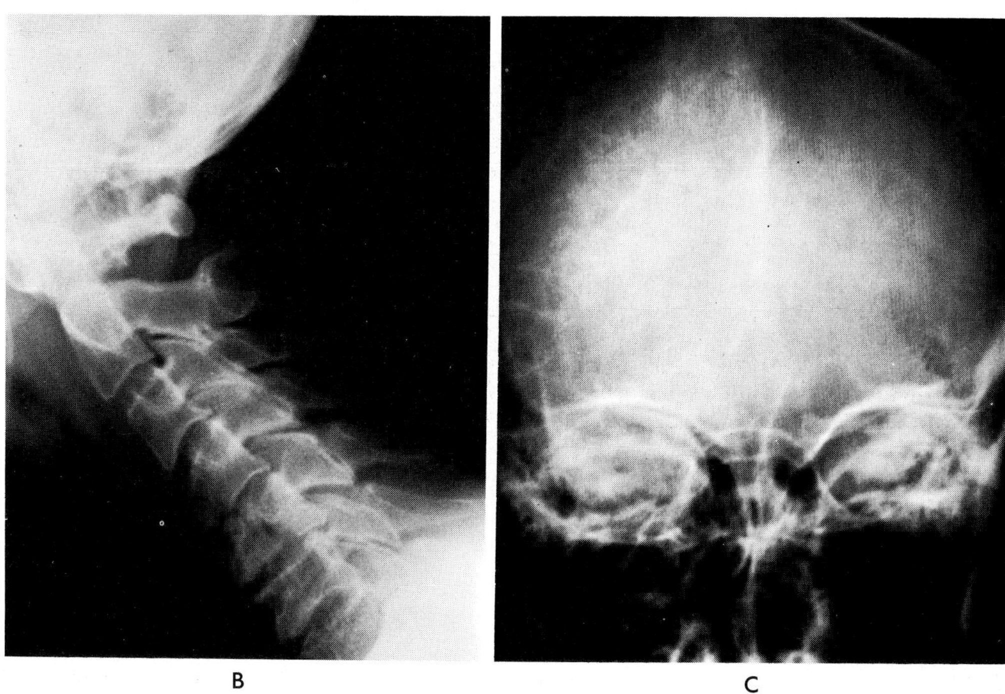

B C

Figure 6–1 *A*, Radiograph of the skull, lateral view. Irregular, linear fracture, running through the middle meningeal vascular groove. *B*, Radiograph of the cervical spine (lateral view) of the same patient, showing compression-fracture with multiple dislocations at C5-C6 and C7. *C*, Right carotid angiogram, anteroposterior view, capillary phase. An epidural hematoma of considerable size is demonstrated as an avascular area between the internal table and cerebral cortex over the right hemisphere.

GENERAL EXAMINATION

Careful examination should be performed to determine the existence of injuries to other organs and systems. The acute head injury is a multidisciplinary problem. Respiratory, cardiovascular and abdominal implications, metabolic disturbances, wounds of the accessory cranial sinuses, complicating injuries of the cervical spine and limb fractures form the most essential parts of a broad spectrum.[72] Judgment in assigning priorities within a cooperative team is essential to handle such complex situations. These aspects are discussed in detail in other sections of the book. Inspection of the whole body after removal of all clothing is mandatory. The recognition and immediate treatment of shock should precede other system evaluations and treatment of the head injury. If there are signs of aspiration or choking, immediate intubation or tracheostomy and clearing of the airway must be undertaken before further examination of the patient.

The patient with a head injury should be placed immediately on a special "head chart" regimen, with frequent recordings of pulse rate, blood pressure, respiratory rate and temperature. It is important to remain alert to the possibility of progressive signs that may be caused by gradual increase of intracranial pressure, even in the presence of concomitant and apparently severe injuries to the extremities or to other organ systems. Oversight in this regard can have a tragic result if dangerous but remediable hemorrhages such as an epidural hematoma are overlooked because of concentrated efforts to deal with a compound fracture of a femur or a pneumohemothorax.

Careful examination of the scalp, head, face and neck should precede special neurological tests. Abrasions, contusions, subcutaneous hematomas and lacerations should be recorded. Gentle palpation of the head may reveal the existence of subcutaneous hematomas or fractures of the calvaria. Palpation must be done with care, however; in some instances of skull fracture, brain substance may be extruded through a torn dura, and undue pressure on dislocated bone fragments may cause further neurological damage.

Hematomas in the periorbital and perinasal areas, or along the neck musculature, are suggestive of possible underlying and more profound damage. Cerebrospinal fluid leak through the nose (rhinorrhea) or through the ear (otorrhea) should be recognized at an early stage of the examination. Fractures of the skull base, quite often not recognizable on routine x-ray examination, may produce "hematomas-at-distance," which usually occur around the eye, in the eyelids and over the mastoid processes. Such hematomas, together with the presence of rhinorrhea or otorrhea, are highly suggestive of basal skull fracture, even in the absence of radiographic confirmation.

If, after thorough search, doubt exists about the presence or the extent of hematomas or lacerations in the area of the scalp covered by hair, the entire head should be shaved to permit a more complete and reliable assessment at the time of the first inspection.

NEUROLOGICAL EXAMINATION

It is outside the scope of this chapter to describe the various stages of a complete neurological examination. Most physicians who are not regularly engaged in diagnosis of neurological diseases have an understandable but unfounded aversion to assessment of disorders within the central nervous system. It is, however, usually not necessary to apply the rigorous rules of a highly specialized neurological evaluation to reach a correct diagnosis. As Klingler[33] has pointed out, the following aspects should be covered in evaluating the condition of a patient with head injury who is admitted to the emergency room:

1. Assessment of the level of consciousness.
2. Assessment of posture and movements (motor system), including reflexes.
3. Evaluation of eye movements and pupils.
4. Evaluation of gross focal neurological deficit.

Assessment of the Level of Consciousness

A clear definition of unconsciousness is still debatable. Russell states: "The state of full consciousness is that in which any occurrence in which the patient is actively or passively concerned, makes an impression on the memory, and can be subsequently called to mind. Any state of consciousness less than this is to be regarded as a grade of unconsciousness."[56]

Symonds[66] points out, however, that the only practicable criterion of "recovery of consciousness" is awareness of external environment and accessibility, as proposed by Mapother.[40] As stated in the introduction, the terms coma, semicoma, stupor, lethargy and drowsiness have been used with various connotations in the past. For practical purposes, an operational description is more valuable. According to Rowbotham,[53] the depth of consciousness may be judged by the reactions of the patient to external stimuli, on various levels.

Unconsciousness. The patient may be completely unconscious, without any psychologically understandable responses either to external stimuli or to inner needs. Although corneal reflexes, swallowing or some of the tendon reflexes may be present, in deep coma they are generally absent, which indicates severe damage to the brainstem. Urinary retention is common.

Response to Stimuli. A patient may respond to painful stimuli. Occasionally, there is some purposeful defense-reaction, expressed by grimacing or hand movements to push away the examiner's hand. The primitive reflexes are all present. The bladder will empty reflexly whenever it becomes distended. No meaningful response can be obtained on questioning.

Confusion. There is little uniformity in describing the state of confusion. A patient may be disoriented in place, time or person. He may present some trend of thought that quite often may be suddenly interrupted, giving way to inappropriate statements or behavior. The Medical Research Council of England[78] proposed a classification, which was adopted during the Second World War and consists of three categories.

SEVERE CONFUSION. These patients generally show loss of touch with their surroundings. However, on repeated stimuli, occasionally reinforced by painful stimuli, they are able to perform simple orders (open eyes, put out the tongue, and so forth).

MODERATE CONFUSION. The patients are generally out of touch with their surroundings, but with some insistence they may give relevant answers to simple questions (inquiries about their age, domicile, type of work).

MILD CONFUSION. The patient is generally capable of coherent conversation and appropriate behavior.

Assessment of the level of consciousness at the time of arrival at the emergency room should always be considered in the light of the information obtained by the history. If the patient was unconscious for only a short period of time, with a subsequent relatively lucid interval followed by progressive clouding of consciousness again, the possibility of an increasing hematoma inside the intracranial cavity, usually extradural in location, is the best working diagnosis. If the patient was found only mildly confused at the time of injury, but during the following hours a gradual decrease in the level of consciousness occurred, progressive shift of the intracranial contents can be assumed, caused either by increasing edema or by collection of blood in the subdural space or in the cerebral parenchyma. On the other hand, if the level of consciousness shows definite evidence of clearing, the patient probably is on the way to recovery from the initial derangement of cerebral function and will not need surgical intervention. Only about 10 to 15 per cent of patients who suffer from head injury will require operation.

From the practical point of view it should again be emphasized that, in evaluation of the involvement of consciousness, the "time-profile" is important. Evidence of progressive deterioration should alert the examining surgeon to the possible need for immediate action. These patients may require special diagnostic studies or, in cases of extreme emergency, immediate exploration. Unnecessary delay in diagnosis and treatment may result in irreversible secondary damage to the brainstem from massive herniation of the cerebral hemisphere and pressing of the brainstem against the sharp edge of the tentorium or from secondary vascular compression inside the tentorial notch.

Assessment of Posture and Motor Function

Complete flaccidity of all limbs and a flaccid jaw are usually exhibited when the patient is still in the initial state of severe shock. If such general flaccidity persists, the prognosis is poor.

The term "decerebrate rigidity" is used to describe the signs that generally indicate severe injury to the brainstem, usually below the red nucleus. The patient shows extensor rigidity of all four limbs, with adduction and rotation of the upper extremities on painful stimuli. The ankles are generally plantar flexed, the hips and knees are fully extended. Passive movements are difficult to elicit, and severe spasm usually is present. No reflexes can be elicited. In extreme cases, in addition to the rigidity of the extremities, opisthotonus can also be found. This situation is compatible with primary brainstem injury, although occasionally a rapidly developing hematoma can cause similar postural changes, indicating additional secondary damage to the stem.

The most common motor sign is evidence of a hemiparesis or hemiplegia. Only occasionally is a monoparesis present. In a comatose patient the hemiplegic limbs can usually be recognized by their decreased tone, the muscles taking the position determined by gravity. The lower extremity is externally rotated, the foot is slightly dropped and turned outward. When elevated by the examiner, the arm or leg is usually hypotonic, especially in the early period after the injury. By use of painful stimuli (a pinprick or pinch) some movement of the limb may be elicited and the degree of paretic involvement assessed. If, in addition to the hemiparetic syndrome, contralateral involvement of one or several cranial nerves is present, the diagnosis of localized brainstem injury can be made, the clinical picture being that of "alternating hemiplegia."

In a few instances, when the lesion is below the vestibular nuclei, marked spasm of the flexor muscles occurs, causing acute flexion of the limbs and body (Fig. 6–2).

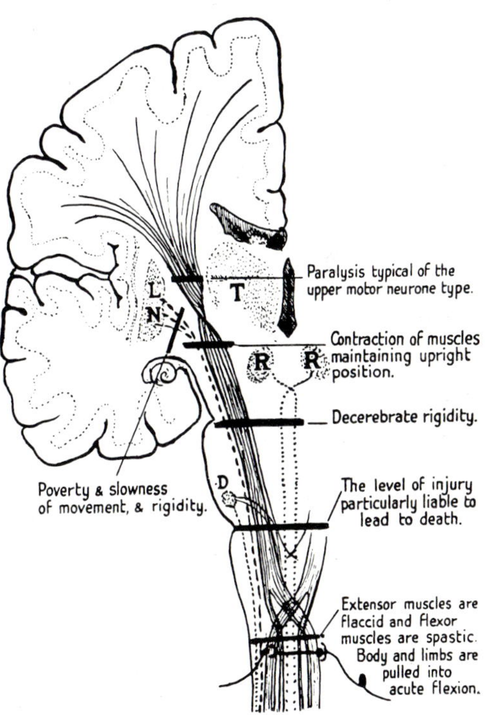

Figure 6–2 The pyramidal and extrapyramidal pathways. According to the level of interruption of these pathways different nervous phenomena ensue. This is one of the main reasons why the clinical pictures in head injuries are so variable. *LN*, Lenticular nucleus; *T*, optic thalamus; *R*, red nucleus; *D*, Deiters' nucleus.

The motor weakness usually also involves the muscles of the face. In moderate disturbance of consciousness that produces various degrees of confusion, some information may be obtainable from the patient about any sensory involvement, including visual fields. If a combination of motor, sensory and hemianoptic visual-field defects is present, the lesion is in all probability in the region of the internal capsule and indicates an intracerebral hematoma or severe interruption of the fiber tracts at this level.

If the patient also has signs and symptoms indicating poverty or slowness of purposeful movements, various degrees of tremor or rigidity, concomitant involvement of the subcortical nuclei can be assumed. The reflexes may be hyperactive, and pathological reflexes may be present. However, in most cases the patients are not seen until a few hours after the acute injury, at which time these reflex changes may not be manifest.

Evaluation of Eye Movements and the Pupils

Eye Deviation. Conjugate deviation of both eyes toward the paralyzed side indicates a lesion of the frontal adversive fields. Spontaneous nystagmus may be present from damage to the cerebellum or the vestibular connections. Skew deviation of the eyes occurs in injuries to the brainstem. Frequently, uncoordinated movements of the eyes, without fixation, can be observed on careful observation, another sign of severe brainstem involvement. Local damage to the orbit or to the eye muscles can also be responsible for deviation of the eyes from the axis. A common finding in severe head injuries is involvement of the third or sixth cranial nerves, and recognition of this is highly important. Since the third cranial nerve innervates all the eye muscles except the superior oblique and the external rectus, paralysis of the third nerve will result in an external deviation of the eye, with slight downward rotation. If there is complete interruption of third nerve function, the pupil will also be dilated and fixed. If the sixth cranial nerve is involved alone, pupillary reaction will not be involved; but the eye will be deviated inward by the other intact muscles innervated by the third and fourth cranial nerves.

Pupillary Reaction. The examination of the pupils is of great importance. If one pupil is dilated and fixed from the very beginning of the injury, this generally means either direct trauma to the third nerve or a very sudden increase of intracranial pressure, as can occur in intraventricular hemorrhage. However, if the pupils were noted to have been of the same size just after the injury, but during the subsequent hours one pupil starts to dilate, a progressive lesion is present that requires immediate diagnosis and treatment. Since the third cranial nerve can be damaged at any point in its entire course from the upper brainstem to the eye bulb, the exact clinical significance of the involvement of the third nerve can be more correctly evaluated if it is considered together with the changes in the level of consciousness.

If the patient is fully awake and oriented, third nerve involvement generally means damage to this nerve in the orbit, in the superior orbital fissure or in the cavernous sinus. If, however, the level of consciousness is definitely involved, or the patient is in a coma, third nerve involvement by compression through a transtentorial herniation is more likely. Rapid progressive involvement of the third cranial nerve requires immediate measures; no time should be wasted with unnecessary diagnostic studies, since the probability of an epidural or acute subdural hematoma is high. Frequent careful observation of the pupillary size and reactions and the position of the eyes is mandatory; these should be checked as frequently as possible, with the recording of the vital signs.

A very small, nonreactive pupil in a patient who is in coma or semicoma is generally indicative of primary involvement of the brainstem. This is also the case if sudden changes in the pupillary size are noted within a relatively short period of time. Sudden pupillary constriction, or sudden dilation of one or both pupils in irregular fashion, is a severe sign and generally indicates a poor prognosis. The consensual reaction of the pupils should also be investigated. Occasionally, a pupil does not react to direct stimulus by light because the optic nerve is damaged; however, good contraction can be elicited when light is thrown into the opposite eye. This means that the damage is in the afferent part of the reflex arc (the optic nerve) and not in the efferent limb (third cranial nerve).

Fundus Examination. Examination of the "eyegrounds" (fundus) may be of some value, although development of significant papilledema within a few hours of cerebral injury is infrequent. The presence of hemorrhages, especially subhyaloid hemorrhages, is indicative of severe head injury with subarachnoid bleeding. A warning should be given to avoid drugs such as homatropine to dilate the pupils for a better view of the eyegrounds. Paralysis of the iris constrictor muscles by miotics prevents careful observation of the pupillary reaction for signs of progressive involvement of the third cranial nerve.

Focal Neurological Deficit. Certain focal neurological deficits can be established even by surgeons or residents who are not familiar with the intricacies of detailed neurological examination. The possible presence of aphasia should be checked if the patient is fully conscious or only mildly confused. *Expressive aphasia* is an inability to formulate words because of lesions of the dominant hemisphere, mostly in the area of the third frontal convolution or within the insular region affecting the intercortical connections of the various speech centers. *Receptive aphasia* is an inability to understand spoken or written words; this indicates a more posterior lesion of the dominant hemisphere, in the neighborhood of the angular gyrus in the lower parietal area. (It is important for the examiner to distinguish between an aphasic patient and one who has a severe degree of confusion or is in semicoma.)

Marked parietal damage in either hemisphere may result in various degrees of apraxia, a condition in which the patient is not able to use the contralateral limbs; this should not be confused with the presence of hemiparesis or hemiplegia. Extrapyramidal motor disorder may be present and indicates focal involvement of the basal ganglia. Marked ataxia of the peripheral type (as manifested in the finger-nose or knee-heel test), or of the more central type (as manifested in truncal ataxia or inability to walk), may indicate involvement of the cerebellum or its connections.

Occasionally, damage to the lower cranial nerves can be established; the patient may show inability to swallow, difficulty of phonation from involvement of the vocal cords and weakness of the sternocleidomastoid and trapezius muscles from injury to the eleventh cranial nerve. Deviation of the tongue and the uvula indicates injury of the twelfth cranial nerve. In cooperating patients, the finding of complete homonymous hemianopsia (or occasionally quadrant hemianopsia) can provide strong evidence that the lesion is located in the optic radiation, either in the posterior limb of the internal capsule or in the temporal lobe near the occipital cortex.

A focal seizure discharge occurs infrequently but may be of diagnostic value in locating a lesion. However, it should be emphasized that postictal involvement of the corresponding contralateral limbs should not be misinterpreted as indicating permanent hemiparesis or hemiplegia. Focal, or occasionally generalized, epileptic discharges may be observed starting a few hours after the head injury. This generally indicates that the lesions—from cerebral concussion or laceration, mostly related to compound fractures or penetrating injuries to the brain—are located in the area of the motor strip or in its immediate vicinity. The more marked participation of one limb (leg versus arm) or even the face may facilitate a more exact focal diagnosis.

SPECIAL DIAGNOSTIC AIDS

Various special diagnostic methods are of value in assessing more accurately the type and site of head injury and its intracranial complications. Although these techniques are valuable, they should be used with judgment and discretion. In most cases, plain skull x-rays and perhaps echoencephalography will be sufficient as a screening technique.

X-ray Examination. Routine x-ray examination of the skull should be performed after the general and neurological examination have excluded the possibility of cervical spine fracture, dislocation of the atlanto-occipital joint (with or without fracture of the odontoid process) and other conditions in which any excessive movement including the necessary flexion or extension of the head to obtain the desired quality of radiograph, is contraindicated. The routine films should include:[21]

ANTEROPOSTERIOR VIEW. This should be taken with the patient lying face up on the radiography table, with the orbitomeatal line perpendicular to the table and the tube inclined 25 degrees caudally.

HALF-AXIAL VIEW. (Towne's projection.) This is made with a 35 degree inclination of the tube caudally (using the same position of patient as previously).

POSTEROANTERIOR VIEW. The patient is in the face-down position with the tube inclined 25 degrees caudally, and the orbitomeatal line perpendicular to the table.

LATERAL VIEWS. Right and left lateral views are taken with the patient in the supine, brow-up position and with the central beam horizontal, entering a point approximately 1 cm. above the external auditory meatus.

BASAL VIEWS. If the clinical and neurological examinations indicate a possible *basal skull fracture*, a basal view (and possibly oblique views of the petrous pyramids) should be obtained. The recognition of a basal fracture on the routine films, including the basal and oblique views, is occasionally very difficult; probably in a majority of cases such a fracture cannot be seen on the radiograph obtained in the emergency room. On the other hand, the presence of a skull fracture (or even several fractures) does not necessarily indicate the exact severity of a head injury;[71] multiple linear fractures may be present without any significant neurological involvement. However, the recognition of linear fractures has significance, especially if there is indication that the fracture line is crossing some of the important vascular channels, particularly the middle meningeal artery or its ramifications, or some of the large venous sinuses (Figs. 6–1, 6–3, 6–4, and 6–5).

The recognition of a *depressed fracture* has more importance (Fig. 6–6). If there is radiographic evidence of depressed fracture that shows displacement more than 4 mm. in depth, surgical intervention (elevation of the fracture) is indicated, even in the absence of neurological deficit or altered consciousness. The importance of skull radiographs in cases of *compound fracture* is evident. The same is true of *penetrating injuries* from missiles. The location of the bullet, the assessment of the trajectory and the possibility of concomitant injuries to the sinuses should be evaluated on the basis of the appropriate radiographs (Figs. 6–7 and 6–8). Plain radiographs of the skull may be of significant value in assessing the presence of a *space-occupying lesion* inside the

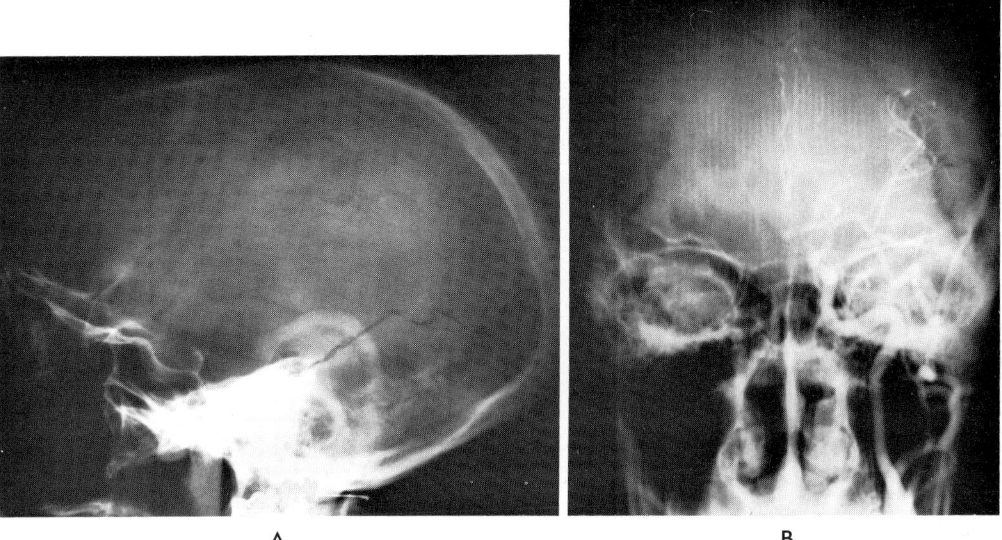

Figure 6–3 *A*, Radiograph of the skull, lateral view. Temporo-occipital linear fracture, crossing ramifications of the middle meningeal vessels. *B*, Left carotid angiogram, anteroposterior view, showing elevation and inward displacement of the middle cerebral artery and mild shift of the anterior cerebral artery, caused by an extradural hematoma, originating underneath the fracture line.

cranial cavity. Since the pineal gland is calcified in about 70 per cent of the population beyond the age of 20, displacement of the calcified pineal gland indicates the presence of a space-occupying lesion, in the form of localized or diffuse cerebral edema or epidural or subdural hematomas (Fig. 6–9). Occasionally, displacement of a calcified choroid plexus may be of some value also (Fig. 6–10).

Plain skull radiographs may show the presence of a pre-existing abnormality inside the cranial cavity. As mentioned before, head injuries may occur as a result of decompensation

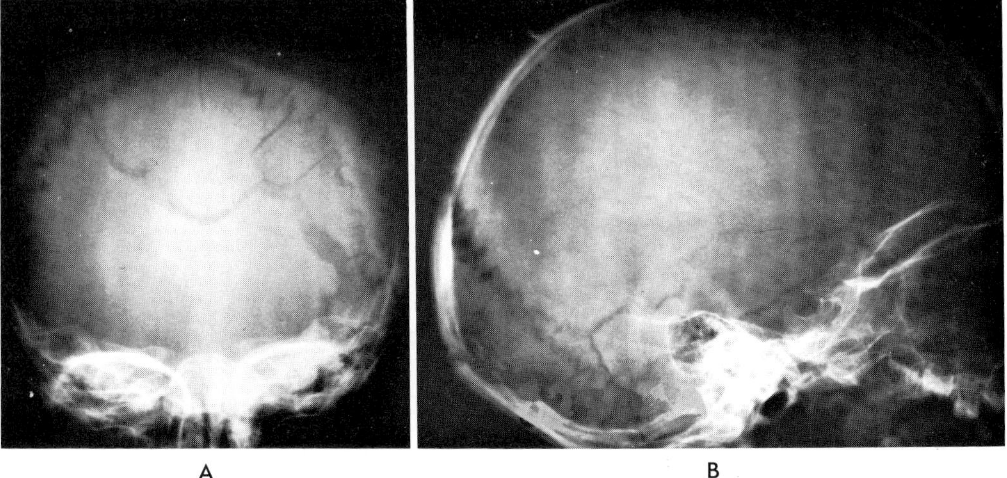

Figure 6–4 Radiograph of the skull (*A*, anteroposterior view; *B*, lateral view), showing multiple linear fractures and widening of the suture lines.

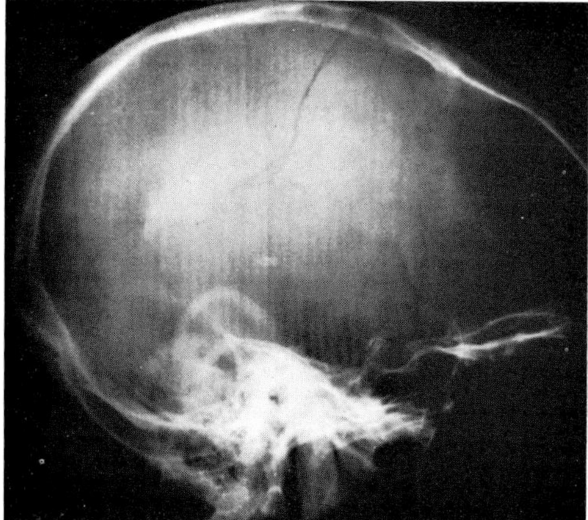

Figure 6–5 Radiograph of the skull, lateral view. Linear fracture line can be seen crossing the superior longitudinal sinus. Pineal gland is calcified but not displaced.

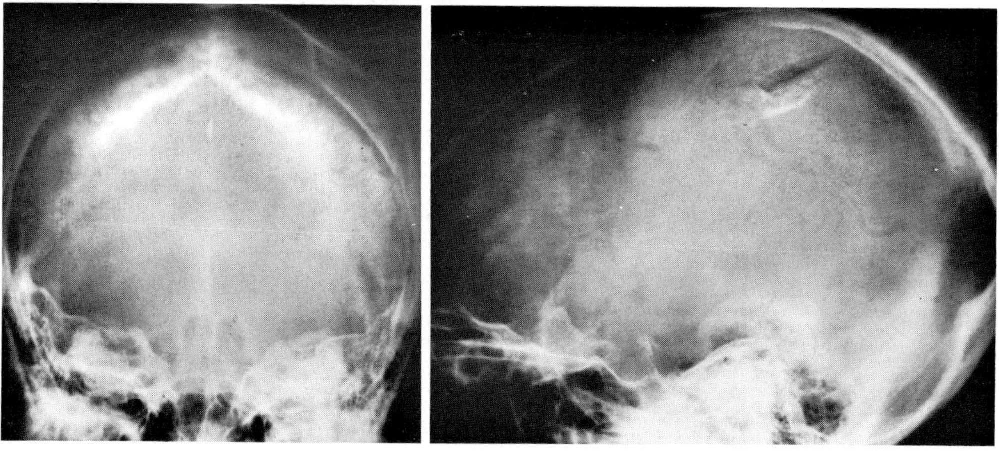

A B

Figure 6–6 Radiograph of the skull (*A*, anteroposterior; *B*, lateral view), showing a healed depressed fracture which has *not* been surgically elevated. This patient developed focal seizures starting eight months after the injury.

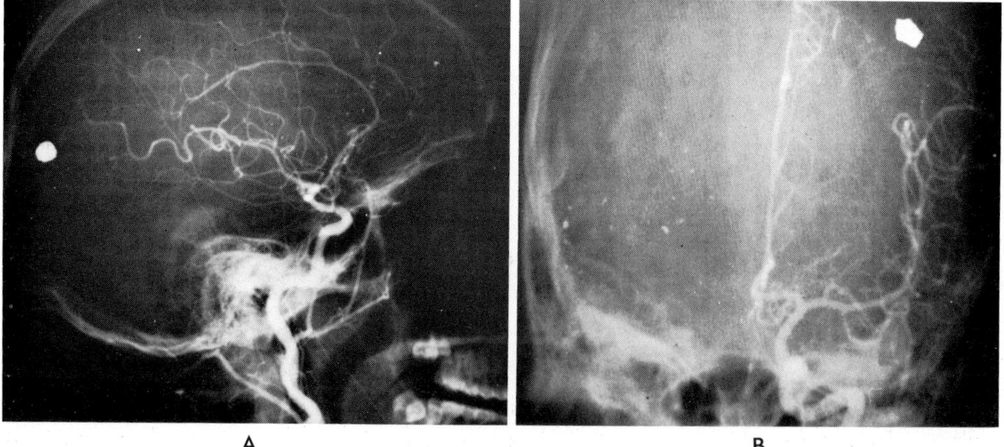

A B

Figure 6–7 Left carotid angiogram (*A*, lateral projection; *B*, anteroposterior projection) in a patient who received gunshot injury. The bullet can be seen in the occipital region. Although the posterior cerebral artery is not visualized, no displacement can be seen in the course of the other intracranial vessels. The trajectory of the bullet can be recognized; the entrance was in the *right* frontal region.

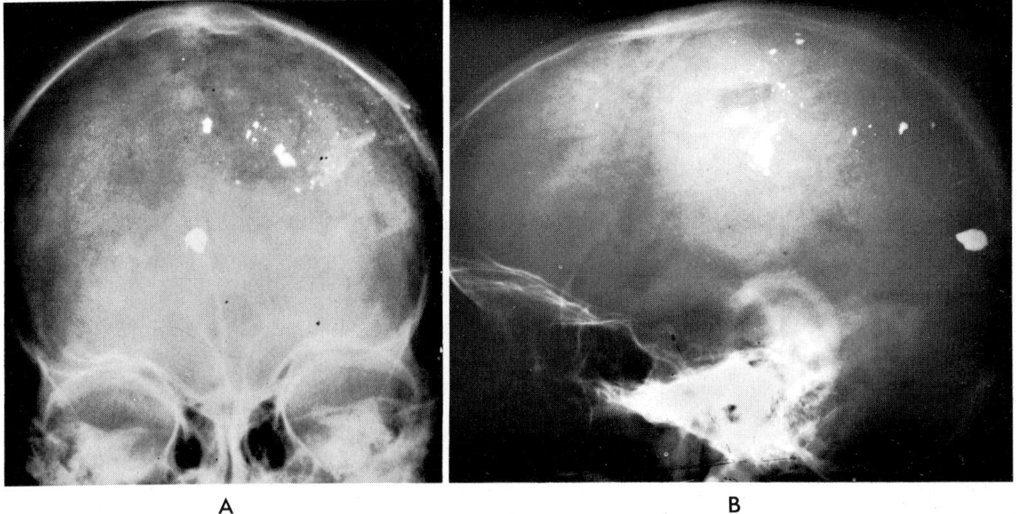

Figure 6–8 Radiograph of the skull (*A*, anteroposterior; *B*, lateral projection), showing multiple fragmentation and the final lodgment of a high-velocity bullet with entrance in the left parietal area.

and sudden hemorrhage into such lesions. Increased vascular grooves on one side of the skull may be of importance on the x-rays. Similarly, abnormal intracranial calcifications in a tumor, or occasionally in a chronic hematoma, will help to establish the correct diagnosis (Fig. 6–11). Separations of the sutures or increased digital markings of the internal table are indicative of pre-existing increased intracranial pressure (Fig. 6–4). In a few instances, fractures through the frontal sinuses may result in communication with the subarachnoid space or the ventricular system, and the x-rays will show air in the subarachnoid space or inside the ventricular cavity.

Occasionally, in addition to the routine projections, tangential views may be useful to visualize small linear fractures or minimal depressed frac-

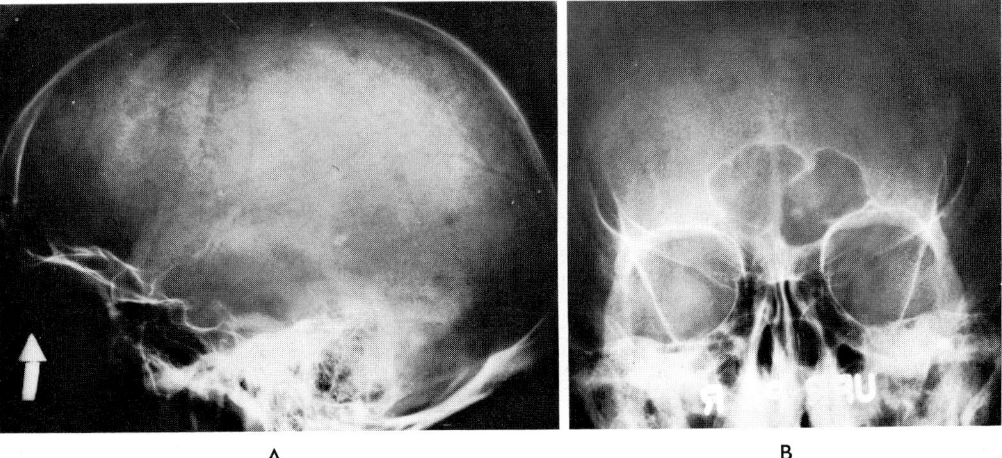

Figure 6–9 Radiograph of the skull (*A*, lateral; *B*, posteroanterior projection) showing displacement of the calcified pineal gland from right to left and inferoposteriorly by a proven subdural hematoma.

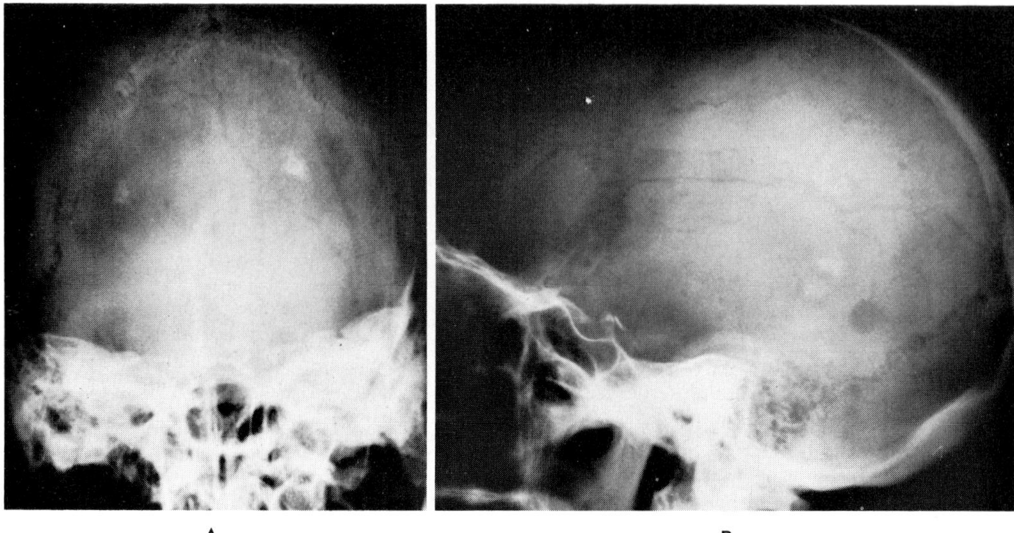

Figure 6–10 Radiograph of the skull (*A*, anteroposterior; *B*, lateral projection), showing calcified choroid plexus bilaterally. The right is displaced downward and posteriorly by a subdural hematoma.

tures in the cranial vault. Such views are generally obtained on an elective basis and are not a routine procedure in emergency room situations.[41]

Lumbar Puncture. Several reports are available about the use of lumbar puncture in the diagnosis of head injuries.[48, 55, 65] In most cases, lumbar puncture reveals either increased intracranial pressure or blood-stained fluid, or both. However, lumbar puncture is not usually a major aid in the diagnosis of head injuries. The confirmation of the fact of increased pressure or of a variable amount of blood in the cerebrospinal fluid does

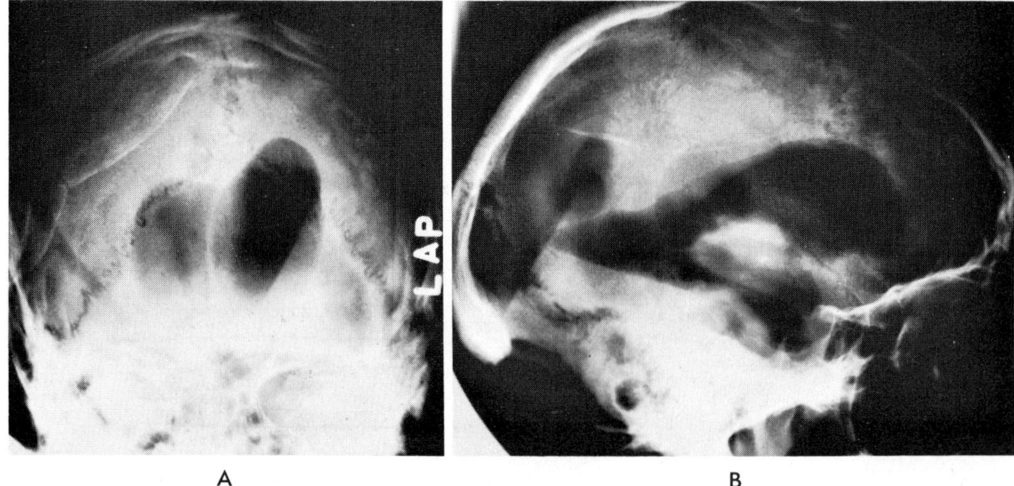

Figure 6–11 Ventriculogram, anteroposterior (*A*) and lateral view (*B*), showing displacement of the ventricular system by a large subdural hematoma. This patient underwent a craniectomy of the posterior fossa years before, when an astrocytoma of the cerebellum was removed. The calcification of the membrane of the subdural hematoma can clearly be seen in both views.

not add significant information for a correct diagnosis. On the other hand, if the lumbar puncture is performed improperly, a sudden herniation of the medial temporal lobe into the tentorial notch, or of the cerebellar tonsils into the foramen magnum, is a real danger. Occasionally, when the history is not clear and the possibility of a concomitant infection (meningitis) exists, lumbar puncture may be performed using a very fine needle with a stylet and withdrawing only the small amount of fluid necessary to count cells and to send a sample for culture.

Echoencephalography. Since the introduction of ultrasonic techniques by Leksell,[34] several reports have been published about the use of echoencephalography in acute head injuries.[28,35,58,70] The method used varies in different treatment centers. The apparatus is basically an ultrasound generator and receiver, displaying the echoes on an oscilloscope, with a camera attachment for permanent recording. A 2.25 MG transducer with a 10 mm. barium titanate crystal is most frequently used.

The examination should be made with a constant intensity of ultrasound. The patient is placed on his back, if possible, and the head is kept motionless. The region of the skull to be investigated is moistened with water or lubricating jelly before the transducer is applied; the transducer's face is in apposition to the scalp and the shaft is at right angles to the sagittal plane. To detect the midline echo, the optimal place for application of the transducer is 4 to 5 cm. above (and slightly in front of) the external auditory meatus. The temporal placement of the transducer can demonstrate a midline shift (Fig. 6–12) or a temporal hematoma (Fig. 6–13). Placement in the frontal, parietal and occipital regions confirms the midline shift and can be used to check ventricular asymmetry. Important observations can be made from echoes reflected from the subarachnoid space, the inner or outer tables of the skull, the subcutaneous tissue and the scalp surface on the side opposite the transducer.

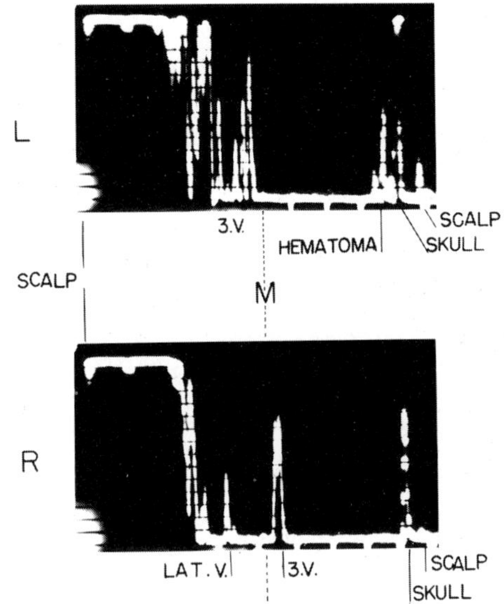

Figure 6–12 Echoencephalograph tracing from the left and right temporal region, showing a significant displacement of the midline echo (third ventricle) by a large hematoma.

Uematsu and Walker[70] commented on the great practical significance of this diagnostic tool. In patients with acute head injury, echograms may detect within a few minutes' time the presence of an epidural hematoma

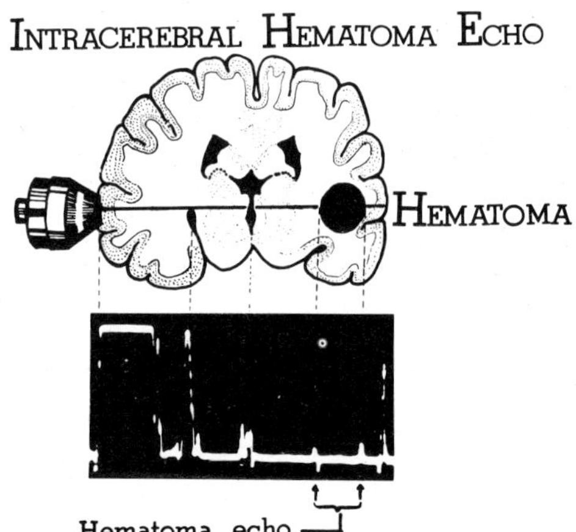

Figure 6–13 Schematic representation of the placement of the transducer and a small intracerebral hematoma. The tracing below shows the corresponding echogram.

(Fig. 6–12) or an intracerebral hematoma (Fig. 6–13). The finding of a midline shift is important of itself, as it gives accurate information about the extent of the space-occupying lesion (hematoma, rapid increase in cerebral edema, subdural collection) in the involved hemisphere. The accuracy of the midline shift is about 98 per cent according to a report by White and Blanchard.[76] Children with head injuries are particularly suitable for echoencephalographic studies because of the ease with which ultrasound is transmitted through the thin skull. Repeated echoencephalography and repeat neurological examination can be used as a reliable combination to establish the progression or regression of a lesion caused by acute head injury.

Rheoencephalography. This technique was introduced and popularized by Jenkner[30] in certain Central European clinics and more recently in some centers here in the United States. Use of this aid has been advocated in the diagnosis of extradural or subdural hematomas in acute head injuries. The main information obtained by rheoencephalography (REE) is the cerebral vascular alteration as reflected in changes of electrical conductivity. In patients with head injury the presence of cerebral hemorrhage or subdural or extradural hematomas causes an increase in peripheral vascular resistance. However, it is not possible to distinguish between them by rheoencephalographic technique. In these cases, the rheoencephalography tracing will have the characteristics of a compression: the angle of inclination is smaller than normal, the amplitude is somewhat lower than normal, and the details of the tracings are not so clearly visible. The changes occur in that order with increase in size of any hematoma. They are more characteristic if they are present on one side and can be compared with a relatively normal tracing of the other side (Fig. 6–14). Although this technique is still experimental clinically and further assessment of its reliability is desirable, it may provide a relatively simple technique to help to confirm the presence of a surgically amenable lesions after acute head injury.

Radioactive Brain Scan. Recent experience seems to indicate that, with further improvement, the radioactive scanning technique will be a useful aid in the diagnosis of intracerebral hematomas and, in some cases, subdural and extradural hematomas. The material used in radioactive scintiscan is mercury 203 or, more recently, technetium-99 (Tc-99). The isotope is injected intravenously and (in the case of technetium) the corresponding biplane scan can be performed within an hour's time. In elective cases (especially in subacute and chronic head injuries) this technique may be of considerable value (Fig. 6–15).

Cerebral Angiography. Since the introduction of cerebral angiography by Moniz in 1927, many reports have

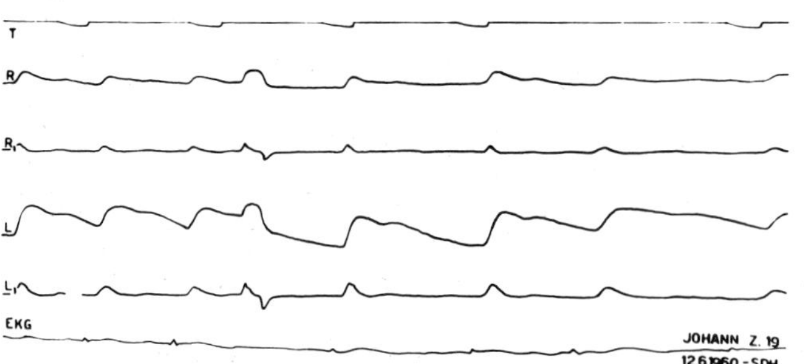

REG in subdural hematoma on the right side (200 milliliter).

Figure 6–14 Tracing from a rheoencephalographic investigation. (From Jenkner's Rheoencephalography.)

A

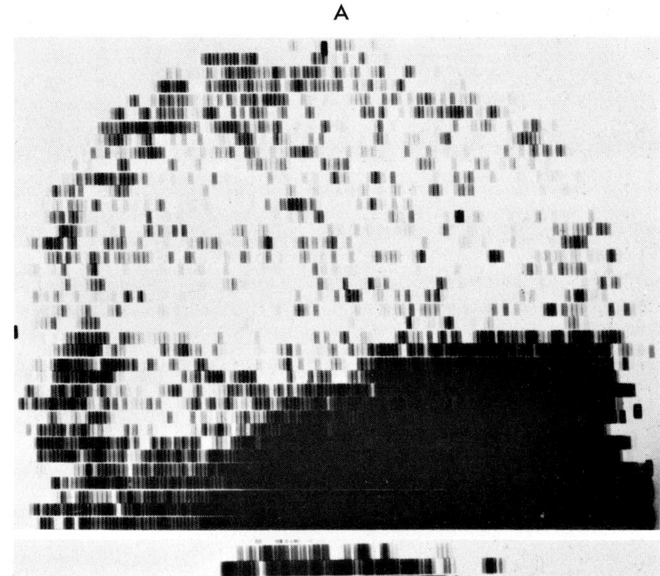

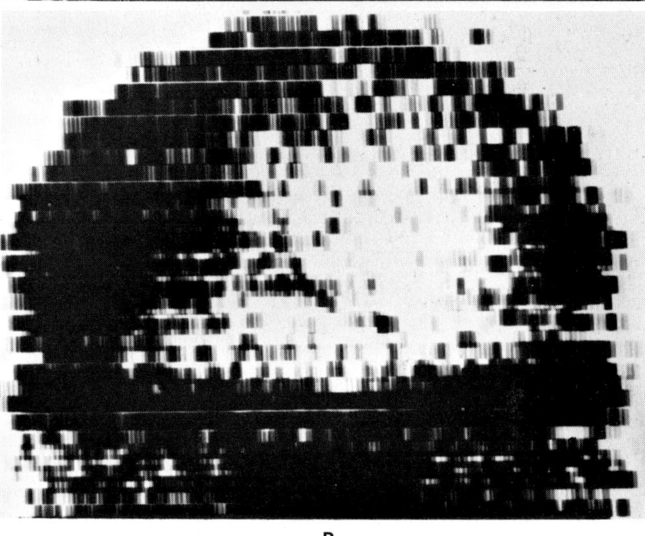

B

Figure 6–15 Brain-scan with technetium-99 (*A*, Left lateral projection, normal appearance; *B*, right lateral projection), showing markedly increased uptake of the isotope along the whole right hemisphere in a distance of 2 to 3 cm. from the internal table. This patient had a huge subacute subdural hematoma.

emphasized its value in indicating the presence and exact location of space-occupying lesions in acute and chronic head injuries.[7, 10, 24, 25, 44, 68, 69] Cerebral angiography can be performed by subcutaneous puncture of the common carotid arteries and injection by hand of 10 to 12 cc. of 50 per cent Hypaque or 60 per cent Renografin. At least three films should be taken in the anteroposterior position and three films in the lateral position. A biplane serial angiograph requires only one injection; simultaneous anteroposterior and lateral views can be obtained, showing the vascular structure in two planes at the same time. If possible to obtain, a right percutaneous retrograde brachial angiogram will be of additional value because it permits visualization not only of the right carotid system but also (via the right vertebral artery) of the posterior circulation. In addition to this right brachial angiogram, a left carotid angiogram should be performed if there is any question of involvement of the other hemisphere. The amount of dye used in the brachial artery is 40 cc. of 60 per cent Reno-

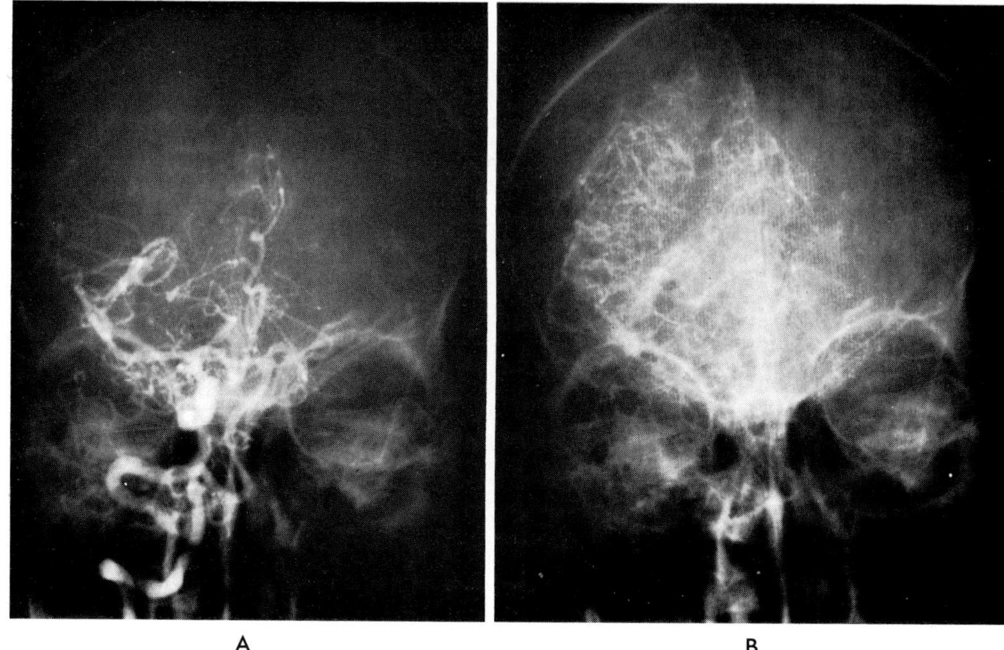

Figure 6–16 Percutaneous right retrograde brachial angiogram. *A*, anteroposterior view, early arterial phase, showing displacement of the anterior cerebral artery from left to right with concomitant shift of the posterior cerebral and middle cerebral arteries. *B*, anteroposterior view, capillary phase, indicating clearly the avascular area between the internal table and cerebral cortex, which corresponds to a large collection of subdural hematoma.

grafin. The puncture is done in the cubital fossa with a Seldinger needle; the sharp end of the trocar can be withdrawn and the needle itself (with a blunt end) can be threaded into the artery. The injection is made by pressure injector at about 120 to 180 mm. of pressure per square inch.

The arterial phase of the cerebral angiography may reveal a displacement of the anterior cerebral artery across the midline, indicating a space-occupying lesion (Fig. 6–16). The cause may be increased cerebral edema, an intracerebral hematoma (Fig. 6–20) or a subdural or extradural hematoma (Fig. 6–16). The capillary phase is more diagnostic for subdural and extradural blood collections. The small arterioles and capillaries usually extend to the internal table since they are lying on the surface of the brain substance just beneath the dura. If there is any collection of blood between the cerebral cortex and the dura mater (subdural hematoma) or between the dura and the internal table (extradural hematoma), displacement of the capillary blush can be visualized in the anteroposterior view (Figs. 6–16 and 6–17). In the lateral views the detection of subdural or extradural collection is much more difficult, although occasionally displacement of the capillary shadow in the anterior fossa and in the anterior portion of the temporal fossa can be detected in the form of an avascular area. Bilateral subdural collections can be detected by angiography, not by displacement of the large vessels, because they remain in their normal position, but by the meniscus-like avascular shadows over both hemispheres in the capillary phase (Fig. 6–18).

The venous phase of the angiograms may show an obstruction of the venous

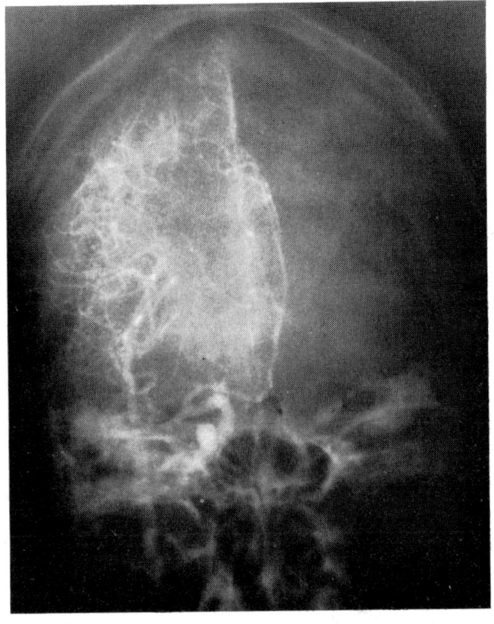

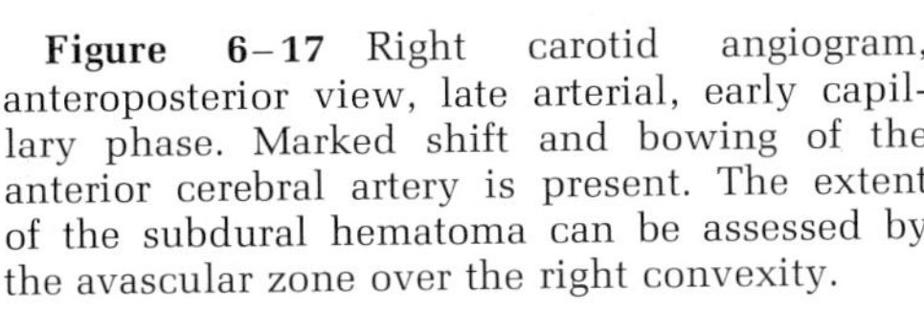

Figure 6–17 Right carotid angiogram, anteroposterior view, late arterial, early capillary phase. Marked shift and bowing of the anterior cerebral artery is present. The extent of the subdural hematoma can be assessed by the avascular zone over the right convexity.

sinuses by fracture fragments. Displacement of the deep cerebral veins, and occasional shift of the bridging veins, may indicate posteriorly placed intracerebral hematomas. Occasionally, cerebral angiography may reveal partial or complete occlusion of the carotid artery as it penetrates the dura (Fig. 6–19).

Angiography should be performed

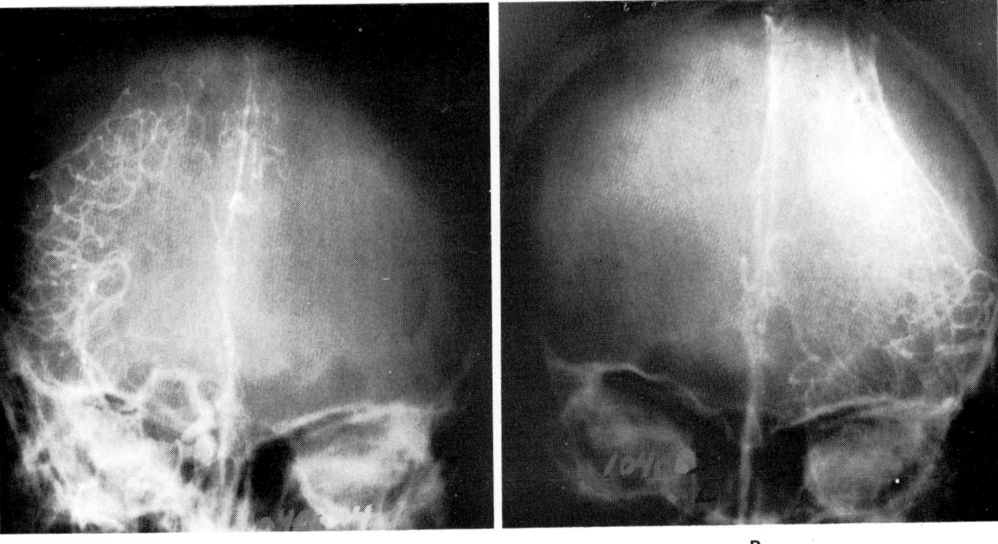

Figure 6–18 Right carotid angiogram, late arterial phase, anteroposterior view (*A*), and left carotid angiogram, capillary phase, anteroposterior view (*B*), showing the presence of a large subdural hematoma left and of a smaller one right. Note: There is only a minimal shift of the anterior cerebral artery from left to right.

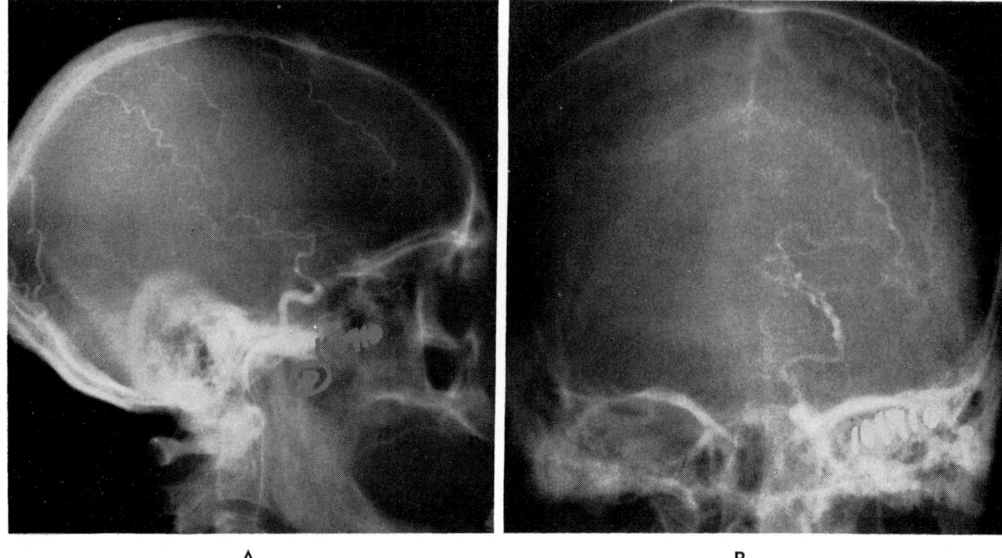

Figure 6–19 Right carotid angiogram (*A*, lateral view; *B*, anteroposterior view), showing severe narrowing of the internal carotid artery at its penetration of the dura. Only a small amount of dye entered the markedly displaced middle cerebral artery. The patient harbored a huge (250 cc.) subdural hematoma and demonstrated signs of extremely severe increased intracranial pressure.

only in those treatment centers in which these procedures are done on a routine basis; otherwise, in acute head injuries with a possible extradural hematoma and rapid clinical deterioration, valuable time may be wasted in trying to perform an angiography inexpertly, perhaps in the middle of the night, with insufficiently trained technical personnel or by residents who do not do this type of diagnostic study routinely. On the other hand, if well-trained personnel are available, the routine cerebral angiography generally can be obtained within 20 to 30 minutes, a reasonable proposition even in the acute situations. However, the value of angiography is greater in the detection of subacute and chronic hematomas.

Widening of the distance between the anterior and middle cerebral arteries in the anteroposterior view suggests the possibility of a deep intracranial clot (Fig. 6–20). Elevation of the middle cerebral artery indicates the presence of a hematoma in the temporal lobe (Fig. 6–21). In patients in whom the head injury resulted from a sudden hemorrhage, angiography is also of value in establishing the possibility of a pre-existing arteriovenous malformation, intracranial aneurysm or, occasionally, intracerebral tumor.

Ventriculography and Pneumoencephalography. With the advent of newer and safer diagnostic techniques, the use of air studies in acute head injuries has decreased considerably. There is almost no indication to perform this type of study if any of the other studies previously mentioned can be obtained, singly or in combination, in addition to the clinical and neurological evaluation. In a few instances, however, in cases of intracerebral hematomas and occasionally in chronic subdural hematomas, ventricular puncture with injection of air into the lateral ventricles can be performed just prior to the operative procedure to establish more accurately the extent of the hematoma by displacement of the ventricular shadow (Fig. 6–11). However, this type of diagnostic procedure is generally done when the decision has already been made to explore the patient surgically.

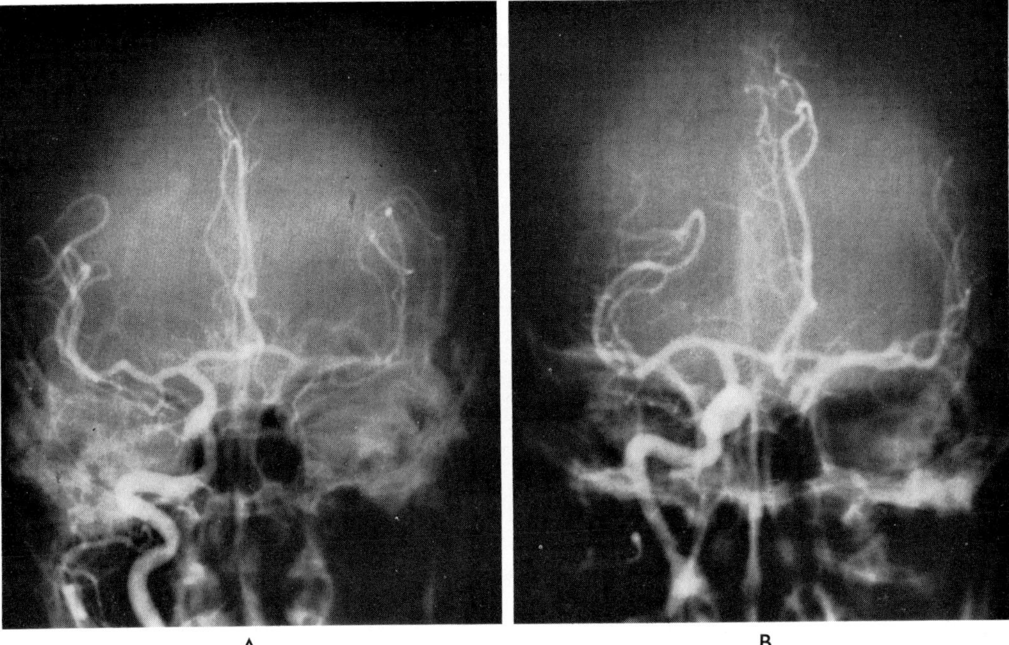

Figure 6–20 Right carotid angiogram with simultaneous compression of the left carotid artery in the neck in a patient with a deep intracerebral hematoma (*A*). Note the increased distance between the right middle and anterior cerebral arteries. Similar investigation (right carotid angiogram with simultaneous compression of the contralateral carotid artery) in a patient with a large subdural hematoma (*B*). Note the marked shift of both vessels, anterior and middle cerebral arteries, from right to left. The Sylvian point is depressed in contrast with *A*.

In a few specialized neurosurgical centers, fractional pneumoencephalography is performed on head injury patients.[54] However, this type of investigation requires highly specialized personnel. Even if all precautions are taken in performing the lumbar puncture and exchanging fluid with air in such manner that the intracranial pressure will not be altered, the risks probably outweigh the advantages. The use of subdural air studies in the diagnosis of subfrontal fractures, especially in cerebrospinal fluid rhinorrhea, has been emphasized by Jefferson and Lewtas.[29] This is a selective technique and generally is performed in a specialized neurosurgical department, not forming part of the routine diagnostic examination of an acute traumatic head injury. The technique can be combined with tomography to provide more accurate information about the site of the leak, by means of the interruption of the air shadow in the subdural space.

Electroencephalography. The value of electroencephalography in head injuries was emphasized first by Williams and Gibbs[75] and later reports confirmed their observations.

Since the electroencephalogram records electrical activity originating in the cell bodies (somata), dendrites and axons of cortical cells and of cells in subcortical gray matter, damage to this tissue may result in a change of electrical activity.

The EEG abnormalities consist mainly of localized or diffuse slow-wave activity, with a high incidence of paroxysmal bursts. These changes generally are more prominent if the trauma was severe and the unconsciousness prolonged. However, electroencephalography cannot indicate the exact nature of the pathology—i.e., whether it is an extradural, sub-

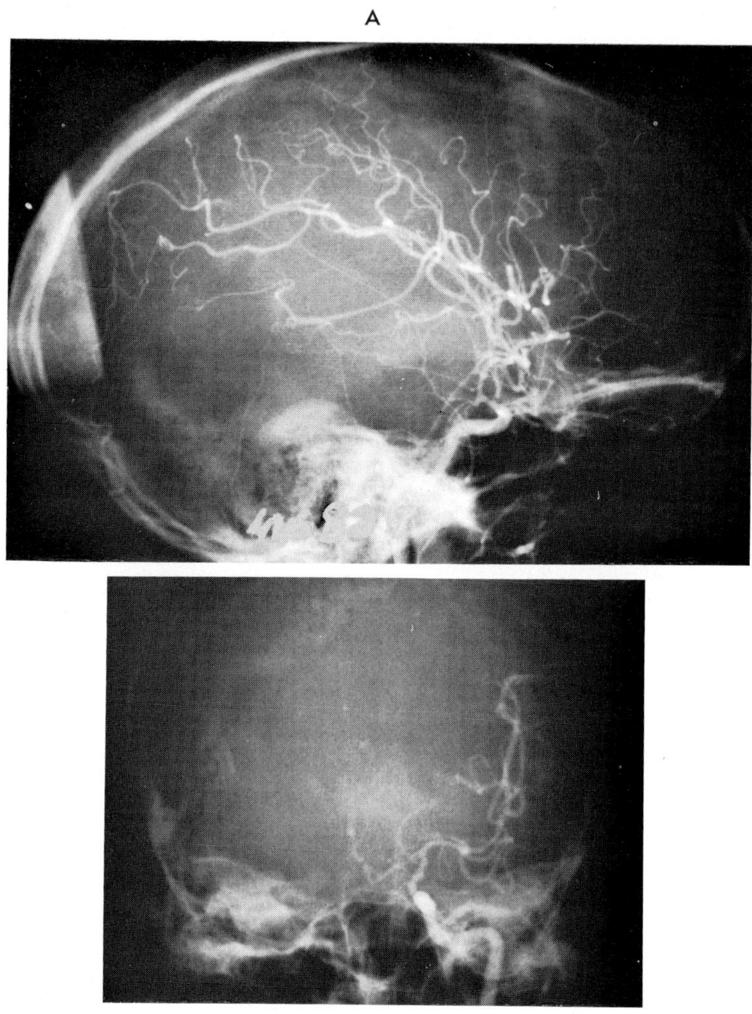

Figure 6–21 Left carotid angiogram, lateral (*A*) and anteroposterior (*B*) views. The middle cerebral artery is elevated, with upward-bowing. Severe spasm can be observed in the internal-carotid and anterior cerebral arteries. The patient had a large intratemporal hematoma.

dural or intracerebral hematoma, or even increased cerebral edema. Its use is limited to cases that are of subacute or chronic character and, in general, the electroencephalography findings are only of auxiliary value. Coma and various degrees of confusional states are generally accompanied by slow waves, with slightly higher voltage in coma and increasing frequency in states of confusion.[26] In a few cases, the electroencephalographic finding will confirm the previously suspected presence of lesions from acute head injury. However, this technique is generally used only on an elective basis and not in patients who arrive at the emergency room in acute distress.

In severe head injuries with clinical evidence of deep coma, the biological activity of the brain may be so much reduced that the EEG will show only a "flat record." Although recovery from such conditions is extremely rare, care should be taken before a conclusion of "cerebral death" is reached. A nationwide survey of this important ethical and biological problem is on the way.[73] An on-line technique of rapid determination of cerebral blood-flow and oxygen consumption may provide more reliable information for prognosis.[49]

Exploration by Trephination. Although any of the foregoing diagnostic methods, alone or in combination, may provide a highly accurate diagnosis, in a few cases the sequence of events is so rapid that no time can be lost in performing special diagnostic studies. If the neurological status suggests a fast deterioration, simple twist-drill openings (made with a sterile stainless steel twist burr, as proposed by Burton and Blacker[6]) may be of considerable value. The twist-hole openings can be introduced into the epidural or subdural space or into the brain substance, relieving the rapidly increasing pressure caused by an extradural or acute subdural blood collection.

The most expedient method in such cases, however, is to take the patient into the operating room, place six routine burr holes, confirm the presumed diagnosis and, at the same time, drain the epidural, subdural or intracerebral hematomas.

Summary and Conclusions

Although there are no precise rules for the selection of diagnostic studies under various conditions, the following statements can be made from previous experience.

Extradural Hematomas. In extradural hematomas, which by their nature may be of rapidly progressive character, the procedures of choice are:

1. *X-rays of the skull* with special emphasis on displacement of the calcified pineal or calcified choroid plexus; assessment of the presence of fracture lines crossing the grooves of the middle meningeal artery and veins, or of the posterior fossa.
2. Echoencephalography.
3. Twist burr-hole opening, with evacuation of the extradural clot if the development is very rapid.
4. Burr holes in the classical fashion, with confirmation of the diagnosis and evacuation of the clot.
5. Cerebral angiography may be done to confirm the diagnosis, but only if experienced personnel are present and the technical facilities are such that the angiographic studies can be performed in about 20 minutes' time.

Subacute and Chronic Hematomas

1. Skull x-rays.
2. Echoencephalography.
3. Radioactive scintiscan.
4. Cerebral angiography.
5. Electroencephalography, possibly.

Intracerebral Hematomas and Possible Progressive Intracerebral Edema

1. Skull x-rays.
2. Echoencephalography.
3. Radioactive scintiscan.
4. Cerebral angiography.
5. If necessary, ventricular puncture and air ventriculography.

The previous comments have been made in analyzing the diagnostic techniques in head injuries in adults. Although there is not much difference in the mechanisms and the clinical presentation in children, it should be mentioned that a substantial amount of intracranial hemorrhage can accumulate in children before focal or generalized cerebral damage can be established on clinical examination because of the expandability of the skull.

The general clinical examination and the neurological evaluation of children is similar to that of the adult, although in small babies the presence of a neurological deficit is more difficult to assess. Among the diagnostic techniques, echoencephalography is especially suitable because of the thin skull of children. The subdural space can be tapped easily through the lateral corner of the fontanelle, allowing an easy confirmation of the presence of subdural hematomas.

Finally, to illustrate the course of events in investigating subacute head injury, the following case history and the various steps of investigation are recorded.

(F. K., JHH #116 64 06.) The patient, a 55 year old businessman, underwent radical extirpation of a carcinoma of the colon and had a colostomy performed. His postoperative progress was satisfactory and he was discharged home. However, just two days prior to his readmission he had fallen in the bathtub and had been unconscious for about 45 minutes. When he regained consciousness he had a mild left hemiparesis and was admitted to the hospital. His level of consciousness was surprisingly clear. There was no evidence of laceration or abrasion over the scalp or over the body. The funduscopic examination revealed a mild degree of papilledema. Neurological examination revealed slight left hemiparesis. The x-rays of the skull showed definite displacement of the pineal gland (Fig. 6–9). Because of the previous history, it was thought that he might very well have a cerebral metastasis that may have been the cause of his fall. Further diagnostic studies were performed. The echoencephalography showed a midline shift of 11 mm. from right to left (Fig. 6–22). The EEG revealed definite evidence of slow-wave depression over the right hemisphere (Fig. 6–23). Radioactive scintiscan demonstrated increased uptake over the right hemisphere, suggesting the presence of a subdural hematoma (Fig. 6–15). Right percutaneous retrograde brachial angiography revealed a classic picture of a large subdural hematoma, with corresponding shift of the anterior cerebral artery from right to left through the midline (Fig. 6–24).

After all these diagnostic studies the patient was taken to the operating room, and through routine burr holes the subdural hematoma (which was mostly liquid) was evacuated. There was already a thin membrane present.

One week postoperatively the patient's neurological deficit disappeared completely. Echoencephalography showed a shift of only 6 mm.; two weeks after the operation the echo showed almost complete disappearance of the shift. We have to assume that this shift resulted from cerebral edema. Clinical impovement continued, and the patient was discharged almost symptom-free.

This particular case illustrates the various diagnostic techniques and their contribution to the positive finding of subacute subdural hematoma, despite the fact that the clinical history and the previous condition of

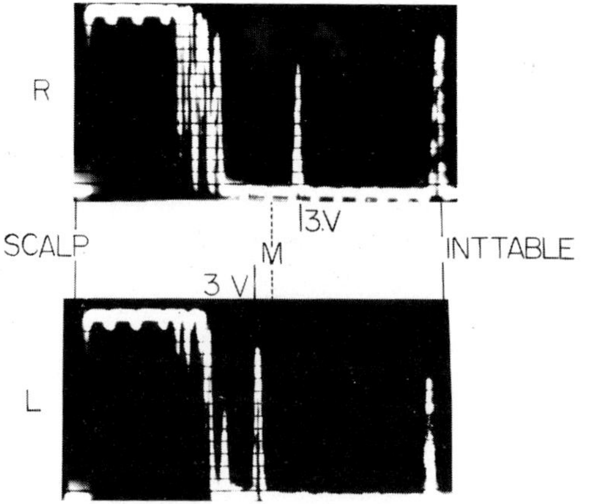

Figure 6–22 Echoencephalogram showing displacement of the midline echo from right to left.

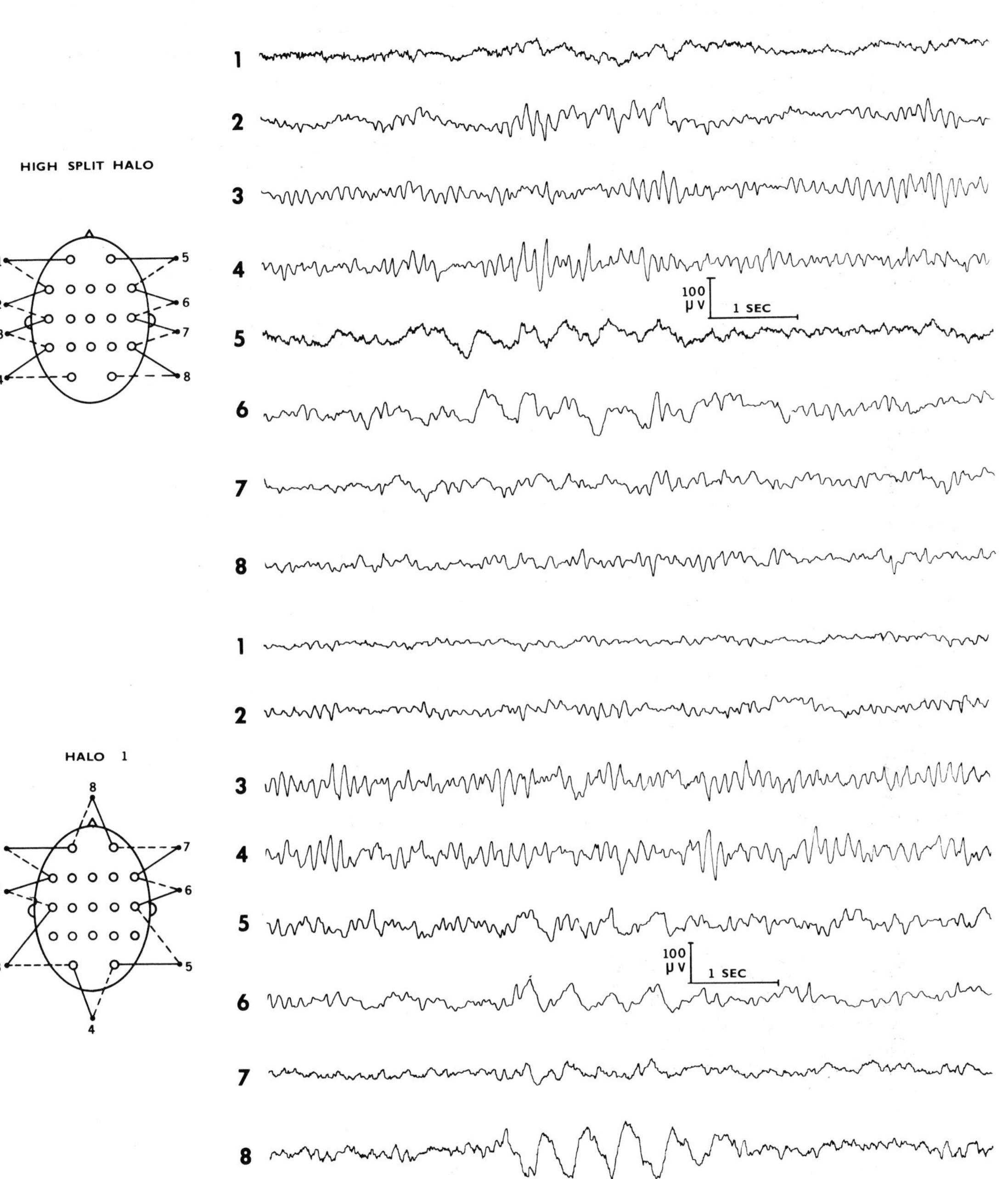

Figure 6–23 Electroencephalogram on the same patient, showing the slow-wave, low-amplitude activity over the right hemisphere.

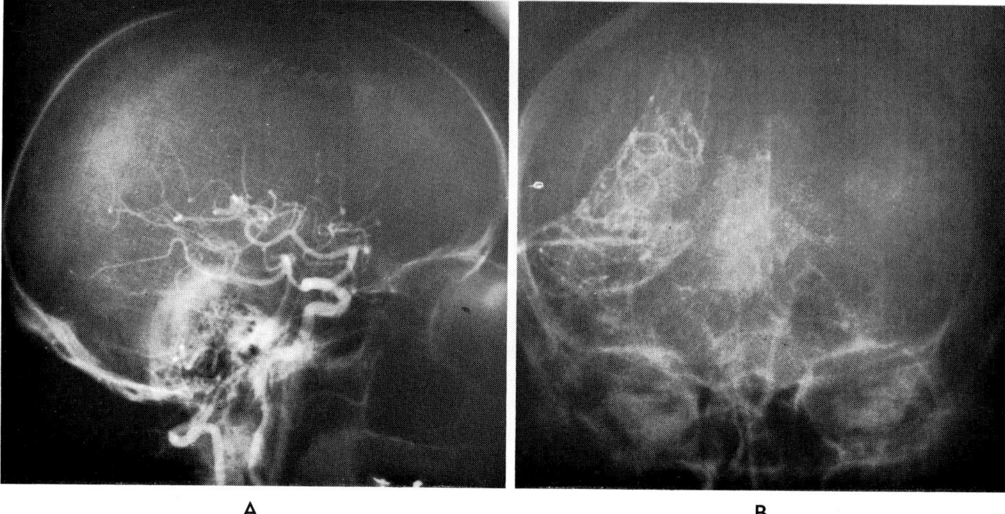

Figure 6–24 Right percutaneous retrograde brachial angiography, lateral (*A*) and anteroposterior (*B*) views, showing the extent of the huge subdural hematoma.

the patient led to the assumption of a different type of pathology. We do not propose that such an exhaustive diagnostic work-up should be performed routinely, even on those patients in whom the possibility of a surgically amenable lesion exists. In many instances a more limited use of these techniques will be sufficient to establish the correct diagnosis.

THE TREATMENT OF CRANIOCEREBRAL INJURIES

J. Donald McQueen, M.D.

MANAGEMENT IN THE EMERGENCY ROOM

Craniocerebral trauma, including scalp injury and brief traumatic unconsciousness, normally constitutes 10 to 15 per cent of the accident room trauma burden. Of these cases, about one-fifth present serious problems and are primary considerations here. Certain aspects of symptomatic treatment are handled before decisions are made on neurosurgical interventions. These include respiratory insufficiency and shock.

Initially, attention is directed to the maintenance of a free airway. The collar is loosened, the mouth is searched for loosened teeth or foreign material and the pharynx is suctioned assiduously. Obstruction from a lax, mislocated tongue is common in the unconscious patient. Bronchial secretions are not cleared and may form excessively as a result of upper brainstem stimulation. Occasionally, frank pulmonary edema ensues. It is therefore wise to consider tracheal intubation for patients in whom tongue traction or positioning and the use of an airway fail to alleviate respiratory obstruction. This is perhaps the single most important decision in the management of these patients; the lowered mortality rates during the past two decades may be traced to this rather than to the use of specific operative techniques or the use of such adjuncts as hypothermia or intravenous hypertonic fluids. Clinically it is often difficult to be sure of the exact contribution of upper airway obstruction to brain swelling; the profound deterioration after aspiration is usually clear, and vomitus and blood are commonly demonstrated in the lungs of head injury victims on postmortem examination. Therefore, equal consideration should be given to the aspiration of gastric contents, and a nasogastric tube should be retained in this group of patients. This problem is especially common in intoxicated individuals.

With acute head trauma, signs of shock point to associated injuries. Sustained neurogenic shock is an entity with spinal cord injury but not with brain injury except in terminal states. Occasionally, a large extradural hematoma will induce incipient shock in an infant because of a disproportionately large head, the adaptability of the brain and the compliance of the skull. The blood pressure levels are usually normal even in this instance, and the diagnosis is made primarily from the combination of pallor and listlessness. However, this is an exception and extracranial trauma must be assumed in the presence of established shock.

About one-third of cases of serious head trauma have other significant injuries. Fractures of the long bones and facial bones, abdominal and chest injuries are relatively common. These diagnoses are often difficult to make in the unconscious patient. A retroperitoneal hematoma, in particular, may be hard to discern in this circumstance. In general, the arrest of hemorrhage from a ruptured spleen or liver will be given priority over neurosurgical procedures, although trephine openings may be placed at the time of the laparotomy. General anesthesia is not contraindicated with acute head injury; however, great emphasis should be placed on (1) the avoidance of hypercarbia and (2) the use of such agents as halothane and ether since the consequent cerebral vasodilation may not be tolerated in a crowded cranium. Similarly, adequate oxygen therapy and deft tracheal intubations and extubations should be stressed.

Concurrent chest and head injuries constitute a particularly unfavorable combination because of the possible aggravation of brain injury by hypoxemia and hypercarbia. Here again, respiratory control is the prime consideration; present-day management, especially with the use of respirators, has greatly improved the prognosis of patients in this group.

With all of these injuries, one or more cannulae are placed in appropriate veins, blood is withdrawn for matching, intravenous fluids are started and blood is replaced. Vasoconstrictors are used very sparingly in order not to mask hemorrhage.

Special effort is required in obtaining the details of the history of these patients because of obvious problems in communication. Knowledge of the previous status of the patient is important in many ways; for example, the prior blood pressure levels should be known since temporarily induced neurogenic hypertension is common with head trauma. A record of cerebrovascular disease may suggest the cause of the injury; one of alcoholism may aid in recognition of a subdural collection. Similarly, an accurate description of the accident may help in locating a depressed fracture, in diagnosing suspected transorbital or infratentorial damage and in mapping sites of contrecoup injury. Information on the sequence of events after the impact is most important. A progressive deterioration of the state of consciousness, with or without a lucid interval, is an indication for neurosurgical intervention. The long-term use of anticoagulants should be determined because of the added risk of intracranial hematoma formation and patients with trivial head trauma who are receiving such agents should be detained or followed closely. These are elementary points; however, they should be stressed since the search for pertinent information in the accident room is commonly deficient.

Certain fundamental clinical findings that bear on neurosurgical interventions are noted here. The essentials are: depression of the level of consciousness, slowing of the pulse, pupillary changes, loss of muscle power, reflex alterations and local changes about the head. A deterioration in the state of consciousness is always the pre-eminent sign and is seldom misleading, although patients with chronic subdural hematomas and other longstanding lesions may become more responsive from time to time as the brain accommodates to the mass. When there is a known head injury, the prime indications for burr-hole explorations are : (1) deep coma, (2) a progressive lowering of awareness or (3) a lucid interval. With the exclusion of hopeless high-velocity missile injuries, explorations should be carried out quickly if the depression of the level of consciousness is sustained and reaches the point where only limited reactions to painful stimuli remain. This exigency is uncommon, and a period of close observation is usually possible. Arteriography should be strongly considered and completed with proper indications and when time permits.

A fixed, dilated pupil is a reliable sign. Misjudgments may occur because of orbital trauma, and transient pupillary changes may be associated with irritation of the frontal eye fields and with seizures. The third nerve is stretched by displaced medial temporal lobe structures which are thrust down by a hematoma or with brain swelling. This process usually occurs bilaterally, and fortuitously, there may be greater involvement on the opposite side in about 20 per cent of cases. This false lateralization is one of the many reasons for the inflexibility of the rule governing the use of bilateral trephine openings or arteriograms.

Slowing of the pulse rate is a helpful sign in the diagnosis of an intracranial hematoma, but it is not reliable as an isolated finding since it is often found without brain compression. The presence of a heart block or intraocular hypertension should be considered.

Hemipareses and reflex changes are valuable localizing findings, although an expanding lesion may be on the same side as the motor loss. Here, the brainstem is displaced so that the contralateral motor fibers are impinged upon the sharp, tentorial edge. Changes in motor power and tone per se are not indications for trephinations and occur commonly with contusions.

Twist drill openings are placed infrequently in the accident room because of the danger of missing significant collections of clotted blood which are unable to pass through small-bore needles. However, such openings are placed in a few instances. One example is that of the unresponsive patient with a suspected massive intraventricular hemorrhage. Another example is the older patient with combined cerebrovascular disease and trauma who presents in such a way that the indications for a full set of trephine openings are meager. Under such circumstances small frontal holes are placed and a ventricle is tapped. Intraventricular hemorrhage is first assessed; if absent, a small 20 to 30 ml. air bubble is injected and films are taken to rule out large collections of blood under or over the dura. The Burton-Blacker instrument is shown in Figure 6–27.

Intravenous hypertonic mannitol infusions are commonly used for the alleviation of brain swelling; except in extreme circumstances their use before burr-hole explorations is contraindicated because of the facilitated expansion of intracranial hematomas.

The corticosteroid derivatives are used very commonly at the present time but are reserved for serious injuries in which the outcome is in question and those causing such states as persistent unresponsiveness and decerebration. If corticosteroid injections are to be given, they should be used soon after the initial evaluation in the accident room or held for later use in patients with regressions. Methylprednisolone compounds are popular; the dosage of dexamethasone is 10 mg. immediately and 4 mg. every 6 hours, either intravenously or intramuscularly.

There are three types of open head wounds; blunt injuries with compound depressed fractures and high- and low-velocity penetrating wounds. All patients with injuries in the first category should be taken promptly to the operating room; initially, the wound is inspected but is not thoroughly irrigated. Routine skull films are obtained and a snug head bandage is applied.

Many injuries from high-velocity missiles are irrecoverable. For example, in a study by Goodman and Kalsbeck[20] 70 per cent of the self-inflicted gunshot wounds were fatal. The force that is expended in the brain varies as the square of the velocity (or the cube at very high speeds) and is sufficient per se to burst the skull. In addition, the bullet commonly traverses the skull and often ricochets about with added damage. These victims arrive in the accident room in deep coma with fixed and dilated pupils. Roentgenograms are made to demonstrate the missile path but specific therapy should be withheld.

Often bullets are slowed or deflected by bone and skirt the brain or enter it at low velocity. In these instances patients may display varied cranial nerve palsies and/or limited brain damage. Adequate antibiotic therapy is instituted; operative intervention is delayed when the major objective is missile removal but is prompt in other instances. Other low-velocity injuries include trauma from perforating knife and fan blades, ice picks, rods and shafts. Patients suffering this type of trauma are taken directly to the operating room, where the undisturbed penetrating object is "prepped" in the field.

OPERATIVE MANAGEMENT

Operative procedures may be divided into three main groups: trephinations, explorations for the elevation of depressed fractures and explorations for debridement of the brain.

Intracranial hematomas are usually evacuated through trephine openings. These holes are routinely enlarged in the temporal areas and are sometimes widened elsewhere in the presence of a large extradural clot. Craniotomy flaps are not turned routinely and only (1) when it is necessary to remove the membranes enclosing chronic subdural effusions in infancy or (2) when it is impossible to retrieve all of the clotted material through small openings.

The head is fully shaved in the anesthetic room, and a second search is made for local signs of trauma. Subgaleal hematomas are of particular importance when over fractures since this fluid may constitute drainage from an extradural collection.

General anesthesia is preferred over local blocks because of the necessity of immobilizing the head during operative procedures. Anesthesia is induced with Pentothal in such a way that struggling is minimized and cerebrospinal fluid pressures are not unduly elevated. The patient may then be curarized, intubated and ventilated with nitrous oxide and oxygen. Nitrous oxide may be eliminated in some cases; halothane and ether should be avoided since they induce vasodilatation and hence augment intracranial crowding. The trachea is intubated as coughing or other airway obstruction will intensify brain swelling and displace intracranial contents through dural openings.

The patient is placed on a Light-Veley headrest for routine trephinations. This supports the head and exposes the vault so that bilateral burr holes may be readily placed in frontal, temporal and parietal regions (Fig. 6–25). The shoulders are supported on pads and the head of the table is elevated a few degrees. The vertical position is not used since shock may be a concomitant problem. Adhesive surgical drapes are valuable because immoderate amounts of irrigation fluids are often used.

The placement of six supratentorial openings is a good routine practice.

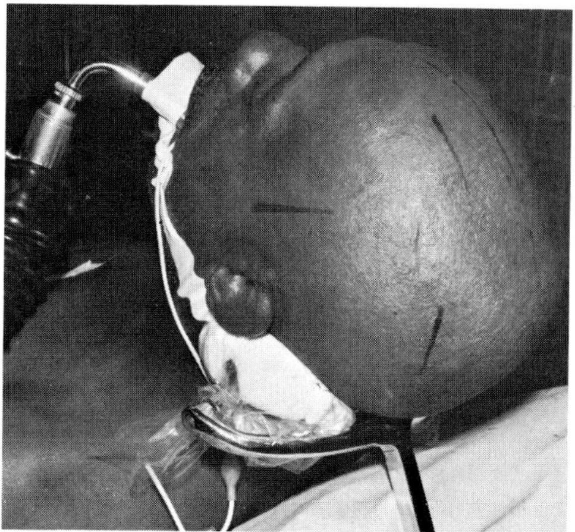

Figure 6–25 Burr-hole sites. The patient is positioned on the Light-Veley headrest so that bilateral openings may be placed in the frontal, temporal and parietal regions.

However, some of these may be eliminated if the brain is slack enough for the free passage of a catheter in the subdural space. The temporal openings are placed first because of the preponderance of clots over and under the temporal lobe. In grave situations bilateral holes are drilled concurrently (Fig. 6–26). A 2.5 inch vertical skin incision is extended within the hairline from the upper border of the zygomatic arch. Branches of the superficial temporal artery are cauterized and Weitlander self-retaining retractors are inserted to expose bone down to the level of the floor of the middle fossa. A cone-shaped opening is drilled through the bone with a McKenzie perforator and is enlarged to a hole of five-eighths inch diameter with a burr. The instruments are shown in Figure 6–27; they should be fashioned from steel that has high degrees of ductility and strength. Motorized units including a perforator such as the Smith drill may be used; however, the important points are the quality of the metal and the sharpness of the cutting edge rather than the choice between individual perforators. The temporal hole is routinely enlarged to the size of a silver dollar. This is done because of the necessity for explorations beneath the temporal lobe and because of the opportunities for small, muscle-protected decompressions and limited temporal lobe resections. The temporal squama is very thin; it is rongeured rapidly and then waxed. Small, self-retaining mastoid retractors are used for the frontal and parietal openings, which are usually not enlarged.

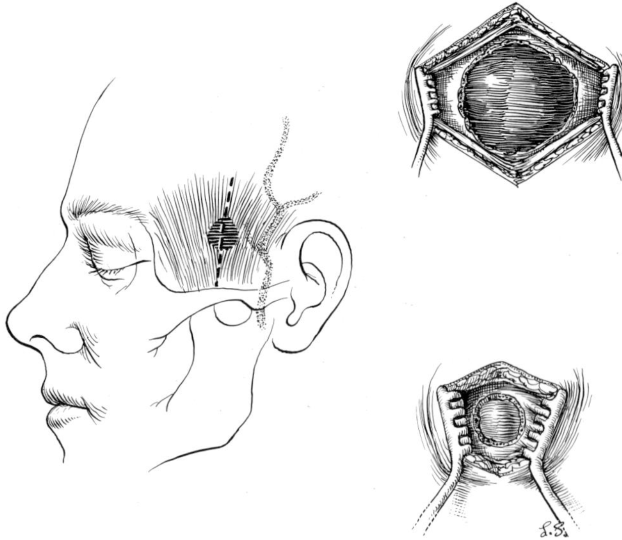

Figure 6–26 Trephine openings. The site of the common temporal opening is shown to the left. This defect is enlarged to the size of a silver dollar as noted in the upper right. The smaller frontal or parietal opening is depicted in the lower right.

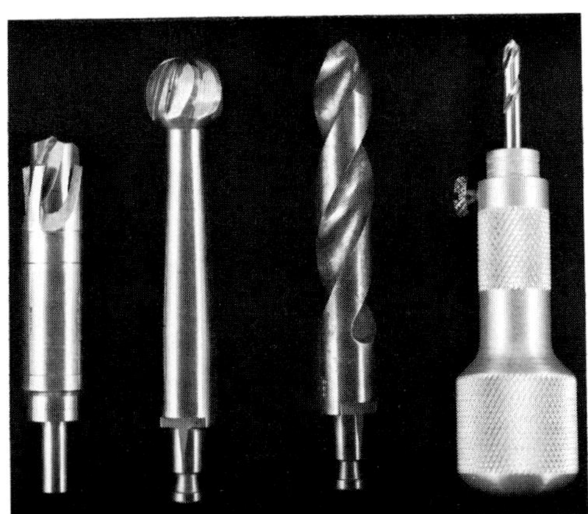

Figure 6–27 Instruments for burr-hole and twist-drill explorations in acute head trauma. From left to right these are: a motor-driven Smith perforator, a burr, a McKenzie perforator and a small hand drill.

Extradural hematomas are readily apparent as the perforator exposes black clot in breaking through the inner table. The torn middle meningeal vessel is nearly always marked by a fracture, which is commonly linear. It is wise to expose all of the collection with a craniectomy before aspirating deep portions of clot. The meningeal vessel is cauterized at the site of the rent and extensively along its course. It is necessary, on occasion, to follow the artery down to the base of the skull and to insert a small cottonoid sliver into the foramen spinosum with a right-angle hook. Numerous other areas are cauterized because of the secondary oozing that occurs as the hematoma lifts the dura mater from bone.

According to Gurdjian and Thomas[23] varied combinations of extradural, subdural or parenchymatous hematomas may be expected in about 17 per cent of cases. The dura mater is therefore opened transversely near the base to rule out a concomitant subdural collection and to inspect the temporal lobe. If this lobe is significantly displaced and remains so over a reasonable period of time, it is helpful to elevate it with a flat brain spatula and then to tease the herniated medical temporal lobe structures back from the tentorial notch. Fine silk sutures are used to close the dura mater and to tack it to the bony edges. An extradural catheter drain is placed. Since the worldwide mortality rate from extradural hematomas remains high, it is worthwhile stressing the dispatch that is required in all phases of their management. The lesion is depicted in Figure 6–28.

To evacuate a subdural hematoma, the darkened dura mater is thoroughly cauterized; a cruciate incision is then made with a small hook and knife. The opening should be wide enough to avoid the dangers of incising or inadvertently tearing the cortical veins that are turgid under states of intracranial hypertension. Membranes are present around chronic subdural hematomas, and the dural incision must be deep enough to nick the exterior covering. The contents—black liquefied blood and clot—are released under raised pressure and are expelled with the respiratory and vascular pulsations of the brain. A catheter is introduced between two holes for saline irrigations. In an adult, it is usually not necessary to turn a craniotomy flap to remove the residual clot or membrane, although there are exceptions as noted earlier. The cortex sometimes re-

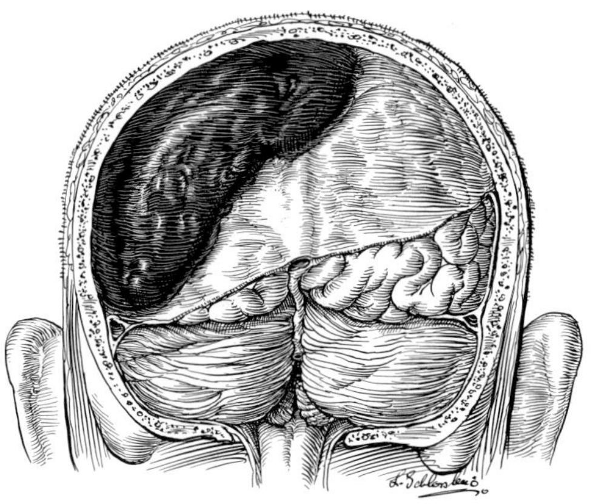

Figure 6–28 A massive extradural hematoma which was first uncovered by the medical examiner.

mains sunken after these evacuations and may not return to its normal position. Many neurosurgeons attempt to expedite this return by directly inflating the ventricular system with saline or mock CSF, although it is not certain that the expansion persists after the added saline has been absorbed. Recurrent hematomas are relatively infrequent in adults, and a subdural catheter drain may be used over a period of 18 hours as an alternative.

In these chronic lesions, the significant space-occupying component is the hematoma; in an acute subdural hemorrhage, the clot is relatively unimportant, but the underlying laceration and edema are significant. The mortality rate from these acute lesions is high and usually little can be accomplished. Exceptionally, the brain may not be lacerated and, with luck, torn bridging temporal veins may be isolated. The bleeding is then controlled by tamponade, cautery and the application of silver clips. An acute subdural hematoma is shown in Figure 6–29.

An intracerebral hematoma will often be located by arteriography or, more clearly, in the chronic stages following air injection. Sometimes the diagnosis is made when a temporal clot ruptures through the cortex during a subdural exploration. In all these instances a blunt ventricular needle is passed into the hematoma cavity for gradual drainage, and a dime-sized cortical window is then made to sluice away the larger clots. Excellent results are obtained in treating these lesions if they are well-contained and if they are polar.

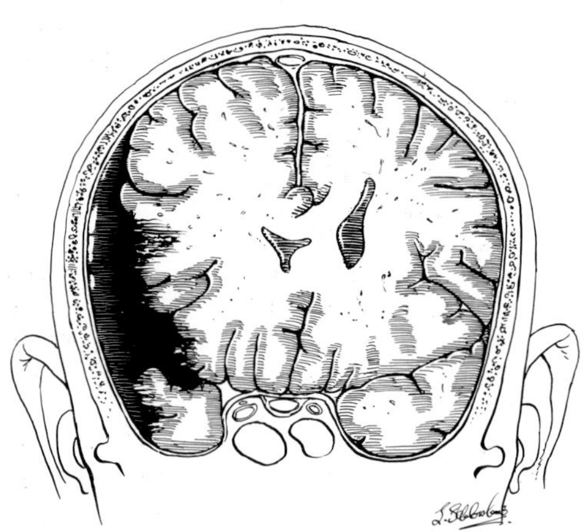

Figure 6–29 An acute subdural hematoma. Note the laceration and swelling of the brain and the subfalcial herniation.

Unfortunately, brain swelling is the major finding in many instances. Some neurosurgeons perform large craniotomies to provide decompression. Bifrontal bone flaps may be removed or bony openings provided over one hemisphere (and sometimes both). A remarkable release of brain tissue occurs; however, harm may ensue from this expansion and herniation. A more conservative plan should be used in most cases.

Similarly, the so-called internal decompression which, in practice, constitutes a partial temporal lobe resection is often used. When edematous cerebral tissue pouts from all burr holes, one has a reasonable indication of substantial, generalized brain swelling; little chance of gain is offered with these extirpations. Contrarily, striking improvement often follows the use of these limited resections when the fullness is limited to one temporal lobe. On *a priori* grounds, a section of the tentorium should give relief from the pressure effects that are so devastating to the upper brainstem with generalized brain swelling. Unfortunately, it is difficult to reach the edge of the tentorium when such a section is needed because of swelling of the temporal and occipital lobes. Conversely, when ready access is possible, the procedure may be unnecessary. These sections may be facilitated by the use of intravenous hypertonic agents. They are performed infrequently and their efficacy is debatable. The crucial area is indicated in Figure 6–30.

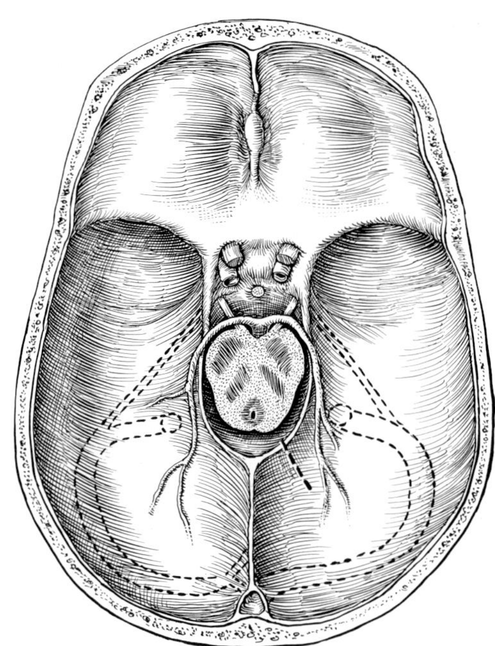

Figure 6–30 The incisura tentorii. Transtentorial herniations may occur from above or below to cause circulatory embarrassment in the distribution of the midline perforating vessels. The brainstem may be displaced against the sharp tentorial edge; the posterior cerebral artery may be kinked over it. The position of a tentorial section is indicated.

Excessive brain needling is often demonstrated on postmortem examination. In general, it is best to restrict these taps to single punctures of zones that are indicated by diagnostic films or which lie under cortical swellings that bulge disproportionately.

Posterior fossa trephinations are not regularly performed in the absence of localizing findings. The indications are more difficult to define but include: (1) a venous sinus-traversing fracture of the occipital squama in association with a substantial neurological deficit, (2) the existence of a blood dyscrasia or the use of anticoagulants in a patient in whom subdural hematomas have been searched for and ruled out supratentorially, and (3) local cerebellar and brainstem signs. For these, it is necessary to place the patient in the cerebellar headrest and to prep and drape anew. Either a long midline incision or two small longitudinal paramedian incisions may be used; in either case, the muscle is quickly split to bone, and self-retaining retractors are placed. A cerebellar extension is added to the Hudson brace. Hematomas occur in the same extra- and subdural compartments and within the cerebellum. Subdural hygromas are also found here and simulate cisternal collections that develop high pressure when the brain swells above and herniates through the tentorial notch to impede the free flow of cerebrospinal fluid.

Exploration for depressed fractures is carried out without delay if the injury is compound or if the depression is pronounced. A few cases are dismissed because of insignificant depressions; the remainder are operated upon within a period of about 24 hours. If there is no laceration, a skin flap is preferred rather than a linear incision. The sunken bone may be elevated in several ways. It is often easy to retrieve the depressed pieces of bone with a rongeur after inserting this instrument through a small hole that has been nibbled in the margin of the intact bone. Sometimes the impinging fragments can be grasped directly or elevated with a dissector that is introduced from an adjacent burr hole. The bone may be retained if reasonable stability can be achieved. However, bony defects usually remain and cranioplasties are required. These may be carried out immediately if there is no contamination but are more frequently performed as secondary procedures. If the dura mater is intact, it is opened only with specific indications.

Although all debridements should be done fastidiously, special care is required for those of the brain since the penalties that accrue from the retention of devitalized brain tissue, bony spicules and other foreign material are severe and include the formation of abscesses and the establishment of epileptogenic foci.

The scalp edges are trimmed and the pericranial tissues are washed with saline. The bone edges are rongeured in the case of a limited injury; a craniotomy flap is opened for an extensive one. Arterial dural bleeding is arrested with the cautery; hemorrhage from rents in venous sinuses is controlled with fingertip pressure over pledgets of absorbable gelatin or cellulose. Attempts are made to completely remove the devitalized brain, using suction and excessive amounts of warm saline. The venous oozing in the depths of these resections is usually handled with gentle tamponade from a loose, cotton "fish." Dural defects are common; in most instances they are closed with grafts of pericranial tissue. Fascia lata may be used, but plastic materials should be avoided. Local antibiotics are not instilled and drains are not placed. Fine wire or plastic suture material is used throughout. The results of this procedure are usually quite satisfactory, and it is perhaps worthwhile to emphasize the painstaking effort that should be expended in the care of such patients because of the focal nature of their injuries.

EARLY MANAGEMENT IN THE INTENSIVE CARE UNIT

An endotracheal tube should not be retained for long postoperative periods. If needed, a tracheostomy should be performed within a few hours after the patient is taken from the operating room. Thereafter, careful and frequent suctioning is carried out with a sterile catheter to remove stationary and excessive secretions.

Oxygen therapy is valuable if there is any suspicion of ischemia of the brain; carbon dioxide inhalations augment cerebral blood flow but are not commonly used because of the attendant vasodilation and because of the fact that the increase in perfusion is in normal brain. In the absence of shock, the head of the bed is elevated 20 to 30 degrees to facilitate venous drainage.

Fluids are given parenterally at first and via a stomach tube after four to five days if the patient cannot swallow. When there is established brain swelling, the fluid intake is usually restricted for several days. Hypertonic intravenous infusions are often used to accomplish a more abrupt and drastic dehydration. Because of the osmotic effect, these agents induce a temporary fall in intracranial pressures and a decrease in brain bulk, as shown in the classic study of Weed and McKibben.[74] There is also a possible long-term benefit from the loss of water with the diuresis and a possible detrimental action as cerebrospinal fluid pressures rise secondarily. Mannitol is currently popular and in comparison with urea offers a relatively long relaxation period (and minimal rebound) because of its nonpenetrating characteristics. It is given quickly in a 20 per cent solution in a dosage range of 1–2 g. per kg. It may be used occasionally after operations (or diagnostic procedures) when the patient worsens suddenly—as with decerebration or pupillary dilatation or when measured intracranial pressures rise precipitously during pressure waves.

General hypothermia was first used for head injury problems by Fay[14]; however, the technique did not become popular until Bigelow et al.[2] demonstrated the specific depression of metabolism during cooling. A cooling blanket is used, and its temperature is conveniently regulated within a range of one to two degrees by a temperature controller and a rectal temperature probe. If the temperature is lowered more than a few degrees below the normal level, shivering and restlessness are provoked; these add serious problems in management and, although they can be influenced by Phenergan, they are usually incompletely suppressed unless the patient is curarized. There is also an increased incidence of pulmonary infection in the lower temperature range (30 to 32°C.) because of depressed ciliary action in the tracheobronchial tree. Because of these drawbacks and the fact that cooling is usually instituted sometime after the injury, this measure is usually reserved for combating hyperthermia and holding temperatures at or a little below the normal level.

Corticosteroid derivatives are used empirically; however, they are viewed more optimistically than the other techniques at the moment. Their initial or continued usage will have to be re-evaluated in the recovery room. An antacid regimen should be employed and the dosage should be tapered off as quickly as possible.

Excessive motor activity is frequently a major problem in the recovery room. A minor degree of restlessness is common and requires only restraint. Agitation is found less frequently and is often inadequately controlled. Paraldehyde is the drug of choice, but its use should be restricted so that the patient's condition is not jeopardized by loss of the opportunity to follow changes in the state of consciousness. The adult dosage is 10 ml., which is given via a gastric tube or as a small retention enema. If initially ineffective, the dose may be repeated with caution; as in the management of status epilepticus, large amounts may be tolerated. In a few instances, violent activity is encountered and Pentothal anesthesia is needed for control; such patients include those with meningeal irritation caused by sizable subarachnoid blood deposits and those with allied states such as asphyxia.

Seizure activity in the recovery room is relatively uncommon with acute head injury, but it should be anticipated when gross brain damage has been noted in the operating room. Diphenylhydantoin sodium is used with an adult dosage of 100 mg. intramuscularly three times a day. This drug should be given routinely in the early stages of recovery from such trauma.

Except for respirator assistance, as in combined head and chest injuries, the continued use of artificial ventilation leads to one of the most trying situations in the recovery room. The prolonged administration of vasoactive drugs in terminal states similarly entails perplexing decisions. It is important to carefully scrutinize and limit the indications for initiating their use. They are sometimes required when a renal donation is under consideration, and here the need for early EEG recordings and for the repeated documentation of peripheral and brainstem reflex activity is stressed.

Samples for serum and urine electrolyte determinations should be obtained in the accident room, repeated frequently in the postoperative period and recorded on detailed fluid balance sheets. This is of particular importance for neurosurgical patients with multiple injuries who may become hyponatremic and develop water intoxication after the administration of excess fluid at the same time that unusual amounts of ADH are being secreted.

Similarly, serial blood gas determinations are mandatory in patients with depressed responsiveness and particularly those who require respiratory support.

Fat embolism with complications from intracranial deposits or pulmonary lesions with secondary cerebral effects should be considered in all patients with major injuries. Chest roentgenogram, cryostat frozen sections of clotted blood, blood gas studies and the search for petechial hemorrhages are stressed. Positive findings add special indications for steroid therapy as well as particular care in ventilation.

CRANIOCEREBRAL INJURY: CLASSIFICATION, PHYSICAL MECHANISM AND UNDERLYING PATHOLOGY

Charles D. Ray, M.D.
and
Edward R. Laws, Jr., M.D.

Head injuries account for approximately three-fourths of all injuries sustained in automobile accidents. Since a knowledge of the tolerance of the nervous system to various stresses is essential in the prevention of injury and subsequent damage, a great deal of study and experimentation has dealt with the nature of injuries produced by various types of trauma. In order to reduce the likelihood of death from head injuries, the surgeon must have an adequate working knowledge of the mechanisms and consequences of craniocerebral trauma to aid in the diagnosis and treatment of brain injury.

Since the brain is an endoskeletal organ lying within a "closed-box cavity," injuries and their consequences must be considered somewhat differently from trauma inflicted elsewhere on the body. Other than direct destruction of brain substance, the most important physical mechanism to be considered is the *development of pressure.* As pressure rises and the brain substance is compressed, secondary phenomena occur which may lead to death. As one learns in medicine, there are relatively few *true* emergencies. However, an expanding lesion within the cranial cavity requires prompt diagnosis and surgical relief to avert death.

ANATOMICAL CONSIDERATIONS

Injuries of the head involve more than just the brain. The *scalp* acts as a protective covering for the head and is able by deformation and stretching to absorb and cushion a certain proportion of the energy imparted to the head. Injuries to the scalp may produce: (1) a contusion or bruise; (2) a laceration; (3) hemorrhage which may be copious, or if the bleeding is confined, a subgaleal hematoma.

The *skull* provides the brain with more substantial and more rigid protection. Injuries to the skull may produce: (1) periosteal contusions or lacerations; (2) transient deformation and distortion of the skull, transmitted to the brain substance; or (3) fracture, which may be either linear or fragmentary with a simple separation of the tables or a depression of both cranial tables. Depressed fractures are usually quite fragmentary and they may also be communicating ("compound") with an associated injury of the dura and underlying brain.

The *meninges* contain the thin layer of cerebrospinal fluid which covers the surface of the brain and acts to a certain extent as a hydraulic shock-absorber. Injury to the meninges may produce: (1) a stretch; (2) a tear, as may be associated with a fracture; (3) hemorrhage, which may occur from disruption of a meningeal artery or injury to a dural sinus—these hemorrhages may collect (and dissect) in the epidural space or the subdural space; or (4) cerebrospinal fluid leak.

Injuries to the *brain* are far more complex, however: (1) a localized cortical injury usually produces little direct clinical effect; (2) trauma to underlying glia in most cases produces only local edema; (3) injuries to surface vessels usually produce only a local hematoma, although there may be secondary ischemic changes; (4) subcortical injuries are more devastating and involve larger structural masses leading to more complex syndromes; and (5) there may be deep injuries to brain substance as a result of shearing forces that inflict distortions and disruption of brain substance. Severe contusion, hemorrhage and/or death follow. Subcortical injuries may produce local and widespread interruption of conduction, the phenomenon of "cerebral shock" (an inhibition of function produced secondarily from a remote injury in regions interconnected by fiber tracts).

Since the scalp is highly vascular, a scalp laceration that has bled but is now stopped should not be extensively examined until the physician is adequately prepared to cope with the severe reactivation of hemorrhage that will likely follow. Not infrequently, a subgaleal hematoma will exhibit a firm rim and have a soft center that feels like a depression. Sooner or later every examiner, convinced that some patient has sustained a depressed skull fracture, will be surprised on x-ray examination to find that none exists.

THE MECHANICS OF CRANIOCEREBRAL TRAUMA

At the moment of initial impact and for the immediate period that follows, trauma is a problem in pure physics. By definition, the injury is produced by a mechanical or physical change of the head with respect to its environment. For many years there have been numerous investigations of brain changes subsequent to trauma, and the problem is still not settled. Holbourn describes the brain, from a physical point of view, as a substance relatively uniform in density, quite elastic and essentially incompressible.[27] Blood, spinal fluid and the basic solid structures of the brain have essentially the same density as water and as such would require tremendous pressures to evoke small changes in volume. In contrast to brain elasticity, the skull is quite rigid. Models of the brain and skull have been made in order to investigate the physics of trauma. They generally involve a fluid or gelatin contained in a transparent case having the shape of the skull. Using high-speed photography and a variety of blows directed from different locations, Edberg and his associates have measured the propagation of fluid movement, shock waves and shearing forces of the "brain" within the transparent "skull."[13]

Figure 6–31 shows the basic types of injuries that are being considered here.

Table 6–1 gives a résumé of the various studies regarding the physics and pathology of head injury. Several concepts are presented in this summary.

When an object is in motion, any sudden change in this motion will be expressed as an acceleration or deceleration. Sellier and Unterharnscheidt have shown that when the head is struck and its velocity is changed to about 1.7 meters per second, or roughly 38 miles per hour, a positive pressure of about one atmosphere will develop at the percussed side of the brain-skull interface and, simultaneously a *minus* one atmosphere at the opposite pole.[63] This effect lasts only about five milliseconds. Thus, when the moving head strikes a fixed object there will be a transient negative pressure produced at the brain-skull interface on the opposite side of the head. This vacuum (minus one atmosphere) produces cavitation (gas bubble formation) within the brain substance and probably is a significant contributing factor in so-called contrecoup injuries. A second major result of force is produced by a sliding or rotary motion of the brain's substance within the cranial vault. This has been demonstrated by Pudenz and Shelden, who used a transparent plastic skullcap on monkeys.[50] The analogy is well taken that if one suspends a floating object in a bucket of water, linear motions of the bucket will not alter the relationship between its walls and the object. How-

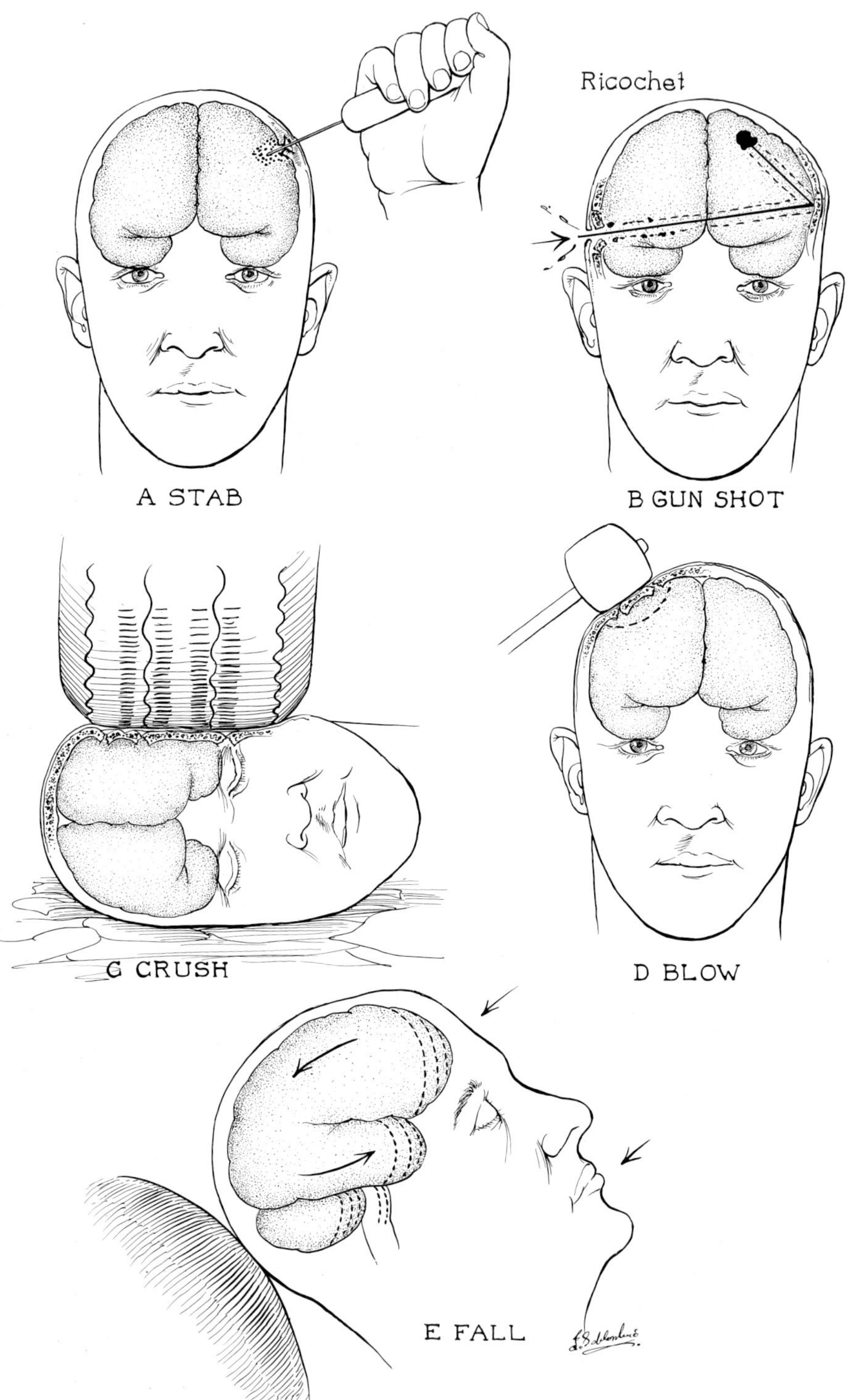

Figure 6–31 Common types of craniocerebral injuries and means by which they are often inflicted.

Table 6–1. Physics and "Typical" Pathology of Head Injury

	INJURY				RESULTS					
					Damage to:					
Type	*Impact Velocity*	*Forces* Momentum*	*Velocity Imparted† (Change)*	*Shear-strain‡*	*Scalp*	*Bone*	*Vessels*	*Brain*	*Stem*	*Clinical Effects*
Stab	Low	Low	Small	Linear+	++	+	+	Local, mild	0	Specific, mild
Gunshot§	High	Low	Small	Linear+	++	++	Deep+++	Specific, variable	0	Specific, variable
Crush	Very low	Very low	0	Linear+	+++	++++	+	Diffuse, mild	0	General, mild
Blow, mild	Low	Low	Small	Linear+ Rotary+	+	+	+	Local, mild	+	General, moderate
Blow, severe	Mod.	High	Large	Linear++ Rotary+++	++	+++	++	Contrecoup	+++	General, moderate to severe
Fall, mild	Low	High	Large	Linear++ Rotary+++	+	+	++	Contrecoup	++	General, moderate to severe
Fall, severe	Low	Very high	Very large	Linear+++ Rotary++++	+++	+++	Surface+++	Diffuse, severe	++++	General, severe

*Impact forces are for moving object striking head (producing acceleration) or for head in motion striking object (producing deceleration).
†Velocity change for skull and brain relative to velocity before impact.
‡Shear-strain force is movement of brain relative to skull.
§Variability of injuries associated with gunshot wounds precludes exact rules. Extent of damage is predominantly dependent on the impact velocity (kinetic energy) of the bullet.

ever, a very slight rotation of the bucket will produce a swirling of the contents and a marked change in the relationships. Since the internal landmarks of the skull are not uniform and show definite prominences that may "trap" the brain during its rotation, certain areas will show the greatest damage when a complex force is applied to the skull. Such factors, presented in Table 6–1 under the column marked shear-strain, are well described by Holbourn.[27] Compressive forces generated within a nonfractured skull tend to be focused at the foramen magnum where tremendous forces may be exerted on the brainstem and cerebellar tonsils.

There are other interesting factors that emerge on careful examination of Table 6–1. *It is less the velocity of the impact force than the momentum imparted to the head and brain that dictates the type and degree of injury.* It is this momentum that suddenly changes the position of the head and also of the brain relative to the skull. It is known that most blows and falls result in complex movements involving both linear and rotary changes in brain position. Rotary shear-strains produce the most damaging effects. An interesting illustration of this in experimental form is reported by Ommaya et al.[46] They showed that a sudden blow from a hard rubber hammer to the occipital area in a lightly anesthetized monkey will produce traumatic unconsciousness when the cranial velocity change is about 35 miles per hour in the freely movable head. However, when the neck is placed in a plaster jacket resembling a neck brace or collar, approximately twice the force is required to produce concussion since head movement is now less rotary and more linear.

From the table we can see that a severe fall injury results in considerable damage to the brain. The head is in motion and is brought to a sudden standstill as it encounters a solid object. This is essentially the set of circumstances in which the head strikes a dashboard, windshield or the ground following a head-on automobile collision. In such instances, sudden deceleration of the head produces a snapping forward of the brain within the cranial vault, resulting in abrupt negative pressure on the opposite pole of the brain. Such negative pressures may lead to cavitation of brain substance. However, the situation is more complex because of the fact that rotary shear-strain will add decidedly to the injury and lead to laceration in areas of relative anatomical entrapment. The frontal and temporal lobes are not so free to move because of intracranial bony prominences and the falx. Courville has emphasized that, regardless of the direction of the blow, these areas will receive greater contusion and laceration than the remainder of the cortical substance.[9]

As the brain slides around inside the cranial vault traction occurs, with rupture of small vessels perforating the brain substance. Many of the consequences of head injury are the result of disruption of these vessels, rather than the direct effect of the physical forces on brain substance. Some of the cranial nerves are especially vulnerable to traction injuries as the brain moves in the skull, particularly the first, second, third and eighth nerves. This problem will be discussed later. When the skull itself has been bent or distorted, the injuries are usually more superficial. This gives rise to the seeming paradox that one patient who has a depressed skull fracture may show little clinical change, yet another patient with no fracture at all may exhibit profound unconsciousness.

It is the velocity of the injuring object that will determine the type of skull fracture produced. Linear fractures are usually produced by low-velocity injuries and depressed fractures by higher velocities. Experiments by Gurdjian and associates show that a steel pellet three-fourths of an inch in circumference traveling at 50 feet per second will produce a linear fracture on striking the exposed skull of a cadaver.[22] The same pellet traveling at 90 feet per second will produce a perforation of the skull with a depressed fracture. Approximately 500 or more inch-pounds of pressure are required to produce a linear fracture. Only 0.05 second is needed for this impact to produce a maximum deformation. The scalp is deformed in about 0.002 second and the skull in about 0.004 second after onset of impact. The extent of a linear fracture may, therefore, be taken as a relatively good index of the severity of the blow and a rough measurement of the severity of traumatic unconsciousness.

Some other interesting points may be observed in Table 6–1. Holbourn points out that a 10-gram bullet traveling at a velocity of 400 meters per second when completely stopped by the head would produce a rotational velocity no greater than that which would occur from the head's striking an object moving at only two miles per hour.[27] Although the bullet has a considerable amount of kinetic energy, it imparts very little momentum. The tract of injury of the bullet is principally dependent upon the kinetic energy, and the resultant rotational factors may produce the widespread damage often seen. Low-velocity bullets usually do not produce traumatic unconsciousness.

A static type of crush injury to the head, unless it is so extensive that it disrupts or avulses neural structures, usually produces no unconsciousness, and the prognosis is quite good. Small children whose heads have been run over by automobiles will often make remarkably good recoveries. In marked contrast, a fall or a blow such as a boxer's uppercut imparts high momentum, produces a sudden change in velocity and causes a complex rotation of the head, resulting in far greater damage than if the blow had been applied in a more linear manner.

The most severely damaging blow commonly encountered occurs in sudden deceleration injuries, as when the head strikes the dashboard of a car. The patient may remain unconscious for a matter of days or months. This unconsciousness, however, is rarely the result of direct cortical brain damage alone but rather is due to changes within the brainstem. Nearly one-third of the patients sustaining such brainstem injuries die instantly. Of those who survive, approximately one-half succumb to delayed effects. Most of these patients simply never wake up.

CAUSES OF DEATH: A CLASSIFICATION

In trauma to the central nervous system death may be attributed to the following factors:

Immediate Causes

1. Direct brain injury (especially vital brainstem centers)
2. Indirect brain injury:
   a. "Neural paralysis"—local ininjury with local and remote depression or inhibition of neural function
   b. Vascular disorders: disruption—tearing of large or small nutrient vessels, occlusion—thrombosis from injury or spasm, compression—formation of expanding hematoma
   c. Brain swelling with compression from cerebral edema
3. Systemic causes: hemorrhage and shock, hypotension with ischemia and thrombosis
   a. Respiratory obstruction—ischemia
   b. Air embolism into the circulation of the brain
   c. Cardiac complications—arrhythmias, pulmonary edema secondary to left heart failure

Delayed Causes

1. Direct brain injury, as above

2. Indirect brain injury, as above, plus cellular-metabolic changes
3. Infection within cranium, meningitis or abscess (depressed communicating fracture, cerebrospinal fluid leak)
4. Systemic causes, fluids, electrolytes, metabolites
5. Respiratory factors
6. Fat embolism
7. Systemic infection, toxins

COMPLICATIONS IN THE MANAGEMENT OF THE UNCONSCIOUS PATIENT

The following are some of the difficulties which may occur following head injury:

1. Airway (aspiration, obstruction, atelectasis)
2. Fluid and electrolytes (inappropriate ADH secretion, "cerebral salt wasting")
3. Infections (central nervous system, respiratory, urinary, open fractures, decubitus ulcers)
4. Gastrointestinal distention
5. Bladder distention
6. Agonal (Cushing) ulceration and hemorrhage from the gastrointestinal tract
7. Hormonal stress reactions
8. Seizures
9. "Vegetative" phenomena (management of abnormal respiration, blood pressure and temperature)
10. Metabolic (acid-base problems, usually a combination of metabolic acidosis and respiratory alkalosis)
11. Abnormalities in CSF flow and absorption (hydrocephalus, either acute high-pressure or more chronic low-pressure syndromes)

As will be explained in more detail later, the electrical rhythms and synchrony of the brain (electroencephalogram) may be affected by brain injury. Whereas focal asynchronism may be produced by pathological changes in the cortex, diffuse asynchronism and generalized dysrhythmia probably result from injury to deeper centers. The reticular substance of the upper brainstem and the posterior hypothalamic regions have been particularly implicated. Such injuries are also usually associated with loss of consciousness.

CONSEQUENCES OF HEAD INJURY

Details of diagnosis and treatment were discussed in previous chapters. It seems to be important here to present a generalized classification of the series of events that are usually seen in association with various pathological entities.

In Figure 6–32 the time sequence of five clinicopathologic conditions of head injury are shown: (A) a disruption of vital centers leading promptly to death; (B) an acute epidural hematoma with compression of underlying brain; (C) contusion of brain substance with subsequent formation of edema; (D) a chronic subdural hematoma that produces compression as the trapped blood undergoes autolysis, absorbs fluid and expands; and (E) simple traumatic unconsciousness without specific pathologic changes. The time base shown is roughly logarithmic. Below the time base are given approximate durations of the mechanisms responsible for the effects seen in each clinical condition. Probabilities are also implicated; e.g., death within the first few days following injury is probably due to compression from edema, which exhibits its maximum effects within a few hours to a few days.

A few points are worth stressing in the consideration of compression syndromes. Although not indicated in Figure 6–32, subdural hematomas fall into three types: acute, subacute and chronic. This classification is primarily based on the time between injury and the onset of clinical signs—namely, less than 24 hours, up to a

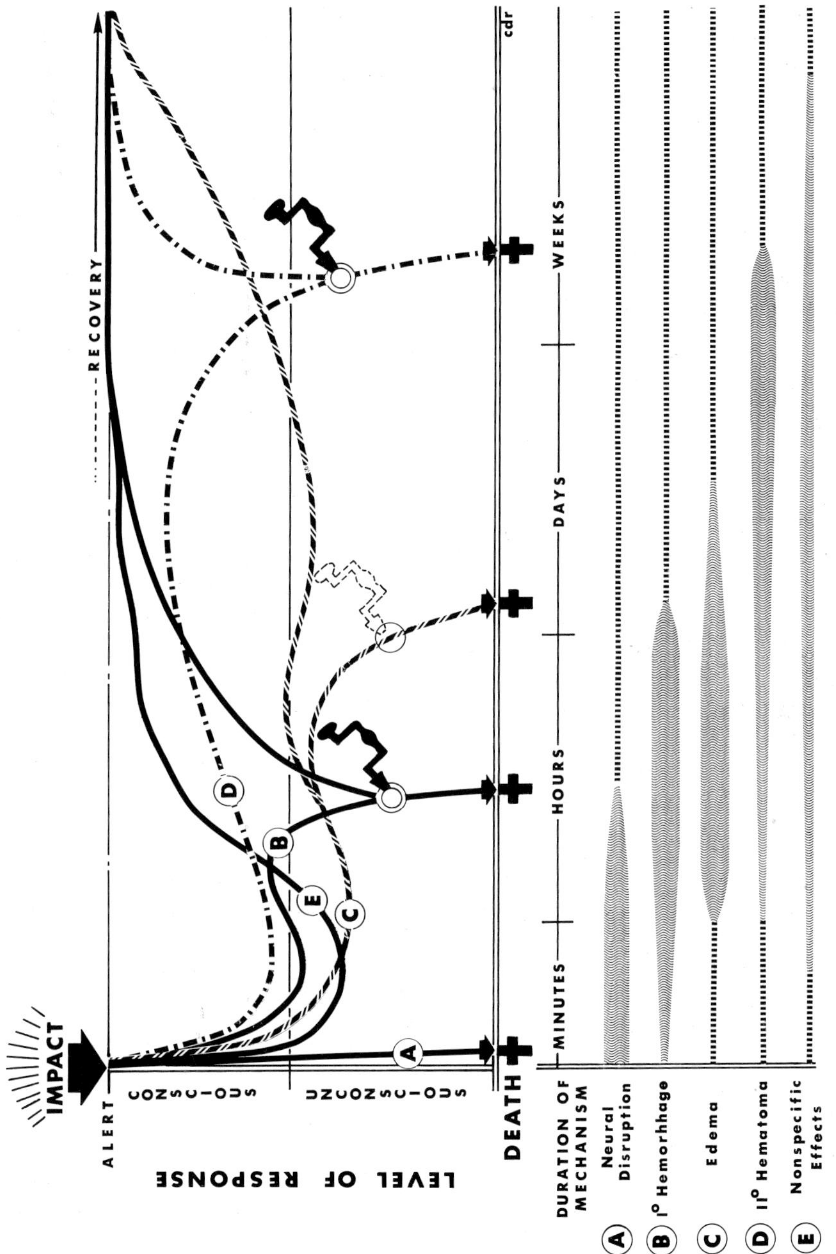

Figure 6–32 Diagram of five common clinicopathologic conditions resulting from craniocerebral injury and their frequently observed sequence of events.

week or two, and those appearing thereafter. Not so obvious, however, are the degrees of severity associated with different types. About 60 per cent of patients with acute subdural hematoma will die despite surgery, about 20 per cent of these with subacute and about 10 per cent of these with chronic. The relative occurrence of the different types of subdural hematomas is about the reverse of these mortality rates; i.e., 20 per cent are acute; 30 per cent, subacute; and 50 per cent, chronic. A patient who arrives in the emergency room with a hematoma and who had no "lucid interval" after injury and is in a deep unresponsive state will probably soon die, regardless of the type of hematoma; by this time, the effects of compression have become essentially irreversible. Subdural collections are more common in the very young, although similar mortality statistics apply as given above for adults. Chronic subdural hematoma is a disease of infants and aged persons. Subdural hematomas of all types occur in a significant percentage of all major head injuries.

The immature nervous system of the very young reacts to injury with a rather intense degeneration; however, both functional and structural adaptability are remarkable.

When the mechanism of compression is contusion with edema, the patient may show a gradual decline in responsiveness within a few hours. As indicated in Figure 6–32, surgery, if performed for decompression, is generally of little value; if other methods of reducing intracranial pressure are unrewarding, death may ensue.

Most cases of epidural hematoma are of a rather violent origin (head-on collision, motorcycle accident, etc.), and the patients die abruptly. Further, most are associated with bleeding of the middle meningeal artery, occur most frequently on the right side (seldom bilaterally) and are rarely seen without a fracture (except in the very young). Most have homolateral dilation of the pupil and contralateral body weakness or paralysis. Although less than 2 per cent of all significant head injuries will have an epidural hematoma, the mortality rate is quite high in unoperated cases (see Fig. 6–33A).

Pathological Changes

As noted, the skull is relatively resistant to compression, although the brain is highly subject to local and widespread effects from jarring of the head. Such jarring of the brain may occur even in the absence of skull fracture and is often more lethal than actual brain laceration. Classically, injuries to brain substance have been classified as *concussion, contusion* and *laceration.*

Concussion. Concussion implies a traumatic event resulting from a relatively minor injury process and is manifested by a transient loss or change in consciousness from which the patient will make a relatively quick and satisfactory recovery. However, the term concussion is often used to suggest a definite process, lesion or change in behavior; no such specificity exists in clinical practice or pathological study. Unconsciousness that persists for more than a few hours is related to more definite organic lesions, probably also involving the brainstem, posterior thalamus and/or temporal lobes. In experimental work it can be shown that a variety of pathological changes are found in the presence of reversible traumatic unconsciousness, but they are not the same from experiment to experiment and show considerable tissue variation by light microscopy. The electron microscopic and metabolic cellular studies show local and widespread changes but are again variable. Nonetheless, whatever the lesions are, they are considered to be reversible.

Contusion. Contusion, on the other hand, is an anatomical and pathological change that can be found on a microscopic and macrocellular level in brain tissue. There is a bruising of

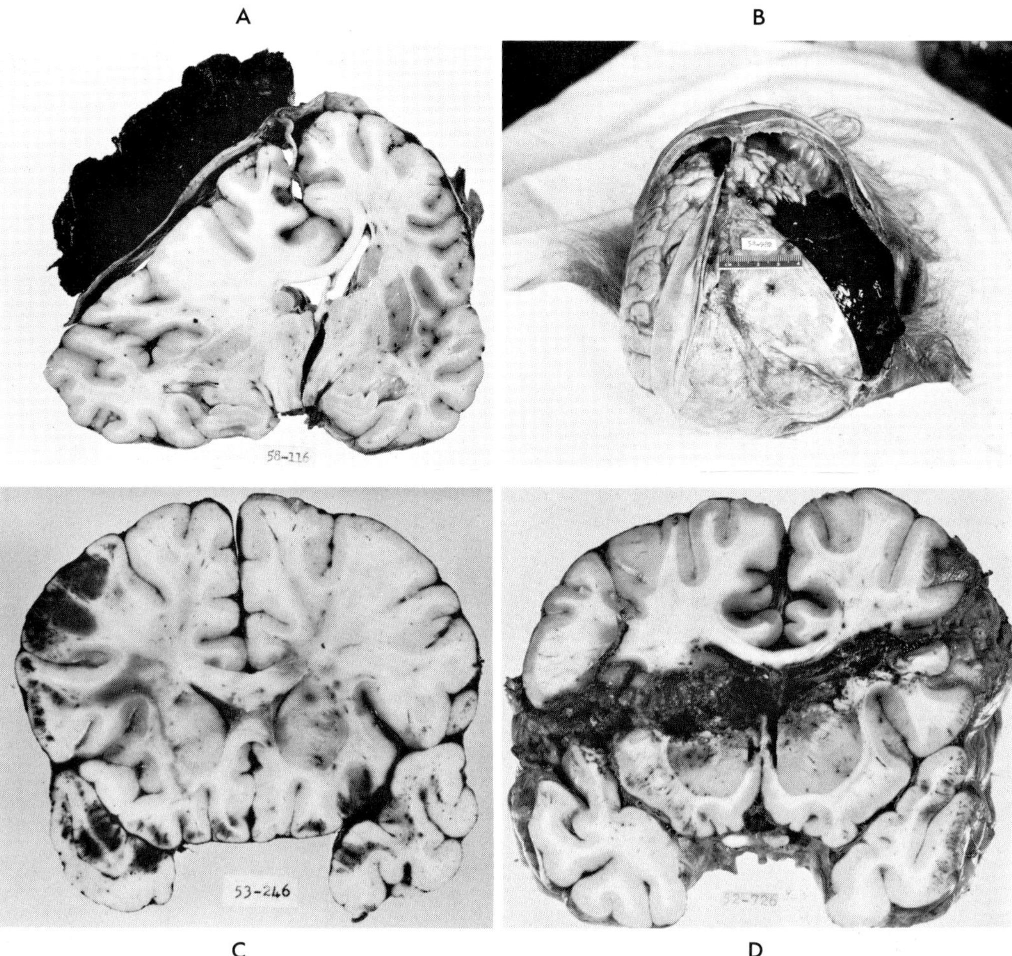

Figure 6–33 Gross pathologic changes following brain injury. *A*, Epidural hematoma. Note displacement of intact dura and underlying brain. *B*, Subdural hematoma. Note firm organization of the clot. *C*, Cortical contusions. Note principal involvement of crests of convolutions. *D*, Gunshot wound. Changes due to widespread contusions are also seen. (Photographs courtesy Dr. Richard Lindenberg.)

the brain substance that results in an injury to vessels and a consequent diapedesis of cells (see Fig. 6–33C).

Laceration. Laceration of brain substance results from open or closed fractures and is a tearing of the substance of the brain by a sudden movement against a relatively fixed intracranial landmark.

Unconsciousness. The immediate onset of traumatic unconsciousness results from a transient and more or less complete inhibition of neural activity on a local or widespread basis. If the brainstem vital centers are involved, respiration will stop and death will occur. Neural elements may receive a sudden intense stimulation which may then be followed by inhibition. Lindenberg and Freytag report that interesting pathological findings are seen in patients who receive relatively uncomplicated head injuries and yet remain in a state of extreme dementia, exhibiting considerable neurological abnormality, and finally expire.[37] Severe and widespread degeneration of the white matter occurs but the gray matter is generally unaffected. This suggests that a secondary degeneration results from the stretching or tearing of fibers at the time of the accident.

Delayed Effects. EDEMA. Most studies, and for that matter actual clinical observation, on patients with head injuries show that the delayed effects of injury are the more problematic. Without question the most important aspect of delayed response to injury is swelling of the brain, or edema, which may occur even in the absence of hemorrhage. The enlargement of the cranial contents produces a rising pressure that eventually leads to widespread effects. There may even be an extrusion of brain substance through the foramen magnum with subsequent cessation of respiration.

In one way or another the problem of edema is related to changes in permeability of small vessels and brain substance. Changes in permeability have been studied by various tracer techniques, notably the use of a fluorescent material placed in the blood stream. The distribution and severity of the permeability are clearly demonstrated by the appearance of fluorescence, which stains the tissues. It can be shown experimentally that even minor injury to the brain may lead to generalized swelling lasting perhaps for days or weeks. Recent intensive electron microscopic studies and histochemical preparations show an actual change in the blood-brain barrier that subsequently permits fluid leakage from the vessels into the brain substance. These changes apparently occur on a molecular basis.

Cerebral edema is the result of hygropic swelling of the astrocytes and of a major expansion of the extracellular space in the white matter. There is evidence that the altered uptake and transport of serum protein by glial elements may be representative of an enzymatic variation within the cells, resulting in the edema.

Experiments by Rockoff and Ommaya have shown that there is a slowing of the cerebral circulation that may contribute to the breakdown in blood-brain barrier and development of edema.[52] The circulatory slowing may be a primary change, in direct response to trauma, which may then secondarily lead to edema.

Of more importance is the recently demonstrated loss of autoregulation of the circulation of the brain which may occur after any significant head injury. Under normal circumstances, the cerebral blood vessels automatically adjust caliber and flow rate to keep cerebral perfusion relatively constant despite wide variations in systemic blood pressure. After trauma, this capacity for regulation may be lost, and, if systemic blood pressure rises in response to increasing intracranial pressure, the hydrostatic pressure in the arterial side of the cerebral circulation will also rise, producing more hydrostatic edema and creating a vicious cycle which will have a fatal outcome unless terminated.

BLUNT FORCE INJURIES. As indicated above, the neurologic syndrome resulting from brain injury is in many cases consequent to injury of the *brainstem.* Contusion hemorrhages in the substantia nigra are not rare. Such contusions may involve the uncus and the entire length of the hippocampus. Post-traumatic amnesia and parkinsonism have been attributed to such changes. Freytag, in a recent report on nearly 1400 cases of brain injuries from blunt forces that had resulted in death (collected over a period of ten years) showed that nearly half of the accidents were the result of falls.[17] About one-fourth were traffic accidents involving pedestrians; in less than 10 per cent was the victim a passenger or driver of a car. In approximately one-fourth of the cases the use of alcohol was connected in some way with the accident. Over one-half of the patients died within 24 hours, and one-fourth survived from one day to one week. Ten per cent lived from one month to six months and only 6 per cent lived longer. Age distribution showed essentially equal representation for each decade of life, except that the second decade had the lowest number of cases.

Over one-third of the patients died in spite of cranial operation. Seventy per cent had skull fractures, with the smallest number of fractures occurring in children under 10 years of age. It is interesting to note that approximately one-fourth of these patients died from epidural hematomas, yet only a small percentage of the *treatable* patients arriving at the emergency treatment room will have epidural hemorrhages. Obviously, most patients with such bleeding never reach medical hands. Two-thirds of the cases had subdural bleeding, of which less than half had skull fractures. Massive subarachnoid hemorrhage was the most frequent finding in all deaths. Generally, this bleeding was poorly developed and probably of venous origin; as such, it therefore may or may not be of clinical significance. Table 6–2 gives the summary of causes of death.

From this work we may draw some important conclusions: Secondary lesions of the midbrain and pons appear to be the most frequent factors leading to death (respiratory collapse) from head injuries. Such secondary lesions may develop within a matter of minutes and may explain why acute subdural hematomas bear such a poor prognosis. Interestingly, this situation is practically absent in infants. Epidural bleeding rarely occurs without skull fracture, but subdural bleeding may occur with or without skull fracture. Particularly notable is the fact that massive subarachnoid hemorrhages of a fatal nature may occur without obvious contusion of the brain. Commonly, brain surface contusions are associated with contusions of deep structures. All traumatic lesions of the cortex may be considered contusions when the dura and head are intact. Pathologically, contusions of the cortex consist of hemorrhages and/or necrosis. Both of these originate from the moment of impact and involve principally the anatomical crest of the convolutions. These lesions may be solitary but are generally multiple and streaky and occur in clusters. The necroses are wedge-shaped and involve both gray and white matter (Fig. 6–34). There may be isolated zones of necrosis which result in cystic change. It appears that the mechanical factors involved in the injury produce these changes rather than secondary changes such as anoxia or vascular stasis.

FIREARM INJURIES. Findings in head injuries resulting from the use of firearms, based on a series of 254 autopsy cases, are discussed by Freytag.[18] In this series the number of suicide cases accounts for better than half the total. Two-thirds of the patients were dead on arrival at the hospital and only 10 per cent lived longer than one day. Most bullet

TABLE 6–2. CAUSE OF DEATH FOLLOWING BLUNT HEAD INJURIES*

(1367 cases)	*Per Cent*
Concussion of vital centers (leading to acute dysfunction without morphologic changes)	6
Contusion of vital areas	8
Secondary involvement of vital areas by edema	25
Secondary involvement of vital areas by hemorrhage and necrosis	24
Meningitis	2
Severe generalized body injuries	11
Disease related or unrelated to the injuries	24

*Based on information in Freytag, E.: Arch. Path. 75:402–413, 1963.

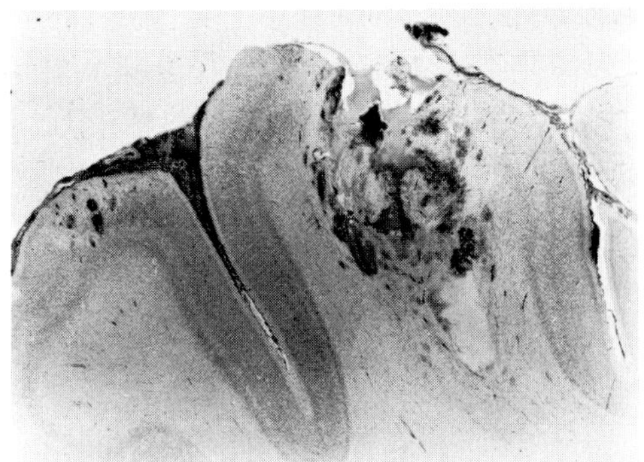

Figure 6–34 Microscopic changes in cortical contusion. The lesion is essentially wedge-shaped, involving hemorrhagic necrosis of both gray and white matter. (Courtesy Dr. Richard Lindenberg.)

wound canals correspond to the size of the slug and generally maintain an even diameter throughout their length. Tumbling or snubbing of the bullet nose results in a widening of the canal as it progresses. A ring of contused tissue surrounds the path of the bullet (see Fig. 6–33D). Remote contusions are sometimes also seen far from the injury tract; e.g., in the cerebellar tonsils. Delayed hemorrhagic processes may also lead to compression of brain substance. All who did not die instantly showed secondary lesions. Edema and often hemorrhage in the midbrain and pons represented the principal causes of death. In the few who survived for relatively long periods of time (up to a few months), secondary lesions of the above character were not found.

Final Outcome

A brief note on follow-up of patients with severe head injuries gives one additional insight into the overall problem. Although a majority have some persistent difficulties, those who survive the immediate accident and subsequent few days or weeks rarely die as a direct consequence of the head injury. The listing of *delayed* causes and complications given previously presents the more common factors.

After the patient has recovered from the acute clinical phases of head injury, the following signs, which represent managerial problems for the patient and his family, may be present. Miller and Stern report the more common sequelae as amnesia, dyspraxia, dysphasia and dysgnosia (i.e., changes in memory, difficulty in performing practical tasks, difficulty with speech and with recognition of objects).[42] There may be paresis or paralysis of a mixed or unilateral type, usually accompanied by spasticity. Most cases of spastic paresis will show an unexpectedly good recovery. Cranial nerve changes may persist, especially anosmia, visual changes such as double vision and discoordinate eye movements, decrease in hearing, ataxia and vertigo. Anosmia increases with the severity of the head injury, the overall incidence being about 75 per cent. There is a high incidence of temporary anosmia in patients with minor head injuries. Most cases do recover, however. Post-traumatic dysphasia and cranial nerve lesions have a good prognosis except for those involving the first, second and eighth nerves. Perhaps the most sensitive and reliable index of severity of injury for cases without signs of focal damage (such as a depressed fracture of intracranial hemorrhage) is post-traumatic amnesia. The duration of amnesia increases with each age group (usually lasting about two weeks). Indeed, the persistence of most clinical sequelae of head injury increases with age.

About 20 per cent of the patients will have some persistent psychiatric or behavioral problems and a similar number will show epilepsy. In most cases, the epileptic seizures begin within two years following the injury, and most of these patients are still subject to seizures after five years. Persistent headache, visual disturbance and vestibular dysfunction comprise a post-traumatic syndrome which may be troublesome for long periods of time after the injury. Approximately half the patients will not show any loss of occupational capabilities, about one-third will not be able to perform as satisfactorily on the job, and 10 per cent or more will be totally disabled. Recent reports of long-term follow-up of patients with severe head injuries indicate that the outcome has generally been more favorable than had been expected or predicted from earlier studies. Such a favorable outcome is doubtless related to an improvement in immediate and subsequent medical care.

INJURIES OF THE VERTEBRAL COLUMN AND SPINAL CORD: MECHANISMS AND MANAGEMENT IN THE ACUTE PHASE

Perry Black, M.D., C.M.

Few nonfatal injuries match the devastating physical and psychological disability caused by severe spinal cord trauma. With improved techniques in management over the past half century, there has been a steady decline in the mortality and morbidity of those who survive the initial injury. The question of the indications for surgical exploration of closed spinal wounds continues to be a controversial subject among neurosurgeons. There is considerable agreement, however, regarding those aspects of patient care that relate to protection against increase in the neural damage, the prevention of complications and the promotion of an optimistic attitude toward rehabilitation. Careful attention to several relatively simple principles in management can sometimes convert a potentially serious outcome into a gratifying result. What is done in the first few hours after spinal injury—at the scene of injury, transportation to hospital and management in the emergency department—can be more important than all subsequent efforts. Although many patients face the grim prospect of permanent paraplegia or quadriplegia, much progress has been made in the social and economic rehabilitation of these patients to happy, useful lives.

This survey outlines various mechanisms of injury and principles of management with emphasis on the acute period.

MECHANISMS OF INJURY

Spinal trauma in civilian practice is generally of the *closed* variety and results from traffic accidents and falls. *Open* wounds due to missiles predominate among battle casualties, but are not uncommon in civilian life. The critical factor in spinal trauma is damage to the neural contents of the spinal canal; the vertebral injury itself is secondary. Consideration in long-term management must also be given, however, to restoration of vertebral column function; this consists of a delicate balance between mobility and stability of the neck and trunk, as well as protection of the neural contents. A knowledge of the mechanics of the injury in each patient is helpful in evaluating the extent of the trauma and may influence management and prognosis.

Closed Injuries

The regions of the vertebral column that allow the greatest mobility are also characterized by relative instability. Their muscular and articular supports are insufficient to resist violent forces. Although all portions of the spine are subject to injury, the junctional region between the rigid thoracic spine and the lower three cervical vertebrae is the most vulnerable. The thoracic spine is infrequently subject to closed injury by virtue of its minimal

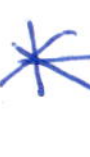

motion and its support by the rib cage. The thoracolumbar junction, however, allows free movement and is consequently a common site of injury. The lower lumbar region, which is quite flexible, is similarly affected near its junction with the fixed sacrum.

Hyperflexion Injuries. Most closed spinal injuries are the result of *indirect* violence that produces extreme movement of a portion of the spine beyond its normal range. To illustrate, a dive into shallow water, or sudden deceleration in a head-on auto collision, causes extreme neck *flexion*, which is the most common mechanism of serious spinal injury (Figs. 6–35, 6–36 and 6–37). The wedging force on adjacent vertebrae may crush one of the bodies, and bone fragments may be driven posteriorly into the spinal canal. Depending on the direction and intensity of the forces, there may be associated fracture of the pedicles or laminae. The fracture may be further complicated by forward dislocation of the upper vertebrae on the lower, if the powerful posterior longitudinal ligament or the articular ligaments are torn. Disruption of the intervertebral disc may result in extrusion into the spinal canal. The extent to which the deranged spine encroaches upon the canal

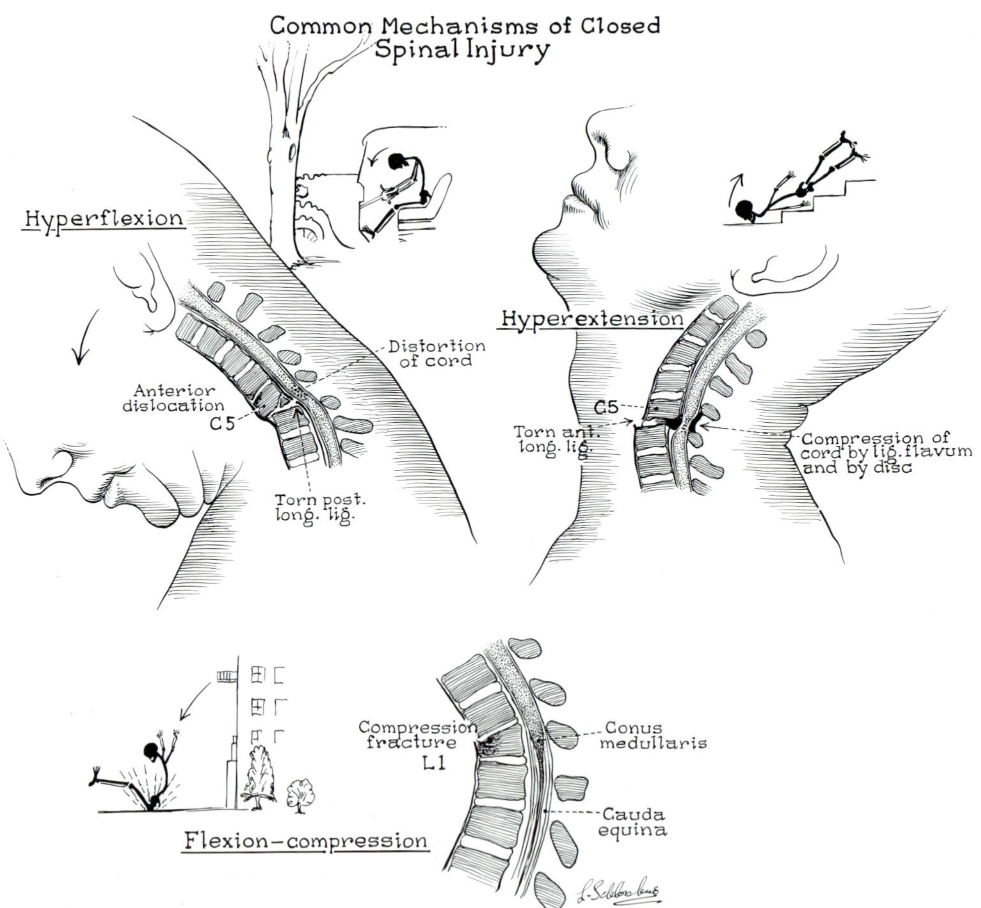

Figure 6–35 Schematic illustrations of closed spinal injury mechanisms. The cervical hyperflexion and hyperextension diagrams represent a composite of possible factors, any number of which may occur in a particular case.

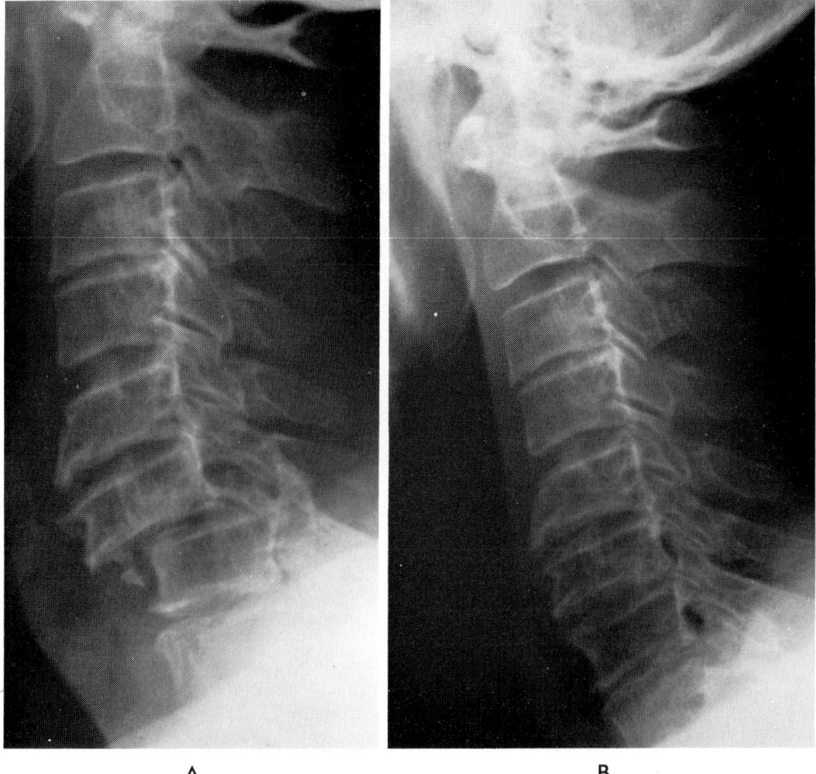

Figure 6–36 *A*, Lateral projection radiograph of cervical spine after hyperflexion injury, showing fracture at C.6–7 with forward dislocation. Encroachment of spinal canal resulted in severe cord compression with paraplegia and partial involvement of upper extremities. *B*, Radiograph of same patient after closed reduction had been achieved by skeletal cervical traction with tongs. If fracture site is stable, traction may be maintained for 6–8 weeks of stabilization until spontaneous fusion occurs. Although, as often occurs in severe spinal cord injuries, this patient did not recover neurological function, it is important to avoid additional neural injury which might jeopardize patient's few remaining capabilities.

determines the degree to which the cord is compressed. Adjacent nerve roots may be similarly compromised within the intervertebral foramina. The suddenness and force of the impact contribute to the severity of the injury.

Hyperextension Injuries. In cervical extension injuries, the spinal cord may be stretched against the forward bulging ligamenta flava, which may contuse the dorsal columns. In extreme cases, posterior dislocation occurs (Fig. 6–35). Older individuals are particularly prone to cord injury during hyperextension (e.g., under anesthesia or in a fall, striking the forehead or chin) because of pre-existing thickening of the ligamenta flava and narrowing of the spinal canal by osteoarthritic spurs. The cord is "squeezed" between the wrinkled ligamentum flavum posteriorly and the spurs anteriorly. The main stress in such an injury is in the center of the cord, resulting in the *syndrome of acute central cervical cord injury*,[60] the clinical features of which are described under "Pathophysiology of the Neural Lesion." The syndrome may also be produced by insufficiency of the blood supply to the cervical cord in hyperextension injuries.[62] These two mechanisms—contusion

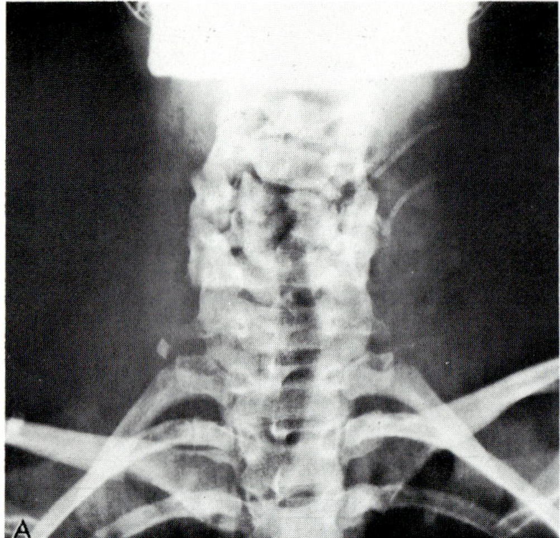

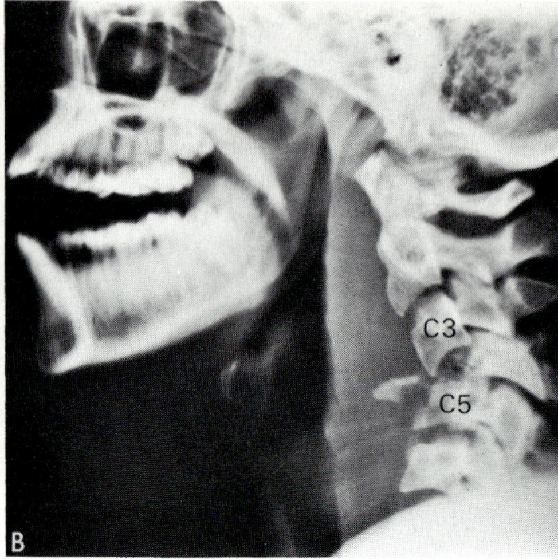

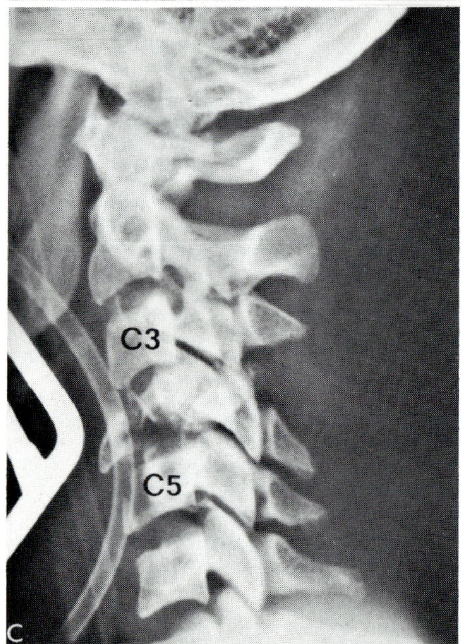

Figure 6–37 Cervical spine radiographs of 17-year-old girl with severe hyperflexion fracture-dislocation sustained in auto crash. *A*, Antero-posterior projection. Note disruption of vertebral elements at C.3,4 and 5. *B*, Lateral projection showing complete shattering of C.4 vertebral body and angulation of spine. Note pre-vertebral swelling due to hematoma formation; in retropharyngeal area, such hematomas can obstruct the airway. *C*, Lateral projection after closed reduction by means of skeletal traction with tongs. Patient was immediately quadriplegic, with motor and sensory level at C.4. There was respiratory embarrassment with right diaphragmatic paralysis owing to partial involvement of phrenic outflow; tracheostomy and respirator were necessary for 6 weeks. Two months after injury, anterior and posterior fusions (in two stages) were performed because of likelihood of instability associated with the severe disruption of the bony and ligamentous spinal elements. Despite permanence of the quadriplegia, some rehabilitation proved possible.

and vascular insufficiency—illustrate how serious cord injury can occur without fracture or dislocation; the possibility of transient, spontaneously reduced dislocation should also be borne in mind.

Dislocations. Dislocations are usually associated with fractures. Displacement into the spinal canal occasionally occurs without producing spinal cord injury. This is explained by the fact that the cord occupies approximately half the spinal canal; the cord may thus be spared. This observation accounts for the survival of some patients with atlantoaxial dislocation, which is often fatal because of compression of the vital cardiac and respiratory centers in the medulla oblongata.

Acceleration ("Whiplash") Injuries of the Neck. Varying degrees of cervical injury may occur when the head suddenly accelerates in relation to the trunk, as in the so-called *whiplash* injury of rear-end automobile collisions.

The extension component of the recoil or oscillating neck motion is the significant mechanism in these injuries,[39] which are usually milder than those which result from a direct impact on the head. The large majority of cases involve a non-complicated cervical muscular or ligamentous "sprain." Occasionally, there is associated disc or nerve root injury, subluxation due to stretching or tearing of ligaments, or fracture.[15] Symptoms such as blurring of vision, vertigo, tinnitus and nystagmus have been ascribed to vertebral-artery spasm or cervical sympathetic irritation, but the evidence for this viewpoint remains controversial.[39] Some authorities believe that mild brain injury (with transient unconsciousness) can occur in whiplash injuries as a result of acceleration-deceleration of the brain, despite the absence of a direct blow to the head.[19, 45]

Falls. Falls from a height, with the patient landing on the feet or buttocks, can cause compression fractures of the lower thoracic and lumbar regions (Fig. 6–35 and 6–38). Consideration should be given to the possibility that an apparent traumatic compression fracture may be *pathological* in nature; the differential diagnosis includes osteoporosis, neoplasm (myeloma or metastasis most likely) and osteomyelitis. Dislocation in the lower vertebral column is less common than in the cervical spine because of less mobility and greater muscular and ligamentous support in this region.

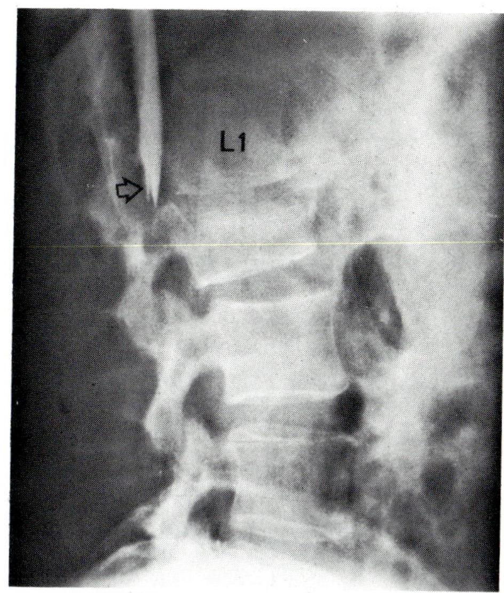

Figure 6–38 Lateral projection myelogram of lumbar region in middle-aged man who fell down flight of stairs, landing on buttocks. Note compression fracture of L.2 vertebral body with bone fragment displaced backward into spinal canal. Compression of conus medullaris and cauda equina caused immediate loss of bladder function (retention) and moderate paraparesis with motor and sensory level at L.1. On lumbar puncture, there was inadequate flow of cerebrospinal fluid, suggesting a manometric block. Contrast medium for myelogram was introduced into spinal subarachnoid space via cisternal puncture. Film shows failure of contrast medium to flow below L.2, despite upright position of patient. Since major defect at level of block (arrow) was ventral (anterior to conus and cauda equina), surgical decompression and fusion were carried out by an *anterolateral* approach. Patient regained bladder function in one month and virtually full use of legs within six months, with minimal residual spasticity. This case illustrates that prognosis for eventual recovery is often good, if, on initial examination, some neurological function is preserved below level of injury.

Combined Craniospinal Injuries. Injuries of the spine are often associated with injuries to other parts of the body, especially in high-speed traffic accidents. Multiple injuries may include one or more of the following: fractured long bones, head, chest, pelvis and abdomen. Since the cervical spine serves as a fulcrum for the relatively heavy head, it is not surprising that injuries of head and neck are commonly associated.[12] Direct impact injuries on the *vertex* of the head—as in falls from a height or blocking with the head in football—represent one serious and often fatal type of combined brain and cord injury. Schneider et al. have postulated that the severe impact force on the vertex causes the brain to herniate through the tentorial notch and foramen magnum, resulting in massive cerebral edema.[61] The force is also transmitted to the medulla and upper cervical spine. There may be associated vascular insufficiency due to compression of the vertebral arteries by the occipital condyles against the laminae of the atlas. An additional stress is said to occur at the cervicomedullary junction, owing to the disparity between the relatively mobile brain and the limited mobility of the upper cervical cord which is held by the dentate ligaments.

Open (Penetrating) Injuries

Missile Injuries. Bullet and shrapnel wounds of the spine may injure the cord by direct penetration into the spinal canal (Fig. 6–39). Complete cord transection is more apt to occur by this mechanism than by indirect closed injury. The missile impact may also drive bone fragments into the cord or nerve roots. A high-velocity bullet may produce transient or permanent paralysis, presumably as the result of a pressure wave in the wake of its passage in proximity to, but without penetrating, the spinal cord. A similar shock-wave phenomenon occurs in cord injury as the result of a nearby explosive blast in which there is no demonstrable vertebral or gross neural damage.

The missile trajectory may be estimated by inspection of the wounds of entrance and exit combined with roentgenographic evidence of the location of metallic fragments. If the missile lodges on the same side of the midline as the wound of entry, it may be inferred that the missile did not pass through the spinal canal. The bullet may initially strike a rib, then ricochet along the rib curvature and finally penetrate the spinal canal via the intervertebral foramen. Through-and-through perforation of the spinal canal

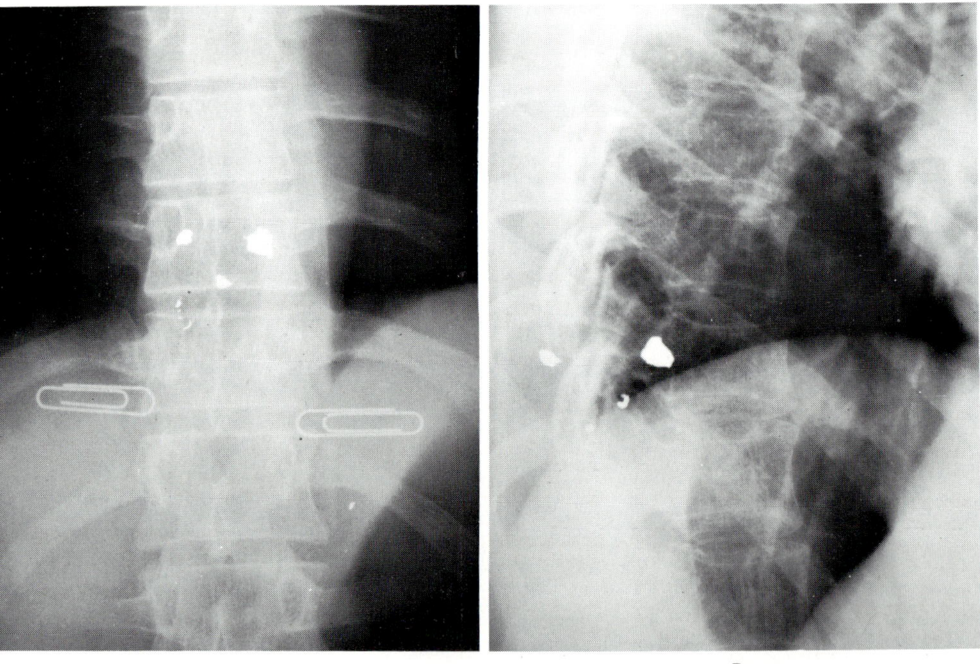

A B

Figure 6–39 Anteroposterior and lateral radiographs of thoracic spine showing bullet injury at level of T.10 and 11. The missile entered from the back and fragments are seen lying within the spinal canal. Paper-clip markers were attached to the patient's skin to aid in localization for subsequent surgical exploration. In general, penetrating injuries of the spinal canal should be explored early for debridement. Priority is, however, given to associated penetrating injuries of the chest or abdomen which may be more immediately life-threatening.

and cord has probably occurred when the sites of entry and of exit are on opposite sides of the midline.

By comparison with closed injuries, spinal trauma due to missiles is often more destructive of the spinal cord but less disruptive of the ligaments supporting the spine. For this reason, there is less tendency to dislocation.

Stab Injuries. Stab wounds of the spine are fairly common in civilian life. These injuries frequently occur in the thoracic region. They may be associated with a nondisplaced fracture of the neural arch, or the tip of the weapon may slip between adjacent neural arches. Classically, half the cord is traumatized, resulting in the Brown-Sequard hemisection syndrome.

PATHOPHYSIOLOGY OF THE NEURAL LESION

Transient Traumatic Paralysis, Contusion and Laceration

Cord injuries range in severity from transient physiological interruption to the permanent paralysis of anatomical cord transection. *Transient traumatic paralysis* is recommended as a substitute for the term "spinal concussion," which has vague connotations. The temporary paralysis from which the patient recovers fully may be accompanied by edema or ischemia of several cord segments. *Contusion* follows a blunt impact against the cord and is characterized by petechiae, edema and focal cellular and tract destruction at one or more segments. Healing is by gliosis, and partial return of function is possible. *Laceration* of the cord is commonly the result of penetrating injuries but may also follow fracture-dislocation. In extreme cases, there is total structural transection of the cord.

Hemorrhage

Bleeding may occur in the epidural and subdural spaces in the spinal canal as well as in the substance of the cord. Whereas epi- and subdural hematoma are frequent causes of brain compression in head injury, extramedullary bleeding in the spinal canal rarely causes serious cord compression. Subarachnoid bleeding may cause meningeal irritation (headache, stiff neck, fever). Blood in either the cranial or spinal *subarachnoid* space, however, does *not* accumulate locally to compress the brain or cord. On the other hand, hemorrhage into the cord itself is of major consequence, due to local destruction of neural tissue and not to the loss of blood-volume which is negligible. The extravasation, which may vary in degree from petechiae to frank hematoma at the site of injury, is usually confined to the central gray matter. Proximal and distal extension of the bleeding, hours or days after the injury, may account for the progression of neurological deficit that occurs in some cases. Thrombosis of damaged blood vessels may also contribute to an advancing deficit.

The *syndrome of acute central cervical cord injury* (Schneider[60]) is often associated with central cord hemorrhage and variable surrounding edema. The striking feature of the syndrome is the greater motor impairment of the upper limbs as compared with the lower. This disparity is explained by the proximity to the damaged corticospinal (pyramidal) motor fibers destined for the upper limbs (Fig. 6–40). The more peripherally situated lower limb fibers tend to suffer less damage. Bladder dysfunction and varying degrees of sensory loss also occur. Partial motor and sensory recovery may ensue spontaneously (without surgical intervention) as the edema subsides, but recovery is limited by the extent to which the central cord has been permanently damaged.

Cord Compression

The effects of compression are those of mechanical distortion of the neural tissues combined with local cord ischemia and contusion. The cord can

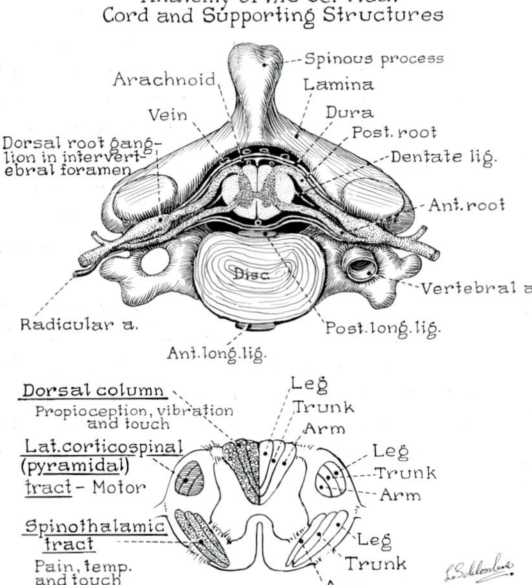

Figure 6–40 *Upper,* Anatomical relationships of the sixth cervical vertebra viewed from above. *Lower,* Outline of the major motor and sensory tracts in the white matter of the cervical spinal cord.

withstand gradual compression over a period of days or weeks, as in the case of slow-growing tumors, but acute compression is tolerated poorly. It has been shown in animal experiments that, if recovery of function is to occur, severe compression of sudden onset must be relieved in minutes (Tarlov[67]). The neurological loss associated with *mild* compression can be reversed, providing the pressure on the cord is removed within two hours. The conus medullaris and the nerve roots of the cauda equina can tolerate longer periods of compression. Unfortunately, in clinical practice, decompression is often impossible within these time limits. Experience has shown, however, that partial recovery from *incomplete* lesions caused by acute compressive forces can occur if surgical decompression is performed even days or weeks after the onset.

It is sometimes possible to determine from the clinical examination and radiographs whether the compression is mainly anterior or posterior. This will determine the surgical approach in decompressing the cord. *Anterior (ventral) cord compression* is suspected when there is motor paralysis and loss of spinothalamic tract function (pain and temperature sense) below the level of the lesion, with preservation of dorsal column sensation (touch, position, vibration) (Fig. 6–40). Anterior cord compression is particularly apt to be associated with a "tear-drop" fracture of a vertebral body in cervical flexion injuries; the anterior fragment slides forward while the posterior vertebral fragment impinges against the anterior cord. Similar compression may result from a ruptured disc, but since the radiolucent disc cannot be demonstrated by plain radiographs, the diagnosis in this case must be made on clinical grounds or by myelography.

Loss of dorsal column sensation, with preservation of other sensory or motor functions, would suggest *posterior cord compression* or contusion (Fig. 6–40).

Vascular Insufficiency of the Cord and Brainstem

The vertebral arteries ascend in the neck via the foramina transversaria of the cervical spine and enter the posterior fossa at the lateral margins of the foramen magnum. Before uniting to form the basilar artery, they each give off a posterior inferior cerebellar artery and a branch which passes caudally to become the anterior spinal artery. The latter unpaired vessel is joined by collaterals (radicular arteries which accompany the nerve roots) from the subclavian, intercostal and lumbar arteries. Collateral supply is poorest in the upper three cervical segments, at T.4 and at L.1; the capability of compensation for vascular insufficiency in these three zones is therefore deficient.

Fractures or dislocations of the spine or contusions of the cord may impair the local blood supply as a result of direct compression; alternatively, spasm or thrombosis may follow arterial contusion.[62] In the cervical region, bilateral injury of the vertebral arteries, in their foramina or at the craniocervical junction, may cause ischemia in the distribution of the anterior spinal artery. The resulting neurological disability may be reversible or permanent. In cases *without* fracture or dislocation, it is difficult to determine whether a neurological deficit is secondary to direct contusion of the cord or to vertebral artery insufficiency; either of these may occur in cervical hyperextension injuries *with or without dislocation.*

Vertebral insufficiency, with reduced flow to the posterior inferior cerebellar arteries or to the basilar artery, may produce brainstem dysfunction. Symptoms include nausea, dizziness, nystagmus, dysarthria, blurred vision and impaired consciousness (which may vary in individual cases from confusion to coma). These vascular manifestations are, however, difficult to distinguish from brainstem contusion or compression.

Spinal Shock

A state of "spinal shock" immediately follows cord injury and consists of a relative loss of motor, sensory and reflex function in those parts of the body innervated by the cord distal to the lesion. Bladder and rectal function are also interrupted. This acute phase may subside within days but commonly persists for three weeks or longer. If the pathological lesion is not severe, normal cord function is at least partially restored as the shock phase recedes. In severe, irreparable lesions, spinal shock is replaced by a state of hyperactive and pathological spinal reflexes, but the sensory loss and the paralysis of voluntary motor function continues. Because all cord lesions initially exhibit some degree of spinal shock, it is not possible to distinguish clinically in the acute phase between an anatomical and a physiological lesion. Hence, it is important to assume the possibility of recovery until proved otherwise.

Regeneration

Damage to the neural cells and tracts of the cord is reversible if the injury is of mild degree. When the damage is beyond the limit of tolerance, the involved cord tissue degenerates and is replaced by glial scarring. Regeneration of nervous tissue cannot occur to any practical degree in the brain and spinal cord in man. For this reason, surgical approximation of the severed ends of a structurally divided cord is futile. Sensory roots may be considered part of the central nervous system because their cell bodies lie distally in the dorsal root ganglia in the intervertebral foramina (Fig. 6–40). By contrast, motor roots, originating in the anterior horn cells, are theoretically comparable to peripheral nerves in regenerative capacity. This applies to clean cuts which do not greatly distort the fiber pattern, but effective regeneration does not generally follow approximation of torn or shredded nerve roots.[11]

Prognosis

In cases with or without continued cord compression, immediate *complete* loss of function below the level of the lesion is usually an ill omen if the total loss persists longer than 24 hours.

The presence of some voluntary motor function—perhaps only a flicker of movement—often signifies that, barring complications, the patient may eventually walk unaided. Complete motor loss with some preservation of sensation is less promising, carrying a 50 to 60 per cent chance of useful motor recovery; motor control may begin to appear days to months following injury.[64] Although some fortunate cases with physiologically incomplete lesions may show gratifying return of function in a relatively short time, the recovery process is generally slow; a plateau of maximal recovery may not be reached until about two years after injury. As in brain injuries, the prognosis for spinal cord trauma is better in younger individuals. The outlook for both survival and recovery of function declines for each decade beyond the age of 40.

The gross appearance of the spinal cord at the time of surgical exploration is often of little prognostic value. Only if the cord is anatomically transected or is severely contused can a definite prediction of permanent paralysis be made. However, a cord grossly normal on the surface may conceal serious intramedullary destruction with a correspondingly poor prognosis.

The electrophysiological technique of evoked response has recently been employed in preliminary trials in humans for early prediction of eventual physiological conduction in a damaged spinal cord. A favorable prognosis is tentatively suggested if an electrical stimulus applied to the skin overlying a peripheral nerve in the leg evokes a scalp EEG response. A satisfactory response implies electrical conduction across the injured portion of the cord.

FIRST AID AT THE SCENE OF ACCIDENT

Recognition of Injury

Spinal trauma is suspected if the patient has any difficulty in moving the lower extremities on command. Similar motor difficulty in the upper limbs indicates cervical cord involvement. The presence of a sensory level on pinprick testing confirms the suspicion of cord or nerve root injury. The patient may complain of local pain in the neck or back. Gentle palpation by sliding the fingers along the spine (without moving the patient) may reveal gross deformity or tenderness. When spinal injury is suspected, special precautions are taken in handling the patient, even in the absence of motor or sensory loss. In the management of an *unconscious* accident victim, consideration is given to the possibility that both head injury and cervical spine trauma have occurred. A bruised forehead or facial lacerations suggest the possibility of a hyperextension injury of the neck. Penetrating spinal injuries are easily identified by inspection and by the accompanying neurological signs. The open wounds are covered with a sterile dressing. Fractures of long bones are splinted in the usual manner.

Respiration

In all patients immediate attention is directed to the airway. Patients with injuries to the upper half of the cervical cord are subjected to respiratory embarrassment because neural control of both the intercostal muscles and the diaphragm is impaired. (The diaphragm is innervated by the phrenic nerve which is derived from the third, fourth and fifth cervical cord segments.) In lower cervical injuries, the intercostal muscles are paralyzed, but the diaphragm remains functional. Airway obstruction due to secretions is cleared by suction, if the apparatus is available. Provision of a pharyngeal airway for unconscious patients is helpful. If a skilled person is available at the scene of the accident, introduction of an endotracheal tube or an emergency tracheostomy with assisted respiration can be lifesaving in cases of high cervical cord injury. Narcotics for pain or restlessness are avoided in cervical cord injury in view of their respiratory depressant effect.

Arterial Hypotension

Unless there is blood loss from other injuries, hypotension after spinal injury is usually due to vasodilatation. If this occurs, venous return to the heart may be increased by elevating the legs.

Oxygen Administration

Lactate accumulates at the site of spinal cord injury, reflecting local ischemia.[38] Cord lactate is also increased in response to anoxia, although the spinal cord is more resistant to anoxia than cerebral tissue. Administration of oxygen (preferably humidified, to prevent drying of the tracheobronchial lining) may therefore have some protective effect on the injured cord, especially if there is respiratory embarrassment or hypotension.

Transportation to Hospital

The cardinal principle in moving a patient with suspected spinal injury is the prevention of any spinal motion that can further damage the cord or nerve roots. The neck should be the single most important consideration in the mechanics of removing an injured person from a car or other confined space. The head and neck must be supported at all times, whether the patient is conscious or unconscious. One rescue worker firmly grasps the head and applies longitudinal traction to bring the head and neck into neutral position, while other rescue personnel ease the trunk and extremities out of the vehicle. In transfer of a patient from the ground to a stretcher, he is lifted "like a log" with spinal alignment maintained by several persons. The individual most responsible for the transfer exerts firm, steady traction on the head and neck (Fig. 6–41A). The patient is placed *supine* on the stretcher, and sandbags are placed on either side of the head to prevent rotation. Canvas halter traction for temporary neck immobilization during transport is desirable. A commercially available constant-tension spring attached to the halter and stretcher is ideal for maintaining immobilization. Alternatively, a 5-lb. weight may be suspended from a rope which is hung over the end of the stretcher (Fig. 6–41B). If a standard head halter is not available, a makeshift emergency neck-traction sling can be made at the scene of the accident from a piece of cloth (Fig. 6–42). Immobilization of the neck is, of course, not necessary in thoracolumbar injuries. However, if there is any doubt regarding the exact level of spinal injury, the safe approach is to handle the patient as a cervical injury. An attendant should accompany the patient in the ambulance during the trip to hospital, with constant attention to the airway (suction as necessary) and to maintenance of neck stability.

If the trip to the hospital will be longer than several hours, an indwelling urethral catheter is introduced to prevent the irreparable damage of an overdistended flaccid bladder. The catheter is allowed to drain freely.

Protection of the denervated skin against the development of decubitus ulcers begins during transport to the hospital. A smooth, dry sheet is used on the stretcher; bony pressure points such as sacrum and heels are padded. The sheet may be used later to lift the patient on arrival at the hospital.

When possible, the hospital is notified in advance of the patient's arrival. In this way, necessary personnel (neurosurgeon, orthopedic surgeon, anesthesiologist, radiology staff) and equipment (e.g., respirator, canvas head halter, tongs for cervical traction, Stryker turning frame, lumbar puncture set) may be prepared for service when the patient arrives.

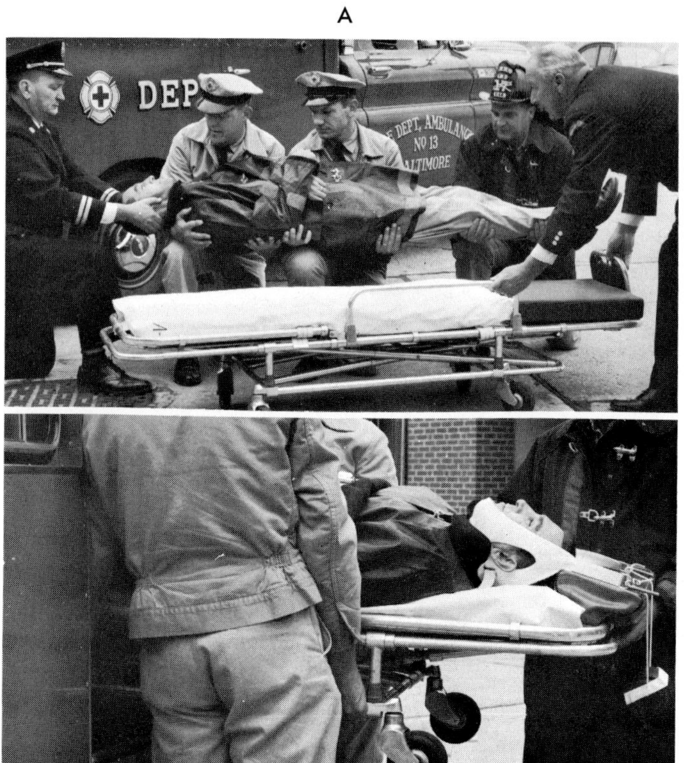

Figure 6–41 *A,* Method of lifting patient with injury of cervical spine, illustrating the maintenance of spinal alignment to prevent further damage to the spinal cord or nerve roots. Steady traction is applied to the head and neck, which is held in neutral position. This technique is employed even if there is only slight suspicion of spinal injury. *B,* Canvas halter traction (or emergency sling shown in Figure 6–42) for temporary immobilization during transport. A 5-lb. weight (shown in photo), or a constant tension spring, is attached. (Courtesy of Ambulance Service, Baltimore Fire Dept.)

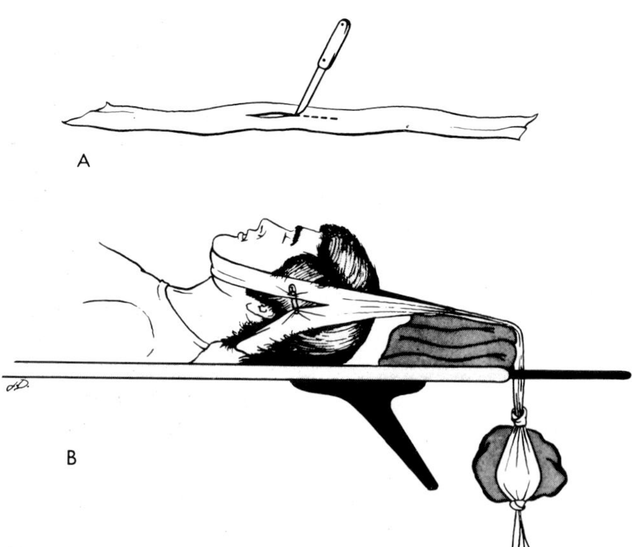

Figure 6–42 *A,* Makeshift emergency neck-traction sling, which can be made at the scene of the accident, from a muslin sling, bandage roll or other heavy piece of cloth about four feet long and six inches wide; a 10-inch longitudinal slit is cut in the middle for the head to slide through (Lewin, 1930). *B,* The slit is held snugly with a safety pin above each ear to prevent slipping off the occiput. The free ends are tied to a 3–5 lb. weight for traction.

Transfer to Another Hospital

Summary notes should accompany a patient being transferred from one hospital to another. The notes should include time and nature of injury, neurological status with emphasis on changes since first examination, associated injuries, medications administered and course of vital signs (level of consciousness, respiration, pulse, blood pressure). Before transfer, temporary neck immobilization should be applied, an intravenous infusion started and an indwelling urethral catheter inserted. In cases with depressed level of consciousness or impaired respiratory function, a pharyngeal airway, endotracheal tube or tracheostomy should be added.

Balance Between Speed and Caution

Ambulance personnel are the first major link in the chain of care for the seriously injured patient. They are frequently faced with difficult emergency situations requiring judgment and ingenuity. There can be no question that speed is important in getting the patient to the hospital so that definitive care can begin. An extra few minutes, however, in preparing the patient for transport can help to prevent unnecessary complications. This includes removal of the victim from the site of the accident with particular attention to the neck, cautious transfer to the stretcher, assurance of the airway, splinting of limb fractures and administration of intravenous fluids where indicated. The same principles apply equally in cases where speedy transportation by airplane or helicopter is available.

MANAGEMENT IN HOSPITAL DURING THE ACUTE PHASE

Immediate Care

On arrival in hospital, the patient is transferred to a portable lightweight x-ray penetrable lifter to which cervical traction can be attached.* The vital signs are checked, and appropriate resuscitation is promptly instituted. Adequacy of respiration is determined. Tracheostomy to permit suctioning is performed when there is doubt of the patient's ability to cough up secretions or when mechanically assisted respiration is necessary to prevent hypoxia. Following cord injury, the blood pressure may drop temporarily to the lower normal range because of loss of sympathetic vasomotor tone. This may be corrected by elevation of the legs; blood replacement is unnecessary since there has been no loss of volume. The absence of tachycardia helps to distinguish the hypotension of "spinal shock" from that of "surgical shock." If the blood pressure is unduly low, and particularly if this is associated with tachycardia and falling hematocrit, suspicion is aroused of hemorrhage from concomitant injury within the thorax, abdomen or long bones.

After the patient's vital processes have been stabilized, a rapid evaluation is made of the total situation. The spinal lesion is identified in broad terms and a cursory examination of other systems is carried out to identify quickly any associated trauma. Specialty consultations are requested as indicated, and decisions are made regarding priority in the management of the various problems. Apart from cardiorespiratory difficulty in high cervical trauma, cord injury itself is not generally immediately life-threatening. Priority is given, therefore, to any cerebral, thoracic or abdominal injuries, the delayed treatment of which may endanger survival. It is often feasible for separate surgical teams to perform procedures simultaneously.

When cervical spine trauma is evi-

*Lying on this lifter, the patient may be safely transferred from one stretcher to another or to an x-ray table without disturbing the traction or spinal alignment. To further minimize handling the patient, it would be desirable for such lifters to be employed in ambulances and exchanged with a similar lifter on arrival in hospital.

dent or suspected, halter traction is applied if this has not already been done as a first-aid measure at the scene of accident. The patient is asked to void to test micturition. If paraplegia is present, an indwelling urethral catheter is inserted and the quantity of residual urine noted.

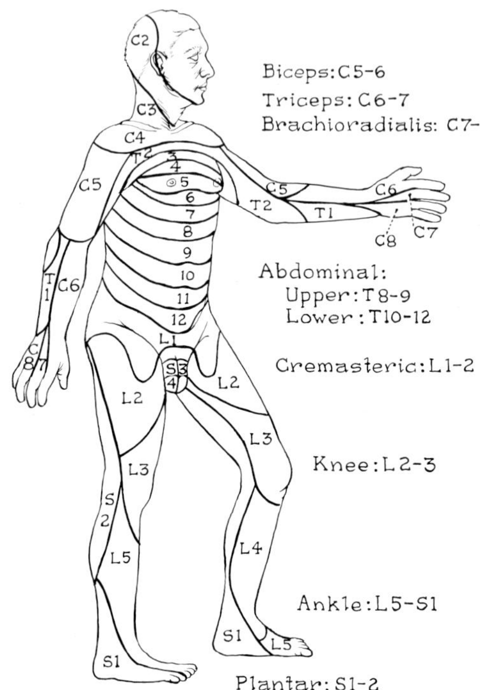

Figure 6–43 Sensory dermatomes and spinal cord segmental reflex innervation. This is helpful in localizing area and level of cord injury.

Detailed Clinical Evaluation

Having attended to the patient's immediate needs, the physician carries out a thorough general physical and neurological examination. A search is made for associated injuries, including head trauma. A brief description from the patient or from witnesses of the circumstances surrounding the accident may indicate the mechanism of injury. A distinction can sometimes be made between a physiologically complete or an incomplete lesion on the basis of the rate of onset of the neurological deficit. If power and sensation were completely lost immediately, then the outlook for recovery is not so favorable as in cases in which the functional loss occurred over a period of minutes or hours. Progressive neurological loss may reflect continued or increasing cord compression which may be remedied by traction (in cervical injuries) or by surgical decompression. Progressive loss, however, may also result from extension of intramedullary edema or hemorrhage or from local cord ischemia. Enquiry is made regarding previous illnesses, such as diabetes, coronary insufficiency or epilepsy, since they may affect the general care of the patient.

The neurological examination at this time is recorded as a baseline for all subsequent examinations in assessing progression or regression of the functional deficit. Ideally, the same examiner carries out the serial evaluations. In addition to localizing the site of the lesion by the sensory and motor level, a check is made of all sensory modalities throughout the affected dermatomes, including the perineum, in search of islands of residual sensation (Fig. 6–43). Motor function is similarly tested, since preservation of even minimal voluntary motor or sensory function has favorable prognostic significance. The level of the motor loss, except in thoracic injuries, is a somewhat more reliable indicator of the cord segment involved than is the sensory level. Paralysis is flaccid in character during the phase of spinal shock. Some spasticity often appears later in the chronic convalescent phase. Pathological reflexes, such as the extensor plantar response (Babinski), signify damage to the pyramidal tract in either or both the brain and spinal cord. In the acute phase, all reflexes below the level of cord injury are usually absent, and even the Babinski response may not appear until the spinal shock recedes. Priapism is also occasionally seen during the acute period.

The brachial plexus is derived from segments C5 to T1. Thus, if the arms as well as the legs are paralyzed (quadriplegia), the cord lesion is situated at or above the C5 segment. When some function is retained in the upper limbs, the segmental level is determined by the specific muscle groups, reflexes and dermatomes affected.

If the upper limbs are spared, the lesion lies below T1. A sensory level on the chest or abdomen is the most useful localizing sign in thoracic cord injury. The abdominal reflexes may help in localization since their innervation originates from segments T8 to T12.

The tapered lower end of the spinal cord, known as the conus medullaris, lies opposite the first lumbar vertebra (Fig. 6–35). Trauma of the lumbosacral spine may damage the conus or the cauda equina, but the spinal cord above the conus will escape injury. The lumbar and sacral nerve roots of the cauda equina are loosely arranged in the spinal canal. Injury to the roots is, therefore, often irregular, giving rise to patchy and asymmetrical motor and sensory loss in the lower limbs. By comparison, injuries of the lower spinal cord may be identified by a more complete and symmetrical distribution of neurological signs. If it is present, a Babinski response confirms cord involvement but does not exclude nerve root injury.

In patients unconscious from head trauma, spinal cord injury is suggested by absence of reflexes below the level of cord injury, or by the finding of a sweat-level on the trunk. In semicomatose patients, a sensory level to pinprick may be identified by the absence of a withdrawal response below a given dermatomal level.

Radiographic Evaluation

When the vital signs are stable, anteroposterior and lateral radiographs are taken of the affected region of the spine. To avoid unnecessary movement, the patient remains on the stretcher; if transfer to an x-ray table is essential, manual or halter traction is maintained in cases of cervical injury.[36] The study is supervised directly by a physician.

In cervical injuries, an open-mouth view of the atlantoaxial articulation is obtained to visualize the odontoid process, fractures of which may be missed on routine projections. Visualization of the lower cervical spine on lateral projections is often obscured by the shoulders. This can be avoided by depressing the shoulders or employing the "swimmer's position," which consists of placing one arm of the patient over his head and depressing the other shoulder.

If the routine anterior and lateral views are normal, as in cases of cervical sprain from whiplash injury, right and left oblique views are made to visualize the neural foramina. In addition, lateral views in flexion and extension help to exclude subluxation. Skull films are also obtained in patients with neck injury in whom there is any suspicion of cranial trauma.

In correlating the films with the clinical findings, it should be remembered that, except in the lumbar region, a particular cord segment lies approximately two spinous processes higher than its correspondingly designated vertebra. The films may not reveal the full extent of the damage; dislocation may be transient and may have reduced spontaneously, so that subsequent roentgenographic evidence is lacking. Furthermore, the films do not reveal radiolucent soft tissue, such as a herniated intervertebral disc or torn ligaments.

The combination of clinical features, plain films and lumbar puncture usually suffices to clarify the problem. A *myelogram* may be performed in occasional cases requiring additional information regarding the question of surgically remediable compression of the cord or nerve roots (Fig. 6–38).

An oily radiopaque solution (Pantopaque) is injected into the spinal subarachnoid space through a lumbar puncture needle. Defects or obstruction in the flow of the "dye" column are observed fluoroscopically. In the thoracic region, a marker is attached to the skin to aid the surgeon in placing his incision if the patient is to be subsequently explored. Although myelography is reasonably safe in lumbar or thoracic injuries, particular caution is exercised in cervical myelography, owing to the neck manipulation necessary in carrying out the procedure. When there is known cervical fracture or dislocation, myelography in this region is avoided, unless cervical traction can be maintained.

Traction for Cervical Injuries

All cases with cervical fracture and/or dislocation are best treated with some form of traction, regardless of the extent of neural involvement and regardless of whether surgery will also be performed (Figs. 6–41, 6–42 and 6–44). (Exceptions to this statement are fractures of the transverse or spinous processes that require only stabilization with a Thomas collar and symptomatic care.) Patients with cervical cord neurological deficit, but *without* fracture or dislocation, are also best placed in traction, at least initially, until the situation is clarified. The stabilization can do no harm and may prevent an unrecognized subluxation or reduce further injury from a herniated disc or thickened ligamenta flava. Young children can often be managed with a head halter, but adults better tolerate skeletal traction employing Crutchfield tongs or other modification, such as the Cone, Gardner-Wells or Vinke skull calipers. The primary purpose of traction is immobilization; in cases of dislocation with or without fracture, traction is also usually capable of realigning the

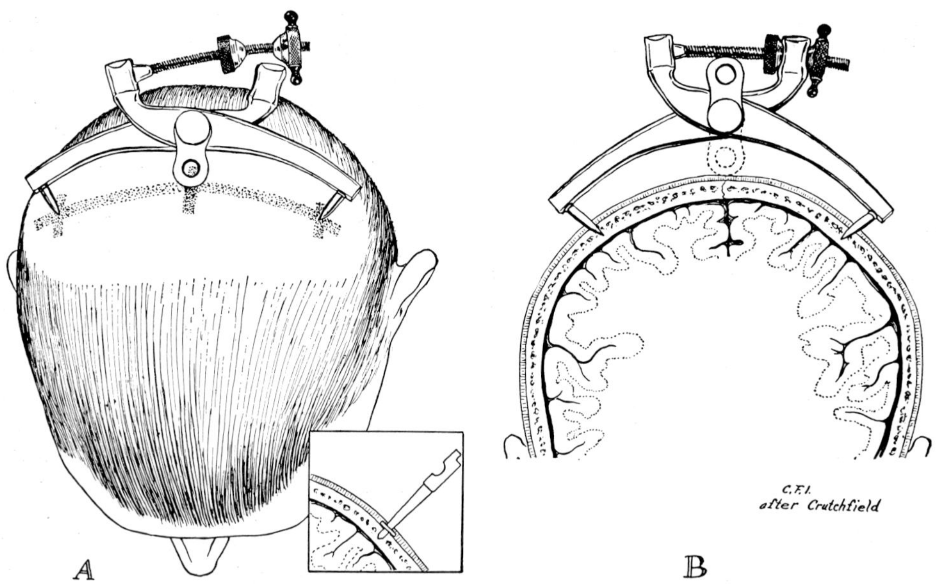

Figure 6–44 Application of Crutchfield tongs for cervical traction. In *A* the tongs are positioned on the head so that the points are spread 10 to 11 cm. *Inset* shows protective flange on drill to prevent excessive penetration. The drill bit should be same diameter as the tong points. In *B* the points are shown lying approximately 4 mm. deep, between the inner and outer table of the skull. (From Smith, H.: Fractures. *In* Crenshaw, A. H. (ed.): *Campbell's Operative Orthopaedics*. 4th Ed. St. Louis, The C. V. Mosby Co., 1963.)

displaced spine. Apart from decompressing the neural elements, traction may correct impingement of the vertebral arteries which supply the spinal cord and brainstem.

Application of Tongs. Crutchfield tongs may be applied in the emergency department or in the operating room. The scalp between the ears is shaved and cleansed. Aseptic technique is essential since local infection, including osteomyelitis and epidural abscess, is a potentially serious complication. A mark is made on the scalp in line with the tips of the mastoid processes, which correspond to the plane of the cervical articulations. Two points, one each on opposite sides and 5.0 to 5.5 cm. from the midline, are deeply infiltrated with local anesthetic. This will provide the desired spread of 10 to 11 cm. between the points of the tongs. Through stab incisions at these points, perforations 3 to 4 mm. deep are made with a drill through the outer table of the skull. A protective flange on the drill prevents overpenetration. The tong points are seated in the perforations and locked. Antibiotic ointment may be applied around each point, and the area should be checked daily for signs of infection.

Amount of Traction. For purposes of stabilization in nondisplaced injuries, only 5 to 10 lbs. traction are needed. If reduction of a dislocation is necessary, 10 to 15 lbs. are initially applied. The head end of the Stryker turning frame or bed is elevated on blocks about six inches to allow countertraction by the weight of the patient. Serial radiographs are made every two hours, and additional traction up to a maximum of 40 to 45 lbs. for muscular individuals is applied with careful monitoring of the patient's neurological status.

Because of greater muscular resistance in the lower cervical spine, more traction is generally required for dislocations here than in the upper cervical region. Muscle relaxants can facilitate reduction, especially in the presence of muscle spasm. Gradual addition of weights, with check x-rays, helps to avoid excessive traction which can cause distraction of the vertebrae, spinal cord or vertebral arteries. When reduction is achieved, traction is decreased to a maintenance level of 5 to 10 lbs. The weights are checked frequently to assure that they hang freely.

Traction Precautions. Tongs of the Crutchfield type are tightened daily (about one-tenth turn) to prevent the points from slipping out. Skull films are obtained every 10–14 days to detect possible penetration of the points through the inner table. A canvas band or padded face mask should be fitted across the Stryker frame at all times to support the patient's head, when in the supine and prone positions, to prevent further injury to the cord if the tongs should accidentally slip out.

Failure of Reduction. If reduction fails to occur within 12–18 hours after instituting traction, this is probably due to locking (overriding) of dislocated facets of the lateral intervertebral joints. In such cases, closed reduction can sometimes be accomplished by altering the angle of traction to slight flexion or extension, depending on the angulation of the locked facets. With the patient supine, a folded sheet under the head causes slight flexion of the neck; a sheet under the shoulders results in slight extension.

Traction beyond 24 hours in an effort to reduce locked facets is not likely to be successful. Consideration is then given to *open* reduction. *With the cervical traction maintained during the operative procedure,* the site of dislocation is explored and the facets unlocked by gently prying with bone instruments under direct vision. Open reduction is far safer than *closed* manual manipulation, which should never be done.

Alternative Traction Methods. Other methods may be employed if tongs are not available or if their use is precluded by a thin skull (as in young children), extensive skull fractures or contaminated scalp lacerations.[59] For example, two burr holes may be placed about 2 cm. from the midline on each side of the skull. On each side, a wire is passed epidurally between the anterior and posterior trephines which are 4–5 cm. apart. The two wires are attached to a weight as in the use of tongs. Alternatively, traction may be applied via a large fish hook (with the barb removed) inserted percutaneously beneath the anterior third of the zygomatic arch bilaterally.

Lumbar Puncture and the Queckenstedt Test

Lumbar puncture is performed as soon as the site of spinal injury has been stabilized and radiographs obtained. In cervical injuries, traction is applied, after which the patient is turned prone on the Stryker turning frame for lumbar puncture. The chief value of lumbar puncture in spinal injury is in the detection of a spinal fluid block which, when present, suggests cord compression. The Queckenstedt test consists of compressing the jugular veins for 10 seconds and observing the rise and fall of the cerebrospinal fluid in the manometer attached to a lumbar puncture needle. By impeding venous return from the brain, jugular compression normally produces a transient increase in intracranial pressure, which is transmitted to the cerebrospinal fluid. The fluid in the manometer promptly rises when the jugular compression is applied and falls with release of compression. In the event of a mechanical obstruction in the spinal canal, the cerebrospinal fluid pressure is not transmitted to the manometer during jugular compression, or it may be delayed. A positive Queckenstedt test is confirmed by manual compression of the abdomen, whereby the increased intra-abdominal pressure is transmitted to the spinal fluid via the epidural veins. If the lumbar puncture needle communicates with the subarachnoid space, the increased abdominal pressure produces a rise in the fluid in the manometer, even in the presence of a spinal block. A manometric block is thus confirmed by a differential response between jugular and abdominal compression.

Bloody spinal fluid indicates subarachnoid bleeding, which may occur in both mild and severe injuries. Xanthochromia appears as the red blood cells disintegrate. In penetrating injuries, the fluid is examined for signs of infection; the examination includes a white cell count, culture, and glucose determination.

Operative Treatment

Operation is undertaken only after the patient's general condition is satisfactory; the mortality is unduly high in the presence of surgical shock or respiratory distress. For cervical injuries, *skeletal traction is maintained during and following operation,* which is performed with the patient on the Stryker turning frame. Endotracheal intubation in cervical trauma is cautiously performed to avoid neck manipulation; alternatively, local anesthesia adds a measure of safety by enabling monitoring of neurological status during the operation.

Surgical intervention is undertaken for one or any combination of the following three purposes: decompression, fusion (internal stabilization), or debridement.

Decompression. The principle indication for surgical intervention is mechanical compression of the spinal cord or nerve roots which cannot be relieved by traction. Any of the following circumstances warrant a decompressive procedure:

1. Progression of the neurological deficit.
2. Manometric (Queckenstedt) or myelographic block.
3. Radiographic evidence of bone fragments projecting into the spinal canal. A radiolucent herniated disc is

suspected when the clinical signs indicate injury of the anterior portion of the cord.

4. Injuries of the conus medullaris or cauda equina.

Several methods of decompression are available. An anterolateral approach for discectomy or corpectomy is employed when the neurological or radiographic findings suggest *anterior* cord compression; fusion is carried out by replacing the surgical defect with a bone graft (Fig. 6–45). Figure 6–38 illustrates a lumbar fracture for which an anterolateral approach was employed for decompression and fusion. *Posterior* compression of the cord is relieved by laminectomy; the dorsal bony arch is resected, leaving the articulations intact to prevent spinal instability (Fig. 6–46). If there is associated instability, a fusion is also carried out if the patient's general condition permits, or fusion may be postponed to a second operation several weeks later.

A few neurosurgeons advocate exploration in patients with complete neurological loss even in the absence of evidence of cord compression.[16] Incision of the cord to aspirate a hematoma is also performed by some surgeons; the current consensus, however, suggests that the hazard of adding cord damage is too great to justify aspiration, since many patients show partial spontaneous recovery.

Fusion. Bed rest and immobilization in a body cast are often adequate as definitive treatment for thoracolumbar injuries. Similarly in the cervical region, external stabilization with skeletal traction alone often results in *spontaneous* fusion over a 6–8 week period, obviating the need for *internal* (operative) stabilization. Operative fusion is performed when there is a risk of later dislocation resulting from spinal instability when the traction is discontinued. Among the types of lesions for which fusion is indicated are comminuted or teardrop fractures of a

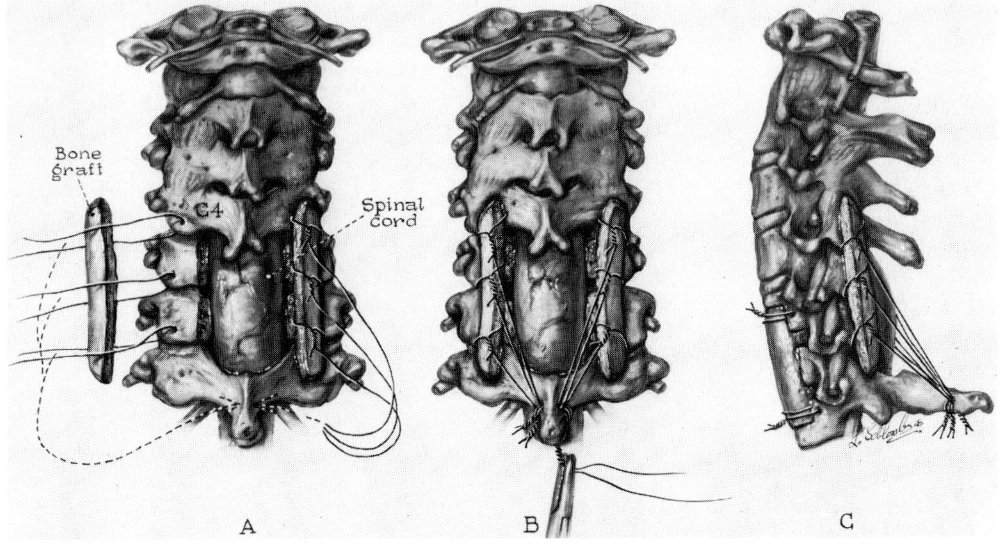

Figure 6–45 Anterolateral approach to the spine for relief of anterior cord compression and fusion. This sketch illustrates technique of vertebral corpectomy and interbody strut fusion in the cervical region. (Although wire is shown in this sketch to hold the bone graft, a soft suture material for *anterior* cervical fusions is preferable, to avoid injury to the adjacent esophagus). (From Schmeisser, G.: Orthopedic aspects of spinal cord injuries. *Md. State Med. J.* 19:95–99, 1970.)

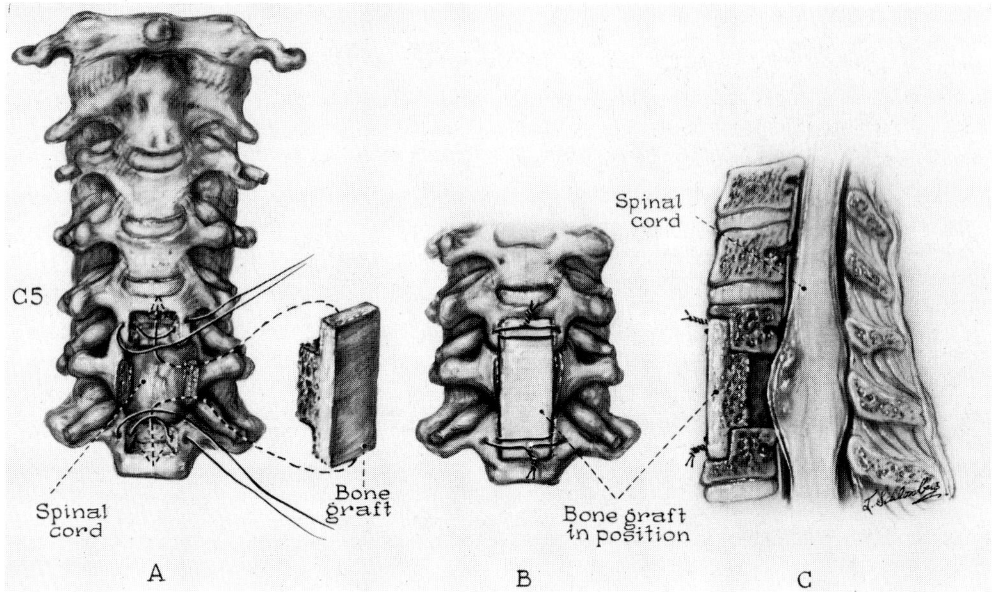

Figure 6–46 Posterior approach to the spine for decompression or fusion. A laminectomy decompression is carried out when there is *posterior* impingement on the spinal cord. If there is associated spinal instability, a bilateral strut fusion with wire check reins is also performed; in the absence of the spinous processes and laminae, the bone struts are wired to the articular facets. In cases with instability but *not* requiring decompression, fusion may be achieved by fastening the spinous processes together with wire and bone grafts. Lateral view, *C*, shows combined anterior and posterior fusions performed in cases with severe instability. (From Schmeisser, G.: Orthopedic aspects of spinal cord injuries. *Md. State Med. J.* 19:95–99, 1970.)

cervical vertebral body; such fractures tend to heal by fibrous union, posing a risk of instability and cord compression months or years later.[60] In evaluating other types of lesions, a useful guide in determining the need for operation is the ease or difficulty with which a dislocation is reduced by skeletal traction. Rapid reduction often signifies considerable ligamentous disruption, making fusion advisable.[51] An *anterior* or *posterior* approach is used, depending on the site of instability, and the operation may or may not be combined with a decompressive procedure (Figs. 6–45 and 6–46). Extensive spinal disruption may require both anterior and posterior fusions, as illustrated by the case shown in Figure 6–37.

Operative fusion offers the physical and psychological advantage of early mobilization of the patient and permits an earlier start of intensive rehabilitation. Some form of *external* stabilization, however, must be continued during the 6–8 week postoperative period until the fusion is solidly healed. External stabilization of the cervical spine can be accomplished by the *halo* fixation apparatus which permits sitting or ambulation (Fig. 6–47). The halo may also be employed for patients who would otherwise be immobilized by skull tong traction alone, without internal fixation.

Debridement. Penetrating wounds with retained foreign bodies in the spinal canal should be explored by laminectomy (Fig. 6–39). Early debridement offsets the development of scarring which may produce pain as well as increase the neural damage.

Surgical indications are less clearcut in cases *without* radiopaque foreign bodies. For example, in stab wound cases with stable or improving neu-

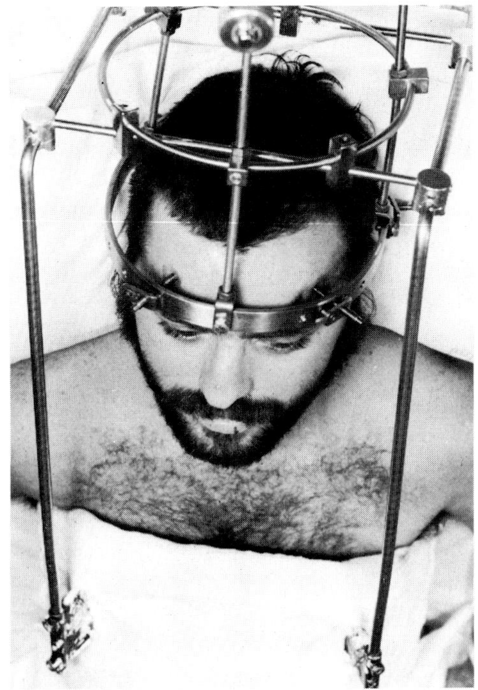

Figure 6–47 The halo fixation apparatus provides secure external immobilization of the cervical spine but permits sitting and ambulation. The skull is held by four pins projecting from a steel ring which is fastened by rods to a body jacket. In patients with sensory loss in whom there is risk of skin irritation, the body cast may be substituted by a steel pelvic hoop pinned to the iliac crests and connected by rods to the halo.

rological deficit, exploration is probably not necessary, except perhaps in an attempt to reapproximate severed motor nerve roots. On the other hand, a bullet passing through the spinal canal may carry fragments of clothing and generally causes considerable tissue disruption for which debridement is desirable.

In any event, penetrating injuries of the chest or abdomen, which may be more immediately life-threatening, take precedence over the spinal injury. Although early exploration is desirable, it can be safely delayed several days. Exploration becomes more urgent, however, if there is suspicion that the penetrating spinal injury is associated with cord compression.

Supportive Care for Major Injuries

Respiratory Function. Administration of oxygen in the early stages may help to reduce anoxic damage to the injured cord. Blood gases are determined if there is a question of adequacy of ventilation. Mental confusion is difficult to evaluate; it may be related to associated head injury, cerebral anoxia due to impaired ventilation or to vertebrobasilar arterial insufficiency.

Patients with spinal cord injury are prone to *pneumonia* owing to reduced ventilatory effort, immobilization and failure to clear secretions from the upper respiratory tract. A respirator or simple blow bottles help to maintain lung expansion, and frequent turning of the patient reduces hypostasis. These patients are also subject to *pulmonary embolus;* this risk may be reduced by the use of elastic stockings and elevation of the legs on a pillow to prevent venous stasis in the lower extremities.

Nutrition. Protein depletion with loss of body weight is one of the serious systemic effects of paraplegia. Examination of the serum protein level may reveal the negative nitrogen balance only in the later stages. Anemia resulting from protein loss appears as early as one week after trauma. Protein deficit plays a major role in susceptibility of paraplegics to urinary tract infection and to the development of decubitus ulcers. Vigorous feeding encouragement is given these patients in whom apathy is commonly encountered. Tube feedings may be necessary. A reasonable daily intake for an adult paraplegic is 3500 calories, which should include a minimum of 125 gm. of protein and added vitamins. The fluid intake is aimed at 4000 cc. to promote "irrigation" of the urinary tract.

Skin. Local care of the skin, in addition to dietary measures, makes ulceration an avoidable complication. Skin maceration is minimized by keeping the linens clean and dry. Turning of patients with cervical injuries on the Stryker frame is carried out every two hours day and night in order to avoid prolonged pressure on bony prominences. Patients with stable compression fractures of thoracic or lumbar spine may be nursed on a regular hospital bed and rolled "as a log" for turning. A pneumatic mattress or a waterbed is useful in protecting the skin, but these devices are not a substitute for frequent turning.

Bladder. Loss of detrusor muscle tone is one of the manifestations of the acute phase following cord trauma. An indwelling urethral catheter prevents excessive stretching of the bladder wall. A cystometrogram is obtained as early as feasible in the acute phase as a baseline for subsequent evaluation of bladder function. For most hospital settings, *continuous* catheter drainage is recommended in preference to either tidal or intermittent drainage. If, however, facilities and personnel are available for rigorous bladder care, *intermittent* catheterization is probably the most effective regimen for the prevention of bladder complications and the promotion of bladder training.[4] Regardless of the method of drainage, the bladder is irrigated twice daily with .25 per cent acetic acid.

As spinal shock recedes over a period of days or weeks, *automatic* or *reflex* micturition gradually appears if the bladder has not been damaged by overdistention or infection. This phase is characterized by vigorous involuntary voiding at intervals of 1 to 3 hours; the catheter may then be removed. In complete cord lesions, automatic micturition will be permanent, but return of voluntary control is possible in less serious injuries. When sacral segments or nerve roots S2 to S4 are destroyed, the bladder remains permanently *atonic;* evacuation in these cases is achieved by manual compression (Credé maneuver). Some patients with urinary stasis and risk of infection may eventually require operative urinary diversion, such as the ileal-loop procedure.

Gastrointestinal Function

Oral feeding is withheld immediately following injury until it is clear that paralytic ileus will not pose a problem. If ileus occurs, nasogastric suction, rectal tube insertion and enemas are employed to decompress the bowel. Injections of neostigmine may help to restore intestinal tone. When the acute stage has passed, enemas are given regularly to avoid fecal impaction.

Stress Ulcers. Spinal cord injury, like any severe stress, may trigger an as yet poorly defined neurohumoral mechanism which results in gastric ulceration, followed by hemorrhage or perforation.[8] Stress ulcers occur more frequently during the first week after injury and affect all age groups. Hemorrhage or perforation occurs silently, without pain or distress; there may be sudden deterioration in the patient's condition, such as shock. *Prevention* of stress ulceration consists of a prophylactic ulcer regimen, including antacids, during the initial phase. Monitoring of vital signs and stool guaiacs are helpful for early detection. Because sepsis from any source increases the incidence and morbidity of stress ulceration, infection should be treated vigorously.

Rehabilitation

Physical and occupational therapy are begun soon after the patient's general condition has stabilized, usually within a few days after injury. To prevent contractures, all limb joints are ranged daily. When at rest, paralyzed hands are splinted in a functional position with the thumb-web stretched, and the shoulder is placed in abduction and moderate external rotation. A vertical foot board is used to prevent foot-drop deformity. The patient is placed in the sitting position as soon as spinal stabilization is secure.

An optimistic, yet realistic approach is adopted in planning the patient's future. The participation of a skilled medical social worker can be invaluable in helping the patient and his family adjust to the new demands imposed by the disability.

New Therapeutic Possibilities

A number of potential treatments for spinal cord injury are currently under investigation. Trials in laboratory animal models suggest slight benefit from the intramuscular administration of *corticosteroids* for 1–2 weeks.[3] The use of corticosteroids on a trial basis in humans therefore seems warranted. Corticosteroids, however, reduce secretion of gastric mucoprotein and may thereby increase the risk of stress ulceration;[8] the risk may be minimized by the use of antacids and anticholinergic agents.

Local hypothermia by application of cold saline to the injured cord in animals also appears promising,[1] but the results of limited trials in humans thus far have been inconsistent. Additional possibilities under investigation, but not yet studied in man, include: (1) *osmotic diuretics,* such as urea[31] and mannitol; (2) agents to *block synthesis of norepinephrine,* local accumulation of which is thought to produce hemorrhagic necrosis at the site of spinal cord injury[47] and (3) *hyperbaric oxygenation*[32].

Management of Minor Spinal Injuries

Acceleration (Whiplash) Injuries of the Neck. For cervical sprains (neck pain and muscle spasm), but without neurological or radiographic abnormality, several days of bed rest at home are prescribed, followed by gradual ambulation. Analgesics, muscle relaxants and mild heat to the neck are helpful. A light cervical collar (a folded towel may suffice) affords mild immobilization, but its use should be tapered off after 1–2 weeks to avoid loss of muscle tone. Not uncommonly, the symptoms first appear or are aggravated several hours or days after the injury. The large majority of patients with simple cervical sprains recover over a period of 3–6 weeks without residual difficulties. A psychoneurotic response to the injury, with prolongation of symptoms, may be avoided by the physician's careful explanation of the condition, the plan of treatment and the expected course of recovery.[15, 19] Patients whose convalescence is prolonged require neurosurgical or orthopedic evaluation in search of complicating factors, such as disc injury.

Acute Lumbosacral Sprain. Musculoligamentous sprains sustained in falls, heavy lifting or bending represent the commonest cause of acute low back pain. The possibility of referred pain from pelvic or abdominal lesions is considered in eliciting the history. Radiographs of the lumbosacral spine are obtained to visualize the vertebral bodies, intervertebral disc spaces and the apophyseal joints. The radiographs also help to exclude unexpected lesions such as pathological fracture, osteolytic defects or abdominal psoas shadows. On physical examination, sciatica, with limitation of straight-leg raising, suggests nerve root irritation, making disc herniation (protrusion) a possibility. In most cases, symptoms of either back sprain or disc herniation resolve spontaneously on bed rest (with board under mattress) for a few days to several weeks. Analgesics, muscle relaxants and local heat are added. Bladder dysfunction (frequency or retention) or rapidly progressing loss of strength (such as foot drop) signify serious nerve root compression for which neurosurgical intervention may be urgently required. If bladder function is in doubt (as in the question of overflow incontinence), a cystometrogram may clarify the situation.

SUMMARY

When a patient presents in the emergency department with major trauma, priority decisions must be made rapidly in determining the steps of appropriate action. When spinal injury is suspected, the following sequence of attention to presenting problems is suggested:

1. Vital signs, resuscitation
2. Rapid evaluation of problem, including search for associated injuries.
3. Head-halter traction for evident or suspected cervical injuries
4. If spinal cord injury is likely, start corticosteroids, first dose I.V., with subsequent maintenance by I.M. route for 1–2 weeks. Give antacids and possibly an anticholinergic agent to protect gastric mucosa against stress ulceration.
5. Request for specialty consultations as indicated
6. Indwelling urethral catheter
7. Detailed clinical evaluation
8. Radiographic evaluation
9. Skeletal (e.g., Crutchfield) traction for cervical injuries
10. Lumbar puncture to test for spinal block (Queckenstedt test).
11. Decision as to further management, e.g., decompressive laminectomy.
12. Supportive care—respiratory function, nutrition, skin, bladder, G-I function, rehabilitation.

REFERENCES

1. Albin, M. S., White, R. J., Acosta-Rua, G., and Yashon, D.: Study of functional recovery produced by delayed localized cooling after spinal cord injury in primates. *J. Neurosurg.* *29*:113–120, 1968.
2. Bigelow, W. G., Lindsay, W. K., Harrison, R. C., Gordon, R. A., and Greenwood, W. F.: Oxygen transport and utilization in dogs at low body temperatures. Amer. J. Physiol. *160*:125, 1950.
3. Black, P., and Markowitz, R. S.: Experimental spinal cord injury in monkeys: Comparison of steroids and local hypothermia. Surg. Forum *22*:409–411, 1971.
4. Boyarsky, S.: Management of the neurogenic bladder: Current status and recent developments. Clin. Neurosurg. *20*, 1973.
5. Brock, S.: Injuries of the Brain and Spinal Cord and Their Coverings. New York, Springer Publishing Co., 1960.
6. Burton, C., and Blacker, H. M.: A compact hand drill for emergency brain decompression. J. Trauma 5:643, 1965.
7. Carton, C. A.: Cerebral Angiography in the Management of Head Trauma. Springfield, Ill., Charles C Thomas, 1959.
8. Clark, W. K.: Stress ulceration. Clin. Neurosurg. *18*:426–440, 1971.
9. Courville, C. B.: The mechanism of coup-contrecoup injuries of the brain. Bull. Los Angeles Neurol. Soc. *15*:72, 1950.
10. Cronqvist, S., and Kohler, R.: Angiography in epidural haematomas. Acta Radiol. *1*:42, 1963.
11. Crosby, E. C., Humphrey, T., and Lauer, E. W.: Correlative Anatomy of the Nervous System. New York, Macmillan. 1962, p. 61.
12. Davis, D., Bohlman, H., Walker, A. E., Fisher, R., and Robinson, R.: The pathological findings in fatal craniospinal injuries. J. Neurosurg. *34*:603–613, 1971.
13. Edberg, S., Reiker, J., and Angrist, A.: Study of impact pressure and acceleration in plastic skull models. J. Lab. Invest. *12*:1305, 1963.
14. Fay, T.: Observations on generalized refrigeration in cases of severe cerebral trauma. Res. Publ. Ass. Res. Nerv. Ment. Dis. *24*:611, 1945.
15. Frankel, C. J.: Medical-legal aspects of injuries to the neck. J.A.M.A. *169*:216–223, 1959.
16. Freeman, L. W.: Injuries of the spinal cord. Surg. Clin. N. Amer. *34*:1131, 1954.
17. Freytag, E.: Autopsy findings in head injuries from blunt forces. Statistical evaluation of 1,367 cases. Arch. Pathol. *75*:402, 1963.
18. Freytag, E.: Autopsy findings in head injuries from firearms. Arch. Pathol. *75*:215, 1963.
19. Gay, J. R., and Abbott, K. H.: Common whiplash injuries of the neck. J.A.M.A. *152*:1698–1704, 1953.
20. Goodman, J. M., and Kalsbeck, J.: Outcome of self-inflicted gunshot wounds of the head. J. Trauma 5:636, 1965.
21. Gryspeerdt, G. L.: Radiology of acute head injuries. *In* Rowbotham, G. F.: Acute Injuries of the Head. (4th Ed.) Baltimore, The Williams & Wilkins Co., 1964, pp. 361–407.
22. Gurdjian, E. S., Lissner, H. R., Latimer, F. R., Haddad, B. F., and Webster, J. E.: Quantitative determination of acceleration and intracranial pressure in experimental head injury: Preliminary report. Neurology *3*:417, 1953.
23. Gurdjian, E. S., and Thomas, L. M.: Organization of Services for the Treatment of Acute Head Injury in Community and Industrial Practice. Presented at the Third International Congress of Neurological Surgery, Copenhagen, August 1965.
24. Hancock, D. O.: Angiography in acute head injuries. Lancet 2:745, 1961.

25. Hirsch, J. R., David, M., and Borne, G.: An angiographic sign of extradural hematomas. Neurochirurgia 5:91, 1962.
26. Hoefer, P. F. A.: The electroencephalogram in cases of head injury. *In* Brock, S.: Injuries of the Brain and Spinal Cord and Their Coverings. New York, Springer Publishing Co., 1960, pp. 707–732.
27. Holbourn, A. H. S.: Mechanics of head injuries. Lancet 2:438, 1943.
28. Jefferson, A., and Hill, A. I.: Echoencephalography. *In* Progress in Neurological Surgery. (Vol. 1.) Chicago, Year Book Medical Publishers, Inc., 1966, pp. 64–93.
29. Jefferson, A., and Lewtas, N.: Value of tomography and subdural pneumography in subfrontal fractures. Acta Radiol. *1*:118, 1963.
30. Jenkner, F.: Rheoencephalography. A Method for the Continuous Registration of Cerebrovascular Changes. American Lecture Series. Springfield, Ill., Charles C Thomas, 1962.
31. Joyner, J., and Freeman, L. W.: Urea and spinal cord trauma. Neurology *13*:69–72, 1963.
32. Kelly, D. L., Lassiter, K. R. L., Vongsvivut, A., and Smith, J. M.: Effects of hyperbaric oxygenation and tissue oxygen studies in experimental paraplegia. J. Neurosurg. *36*:425–429, 1972.
33. Klingler, M.: Das Schädelhirntrauma. Leitfaden der Diagnostik und Therapie. Stuttgart, G. Thieme Verlag, 1968.
34. Leksell, L.: Echoencephalography. I. Detection of intracranial complications following head injury. Acta Chir. Scand. *110*:301, 1955.
35. Leksell, L.: Echoencephalography. II. Midline echo from the pineal body as an index of pineal displacement. Acta Chir. Scand. *115*:255, 1958.
36. Lewin, P.: Head sling traction technic in cervical spine roentgenography. Am. J. Surg. 8:434, 1930.
37. Lindenberg, R., and Freytag, E.: The mechanism of cerebral contusions. A pathologic-anatomic study. Arch. Pathol. *69*:440, 1960.
38. Locke, G. E., Yashon, D., Feldman, R. A., and Hunt, W. E.: Ischemia in primate spinal cord injury. J. Neurosurg. *34*:614–617, 1971.
39. Macnab, I.: Acceleration injuries of the cervical spine. J. Bone Joint Surg. *46A*:1797–1799, 1964.
40. Mapother, E.: Mental symptoms associated with head injury: The psychiatric aspect. Brit. Med. J. 2:1055, 1937.
41. Mayer, E. G.: Schädelröntgenologie. Berlin, Springer Verlag, 1959, pp. 173–191.
42. Miller, H., and Stern, G.: Long-term prognosis of severe head injury. Lancet. *1*:225, 1965.
43. Monakow, C. von: Die Lokalisierung in das Grosshirn und der Abbau der Funktion durch kortikale Herde. Wiesbaden, Ed. Bergman, 1914.
44. Norman, O.: Angiographic differentiation between acute and chronic subdural and extradural haematomas. Acta Radiol. *46*:371, 1956.
45. Ommaya, A. K., Faas, F., and Yarnell, P.: Whiplash injury and brain damage. J.A.M.A. *204*:285–289, 1968.
46. Ommaya, A. K., Rockoff, S. D., Baldwin, M., and Payne, P. M.: Experimental concussion. A first report. J. Neurosurg. *21*:249, 1964.
47. Osterholm, J. L. and Mathews, G. J.: Altered norepinephrine metabolism following experimental spinal cord injury. Part 2. Protection against traumatic spinal cord hemorrhagic necrosis by norepinephrine synthesis blockade with alpha methyl tyrosine. J. Neurosurg. *36*:395–401, 1972.
48. Paterson, J. H.: Some observations on the cerebrospinal fluid in closed head injuries. J. Neurol. Psychiat. 6:87, 1948.
49. Pevsner, P. H., Bhushan, C., Ottesen, O. E., and Walker, A. E.: Cerebral bloodflow and oxygen consumption. An online technique. Johns Hopkins Med. J. *128*:134–140, 1971.
50. Pudenz, R. H., and Shelden, C. H.: The lucite calvarium—A method for direct observation of the brain; cranial trauma and brain movement. J. Neurosurg. *3*:487, 1946.
51. Robinson, R. A.: Anterior and posterior cervicalspinefusions.Clin.Orthopaed. *35*:34, 1964.
52. Rockoff, S. D., and Ommaya, A. K.: Experimental head trauma: Cerebral angiographic observation in early posttraumatic period. Am. J. Roentgenol. *91*:1026, 1964.
53. Rowbotham, G. F.: Acute Injuries of the Head. (4th Ed.) Baltimore, The Williams & Wilkins Co., 1964.
54. Ruggiero, G.: L'Encéphalographie Fractionnée. Paris, Masson & Cie., Ed. Librairie de L'Academie de Médecine, 1957.
55. Russell, W. R.: Discussion of the diagnosis and treatment of acute head injuries. Proc. Roy. Soc. Med. *25*:751, 1932.
56. Russell, W. R.: Cerebral involvement in head injury. Brain *55*:549, 1932.
57. Sano, K.: The presence of intracranial hemorrhage in medical examiner's cases. Presented at the Third International Congress of Neurological Surgery, Copenhagen, August 1965.
58. Schiefer, W.: Die Echo-Enzephalographie diagnostischer Möglichkeiten. Deutsch Med. Wschr. *89*:1394, 1964.
59. Schneider, R. C.: Cervical traction, with evaluation of methods, and treat-

ment of complications. Internat. Abstracts Surg. *104*:521–530, 1957.

60. Schneider, R. C.: Surgical indications and contraindications in spine and spinal cord trauma. Clin. Neurosurg. *8*:157, 1962.
61. Schneider, R. C., Gosch, H. H., Norrell, H., Jerva, M., Combs, L. W., and Smith, R. A.: Vascular insufficiency and differential distortion of brain and cord caused by cervicomedullary football injuries. J. Neurosurg. *33*:363–375, 1970.
62. Schneider, R. C., and Schemm, G. W.: Vertebral artery insufficiency in acute chronic spinal trauma. J. Neurosurg. *18*:348–360, 1961.
63. Sellier, K., and Unterharnscheidt, F.: Mechanik der Gewaltenwirkung auf dem Schaedel. Excerpta Medica *93*:55, 1963.
64. Suwanwela, C., Alexander, E., Jr., and Davis, C. H., Jr.: Prognosis in spinal cord injury with special reference to patients with motor paralysis and sensory preservation. J. Neurosurg. *19*:220, 1962.
65. Symonds, C. P.: The effects of injury upon the brain. Lancet *7*:820, 1932.
66. Symonds, C. P.: Assessment of symptoms following head injury. Guy's Hosp. Rep. *51*:461, 1937.
67. Tarlov, I. M.: Spinal Cord Compression. Mechanisms of Paralysis and Treatment. Springfield, Ill., Charles C Thomas, 1957.
68. Taveras, J. M., and Wood, E. H.: Diagnostic Neuroradiology. Baltimore, The Williams & Wilkins Co., 1964.
69. Thomson, J. L. G.: Arteriography in head injuries. J. Fac. Radiologists *14*:339, 1961.
70. Uematsu, S., and Walker, A. E.: A Manual of Echoencephalography. The Williams & Wilkins Co., 1971.
71. VerBrugghen, A.: Neurosurgery in General Practice. Springfield, Ill., Charles C Thomas, 1952.
72. Walker, A. E.: The acute head injury: a multidisciplinary problem. Neurologia Medio-Disurgia *9*:7–20, 1968.
73. Walker, A. E.: Personal communication, 1972.
74. Weed, L. H., and McKibben, P. S.: Pressure changes in the cerebrospinal fluid following intravenous injection of solutions of various concentrations. Amer. J. Physiol. *48*:512, 1919.
75. Williams, D., and Gibbs, F. A.: Electroencephalography in clinical neurology: its value in routine diagnosis. Arch. Neurol. Psychiat. *41*:519, 1939.
76. White, D. N., and Blanchard, J. B.: Studies in ultrasonic echoencephalography. IV. Results of an averaging technique to localize the cerebral midline structure. Neurology *15*:1041, 1965.
77. Woodhall, G.: Acute cerebral injuries: Analysis of temperature, pulse, and respiration curves. Arch. Surg. *33*:560, 1936.
78. Medical Research Council: Glossary of Psychological Terms Commonly Used in Cases of Head Injury. M.R.C. (War) Memor. No. 4, March, 1941.

chapter

7

INJURIES OF THE EYE, THE LIDS AND THE ORBIT

David Paton, M.D., F.A.C.S. and Jared Emery, M.D.

The eye and its surrounding structures are subject to serious injury from many forms of head trauma. Treatment of such injuries is the proper concern of an ophthalmologist, but most trauma cases are seen first by the emergency treatment room surgeon or other attending physician. For that doctor, the importance of routine examination of the eye, the lids and the orbit can scarcely be overstressed. Whether or not he must accept the responsibility of treating the injuries himself, he must not fail to suspect or discover their presence. Emphasis here is given to the variety of injuries that the examiner should seek and the primary treatment that the more common ones require.

Chemical burns of the eye are probably the only true ocular emergency. Other lesions of prime concern are lacerations of the globe, intraocular foreign bodies, severe lid lacerations and hyphemas. Prompt attention, however, is a matter of hours, not minutes. There is time for adequate examination and time for an unhurried decision regarding optimal management. Too frequently, lacerations of the globe are undetected because tightly swollen lids are not separated by lid retractors for an adequate view of the eye itself. Surgical correction of facial fractures is sometimes completed without recognition of a "blowout" fracture of the orbital floor that was not visible on routine skull films. Intraocular bleeding is occasionally unidentified if persons with "black eyes" are simply dispatched with cold compresses, and minor lid lacerations are at times repaired without detection of an unsuspected intraorbital foreign body. It is to the credit of emergency room staffs that these oversights do not happen more often.

Further reason for careful evaluation of the eyes in accident cases is the assistance this may give in general appraisal of the patient's illness and in decisions for his referral to consultants. The pupils can give useful clues to the state of consciousness

TABLE 7–1 CAUSES OF ASYMMETRY OF THE PUPILS

1. Antecedent causes of unequal pupils.
2. Traumatic mydriasis or miosis from direct blow to eye.
3. Unilateral blindness.
4. Iridodialysis or rupture of iris sphincter.
5. Unilateral use of topical drugs.
6. Intraorbital trauma to ciliary nerves or ganglion.
7. Horner's syndrome from injury to brainstem or cervical sympathetic pathways.
8. Intracranial third nerve palsy.

and to specific intracranial disorders, but these clues can be interpreted only after consideration of the many reasons for abnormal pupillary size and reactions (Table 7–1). Following accidents, double vision is a frequent complaint, with multiple possibilities to be considered in the differential diagnosis (Table 7–2). Loss of vision following an injury should be diagnosed by thorough evaluation (Table 7–3). The position of the eyes, testing of the corneal reflexes and the presence of nystagmus are well-known observations of neurological importance. Evaluation of carotid artery function is often assisted by determination of the relative central retinal artery pressures through ophthalmodynamometry.[21] Papilledema is of concern in all cases of head trauma; but there are several causes of "blurred" optic nerveheads that must be remembered in appraisal of the fundus appearance (Table 7–4).

It is unreasonable to expect a general surgeon to deal comprehensively with traumatic injuries of the eye, but it is important that the surgeon develop a keen awareness of ocular injuries and a practical knowledge of their management. Table 7–5 sum-

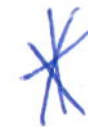

TABLE 7–2 THE DIFFERENTIAL DIAGNOSIS OF DOUBLE VISION FOLLOWING HEAD TRAUMA

1. Orbital fracture (particularly blowout fracture of the floor) causing restricted function of inferior rectus and inferior oblique muscles.
2. Hematoma in orbit and/or ocular muscles.
3. Third, fourth or sixth cranial nerve palsies (orbital or intracranial).
4. Avulsion, contusion or transection of extraocular muscles.
5. Avulsion of pulley of superior oblique.
6. Subluxation of the lens (unilateral diplopia).
7. Edema or detachment of the macula (unilateral diplopia).
8. Decompensation of pre-existing ocular phoria, becoming tropia.
9. "Whiplash" injury, and other diplopias of obscure origin.

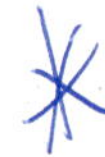

TABLE 7–3 THE DIFFERENTIAL DIAGNOSIS OF POST-TRAUMATIC LOSS OF VISION

1. Lid swelling; blood or foreign material covering cornea; corneal damage.
2. Hyphema; vitreous hemorrhage.
3. Traumatic cataract; luxation of the lens.
4. Central retinal artery or vein occlusion (from markedly increased orbital pressure or embolus).
5. Traumatic retinal edema and hemorrhages of retina from direct or contrecoup blows.
6. Avulsion of optic nerve by lateral orbital wall trauma or contrecoup blow to head.
7. Retinal detachment.
8. Cortical blindness from hematoma, ischemia or anoxia (patient may be unaware of blindness).
9. Intracranial interruption of visual pathways (hemorrhage, foreign body).
10. Acute congestive (angle closure) glaucoma precipitated by emotional trauma of recent accident or from intumescent lens, etc.
11. Hysteria.
12. Malingering.

TABLE 7–4 THE DIFFERENTIAL DIAGNOSIS OF "BLURRED" OPTIC NERVEHEADS

CONDITION	VISION	VISUAL FIELDS	RETINAL VEINS	NERVE-HEAD COLOR	RETINAL HEMOR-RHAGES	PERIPA-PILLARY RETINAL EDEMA	VIT-REOUS CELLS	SYMMETRY OF NERVEHEADS	COMMENTS
Early papilledema	Normal	Normal (except blind spot enlarge-ment)	Slightly distended; early loss of spontan-eous pul-sations	Pink	±	±	–	Often asymmetrical	Rarely: extension of subarachnoid hemorrhages into the eye; headaches
Advanced papilledema	Normal or, at times, some-what reduced	Normal (except blind spot enlarge-ment)	Distended without spontan-eous pul-sations	Very pink to pale	+	+	–	Often symmetrical	Sixth nerve palsies additional clue
Hyperopia and physiological variants	Normal	Normal	Normal	Normal	–	–	–	Often symmetrical	Fundus seen with + lens; central disc-cupping usually present
Optic neuritis	Impaired	Central scotoma, ± periph-eral loss	Distended ± spontan-eous pul-sations	Pink	±	±	±	Unilateral usually	Precipitous onset; may have pain with ocular motility
Optic nerve avulsion	Blind eye	Absent	Sludged	Pale	±	–	±	Contralateral eye normal	Contrecoup or direct trauma
Hyalin bodies of nervehead	Normal	Normal (rarely binasal field cuts)	Normal	Normal	–	–	–	Often symmet-rical; hyalin bodies some-times seen at disc margins in one eye only	Often familial (examine parents and siblings)
Hypotony of eye (after trauma)	Slightly impaired	Usually normal	Distended	Pink	±	Peripheral edema	–	Unilateral	Soft eye; commotio retinae

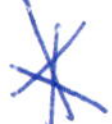

TABLE 7–5 EMERGENCY ROOM EVALUATION OF TRAUMA AFFECTING THE ORBIT, LIDS OR EYE

1. Obtain history of previous eye disorders, type of chemical burn or nature of injuring object, and tetanus immunization.
2. Determine visual acuity and screen visual fields by confrontation with test object.
3. Differentiate partially penetrating and completely penetrating (perforating) injuries of cornea and sclera. Use lid retractors. Note uveal prolapse.
4. Note hemorrhages and infections of orbit, lids and conjunctiva. Account for chemosis.
5. Investigate depth of all lid lacerations, noting fat in wound. Seek foreign bodies under lid: evert lid and sweep fornix with cotton swab after use of topical anesthetic.
6. Palpate orbital rim; feel for crepitus through lids; test facial and corneal sensation; auscultate for orbitocranial bruit.
7. Appraise real or apparent anterior, posterior or vertical displacement of globe.
8. Characterize diplopia by analysis of ocular ductions and versions; attempt forced-duction test using forceps and topical anesthetic.
9. Record pupil shapes, sizes and reactions, accounting for asymmetry.
10. Inspect for hyphema, iridodonesis and iridodialysis.
11. Examine cornea for opacities, ulcers, foreign bodies, rust rings and abrasions (use fluorescein paper). Avoid steroid-containing medications.
12. Use loupe or slit lamp to detect foreign body paths in cornea, iris and lens.
13. Estimate comparative depth of anterior chambers for evaluation of intumescent cataract, displaced lens and recessed chamber angle.
14. If traumatized globe is intact and cornea undamaged, measure intraocular pressure with tonometer.
15. Ophthalmoscope: Differentiate various types of intra-ocular hemorrhages. Record appearance of nerveheads, maculae and retinal circulation. Visualize foreign bodies if possible.
16. Get x-rays in all cases of possible retained foreign body in globe or orbit, and whenever orbital fracture is conceivable.
17. Consider value of photographing all injuries.

marizes the considerations that should be kept in mind for "work-up" examination of various types of injuries of the eye and its adnexa. Figure 7–1 shows a minimal set of equipment essential for emergency room evaluation of ocular trauma.

INJURIES OF THE LIDS

The first step in caring for an injury of the lid is to determine the extent of the injury, with particular attention being given to the underlying globe. Small lacerations should be gently probed and, at times, explored; large ones can simply be laid open. Prophylactic antibiotics, tetanus immunization and hemostasis are so routine in general surgery that further comment is unnecessary. The same is true of most burns, but more is said about these later.

For lacerations of the lid, the surgeon should perform a meticulous primary repair, employing instruments and sutures suitable to the delicacy of the task. Many months should then elapse before plastic revision for cosmetic correction of any residual deformities is undertaken; it is remarkable how often a primary repair produces an excellent final result after a year or more of gradual improvement. Permanent deformity of the eyelids is not only of major functional significance to the eye, but it may also entail a major catastrophe to the psyche of the patient. Vanity in these matters far transcends the group of supersensitive females preoccupied with appearance. Surely few other areas of the body require more attention to careful reapproximation of tissue planes and precise reconstruction of defects to assure satisfactory results. However, rarely is scrupulously performed surgery so well rewarded—the rich blood supply of the eyelids, the thinness and laxity of the lid skin and the

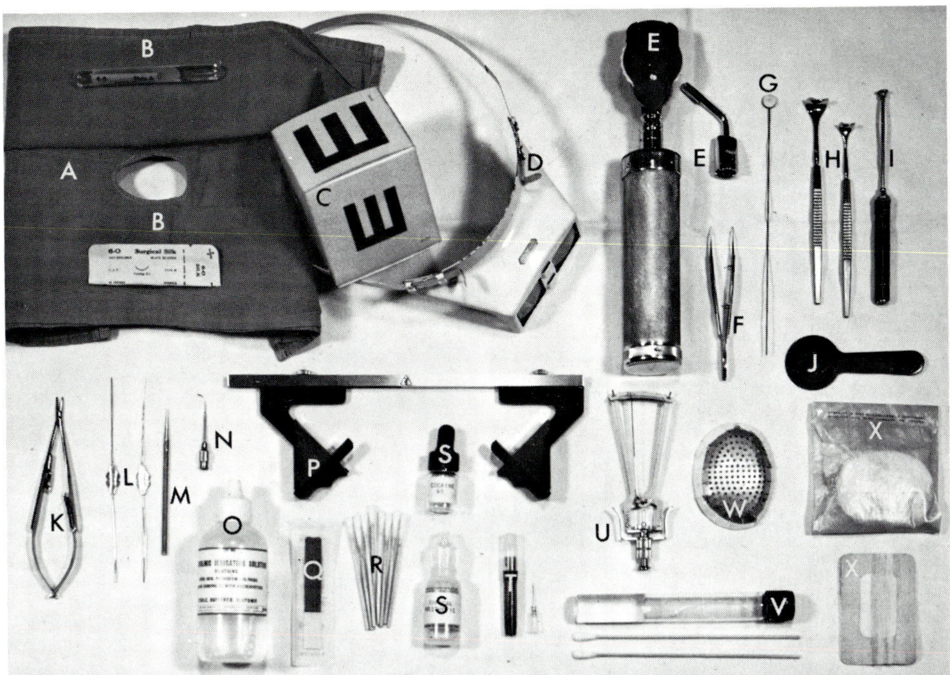

Figure 7–1 Equipment essential for emergency room evaluation of ocular trauma. *A,* Drape for minor lid laceration repairs; *B,* ophthalmic 6-0 catgut and silk sutures; *C,* "E box" for visual acuity testing; *D,* loupe; *E,* hand ophthalmoscope and transilluminator; *F,* fine, toothed forceps; *G,* test object for visual field examination; *H,* lid retractors; *I,* ophthalmodynamometer; *J,* pin hole disc for acuity measurement; *K,* needle holder for ophthalmic sutures; *L,* lacrimal probes; *M,* punctum dilator; *N,* curved, blunt lacrimal irrigation needle; *O,* squeeze bottle for sterile saline irrigation; *P,* exophthalmometer; *Q,* fluorescein paper strips in sterile envelope; *R,* cotton applicators; *S,* topical anesthetics; *T,* disposable No. 25 needles; *U,* tonometer; *V,* culture tube; *W,* protective metal shield; *X,* eye patches.

infrequency of infection all provide an ideal tissue for plastic refurbishing.

Surgical Anatomy of the Eyelids. A comprehensive review of lid anatomy cannot be included here, but selected features of particular importance in surgical repairs will be mentioned. *The lids should be regarded as double-layered structures: the anterior layer is composed of the skin and orbicularis muscle and the posterior layer, of tarsus and palpebral conjunctiva* (Fig. 7–2). Examination of the lid margins reveals a faint, linear demarcation between these two layers: the "gray line," or mucocutaneous junction. Each of the two surgical layers of the lids should be separately closed in all lid lacerations that transect the tarsus. Another important aspect of the two surgical layers of the lids is the inherent convenience of splitting the lids along the gray line so that a sliding flap of skin-muscle can be used to fill a post-traumatic lid defect. Undermining the anterior surgical layer is readily performed; and because of the abundance of skin in the vicinity of the lids, large defects can usually be closed by such flaps, which are brought over the relatively fixed posterior layer. Defects in the posterior layer of tarsus and palpebral conjunctiva can be filled by bringing across the lid-fissure portions of the same layer from the opposing lid—deficiency of which, if not total, will make little difference to the uninjured tissue from which it is removed.

The conjunctiva is a mucous membrane lining for the entire posterior

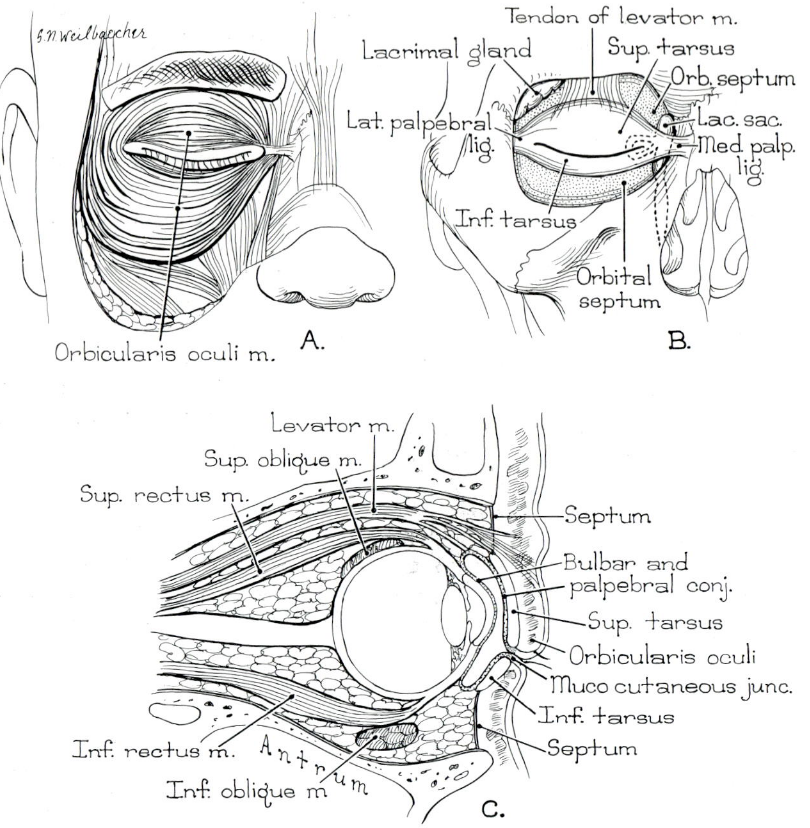

Figure 7–2 The lids and orbit.

surface of the lids, reaching from canthus to canthus and fornix to fornix, forming a sac that is open anteriorly at the lid fissure and closed at the limbus (Fig. 7–2*C*). The conjunctiva is a distinct tissue layer except where it is firmly adherent to the tarsus of the lids; it has generous recesses (the upper and lower fornix) whose loose folds permit marked lid and eye mobility. Like the skin of the lids, its natural laxity permits extensive mobilization for surgical repairs. Like other mucous membranes, its mucocutaneous junctions are abrupt, smooth boundaries that cannot be emulated by surgical apposition of conjunctiva to skin. Consequently, it is important to salvage as much natural lid margin as possible in lid reconstructions. Mucous membrane grafts *within* the conjunctival sac do exceptionally well. Customarily, they are taken from the contralateral eye or the buccal cavity.

The tarsal "plates" provide the strength and curvature of the lids. The tarsus is dense fibrous tissue containing the meibomian glands whose orifices are posterior to the gray line. There is no cartilage in the lids. Peripheral to the tarsi is the orbital septum, of which the upper and lower tarsi are merely thickened portions in the same fascial plane. The orbital septum attaches to the periosteum at the orbital rim throughout its circumference and forms the anterior barrier between orbital contents and the skin-muscle layer. *If a lid laceration contains fat, the examiner knows that the orbital septum has been perforated.* Superiorly, the septum is pierced by the tendon of the levator palpebrae muscle, which courses from the orbital apex to the skin of the upper lid, inserting near the upper margin of the tarsus and producing the upper lid fold. Traumatic damage to the levator muscle may therefore be signaled by the absence of lid fold as well as by ptosis of the lid. Lacerations involving the superior portion of the orbit, particularly in its medial third, sometimes involve the aponeurosis of the levator tendon; this must be recognized and repaired.

The lacrimal gland is located at the lateral aspect of the superior orbital margin. During orbital explorations from lateral or superior approaches, the surgeon must avoid damage to both the gland and its ducts, which enter the conjunctival fornix superotemporally. The eyelids contain the canaliculi of the lacrimal drainage apparatus (Figs. 7–2, 7–11 and 7–12). In repair of lid lacerations, attention should be directed to the functional role of the lids—not only to the fact that the lid must be able to close fully to protect the eyeball, but also to the part the lids play in distribution and drainage of the tears.[15] Blinking does more than moisten the cornea with tear film. The gentle squeeze of eyelid closure brings the lacrimal puncta of the lids into close contact with the pooled tear fluid of the eye; the contraction of the orbicularis fibers assists in the propulsion of tears into the canaliculi and compresses the lacrimal sac itself, causing the tear flow to proceed into the nose via the nasolacrimal duct. The orbicularis fibers of the lower lid, in particular, should be given great respect at the time of injury repair; surgical skin-muscle flaps or superficial tissue deformity from primary trauma itself can cause irreversible loss of function of the lacrimal drainage passageways, even though the drainage structures themselves were spared from the original trauma.

Finally, it is useful to recall that the orbit has no lymphatics, whereas the lymphatic drainage of the eyelids is divided into two main pathways. The medial two-thirds of the lids drain to the submaxillary glands and the lateral one-third to the preauricular glands. Inflammation of the eyelids is often associated with palpable enlargement of these glands.

Ecchymoses of the Lids. Direct blows to the eyelids may cause ecchymoses from the plentiful blood supply of the lids themselves. Often there is an associated orbital hemorrhage with proptosis of the eye and hemorrhage under the conjunctiva. What is a unilateral "black eye" one day may spread to the other side in ensuing days, as the blood within the lids seeps subcutaneously across the nasal bridge.

Hemorrhage within the lids is of no consequence per se, but it can signal other more serious injuries to orbital contents. For example, fracture of the roof of the orbit is not infrequently followed by dissection of hemorrhage along the levator muscle, producing subconjunctival hemorrhage superiorly and also ecchymosis of the upper lid. Orbital floor fractures may be associated with hemorrhage in the lower lid and inferior portion of the orbit. As will be described more fully later, there are also various contusion injuries within the eye that can accompany hematomas of the lids.

Treatment of lid ecchymoses themselves is usually limited to initial cold compresses, subsequent hot compresses and the use of sunglasses for a fortnight.

Traumatic Ptosis. It is important to identify the levator muscle during repair of upper lid injuries so that the tendon can be sutured to the upper margin of the tarsus and the muscle function restored (Fig. 7–9C).

Any upper lid swelling is associated to some degree with a drooping of the upper lid or narrowing of the lid fissure. Most often that type of ptosis resolves as the edema subsides, and lid function returns to normal. Any persistent soreness or photophobia of the eye will produce a partial "protective" ptosis that will persist as long as the irritation remains. There are times, nevertheless, when a blow to the eye is followed by a prolonged ptosis of the upper lid without evident damage to the third cranial nerve, without evident avulsion of the levator palpebrae muscle and without abnormality of the eye itself. Once the examiner is satisfied that there is no clinical evidence of mechanical interruption of the levator muscle, the only recourse is to wait an extended period of time before surgical repair is considered. Spontaneous correction of traumatic ptosis may require a year or more; thus, ptosis operations must not be considered for many months following such injury.

Anesthesia for Repair of Lid Injuries. The majority of lid lacerations can be repaired under local anesthesia if the patient is cooperative. Figure 7–3 shows the customary sites of injection for those branches of the fifth and seventh cranial nerves which serve the periocular tissues. It is preferable to give retrobulbar anesthesia when lacerations involve the conjunctiva and when orbital hemorrhage or lacerations of the globe do not contraindicate increased intraorbital pressure by addition of the anesthetic solution. Topical instillation anesthetics are useful adjuncts, particularly when the effect of the infiltration anesthesia is waning.

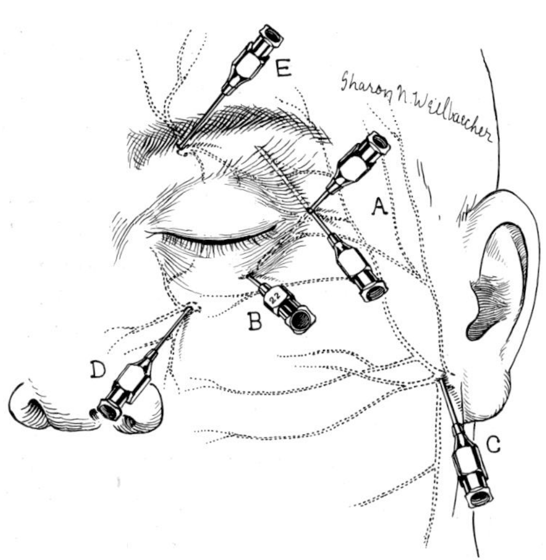

Figure 7–3 Sites of anesthetic injection for repair of lid lacerations.

Lidocaine (Xylocaine) in 2 per cent solution is currently a favored agent for infiltration anesthesia; longer effect and reduced bleeding are achieved by the addition of 2 drops of 1:1000 epinephrine per 10 ml. of the anesthetic. The amount of lidocaine injected may not exceed 500 mg. if used with epinephrine, or 300 mg. if used without epinephrine. This dosage must be reduced for children and for elderly or debilitated patients. Topical anesthetics that can be dropped onto the eye and the conjunctivae include cocaine 4 per cent, proparacaine hydrochloride (Ophthaine) 0.5 per cent, and others. Cocaine is probably the most effective but has the occasionally undesirable side effect of temporarily reducing corneal transparency.

TECHNIQUES. Paralysis of the orbicularis muscle can be obtained by the O'Brien technique. The zygomatic arch is located and followed back to a point just above the tragus of the ear; the condyloid process of the mandible is felt to slip forward under the finger as the patient opens his mouth. The patient is directed to close his mouth and the injection is made just anterior to the condyloid process, not in the joint itself. At this site, only 2 or 3 ml. of 2 per cent lidocaine is required for good lid akinesia (Fig. 7–3*C*). This injection does not provide anesthesia of the lids or globe; but, when used in combination with retrobulbar injection, it helps in avoiding excessive lid swelling when reapproximation of tissues can be facilitated by minimizing edema. Supplementary injections at the supraorbital notch and infraorbital foramen augment anesthesia of the lids (Fig. 7–3*D* and *E*).

The Van Lint technique of akinesia and anesthesia of the eyelids employs local injection of the anesthetic into the deep subcutaneous tissues of the orbital margins (Fig. 7–3*A*). As much as 10 ml. of lidocaine with hyaluronidase and epinephrine can be used in this manner. Hemorrhage from the injection can occur but rarely complicates surgical repairs.

Retrobulbar injection of local anesthetic is a useful and sometimes essential adjunct to repair of lid lacerations, particularly when the bulbar conjunctiva requires surgical manipulation or when ocular motility is undesirable. The technique is simple, but the injection should be made by someone familiar with orbital anatomy (preferably an ophthalmologist) because hemorrhage, damage to the globe and inadequate akinesia can result from improper placement of the needle. A 23 gauge by 35 mm. Atkinson retrobulbar needle with a special sharp but rounded point reduces the possibility of orbital hemorrhages. After the skin has been cleansed and a wheal of anesthetic has been produced at the injection site, the patient is directed to look upward and toward his nose. The needle is introduced through the skin just above the junction of the middle and lateral third of the inferior orbital margin (Fig. 7–3*B*). The needle is passed through the orbital septum and then directed obliquely upward and slightly inward toward the apex of the orbit. The plunger is retracted to determine whether a vessel has been penetrated; if not, 1 to 3 ml. of anesthetic is injected. It is important not to wag the needle tip, as this is the chief cause of retrobulbar hemorrhage. Some surgeons prefer to inject into the muscle cone just posterior to the globe, whereas others insert the needle farther into the apex of the orbit.

A surgeon unaccustomed to lid surgery will too often forget that abrasions of corneal epithelium may occur from contact with instruments, sutures or sponges. Undetected and unattended corneal abrasions can proceed to corneal ulcerations and will create severe discomfort for the patient when the anesthetic has worn off.

Preoperative Preparation for Repair of Lid Wounds. EYELASHES AND BROW. Eyelashes may be trimmed if desired; they regrow promptly, regaining their normal length in 4 to 6 weeks.

In contradistinction, the brow hair should not be shaved, for in rare cases this hair does not regrow and at times the pattern of new brow hair is irregular. Unusual though these misfortunes may be, the advantages of shaving the brow are slight and do not warrant the possible complications.

CLEANSING THE SKIN AND CONJUNCTIVA. Many techniques for cleaning the skin are acceptable preoperative routines. Preliminary use of liquid green soap is time-honored. The soap (and all other antiseptic agents) should not be used within the conjunctival sac but should be applied only to the skin and the surrounding surgical field. Detergents containing iodine compounds are also used in this manner and are probably superior to soap. Irrigation is the key to adequate wound cleansing. An intravenous set with a suspended 500 ml. bottle of sterile saline is a convenient way to "hose down" the injured region, combining lavage with tissue separation to wash away particulate foreign material. The conjunctival sac is also thoroughly irrigated with saline, and cotton swabs are used to assure absence of foreign bodies in the fornices of the conjunctiva. Alcohol is then used on the skin following completion of the irrigation.

DRAPING, LIGHTING AND MUTUAL COMFORT. Draping of the wound for sterile repair will depend upon the site of the lesion. In all cases, a head towel should be used, and it is considerate to recall that the ear is not a comfortable repository for drainage of blood, saline or tears. It is customary to employ an "eye sheet" with a central 3- to 4-inch round opening when only a small area of exposure is required.

The necessity for a strong, well-directed operating light is obvious. The general surgeon is reminded of the advantages of wound repair from a sitting position. Arm's-length surgery is less conducive to precise manipulations.

Simple lacerations of the Lids. After debridement, search for foreign bodies and control of bleeding, the actual repair of lid lacerations is similar to wound repair elsewhere *except for the particular importance of separate layer closure and the need for fine suture material.* Prevention of contracture deformity of the lid contours is of vital concern. Poor wound closure can result in abnormally thin or thick scars and resultant impairment of lid functions. Ragged wound margins should be trimmed, but as much tissue as possible should be preserved. Healing is surprisingly excellent despite a patchwork of suture lines at the time of primary closure. Hawsers of 4-0 black silk have no place in repair of the lids; 6-0 or 7-0 gut, and 7-0 or 8-0 silk are the mainstays of lid surgery. It is unnecessary to discuss the advantages of interrupted sutures, a symmetrical placement of the suture needle in the skin edges and the eccentric placement of suture knots so that these do not override the wound itself.

Basic to repair of lid lacerations is the technique of incision along the gray line to obtain mobilization of the skin-muscle layer when a sliding flap is needed. The lid is grasped firmly with forceps and a knife blade tip begins the gray line incision, extending only to a depth of about 3 mm. Separation of the skin-muscle layer from the tarso-conjunctival layer is then completed to the full depth desired by the use of fine blunt scissors, which are used by spreading the blades and obtaining the plane of dissection without injury to the tarsus or the vascular orbicularis muscle (Fig. 7–4). Wounds are rarely as sharp and simple as diagrammed in textbooks. Not infrequently, the tarsus is raggedly torn and needs restoration of neat contours prior to closure. Yet, excision of any portion of the tarsus causes much greater wound stress than does comparable excision of the loose skin-muscle layer, which can be undermined and mobilized readily. Thus, to avoid postoperative notching of the lid margin, the surgeon can trim the ragged margins of the transected tarsus in a slightly curved fashion so that when these curved margins are brought together vertically the straight line of closure will afford slightly greater tarsal width than before the injury (Fig. 7–5). This slight overcorrection (pouting of the lid margin at the site of repair) can produce a smooth-contoured lid when scarring ensures.

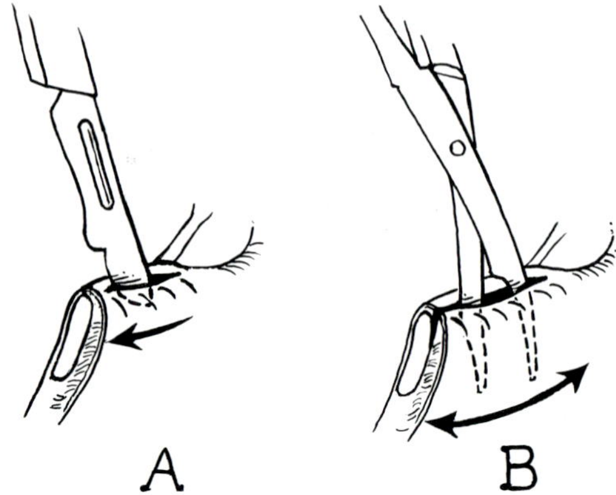

Figure 7–4 Technique of lid splitting along the gray line.

For lacerations involving the lid margin, Fox's modification[7] of Minsky's[18] figure-8 splinting suture is a useful means of assuring good closure of the marginal wound and prevention of lid notching. An intermarginal suture of 4–0 silk is passed into the tarsus within the wound to emerge in the gray line on either side (Fig. 7–6*A*). The tarsoconjunctivita is closed with interrupted 5–0 or 6–0 chromic gut sutures tied such that the knots lie on the anterior tarsal surface and will be buried within the wound (Fig. 7–6*A*). The intermarginal suture is then tied

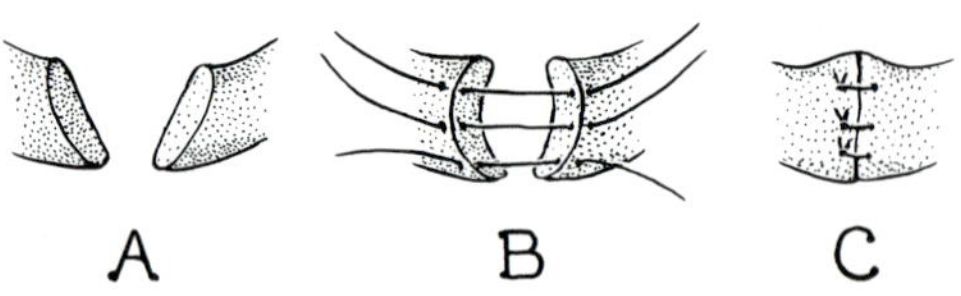

Figure 7–5 Repair of tarsus to prevent lid notching.

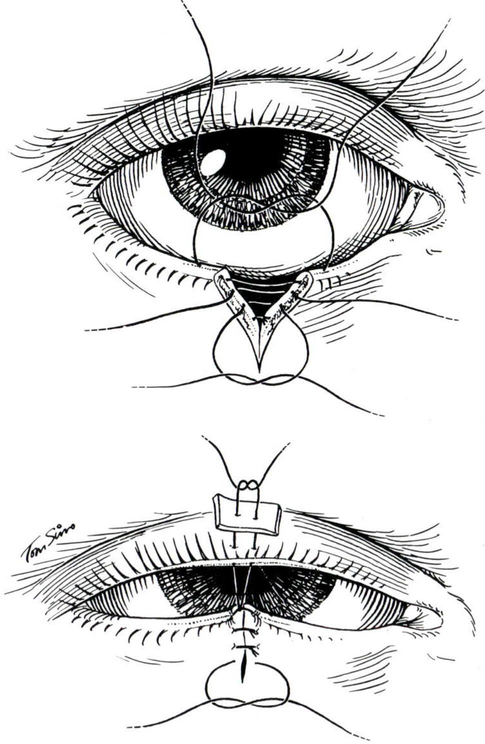

Figure 7–6 Fox's modification of Minsky's figure-8 splinting suture for lid laceration repair.

and passed through the gray line of the opposite lid margin to emerge in the skin where it is tied over a peg (Fig. 7–6*B*). The skin at the laceration site is closed with 6–0 or 7–0 interrupted silk sutures (Fig. 7–6*B*). The skin sutures are removed after 5 days and the intermarginal suture after 10 days.

Avulsions of the Lid. Glancing blows can avulse a lid which then dangles free like a pedicle flap, having little or no loss of its substance (Fig. 7–7). The most important factor in repair of such injuries is identification of the stump of the canthal ligament* from which the lid has been torn so that lid and ligament can be reapproximated, either with synthetic nonabsorbable suture material or fine wire (Fig. 7–8). Because these tissues are edematous at the time of this injury repair, the essential role of the canthal ligaments is not readily appreciated, and it may be weeks before the effect of failure to repair an avulsed ligament is noticeable. Fractures of the orbital walls, particularly the lateral one, can tear the canthal ligament from its bony insertion; this, too, must not be overlooked when the bones themselves are realigned. Clues to the injury are a droopy appearance of the lateral canthus and undue laxity of the lid. At the medial canthus, lid avulsion necessarily involves damage to the lacrimal canaliculi; repair of these will be discussed later.

*Since the canthal "ligament" unites muscle to bone, it should be referred to as a *tendon*, but the conventional nomenclature is used here.

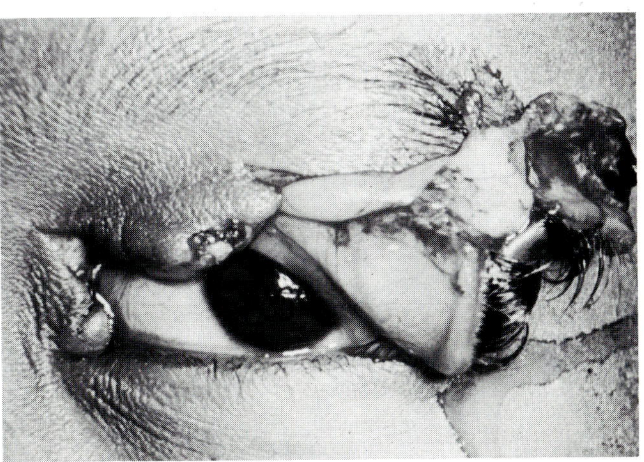

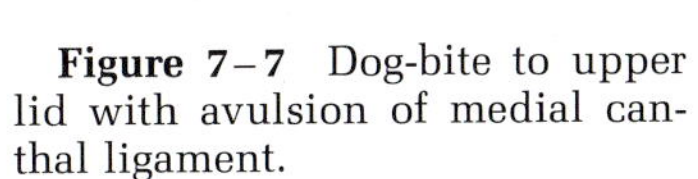

Figure 7–7 Dog-bite to upper lid with avulsion of medial canthal ligament.

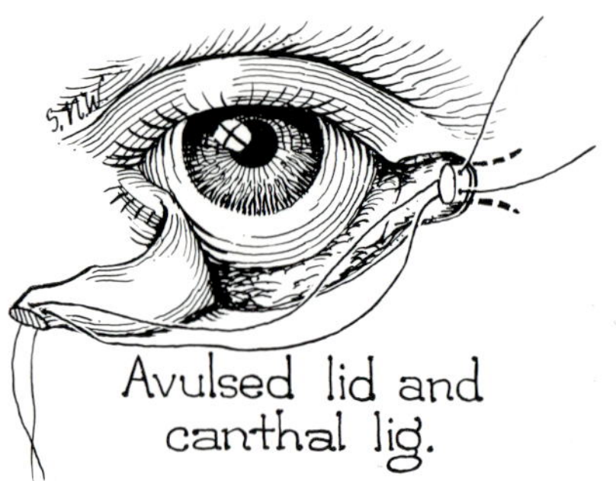

Figure 7–8 Diagram to illustrate the importance of identification and repair of lacerated canthal ligament.

Extensive Lid Lacerations with Loss of Tissue. The majority of lid lacerations associated with loss of tissue can be repaired by judicious construction of flaps and free use of lid-splitting along the gray line. Only rarely are free grafts required. The two-layered closure of lid wounds is the basic principle of the surgical approach.

At first glance in an emergency treatment room, lid trauma can produce a startling disfigurement (Figs. 7–7, 7–9*A*): a scrambled mass of tissue with areas of unnaturally exposed eyeball, twisted lid fragments containing eyelashes displaced toward the brow, sections of exposed and everted tarsus, particles of foreign material throughout the wound and profuse bleeding. Once the injured area has been cleansed and bleeding controlled, the pieces can usually be replaced with surprising completeness, but a logical plan of repair must be formulated. Assuming that the eye has not been injured and that x-rays have failed to disclose a retained foreign body, the surgeon should give attention to the integrity of the lacrimal drainage apparatus, the levator palpebrae tendon and the orbital septum. Repair of lacrimal canaliculi is discussed in a subsequent section.

Reference has already been made to the importance of suturing a severed levator tendon to the upper margin of the tarsus. The fascial layer of septum, tarsus and canthal ligament must be organized and realigned first. Attention is then turned to the lid margins at the angles of the lid fissure. Despite extensive damage to the lateral or medial canthus, there is usually a remnant of the lid angle attached to the canthal ligament which is a vital landmark upon which to build the reconstruction. Usually, most of the tissue fragments can be drawn back into their natural position, and denuded strips of tarsus can be salvalged; thus, the tarsoconjunctival layer can be reformed piecemeal by laborious tissue identification and suturing.

A *lid needs continuous tarsus at its margin for stability of its contour.* This is the most important principle of surgical repair of the tarsus. All but a 2 mm. strip of lid-margin tarsus can be excised (as is commonly done in many parts of the world for trachomatous scarring) without significant residual deformity of the lid contour; however, a continuous strip of tarsus must be retained at the lid margin if deformity is to be prevented. If there is absence of tarsus, a wedge or tongue of the tarsoconjunctival layer can be slid into the defect from the opposing lid (Fig. 7–9*B* and *C*), constituting a tarsorrhaphy at this site (which is advantageous in cases of extensive lid trauma). When, after several months, the lids are separated, the defect in tarsus in the uninjured lid will cause no cosmetic deformity. Damage to the meibomian glands is of no practical consequence.

Once the posterior surgical layer has been reconstructed by securing an avulsed canthal ligament, suturing of orbital septal defects and repair of tarsus, the skin-muscle layer is separately closed. There is marked variation in the laxity of this layer, with slackness more pronounced in the elderly. Simple undermining of the skin-muscle layer is generally sufficient for mobilization and closure of tissue defects that do not include the lid margin. When skin-muscle defects *do* include the lid margin, wide incision along the gray line is often necessary to obtain a sliding flap. Extensive gray line incision has

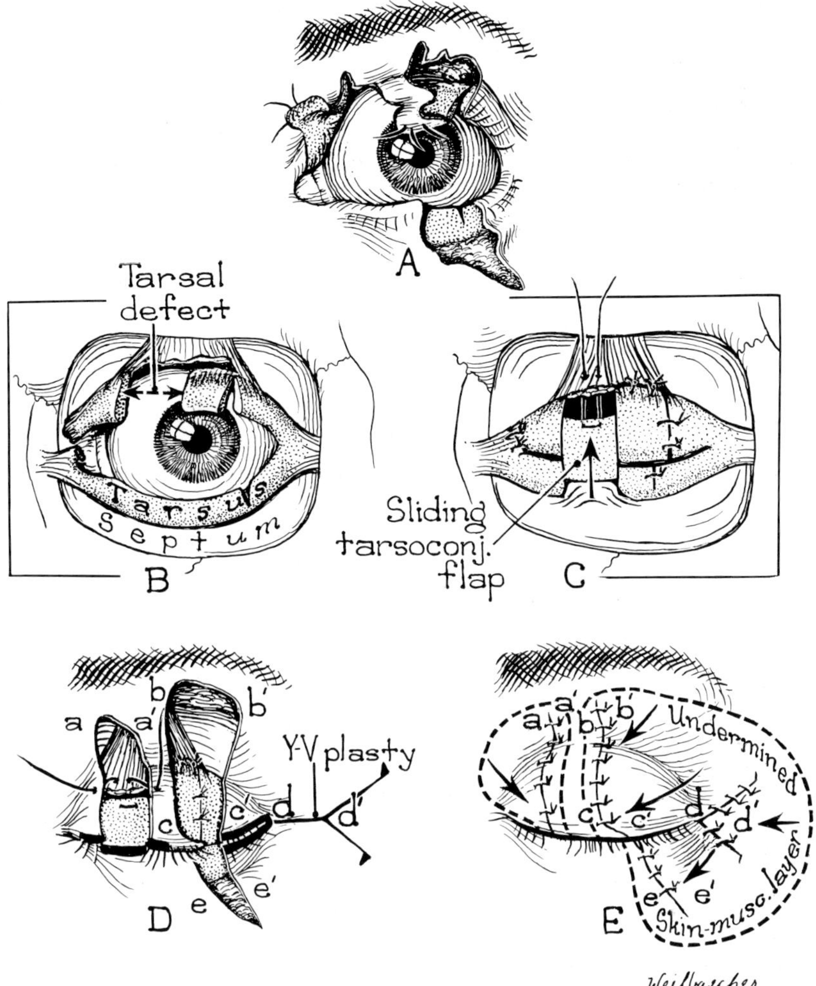

Figure 7–9 Diagrammatic illustration of the steps necessary for repair of extensive lid lacerations. *A*, Appearance of the original injury. *B* and *C*, The skin-muscle layer has not been shown in order to demonstrate repair of the tarsoconjunctival layer. *D*, Heavy lines at the lid margins indicate where gray-line splitting is required for mobilization of skin-muscle sliding flaps. *E*, As in most cases of lid lacerations, the skin-muscle layer can be closed without use of skin grafting if sufficient mobilization of the anterior layer is accomplished.

no disadvantages if the surgeon is careful to find a proper plane and does not split the tarsus itself or damage the muscle by excessive use of the knife blade.

Sliding flaps of skin-muscle are best mobilized from the lateral regions of the lids and the tissue overlying the temporal fossa. Gray line incision and two-layered separation can be extended all the way to the lateral canthus, followed by a partial cantholysis to free the orbicularis insertion from the canthal ligament. A flap of undermined skin and muscle can be brought medially, with or without auxiliary incisions, to prevent lateral skin traction tending to withdraw the flap (Fig. 7–9*D* and *E*). The use of Z- and Y-plasties is often of great convenience in repair of extensive lid lacerations; since these represent well-known surgical maneuvers, they need not be discussed in detail here. It is important, however, to avoid tension on a flap. The sutures should do little more than hold the tissue margins together. When the superficial tissue defect to be filled does not include the lid margin, the sliding flap of skin-muscle need not involve the lid margin; therefore, incision along the gray line is unnecessary.

Unless there is extensive loss of lid tissue and a large field of surrounding trauma, plastic pedicle flaps are rarely needed at the time of primary repair. Efforts to simulate a natural lid margin by a pedicle flap containing brow hair are rarely successful and should not be done at the time of accident room surgery, if at all.

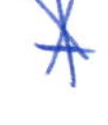

It is seldom necessary to perform free skin grafts for treatment of lid injury, but extensive loss of lid substance occasionally requires them. If the tissues are clean, the results can be excellent. The best site of full-thickness donor skin for lid grafting is the lax skin fold of the contralateral upper lid. No other skin of the body provides so good a color match or is so thin. Possibly another excellent donor site would be the skin of the prepuce or penis, but the usual donor is not enthusiastic about use of this site. Thus, the next best donor sites are the cephalo-auricular angle, and the supraclavicular fossa (if it is not hair-bearing). When defects between the medial canthus and the bridge of the nose are grafted, the surgeon should be especially careful to get good apposition of the graft to the deep underlying tissues; this is facilitated by stab incisions in the graft and by a tightly applied postoperative dressing. Split thickness skin grafting is an occasionally useful and at times necessary adjunct to the treatment of severe lid burns or denuded skin areas where granulation tissue has already formed. The principles and techniques of skin grafting are not specific for eyelid injuries.

Traumatic Loss of the Lids. In the event of almost complete loss of the eyelids, priority attention must be given to protection of the globe, which may be completely spared from the devastation that has destroyed the eyelids. Effective protection of an exposed but uninjured globe, prior to the extensive plastic surgery necessary for rebuilding the eyelids, can be obtained in several ways. The ophthalmologist will usually incise the bulbar conjunctiva around the limbus of the eye and undermine this tissue peripherally so that it can be brought over the cornea either as an apron or bridge flap. Surgeons without training in ophthalmology would not want to undertake this dissection of tissue on the globe itself. An alternative method utilizes the laxity of the conjunctiva of the upper and lower fornix.[10] *Without any dissection,* the conjunctiva can be grasped at the upper fornix with forceps and a suture passed through it and then brought through a similar fold from the lower fornix, in the same vertical line. Thus, by using multiple interrupted sutures, a double thickness of conjunctiva can be brought over the globe and a horizontal straight line closure of conjunctiva across the cornea can be obtained (Fig. 7–10). These sutures will not hold for more than a few days, but this is more than enough time for accomplishing plastic revision of the lids. Rebuilding a lid often requires large pedicle flaps, sliding flaps and mucous membrane grafts—the details of which are not appropriate here, since that is clearly the responsibility of specialists.

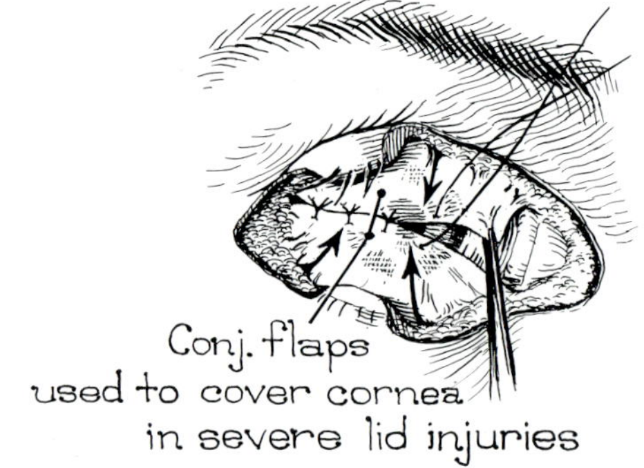

Figure 7–10 A simple method of providing temporary protection to an exposed globe by double thickness flaps of undissected conjunctiva.

Injuries of the Lacrimal Apparatus. The anatomy of the lacrimal drainage apparatus is illustrated in Figure 7–2*B*. Lacerations within the medial fourth of the lids may impair tear drainage to the nose by direct injury to the puncta, the canaliculi, the lacrimal sac or the nasolacrimal duct. Lid injuries may also disrupt lacrimal drainage indirectly if lid deformity causes poor pumping by the orbicularis muscle or poor apposition of the punctum against the eyeball. Thus, in repair of such lid lacerations, attention must be directed to the normal conformity of the lid as well as to the severed canaliculus.

Repair of a canaliculus is not always successful, but it is well worth undertaking. If only the upper canaliculus is injured, there is little likelihood that epiphora (spillage of tears over the lid margin) will result. Some persons whose lower canaliculus has been irreversibly damaged, get along well with the upper canaliculus alone, but this is unusual.

For surgical repair, the following procedures are employed. After instillation and injection of local anesthetic, a punctum dilator is used to widen (but not split) the aperture to the canaliculus, permitting passage of probes. The Worst pigtail probe[22] is passed through the upper lacrimal canaliculus around to the lower canalicus where it appears within the wound (Fig. 7–11*A*). A silk suture is then attached to the probe which is reversed (arrow, Fig. 7–11*A*), drawing the suture through the canaliculus (Fig. 7–11*B*). The pigtail probe is then passed through the lower punctum, and the suture is drawn through the remainder of the lower canaliculus (Fig. 7–11*B* and *C*). The suture is then used to draw a small polyethylene tube through the canicular system as illustrated in Figure 7–11*C*. The ends of the lacerated caniculus are sutured together with

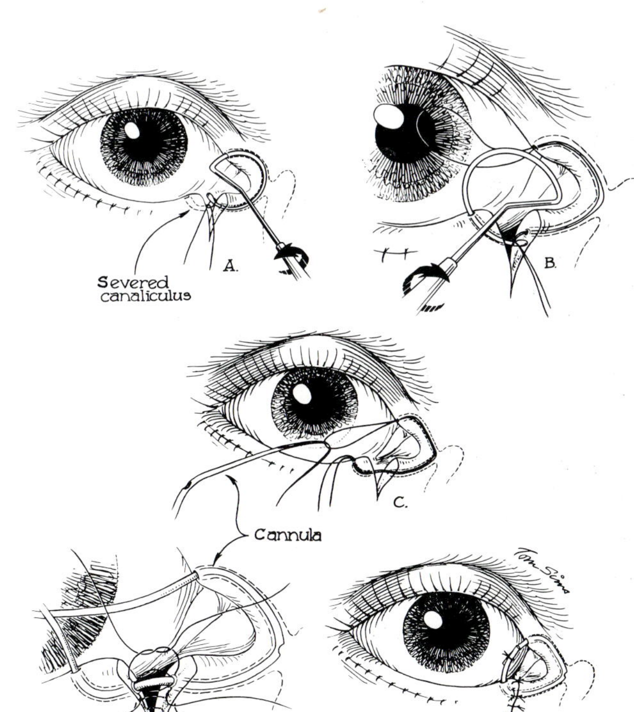

Figure 7–11 Worst's method of identifying and repairing a severed canaliculus.

10–0 nylon or 8–0 virgin silk sutures (Fig. 7–11*D*), with the aid of the operating microscope. The lid margin, deeper tissues and skin are sutured (Fig. 7–11*E*). The polyethylene tube is left in place for several weeks.

Occasionally, it is not possible to pass the pigtail probe through the canicular system, in which case the proximal portion of the canaliculus may be identified by injection of sterile milk through the upper canaliculus while applying pressure over the lower part of the lacrimal sac with a cotton-topped applicator (Fig. 7–12*A*). An alternative method is to pool sterile saline in the wound and then watch for bubbles while injecting air into the upper canaliculus. Once the proximal opening of the severed canaliculus is identified, canalicular anastomosis remains the greatest challenge; many methods of repair have been advocated.[6] Perhaps the simplest means is to thread a fine polyethylene tube over a lacrimal probe and pass these two through the punctum, through the distal portion of the canaliculus, and then through the proximal portion of the canaliculus (Fig. 7–12*B*)—a final step that is more easily described than performed. If the lacrimal sac has been lacerated or exposed in the dissection, it is sometimes easier to make an incision in the sac and introduce the polyethylene tube (or whatever stent is used) from the retrograde direction and thereafter to the distal portion of the canaliculus. Once the tube or similar stent is in position, the two portions of the canaliculus are sutured to each other as described above.

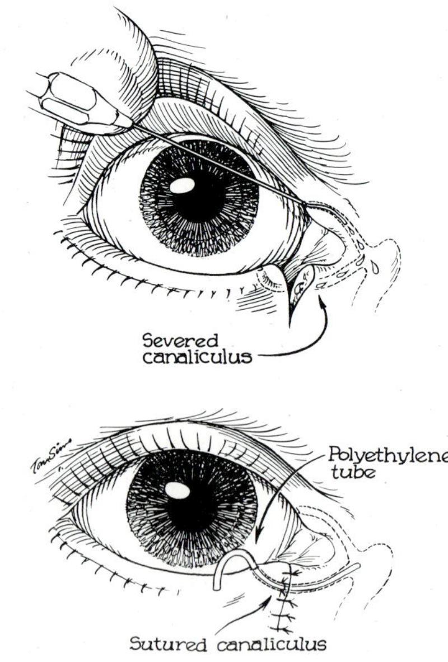

Figure 7–12 Method of identifying and repairing a severed canaliculus.

INJURIES OF THE ORBIT

Fractures of the Orbit. Facial fractures frequently include damage to the walls of the orbit and resultant injury to intraorbital contents; consequently, they are of importance to the ophthalmologist. In particular, blowout fractures of the orbital floor are of prime concern to the eye specialist because of the frequent impairment of ocular motility that results when orbital tissue is extruded into the maxillary antrum.

Orbital trauma is typically signaled by ecchymosis and swelling of the lids, and by mild to severe proptosis and ophthalmoplegia from hemorrhage within the orbit. In addition, there may be subcutaneous emphysema (crepitus, palpable through the lids) from fractures of sinuses, and localized anesthesia of the skin in areas innervated by the supraorbital and infraorbital branches of the trigeminal nerve along the roof and floor of the orbit, respectively. Defects in the orbital rim can sometimes be detected clinically.

Fractures that cannot be diagnosed until special x-ray views are obtained can be suspected from a variety of clinical signs. For example, fractures of the roof of the orbit are often followed by hemorrhage into the upper lid and subconjunctival hemorrhage on the lateral aspect of the globe. Lateral wall fractures are the ones more apt to be associated with avulsion of the optic nerve and profound loss of vision. Medial wall fractures usually produce orbital emphysema which, even if not palpable, is frequently visible in x-rays. Systemic antibiotics are indicated, but surgical repair is not necessarily undertaken if there is no damage to the orbital contents. The patient must avoid nose-blowing or muscular straining if an orbital fracture into one of the sinuses is suspected.

The percentage of accurate diagnoses is greatly increased by well-planned, technically excellent x-rays (Table 7–6). Tomography and the use of intraorbital radiopaque contrast material are sometimes valuable adjuncts to x-ray studies. References to pertinent literature on this subject have been given in the table.

Blowout Fractures of the Orbital Floor. The alert surgeon will usually diagnose the majority of orbital fractures at the time of his initial evaluation of an injury. The one fracture that he is most likely to overlook is the blowout fracture of the orbital floor, which is often unassociated with fractures of the orbital rim or other facial bones.

When the force of a blunt object (such as a fist or baseball) is exerted upon the orbit, there is compression of orbital tissues; the markedly increased hydraulic pressure within the orbit may result in a blowout at the site of the weakest portion of the orbit, the floor. Orbital fat may prolapse into the maxillary antrum, and the inferior rectus and inferior oblique muscles are often included with the incarcerated tissues (Fig. 7–13). When these two ocular muscles are caught in the incarceration, not only is their function restricted but they also serve as limiting bands that prevent full range of contraction of other ocular muscles not involved in the fracture. As a result, downward gaze may be reduced because of a pinched inferior rectus, but *upward gaze is often more impaired.* This occurs not only from incarceration of the inferior oblique but also because the superior rectus cannot elevate the globe against the short rein of the trapped muscles beneath the globe.

It is not necessary to obtain a definitive diagnosis of orbital floor fracture at the time of emergency room examination; other injuries may take precedence, and the surgeon often must wait several days until orbital swelling has subsided before adequate clinical examination can be performed. A blowout fracture is never an emergency, whereas simultaneously incurred globe injuries frequently are.

Clinical suspicion of a blowout fracture is based on one or more of the following findings: anesthesia of the ipsilateral side of the nose and skin of the lower lid; diplopia, from limitation of the inferior rectus and inferior oblique (Figs. 7–14 and 7–15); positive forced-duction test of the inferior rectus (see later); or, several weeks after injury when orbital swelling has resolved, downward and inward displacement of the globe with increase in the supratarsal sulcus (Fig. 7–15). Confirmation can be obtained by x-ray studies in more than 90 per cent of cases if the proper special views and techniques are employed.[4]

When upward gaze is impaired following trauma, it is helpful to determine the site of injury by the forced-duction test. After topical anesthesia, a forceps is used to grasp the eye at the insertion of the inferior rectus muscle, about 7 mm. above the limbus. The patient is requested to look up and the eye is rotated upward by the examiner; if it then shows full range of motility, the superior rectus or inferior oblique may be paretic. If it does not elevate even with manual force, the eye is being restrained by something—usually the incarceration of tissue in an orbital floor fracture. Of course, the forced-duction test can be used to test the motility of the other rectus muscles as well. When using forced duction, the inexperienced examiner should not mistake posterior displacement of the

TABLE 7–6 SUGGESTIONS CONCERNING RADIOGRAPHIC PROJECTIONS FOR ORBITAL INJURIES*

ANATOMICAL SITE	OPTIMAL RADIOGRAPHIC PROJECTION	ADDITIONAL STUDIES
Orbital roof Superior orbital rim	Caldwell (15° PA)	Tomography: particularly suitable to show isolated fractures of the orbital plate or damage of cribriform plate (preferably pluridirectional)
Medial wall		
upper half	Caldwell	Hypocloidal Polytomography
lower half	Special View I (Fueger)†	
Orbital floor		
"en face"	Waters	Hypocloidal Polytomography
profile	Special View I (Fueger)† Special View II (Fueger)‡	
Lateral wall	Caldwell Rheese Special View II (Fueger)‡	Usually not necessary
Infraorbital rim	Waters	Usually not helpful
Optic foramina	Rheese	Tomography (preferably pluridirectional)

*A facial bone survey should always be obtained to determine the extent of facial trauma. A lateral projection should be included to show the facial bones in a second plane. Special projections with narrow collimation should follow the facial bone survey. Technical excellence is necessary. There must be no motion. The density range should be long.

†Fueger I. Forehead-film-position, C/R 30 degrees caudad, to exit one to one and a quarter inches below nasion.

‡Fueger II. Oblique position, sagittal plane rotated 20 degrees, C/R 35 degrees caudad; through affected orbit, to exit one inch below infraorbital rim.

For further information see references 17, 19 and 21.

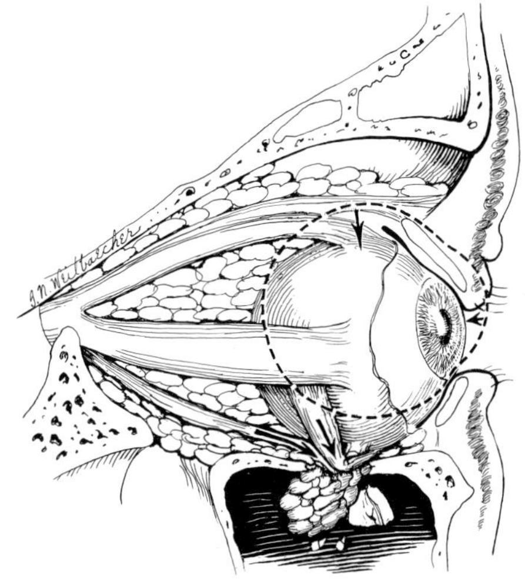

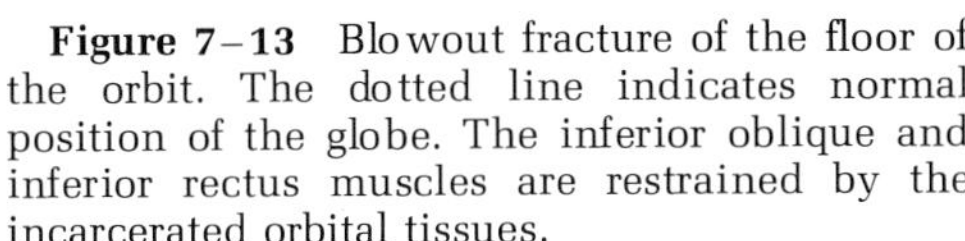

Figure 7–13 Blowout fracture of the floor of the orbit. The dotted line indicates normal position of the globe. The inferior oblique and inferior rectus muscles are restrained by the incarcerated orbital tissues.

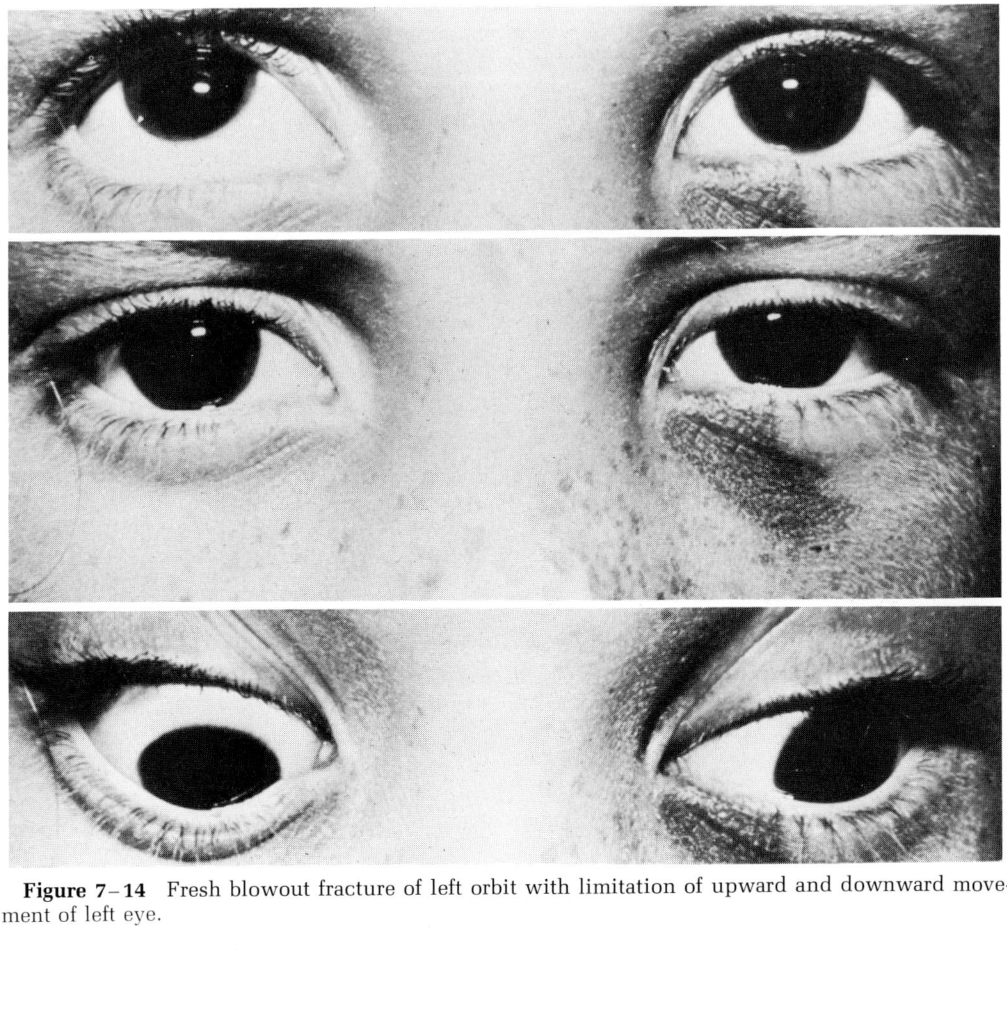

Figure 7–14 Fresh blowout fracture of left orbit with limitation of upward and downward movement of left eye.

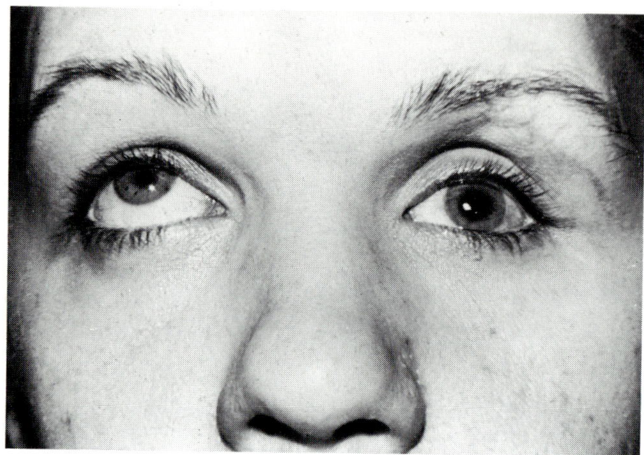

Figure 7–15 Old blowout fracture of left orbit with enophthalmos and limited upward gaze of left eye.

eyeball for improved ocular motility. Because of lid swelling and the discomfort of forced motility, this test is not always useful for preoperative diagnosis.

Surgical Technique for Repair of Blowout Fractures. Floor fractures should be repaired when incarcerated orbital tissues cause restriction of movement of the globe with significant diplopia or when extensive bony defects are present on x-ray. Small fractures without incarcerated muscles do well without surgery. It is preferable to operate between five and fifteen days after injury, when orbital edema has subsided, and significant fibrosis of the fracture site has not yet occurred.

The usual surgical approach is accomplished by a lower eyelid incision through skin and orbicularis, followed by incision of the periosteum below and parallel to the inferior orbital rim. The periosteum is then elevated, the orbital floor exposed, and the extent of the fracture is determined. Any incarcerated orbital tissues are carefully removed from the fracture site. *It is important to demonstrate full range of all ocular ductions at the time of surgical repair.* Bony fragments or hinged flaps are restored to their original positions whenever possible. If the restored floor is of inadequate strength or if a defect remains, the floor is reinforced by a sheet of alloplastic material such as Supramid or Teflon. Periosteum and then skin are closed.

In some cases incarcerated orbital tissues cannot readily be freed by the trans-eyelid approach described above. On those infrequent occasions, further exposure must be gained by utilizing the Caldwell-Luc approach in combination with the trans-eyelid approach. The upper lid is retracted, and an incision is placed in the gingivolabial fold between the second molar and the canine teeth. The maxilla is then exposed in the region of the anterior wall of the maxillary antrum. A bony opening large enough to admit a finger into the maxillary antrum is then chiseled out. This permits exposure of both the superior and inferior aspects of the orbital floor, and simultaneous manipulation of fracture fragments and incarcerated tissues from above and below allows release of the entrapped tissues with the least possible trauma. The Caldwell-Luc approach is best performed by an otolaryngologist. Pre- and postoperative management and orbital surgery are best performed by an ophthalmologist.

Orbital Hemorrhage. Blunt trauma to the orbital region may result in extensive hemorrhage with proptosis and limitation of ocular motility. Occasionally, blood may dissect forward beneath the conjunctiva to produce a firm

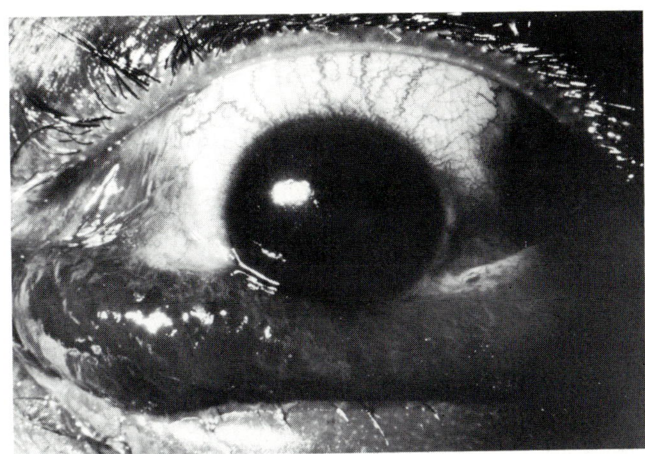

Figure 7–16 Orbital hemorrhage with proptosis and large subconjunctival hematoma preventing lid closure.

red mass that interferes with lid closure (Fig. 7–16). In extreme cases, the orbital swelling may cause a serious rise in intraocular pressure, requiring lateral canthotomy and possibly intraorbital injection of hyaluronidase (150 units in 1 cc.). An ophthalmologist should examine such an eye as soon as possible.

INTRAOCULAR AND INTRAORBITAL FOREIGN BODIES

With any puncture wound of the lids or ocular tissues the surgeon should make every effort to exclude the possibility of a retained intraorbital or intraocular foreign body. He should obtain x-rays if the presence of a foreign body is even remotely suspected. However, glass, plastics and a host of other materials are often not visible on the films. Intracranial injuries from transorbital foreign bodies are infrequent but are potentially quite hazardous (Fig. 7–17*A* and *B*).

Common sites for lodgment of foreign bodies within the eye and beneath the lids are shown in Figure 7–18. Eversion of the upper lid is extremely important in routine search for small missiles that have struck the eye. To get optimal x-ray views of the anterior segment of the eye, a dental film can be placed deeply near the bridge of the nose, and an oblique x-ray of the anterior ocular segment can be obtained that is free of bony markings. Several exposures should be made so that artefacts on one film are not misinterpreted as small foreign bodies.

The majority of metallic chips that enter the eye are from a metal-on-metal blow or from a grinding-wheel injury. The generated heat of the struck metal particle probably accounts for sterility, for endophthalmitis is the least likely complication. Iron-containing foreign bodies eventually cause siderosis within the eye, and copper-containing metals produce chalcosis. All foreign bodies within the eye create the strong possibility of functional loss of the eye from mechanical damage or secondary inflammation. A safe generalization is that intraocular and intraorbital foreign bodies should be removed as soon after the injury as possible, before they cause damage by disintegration products or become encapsulated by fibrous tissue.

When scout films of the orbit demonstrate a radiopaque foreign body (Fig. 7–19*B*), there are several techniques for determining whether it is located within the globe and, if so, at precisely what location. The Sweet's

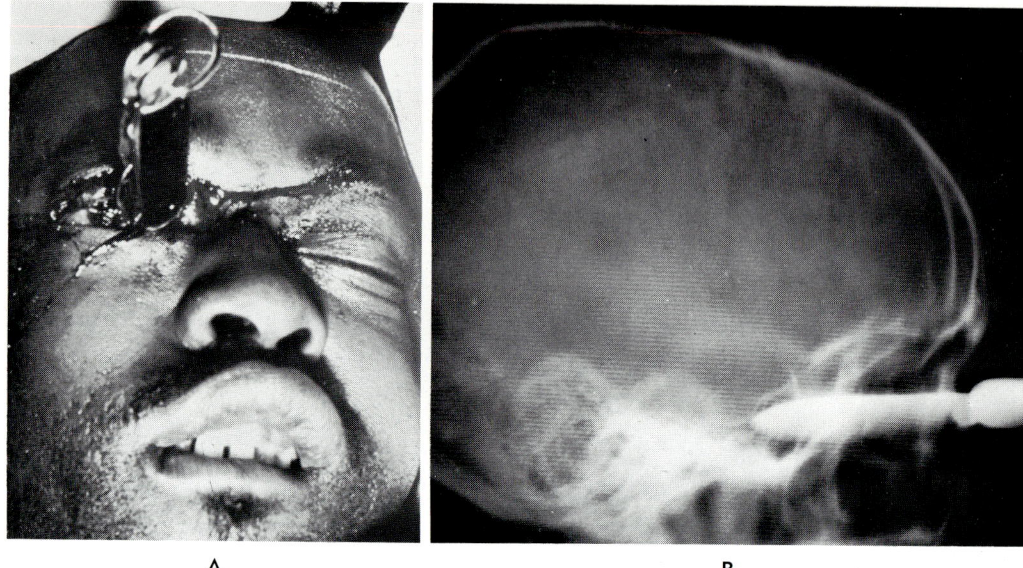

Figure 7–17 *A,* A 35-year-old male with pen knife embedded to the hilt in the right orbit. There was no light perception of the right eye and total ophthalmoplegia. The globe itself was intact. *B,* X-ray showing the tip of the blade next to the sphenoid sinus. The knife was removed by simultaneous right frontal craniotomy and orbital exploration. The knife had not entered the dura, but severed the optic nerve and the medial rectus muscle. Except for ophthalmoplegia and loss of vision, the patient's recovery was uneventful. (Case reported previously and photographs published with permission of Dr. David Paton and the authors: Bard, L. A., and Jarrett, W. H.: Intracranial complications of penetrating orbital injuries. Arch. Ophth. *71*:322, 1964.)

localization procedure is a classic example,[12] other methods employ a contact lens with radiopaque markers, ultrasound[2] or an electromagnetic sounding device such as the Berman locator (which is primarily of use at the time of operation). The problems and methods of removing these retained foreign bodies are so clearly the responsibility of the ophthalmologist that they will not be discussed here.

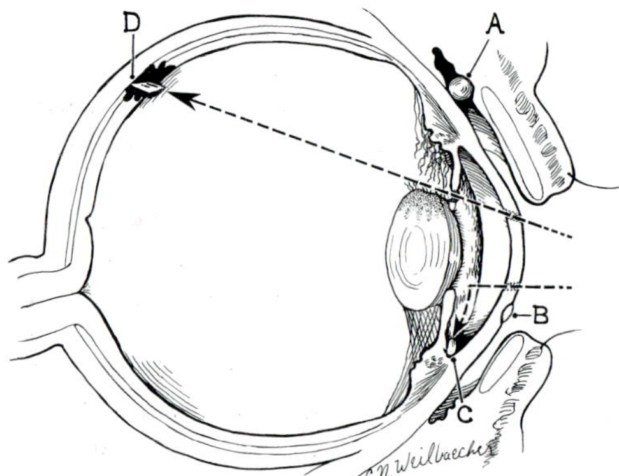

Figure 7–18 Common sites of foreign bodies. *A,* BB pellets and even contact lenses may be retained in the conjunctival fornix of the upper lid. *B,* Corneal foreign bodies are usually found within the lid fissure. *C,* Small sharp fragments such as glass may pass through the cornea and sink into the angle of the anterior chamber inferiorly. *D,* Metallic missiles may pass through the cornea, iris and lens and lodge in the posterior wall of the eye or remain within the vitreous cavity. Less frequently, they pass entirely through the eye and remain within the orbit.

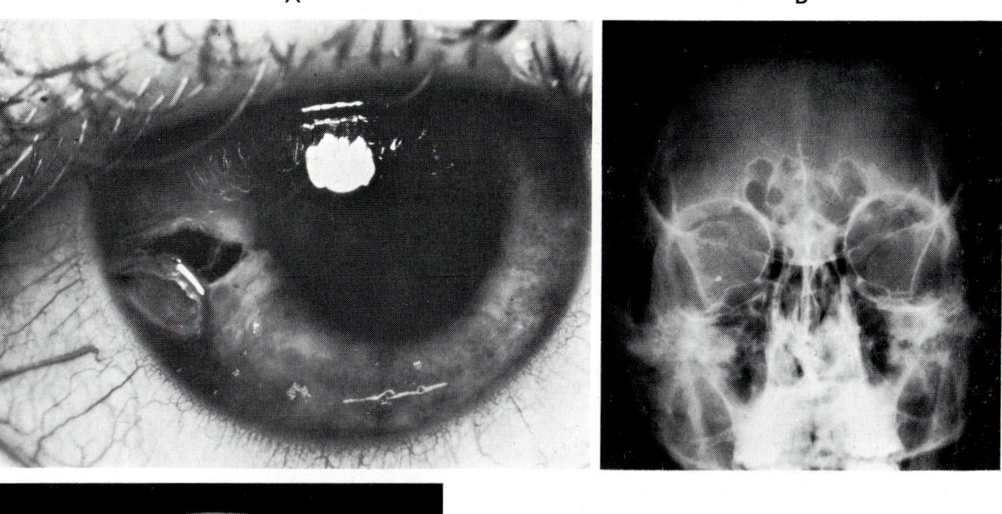

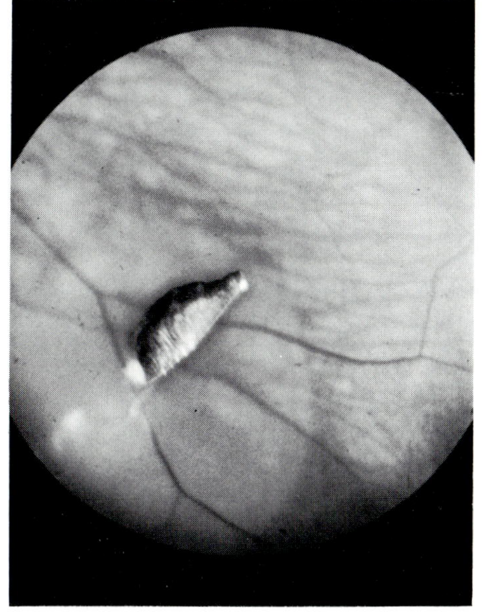

Figure 7–19 A metal fragment has passed through the cornea and iris with little gross evidence of ocular damage (*A*). The foreign body is seen by skull x-ray (*B*) and, in this case, can also be visualized with the ophthalmoscope on the surface of the retina (*C*).

BURNS OF THE EYE AND ADNEXA

Chemical Burns of the Eye. Burns of the eye by alkali or acid are the most urgent of all ocular emergencies. The extent of permanent injury is not only related to the nature and concentration of the chemical, but also to the time lapse before decontamination.[16] Strong alkalis such as lye and lime cause ischemia and necrosis of conjunctiva and sclera and rapid opacification of the cornea (Fig. 7–20). Unless irrigated within moments, the eye may eventually be lost.

With the rare exceptions of chemicals that react violently with water, the immediate treatment of chemical burns must be copious irrigation of the eyes, using the nearest source of water. The victim's face should be placed under a foreceful stream of water from a shower, drinking fountain,

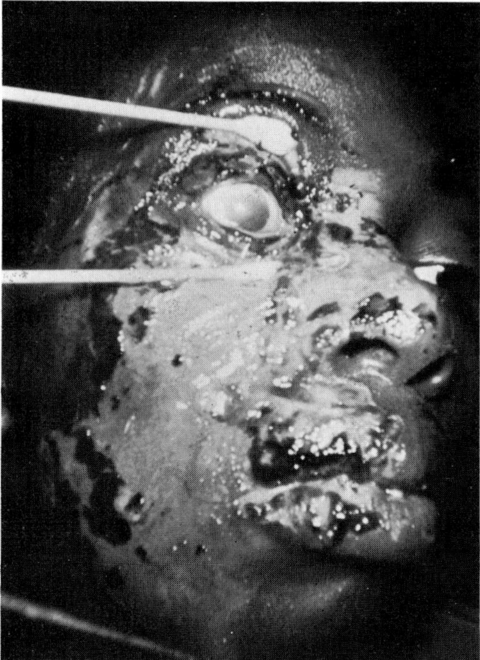

Figure 7–20 Alkali burn to right eye and skin of face.

hose or bathtub faucet. The lids must be held apart, for severe orbicularis spasm might otherwise prevent the beneficial effect of the irrigation. Particulate matter of the chemical should be promptly removed with cotton swabs: the lids should be everted and cotton applicators used to sweep the fornices of the conjunctival sac.

After initial lavage, early use of topical anesthetic will greatly facilitate the emergency measures by easing the patient's discomfort. Systemic analgesics are also valuable. As soon as possible, irrigation should be continued with a reservoir of isotonic saline connected to an intravenous tubing set; this should be continued for a minimum of 20 minutes.

Neutralizing solutions have not been found effective in the treatment of chemical burns. There are only a few specific antidotes of proved value in burns with common chemicals. For example, mortar and plaster (which contain calcium hydroxide) are removed with greater ease by the use of 0.01M solution of neutral sodium edathamil (EDTA).[9]

After lavage, mydriatics are instilled to reduce iris adhesions to the lens (atropine is favored because of its prolonged action); it is customary to start treatment with topical steroids to reduce iritis. Cysteine or other collagenase inhibitors may be useful in preventing loss of corneal stroma by the action of collagenase liberated by injured corneal epithelium. In rare cases, severe chemical burns are treated by emergency corneal grafts to preserve the eye when corneal destruction is so extensive that its eventual slough can be predicted. The prognosis for such grafts is poor; therefore, surgery is usually deferred until perforation of the cornea is imminent. Both moderate and severe chemical burns by alkali or acid may lead to scarring of the conjunctiva, with resultant adhesions between the lids and the globe (symblepharon). The use of steroid ointment and a plastic contact lens or other conformer fitted into the fornices within the lids is a means of reducing this scarring, which can be a late complication of great severity.

Thermal Burns. Thermal burns of the lids are treated in much the same way as elsewhere on the body. Marked edema and tissue necrosis are usually present, making examination of the globe dependent upon the use of lid retractors. Tarsorrhaphy is often impossible because of friable lid tissue; exposure of the globe must be prevented in succeeding days, and treatment with artificial tear solution or an ophthalmic ointment is then essential. Thin split-thickness skin grafts (of 0.005 inch thickness) are sometimes required. A convenient donor site is the medial surface of the upper arm. A common late complication of lid burns is cicatricial ectropion, eversion of the lids by scar tissue.

Radiation Burns of the Eye. Ultraviolet radiation is the most common form of radiant energy producing ocular injury; the chief sources are welding arcs, "sun-tan" lamps and carbon arcs. There is an interval of six to 10 hours after exposure before symptoms begin; the patient first notes an irritated sensation of the eyes that progresses to severe photophobia, pain and blepharospasm. Examination shows mild chemosis; topically applied fluorescein produces a punctate staining of the cornea. Treatment consists of mydriatic drops, topical ophthalmic ointment and a semipressure eye dressing that restricts lid blinking. Sedatives and analgesics are often required. The eye patches remain in place for at least 24 hours; by then, the corneal epithelium is usually restored and the symptoms gone.

Infrared flash burns are usually of little consequence; the lids develop an immediate temporary erythema, but the eye itself is unharmed. However, prolonged exposure to the shorter wavelengths of infrared is responsible for the development of heat cataracts. In the past, glassblowers and metal-furnace stokers, who were improperly protected from the radiation, developed cataracts after many years of such employment.

Cataract is a late result of ionizing radiation of various types; high speed neutrons from cyclotron exposure or from atomic blasts are the most typical sources. Beta radiation will also cause cataracts if the eye is exposed to excessive doses; the latent period for development of such lens changes is usually two and a half years.[19]

Changes in the posterior portion of the globe from radiation exposure are rare. Viewing of a solar eclipse is the most notable exception; irreversible damage to the macula can result from failure to protect the eye from the excessive brightness. Since there is no emergency treatment for radiation burns of this nature, further discussion will not be included.

INJURIES OF THE CONJUNCTIVA

Conjunctival Hemorrhage. Conjunctival hemorrhage is the most common accompaniment of ocular trauma but is, in itself, of no consequence. Spontaneous hemorrhages of the conjunctiva occur in adults of advancing age, and in others without apparent reason. No known medication will effectively speed resorption of the hemorrhage, but all traces of it should be gone in a week or two. Subconjunctival hemorrhage from orbital bleeding is sometimes so severe that the conjunctiva balloons out between the lids and must be kept lubricated with ointment until the swelling subsides and the conjunctiva returns within the lid fissure. Use of a rubber glove filled with crushed ice is a good way to hasten regression of the swelling.

Chemosis. With or without hemorrhage of the conjunctiva, chemosis is often of serious portent (Fig. 7–21). Benign causes of conjunctival edema are ultraviolet exposure and various forms of allergic conjunctivitis. Chemosis is often characteristic of endocrine exophthalmos, pseudotumor of the orbit and trichinosis. *Following injury, acute chemosis with hemorrhage of pronounced or minimal amount may be caused by a retained intraorbital foreign body, fracture of the orbit, scleral rupture, carotid-cavernous fistula or traumatic asphyxia.*

Lacerations of the Bulbar Conjunctiva. Every conjunctival laceration should be carefully explored after use of topical or retrobulbar anes-

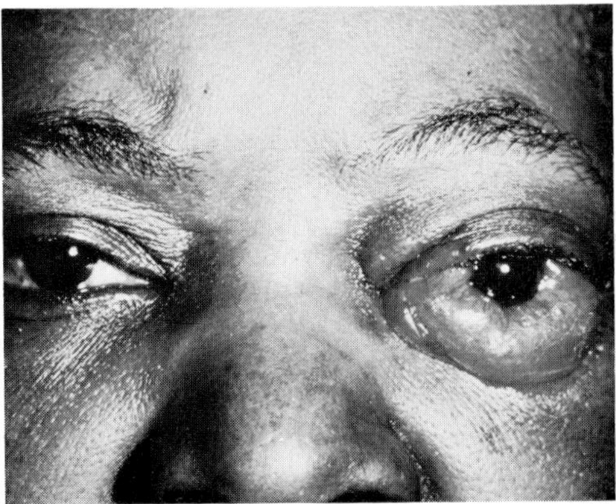

Figure 7–21 Chemosis in this case was due to traumatic carotid-cavernous fistula. There was an orbital bruit and proptosis of the left eye.

thetic. Again, the possibility of the presence of occult foreign bodies must be considered. Repair of a conjunctival laceration is not necessary unless it is more than a centimeter in length. Interrupted 7–0 or 8–0 gut sutures are sufficient; the only precaution necessary is care that conjunctival edges are properly recognized and that Tenon's capsule (the fascia beneath the bulbar conjunctiva) is not confused with the thinner and more superficial layer.

INJURIES OF THE EXTRA-OCULAR MUSCLES

Hematoma of the extraocular muscles is not uncommon following contusion injuries to the orbit or lacerations by a foreign body. These hemorrhages are visible only at exploratory operation, except when they extend along the muscle sheath to the insertion of its tendon on the globe. The only significant consequence of such hemorrhages is the transitory limitation of the muscle's action and the problems in differential diagnosis raised thereby.

The ocular muscles are not often avulsed, but foreign bodies entering the orbit can sever the muscles and render them functionless (Fig. 7–17). See also the earlier section on fractures of the orbit.

INJURIES TO THE GLOBE

Techniques of Examination. Corneal abrasions are often due to a foreign body caught under the upper lid. Every physician should know how to evert the lid, for he will be called on to remove "cinders" or "trash" from the inner aspects of the lids throughout his professional life. The patient should be conveniently seated and directed to look down; the upper lid is grasped by its central lashes and pulled downward and slightly outward; the examiner then presses with a finger or cotton applicator at the upper margin of the tarsus and maintains this gentle pressure while the lid is flipped into the everted position. Key assistance in this maneuver is gained by a cooperative patient who maintains downward gaze and does not squeeze the eyelids. A drop of topical anesthetic should be used beforehand if the eye is painful.

When the eye has been lacerated, pressure on the globe must be avoided. Upper lids can be retracted with the examiner's thumb on the superior orbital rim. If the view is still inadequate, a topical anesthetic is instilled and lid retractors are employed.

Corneal Abrasions and Foreign Bodies. There is hardly a person who does not know the anguish of a corneal abrasion. There is sudden onset of pain, lacrimation and blepharospasm; blinking and motions of the eyeball serve to aggravate the pain. Eyes so injured are not easily examined until the patient is afforded relief by a topical anesthetic such as proparacaine hydrochloride 0.5 per cent. The cornea should be inspected with a bright hand light, using oblique illumination. If no foreign body is seen, the upper lid should be everted (as described previously). The foreign body is often a tiny piece of grit lodged on the palpebral conjunctiva (Fig. 7–22); this can be removed by a light touch with a moistened cotton applicator.

If no foreign body is found and no corneal abrasion is seen with the hand light, fluorescein dye is an infallible means of demonstrating epithelial injury or denudation. The sterility of aqueous solutions of fluorescein is not readily maintained, and they afford an excellent culture medium for pseudomonas; sterile strips impregnated with fluorescein are now in widespread use. A drop of sterile saline is placed on the paper and its tip is touched to the palpebral conjunctiva. Blinking spreads the dye over the cornea; the eye is then irrigated with sterile saline from a plastic squeeze bottle.

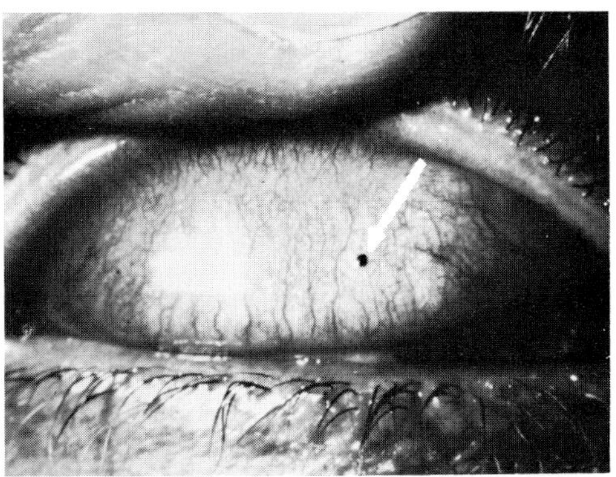

Figure 7–22 A common lodging site for air-borne dust particles is the tarsal conjunctiva (arrow). Vertical "scratch marks" on the cornea are brought out with fluorescein staining and suggest the location of the foreign body as well as account for the marked discomfort that it produces.

Green dye remains wherever corneal epithelial cells have been damaged or lost by abrasion.

Once the "cinder" has been removed and the abrasion identified, treatment is primarily that of putting the eye at rest until the corneal epithelium covers the defect. The corneal epithelium, composed of stratified squamous cells, is separated from the corneal stroma by Bowman's membrane. If a foreign body has not entered the stroma, no corneal scarring will result. A short-acting "pupillary dilator" such as homatropine 5 per cent will make the eye more comfortable and reduce the effects of secondary iridocyclitis. A broad spectrum antibiotic ointment is customarily used to prevent infection, and a semipressure patch is applied for eight to 48 hours, depending on the severity of the injury (Fig. 7–30). The patient should *never* be maintained on topical anesthetic; it can retard healing, aggravate the keratitis and cause addiction.

Metallic foreign bodies (from grinding wheels, hammering metal on metal, etc.), sometimes lodge in the cornea; if allowed to remain, iron-containing particles will become surrounded by a rust ring within two days of the injury. After use of topical anesthetics, the metal fragment can often be removed by a small jet of ophthalmic irrigating solution applied with a plastic squeeze bottle, or by a gentle rub with a moistened cotton applicator. If this is unsuccessful, the foreign body should be removed by an opthalmologist as follows:

The patient's head is placed in a comfortable position (with the patient either supine or sitting at a slit lamp) and the foreign body is removed with a dental burr or similar instrument. Deeply lodged foreign bodies must be removed in the operating room by the use of shelved corneal incisions and with proper precautions to avoid collapse of the anterior chamber or loss of the foreign body within the anterior chamber. Rust rings should also be removed, either at the time of the first examination or several days thereafter when they can be more easily curetted with a dental burr.

Fragments of glass, thorns, caterpillar hairs and similar splinter-shaped objects are often difficult to detect without the magnification of a slit lamp. For this reason, the patient who feels that he has a foreign body in his eye should not be treated casually if gross examination is negative. Herpetic corneal ulcers sometimes begin with a scratchy sensation in the eye and can be detected only by fluorescein stain, which displays a characteristic dendritic pattern. Not only can the discomfort of herpetic keratitis simulate a foreign body in the conjunctival sac, but this viral infection may follow a corneal abrasion. Presumably, the herpes simplex virus gains entrance to the cornea at the site of epithelial damage. It is well known that steroids are contraindicated for superficial herpetic infections of the cornea; therefore, *no medication containing a steroid should ever be used in eyes with a corneal abrasion.*

Corneal and Scleral Lacerations. In all cases of post-traumatic lid swelling, deep laceration or damaged periocular tissues, the globe itself should be carefully examined with a determination inversely proportional to the ease of the examination. The only way to see the globe in the presence of severely swollen lids is to separate the lids forcefully with lid retractors.

The appearance of a corneal or scleral laceration needs little description. Occasionally, the signs of trauma are mild (Fig. 7–19A), but usually injury to the globe is readily apparent (Fig. 7–23). The anterior chamber is often flat, and the iris or the ciliary body may be incarcerated in the wound or prolapsed through it. Frequently there is external bleeding from the injured sclera and internal hemorrhage within the anterior chamber (hyphema, described later). It is not always easy to determine whether the lens has been damaged: hemorrhage may obscure an adequate view, and *rapid accumulation of fibrin in the pupillary space is sometimes indistinguishable from flocculent lens cortex.* The entire lens, along with some of the vitreous, can be extruded through the wound; it may be wiped away when the injury is first inspected. If this is the case, such information must be recorded on the patient's record, as it may be of assistance to the ophthalmologist in deciding future management of the injured eye.

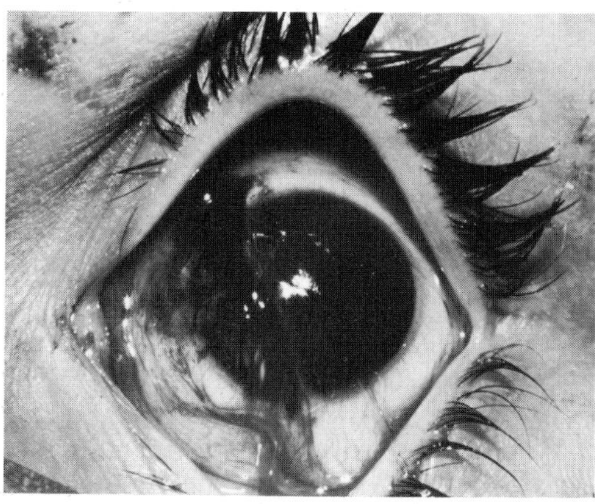

Figure 7–23 Corneoscleral laceration.

Until the time of surgical repair, a lacerated eyeball should be protected from further damage by relief of blepharospasm with analgesics (or facial nerve block if necessary), topical antibiotic *drops* (not ointment) and a protective shield taped over an eyepad. The patient should be prepared for general anesthesia; he should receive nothing by mouth, be sedated, have x-rays of the orbit for possible foreign body and receive tetanus immunization. Broad spectrum systemic antibiotics should be started promptly, even if surgery must be delayed until other injuries have been investigated.

Cataract from Perforating Injury of the Globe. Hatpins, darts, needles and other sharp objects can cause puncture wounds of the eye with scarcely any residual evidence of the site of entrance other than rapid development of a cataract. Any injury to the lens capsule has a strong likelihood of producing a cataract, which may develop within minutes or within months. Swelling of the lens may ensue, causing shallowness of the anterior chamber and, at times, glaucoma as a result of closure of the chamber angle from the anteriorly bulging cataract; early surgery for lens removal is then indicated. It is true that some small foreign bodies can remain within the lens or pass entirely through it and cause only localized opacity of the lens fibers, but such cases are exceptional. Usually, once there is partial opacity, the entire lens becomes cataractous. A discussion of the management of cataracts is not apropos here, but it is important to recognize injury of the lens. Markedly "swollen" (intumescent) cataracts require early surgery. The degree of intumescence can be estimated by appraisal of the anterior chamber depth.

General Information about Repair of Wounds to the Globe. Many of the problems of surgical repair of a lacerated globe are of concern only to the eye specialist. However, there is one standard practice of ophthalmologists that is pertinent here since it represents a general philosophy about the necessity for wound repair in seemingly hopeless cases. Unless there is no light perception and almost total destruction of the eyeball, an ophthalmologist will usually make every effort to repair the eye as carefully and completely as possible. Of prime importance is the fact that occasionally some vision can be salvaged. Second, the patient himself will know that every effort was made to save his eye; and if it must be removed in later days, he is more prepared to accept this decision. Finally, there are many times when the injured person is either disoriented, inebriated or irrational; this is a difficult time to request consent for enucleation of the damaged eye. It is better to attempt salvage of every eye, except those with extensive extrusion of intraocular contents and a degree of laceration that defies repair.

Any perforating injury of the eye (especially with prolapse of iris or ciliary body) has a slight but significant chance of inducing sympathetic ophthalmia. This is a bilateral, granulomatous uveitis originating from unilateral injury and probably resulting from injury-induced autosensitivity to uveal pigment. In trauma cases in which iris or ciliary body prolapse has not been treated (or the eye enucleated) within several weeks of the injury, the incidence of sympathetic ophthalmia may be as high as 3 to 5 per cent of cases.[13] The frequency of this dreaded disorder has diminished greatly in recent years because of prompt treatment of injuries, early enucleation when necessary, and possibly also from the use of systemic steroids. But sympathetic ophthalmia remains a threat to be considered with every eye injury.

Sympathetic ophthalmia may occur from 10 days to many years following the initial injury. Its usual onset is within the first two months after injury to uveal tissue. It is important to decide within the first 10 days whether the patient's repaired eye has a fair chance of providing useful vision; if it does not, enucleation is advisable. Inflammation in the second (uninjured) eye does not occur if the injured eye has been removed prior to the earliest evidence of inflammation in the uninjured eye. Once the second eye is involved, it is doubtful whether enucleation of the injured eye is beneficial. Frequently the sympathetic ophthalmia is so severe that the eye originally injured is eventually the patient's better eye.

Phacoanaphylaxis is probably similar to the pathogenesis of sympathetic ophthalmia. Subsequent to injury to the lens, an eye will sometimes develop a delayed inflammatory reaction and granulomatous uveitis alike in many respects to sympathetic ophthalmia. In rare cases, the uninjured eye may also develop uveitis from sensitivity to lens protein. Sympathetic ophthalmia and phacoanaphylaxis sometimes occur in the same eye.

The use of systemic steroids has been a great boon in the treatment of these two postinjury disorders. Sympathetic ophthalmia can be suppressed by steroid therapy, but if its incidence is decreased by the use of steroids its occurrence is not entirely prevented. Steroid therapy has undoubtedly saved many eyes from complete loss; but it usually must be continued for many years, and the inflammation may become low grade and indolent despite its use.

INTRAOCULAR CONTUSION INJURIES

A clenched fist and a multitude of other missiles can strike the eye and cause havoc with its contents. The examiner should take careful stock of the damages (Fig. 7–24).

Hyphema. Hyphema refers to hemorrhage within the anterior chamber. BB shotgun pellets, stones and

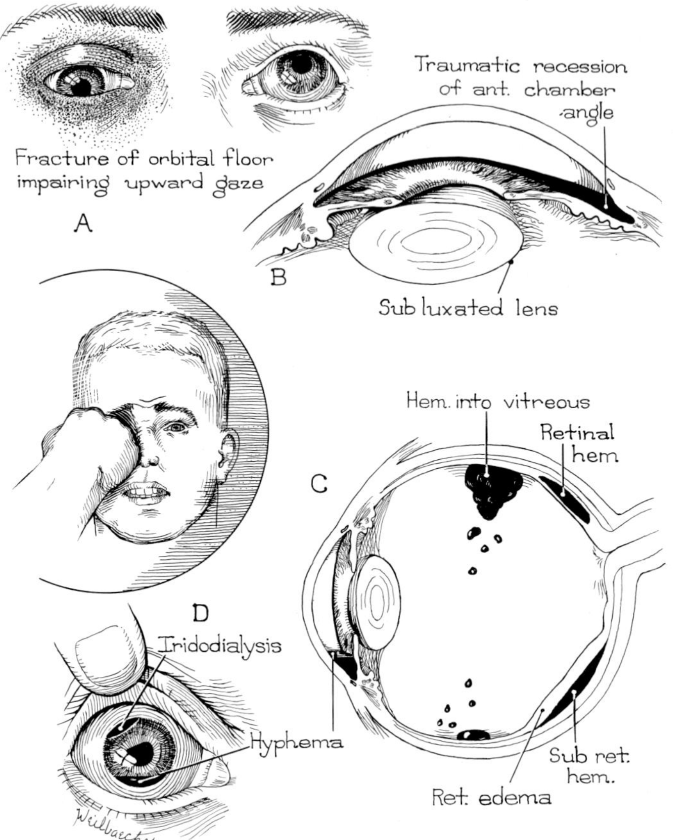

Figure 7–24 Common contusion injuries.

fists are notorious causes of hyphema. Some hyphemas fill the entire anterior chamber, but most are less in amount and settle inferiorly where they can usually be seen with a hand light (Figs. 7–24*C* and *D* and 7–25). An *iridodialysis* is sometimes associated with contusion hyphemas; this is a traumatic disinsertion of the iris from the ciliary body (Fig. 7–26) and indicates the site of bleeding. Hyphema without iridodialysis is commonly caused by rupture of the arterial circle of the ciliary body located near the angle of the anterior chamber.

It is not commonly realized that the presence of blood in the anterior chamber can cause marked somnolence through reflex mechanisms that are poorly understood. Particularly in children, hyphemas can produce such drowsiness that, when coupled with the history of trauma, they will often lead a surgeon to put these patients on a head chart. It is significant that the hyphema alone may account for the lack of alertness, although possible head injury must still be considered.

The management of hyphemas should be conservative. *Patients should be hospitalized and put to bed; both eyes should be covered until the hemorrhage has resorbed.* No miotic or dilating drops should be used in the eye; the only indicated systemic medication is a sedative if this becomes necessary. Unless a hyphema entirely fills the chamber it is not a danger to the eye. However, within the first five days following injury, spontaneous rebleeding is common.

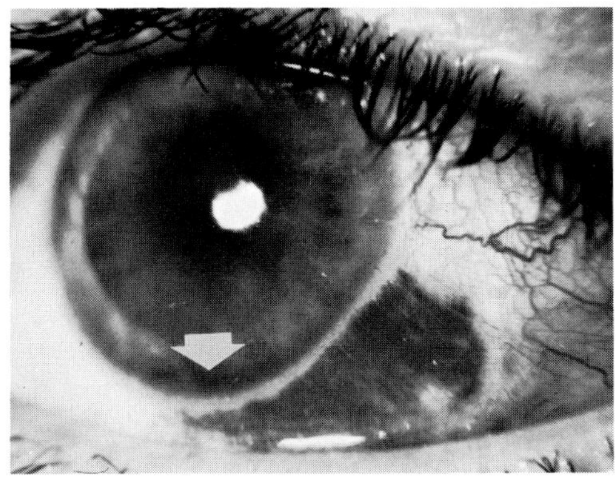

Figure 7–25 The photograph shows a conjunctival hemorrhage which is of no consequence per se; the arrow indicates a small hyphema which could easily escape cursory examination but may have serious prognostic significance.

Rebleeding frequently fills the entire chamber and may cause secondary glaucoma. If the hemorrhage does not resorb promptly, blood pigment enters the cornea where it causes prolonged brownish "blood staining."

After a few days, a total hyphema changes from red to black in color (an "eight ball" hyphema); the intraocular pressure is invariably elevated and the prognosis is guarded. Oral carbonic anhydrase inhibitors such as acetazolamide (Diamox) are used to reduce the intraocular pressure; if the hemorrhage does not promptly resorb, surgical intervention is indicated. The anterior chamber is opened via a cataract-type incision at the limbus, and the clotted hyphema is removed as extensively as possible without trauma to the ocular structures. Generally, surgery is avoided in cases of hyphema unless total hyphema with secondary glaucoma is not self-limited within a few days. One indication for surgery is the onset of corneal blood staining, detected by slit-lamp examination.

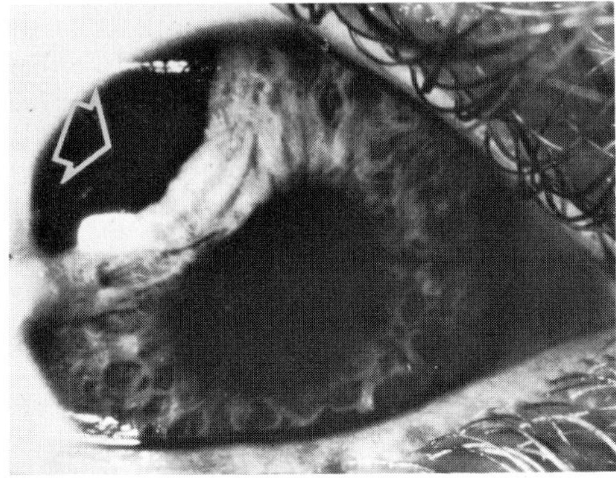

Figure 7–26 Following blunt trauma, there is not only a hyphema but flattening of the pupillary contour owing to a large iridodialysis (arrow). The cornea is intact and the damage to the iris is not discovered unless the upper lid is properly elevated.

Traumatic Mydriasis and Miosis. Almost any trauma to the eye may be followed by a mild inflammation of the iris and ciliary body; the intraocular pressure is lower than normal in the early post-traumatic period, and the aqueous humor contains cells and fibrin. More severe blows will, in addition, be accompanied by dilation or constriction of the pupil, a traumatic mydriasis or miosis that may persist for several days. The pupil reacts minimally and is often slightly irregular. Hard blows to the eye can produce a rupture of the iris sphincter and cause permanent deformity of the pupil. The causes of pupillary asymmetry following trauma are listed in Table 7–1.

Traumatic Recession of the Anterior Chamber Angle. It is now recognized that blunt trauma to the eye is a frequent cause of a unilateral glaucoma that may develop months or years following the injury. The blow causes a cleft in the tissues at the anterior chamber angle, the most important site of aqueous drainage from the eye (Figure 7–24*B*). Follow-up studies on eyes with traumatic hyphema indicate a glaucoma incidence of about 7 per cent. Thus, all patients with hyphema should be referred to an ophthalmologist, who should perform studies of the intraocular dynamics, examine the angle of the anterior chamber with a gonioscope and provide long-term follow-up observations.[1, 14]

Contusion Cataract. Even when

there is no detectable damage to the lens capsule, contusion injuries can lead to secondary cataract. (Cataracts secondary to perforating injures were discussed earlier.)

Subluxation and Luxation of the Lens. Blunt trauma to the globe can break the zonular fibers that encircle the lens radially and anchor it to the ciliary body. When 25 per cent or more of these fibers are broken, the lens is loosened and is no longer held as firmly against the posterior surface of the iris (Fig. 7–24*B*). Thus, with subluxation of the lens, the anterior chamber deepens; there is also a shimmering of the iris (iridodonesis); both of these signs can be detected by handlight examination of the patient. Certain diseases predispose to zonular fiber disintegration, which can be further increased by relatively minor trauma; Marfan's syndrome and syphilis are the most common examples. Therefore, routine examination of the traumatized eye should include appraisal of the depth of the anterior chamber and a search for iridodonesis. The lens may be loose in situ or entirely luxated, either into the vitreous cavity or into the anterior chamber; only in the latter instance is emergency surgery required. Removal of a subluxated or luxated lens is not undertaken without careful evaluation of the risks involved; this is beyond the scope of this chapter.

Scleral Rupture. Blows to the eye sometimes produce rupture of the globe. The most common sites are: in an arc circumferential to the corneal limbus, opposite to the blow impact site; at the insertion of the rectus muscles on the globe; or at the equator of the eyeball. Thus, a scleral rupture can be present without being visible to the examiner. Suspicion of rupture is aroused when the anterior chamber is filled with blood, the eye is soft (as determined with a tonometer) and there is marked hemorrhagic chemosis of the conjunctiva disproportionate to other evidences of injury. A ruptured globe is rarely salvaged by surgery, but the attempt to repair it is almost always justified, particularly if it is the patient's better eye.

Contusion and Concussion Injuries to the Posterior Segment of the Eye. VITREOUS HEMORRHAGE. Vitreous hemorrhage from trauma is usually caused by damage to a retinal vessel. Loss of vision may be sudden and profound; and the site of retinal pathology may be obscured from the examiner's view. The examiner will note a loss of the usual "red reflex" when using the hand light. Often no fundus view is possible with an ophthalmoscope. Patients with eyes with a predisposition to hemorrhage are particularly vulnerable; persons with hypertension, arteriosclerosis, diabetes and sickle cell diseases are examples. The treatment of vitreous hemorrhage is expectant; most vitreous hemorrhages eventually resorb, and the underlying pathology can then be detected and sometimes treated.

TRAUMATIC RETINAL DETACHMENT. Retinal detachments resulting from ocular trauma are usually late sequelae of the original injury. When the retina detaches soon after contusion of the eye, the detachment is generally due to antecedent vitreoretinal pathology which, after blunt trauma, leads to tears in the retina and the detachment.

A retinal detachment is suspected when there is a history of floating black specks, "light flashes" and a curtain-like defect in the peripheral field of vision. Examination with an ophthalmoscope often reveals a billow of whitish retina which shifts with change in the patient's position. Typical traumatic retinal detachments are usually the result of far peripheral retinal tears which cannot be seen with a hand ophthalmoscope.

Since vitreous hemorrhage damages the vitreous structure and can lead to vitreous bands pulling on the retina, it is easy to understand why retinal detachment can be a late sequela of traumatic vitreous hemorrhage. But contusion injury alone, without hemorrhage into the vitreous, can also cause microdestruction of the vitreous structure and facilitate the late occurrence of retinal detachment. These factors are very difficult to appraise but have medicolegal implications of such importance that they constitute another reason for referral of patients with eye trauma to an ophthalmologist.

RETINAL HEMORRHAGES AND EDEMA. Either direct blows to the eye or contrecoup trauma from blows to the back of the head can produce retinal edema, with or without reduction in vision, depending upon the location. If the examiner is uncertain whether there is retinal edema, comparison with the other eye is helpful.

A short time after concussion injury to the eye, large subretinal hemorrhages may be found (Fig. 7–27); these are often accompanied by intraretinal and superficial retinal hemorrhages, which appear a brighter red than the grayish blue of deep hemorrhages. Macular vision is not necessarily affected unless macular hemorrhage or edema occurs (Fig. 7–28) or unless in the ensuing days hard retinal exudates form in a star configuration at the macula (when the prognosis for macular function is poor). Traumatic edema and hemorrhages of the retina are usually referred to loosely as commotio retinae. The chance of recovering vision is generally good, but coincident contusion injuries of the anterior segment of the eye may account for late onset of glaucoma that eventually affects retinal function if the intraocular pressure is not adequately controlled.

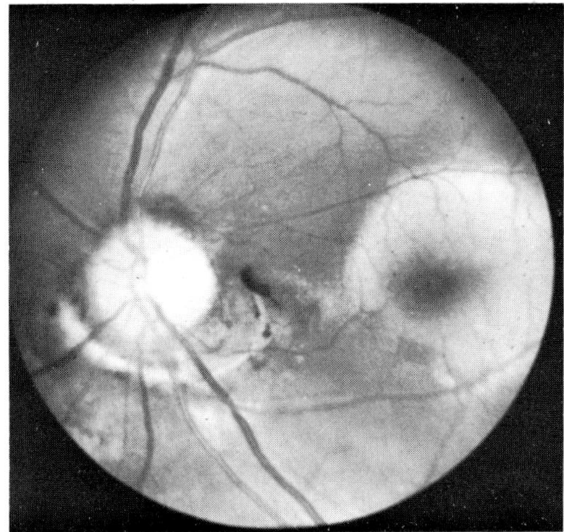

Figure 7–28 Edema and hemorrhages surround the optic nerve head, and there is edema of the macula in this eye which has sustained blunt trauma.

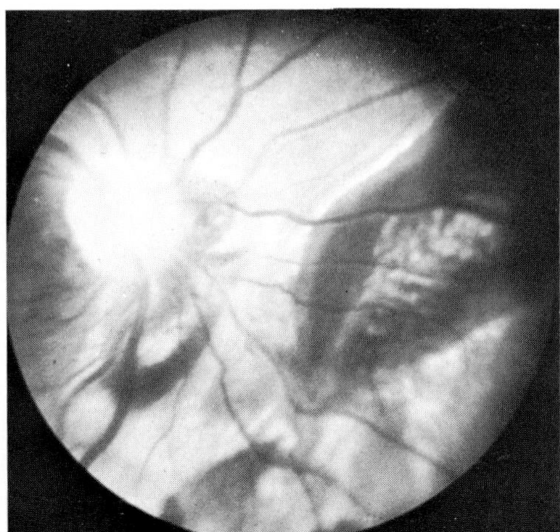

Figure 7–27 Traumatic retinal and subretinal hemorrhages characterize "commotio retinae." In this case, traumatic recession of the chamber angle led to eventual loss of all vision through failure of the patient to take medications prescribed for secondary glaucoma.

RUPTURE OF THE CHOROID. Severe concussion injury to the globe can produce a rupture of the choroid that, at the time of the emergency treatment room examination, appears as a large retinal hemorrhage at the posterior pole of the eye, often breaking through into the vitreous. Late clearing of this hemorrhage then permits view of a vertical yellow-white scar, which often transects the macula and causes permanent impairment of vision (Fig. 7–29).

CENTRAL RETINAL ARTERY OCCLUSION. Prolonged compression of the eye from external pressure or from severe intraorbital swelling sometimes occludes the central retinal artery. Operating on a patient in the face-down position is one way that this intraocular tragedy can occur; the

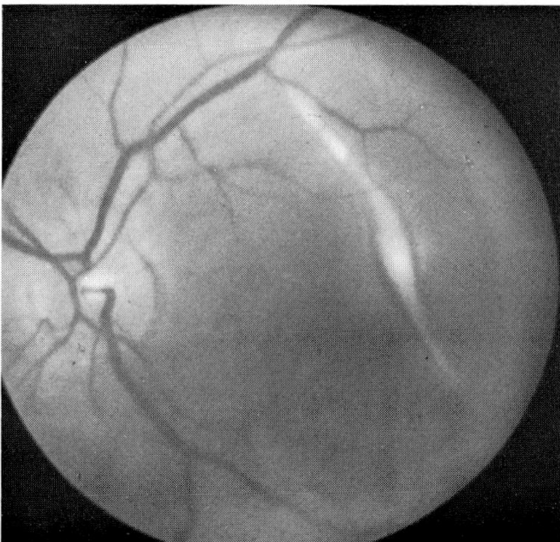

Figure 7–29 Six months following a blow to the eye, vitreous and retinal hemorrhage have cleared. A spindle-shaped scar of choroidal rupture is seen at the posterior pole, damaging macular vision.

surgeon must, therefore, be careful to see that the eye is not being pressed upon. The optic nervehead appears pale; the arteries are narrow; and vision is either absent or extremely slight. Edema of the retina ensues, leaving a "cherry red spot" at the macula, where retinal thinness and absence of edema permit transmission of normal fundus coloration from the choroid. Central retinal artery occlusion from trauma is fortunately rare, for treatment is not particularly effective. The patient is directed to breathe from and exhale into a paper bag to attain vasodilation by increase in the carbon dioxide content of the inhaled air; intravenous and oral carbonic anhydrase inhibitors such as acetazolamide are given; and retrobulbar vasodilators such as aminophyllin or tolazoline hydrochloride (Priscoline) are sometimes used. An effort must be made to relieve intraorbital pressure if it exists; a canthotomy may be helpful, and retrobulbar injection of hyaluronidase may be tried.

Long-bone fractures can be followed by fat emboli that may pass through the pulmonary circulation and appear as small yellowish spots within the retinal artery branches. Large emboli are potential causes of occlusion of the artery itself.

SWELLING OF THE OPTIC NERVEHEADS. Any patient with a history of head trauma, loss of consciousness or suspected intracranial hemorrhage should have an examination of the optic nerveheads, and a description of the findings should become part of the hospital record. It is sometimes very helpful to know the initial appearance of the nerveheads soon after an accident, to detect later the presence of early papilledema. *Papilledema does not occur rapidly.* When "swollen" optic nerveheads are seen immediately after trauma, antecedent causes should be suspected. Factors in differential diagnosis have been listed in Table 7–4.

TYPES OF EYE DRESSINGS

All surgeons know how to apply a simple gauze eye patch or a pressure head dressing, but the common *semipressure dressing* does deserve mention. When eyelid blinking is to be avoided and the injured eye protected from contamination, a firm dressing is highly desirable and should be routinely employed. Two oval eye patches are removed from their sterile envelopes and placed over the closed lids. Strips of paper tape, which hold securely but leave virtually no residue in contrast to regular adhesive tape, are then placed over the soft gauze patches in a diagonal and slightly arcuate line, so that their ends overlap on the central forehead and lower portion of the cheek, respectively (Fig. 7–30). Increased firmness of the dressing is obtained by applying the tape first to the forehead and then *pulling* it firmly toward the cheek before applying the remaining tape end. Generous use of diagonal tape strips affords a good protective dressing that will not come off; horizontal and vertical

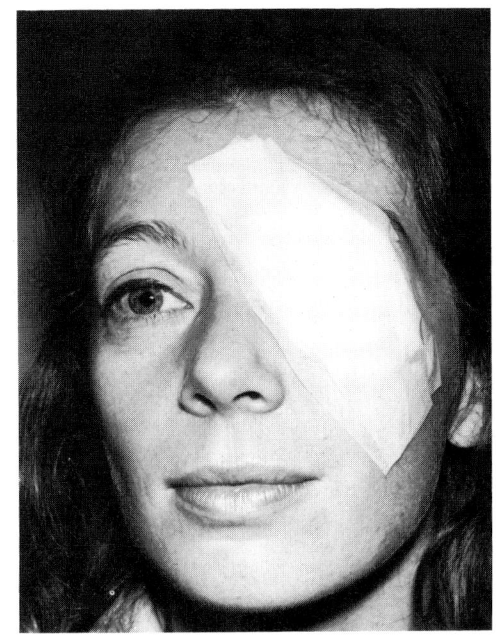

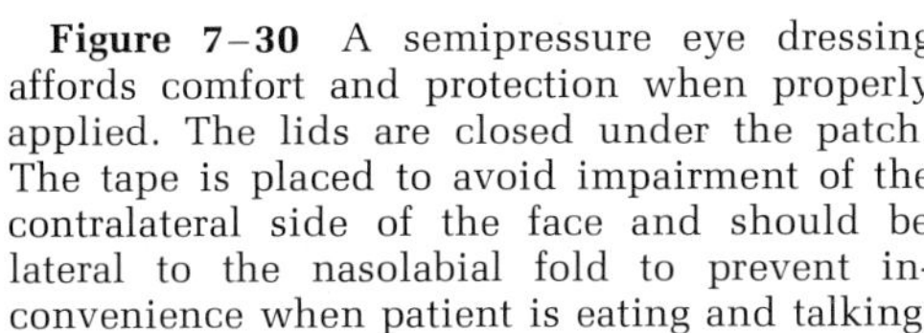

Figure 7–30 A semipressure eye dressing affords comfort and protection when properly applied. The lids are closed under the patch. The tape is placed to avoid impairment of the contralateral side of the face and should be lateral to the nasolabial fold to prevent inconvenience when patient is eating and talking.

tapes are unnecessary and uncomfortable. When added protection against trauma to the eye must be guaranteed, a metal eye shield can be used over a single eye patch (Fig. 7–1W). The shield is taped so that its margin touches the brow and cheek. Remember that when an eye dressing is removed it should be done with great gentleness and care.

REFERENCES

1. Blanton, F. M.: Anterior chamber angle recession and secondary glaucoma, a study of the aftereffects of traumatic hyphemas. Arch. Ophthalmol. 72:39, 1964.
2. Bronson, N. R., II: Non-magnetic foreign body localization and extraction. Am. J. Ophthalmol. 58:133, 1964.
3. Brown, S. I., Weller, C. A.: The pathogenesis and treatment of collagenase-induced diseases of the cornea. Trans. Am. Acad. Ophthalmol. .Otolarngol., *74*:375–383, 1970.
4. Emery, J. M., von Noorden, G. K., and Schlernitzauer, D. A.: Orbital floor fractures: Long-term follow-up of cases with and without surgical repair. Trans. Am. Acad. Ophthalmol. Otolaryngol. 75:802–812, 1971.
5. Emery, J. M., von Noorden, G. K., Schlernitzauer, D. A.: Management of orbital floor fractures. Am. J. Ophthalmol. *74*:299–306, 1972.
6. Fasanella, R. M.: Pitfalls and complications in surgery and trauma of the lacrimal apparatus. *In* Fasanella, R. M. (ed.): Management of Complications in Eye Surgery. (2nd Ed.) Philadelphia W. B. Saunders Company, 1965, 1965, pp. 110–148.
7. Fox, S. A.: Lid Surgery: Current Concepts. New York, Grune & Stratton, 1972, pp. 18–21.
8. Fueger, G. F., Milauskas, A. T., and Britton, W.: The roentgenological evaluation of orbital blowout injuries. Am. J. Roentgenol. 97:614, 1966.
9. Grant, W. M.: Toxicology of the Eye. Springfield, Ill., Charles C Thomas Co., 1962.
10. Haik, G. M.: A fornix conjunctival flap as a substitute for the dissected conjunctival flap, a clinical and experimental study. Trans. Am. Ophthalmol. Soc. 52:497, 1954.
11. Hanafee, W. N. (ed.): Symposium on Radiology of the Orbit. Radiol. Clin. N. Amer. *10*:1–182, 1972
12. Hartmann, E., and Gilles, E.: Roentgenologic Diagnosis in Ophthalmology. (G. Z. Carter, trans.; C. Berens, ed.) Philadelphia, J. B. Lippincott Co., 1959.
13. Hogan, M. J., and Zimmerman, L. E. (eds.): Ophthalmic Pathology. (2nd Ed.) Phil-

adelphia, W. B. Saunders Company, 1962.
14. Howard, G. M., Hutchinson, B. T., and Frederick, A. R., Jr.: Hyphema resulting from blunt trauma. Trans. Am. Ophthalmol. Otolaryngol., *69*:294, 1965.
15. Jones, L. T.: An anatomical approach to problems of the eyelids and lacrimal apparatus. Arch. Ophthalmol. *66*:111, 1961.
16. Leopold, I. H., and Lieberman, T. W.: Chemical injuries of the cornea. Fed. Proced. *30*:92–95, 1971.
17. Merrill, V.: Atlas of Roentgenographic Positions. St. Louis, The C. V. Mosby Co., 1949.
18. Minsky, H.: Surgical repair of recent lid lacerations: Intermarginal splinting suture. Surg. Gynec. Obstet. *75*:449, 1942.
19. Newell, F. W.: Radiant energy and the eye. *In* Industrial and Traumatic Ophthalmology; Symposium of The New Orleans Academy of Ophthalmology. St. Louis, The C. V. Mosby Co., 1964, pp. 158–187.
20. Paton, D., and Goldberg, M. F.: Injuries of the Eye, the Lids, and the Orbit: Diagnosis and Management. Philadelphia, W. B. Saunders Company, 1968.
21. Weigelin, E., and Lobstein, A.: Ophthalmodynamometry. (Daily, R. K., and Daily, L., trans.) New York, Hafner Publishing Co., 1963.
22. Worst, J. G.: Method for reconstructing torn lacrimal canaliculus. Am. J. Ophthalmol. *53*:520, 1962.

chapter

8

EMERGENCY CARE OF MAXILLOFACIAL AND NECK INJURIES

Milton T. Edgerton, Jr., M.D.

The modern background to treatment of facial fractures may be traced to World War I when a high incidence of facial injuries required the development of basic principles of surgical management. Varazted Kazanjian, Vilray Blair and John Staige Davis were pioneers during that era. Further experiences with large numbers of facial injuries from automobile accidents, and later from World War II, have led surgeons to replace the use of complex external apparatus with direct open reduction and wire fixation of fractured bone. Modern plastic surgery techniques of soft tissue wound management, antibiotics, improved anesthesia, better provision of a nonobstructed airway and appropriate use of blood transfusions have greatly improved the care of these injuries.

The human face is the center for the vital functions of speech, eating, smell, taste, vision and hearing; it is also the most conspicuous part of exposed anatomy. Facial expressions give man a vast international nonverbal language that conveys both ideas and emotions to his neighbors. Indeed, the appearance of the face is the largest single element in an individual's sense of identification or body image. It is the face that allows us to recognize one another and we often attempt to judge another's intentions or character by looking at his face. Consequently, deforming injury in this area creates complex and severe stresses in the patient's life.

Surveys of automobile accidents indicate that the head is injured in over 72 per cent of all accidents and the neck and cervical spine in an additional 8.7 per cent. Recent federal legislation is aimed at improving the mechanical safety of automobiles. Although this is desirable, new safety features on cars will not alter the fact that emotional turmoil of the driver, just prior to an accident, plays a big role in many of the investigated high speed crashes on our modern expressways. Alcohol is an additional factor in the cause of over 50 per cent of these automobile casualties. The doctor must always consider the possibility of intoxication in any patient with facial injury. Facial fractures involve males three and a half times as often as females; such injuries are relatively uncommon in older people and young children.

INCIDENCE, ETIOLOGY AND SIGNIFICANCE OF FACIAL INJURIES

Incidence. Maxillofacial and cervical injuries are more common with high speed travel, fast moving machine parts in industry and high speed missiles in warfare. As Americans, and indeed people all over the world, have taken to the highways, facial impacts against windshields and dashboards have multiplied the number of injuries alarmingly.

Other major causes of facial injuries are fist fights, motorcycle and bicycle accidents, falls, epileptic seizures and a variety of athletic and recreational activities.

The recent popularity of the Snowmobile in the northern states and Canada has presented surgeons with a new cause for facial injury. In traveling across country, the rider may be struck by low branches, wire fences and other unexpected obstacles. When wearing goggles, fragments of the latter are not infrequently driven into the soft tissues of the face at the time of impact. Neck injuries have been unusually common in these cases.

Individual Facial Fractures. Approximately two-thirds of facial fractures involve the mandible alone, one-fourth the maxillae and associated bones and one-tenth both the mandible and maxillary complex (thus, the mandible is involved in three-fourths of all facial fracture cases). The middle third of the face is involved in one-third of the facial fractures. Nasal bones alone are fractured in one-fourth of facial injuries. These figures, of course, vary significantly, depending upon the occupations, ages, climate and living conditions of the population serviced by any given hospital emergency room.

Etiology. Recent investigations have shown that 75 per cent of all deaths and injuries in crash decelerations are a result of maxillofacial injuries caused by the head striking a nonyielding object. The Federal Aviation Agency carried out experimental studies in 1965 to determine the tolerances of the human face to crash impact. In most automobile and aircraft crashes, the head is usually thrown against an object that has some degree of "deformation yield." Such yielding increases deceleration time and allows a larger area of the face or head to receive the shock of the blow. It was of obvious importance to determine what force individual face bones would sustain without fracture in the human skull.

When man is traveling at a high speed, he is usually surrounded by nonyielding rigid knobs, door posts, rigid tubes and other instruments designed to create a small area of impact if struck by the moving head or face. If this surface could be constructed of medium weight deformable metal and padded with two inches of "slow return" material, the impact load would be distributed over the available area of the face. Such changes would reduce or almost eliminate maxillofacial fractures in crash impacts. If the deceleration force is measured in "g's," the following impact forces will produce fractures on the human face:

Nasal bones	35–80 g's
Zygoma	50–80 g's
Mandibular condyles (applied on the chin)	70–110 g's
Central maxilla	150 g's

Frontal bone 120–180 g's

Studies also show that blows to the face in excess of 30 g's will produce unconsciousness lasting from 15 minutes to two hours, with or without associated fractures. If design engineers will produce vehicles with dashboards that would deform with head impacts of 40 feet per second, a tremendous reduction in the number of maxillofacial injuries will occur.

Significance. The physician treating maxillofacial injury has responsibility to:

1. Save life.
2. Restore function.
3. Prevent and correct resultant deformity.

Injuries to the neck and cervical spine are particularly important as over 15 per cent of them are fatal and over 8 per cent are "dangerous" (Cornell University Study, 1961). A combination of craniocerebral injury and injury to the long bones has been reported as the most frequent type of major automobile crash injury. All doctors are called upon at times to render emergency care to crash victims at the roadside or in a hospital emergency room. *In few injuries is the final outcome so directly dependent upon the early proper care given the patient* as with a severe maxillofacial injury.

Facial injuries disturb the functions of chewing, eating, talking, breathing and seeing. In addition, the more subtle problems of appearance, identity, emotional expression—indeed, basic physiognomy—may be altered by deformity. It is in the appearance of the face that the individual has his greatest source of self-identification. It is small wonder that the management of these injuries demands meticulous *attention to detail.* The failure to handle the patients with skill and competence will produce serious medicolegal problems for physicians and hospitals.

The peculiarities of facial anatomy indicate the use of treatments and techniques that, at first glance, seem very different from methods used to care for injuries to other parts of the body. However, all these techniques are firmly based on sound principles of general surgery. The complex array of headcaps and dental splints that once were widely advocated have caused many to lose sight of the elementary principles involved.

Surgeons dealing with facial injuries must be ever alert to the possibility of occult life threatening injury elsewhere that must be diagnosed and treated before attention is focused upon less urgent aspects of the cervicofacial injury. The proper management of the maxillofacial injury itself will depend upon: (1) an exact understanding of the method of injury, (2) detailed knowledge of the anatomy and physiology of the injured area, and (3) a completely accurate assessment of the injury—this is often obtainable only in the operating room.

TRANSPORTATION OF THE PATIENT WITH FACIAL INJURY

Bleeding from wounds in the head or neck should be arrested by elevation of the head and simple pressure exerted on the bleeding point with the finger against a clean handkerchief or dressing. The airway should be cleared by removing blood clots, dentures and foreign bodies from the mouth. If the patient is unconscious the head should be placed in a dependent position and the tongue pulled forward (Fig. 8–1). A dressing should be used around the head only if needed to stop gross bleeding or to splint obvious loose parts that are painful on movement and easily jiggled. If the patient is conscious, allow him to sit up to control airway and oral mucous secretions. Be particularly careful about moving the head if there is pain or spasm in the neck region or any suggestion of anesthesia or paralysis in the extremities.

In dealing with any medical emergency, it is important that the physician have a pre-prepared plan of

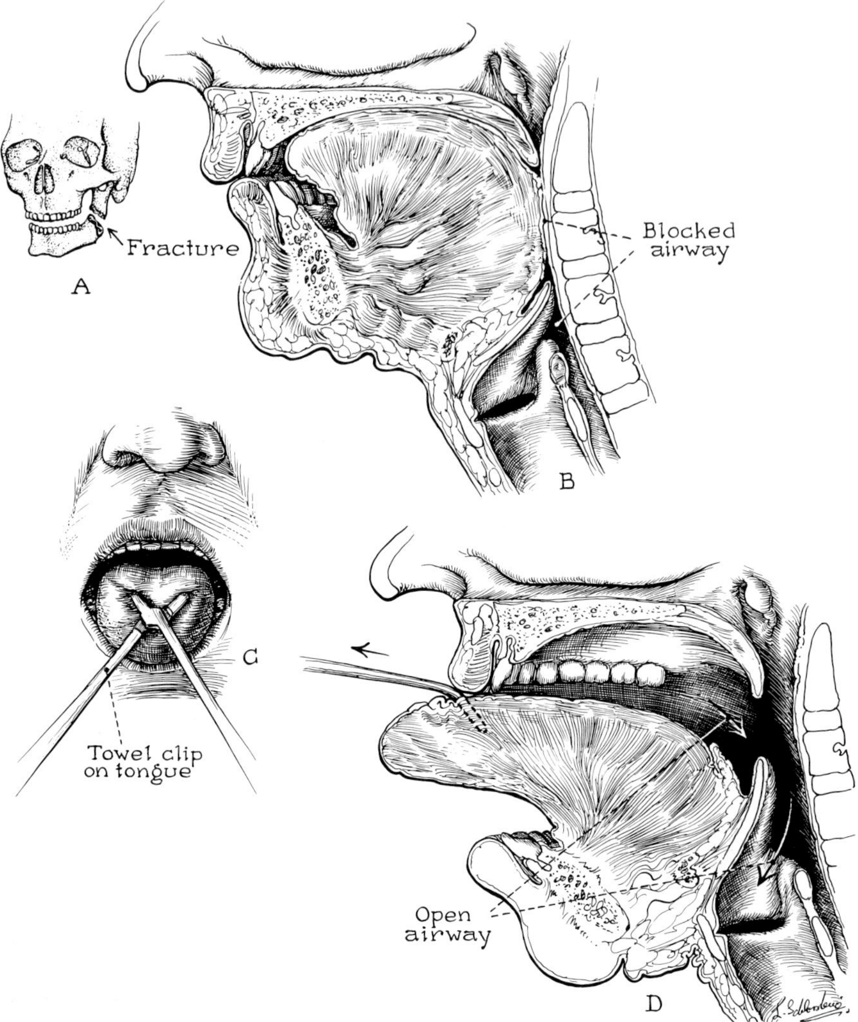

Figure 8–1 When the bony arch of the mandible is fractured in one or more places as shown in the inset *A*, the chin is allowed to drift backward carrying with it the geniohyoid, genioglossus and mylohyoid muscles. The base of the tongue is allowed to settle posteriorly as shown in *B* and obstruct the entrance to the glottis. The patient may be unable to breathe unless the chin is brought forward. It may be necessary to support both the chin and the tongue in a forward position by means of a towel clip inserted near the anterior tongue (*C* and *D*). This produces very little discomfort and may be lifesaving. Rubber shod clamps of various types are generally ineffective in holding the tongue of struggling airway-obstructed patients. This type of respiratory obstruction is particularly common with bilateral fractures involving the body of the mandible.

action, including a definite order of priority in the management of the injury. When confronted by a patient with severe maxillofacial injury, three are three phases in his activity:

1. A period of urgent diagnosis of life-threatening problems, combined with immediate treatment to correct these.

2. A more leisurely period of diagnostic evaluation of the exact extent and nature of the problem.

3. A period of definitive team treatment, which may be carried out with the aid of

surgical specialists working under the supervision of a single responsible surgeon.

URGENT SURGICAL MANAGEMENT

Establishment of Adequate Airway. *The principle cause of death from facial injuries is obstruction to the upper airway.* The number of minutes that a patient may live with a partially obstructed upper respiratory tract varies directly with the percentage of the lumen obstruction and inversely with his myocardial reserve. Attention should be given to the establishment of an airway *even before the arrest of hemorrhage* (except, of course, when there is division of a major arterial trunk with active spurting into the wound).

DIAGNOSIS OF RESPIRATORY OBSTRUCTION. If the patient is conscious, it is important to ask him if he is "having any difficulty getting his breath." Even if he is unable to speak as a result of injury, he may be able to affirm or deny this by a nod of the head. If the patient is unconscious, the airway should be checked carefully. Do not wait for evident cyanosis; this is too late! It is a sign of impending death—not of respiratory obstruction.

Noisy breathing is an important sign. *All noisy breathing is obstructed breathing.* However, if the obstruction is complete, there will be no noise. Rather, one must look for intercostal retraction and paradoxical movements of the lower neck and chest with attempted respiratory movements by the patient. If there is any doubt, the examiner should place the back of his hand or his opened eye near the patient's mouth and nose to detect directly the movement of air with breathing. If the patient is still attempting respiratory movements but has poor color, and if the air movement felt against the eye or hand suggests inadequate exchange, quick check should be made for pneumothorax with chest injury or compression of the larynx or trachea from neck injury. If these injuries are apparently absent, the chin should be lifted forward; it will bring with it the base of the tongue. In the unconscious patient it may be necessary to insert a bite block in order to open the jaws. The examiner's fingers can then be swept quickly back into the pharynx to locate and remove any clots or foreign bodies. At times, the patient's missing denture will be found driven back into the throat. If the mandibular arch has been fractured, it may collapse and allow the base of the tongue to obstruct the entrance to the larynx. In this event a large towel clip or safety pin may be passed through the anterior tongue and traction used to bring both tongue and mandibular arch forward (Fig. 8–1). If this does not produce an immediate gratifying inrush of air, the examiner should check the position of the maxilla and soft palate. These structures may be impacted downward and backward in severe "midfacial mashes" so as to obstruct the entire oropharynx. If this is the case, the fingers should be passed up behind the free edge of the displaced soft palate to attempt forceful forward elevation of the fractured obstructing bone and soft tissue.

Should these measures not *immediately* relieve the obstruction, the tip of a laryngoscope should be inserted behind the tongue base, the vocal cords inspected for damage and an attempt made to pass an endotracheal tube. If the surgeon or anesthesiologist is unable to insert the endotracheal tube promptly, the attempt should be abandoned and a coniotomy performed whenever the obstruction is so severe that time does not permit an ordinary tracheostomy.

Coniotomy has proved to be of great value in the rapidly worsening patient with glottic or supraglottic airway obstruction that requires emergency establishment of an airway below the level of the larynx. It may be performed with only a pocketknife and without a special tracheal cannula to keep the opening patent. Danger from bleeding or pneumothorax is minimal. This very useful procedure was first described by the French surgeon, Vicq d'Azyr in 1805. It consists of a transverse division of the cricothyroid (conic) ligament which runs from the thyroid cartilages inferiorly to insert on the cricoid cartilage. The ligament is near the skin just below the prominence of the larynx and may be quickly opened with little bleeding using no equipment but a knife. A single suture placed in each edge of this incision will keep the soft tissue open (Fig. 8–2). If available, one or more large (13-gauge) needles may be inserted through this ligament preliminary to the coniotomy to give some immediate

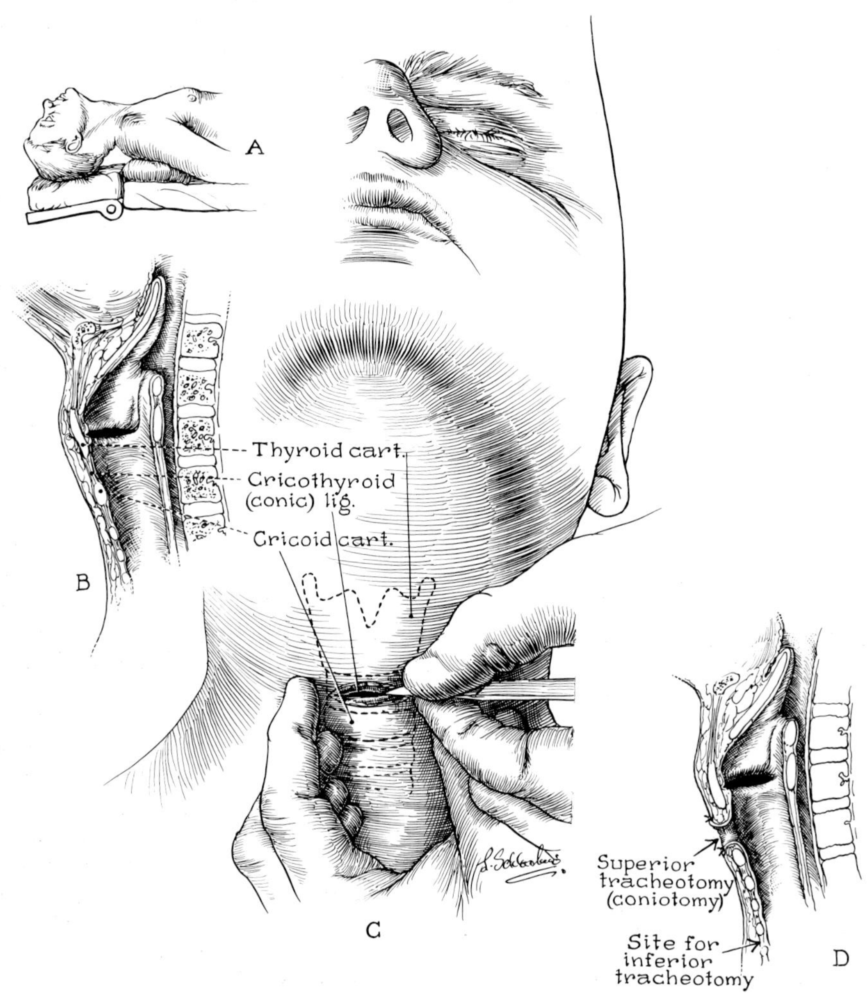

Figure 8–2 Emergency coniotomy. When there is critical blockage of the upper airway, the patient's head may be quickly extended and a short transverse incision made just above the cricoid cartilage. The index finger and thumb of the left hand are used to press the skin laterally and to fix the trachea in the midline. The knife is held with only a small part of the blade showing so as to avoid injury to the posterior wall of the trachea in a struggling patient. One or two stitches will hold the edges of the skin back from the wound until an elective tracheostomy can be performed.

relief while the airway is further enlarged. It is usually wise not to use the coniotomy as a long-term airway. Once the acute air shortage is relieved, the surgeon may perform an elective tracheostomy through the third or fourth tracheal ring, using a transverse skin incision and local anesthesia.

When the airway obstruction is only partial, it is often possible to carry out a tracheostomy as the primary procedure. In such patients it is usually desirable to first insert an endotracheal airway as it will facilitate the tracheostomy and make it a truly elective procedure. Patients who have major burns about the face and neck or who have had blunt injuries to the anterior larynx may be especially susceptible to the sudden closing off of the upper airway at a period several hours after injury. (See Chapter One.) One should remember that in children the apex of the pleural cavities extends well up into the base of the neck and lies close to the trachea on either side. If the pleura is opened in an already "air hungry" patient, a pneumothorax may not be recognized and may produce disaster. In addition, the brachiocephalic vessels come high into the base of the neck in children and must be avoided carefully in performing a tracheostomy.

No patient with questionable airway obstruction should be given any respiratory depressant drugs for the relief of pain. The primary sign of respiratory obstruction is *restlessness.* Any patient with facial injury who thrashes his extremities or struggles to raise his head from the stretcher or bed should be immediately checked for increasing respiratory obstruction.

If the patient is making no attempts at respiratory movements of the chest wall, mere provision of a proper airway will obviously do little good. In such patients, assisted pulmonary ventilation should be instituted immediately with the establishment of airway. This may be achieved by mouth-to-mouth (or mouth-to-tracheal cannula) assistance until an endotracheal tube and positive pressure equipment may be obtained. Any patient lacking a pulse or cardiac sounds on auscultation requires simultaneous external cardiac massage and provision of an unobstructed airway for hope of resuscitation. (This is discussed in detail in Chapter Four.)

Control of Bleeding. Bleeding, next to obstructed airway, is the most common cause of death from facial and cervical injury. Except for instances of direct division of a carotid artery, cervicofacial hemorrhage is usually readily controlled by simple compression applied over sterile gauze (or even a clean handkerchief) directly against the bleeding point. It is both unnecessary and dangerous to attempt instrument clamping of vessels deep within the neck or in the face. Brachial plexus palsies and injuries to the recurrent laryngeal nerve or thoracic duct have followed such efforts. If the patient is unconscious, elevation of the head and shoulders to a 45 degree angle will further reduce bleeding. If excessive bleeding issues from the nasal or oral cavities, some form of gauze packing against the torn mucosa may be required. With stubborn nasal hemorrhage, rubber catheters may be passed through the nasal cavity into the pharynx and then brought out of the mouth. Sutures are attached to the catheter tips and used to draw a tamponading pack up behind the palate so that the gauze presses against the posterior choanae. Often bleeding will cease after the careful removal of clots overlying the bleeding points within the nasal cavity.

Whenever the surgeon suspects that serious blood loss has occurred from the facial injury or into a body cavity, he should immediately start an intravenous infusion with a large-bore needle; and blood should be obtained for baseline hemoglobin and hematocrit determinations, typing and crossmatching. A central venous pressure monitoring system may be established to constantly monitor the infusion.

Arterial bleeding in the head and

neck rarely requires surgical exposure and ligation of the carotid artery. Indeed, this often has little effect on facial bleeding. If the patient shows clinical signs of shock without sufficient facial bleeding to produce it, the physician should be alerted to the possibility of bleeding elsewhere.

Ambulance attendants, family and friends should be carefully questioned as to the *amount of blood lost* at the scene of the accident and en route to the emergency room. Major bleeding may have ceased *only* when blood pressure fell to low levels with such early exsanguination. An attempt should be made to determine if the patient has a history of hypertension. Systolic readings of 120 mm. of mercury may actually represent severe shock in the patient with marked preinjury hypertension.

Management of Intracranial Injury or Bleeding. In patients with facial bone fractures, approximately 13 per cent have concussion, 10 per cent have skull fractures and 8 per cent show cerebrospinal rhinorrhea. If the patient's head and face have been caught between two rigid surfaces, cranial bone fractures are common. A deepening level of consciousness, inequality of the pupils, palpable depressed fragments of skull bone or marked bradypnea and bradycardia are signs that should alert the physician to the possibility of intracranial damage or hemorrhage. In such cases a head chart should be started immediately and a neurosurgical consultation obtained. (See Chapter Six.)

Search for Injuries to Neck, Cervical Vertebrae, Larynx or Trachea. Injury to the neck requires urgent treatment primarily when there are fractures or dislocations of the cervical vertebrae or blows that compress and fracture the larynx or trachea. Some type of neck injury is found in approximately 5 per cent of patients with mandibular or maxillary fractures. Frequently, cervical spine injuries will involve both a fracture and a dislocation in the same patient. Some of these patients will show no localizing neurologic findings, despite spinal cord damage. Cervical spine x-rays will help pinpoint many of these injuries and also will suggest a fracture of the larynx or trachea if they show free soft-tissue air. Tracheal or laryngeal injuries may produce severe mechanical obstruction to the airway. Intubation, coniotomy or tracheostomy will provide rapid relief (Fig. 8–2). Injury to the cervical vertebrae may be suspected if there is stiffness, spasm or pain on movement of the neck. Great care should be taken to avoid excessive movement of the neck and head when transporting such a patient to avoid division of or injury to the spinal cord or related important nerve roots. When the patient is lifted from the street or a stretcher, it is wise to apply manual traction to the neck by placing the hands under the patient's ears or against the temples.

When patients with severe maxillofacial injuries are conscious and seem free of serious neck injury, it is usually wise to elevate the head to improve swallowing of oral mucus and opening of the upper air passage. Head elevation also increases efficiency of cough, reduces bleeding from the facial wounds and aids depression of the diaphragm.

Examination for Distant Major Injuries. The patient should be checked for unsuspected distant major injuries. The abdomen should be checked for rigidity, ileus or fluid wave. A ruptured spleen, kidney, or bowel may accompany facial injuries. A full bladder at the time of automobile impact often causes a rupture of this viscus with the sudden deceleration. There has been some suggestion that the recent increase in injuries to the visceral organs and abdominal vessels with automobile accidents might be related to the old-type seat belt which secures the passenger only across the lap. The newer seat belts with shoulder straps appear to provide additional protection for both abdominal organs and the face.

Fractures of other bones are found in approximately 20 per cent of patients with a facial bone fracture. Rib fractures should be detected and the pain relieved by reduction, splinting or intercostal nerve block in order to improve pulmonary ventilation and prevent pneumonia. Pneumothorax should be relieved by needle aspiration and chest catheter, sucking wounds of the pleural cavity should be closed with tape traction and major long bone fractures of the extremities should be splinted promptly.

Early Check and Recording of Vision. Any patient with evidence of a major blow to the head or face should have each eye carefully checked for both central and peripheral vision. Any loss of visual ability *should* be carefully recorded so that initial surgical manipulations will not be blamed for unnoticed or unrecorded early blindness. Even a conscious patient may not realize that his injury has already produced a major loss of vision in one eye. An attempt should be made to detect diplopia in the four major quadrants of vision in all conscious patients with facial injury. The fundus should be checked for hemorrhage into the vitreous or dislocation of the lens. Any penetration of the sclera demands prompt attention.

When urgent measures to save life (the establishment of airway, arrest of bleeding, the drawing of blood for cross-matching and the starting of intravenous fluid) have been completed, the surgeon may then turn his attention to a more analytical and careful diagnostic study of the patient with the primary complaint of a severe maxillofacial injury.

DIAGNOSTIC STUDIES OF MAXILLOFACIAL AND CERVICAL INJURIES

Complete Details of History—Initial Photography

An attempt should be made to clarify the exact history of the injury to determine the nature of the force producing the deformity and the direction from which it originated. The patient's previous medical history should be carefully assessed for other disease processes. Pre-existing renal, cardiac, vascular or respiratory disorders should be known before starting definitive treatment. Diabetics with hypoglycemia or epileptics often suffer facial injuries when they lose consciousness suddenly and fall. If there is any odor of alcohol, the patient's breath or blood should be tested for alcoholic content. Severe depression of the central nervous system may be partly due to drug or alcoholic ingestion and partly to head injury. This combination of causes is seen often in suicide attempts and may confuse the diagnosis.

Before taking any patient to the operating room, nearest relatives should be contacted and an operative permit secured. Careful photographs should be taken of any significant external deformity before corrective treatment. These should be taken only *after* the clothing has been removed and blood cleansed from around the wounds. Such records have important medicolegal value and are vastly more accurate than verbal descriptions. Patients are frequently too ill or upset to realize the extent of their original disfigurement. Every modern emergency treatment room should be equipped with simple, readily available photographic equipment and personnel should be trained to use it.

Key Points in Physical Examination

OCCLUSION OF THE TEETH. Malocclusion is one of the most accurate diagnostic signs of mandibular or maxillary fracture. The examiner must have a working knowledge of normal dental relationships (Fig. 8–9). In the unconscious patient the jaws may be brought together and the meshing of the cusps of upper and lower teeth may be checked. Even small displacements of tooth positions that result from jaw fractures are readily reflected in these dental relationships. If the patient is conscious he will usually volunteer that his "teeth don't fit right." If dentures are normally worn and have been removed, they may be replaced to check the occlusion. If dentures are broken, the segments may be reinserted to aid in checking for bony displacement.

POINT TENDERNESS AND MOBILITY OF FACIAL BONES AT LINES OF FRACTURES. Fractured facial bones usually show well localized tenderness when palpated. In addition, abnormal mobility or even slight asymmetry may yield a clue to the diagnosis of fracture. To determine bony symmetry, the examining fingers of both hands may be simultaneously used to palpate both sides of the face. The key points of the infraorbital rim, zygomatic arch, the anterior wall of the antrum (with fingers beneath the upper lip), the angles of the jaw and the lower border of the body of the mandible are compared with corresponding points on the opposite side of the face. If this is carried out with the operator standing directly in front of the patient, even small displacements of the facial skeleton may be detected. The upper teeth and the hard palate should be grasped by the operator's fingers and an attempt made to move the upper jaw both up and down and from side to side (Fig. 8–3). Midfacial fractures of the maxilla may often be detected in this way. If the examiner's little fingers are simultaneously placed in both of the patient's external auditory canals while the latter opens and closes his mouth, movements and symmetry of the mandibular condyles may be easily checked.

PALSIES OF THIRD, FOURTH, FIFTH, SIXTH AND SEVENTH NERVES. Careful testing for cranial nerve palsy is important in assessing facial injuries. In particular, anesthesia of the upper lip and central upper teeth suggest fracture of the maxilla near the infraorbital foramen. Palsy of the facial nerve may be revealed by difficulty in closing the eye, elevating the brow or retracting the corner of the mouth. Diplopia or strabismus *may* indicate palsy of extraocular muscles, but the diplopia accompanying facial fractures is much more commonly due to bony deformities of the orbit that displace the origins of the extraocular muscles or trap them in fracture lines. It is common to find double vision upon re-examination several days after injury when it was not detectable at the initial examination shortly after injury. This may result from increasing displacement of the globe by hematoma, resolution of early orbital edema or progressive herniation of orbital fat through fracture lines down into the antrum to produce progressive enophthalmus.

ADEQUACY OF NASAL AIRWAY. (See section on nasal fractures.) A nasal speculum should be used to permit suction of clots and crusts from the nasal cavity and to check the mucosa for lacerations or displaced bone fragments. The position of the nasal septum and the mobility of the nasal bridge should be determined. The patient should be asked to close his lips, and the airway through each side of the nasal cavity may be checked by alternately blocking one nares and then the other with a fingertip as the patient is instructed to inhale forcefully.

PRESENCE OF BLOOD, RUPTURED TYMPANIC MEMBRANE OR BONY INFRACTURE OF THE EXTERNAL AUDITORY CANALS. The external auditory canal should be checked with an otoscope for blood clots or ruptures of the tympanic membrane. Severe blows on the chin will often drive the heads of the mandibular condyles backward with sufficient force to break the bony walls of the external auditory canals. A completely blocked canal with or without bleeding from the ear may then be encountered on otoscopic examination. Middle ear

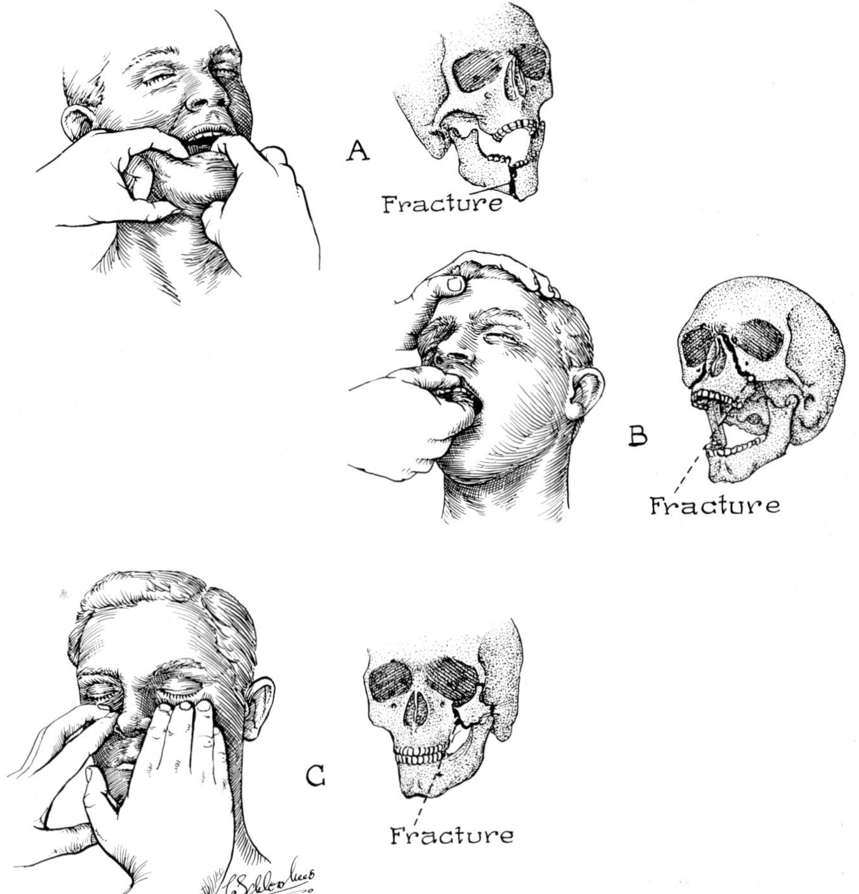

Figure 8–3 Manual examination for diagnosis of fractured bones of the face and jaws; careful examination with bimanual palpation will reveal the vast majority of facial fractures. In *A*, a gentle rocking motion of the fingers will reveal movement or pain at the site of fractures of the mandibular body or symphysis. In *B*, the top of the head is fixed and an attempt is made to move the hard palate by grasping the upper central incisor teeth. Midface fractures will often reveal slight movement or pain. In *C*, the examiner feels for symmetry of the infra-orbital rim, or for a step or "notch" along the normal smooth lateral rim of the orbit.

injuries may also be present and require special radiographs and otologic consultation.

MOBILITY AND CREPITUS AT THE TEMPOROMANDIBULAR JOINT. A finger placed in each external auditory canal will allow the operator to determine the position, shape and movement of the head of the mandibular condyles when the jaw is opened and closed. If one condyle does not move or if it is displaced, tomograms of the temporomandibular joints should be obtained.

CEREBROSPINAL FLUID RHINORRHEA (APPROXIMATELY 8 PER CENT OF CASES). If the patient is placed face down for a short while, any significant leak of cerebrospinal fluid would be detected by the appearance at the nose of a watery nonmucoid liquid. If there is doubt about the nature of this fluid, let some of it dry on a handkerchief. Nasal mucus will stiffen the handkerchief, but cerebrospinal fluid will dry without stiffening. Cerebrospinal fluid will also show glucose on testing.

MENTAL STATUS EXAMINATION INCLUDING RECENT MEMORY AND ORIENTATION. A brief mental status examination should be carried out, including a simple test of the patient's memory for both recent and remote events and his orientation in time and place. Concussion of the brain is one of the injuries most commonly associated with facial fractures. Headache, lethargy, vomiting, dilated or fixed pupils or a positive Babinski reflex all suggest intracranial injury. Many automobile accidents or gunshot wounds to the head occur when the patient is emotionally depressed and are the result of destructive tendencies. Only a careful history and mental status examination will bring to light the need for treatment of the emotional disease underlying the injury.

RE-EXAMINATION OF CHEST, ABDOMEN AND EXTREMITIES FOR DELAYED APPEARANCE OF ASSOCIATED INJURIES. Fractures in other parts of the body are found in over 20 per cent of patients with facial fractures. A fractured spleen, liver or kidney may have continued to bleed slowly or may open a fresh clot following the re-establishment of normal blood pressure levels. Peritonitis may develop slowly from leaks into the intestinal tract, or hemothorax may produce delayed shock or dyspnea. Thus, chest and abdomen must be examined periodically after initial major trauma. Delayed bleeding or extravasation of urine or bile into the peritoneum or retroperitoneal tissues may quickly change the clinical picture.

PERTINENT RADIOGRAPHS AND LABORATORY STUDIES. Laboratory tests should be kept to a minimum; only those leading to more accurate therapeutic management should be ordered. The cost of medical care today makes it incumbent upon physicians to use laboratory facilities with discretion.

A single stereo-Waters (submento-occipital plane) roentgenogram will give almost all the diagnostic information needed in the emergency care of fractures of the facial bones. If there is also clinical evidence of mandibular fracture, posteroanterior and lateral oblique roentgenograms of the bodies of the mandible and, occasionally, tomograms of the temporomandibular joints may be indicated. Nasal bone roentgenograms are virtually useless since they so seldom affect treatment. A nasal fracture seen only in roentgenogram and without accompanying clinical displacement of the external nose or obstruction to the airway does not require surgical reduction. Conversely, nasal fractures with obvious clinical displacement may not show effectively on x-ray but may require surgical reduction. If there is evidence of injury to the cervical muscles or vertebrae, such as neck pain and spasm or tenderness of the cervical spinous processes, roentgenograms should be taken with the neck in positions of extension and flexion.

Urine should be checked for sugar and albumin; and if injuries are extensive, a catheter should be left in the bladder to determine hourly urinary output. Blood smears, hematocrits, and blood volume determinations often give additional knowledge. Continuous venous pressure determinations may be obtained from the subclavian vein and are of particular value in titrating the amount of intravenous fluid that may be tolerated without producing pulmonary edema.

SPECIALTY CONSULTANTS. Diagnostic consultations may be needed. In many large medical centers it is practical to establish a regular maxillofacial team under central supervision. In other hospital emergency rooms, both a general surgeon and a plastic surgeon will have been called upon the arrival of any patient with a severe maxillofacial injury. Both will normally participate in the diagnostic evaluation and emergency care. It may quickly become apparent that consultations are also desirable in otolaryngology, dentistry, ophthalmology and neurosurgery. Each of these specialties may contribute valuable aid in the management of special problems with the facially injured patient. They should be called as early as it is evident that their services are needed.

Once life-endangering injury has been controlled and an analysis made of the extent of damage to the face and cervical region, the question of definitive treatment arises. When there are major abdominal injuries such as a suspected rupture of a hollow viscus or organ, it is usually wise to admit the patient for care and observation on the general surgical service since a sudden change in the abdominal condition might require immediate surgical intervention. Similarly, if there appear to be no abdominal injuries but severe intracranial damage is evident, with loss of consciousness and indications of increasing intracranial pressure, the patient should be admitted on the neurosurgical service for observation and care until the intracranial condition is stabilized. If neither of these conditions exists, it is usually desirable to admit patients with major maxillofacial injuries under the care of a plastic surgeon who has had liberal general surgical training. It is expected that attention will be paid not only to the patient's maxillofacial problems but also to the possibilities of the appearance of shock or of changes in the abdominal, thoracic or pelvic problems.

If the injury is less severe and is confined to localized areas, such patients may be best treated by admission to a specialty service such as ophthalmology, dentistry or otolaryngology. It is important in all cases that the responsibility for coordinating the multiple treatments for facial injury be vested in a single responsible physician. In the case of extensive injuries, this physician should be a surgeon with broad training in the field of general surgery.

DEFINITIVE EMERGENCY SURGICAL TREATMENT

Proper Time and Location of Surgery. General Emergency Operating Procedures. Maxillofacial injuries should not be treated in the emergency room unless they are of a very simple nature. Soft tissue lacerations of the face, not involving nerves, ducts or cartilages, and lesser fractures of the mandible with minimal fragment displacement that do not require open surgical reduction may be readily managed without the use of the operating room. In all such instances, local anesthesia should be employed and careful attention should be given to the principles of wound care.

All patients with major injuries requiring complex operative manipulation, additional incisions for bone fixation or general anesthesia should be transferred to the general operating room where adequate assistance, aseptic conditions, better tools and lighting and complete anesthetic equipment are available. Many times two or even three surgical specialties may be represented as a team in such a definitive emergency reconstruction. The head of such a team must be able and willing to integrate the knowledge and talents of his colleagues in their contributions to the relief of deformity and dysfunction.

Immediate or Delayed Reduction of Facial Fractures. Several factors should be considered in deciding on the time of fracture reduction.

1. Are there significant advantages to the patient or to the injured part in undertaking immediate treatment?

2. Is facial edema already so marked that it would make manipulation of the tissues difficult and disguise landmarks for proper reduction of fractures?

3. What is the general condition of the patient? Is there any evidence of hemorrhagic shock? Is there a history of recent alcoholic intake? Does the injury represent a possible attempt at suicide? What is known of the patient's cardiac status?

4. Is the patient conscious? It is almost never wise to undertake facial bone reductions in an unconscious patient.
5. Is a significant cerebrospinal fluid leak present, indicating a basal skull fracture? Would early reduction of fractures increase or decrease such leakage?
6. Do you have proper operative permit and adequate relationship with the patient and relatives? Is the patient a minor? Does the family wish other consultants called before definitive treatment is started?

Most severe maxillofacial injuries are best managed in two steps. The definite phase of urgent care (described previously) is carried out in the emergency room and is followed by a waiting period of several days, during which time ice compression of the facial area is used to reduce edema. During this period the patient's general condition is evaluated, any additional roentgenograms needed for definitive treatment are obtained, antibiotic therapy is started and further consultations are completed.

The patient with facial fractures should be scheduled for thoughtful elective surgery several days after injury when the facial edema is subsiding. This usually gives results that are superior to middle-of-the-night endeavors.

General Principles of Repair of Soft Tissue Injuries

Blood Supply. Major facial lacerations or avulsions are found in over 40 per cent of patients with facial fractures. Certain differences exist in the management of the facial soft tissue injury when compared with soft tissue injury in other parts of the body. These differences relate primarily to the tremendously rich blood and lymphatic supply to the face, which permits more refined reconstruction and delayed primary repairs. Secondly, the attachment of the delicate mimetic muscles of the face directly into the facial skin produces the subtle facial expressions and creates special problems in surface healing. The repair of skin and subcutaneous tissue without consideration of the small muscles attaching to that part of the face may result in a kinetic deformity that could have been prevented but which is almost impossible to correct later.

Although lacerations in other parts of the body are frequently left open if they are seen over six hours after injury, such treatment is not desirable in the face. Indeed, *clean lacerations of the face may be closed as long as 24 hours after injury with considerable profit to the patient.* Such primary closure is beneficial in minimizing deep cicatrix and distortion of immediately subjacent facial muscles. Extensive facial injuries require protection from tetanus, usually by a booster dose of toxoid; gas gangrene following facial trauma is an extremely rare occurrence.

Experimentally, doses of *Staphylococcus aureus* in the magnitude of 10^8 organisms are usually required to produce abscess formation if inoculated into the skin of a healthy human. Lesser doses result only in temporary localized cellulitis, and recovery takes place without tissue necrosis. If the tissue is first traumatized by crushing, or if a bit of sterile suture or blood clot is experimentally placed beneath the skin, the dosage of bacteria required to produce abscess is reduced *approximately ten thousandfold* (10^4 bacteria). Conversely, if the blood and lymphatic circulation to and from a given area of skin is rich (as in the face), many times more bacteria may be managed by the local cellular and humoral mechanisms without resultant tissue necrosis than in the case of skin with less capillary flow (as the skin of the foot or ankle). This wide variance of bacterial defense in different parts of the body explains both the need for meticulous debridement of all crushed or necrotic tissue and the ability to carry out many delayed or primary reconstructive maneuvers on the injured face.

Cleansing of Skin and Wound Irrigation. The preparation of a facial wound before suturing involves preliminary washing of the surrounding skin with soap and water and an antiseptic with lipolytic qualities. pHiso-Hex, Septisol and other soaps containing 3 per cent hexachlorophene (Gll) have proved quite effective in reducing bacterial flora of skin. Eyebrows should *never* be shaved, as some fail to regrow. Local anesthesia may be painlessly injected directly through the cut margins of the open wound and will reduce the discomfort of cleansing and irrigation. This is significantly less painful than injection of the anesthetic through the intact adjacent skin. Lidocaine hydrochloride (Xylocaine) is longer lasting but procaine hydrochloride (Novocain) is less painful on initial contact with the tissues and its effect is of adequate duration for almost any repair.

Gentle soapsuds washing of the wound and surrounding area should be followed by copious irrigation with isotonic saline. When irrigation with large amounts of saline (one to three liters used to *forcefully* flush out the wound in all its recesses) was instituted in The Johns Hopkins Hospital emergency room as standard treatment for all fresh cutaneous wounds, the infection rate dropped to *one-third* the previous level. Prior attempts to reduce these infections by the use of prophylactic antibiotics, stronger germicides on the surrounding skin or topical antibiotics to the wound had all been unsuccessful. After washing of the wound, the surrounding skin *(but not the wound)* may be prepared with benzalkonium chloride 1:1000 (Zephiran) or povidone-iodine solution (Betadine) to reduce concentration of skin bacteria.

Anesthesia. General anesthesia is occasionally necessary for emergency treatment of extensive compound facial injuries, but its use is generally reserved for reduction of displaced fractures after the facial edema has begun to subside and the general condition of the patient has stabilized and been assessed. Endotracheal anesthesia is invaluable in controlling the airway and in permitting the anesthetic equipment to be placed at some distance from the facial wounds. Halothane (Fluothane) is a valuable agent since it permits the use of the electrocautery without danger of explosion and it reduces greatly the incidence of postoperative nausea and vomiting in comparison with many of the earlier agents. When general anesthesia is used on patients whose jaws must be wired together, it is wise to leave the nasal endotracheal tube in position until the patient is fully reacted to avoid the dangers of aspiration.

Anesthesia may be infiltrated locally or by nerve block, using 1 per cent lidocaine hydrochloride (Xylocaine) containing 1:100,000 parts of epinephrine or 1 per cent procaine (Novocain). With major soft tissue lacerations, it is desirable to do nerve blocks either at the infraorbital foramen, the mental foramen or, at times, to block the second and third divisions of the fifth cranial nerve where they emerge from the base of the skull at the foramina ovale and rotundum.

Minimal Debridement. It is particularly important to carry out minimal debridement of facial skin. Every square millimeter of tissue may be of value to the plastic surgeon in ultimate reconstruction. Even though bits of skin or vermilion may be totally detached and driven into another area, as by high explosive missles, these valuable fragments should be left and may be made to survive as "grafts" in the new location. They may later be returned, by plastic techniques, to their normal location. It is better to err on the side of attempting to save tissue that may ultimately necrose rather than to sacrifice any skin, cartilage or mucous membrane that is viable. The surgeon should remember that, except for the lips, there is no vermilion on the body that can be grafted to replace a missing lip segment. Mucous membrane is the best, but it is an imperfect substitute (Fig. 8–31A and B). When resurfacing of the face is necessary, any skin grafts taken from donor areas inferior to the clavicles will permanently lack the pink "blush" quality of facial skin. At times, facial tissue that is completely avulsed may be replaced as a free graft after careful removal of every vestige of fat clinging to its undersurface. The texture and color of this will be superior to skin grafted from *any other part of the body* at a later date. The inherent vascular pattern gives a ruddy color to the "blush area" which is not duplicated by any other tissue.

If an explosion has produced traumatic tattooing or brush abrasions have discolored the underlying dermis with grit or carbon particles, it is

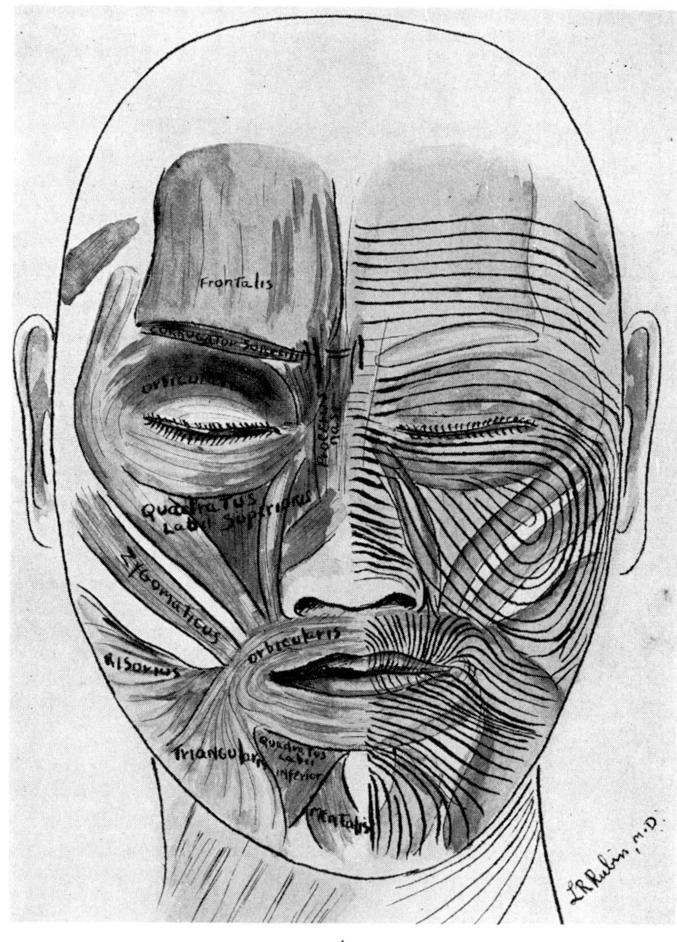

A

Figure 8–4 *A*, This drawing from Rubin[16] shows on the left the position of the major superficial facial muscle groups and on the right the primary lines of skin relaxation produced by the combined effect of these muscles and the elasticity of the skin. Notice that although many of the lines of relaxation are at right angles to the long axis of the underlying muscle, some of the lines are at variance with this principle. In general, any laceration lying directly parallel to one of these underlying lines of relaxation will heal with minimal hypertrophy and thickening, whereas any laceration lying at right angles to one of these functional lines will heal with marked thickening. These lines do not coincide in many instances with the original "lines of Langer."

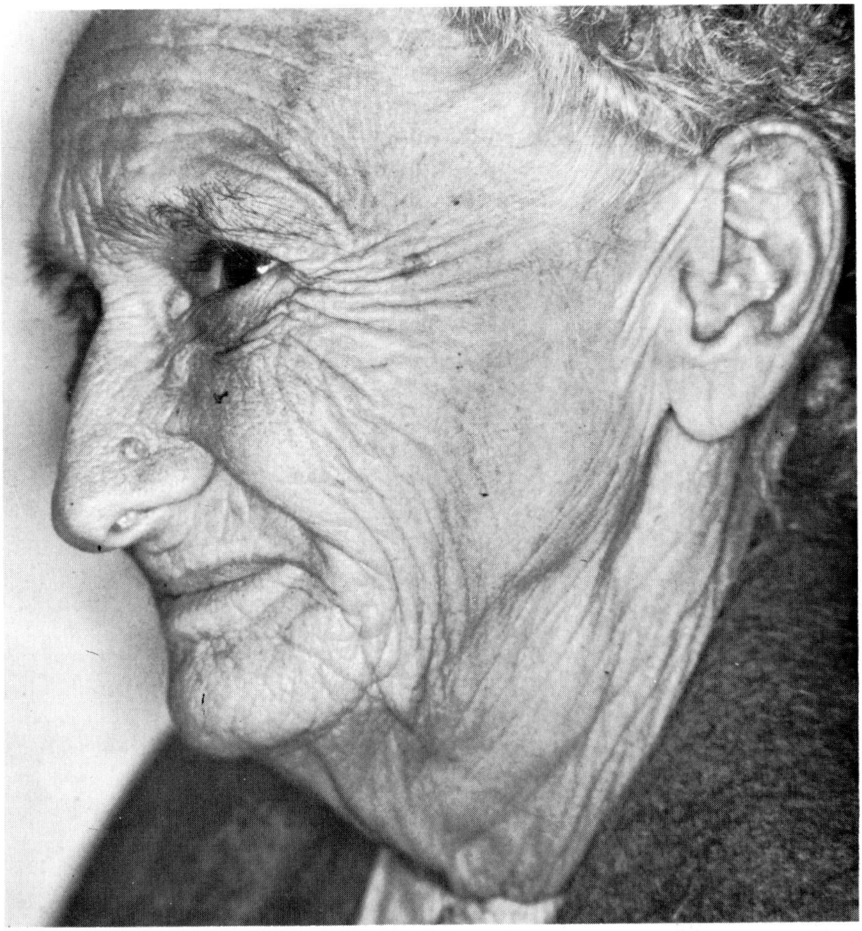

B

Figure 8–4 *Continued.* *B,* The elderly patient often presents a living example of the normal lines of skin relaxation. Notice that most of the creases in this patient's face coincide with the lines of relaxation in *A.* If primary lacerations cross directly over the more important functional creases, the surgeon may rearrange the laceration by proper use of local flaps even at the time of primary injury. Any additional incisions used to reduce underlying bony fractures should, of course, be placed directly in a functional "line of skin relaxation." (Courtesy of the Journal of Plastic and Reconstructive Surgery [*3*:147, 1948].)

important to carry out *immediate* surgical abrasion treatment using a high speed engine and a diamond wheel or wire brush abrasion technique. It may be important to spend hours, if necessary, to remove coal dust, hair or any insoluble pigmented particles. If these are allowed to remain in the skin during healing, hundreds of separate incisions (one over each particle) will be required to remove them later.

Suturing Facial Wounds. Incisions in the face that lie parallel to the lines of the skin relaxation may be counted on to heal in a very kindly fashion, even with minimal skin closure. These lines should not be confused with the lines of skin elasticity described by Langer[13] (Fig. 8–4 *A* and *B*). Patients should be warned of possible unsightly scars when lacerations cut across these lines at right angles. At times immediate Z-flaps may be cut and shifted to prevent later contractures. In some patients the trauma to the skin may make it wiser to plan a later plastic repair.

When lacerations result in beveled or angled cutting of the skin layers, surgical authors formerly recommended debriding these skin margins back to right-angled wound edges. That practice probably should be avoided unless the margins debrided are non-viable because of crush injury. Recent experiments indicate that the oblique slice through the dermis may even provide superior healing if care is taken to gain meticulous apposition of the margins.

Very few subcuticular sutures should be used in the face in the absence of division of underlying muscle bundles. The decision to use subcuticular sutures in the closure of any given facial wound calls for a precise judgment. If the closure will necessitate considerable tension on the skin sutures, it is wise to place subcuticular sutures that may be counted on to secure the wound when the skin sutures are removed. The subcuticular sutures should be placed as deeply as possible within the dermis and with the knots lying in the subcutaneous fat. Skin sutures should be tied loosely and removed in three days to prevent permanent "cross-hatch" suture scars. We have seen this hatching persist, in some instances, when all sutures were removed after only four days. During the first three to four days after closure, the facial wound shows rapid proliferation of and invasion by capillaries, but there is little development of tensile strength. Consequently, the skin margins *must* be supported for several days after the early removal of skin sutures in order to prevent disruption or early spreading of the soft scar. This support can be provided by placing collodion gauze strips or adhesive Steristrips over the incision for four or five days after removal of the sutures. Hydroxyproline concentrations of the healing scar and tensile strength determinations show that the facial wounds are reasonably secure after ten days.

Meticulous hemostasis should be carried out in repairing facial lacerations. This helps to avoid the collection of even small blood clots in the deep recesses of these wounds. Such clots lead to fibrosis and palpable thickening in the postoperative period. If any buried sutures are used, the knots should be tied at the deepest part of the loop and they should be placed in stout fascia well beneath the surface so as not to encroach on oil glands or hair follicles within the dermis. The choice of the type of suture material is not nearly so important as the method and depth of suture placement. The operator should develop the technique of using skin hooks in place of toothed forceps to handle the wound margins when suturing the face. This will avoid the damaging effects of tissue crushing that are seen even with careful use of fine spring forceps. There should be no need to use cuticular sutures heavier than 6-0 silk on the face, and the sutures should be placed within 2 to 4 mm. of the wound margin to avoid inversion of edges. They should be removed usually within three days. Nylon, mersilene, polydek and stainless steel sutures are all well tolerated as facial sutures, but most alloys of stainless steel wire lack the flexibility for perfect coaptation of wound edges.

In small children with modest lacerations of the face, it is usually wise to close these wounds, after proper cleansing, by using only adhesive strips, "butterflies," or some type of synthetic strip with skin adhesive (Fig. 8–5). In many instances, the final result will be superior to suturing. The child also will be spared an unpleasant experience involving injection of anesthetic and placing of sutures. Should further surgical improvement of the scar be necessary, it may be carried out later in an aseptic field with a relaxed and sedated child, with more likelihood of an optimum result. There is little to defend the practice of holding down a crying,

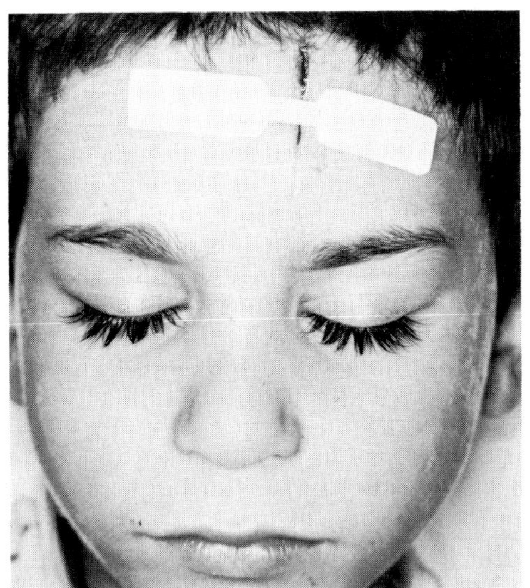

Figure 8–5 This type of simple butterfly dressing may be used to draw together and approximate wound edges of most fresh facial lacerations. The wounds are first cleaned and irrigated, but no local anesthetic injections are necessary. Usually two or three "butterflies" or other type of adhesive skin strip will suffice to hold the wound without dressing change for a four- or five-day period. Many favorably placed lacerations will require no later treatment. Others, such as this vertical laceration of the forehead, may require a later Z-plasty that is best performed on a healed wound. Eyebrows should never be shaved in suturing facial lacerations.

frightened, small child while four or five sutures are placed somewhat awkwardly.

When soft tissue lacerations lie at right angles to the lines of skin relaxation, muscle pull and movement on these scars will usually produce later hypertrophy and unsightly deformity (Fig. 8–6 *A* and *B*). A knowledge of wound dynamics makes it possible for the surgeon to accurately predict most of these complications of healing, and the patient should be warned of these problems at the time of original treatment. Indeed, in many instances, plastic surgeons will resort to primary z-plasty and local flap shifts in order to prevent the almost certain development of these scar hypertrophies. Such "primary flaps" require a knowledge of facial skin circulation and should not be undertaken if the skin has been crushed. When the patient is an Oriental or a dark-skinned Negro, such immediate flaps are more likely to produce true keloids, and a careful history of skin healing of prior wounds will be a valuable guide in choosing treatment.

Dressing Techniques. Pressure dressings are rarely necessary with soft tissue lacerations of the face and are likely to interfere with eating or breathing and be uncomfortable in the postoperative period. Usually, sutured incisions may be left open for frequent cleansing with weak concentrations of hydrogen peroxide or they may be covered with a light greasy protective dressing to avoid dry crust formation that may block wound secretions. Adhesive or synthetic strips may be placed across the sutured incisions to splint the cheek, lip or forehead and to reduce tension on suture lines. It is important to prevent the accumulation of dry crusts on the sutures if permanent pits and irregularities in the surface healing are to be avoided. After each cleansing of the sutures, a coating of sterile white oil will minimize further accumulations. Antibiotics are rarely indicated with lacerating injuries of the face that involve only soft tissues, but are desirable when compound fractures and crushed tissue are also present.

When the eyelid and orbital regions have received an extensive blow, a pressure dressing will be of great value in preventing the development of severe lid and conjunctival edema. If such massive swelling is allowed to occur, some patients will develop exposure and drying of the cornea or permanent skin striae from the irreversible stretching and scarring of lid skin. In the cervical region, large flaps that have been elevated may be dressed with the aid of continuous suction catheters beneath them. This utilizes normal atmospheric pressure in keeping the flaps in contact with the underlying bed.

Proteolytic Enzymes. Many pharmaceutical houses have enthusiastic-

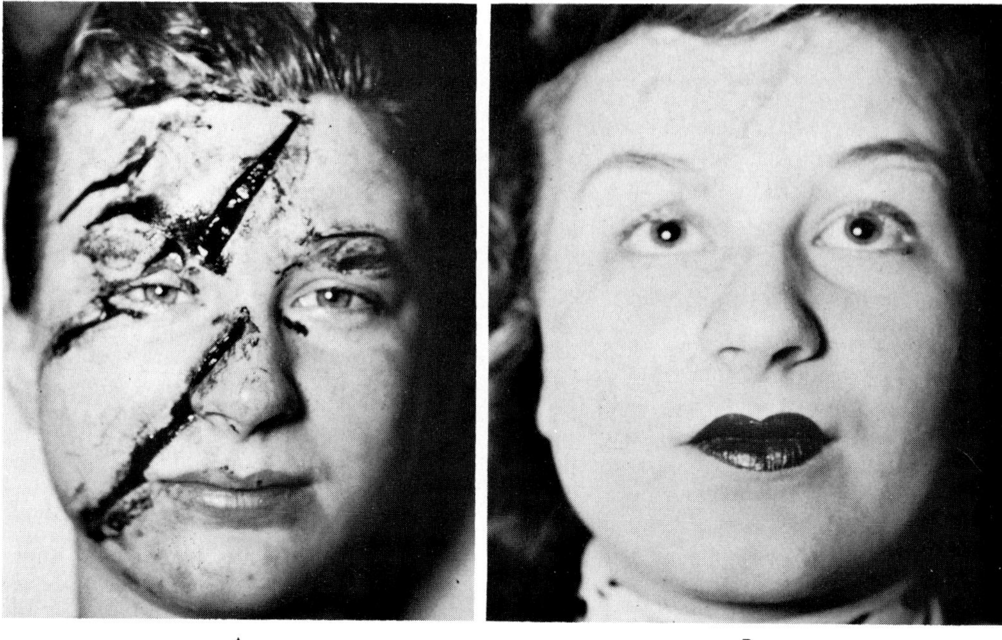

Figure 8–6 *A* and *B*, These lacerations were sustained when the patient's head was thrown against a broken windshield. Many of the lacerations fall along "lines of skin relaxation." The laceration of the central forehead is unfavorably placed and tends to gape more than the others. Part of the levator muscle to the right upper eyelid was also divided. Only a few subcuticular sutures of 5-0 silk were used in the vertical forehead laceration. All other lacerations were closed with fine skin sutures to produce the result shown (*B*) when the patient returned for minor revision of scars three months later. The levator muscle of the right upper eyelid was shortened at the same time. A primary Z-plasty in the forehead scar might also have been used as an alternative method of treatment.

ally promoted proteolytic enzymes for systemic and localized use in increasing fluid absorption from traumatized areas. Controlled studies to date have *not* established that patients receiving these expensive medications ultimately obtain better results than those in control groups. Resolution of experimental hematomas in human volunteers was not significantly accelerated by use of several commercial enzymes widely used by surgeons. Enzyme therapy such as hyaluronidase (Wydase) breaks down hyaluronic acid in the connective tissue and produces some initial resolution of traumatic edema, but "rebound edema" is common and ultimate results are not impressively better than when it is not used. Plastic surgeons *have not* been impressed with the value of these expensive drugs.

In contrast to the general ineffectiveness of enzymes in controlling traumatic edema and eventual healing, it is becoming apparent that some of the newer proteolytic enzymes can be of significant value as *debriding agents*. When applied properly and kept moist, some of these agents have shortened the removal of slough on the face from 22 days to five days, thus greatly facilitating treatment.

General Principles of Treatment of Maxillofacial Fractures

CRANIAL BONE FRACTURES

Cranial bone fractures may be accompanied by depression of a bone fragment requiring early elevation. Rapidly rising intracranial pressure may result from a torn middle meningeal artery and may require burr holes for decompression. A careful neurologic examination will usually reveal any central damage. (See chapter on head injuries.) Cerebrospinal fluid leaking from the nose or mouth may indicate basal skull fracture through the cribriform plate. Such leakage of fluid is no longer considered a contraindication to the careful reduction of other facial bone fractures. Indeed, such reductions are often followed by return of the torn dura to a normal position and a prompt cessation of the cerebrospinal rhinorrhea. Antibiotic therapy in such patients greatly reduces the danger of meningitis. If a patient remains in coma from the head injury, it is wise to wait until consciousness is recovered before proceeding with general anesthesia and reduction of facial fractures. If facial fractures are not reduced within ten days of injury, they become severely fixed in malposition and quite difficult to reduce. Should unconsciousness persist this long, careful manipulations of displaced facial bones may be indicated.

FRACTURE OF CERVICAL REGION

The cervical vertebrae should be checked for dislocations and fractures. Spasm of neck muscles or straightening of the normal vertebral curve as seen in lateral roentgenograms of the neck may suggest fractures of vertebral bodies or dislocation of a facet. In the cervical region the vertebral canal space clearance around the spinal cord is small, and excessive movements of a fractured neck have been known to produce additional neurologic injury and even quadriplegia.

Major injury to the cervical spine is indication for orthopedic consultation, and certain mechanisms of injury should lead the surgeon to suspect difficulty in this area. Forcible hyperflexion of the head on the neck is commonly known to produce crush fractures of the bodies of the fifth, sixth or seventh cervical vertebra. Falls sustained on the top of the head from a height tend to produce fractures of the atlas. In such injuries there is marked spasm of the neck muscles and the patient tends to hold himself as if he were balancing a weight upon the top of his head. Any motor or sensory paralysis of the upper or lower extremities may point to a serious lesion of the cervical vertebrae. In such instances, gentle traction to the head and careful support during transport of the patient are necessary emergency maneuvers.

Compression fractures of the laryngeal cartilages or trachea may be followed by the gradual increase in intraluminal edema, producing a sudden shut-off of the cervical airway some hours after injury. With lesser injuries of this type, steroid therapy may help to maintain the glottic airway. In addition to tracheostomy, the insertion of an inflatable balloon into the infraglottic larynx behind the fractured cartilage may permit reduction, with opening and splinting of the upper airway. If this is not successful, surgical opening of the larynx and even skin grafting to relieve the larynx and trachea may be required.

MANDIBULAR FRACTURES

The large, strong mandibular arch is balanced in position by many strong muscles of mastication. When the jaw is fractured, the mandibular fragments are readily displaced by these same powerful muscles. Thus, strong methods of bone fixation and longer splinting periods are required when the mandible is fractured than in the case of other facial bones. In contrast, the remaining facial bones (the "membranous bones") surrounding the orbit, nose and paranasal sinuses are light in weight and easily comminuted. When fractures of these bones are surgically reduced, the lack of strong muscle pull makes it easier to hold them in the correct positions than to hold mandibular fragments. Membraneous bones of the face also tend to unite quite rapidly.

It is of some interest that the central facial bones are highly efficient energy decelerators. This ability of nasal and parasinus bones to absorb great force prevents vital injury to the brain and spinal cord in many individuals when the face meets any solid object with great speed.

Most simple mandibular fractures may be best treated by the method known as *intermaxillary wiring.*

Intermaxillary Wiring or Elastic Band Fixation. It is a happy anatomical fact that the mandible contains hard white structures that are firmly fixed to it and that emerge through the mucous membrane covering its surface. These mandibular appendages, the teeth, serve as convenient handles to manipulate and control mandibular bone fragments following fracture. Teeth are very helpful both in diagnosis and in fixation of jaw fractures. When each major fractured jaw fragment contains adequate dentition, it is usually a simple matter to reduce mandibular fractures by the application of soft metallic arch bars to each of these fragments. These bars contain small metal pegs and are held in place by passing metal ligatures of stainless steel about the neck of each tooth to encompass the bar. Elastic bands are then applied to these bars in such directions that the teeth (and attached jaw fragments) will be drawn into their normal occlusal relationships. By using *elastic* rather than *rigid* bands, the reduction will continue over a period of several days and successfully overcome muscle spasm that might be present at the initial reduction. This technique is called intermaxillary wiring or, more accurately, intermaxillary elastic band fixation (Fig. 8–7). A mandibular fracture may thus be brought back into normal alignment with an intact upper alveolar arch or, conversely, a fractured maxilla by similar elastic traction may be drawn back into alignment with an intact mandibular arch. These arch bars and elastic bands need to be left in place approximately six weeks for proper healing. When the bands are removed, bone union must be tested by palpation as x-ray changes will not demonstrate callus formation for several additional weeks. When fractures of the mandible result in unfavorable position of the bone fragments, or when both arches are fractured and badly displaced, a more complex arrangement is required.

Open Reduction and Wiring (Transosseous). There are certain circumstances under which intermaxillary elastic band fixation does not offer sufficient fixation for mandibular fractures. These include:

1. Patients with an edentulous mandible or maxilla.
2. Displaced fractures of the mandible in which one or more fragments do not contain healthy erupted teeth.
3. Displaced mandibular fractures in small children with only deciduous dentition.
4. Patients with traumatic disruption of both arches who will need another point of fixation for realignment.

The first known report on the use of interosseous wiring of the mandible is by the surgeon Gurdon Buck.[5] In 1846 he reported an open reduction of the mandible using malleable iron wire for fixation of the fragments. The fracture involved the lower jaw between the first and second incisor teeth on the left side and occurred when a seaman was struck in the face by a block. To accomplish reduction of the fracture Dr. Buck proceeded as follows:

> The lower lip was divided along the median line to the chin, and the flaps dissected up to expose the ends of the bones. The remaining adhesions were divided and a narrow chisel insinuated behind the fragment to be exercised in order to protect the soft parts, while with a metacarpal saw, a perpendicular section was effected. The left middle incisor tooth, being loose in the right fragment, it was removed. The

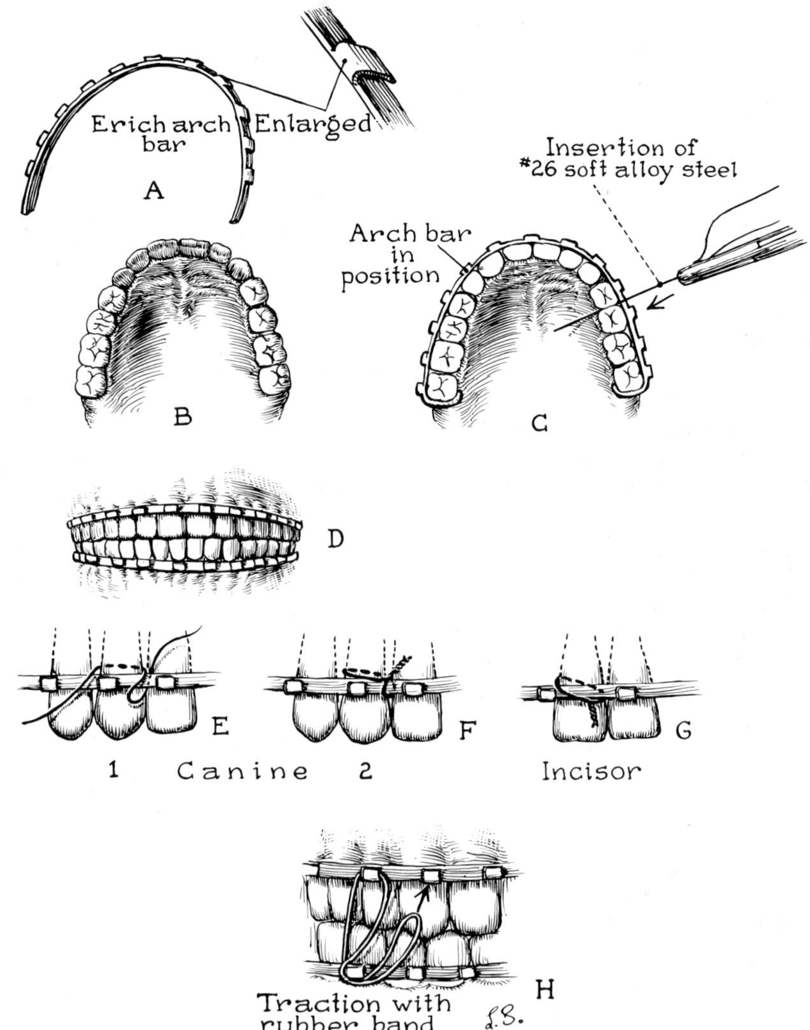

Figure 8–7 Method of applying soft metallic arch bars to upper or lower jaw in preparation for use of intermaxillary elastic band fixation of a fractured maxilla or mandible: The soft metal Erich bar is bent to fit against the dental arch and allowed to curve about the most posterior tooth. Soft steel wires are then passed about the necks of the molar teeth and about the bar to make the latter secure. *E, F,* and *G* illustrate the variations in applying the wire when it is necessary to use a canine tooth as one point of fixation. This method prevents the tendency of such forces to slowly extract the anchored tooth. Once the arch bars are properly attached, elastic bands may be applied to the metal hooks, as shown in *H,* to bring the jaw fragments and teeth into satisfactory occlusion.

ends of the bone now admitted of accurate adjustment, so as to bring the teeth of both sides on the proper level. To maintain them in this position, a hole was drilled near the lower angle in each bone, and a piece of malleable iron wire passed through, with the ends drawn forward and twisted, so as to secure the desired object.

Six weeks later Dr. Buck reported: "the opening through which the wire passed was healed up. Union solid. Discharged cured."

In recent years all plastic surgeons have moved steadily toward an increased use of open reduction and direct interosseous wiring of mandibular fractures.[7] There are numerous advantages to open reduction:

1. It produces immediate and simple reduction.

2. It provides hairline correction of bony displacement.
3. It relieves pain and provides more comfort than other types of appliances.
4. It avoids the need for constant adjustment of oral or external appliances or the danger of displacement of the bony fragments by muscle pull.
5. It reduces the period of total jaw immobilization.
6. It does not interfere with prompt reduction and positive fixation of fractures in other parts of the body.

The only significant disadvantages to open reduction and direct transosseous wiring are the necessity for the surgeon to be thoroughly familiar with the location of the branches of the facial nerve (so as to avoid injury to them during the operation) and the occasional necessity to remove a steel wire from the bone because of late tenderness or drainage. When incisions are properly placed in the lines of skin relaxation (Fig. 8–8), the external scars of open reduction are almost invisible when healed.

Before the reduction of mandibular fractures, the oral cavity should be carefully inspected. Any loose teeth should usually be removed as well as any tooth lying in the fracture line of the mandible. This is especially true if that tooth root shows evidence of root abscess or fracture and might serve as an inciting cause to the development of osteomyelitis. Many times healthy teeth lying in undisplaced fracture lines may be saved, and they will often contribute greatly to jaw fixation and mastication after healing. The mouth should be swabbed and the teeth scrubbed with a small toothbrush, using a mild detergent mouthwash.

Many mandibular fractures are compounded into the oral cavity, and it is important that the tears in the mucous membrane be loosely reapproximated with fine sutures. Such closure will avoid continuing massive contamination of the fracture line by gravitational collections of saliva and oral cavity bacteria in the depths of open mouth wounds. If these "saliva pools" are allowed to lie in direct contact with the fracture line, nonunion and osteomyelitis will commonly result. It is important that surgeons understand the basic principles of dental occlusion (Fig. 8–9). Recognition of the preinjury occlusion of the teeth is necessary in order to re-establish this original occlusion by the reduction of any jaw fractures. Most patients with jaw injuries readily detect even very minor variations in their normal bite relationships and so advise the surgeon. It is usually desirable to check this with some standard reference for normal occlusion.

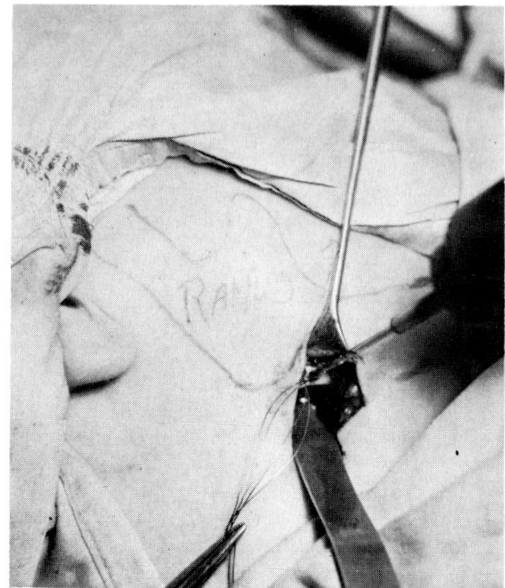

Figure 8–8 This simple type of exposure is ideal for transosseous wiring with open reduction of fractures of the angle of the mandible body or ramus. The incision is made with a knife only through the skin and fat. The remainder of the exposure is then obtained with gentle blunt dissection, going between parallel branches of the facial nerve. The periosteum of the mandible is elevated at the inferior border to reveal the fracture site. Drill holes are placed as shown in this illustration on either side of the fracture line, and doubled strands of No. 26 steel wire may be used to achieve a hair line reduction. The outline of the mandible is drawn on the skin here only for orientation.

Angle's[2] classification of dental

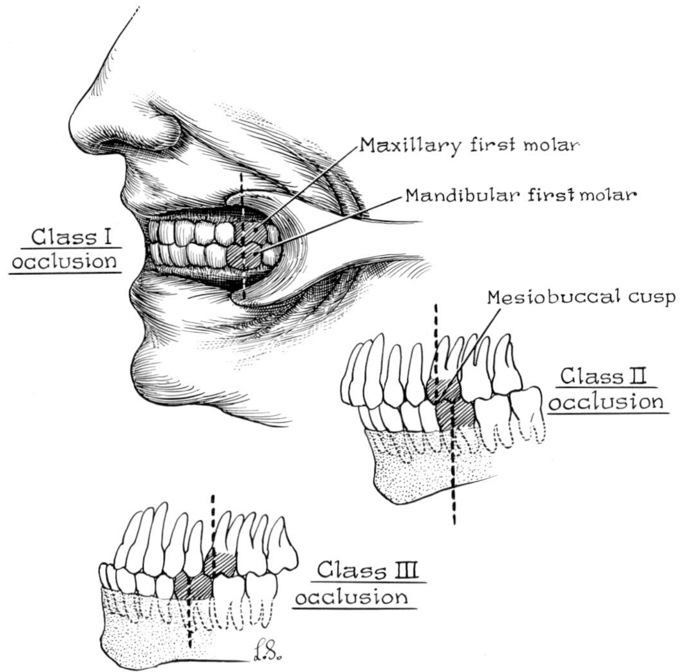

Figure 8–9 Elementary types of dental occlusion as originally described by Angle. The relationship of the mesiobuccal cusp of the maxillary first molar tooth to the mandibular first molar tooth is used as a guide for normal types of occlusion. Class II occlusion is commonly seen in patients with mandibular retrusion; class III occlusion is the type seen with prognathism. In fractures of the mandible or maxilla, the surgeon attempts to re-establish the occlusion present prior to the injury.

occlusion is based on the relationship of the mesiobuccal cusp of the maxillary first molar tooth to the mandibular teeth below (Fig. 8–9). In patients with normal bite relationships, this cusp interdigitates in the mesiobuccal groove of the mandibular first molar tooth. With distoclusion (retroclusion or Class II malocclusion), the mesiobuccal cusp of the maxillary first molar is anterior to the mesiobuccal groove of the mandibular first molar. The reversed displacement is known as mesioclusion (prognathic occlusion or Class III malocclusion). In this instance, the mesiobuccal cusp of the maxillary first molar is in the space between the first and second mandibular molars. Lateral blows to the upper or lower jaw may produce either a unilateral or bilateral crossbite as a result of a horizontal fracture and segmental medial displacement of one or both alveolar processes with their contained teeth. In such instances the full vertical height of the mandible or maxilla may or may not also be fractured.

Fractures of the mandible may be divided for simple classification into four groups:

1. *Fractures of the Condylar Neck.* This is the weakest portion of the mandible and accounts for 35 per cent of the fractures.
2. *Fractures of the Mandibular Angle, Ramus and Coronoid.* This portion of the bone lies beneath the masseter and temporal muscles and accounts for 30 per cent of the fractures of the mandible.
3. *The Body of the Mandible and/or the Alveolar Ridge with Its Contained Tooth Roots.* This accounts for 25 per cent of mandibular fractures.
4. *Anterior Mandibular Fractures.* These fractures involve the symphysis and mandible from midline back to the mental foramen on either side. They account for 10 per cent of mandible fractures (Fig. 8–10).

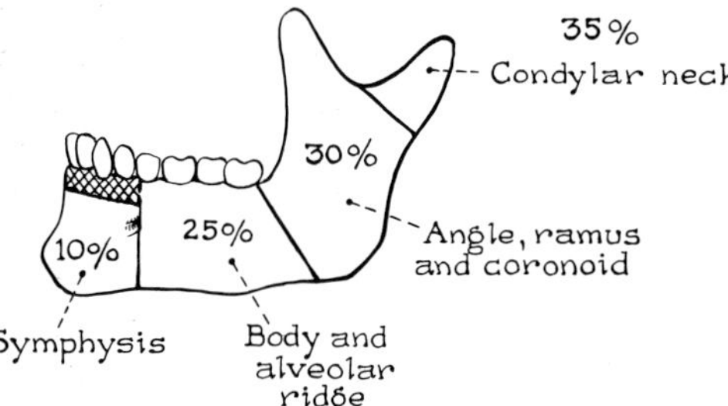

Figure 8–10 A simple classification of mandibular fractures with approximate incidence is shown in this diagram. Note that the masseter and temporalis muscles tend to pull any attached posterior bone fragments strongly upward. The internal pterygoid muscle tends to pull the neck of the condyle medialward and forward when the latter is fractured. The cross-hatched area of the alveolus shown anteriorly merely indicates that this region of bone is involved not only with fractures through the symphysis but also occasionally with fractures of the body of the mandible, including horizontal fractures of the alveolus itself. Slightly differing methods of fixation are required for each of these four major types of mandibular fracture.

Treatment of these fractures depends on an understanding of the action and force of strong muscle groups acting on each of these major segments of the lower jaw. A fractured anterior mandibular segment will be pulled downward and posteriorly by the depressor-retractor group of muscles (the geniohyoid and digastric muscles). A fracture through the body of the mandible will usually show an upward and medial displacement of the posterior fragment due to the powerful force of the elevator muscles (masseter, medial pterygoid and temporal muscles). Such a displacement may fail to occur if the fracture has a "favorable" direction (i.e., if the line of the fracture runs posteriorly to anteriorly through the mandibular body as it descends from the alveolar margin to the inferior border of the mandible. With such a "favorable" fracture line, the muscle forces tend to impact the mandibular fragments against each other. A fracture line that lies at right angles to this favorable direction will allow the muscles to distract the fragments.

Fractures through the angle and ramus of the mandible may show minimal displacement, or the posterior fragment may be displaced markedly forward and upward. This often depends upon the fracturing force since the bone of the ramus is thin, making medial or lateral displacements of fragments common. Fractures through the neck of the condyle are usually accompanied by anterior and medial rotation of the proximal mandibular condyle and neck as a result of "protrusor" action of the lateral pterygoid muscle. Each of these muscles of mastication has great power, and when in spasm following injury, they tend to redisplace the bone fragments after reduction unless strong, well-engineered fixation is used to secure the jaw fragments for four to eight weeks.

Diagnosis of Mandibular Fractures. A fractured mandible can usually be diagnosed on clinical evaluation alone. The cardinal features include complaints of malocclusion of the teeth, mobility of a portion of the mandible on bimanual manipulation (Fig. 8–3), frequent compounding of the fracture into the oral cavity (especially if the body of the mandible and alveolus are involved), pain localized at the fracture site on movement or palpation, inability to chew properly, some degree of trismus and edema or hematoma at the site of fracture. If the inferior alveolar artery was torn by the separation of the fracture line, there is usually discoloration of the overlying skin by ecchymosis.

If the mouth was closed at the time of injury, there may be associated avulsion of one or more of the cusps of premolar or molar teeth. Strong lateral forces not only shear off high points on the teeth, but may also cause exposure of dental pulp. Reimplantation of avulsed teeth may be successful, particularly in young children, whose teeth have open root canals, but such decisions should be left to an exodontist.

Roentgenographic examinations are

of greatest value in determining (1) the position of bone fragments before reduction, (2) the presence of caries, abscesses or broken roots of teeth in the fractured area, and (3) the position of the bone following surgical reduction.

General Principles in Treatment of Mandibular Fractures. Once the diagnosis of mandibular fracture is clearly determined, treatment may be carried out by wiring a section of soft metal arch bar (containing small metal projecting hooks) to the teeth in the upper jaw and to each fractured segment in the lower jaw (Fig. 8–7).

The teeth serve as convenient pegs to which may be wired a separate section of arch bar for each displaced bone and tooth unit. An arch bar is also fixed to the maxillary arch and the mandibular fragments may be drawn into proper position by using small rubber bands (easily made by cutting slices off ordinary soft rubber tubing) to connect the arch bar hooks at corresponding points in upper and lower arches (Fig. 8–7*H*). This method of "intermaxillary elastic traction" may not produce "instant normal occlusion" when first applied, but over a period of several days the gentle gradual pull of the elastic bands overcomes the spasm of opposing muscles, the high points of tooth cusps tend to slide into the proper "valleys" or grooves between the cusps of opposing teeth, and the jaws settle into the desired relationships for healing. When all fracture fragments contain teeth, or when there is minimal displacement of bone, such intermaxillary elastic splinting may be the simplest and best surgical treatment for a mandibular fracture. When there are large bony fragments bearing no teeth, or when tooth-bearing fragments have been markedly displaced and are unstable, other surgical measures are often of value.

Plastic surgeons stress both the simplicity and the effectiveness of direct transosseous wiring of the mandibular fragments (see pp. 277–278). Such wires may be inserted through small (1.5 cm.) incisions, may be left in the tissues permanently and allow the patient to use his jaws at a much earlier postinjury period than in the case of patients treated only by the use of intermaxillary elastic fixation. Open reduction is of special value with displaced fractures of the ramus and with double fracture lines in the region of the symphysis. When direct interosseous wiring is undertaken, the skin incisions should be placed parallel to the lines of skin relaxation (Fig. 8–8); the facial nerve branches may be located just deep to the platysma muscle and bluntly separated. The drill holes should be placed in the bone on either side of the fracture line at a proper angle to anticipate the direction of muscle pull on the bone.

Direct interosseous wiring may be combined with intermaxillary elastic traction or, in the edentulous patient, with circumferential wiring. Such circumferential wires may be passed so as to encircle the overlapping ends of the fractured edentulous mandible or, when the patient's denture is not broken by the injury, it may be positioned against the oral surface of the fractured mandible and the encircling wires allowed to include both denture and mandible.

A French surgeon, Jean-Baptiste Baudens, appears to have been the first to describe the concept of circumferential wiring for mandibular fractures.[3] In 1840 he outlined his treatment of a soldier with an oblique fracture through the region of the angle of the mandible and severe displacement of the proximal fragment. He was "able to hold the fracture securely with one circumferential wire passed around the mandible with a needle. The two ends of the ligature were fixed over a posterior tooth." Baudens was criticized by Professor Roux, who suggested that the pressure of the metal ligature upon the bony tissue might alter the structure of the bone. Baudens pointed out that the wire had "remained in place for twenty-three days and left the bone in a condition of good health."

In 1852 Cesar Robert modified this treatment by passing the circumferential wire over a small lead plate.[15] In modern times a denture or small acrylic shell is used in place of the lead plate.

Most mandibular fractures may thus be managed by a combination of intermaxillary elastic band traction, direct transosseous wiring with open reduction, or circumferential wiring with or without use of the patient's dentures or a dental splint. On occasion an extra plane of fixation is required, particularly in the edentulous mandible and when much destruction of the maxilla has also occurred. Such stability may be gained by drilling a straight steel Kirschner wire through the lower borders of the mandible from side to side after reduction and manual fixation of the arch (Fig. 8–23).

One must remember that the mandible does not produce a dense callus for many months following clinical healing of a fracture line; thus, it is both unnecessary and unwise to wait for radiologic evidence of bony union before stabilizing the jaws in the postoperative period. Clinical bony union is a much more reliable guide as to the time at which jaw function should be resumed. Indeed, mild stress applied to the fracture line in later stages of healing appears to actually accelerate the rate of bony union in some fractures.

Fractures and Dislocations of the Mandibular Condyle. In general, fractures of the condylar neck should be treated conservatively by simply restoring occlusion with intermaxillary wiring for a three-week period. However, when there has been severe displacement of the head of the condyle, particularly in young children in whom growth arrest would create serious deformity, a very gently performed open reduction carried out as a primary or delayed procedure may be of great value. Exposure of the condyle may be obtained with least danger to the facial nerve by an incision *behind* the external ear. This approach divides the postauricular muscle fibers and fascia and the full circumference of the cartilaginous external auditory canal. The operator may then reflect the ear, parotid gland and facial nerve forward and downward to reveal the entire lateral and posterior surfaces of the temporomandibular joint. The dissection should be gentle and carried out so as to preserve as much soft tissue attachment (blood supply) to the fractured condyle as possible. If the bone is exposed too widely, aseptic necrosis may develop postoperatively. If both condyles are fractured and displaced, and if the symphysis and body of the mandible are also comminuted, it may be difficult to maintain an adequately forward position of the lower jaw during healing. In such circumstances open reduction and direct wiring of the symphysis and body fractures may be combined with application of a simple plaster head-cap that contains a projecting metal arm. This arm may be used to permit an elastic forward traction on the condylar fracture lines (Fig. 8–11 *A* and *B*) by attaching it to the mandible with a Kirschner wire or arch bar.

With all compound mandibular fractures, attempts should be made to suture loosely any lacerated mucosa in the area of the fracture. This accelerates wound healing and reduces the incidence of bone infection. With major avulsions and loss of mucosa, drainage should be carried out in a dependent direction through a small submandibular "stab" incision rather than by "uphill" drainage into the oral cavity.

In the case of explosive wounds resulting in loss of large segments of the mandible, it may be necessary to fix the remaining portions in normal position by means of external skeletal pin fixation (Fig. 8–12). This fixation

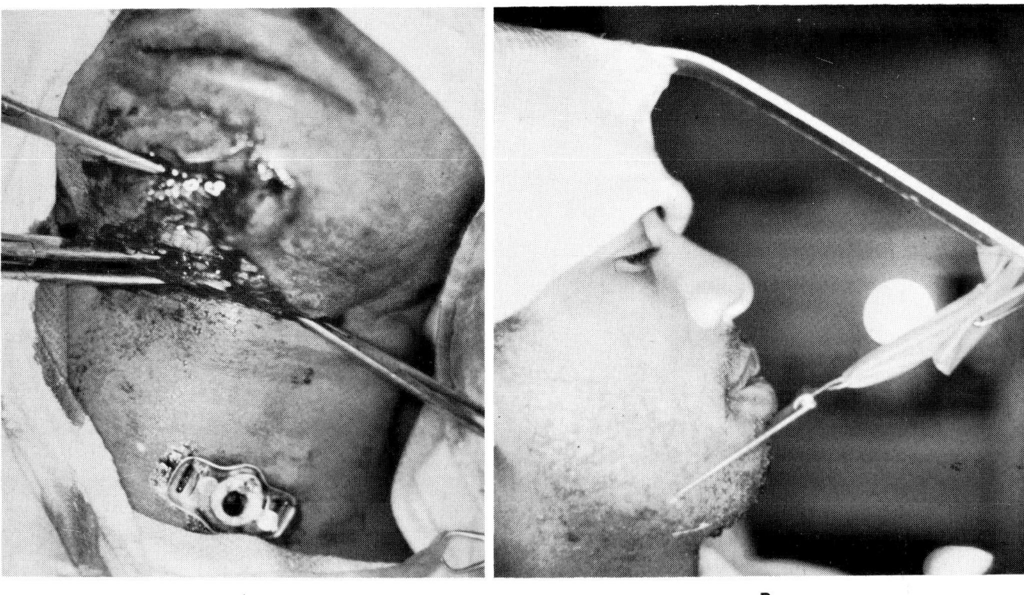

A B

Figure 8–11 *A* and *B*, This patient suffered a severe comminuted fracture of the mandible involving both condyles and both rami, and a triple fracture of the symphysis following a head-on collision in a speeding automobile. Emergency tracheotomy was lifesaving, but transosseous wiring of the mandibular fractures and intermaxillary elastic fixation would not succeed in holding the lower mandibular arch forward in satisfactory position. To restore the arch, a steel pin was passed through the lower border of the body of the mandible and held forward by moderately strong elastic traction supplied by means of a metal rod and plaster head cap as shown in *B*. The dislocated condyles were gently maneuvered back into position when the severe facial edema had subsided. Good mandibular function resulted.

will retain alignment of fragments until soft tissue healing is complete and may be followed by bone grafting and further plastic repair. At times a small buried bone plate may be used to maintain the space caused by the missing segment of bone.

DISLOCATION OF THE TEMPOROMANDIBULAR JOINT

Spontaneous dislocation of the lower jaw may occur as the result of a sudden interruption in the normal jaw-closing action of the muscles of mastication. It may also result from trauma which suddenly forces the condyle out of the fossa. In the absence of fracture, the dislocation always displaces the head of the condyle in an anterior direction. The chin shifts to the opposite side, and the teeth on the side of the dislocation become locked in an open bite position with considerable pain and muscle spasm.

A writer in the Smith Papyrus (written 25 centuries before the time of Christ) gives advice for treatment for dislocation of the mandible: "If thou examinist a man having a dislocation in his mandible, shouldst thou find his mouth open and his mouth cannot close for him, thou shouldst put thy thumbs upon the ends of the two rami of the mandible on the inside of his mouth, (and) thy two claws (meaning two groups of fingers) under his chin, (and) thou shouldst cause them to fall back so that they rest in their places."[17]

W. B. Johnson[10] first reported that local anesthetic (1 per cent lidocaine hydrochloride) injected unilaterally

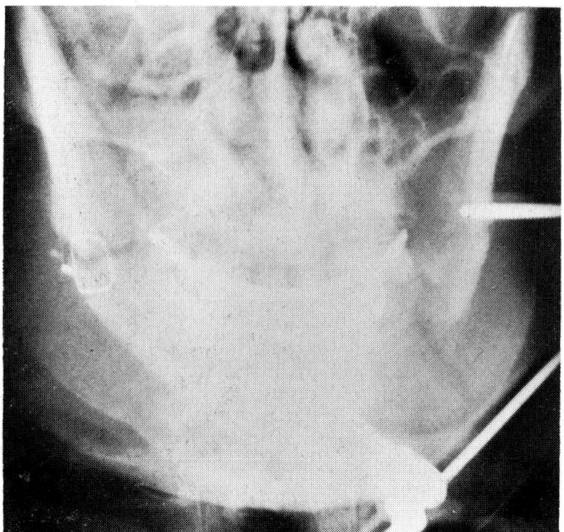

Figure 8–12 This x-ray shows a necessary combination of three methods of fixation for a compound fracture of the mandible. The injury resulted from a shotgun blast with destruction of approximately two inches of the body of the right mandible. Intermaxillary elastic traction has been applied by arch bars to the upper and lower jaw. The fracture of the left angle of the mandible has been reduced by direct transosseous wiring, and external skeletal fixation has been applied across the defect in the right mandible. This large defect in the bone was filled later with an iliac bone graft to retain the lower arch.

into the connective tissue of the torn temporomandibular joint capsule brought about consistent spontaneous reduction of the dislocation. When this excellent method is not successful, manipulation may be undertaken. The operator should face the patient with the thumbs placed inside the mouth and the lower borders of the mandible grasped on both sides with the fingers. The posterior mandible is depressed, and the symphysis is elevated. This position is held gently but firmly until the condyle slips backward over the articular eminence. At times muscle relaxing drugs and general anesthesia may be required to effect reduction. Occasional patients reappear habitually in emergency treatment rooms with a long history of recurrent dislocation of the temporomandibular joint. Such patients may be effectively cured by a simple reconstructive operation that involves the use of a tendon graft to rebuild the torn anterior joint capsule. Many sufferers of chronic dislocation of the jaw are unaware that such relief is available.

FRACTURES OF MEMBRANE BONES OF THE FACE

Central facial bone fractures involve membrane bones which comminute more easily than the mandible when struck, but they are not so difficult to hold in place after reduction because the muscles attaching to them are not of the strength and leverage of those that insert on the mandible. Consequently, reduction usually does not require strong or prolonged fixation. The thinness of membrane bone and the lack of support provided by adjacent paranasal sinuses cause it to respond to a sharp blow by breaking like an eggshell into many tiny fragments that are often difficult to replace. Such fractures occur in well-defined patterns at weak points in membrane bone. They may be considered under the headings of nasal fractures, zygomatic arch fractures, malar compound and orbital bone fractures, and complex transverse middle-face fractures (midface mash).

Nasal Fractures. Diagnosis of a nasal fracture is readily made by such findings as bleeding from the nose, external displacement of the nose, localized bony tenderness, difficulty in breathing or evidence of septal edema and deformity on intranasal speculum examination. Roentgenograms of the nasal bones are of interest but of little value in treatment; they should not be required to determine whether operative reduction of the nose is required. Their importance has been overemphasized since noses that are clinically straight and without septal deformity need no surgical reduction even if roentgenograms show minor fracture lines. In the presence of massive nasal and paranasal edema, treatment should be postponed for seven to ten days. This will permit the swelling to subside and will improve manual palpation of the position of the bones at the time of fracture reduction.

The prominent location of the nose and its relative structural weakness may be responsible for the fact that nasal fractures are more common than any fracture other than fractures of the wrist. Early treatment is quite important since neglect of a nasal bone fracture may result in a deformity that increases slowly over a period of months or years. Such deformities are extremely difficult to correct by later surgery and often require a formal rhinoplasty.

Most nasal fractures should be treated by simple reduction, using only local anesthesia and a lightly padded elevator placed within the nose that will "snap" the bones back into good position. Some fractures are complicated by extensive compound soft tissue wounds or by crushing forces that also destroy the central maxillary bone foundation on which the nose normally rests. Such injuries create difficult therapeutic problems.

Nasal fractures in children are of particular importance because of the danger of growth arrest or delayed nasal deformity that may follow improper treatment. The small external nares and air passages in children make it difficult to visualize and evaluate septal fractures. In general, one should assume that a nasal fracture is present in any child bleeding from the nose after injury. If there is doubt, children with suspected nasal fracture should be given general anesthesia and a topical vasoconstrictor should be applied to the nasal septal mucosa to permit determination of a possible fracture. If a badly displaced septal fracture is discovered in a child, later growth problems and airway obstruction may be expected. With the aid of a small exploratory septal incision, any displaced section of septal cartilage may be discovered, gently elevated back into place and held in the midline by light nasal packs.

Severe frontal forces applied to the nose may flatten the nasal bones and drive the lacrimal bones and internal palpebral ligaments out of position (the "canthal crush" deformity). Obstruction to the nasolacrimal ducts and to the ostia of the ethmoidal sinuses may result. The cribriform plate and the frontal bone may be damaged. Epiphora and dacryocystitis may result. Permanent pseudohypertelorism may remain and cause a great sense of deformity. Fracture of the quadrilateral cartilage of the nasal septum at its junction with the perpendicular plane of the ethmoid may result in a backward displacement and shortening of the nose, with retraction of the columella and flattening of the upper lip. Subcutaneous emphysema may be present and progressive because of the patient's repeated efforts to use his nasal airway, thus spreading air through the subcutaneous tissues.

Diagnosis cannot be adequately made of the extent of damage in the fractured nose without shrinking the edematous nasal mucosa with a vasoconstrictor drug. We prefer to use a 10 per cent cocaine hydrochloride solution applied very *sparingly* (8 cc. will moisten four long cotton applicators) as both topical anesthetic and vasoconstrictor. The patient's history should first be carefully checked for drug sensitivity, and intravenous fluids should be started. Proper supportive anesthetic equipment (oxygen, gas machine, intubation tubes and laryngoscope) should be available in the event of a drug reaction. The development of occipital headache or numbness and tingling in the fingers is indication of toxicity and should be followed by abandonment of the procedure and proper supportive measures.

Treatment of nasal fractures is most easily carried out in the first hours after injury. After the mucous membranes have been shrunk and the extent of damage determined, a blunt elevator covered with a protective thin rubber tubing may be used to raise the depressed or deviated fragments. The thumb may then be used to mold the elevated bones into symmetrical positions. Local block and topical anesthesia is always preferred to general anesthesia except in very young children or for complicated injuries. Simple nasal fractures may often be literally "snapped" back into position and then require no splinting or packing. At times the dislocation of the nasal septal cartilage will be automatically reduced when the external nasal pyramid is lifted into proper position. In addition to a simple elevator, the surgeon usually needs only a pair of Asch forceps, a long bladed nasal speculum and a narrow suction tip. Unless nasal fractures are reduced within the first several days following injury, bony fixation may become quite solid, necessitating a formal rhinoplasty for correction. Fixation of most nasal fractures may be provided by combination of light anterior nasal packing and the application of a thin external splint of plaster of Paris (Figs. 8–13 and 8–14), a dental compound or sheet aluminum covered with adhesive.

It is wise to leave the nose packed with gauze only as long as may be required for fixation of the bony parts. Even gauze impregnated with bland ointment creates secondary irritation and edema in the nasal mucous membranes. If such internal splinting is required for more than four to five days, it is desirable that the gauze be impregnated with an antibiotic in order to minimize the development of infection.

At times the severe comminution of the bridge of the nose requires that perforated acrylic or lead plates be applied to the lateral walls of the nose and attached to one another by wires passed across the nasal cavity and out through the holes in the plates. When these wires are tightened the plates draw the bits of nasal and maxillary bone forward and back to the midline, thus narrowing the width of nose and canthus and preventing collapse of the nasal bridge. Rarely, an additional external plaster head-cap or skeletal fixation to the cranium is required to provide a stable point anterior to the nose that will allow additional traction to this type of crushed-in nose. When lead plate splinting is used, it should be left on for 10 to 14 days, depending on the amount of comminution with the injury.

Cerebrospinal rhinorrhea may accompany severe nasal fractures. In such circumstances neurosurgical consultation is desirable, but this complication is *not* a contraindication to reduction of nasal or other facial fractures. If the surgeon waits for many days in hopes that this leakage will stop, ultimate reduction of the nasal fracture may be difficult and permanently unsatisfactory. Broad spectrum antibiotics should be given as long as spinal fluid leak continues in order to reduce the danger of meningitis.

Hematomas should not be allowed to remain within the tissues of the nasal septum since they may be followed by narrowing of the airway and progressive deformity of the nose. A failure to discover and remove one of these clots may also result in infection, abscess and even septal perforation. There is a tendency for septal hematomas to recur, and the nose should be inspected at reasonable intervals following evacuation of such a clot.

Zygomatic Arch Fractures. Zygomatic arch fractures usually result from direct localized blows just anterior to the ear. When the major part of the malar compound is not fractured, a segment of the arch may be carried inward, producing pain on opening of the jaws and some degree of trismus (Fig. 8–15*A*). Such fractures may be diagnosed on palpation unless there is extensive associated

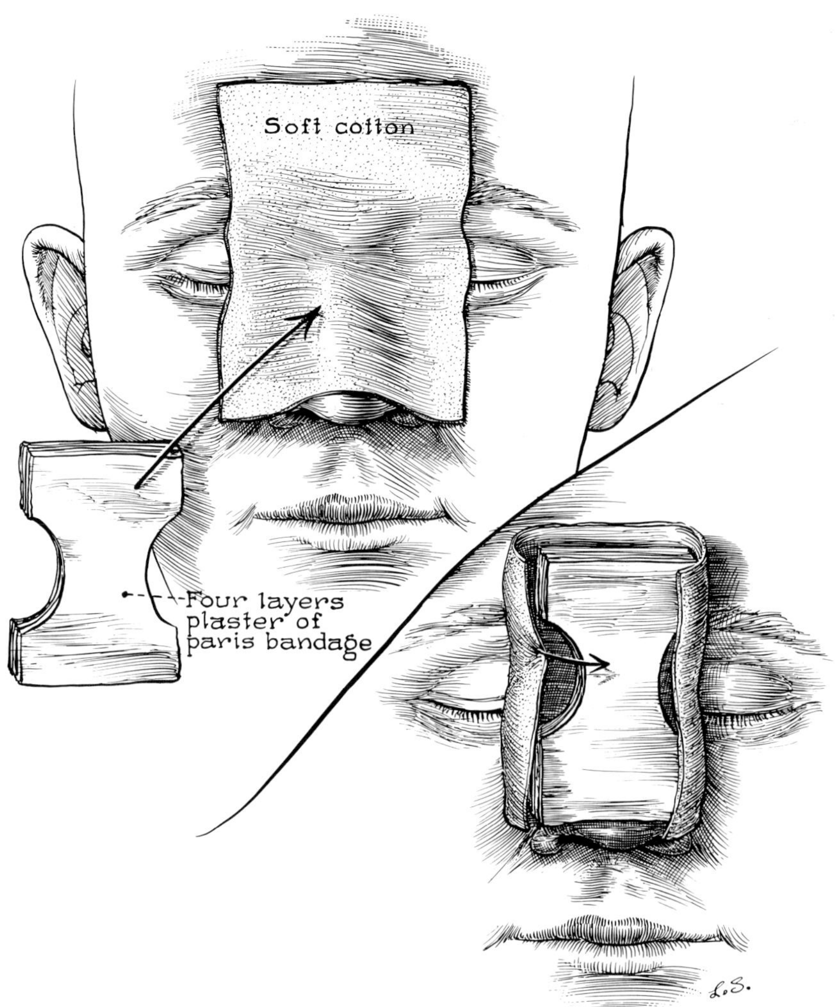

Figure 8–13 Every surgeon should know how to splint the external nose after reduction of a nasal fracture. Simple materials will provide an excellent splint. One or two thicknesses of soft cotton roll are first placed over the nose after reduction of fracture. Four thicknesses of fast-setting ordinary plaster of Paris may then be cut to relieve pressure over the inner canthus of each eye. The wet plaster is then molded gently to the shape of the underlying glabella and nasal bones. The edges of the cotton are turned upward to protect the skin from the edges of the plaster.

hematoma or edema. There is point tenderness over the arch, and the patient has reduced lateral movements of the lower jaw. The roentgenogram most useful to demonstrate this fracture is a submental-vertical projection of the zygomatic arches. The tube is placed beneath the patient's chin, and the emulsion plate is put behind the occiput and held parallel to the zygomatic arches. The film should be deliberately underexposed to obtain the best detail.

The most popular treatment for zygomatic arch fractures is the approach of Gillies, Kilner and Stone.[9] Some of the hair is shaved in the temple region. A one-inch incision is made, down to and including all of the temporal fascia, to expose temporal muscle fibers. A heavy, long elevator is then passed downward

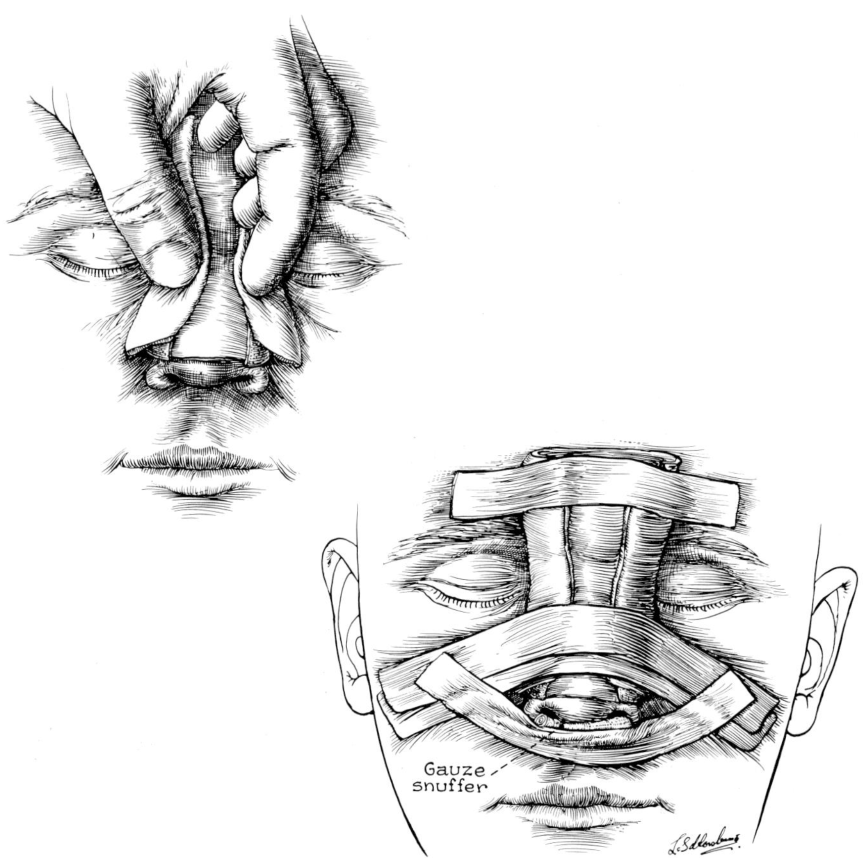

Figure 8–14 If needed, the surgeon may place two more small strips of plaster along each side of the nose for additional strength in the splint. The fingers are then used to support the plaster in proper position against the bridge until the splint becomes firm. Strips of adhesive are used to secure the splint to the cheeks and the forehead, and a removable gauze snuffer is lightly taped across the end of the nose to control any secretions from the nasal packing. This splint is usually left in place five days.

along these muscle fibers until its tip is felt suddenly to dip medially beneath the fractured zygomatic arch. By using a roll of gauze against the side of the head as a fulcrum, the operator elevates laterally the depressed bony fragment; usually he can feel it "click" into place. If a fracture is unstable, it may be retained in a good lateral position by passing a single circumferential wire around the arch and attaching it to a simple rigid suspension bridge that rests on the temporal bone superiorly and the angle of the mandible inferiorly (Fig. 8–15 *B* and *D*). Such support should be maintained for approximately 10 days to establish union. During this period the patient may be allowed to chew soft food.

Fractures of the Molar Compound and Orbital Bones. MALAR COMPOUND. The zygoma or malar compound is a dense bone forming the prominence of the cheek. It has four major "arms" or processes. These articulate with the frontal, maxillary and temporal bones and with the greater wing of the sphenoid bone. The junctions with the sphenoid and zygomatic process of the temporal bone are weak and easily fractured. The medial surface of the zygoma helps to form the greater portion of

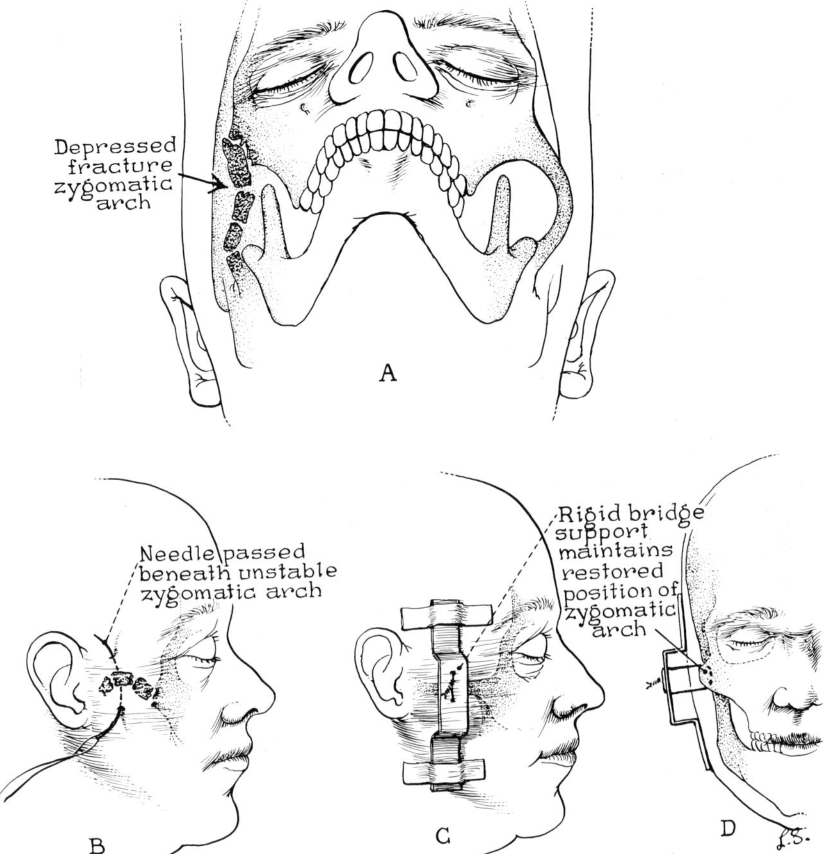

Figure 8–15 Fractures limited to the zygomatic arch usually involve at least three fracture lines. The swelling and displacement may impinge on the underlying coronoid process of the mandible, causing pain when the jaw is opened. Most of these fractures can be reduced simply by the classic approach of Gillies. This involves passing an elevator beneath the fracture by means of a small incision within the hairline. At times the arch fragments will not remain stable in the reduced position, and this simple device using a bridge splint will maintain the position without undue discomfort to the patient. The wire and splint are usually removed after a 10-day period.

the lateral floor of the orbit and contributes to the lateral superior wall of the maxillary sinus. Fractures of the malar bone are present in two-thirds of all middle face fractures. The malar bone is usually fractured along with any adjacent articulating bone. When the zygoma is displaced, it usually produces fractures of the orbit, the anterior and lateral walls of the maxillary antrum, the zygomatic process of the temporal bone, and separations at the zygomaticofrontal and zygomaticosphenoid suture lines.

Knight and North[11] have made a most useful classification of zygoma fractures. Based on their studies, there are six common types of malar bone fractures:

1. One in 20 fractures of the malar compound shows no significant displacement, and treatment is not required.
2. One in 10 involves only the zygomatic arch (Fig. 8–16*A*). In this fracture pattern there are typically three fracture lines of the arch, with a "buckling-in" of the fragments.
3. One-third of malar compound fractures produce unrotated fractures of the body of the zygoma (Fig. 8–16*B*), with

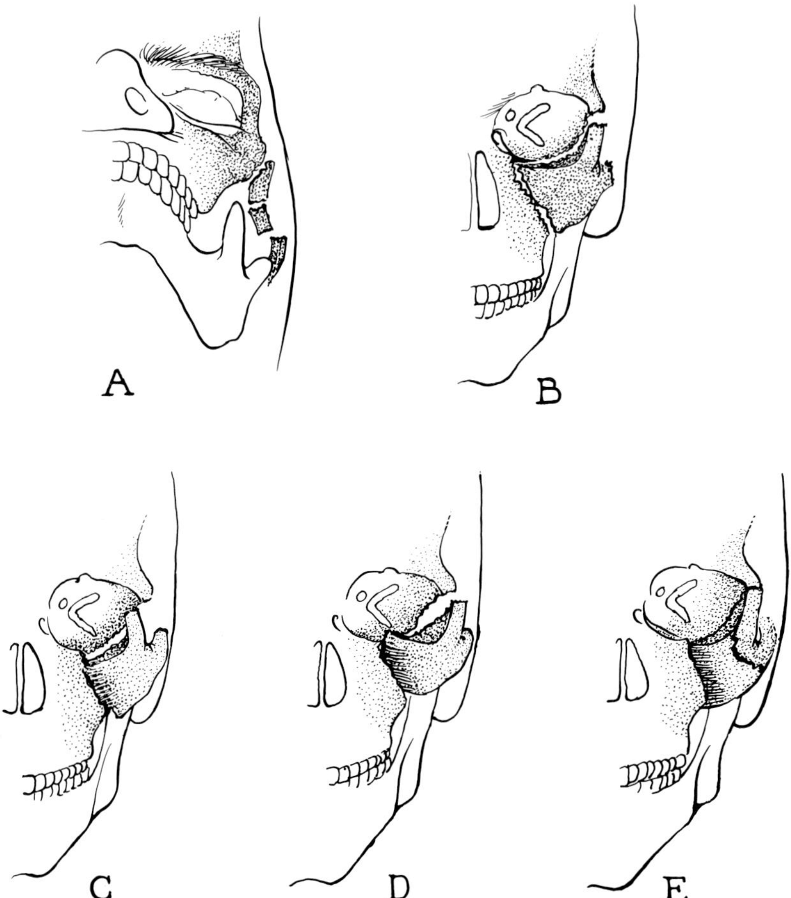

Figure 8–16 Simple classification of displaced fractures of the zygomatic compound: One-tenth involve the arch only (*A*), one-third show inward or downward displacement without rotation (*B*), one-tenth show medial rotation of the upper part of the zygoma toward the midline (*C*), one-fifth are rotated laterally (*D*), and one-fifth are complicated by additional fractures of the central heavy portion of the malar bone (*E*). These various types of fracture may be readily determined on examination and x-ray, and their recognition is of considerable help in planning operative reductions.

displacement directly into the antrum (backward, inward and slightly downward).

4. One in 10 fractures of the malar compound is *medially* rotated (Fig. 8–16*C*). The left malar compound in such injuries is thus rotated counterclockwise (or clockwise in the case of a fracture of the right malar compound) when viewed from the front. Examination of the Waters view roentgenogram shows apparent downward displacement at the infraorbital margin.

5. One-fifth of the malar compound fractures are *laterally* rotated and apparently caused by blows below the horizontal axis of the bone (Fig. 8–16*D*). When such fractures involve the left malar compound it appears to be rotated clockwise when viewed from the front (i.e., away from the midline). On roentgenogram with the Waters view, these fractures often appear to be displaced upward at the infraorbital margin.

6. Finally, about one-fifth of the malar compound fractures are complicated by additional fracture lines through the dense bone of the main fragment (Fig. 8–16*E*).

Most fractures of the zygomatic compound tear the lining of the maxillary sinus and cause hematoma within the sinus cavity. Ecchymosis and subconjunctival hemorrhage are almost pathognomonic of facial bone fracture. The lateral palpebral ligament is attached to the zygomatic portion of the orbital rim. It may be significantly displaced with zygoma fractures and, if the bone is not replaced, a downward and lateral deformity of the external canthus of the eye is produced. Similarly, the orbital septum is drawn inferiorly by any downward displacement of the malar compound and infraorbital rim. This will produce a permanent widening of the eyelids with epiphora and lower lid deformity.

Diagnostic features of fractures of the zygoma include flattening of the cheekbone, depression in level of the globe, diplopia, downward displacement of the lateral palpebral ligament, downward retraction of the lower eyelid, subconjunctival hematoma or unilateral epistaxis. Numbness of one-half of the upper lip and palpable irregularity, displacement or tenderness of the orbital rim (Fig. 8–3*C*) will often be present. If the index finger is passed behind the upper lip and used to palpate the anterior wall of the antrum, bony irregularities may be detected with many zygomatic fractures. A stereo-Waters roentgenogram of the face will usually provide all the needed radiographic information for surgical management of this fracture. Occasionally, tomograms taken through portions of the bony orbital walls will be of help in determining fracture lines or herniations into the ethmoids or antrum. Clouding of the antrum is commonly seen and usually represents collected hematoma. Such clots will usually liquefy and spontaneously drain out into the nasal cavity if the antral drainage is not blocked at the ostium by bone impaction. Anesthesia of the infraorbital nerve with numbness of the upper lip is commonly a diagnostic feature with malar compound fractures. Delay in relieving the pressure of fractured bone on the nerve (often at its emergence from the infraorbital foramen) may result in permanent anesthesia or even severe facial neuralgia.

ORBITAL BONES. Diplopia and orbital floor fractures accompany middle face fractures in over 25 per cent of the cases. "Double vision" will prove to be transient in about one-third, with eye symptoms disappearing within one week along with the absorption of intraorbital hemorrhage and edema; in about one-third the difficulty will persist; and in about one-third the problem will appear late and will persist. Diplopia may result from several mechanisms:

1. Loss of bony support of the floor of the orbit with downward displacement of the origin of the inferior oblique muscle and the globe.
2. Increase in total volume or capacity of the bony orbit, producing relative enophthalmus and ineffective extraocular muscle control.
3. Anchoring of the inferior rectus muscle in a fracture line of the orbital floor, thus limiting eye movement (especially in upward rotation of the eye).
4. Herniation of orbital fat into the antrum through a fracture line in the orbital floor. This herniation of tissue may increase progressively over a period of days or weeks following injury. The movements of the eye seem to massage orbital fat down through the fracture line. Edema or hematoma within the orbital box may raise orbital pressure and help to extrude additional material into the antrum. Serial tomograms of the antrum will show this increasing displacement in some untreated patients.
5. Partial or complete paralysis of cranial motor nerves that supply the extraocular muscles may result, on *rare* occasions, from direct injury of the original trauma.
6. An increase in volume of orbital contents may appear if hematoma and fibrosis develop within the lateral and inferior bony walls of the orbit. This may produce proptosis and marked limitation of eye muscle movement. Such hematomas have also been associated with nerve palsies of the extraocular muscles that recover only after the clot is removed.

All these mechanisms of producing diplopia create some form of muscle imbalance. Merely dropping the level of the globe produces diplopia by causing an associated abnormal stretch, tear, palsy or ankylosis of one or more extraocular muscles. In many instances diplopia associated with orbital floor fractures will not appear until several days, or even weeks, after injury. The initial support of the globe by traumatic edema may mask incipient double vision for as long as six to eight weeks. At this late date, replacement of the fractured fragments is impossible and the eye function and facial deformity may be corrected only by major complex plastic operations involving bone grafting or synthetic implants (Fig. 8–19 *A* to *C*). There is thus good reason to attempt to detect *all* orbit floor fractures during the first few days after injury.

There are two basic types of orbital bone fractures: pure blow-out fractures, and complex orbital fractures associated with middle face fractures.

The simple blow-out is thought to occur from a sudden blow directly on the closed eye, suddenly forcing the globe inward and splintering the thin floor of the orbit by the sudden increase in intraorbital pressure without causing other facial fractures. Although not rare, *this type of fracture is much less common than the orbital fracture associated with other facial fractures.*

There are five cardinal signs that lead one to suspect an orbital bone fracture:

1. Bony deformity and tenderness of infraorbital, or canthal, regions on palpation.
2. Subconjunctival hemorrhage and discoloration of the eyelids.
3. Infraorbital nerve anesthesia of over 24-hours' duration.
4. A measurably lowered position of the center of the pupil of one eye in comparison with the other.
5. Early diplopia (this may disappear after a few hours only to return later). In some patients it may be detected only when the eyes are placed in a single position of gaze.

A surgical exploration of the orbital floor is indicated by the appearance of *any* of the above signs (Fig. 8–17).

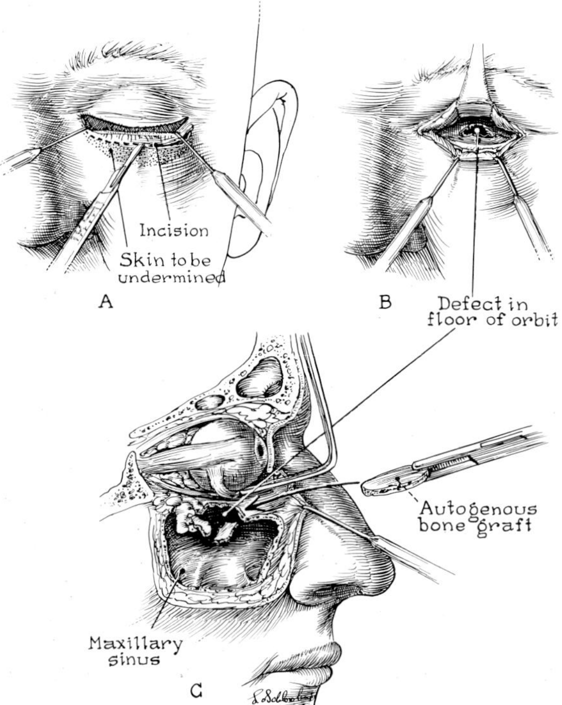

Figure 8–17 This simple method of exploration of the floor of the orbit should be utilized in *all cases with clinical signs suggestive of a possible fracture to the bony floor of the orbit.* The incision should be placed only 2 to 3 mm. below the lash border rather than at a lower level in the eyelid. The orbicularis occuli muscle fibers are gently separated, and the periosteum elevated from the floor of the orbit. An effort should be made not to enter the mucous membrane of the antral cavity. If a defect is encountered in the orbital floor, any completely loose bone fragments in the antrum (C) should be removed and the defect repaired by rotating long orbital floor bone fragments to bridge the opening or by replacement with an autogenous iliac bone graft or a synthetic material such as silicone. Such a procedure will often prevent the late development of diplopia several weeks after injury. If the defect is left unrepaired, movements of the globe tend to cause the migration of fat and other soft tissue into the antrum with resulting enophthalmus.

There are additional diagnostic studies of value:

1. Tomograms of the orbit may show disruptions of the orbital floor or medial wall.

2. Orbitograms may be made by injecting a few milliliters of radiopaque material along the orbital floor and trying to determine if this material leaks through a fracture line. Although of considerable interest, this technique produces both false positive and false negative results. Since orbital floor exploration has proved to be a safe, simple procedure that may be carried out under local anesthesia and with no residual deformity, it remains the most dependable method of establishing the diagnosis of many orbital bone fractures. Certainly the most serious present-day problems associated with zygoma fractures are *associated with the failure to suspect and discover orbital fractures at an early postinjury date.* Routine orbital exploration is advisable in all suspected cases and will uncover many correctable problems. We have twice encountered a sharp bone spicule displaced from the floor of the orbit, standing vertically, and pressing its sharp edge deeply into the sclera. Later perforation of the globe might well have occurred in either or both of these cases had routine exploration not been carried out.

Because of the frequency of missed diagnosis of orbital fractures on clinical and roentgenographic studies, it is now our practice to *expose the orbital floor in all cases of suspected orbital bone fracture.* (See section on treatment.)

TREATMENT OF FRACTURES OF THE ZYGOMATIC COMPOUND AND ORBITAL BONES. Treatment of these fractures varies greatly and depends on the stability or instability of the bone fragments following reduction. Unrotated fractures of the malar compound, like fractures of the zygomatic arch, tend to be relatively stable on reduction. Many will remain in good position as a result of the support offered by normal muscular attachments to the bone and by impaction of the fragments at the time of reduction. Certain types of fractures consistently require supplementary fixation after reduction. These include laterally rotated fractures of the body of the malar compound, fractures involving the dense central eminence of the malar compound, and unrotated fractures with gross medial displacement and extensive impaction and comminution of bone.

Until recent years, support and fixation of zygoma and antral fractures was obtained commonly by the use of folded gauze packing placed within the antrum by means of the traditional Caldwell-Luc exposure. This approach involves an incision behind the upper lip in the canine fossa and the removal of a bony window from the anterior antral wall. Although this method of antral packing gives adequate bony support, the reductions are inexact and morbidity is greater than with newer methods. Late complications that have been reported after antral packing include diplopia, malunion, residual facial deformity on subsidence of edema, and even blindness from pressure of the pack against the optic nerve. Antral secretions tend to be blocked from egress; temperature elevations and persistent facial edema may be related to packing; thin bony fragments of the antral wall or orbital floor are sometimes distracted from one another by overpacking or they may later be pulled out of position by catching on the pack at the time of its removal. Thickening of the antral mucosa is a common sequel of this method of management. Such complications may be largely eliminated by newer methods of direct wire fixation of bony fragments.

Antral packs are of historical interest, but our experience has been similar to that recently reported by Dingman and Natvig.[6] We have also encountered many instances of zygomatic fractures in which antral packing and methods of closed reduction have failed to secure ideal replacement of bony parts. When such fractures are treated by open reduction, it becomes apparent that roentgenographic and clinical examinations frequently fail to reveal the degree of displacement. Open reduction and direct wiring of displacements of the zygoma may be carried out through the associated facial lacerations or small esthetic incisions. This "jigsaw puzzle concept" of replacing facial fractures and attaching each piece of bone to its neighbor with fine wire probably constitutes one of the greatest twentieth century advances in the treatment of maxillofacial injuries. The wiring should be based on some remaining portion of the skull that is stable and unfractured, and the surgeon should then wire the more mobile fragments.

To expose fractures of the orbital floor, a single incision is made about 3 mm. below the lash border of the lower eyelid (Fig. 8–17*A*). Since 1971 the author has explored the orbit by means of an incision made through the *conjunctival* surface of the lower lid. This incision is approximately 3 millimeters below the border of the lower lid and extends across its entire width. A very adequate exposure of the bony floor of the orbit is obtained in this manner. The incision is closed with three 6–0 plain catgut sutures, and the subciliary skin incision shown in Figure 8–17 may be avoided. If actual wiring of fractures along the orbital rim is required, the skin incision in the lid is preferable to one through the conjunctiva. It is a matter of only a few minutes' dissection to separate the orbicularis muscle fibers, incise the orbital septum and elevate the periosteum of the orbital floor (Fig. 8–17*B*). The surgeon may then detect displacements in this region far more accurately than is possible by tomograms, planograms or orbitograms. Such explorations are benign surgical procedures with the fine line scar hidden in a normal eyelid crease.

When large sections of the orbital floor are missing or badly crushed, some support must be provided to prevent ptosis of the globe into the antrum. The use of a thin sliver of autogenous bone from the patient's iliac crest is highly satisfactory (Fig. 8–17*C*). Recently thin sheets of Teflon, silicone, or synthetic collagen have been substituted for the bone. These synthetic materials give adequate support but they have a tendency to migrate or extrude because of their nonadherent surfaces. If used, they should always be perforated and anchored in position to the orbital bone with nonabsorbable sutures. Synthetic implants are best avoided when there are large losses of the mucous membrane lining to the roof of the antral cavity. When they are inserted without adequate soft tissue cover, draining sinus tracts will form, leading into the antrum or orbit or out through the eyelid skin.

With acute simple inward and downward displacements of the malar compound, it is sometimes possible to reduce the fracture by passing a curved metal blunt urethral No. 18 sound through the thin medial bony wall of the antrum in the area just beneath the inferior nasal turbinate (Fig. 8–18*A*). The top of this sound may then be used to elevate the dense central portion of the malar compound, forcing it outward to match the bony contour of the opposite cheek. This will produce effective reduction, especially in the case of an unrotated fracture of the zygomatic compound (Fig. 8–18 *B* and *C*). In most instances, this form of reduction should be combined with small skin incisions placed beneath the lower eyelid and also at the suture line. These incisions permit direct interosseous wiring and secure the fragments in a reduced position.

If reduction is not effected within a few hours, severe facial edema or the condition of the patient may complicate immediate reduction and make it advisable to utilize local hypothermia (ice packs) and defer operation for several days. It is unwise to let the patient go without fracture reduction for more than two weeks

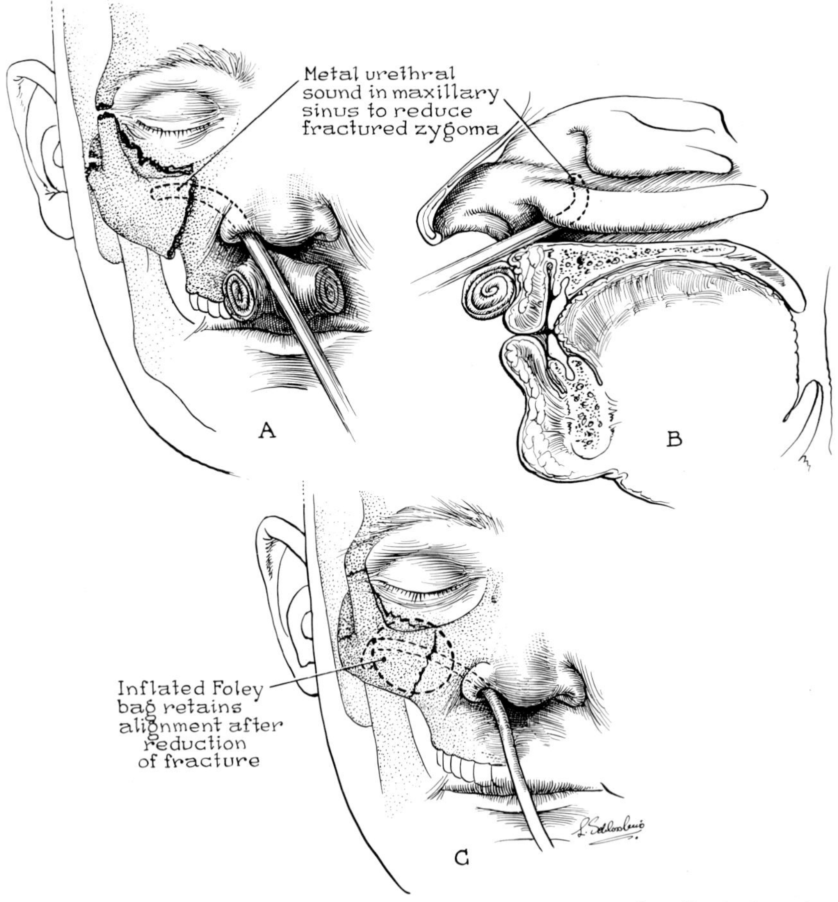

Figure 8–18 Early nonrotated fractures of the zygoma may at times be effectively reduced by the simple insertion of a metal urethral sound through the thin medial wall of the antrum by means of the nasal cavity. The tip of the sound may then be directed up beneath the solid central portion of the malar bone and a leverage action brought to bear against the bone from within. The roll of gauze acts as a fulcrum to protect the upper lip, and strong outward force can then be brought to bear on the zygoma. At times the bone will actually be heard to "click" back into place. If the zygoma does not remain stable in the reduced position, a Foley bag catheter can be inserted by the same route and the bag inflated until the bone receives adequate support.

following injury, lest the zygoma become firmly fixed in a position of malunion. McCoy et al.[14] have wisely pointed out the dangers and disadvantages of using the traditional Caldwell-Luc incision (made through the mucosa of the canine fossa behind the upper lip) and of placing gauze packing into the antrum postoperatively. Most plastic surgeons avoid using this approach whenever possible. Eyebrows should not be shaved nor eyelashes trimmed in carrying out reductions of facial fractures. Occasional patients have considerable difficulty in regrowing these specialized types of hair.

It is frequently possible to reduce bleeding during the reduction of facial fractures by injecting the fracture sites with small amounts of local anesthetic containing epinephrine solution 1:120,000. Once the bone fragments are loosened, fixation of the zygoma should begin with its reattachment to the firm zygomatic process of the frontal bone by a single steel wire placed through holes drilled on either side of this suture line. Attention is then turned to the fracture lines located along the infraorbital rim. Again, small drill holes are made with a power drill on either side of the fracture line and a steel wire loop is placed to fix the medial end of the fragment. The zygomaticofrontal incision may next be used to insert a long elevator behind the zygomaticotemporal process to elevate and further rotate this process outward and upward. If the arch of the zygoma is also fractured with these injuries, it may be reduced with fine wire sutures by means of a small direct transverse incision over the fracture line or by the method shown in Figure 8–15. Fractures of the floor of the orbit are always present when the zygoma is fractured.

At times the collection of blood and bone fragments within the antrum makes it necessary to explore and debride this cavity. In such instances the Caldwell-Luc exposure through the canine fossa is satisfactory. In opening the antrum, an attempt should be made to retain soft tissue attachments to as much as possible of the bone of the anterior antral wall. Careful irrigation of the cavity and removal of clots will often reveal that much of the antral mucous membrane may be preserved.

In former years many complex headcaps were devised for stabilizing zygomatic and nasal fractures. These have proved to be rarely desirable or necessary in reducing fractures of the zygomatic compound. It is the exceptional patient who benefits from this type of fixation today. In the case of zygomatic compound fractures that remain unstable after direct interosseous wiring and reduction, the suspension wire technique originally described by Adams[1] is of great value (Fig. 8–22). When the zygomatic compound is not repositioned within the first two weeks after injury, it is sometimes very difficult to loosen the bone fragments at the time of the delayed operation. In such cases, very complex late reconstructive procedures, including contour bone grafting and multiple osteotomies, may be required. Even then the result is likely to be only partly satisfactory.

In recent years it has been possible to correct double vision in approximately 80 per cent of patients with persistent traumatic diplopia that resulted from improperly reduced zygomatic compound and orbital floor fractures. This has been achieved at The Johns Hopkins Hospital by means of surgical restoration of lost orbital contents and globe support through use of wedges of the iliac bone to lift and position the eye (Fig. 8–19 *A* to *D*). A careful ophthalmologic consultation is desirable to rule out associated paralysis of extraocular muscles before undertaking the correction of "displacement diplopia" resulting from skeletal malposition with "dropped globe" or from fixation of the inferior rectus muscle in the orbital floor fracture line.

FRACTURES OF THE MAXILLAE (MIDDLE-FACE FRACTURES)

Incidence. The upper jaw is formed by the two maxillae and the paired palatine bone. At The Johns Hopkins Hospital, fractures of the upper jaw occur about one-third as commonly as fractures of the mandible. These fractures are known in Canada by the colorful term of "midface mash."[8] The ability of the maxillae to absorb great energy in the process of fracturing offers considerable protection to the cranium and its contents. It is a particularly common injury following crashes in automobiles or planes where the passengers must sit facing forward. There has been a strange reluctance of designers of commercial airplanes to face seats rearward despite increasing evidence that this position will greatly reduce injuries on

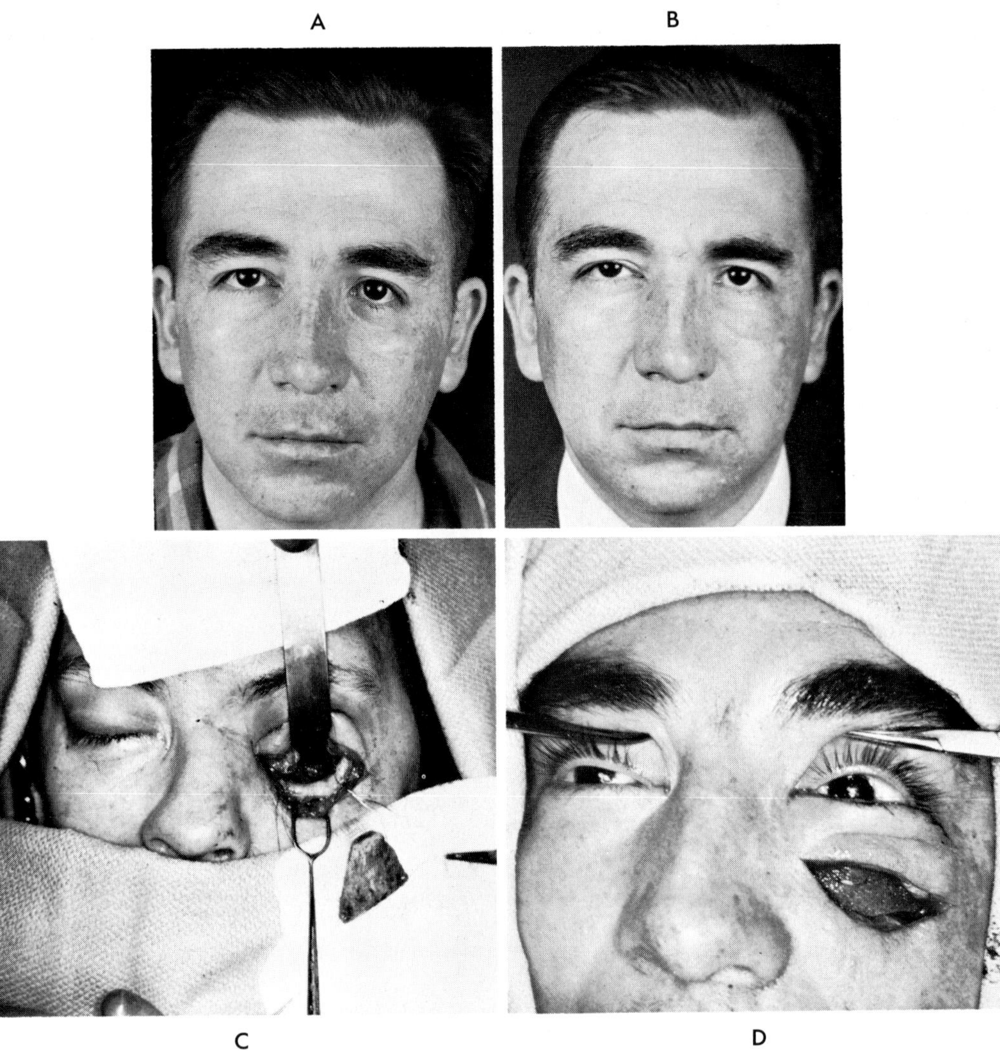

Figure 8–19 This patient had a fracture of the zygomatic compound with incomplete early reduction resulting in the left lower eyelid and dropping of the globe shown in *A*. He had troublesome double vision which prevented him from carrying out his occupation as an airplane pilot. Elevation of the left globe and complete relief of the diplopia was achieved two and a half years after the injury by means of bony reconstruction of the left orbit. *C* shows the badly displaced infraorbital rim at exploration. The periosteum was elevated, and approximately 8 cc. of iliac bone was fitted in along the inferior and lateral walls of the orbit in order to provide additional volume of orbital content. This tends to correct existing enophthalmus and to stretch forward the cone of extraocular muscles once again. It is firmly wired into position with two steel wires. *D* indicates the usual amount of overcorrection allowed in obtaining the level of the globe. Many complex late plastic repairs could be avoided by a more aggressive approach to reconstruction of the bony orbit at the time of the primary injury. The final result is shown in *B*. The diplopia was corrected, and the patient is now active as a pilot.

crash. As with the membrane bones of the face, secondary muscle contraction and spasm play only a very small role in the displacement of maxillary fractures; the original impact produces the entire deformity.

Classification. In 1900 René LeFort[13] carried out classic experiments to determine the portions of greatest weakness within the maxilla. His work has resulted in a classification of fractures of the maxilla that is now widely used.

LeFort carried out over 40 experiments, mostly upon cadavers, inflicting trauma to the face and studying the resulting nature of fractures. He concluded:

> Fractures of the face, although they are not frequent, nevertheless are much less rare than we have thought and most of them are not discovered by the physician. And . . . quite rarely, nevertheless, the base of the cranium is involved in these fractures. This hardly ever occurs except by bilateral compression of the head, that is, by pressure applied not only to the cranium but also to the face. In such cases, the cranium may be fractured. One almost always notices the independence of the cranium from the face at the pterygoid apophyses and at the lateral plates of the ethmoid which, anatomically, being rather to the face than to the cranium, and which adhere to the maxilla. . . . The most frequent fracture which we have obtained in our experiments corresponds to the great transverse fracture of Guérin. It includes the roof of the palate, the alveolar ridge, and the pterygoid apophyses.

Surgeons and dentists alike have tried to treat fractures of the maxilla with a multiplicity of external appliances to hold these bones in position. Only in recent years, with the advent of the surgical publications by Milton Adams,[1] Reed Dingman,[6] Fredrick McCoy[14] and others, has direct surgical reduction replaced the external appliance methods. The most widely used classification is based on LeFort's early studies.

LEFORT I FRACTURES (transverse maxillary fractures of Guérin). This in a transverse fracture in which the fractured segment contains the upper teeth, the palate, lower portions of the pterygoid processes, and a portion of the wall of the maxillary sinus (Fig. 8–20).

LEFORT II FRACTURES (pyramidal fractures). In these fractures the fractured fragment also contains the nasal bones and the frontal processes of the maxilla (Fig. 8–21). The fracture lines usually run through the lacrimal bones and inferior rim of the orbit, continuing downward near the zygomaticomaxillary suture. The fracture line then extends beneath the malar bone toward the pterygomaxillary fossa. This often produces significant widening of the inner canthus of the eyes, epicanthal deformity of the bridge of the nose and destruction of the ethmoidal sinus cells.

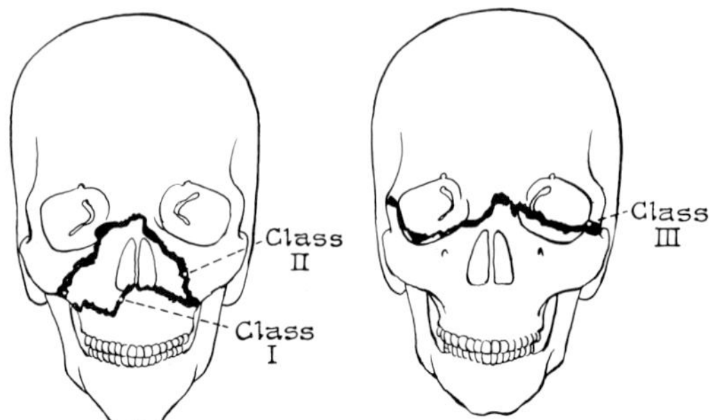

Figure 8–20 The three major patterns of fracture line seen in middle face fractures were first described by LeFort in 1900 and often assume one of the three classifications shown here. The class I fracture is also known as a transverse maxillary fracture or a Guérin fracture. The class II fracture usually includes the nose in the mobile central fragment and is known often as a pyramidal fracture. The class III fracture includes also both zygomatic compounds in the mobile fragment and is referred to frequently as a craniofacial disjunction. At times, fracture lines may exist in two or three of these classic patterns in a single patient. They represent the lines of least strength in the facial bone skeleton.

LEFORT III FRACTURES (craniofacial disjunction). In this fracture, the maxilla, nasal bones and zygomatic compound are all separated as a unit from the cranial attachments (Fig. 8–20). Such injuries usually involve multiple additional fractures within this large mobile segment and, on healing, the patient will be troubled by severe elongation deformity of the central face unless vigorous measures are taken to combat this during early treatment (Fig. 8–22).

In addition to the three major types of LeFort fractures, one may see verti-

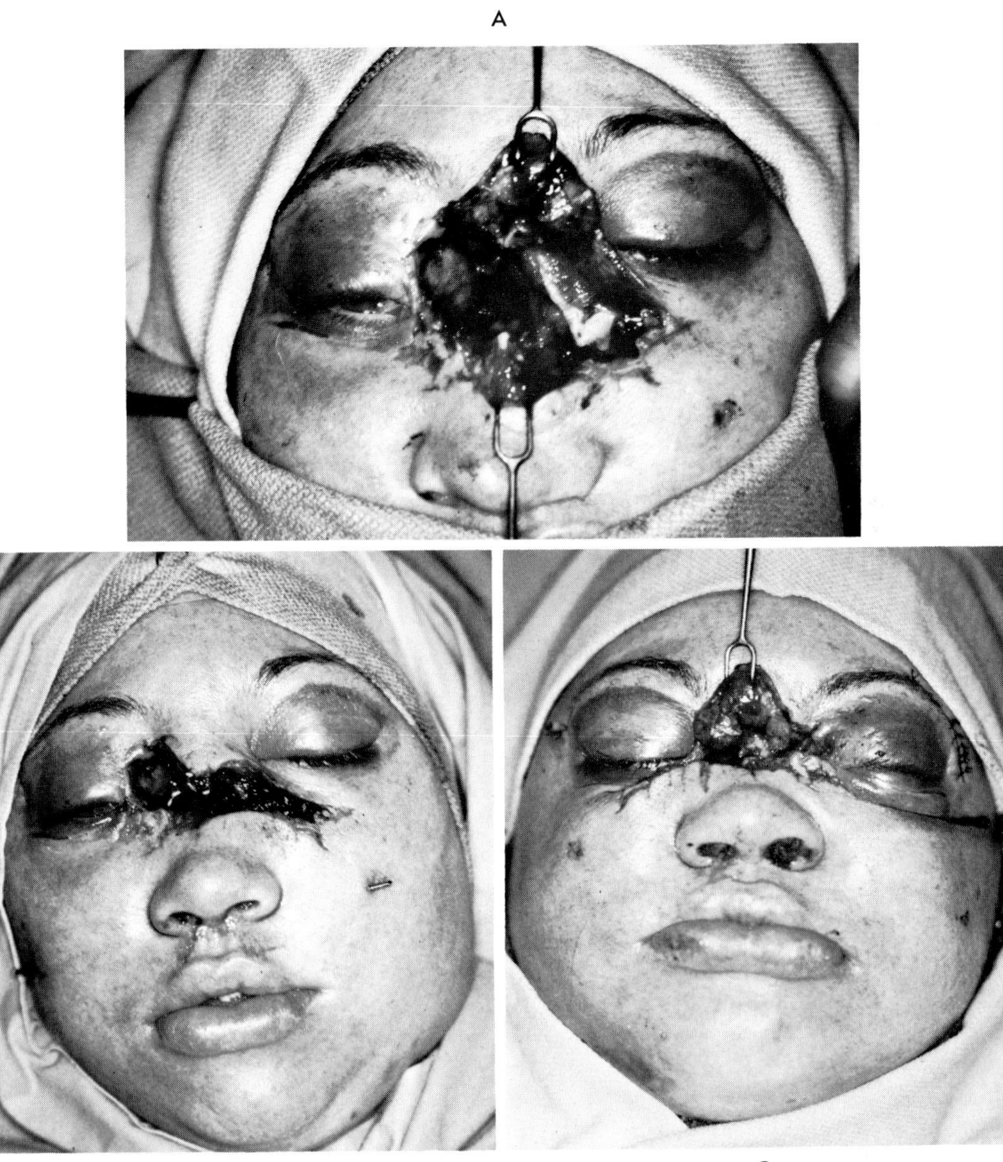

Figure 8–21 This young woman was thrown into the steering post of her car in a head-on collision and suffered a severe midface mash, with pyramidal fractures involving the bridge of the nose and left side of the right eye and the marked loss of bone in the region of the nasal bridge and ethmoids. Initial hemorrhage was difficult to control even with packing. In *B* arch bars have been applied, and the teeth are in good occlusion. The multiple maxillary and antral fractures have been further stabilized by a transverse Kirschner wire pin as advocated by Brown.[4] The eye is still unsupported, and the central face is still elongated. In *C* a craniomaxillary suspension wire has been applied on the right side (see Fig. 8–22), and the mobile central face has been lifted upward to restore the normal relationship between eyes and mouth. The soft tissue wounds were then repaired primarily, and a later bone graft to the bridge of the nose restored facial balance.

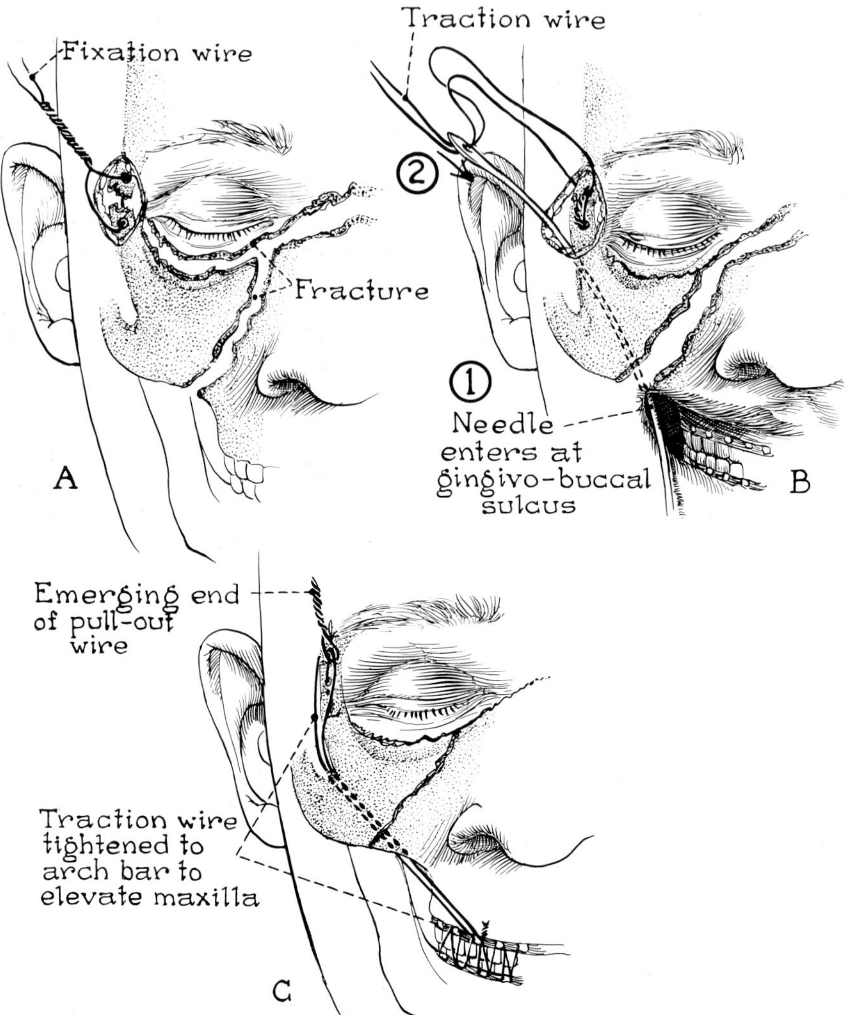

Figure 8–22 For a unilateral or bilateral LeFort III fracture, a method is needed to secure the central face firmly against the base of the skull to avoid facial elongation. This method of craniofacial suspension is of great value. The zygomaticofrontal suture line is first reunited with steel wire and drill holes, fixing the zygoma firmly to nonfractured frontal bone. A double loop of steel wire is then passed through the drill hole in the frontal bone and drawn subcutaneously behind the zygoma to emerge in the buccogingival sulcus as shown in *B*. An arch bar may then be applied to the upper arch, and the two ends of the suspension wire are passed about this arch bar at an appropriate location to provide strong upward and lateral traction to the central bony fragments of the face. After three weeks the ends of the wire are cut free of the arch bar behind the upper lip, and the pull-out wire in the region of the brow is used to withdraw the entire suspension wire loop.

cal or segmental fractures through the maxilla which may separate portions of the central face near the midline. Fractures may also occur horizontally through portions of the upper alveolar ridge, or the entire maxilla may be driven upward and backward into the interorbital space.

Diagnosis. Middle-face fractures often produce dish-face deformities in which the patient develops an elongation of the vertical distance between the lips and the eyes. If the surgeon has not seen the patient prior to the injury he may fail to recognize this facial elongation, especially in the presence of severe facial edema.

Malocclusion, involving open-bite deformity and considerable conjunctival and labial edema, may be seen. Mobility of the maxilla is a cardinal feature of such fractures and may be detected by the examiner's ability to manually move the anterior hard palate and alveolus (Fig. 8–3). Severely impacted fractures may lack this mobility. Malocclusion is not always present, even in the presence of complete craniofacial disjunction, and the surgeon should not be falsely reassured by finding good dental occlusion. The appearance of a watery fluid issuing from the nostrils, and having a salty taste to the patient, should suggest damage to the cribriform plate. Stereoscopic roentgenograms in the Water's position provide an excellent x-ray view for visualizing these fractures. Planograms, using an eccentrically moving source of roentgen rays, may give beautiful bone detail. One should look for disruptions of the frontomaxillary sutures, step irregularities in the infraorbital regions or breaks in the continuity of the lateral wall of the sinus.

Treatment. A severe midface mash may produce severe upper respiratory obstruction by impaction of palatal and maxillary bone posteriorly and inferiorly into the oropharynx; as concomitant edema develops in the supraglottic area, obstruction increases. Emergency reduction of this fracture may be accomplished by the examiner if he will hook his fingers about the displaced posterior border of the soft palate and pull forward the fractured bones of the central face. This maneuver may simultaneously establish both the diagnosis and the patient's airway. Hemorrhage can be severe with maxillary fracture because of rupture of the internal maxillary or greater palatine arteries. Massive bleeding from the nose in these patients is usually from multiple tears in the highly vascular mucous membranes of the septum or nasal turbinates. This bleeding may be controlled by inserting a one-inch diameter gauze behind the soft palate and drawing it forward against the posterior choanae. This pack is placed in the nasopharynx with the aid of two rubber catheters passed through the nasal cavity along each side of the septum to emerge in the oropharynx. The pharyngeal tips of the catheters are then grasped by a clamp and are drawn forward through the lips. Each catheter tip is then secured with a heavy silk suture to one end of a wide postnasal pack. The latter is then pulled into the posterior choanae by traction on the nasal catheters. Additional packing of the nose or even ligation of the external carotid arteries may be required.

Middle-face fractures were formerly managed in many clinics by the use of plaster head-caps, external pin fixation and elaborate dental splints. Greater experience has shown these to be unnecessarily complicated, unsatisfactory in securing reduction and unpleasant to the patient. In recent years, the concept of open surgical exposure and direct fitting together of the pieces of the bony puzzle has gained widespread acceptance. The combined use of interosseous wiring and suspension sling support has markedly improved the results in the treatment of these complex facial fractures. When the mandibular arch is intact, LeFort I (transverse maxillary) fractures may be reduced, and occlusion may be restored, by applying arch bars to upper and lower jaws (Fig. 8–7). To avoid elongation of the middle-face, two wires are then placed through drill holes in each infraorbital rim. The wires are next passed downward through the subcutaneous tissue of the cheeks to emerge in the buccogingival sulcus. The maxilla is firmly pressed superiorly into normal position, closing the fracture lines, and the two suspension wires are tightened about an arch bar previously applied to the upper teeth.

LeFort II fractures (Fig. 8–20) are often displaced posteriorly and require a loosening of the fragments and a bringing forward of the maxillae if the teeth are to regain normal occlusion. Again, intermaxillary wiring and arch bars may be applied if sufficient teeth remain for fixation. In most LeFort II fractures, maxillary suspension wires may be passed downward subcutaneously from anchoring drill holes or wire loops that have been placed through the zygomatic process of the frontal bone. These wires emerge through the mucosa in the sulcus behind the upper lip, and there they may be twisted securely to the upper arch bar. As the wires are tightened, the dental line will rise and the central face will again shorten to its normal length (Fig. 8–22). Small pullout wire loops can be passed around the upper anchor points of these suspension wires to aid in their removal after approximately three weeks. Individual transosseous wire loops may be placed through tiny drill holes at any other major fracture lines (especially along the infraorbital rims or at fracture lines of the lacrimal bones). These provide further security and reduction of the lesser bone fragments.

LeFort III (craniofacial disjunction) fractures require combination methods of fixation because of the multiple fracture lines that involve the nasal bones, the zygoma, the maxillae and, often, the palatine bones. Such combinations make use of the usually intact frontal bone for application of craniofacial suspension wires (Fig. 8–22). If intact, the mandibular arch (or one restored by open reduction and wiring) is used as a guide to positioning of the maxillary fragments for proper occlusion. The surgeon must remember that simple wiring of the teeth in the fractured upper jaw to the teeth in an intact mandible may restore perfect dental occlusion, but *leave uncorrected an associated elongation of the central face.* Edema may obscure this deformity initially, but if not recognized and treated early, the patient will be left with a distressing "dish-face" deformity. *The late correction of this deformity is both complex and unsatisfactory in contrast to the excellent results that may be obtained with good emergency management* (Fig. 8–23).

In the event that the mandibular arch is also fractured, it should be realigned by open reduction and direct interosseous wiring in order to provide a proper lower arch as a guideline for the establishment of occlusion in positioning the upper arch bone fragments. Thus, if the surgeon will follow an orderly plan in facial reductions, working from nonfractured stable bony points to unstable areas, he may be able to replace the pieces of the puzzle quite satisfactorily. In the absence of dentition, if the patient possesses an intact denture, the surgeon may fasten this to the upper or lower jaw by circumferential or direct osseous wiring. The denture may then be drilled to permit the attachment of an ordinary arch bar and utilized much like the patient's remaining natural teeth in securing a normal bite relationship.

WIDE BRIDGE AND EPICANTHAL DEFORMITIES OF THE NASAL AND INFRAORBITAL REGION

With many severe blows to the region of the bridge of the nose, the nasal bridge is comminuted, and the thin ethmoid bone of each medial orbital wall is badly crushed and carried posteriorly.

These injuries are often seen in automobile accidents when the face strikes the dashboard or the steering wheel. If the force of the impact is in the region of the glabella above the nasofrontal suture line, the anterior wall of the frontal sinus is often fractured inward. If the impact is somewhat lower, over the nasal bridge, the major displacement is in the interorbital structures. The frontal processes and nasal bones may then be driven backward as a unit between the eyes. The

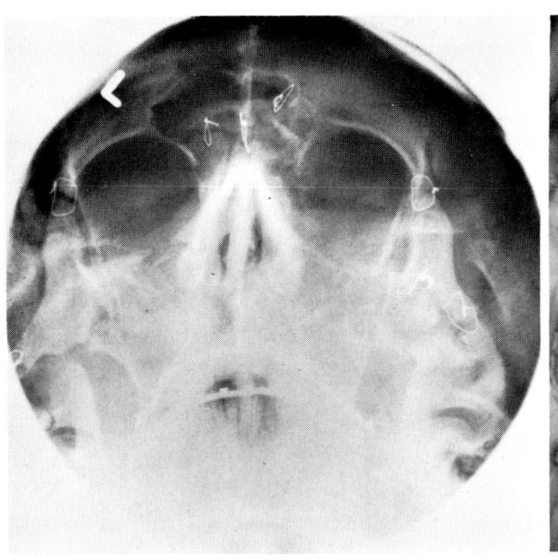

A

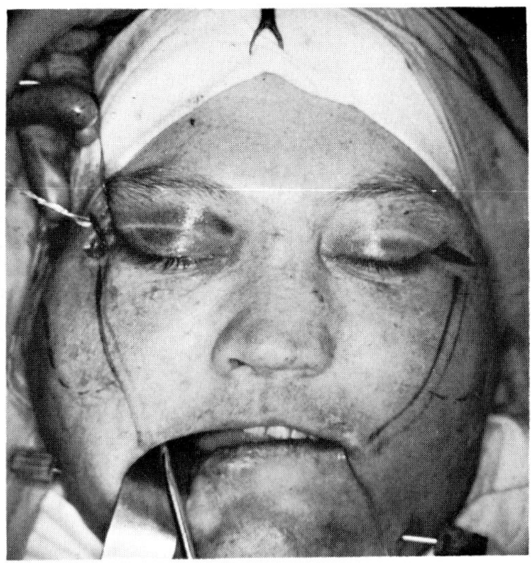

B

Figure 8–23 Complete craniofacial disjunction occurred in this patient when he was forced to make a crash landing in his private plane and was thrown forcefully against a padded panel. The x-ray shows multiple fracture lines involving bilateral class I, II and III LeFort fractures. The nose was also badly fractured. The mandibular arch was broken in three places, but no major facial lacerations occurred! Reduction was secured by the application of arch bars and intermaxillary elastic traction, by multiple transosseous wiring of the frontal and zygomatic bones, and by bilateral craniomaxillary suspension wires attached to the upper arch bar as shown in *B*. Note that additional fixation of the mandibular arch was achieved by a transverse Kirschner wire passed through the lower border of the mandible behind an unstable fracture in the region of the right mental foramen. It was not necessary or desirable to pack this man's antral cavities with gauze through a Caldwell-Luc exposure. In *B* the left craniomaxillary suspension wire has already been placed and may be seen emerging from the left corner of the patient's mouth. A Saunder's fascial needle has been passed behind the right zygoma and is about to be used to draw the right suspension wire along the course marked by ink on the cheek and out of the buccogingival sulcus.

orbital rims are fractured and there is telescoping of the ethmoidal plates and frequently a fracture of the skull base. Cerebrospinal rhinorrhea is common in these injuries. The medial orbital walls are pressed laterally by the force and impinge on the medial rectus muscles. The surgeon's problem is to find a method of reconstructing the bony anterior ethmoidal labyrinth.

In many of these patients the nasofrontal ducts will be obliterated blocking the frontal sinus. The anterior ethmoidal artery may be lacerated and produce extensive hemorrhage. The trochlea of the superior oblique muscle may be displaced or fractured producing diplopia, and a high percentage of such patients are left with a deforming traumatic hypertelorism. This type of fracture is one of the most difficult of maxillofacial injuries to correct; and, on many occasions, the plastic surgeon may wish help of a neurosurgeon to effect correction. In such instances a combined intracranial and extracranial surgical approach may offer many advantages.

If the lacrimal apparatus has been damaged, the discharge of watery tears into the wound may be confused with cerebrospinal fluid as both will give a test for reducing substances. Clarification may be obtained by placing fluorescein dye in the lumbar subarachnoid space and inserting cotton pledgets within the nose in the sphenoid-ethmoidal recess. If these pledgets are examined with a Wood's light, after thirty minutes the presence of spinal fluid leakage and its location may be established. With such "bridge bashes" it is extremely difficult, by ordinary traction devices or even by lashing lead plate splints against the lateral walls of the nose, to re-elevate the nasal bridge to a normal position and regain a normal shape to the inner canthal regions. In such patients it is of significant help to make small longitudinal incisions anterior to the canthal ligament on either side of the nasion (Fig. 8–24). Through these incisions, the periosteum may be elevated along the medial bony wall of each orbit to expose the fractured ethmoid cells. It may then be possible to gently insert an opened, large, smooth, long-bladed forceps, such as

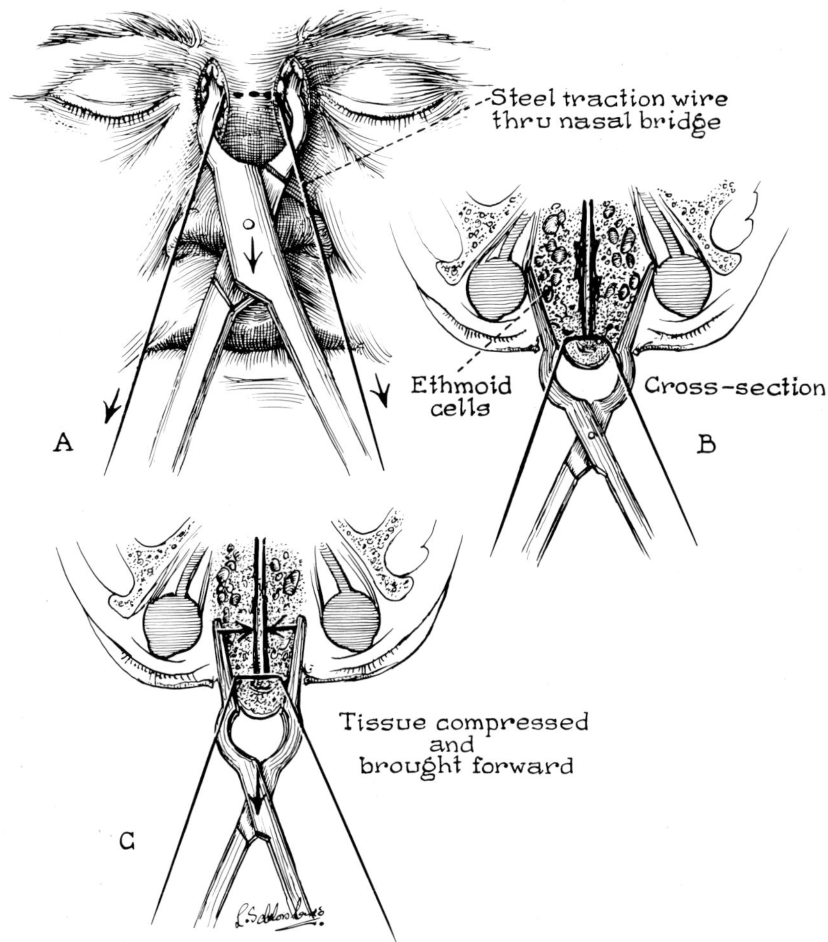

Figure 8–24 When a head-on blow crushes the nasal bridge back into the ethmoid region, aggressive methods of early reduction are necessary to prevent permanent severe deformity about the nose and inner canthi. Bone of the nasal bridge is often forced toward the corner of the eye on either side, and reduction of the nasal fractures may not correct this deformity. Two longitudinal incisions may be made as shown in (*A*), and a heavy traction wire may be passed through the dense bone of the nasion. The periosteum along the medial wall of each orbit may then be carefully elevated for a distance of approximately 3 cm. An assistant is then asked to exert strong forward traction on the steel wire through the nasal bridge while the operator uses a wide-jawed and flat-bladed clamp to gently manipulate the ethmoid bone back toward the midline. In this way, a molding and bringing forward of the bridge of the nose may be accomplished during the first few days after such fractures. It is almost impossible to accomplish this reduction once the bones have healed firmly into position.

the Asche or Walsham forceps, and gently compress the widened ethmoid bones back to the midline. The two blades of the clamp may be placed first superior to the attachment of both internal canthal ligaments and firm pressure then exerted in closing the jaws of the clamp. The maneuver is repeated with the blades of the clamp passed inferior to the canthal ligaments.

The forward reduction of the nasal bridge may be further aided if strong anterior traction is applied to a thin padded elevator placed within the nasal cavity alongside the upper nasal septum. If the inner canthal ligaments have been split away from the bony nose, they may be wired to one another across the midline by use of a small drill hole placed through the nasal bridge. This operative reduction of the bridge bash seems to be effective only if applied to the face within one week after injury. Within that period it can be very helpful in preventing epicanthus deformity and pseudohypertelorism.

FRACTURES OF FRONTAL BONE AND SINUS

In cases of frontal sinus fracture, surgeons formerly recommended that all sinus membrane be removed and that the bony cavity be collapsed inward. This technique of "obliteration of the sinus" is almost always unnecessary and is quite deforming.

When the anterior wall of the frontal sinus has been fractured, care should be taken to reduce it and wire it accurately in place. At the same time, the mucous membrane lining and cavity of the sinus should be explored and irrigated. The nasofrontal duct should be gently probed to be sure that it has not been obliterated by the fracture. The insertion of a metal dilator will often reopen a collapsed nasofrontal duct and, if necessary, a catheter can be placed within this channel as a stent so that one end extends into the nasal cavity. If the posterior wall of the frontal sinus has been fractured, the sinus may still be preserved, provided the patient is protected from the development of pneumatocele (readily detected by postoperative x-ray) and from unrecognized injury to the dura with resultant spinal fluid leak. Over the past 15 years, the author has found it unnecessary to surgically obliterate a single frontal sinus following injury!

In the absence of displacement of the frontal bone, the appearance of an air-fluid level on sinus x-ray several days after surgery is highly suggestive of damage to the nasofrontal duct and suggests further study. If unrecognized, such complications can lead to mucoceles or mucopyoceles.

FRACTURES OF THE FACIAL BONES IN CHILDREN

Every emergency room team is asked to care for children whose faces were injured in automobile accidents. Usually they have been sitting, without protection of seat belt, between parents on the front seat of the family car. The child is usually frightened and uncooperative, and the face is often badly swollen. The mother is sometimes hysterical. Clinical examination of the damaged facial bones of such a child will be difficult. The nasal cavity is so small that it is difficult to insert a speculum or light. X-rays are badly obscured by the multiple unerupted tooth buds present through the upper and lower jaws of all small children. Paranasal sinuses may not yet be pneumatized. A number of deciduous teeth may be missing, and the child may be totally unable to indicate whether his dental occlusion is satisfactory. In the absence of grossly displaced fractures or other injuries, there is a strong temptation for the surgeon to send the child home and to recommend the application of ice compresses to the face and ask the parents to bring the child back to the clinic two weeks later, "when the swelling has subsided." This temptation should be avoided.

Facial bone fractures are relatively uncommon in children, comprising only about 4 per cent of the total number of facial fractures. Fortunately, children have very resilient bone that stands considerable trauma without fracture or, in many instances, with only a greenstick deformity. Young bone is highly vascular and heals very rapidly. It is also more resistant to infection than is adult bone. The paranasal sinuses are small and cause little problem in fractures of the facial bones of children. Several precautions should be stressed in the management of childhood facial fractures; several problems of treatment arise with children that are not seen in adults.

Injury to immature facial bones will sometimes result in the arrest of growth, which may not manifest itself until some years later. This is most likely when the growing suture lines near the base of the skull are displaced. Some surgeons have also reported overgrowth of injured facial bones in children. It is our impression that this is *not* true overgrowth, but rather is the result of early malunion and an increase in asymmetry of the deformity associated with continued growth on the normal side of the face. This is a particularly common problem when a fracture involves the neck of the mandibular condyle. Such a fracture in a small child may be followed by severe progressive asymmetry of the face and by shifting of the chin both backward and toward the side of the injury as the child gets older.

Teeth are small and easily dislodged in children. The roots of deciduous teeth may be partially resorbed at the time of injury. Such teeth may be readily aspirated when dislodged and may produce pulmonary abscesses if they are not discovered and removed. When deciduous teeth are lost prematurely, there is often abnormal underdevelopment of the alveolar bone and adjacent mandible or maxilla. Between the ages of six and 12 children have a period of "mixed" dentition in which the deciduous teeth have such small roots that they will not adequately permit secure attachment of arch bars, and the permanent teeth are likely to be insufficiently erupted to be of value. Tooth buds almost always lie in the fracture line of mandibular or maxillary fractures in small children. If these buds are injured by the fracture or the reduction, dental eruption may be delayed.

Fracture dislocations of the mandibular condyle are so commonly followed in children by severe growth asymmetry that it is usually wise to attempt gentle open reduction and repositioning of the mandibular condyle. This may best be carried out by a retroauricular incision that divides the full circumference of the external canal and permits the surgeon to reflect the ear, parotid gland and facial nerve forward in a single unit in order to expose the fractured condyle. If it is evident that some portion of the face is not developing properly following injury, it may be wise to build up that portion of the anatomy with pedicle flaps and bone or even with various synthetic implants. This will serve to minimize psychologic damage to the child and to keep the soft tissues under sufficient stretch stimulus to provide an adequate pocket for later bone grafting. At adolescence an adult-sized bone graft can be inserted at the time of removal of the synthetic implant.

If the above considerations are kept in mind, the management of facial bone fractures in children will respond well to the methods utilized in the treatment of adults.

INJURIES TO SPECIALIZED FACIAL FEATURES

Eyelids and Orbit. Eyelid skin is the thinnest skin on the surface of the body. As a result, it is difficult to replace it exactly with skin grafting, and the lid is susceptible to massive

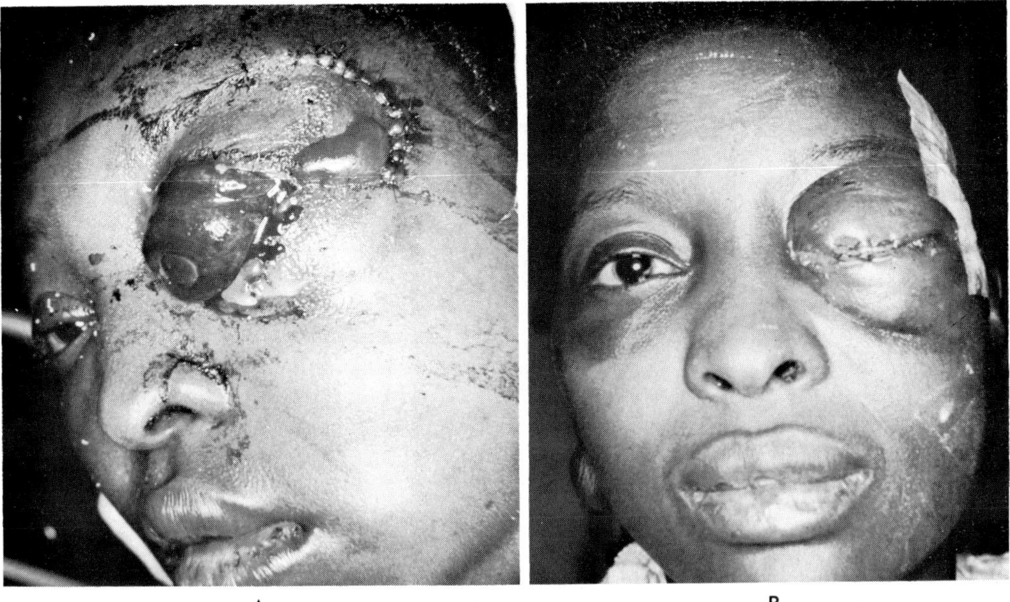

Figure 8–25 *A* and *B*, This patient suffered class III fractures of the frontal bone, orbit and zygoma. Rapidly developing hemorrhage and ocular edema produced the severe proptosis and chemosis of the left eye. A protective double tarsorrhaphy performed earlier would have prevented much of this complication. In order to protect the cornea from drying and ulceration, a full lid closure was carried out as shown in *B*, and a compression dressing was used to further bring about resolution of the severe edema. Loss of a major portion of an eyelid requires urgent reconstruction to protect the cornea from secondary perforation.

edema which may produce stretching and rupture of elastic fibers and permanent lid striae (Fig. 8–25*B*). Eyelid skin withstands thermal injury poorly because of its thinness. Slight displacements of the mobile skin during healing may produce secondary deformities of the lash border, which are very troublesome to the patient from the standpoint of both appearance and function.

Severe injuries to the lids and orbit call for protection of the cornea by early closure of the eyelids with or without suturing and by the application of a firm compression dressing to control traumatic edema. If this is not done, proptosis and severe conjunctival edema may follow, producing disability and deformity similar to that shown in Figure 8–25*A*. Even then, it may be possible to protect the cornea by performing a tarsorrhaphy between the upper and lower eyelids until the traumatic edema subsides (Fig. 8–25*B*). The closed eyelid is also the best possible treatment for corneal abrasions that may have occurred with the original injury. (See Chapter Seven.) At times, lacerations involving the region of the inner canthus of the eyelids may divide one of the canaliculi on its route from the eyelid to the nose. The loss of the lower canaliculus is more important than loss of the upper and is likely to result in troublesome epiphora if not corrected. It is usually possible to find the two ends of a freshly divided canaliculus and repair them by the method illustrated in Figure 8–26. In the past few years the use of microsurgical techniques has greatly improved the reliability of reconstructive methods on small structures such as canaliculi, facial nerves, the parotid duct and small but important blood vessels.

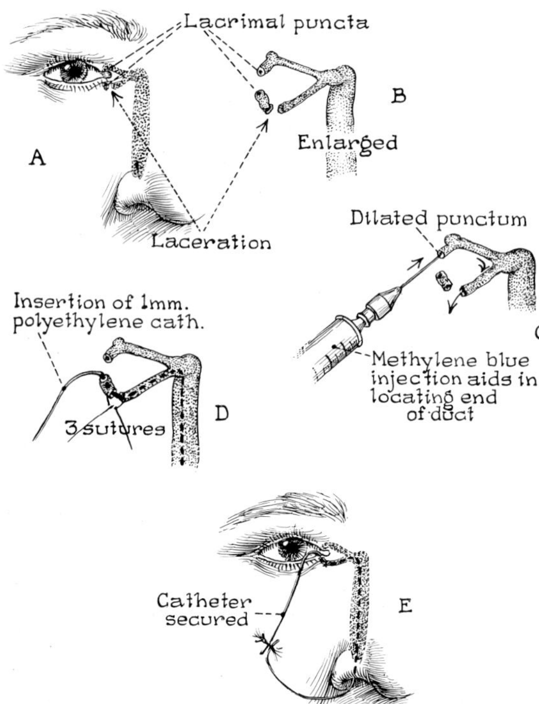

Figure 8–26 Technique of identification and repair of divided canaliculus: The proximal end is located by dilating the punctum with a lacrimal probe and passing it to the point of division. The distal end may be found by injecting a small amount of methylene blue through the noninjured punctum or directly into the lacrimal sac if both have been divided. A tiny polyethylene catheter is then passed through the divided duct into the sac to emerge in the nasal cavity. After closure of the duct with fine sutures, the two ends of the catheter may be sutured together to complete the circle until healing has occurred.

Full Thickness Losses of Portions of the External Nose. Certain injuries to the nose involve full thickness losses of the tip or nasal alae. Many times these can be repaired primarily with a proper appreciation of plastic techniques. A nasal rim that has been sliced off may be replaced if the missing segment is located and brought to the emergency room with the patient. In its absence, a composite graft, consisting of two thicknesses of ear skin and the contained cartilage, may be transferred into the defect to replace the amputated segment (Fig. 8–27). Very careful postoperative splinting is necessary for successful "take" of these thick grafts.

Full Thickness Losses of All or Part of the External Ear. Completely amputated portions of the ear helix or lobule that are less than 1 cm. in thickness or width can often be returned as a composite graft by resuturing the amputated part. The blood supply of the ear is excellent, and very small remaining pedicles of soft tissue will often support long and badly lacerated pedicles of ear skin and cartilage. With larger losses of soft tissue that expose significant amounts of underlying ear cartilage, local pedicle flaps may be designed from the area of the mastoid region or the nonhair-bearing preauricular skin (Fig. 8–28 *A* and *B*). Island arterial flaps may even be removed from the fascia and subcuticular tissue of the temple, moved to the ear and covered with split thickness skin grafts taken from the lateral neck.

Because of the high vascularity of immature bone, there is rapid healing (but also rapid malunion) of facial fractures in children. If these fractures are not reduced within the first few days after injury, it becomes almost impossible to reposition them later. (Delayed reductions may be practical in adults for two to three weeks after injury.) Small anatomical parts, susceptibility to edema and the difficulty in obtaining x-rays add to the problems of diagnosis of facial fractures

Figure 8–27 Moderate full thickness losses of the nasal rim or tip may in some instances be repaired either by resuturing of the amputated skin and cartilage or, when the missing segment is crushed or cannot be located, a primary composite graft can be removed from the antihelix of the ipsilateral ear including the necessary supporting cartilage. Such primary reconstruction should not be undertaken in the case of nasal losses from the dog bite or human bite or when the wound is badly contaminated. The composite graft may be more easily handled if the several layers are first transfixed with sterile pins through all layers and the cartilage.

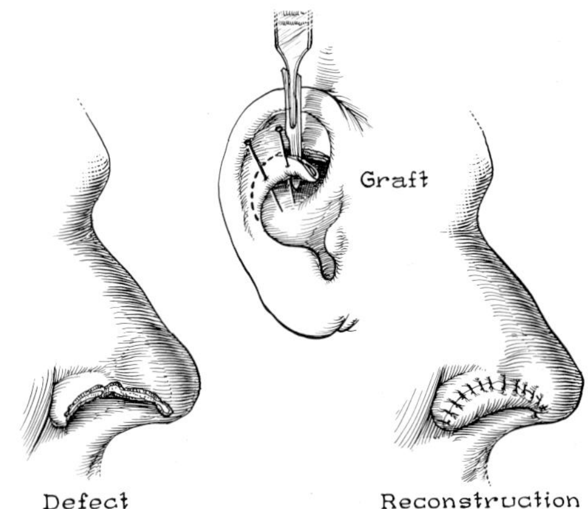

in children; a significant number of nasal fractures are thus unrecognized and untreated. Unreduced nasal fractures may produce progressive deformity with growth. At times the child may have severe nasal obstruction requiring rhinoplastic or septal surgery during adolescence. Children are also susceptible to ankylosis of the temporomandibular joint following trauma to the chin. This is quite common following fractures of the condyle neck. After extensive facial trauma, with craniofacial dysfunction, we have found that some children may have a continuing cerebrospinal fluid leak.

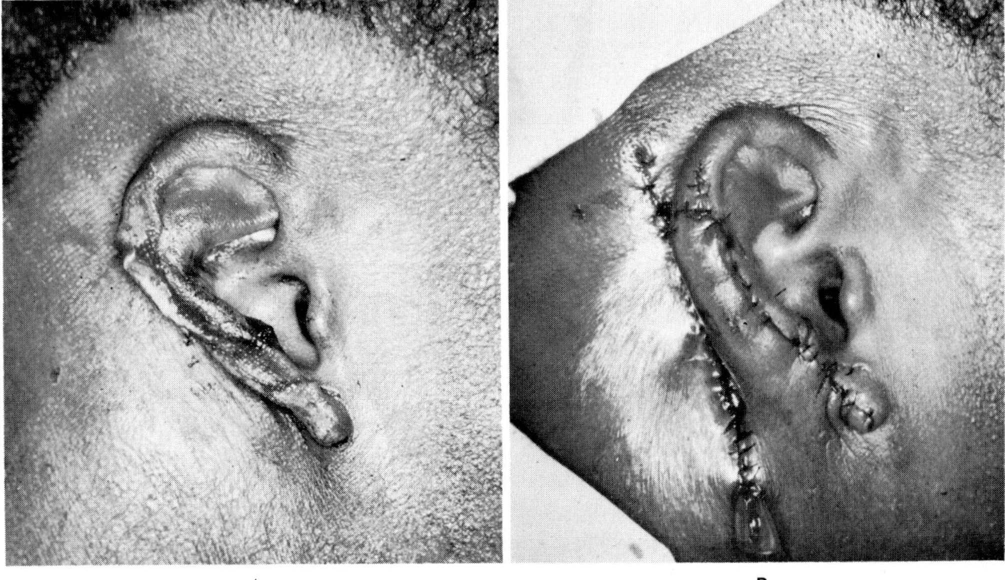

Figure 8–28 (*A*) A knife wound resulted in the loss of approximately 30 per cent of this man's external ear, with marked exposure of the remaining ear cartilage. To facilitate healing, prevent a spreading chondritis and reconstruct the helix of the lower ear, an immediate mastoid flap (*B*) was elevated on an inferior pedicle and brought forward to cover the exposed cartilage. The lower pedicle of this flap was divided later and shaped into an ear lobule. The mastoid donor defect has been closed by undermining and advancement.

This may lead to recurrent bouts of meningitis over a period of months, or even years, until the dural tear is repaired.

Finally, it must be recognized that small children look upon medical treatment with considerable apprehension, and their lack of cooperation in combination with parental anxiety may further complicate the surgeon's task.

What are the therapeutic methods that aid the surgeon in the management of problems encountered with fractures in the faces of children? Both child and parents obviously require gentleness and patience in the examination and the therapeutic manipulations that follow. Local anesthesia may prove very unsatisfactory even for simple fractures in children, and general anesthesia is often more desirable. Even in the removal of arch bars or pull-out wires, it is wise to utilize heavy sedation and local lidocaine (Xylocaine) in mucous membranes in order to gain cooperation and minimize discomfort and anxiety. Children have a tendency to manipulate "tricky" or removable appliances that may be used for fixation. For this reason as well as because of dental immaturity, open reduction is more often indicated in children than in adults. Further support for the use of open reduction of fractures in children comes from the realization that the late adverse consequences of inadequate closed reduction are much more severe in the case of children than of adults.

Because of the difficulties in obtaining exact diagnosis of facial fractures in children, it is often wise to carry out a diagnostic surgical procedure. At times this may require a general anesthetic. An exploratory incision may be made in the septal mucosa to identify a suspected fracture or dislocation of the cartilaginous nasal septum, or an exploration on the floor of the orbit may be indicated for a possible blow-out fracture or a fracture of the zygomatic compound. It is important that reductions of these fractures in children be carried out early to avoid rapid bony malunion.

Loose teeth should be repositioned promptly and carefully splinted for at least three weeks. Many of them will again become secure. In children, this possibility is increased by the presence of open root canals. If teeth appear to be missing and are not found at the scene of the injury, a chest x-ray will rule out the possibility of the patient's having aspirated the missing teeth. When it is difficult to apply arch bars because of mixed dentition in a child, circumferential wires may be applied so as to include the arch bar and the body of the mandible. These wires will secure an arch bar in good position without the danger of extracting teeth. In the upper jaw, an incision can be made in the sulcus behind the upper lip to expose the bony rim of the nasal pyriform opening. Drill holes may be placed in this bony margin and used to attach steel wires. The ends of the wires may be brought out through the incision and attached to the upper dental arch bar.

Careful consideration must be given to possible consequences of injuries to the facial bones in children. The family should be warned of the possible growth asymmetry that may develop. A failure to do so may be followed by great loss of confidence in the surgeon when such deformity appears at a later date.

If the entire external ear is amputated, or some major portion of it, one cannot hope for resuturing to be successful. In such instances, the entire skin and subcutaneous tissue may be removed from the cartilage and the latter may be preserved by burying it primarily beneath the subcutaneous tissues of the mastoid region. In this way, the valuable auricular fibrocartilaginous framework may be preserved for later reconstructive stages.

Lips and Cheeks. The lips are commonly perforated by the patient's own teeth, producing a dirty wound that should be closed very loosely by sutures, if at all. When areas of the vermilion have been lost, they may require later substitution in the form of mucous membrane flaps taken from the inner surface of the lip or from the lateral side of the tongue.

Children commonly suffer severe electrical burns of the lips and tongue when they find an extension cord on the floor that is still connected to the house current but not to a lamp. These extension cord heads are often a chocolate color and invite the child to place them in his mouth. The result is a painful third degree burn involving the commissure of the mouth and tongue, generally requiring delayed and complex plastic surgery to open and shape the mouth properly. Although some surgeons have advocated early resection of the necrotic muscle of the lip in these injuries, most plastic surgeons feel that a better result can be obtained with delayed repair. Secondary hemorrhage may develop in these wounds after 10 or 12 days and may cause profound hemorrhagic shock if it occurs during sleep.

When considerable cheek substance has been lost from electrical or traumatic injury (Fig. 8–29 *A*), repair must be designed not only to provide skin replacement to the cheek but also to replace the missing mucous membrane lining and necessary bulk within the cheek. To avoid unsightly contour depression, it is often necessary to elevate a pedicle flap from the neck or chest and to transfer one end to the defect after lining its undersurface with a skin graft (Fig. 8–29 *B*). Three weeks later the lined flap may be divided and the pedicle returned to the neck. Removal of the excess fat will produce, in such instances, an adequate reconstruction of the cheek and corner of the mouth (Fig. 8–29 *C*).

Parotid Duct. Compound wounds of the face often involve transection of the parotid duct just prior to its entrance into the oral cavity. The surgeon should bear in mind carefully the normal location of the parotid duct. It is usually on a line between the base of the nostril and the lobe of the ear. It emerges from the parotid substance to run across the lateral surface of the masseter muscle and then to dip medially at the anterior border of the masseter to pass between some of the upper fibers of the buccinator muscle. A branch of the facial nerve usually travels with this duct over the proximal half of its course. Thus, injury to the nerve should be suspected whenever the duct is divided. The recent availability of operating microscopes in most surgical operating rooms greatly improves the accuracy of reconstruction of these structures. If the two ends of the duct can be located and a small polyethylene cannula threaded along the lumen, it is possible to carry out careful end-to-end suture of the duct over this indwelling catheter. For the best results care should be taken not to let the sutures enter the lumen of the duct. The catheter tip should be allowed to project into the oral cavity and should be sutured into position for several weeks (Figs. 8–30 and 8–31).

Facial Nerve Injuries. Major lacerations involving the cheek that cross the course of the facial nerve may divide important branches.

In 1972 evidence was presented from several sources to indicate superior results with facial nerve injury if immediate repair is carried out. This is in part due to the ease of finding the divided nerve ends before nerve degeneration has occurred. Muscle contraction on stimulation of the distal nerve fragment is usually lost after one week. Facial nerve repair should probably not be undertaken by any surgeon who is without experience in the use of the operating microscope. Sutures of 9–0 nylon plus a fibrin "fixation" technique will provide a highly reliable degree of nerve recovery. Such microsurgery teams are available in most major medical centers as a standard technique where plastic surgery teams are available for emergency calls. The nerve ends may be located by careful use of a nerve stimulator

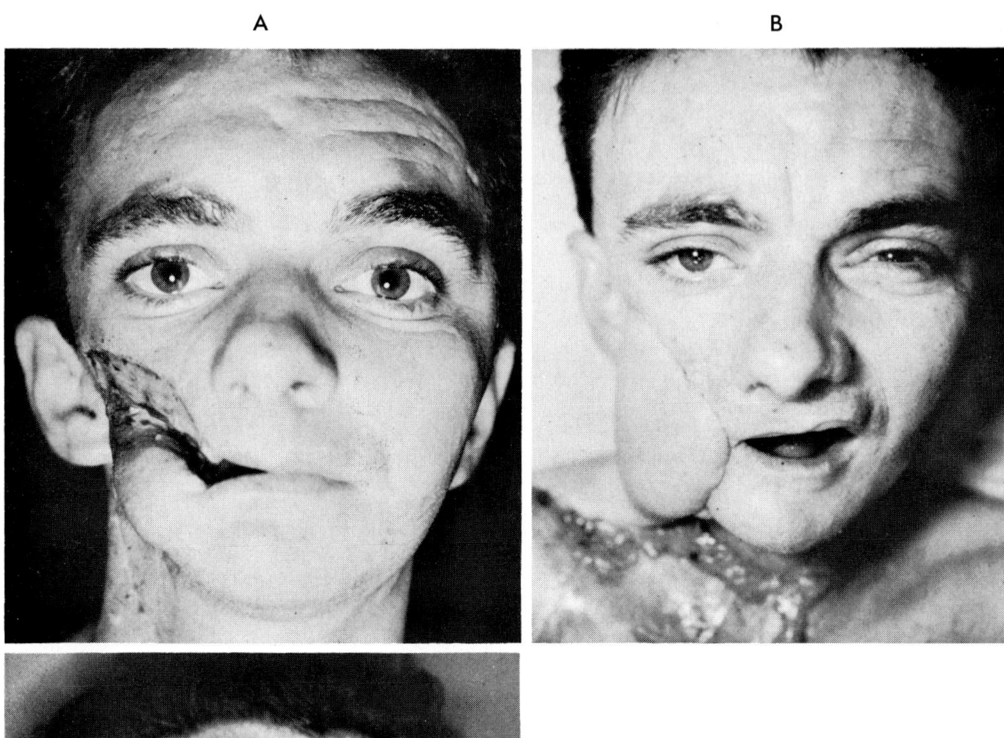

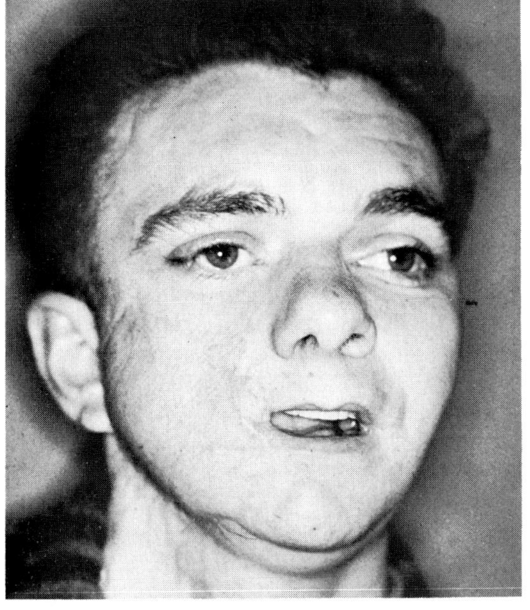

Figure 8–29 *A*, This young man suffered a traumatic avulsion of the full thickness of the right cheek. A split graft has been applied to the defect above and over the mandible to provide the initial healing. Reconstruction requires the transfer of a lined pedicle flap to provide skin mucosal replacement of the cheek and sufficient bulk for contour. In *B* a cervicothoracic flap has been elevated with its base on the right shoulder and with a split thickness graft lining its undersurface. In *C* the flap has been fitted into the cheek, the extra bulk has been removed, and the pedicle has been returned to the shoulder. A free skin graft on the neck replaces the donor flap.

to detect the distal branches and by careful anatomical dissection to locate the proximal branches. Whenever possible, these tiny nerves should be brought together and sutured with one or two very fine sutures of nonabsorbable (7-0) material. Surprisingly good function can be achieved by the resuture of the facial nerve. Indeed, the facial nerve and the digital nerves in the hand seem to be those nerves most likely to obtain good functional results if carefully repaired by suture or nerve grafting following trauma (Fig. 8–32 *A* and *B*).

At times a portion of the facial nerve

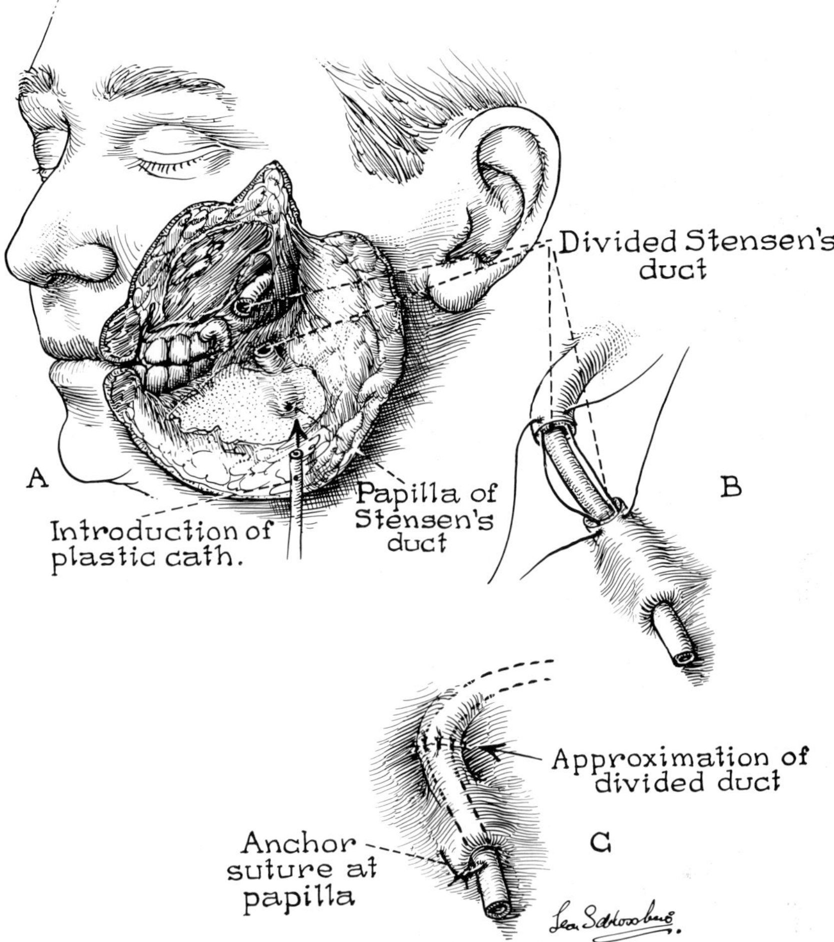

Figure 8–30 Explosion injury to the cheek resulted in multiple fractures with division of the parotid duct approximately one and a half inches before its entrance into the oral cavity. The proximal end of the duct was found at operation and identified by the slow discharge of serious parotid secretion. The distal cut end was found by a retrograde threading of a polyethylene catheter from the duct papilla on the oral mucosa. Six-zero silk sutures were then placed in the submucosa of the duct to carry out fine closure of the divided duct with interrupted sutures. The catheter is anchored to the oral mucosa to prevent its slipping out in the postoperative period and is removed two weeks later.

may be avulsed by a primary injury or a section may be removed because of tumor. In such instances, primary neurorrhaphy may not be possible. Autogenous facial nerve grafting may produce excellent results. We have preferred to use the sensory branches of the great auricular nerve as the most suitable donor nerve. This nerve may be easily exposed through a short transverse incision in the lateral side of the neck, and the number of branches removed can be made to coincide with the number of major distal trunks of the facial nerve to be repaired. It is important for good regeneration that the nerve be placed in the defect without tension and that a bed of rich vascularity be supplied to the graft. When applied to a primary injury, such nerve grafts are likely to be highly successful (Fig. 8–33 *A* through *C*).

Major Compound Injuries of the Face with Gross Loss of Bone and Soft Tissues. In the case of explo-

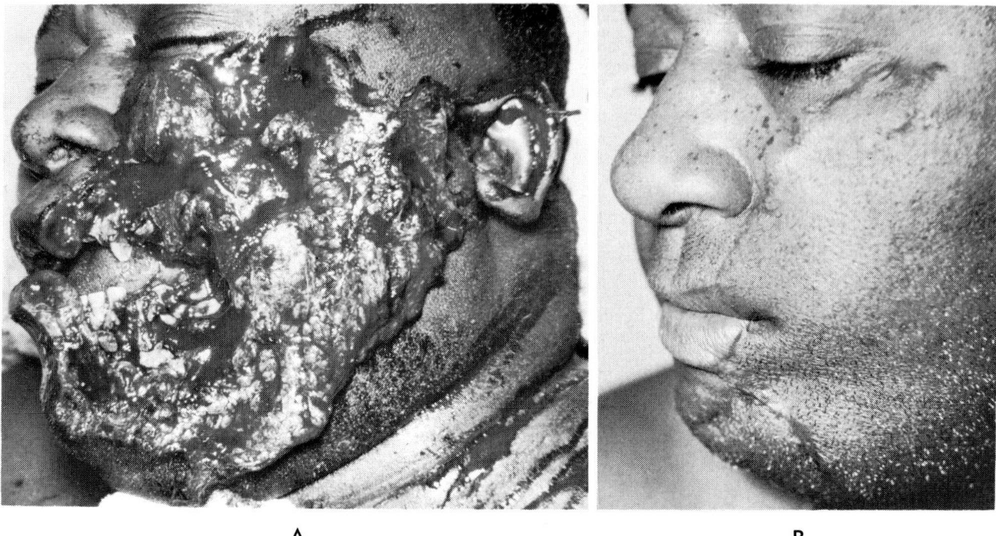

Figure 8–31 *A* and *B*, This patient received an explosive wound of the face with compound fractures of the upper and lower jaw, loss of several teeth, extensive lacerations of the left cheek involving transection of the parotid duct, and loss of vermilion at the left commissure of the mouth. After thorough irrigation and clean-up, arch bars were applied to the upper and lower jaw for intermaxillary elastic traction; and a repair of the parotid duct was carried out as illustrated by the technique in Figure 8–30. *B* shows early result, including a patent left Stensen's duct. The loss of vermilion in the left corner of the mouth is evident and requires a mucous membrane flap from behind the upper lip. The arch bars were left in position for six weeks.

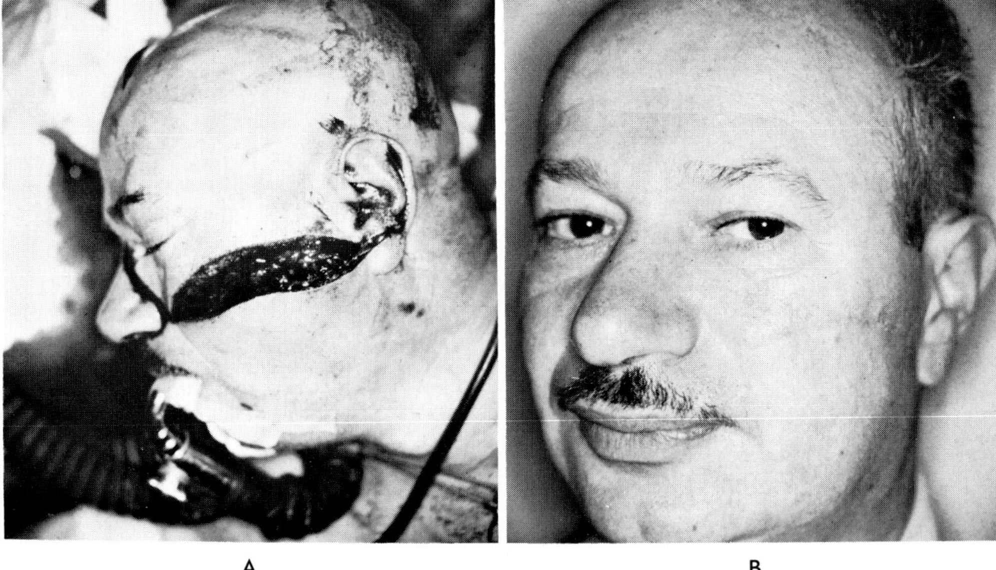

Figure 8–32 *A* shows a deep hatchet wound of the cheek sustained when this grocery store owner was attacked by a hold-up man. Both his parotid duct and three large branches of the facial nerve were divided. Other injuries of the extremities made the use of general anesthesia desirable. Careful repair of the parotid duct and resuture of the three branches of the facial nerve were carried out at primary operation. Four months later, the result shown in *B* indicates a definite return of tone in the facial nerve branches supplying the upper and lower lip. The nerve branches to the forehead and right eyebrow have largely recovered, and there is very little brow ptosis present.

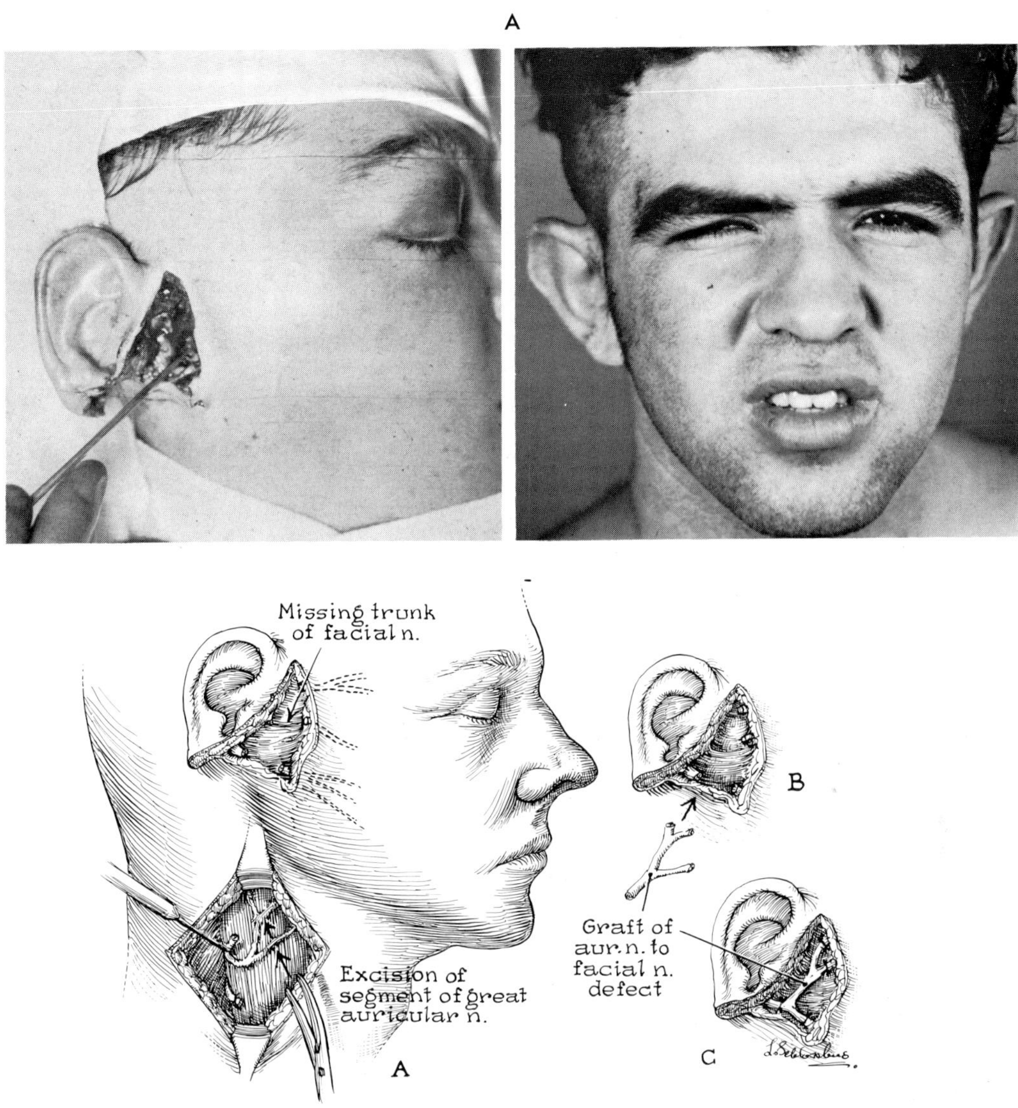

Figure 8–33 *A* shows a rotary blade avulsion injury of the cheek and ear with a missing section of the lower ear and approximately a one-half inch gap in the facial nerve. The distal ends of the nerve were located with a small electrical stimulator, and the proximal trunk was picked up just beneath the external auditory canal. A donor nerve graft of appropriate length was then removed from the great auricular nerve where it crosses the posterior border of the sternomastoid muscle. The technique is illustrated in *B*. The three distal branches of the great auricular nerve graft were each sutured carefully to the three branches of the facial nerve which could be located in the cheek. *C* shows the tone and balance that have returned to the face approximately six months following the primary injury and just prior to a small plastic operation designed to reposition the lateral position of the ear cartilage. If facial nerve repair is not successful by suture or grafting, dynamic muscle transfers will offer the patient considerable relief from the distressing deformity of facial palsy.

sions or high-velocity missile injuries, such as are commonly seen in hunting accidents or in the war-wounded, an entirely different problem in reconstruction may present to the surgeon. Such patients may have lost such an extensive amount of soft tissue that there is little covering material for the damaged bone and a lack of soft tissue substance to rebuild features. Such patients are likely to require a long and complex series of reconstructive steps which, at times, run over the course of one or two years. The initial management should be aimed at control of hemorrhage and the establishment of a safe airway. The control of infection and the preservation of all possible damaged tissue may be of value for later reconstruction. Unlike the construction of a house in which the foundation is built first, the reconstruction of a major portion of the missing face must be carried out from the outside surface, working inward. Thus, the surgeon must first think of providing sufficient skin and lining to the cheeks, lips and oral cavity into which he may later insert proper bone grafts to pro-

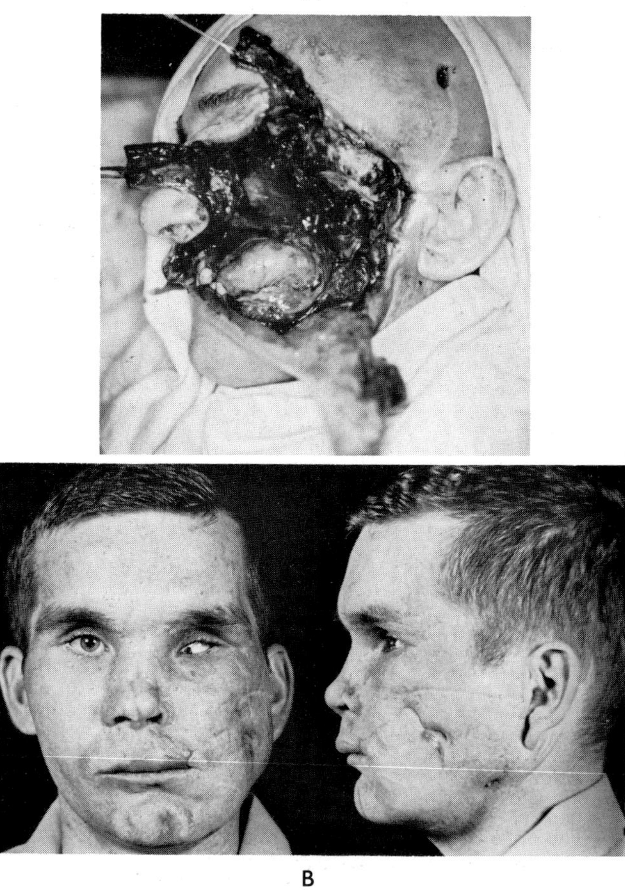

Figure 8–34 *A* shows a young man who looked into a cylinder of highly explosive gas just as it was ignited by the flame of a match. The left eye, the left maxilla, the left zygoma, and the left mandible with parotid gland and much overlying cheek tissue were all badly destroyed. At the time of primary repair, an effort was made to save all remaining tissue after thorough debridement. A plastic conformer was sutured into the left conjunctival sac and a gold implant was placed inside Tenon's capsule to complete the enucleation of the left eye. Portions of the mandible were rewired, and the soft tissue flaps were closed over the wound. Six weeks later, the patient developed swelling and drainage in the left cheek (*B*). It was obvious that the lack of soft tissue attachments and blood supply had resulted

vide stability and, perhaps, a proper ridge on which a denture may be seated. Following the build-up of cheeks and jaw, it may be necessary to bring distant pedicle flap tissue to the face for the reconstruction of an external nose, the building of eyelids or the reconstruction of external ears. The value of proceeding with this multistaged type of reconstruction has been evidenced in considerable numbers of young men injured in World War II and the conflicts in Korea and Viet Nam. Indeed, many of these young men are now supporting families and carrying out successful and creative jobs in the community. The expense of this type of medical care is tremendous and, in the absence of its assumption by some governmental or insuring agency, the private citizen is unlikely to be able to meet the burdensome expenses of this type of care (Figs. 8–34 and 8–35).

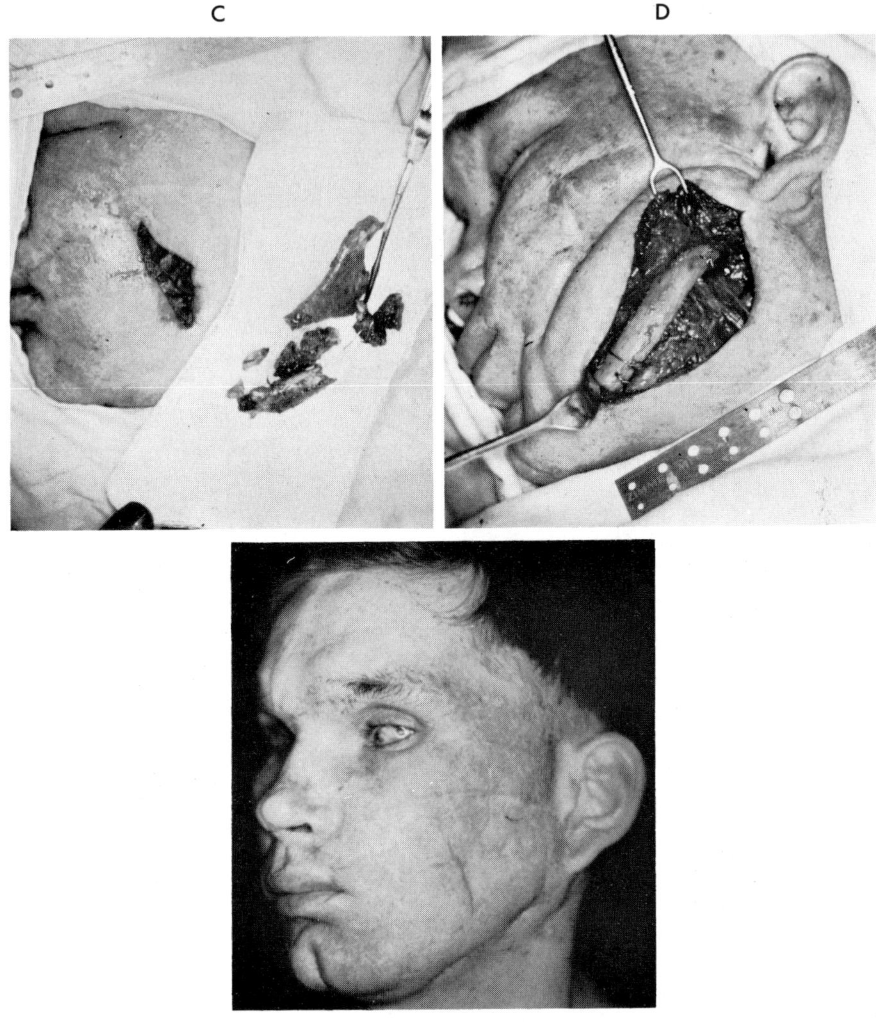

in infection of some bone fragments. Exploration revealed sequestration and osteomyelitis in eight fragments of mandible. These eight fragments were removed (*C*). Six months later a rib graft was inserted to reconstruct the mandible (*D*), and a reasonable repair of the deformity resulted (*E*). This patient has obtained an artificial left eye and is now married and supporting his family despite the magnitude of his original injury.

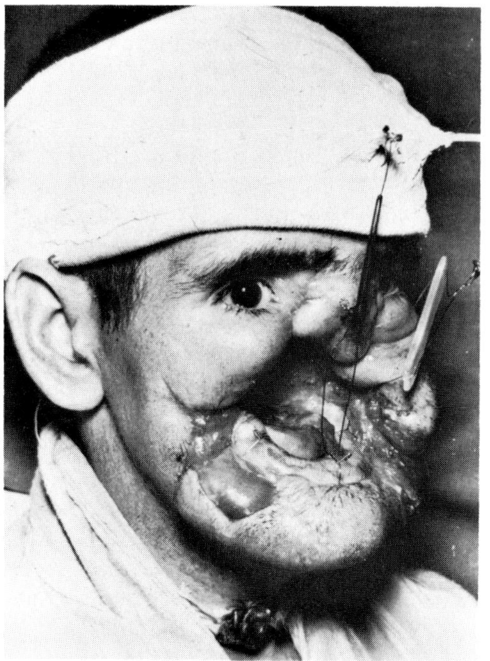

Figure 8–35 This young man sustained a high velocity shell fragment injury of the entire middle face during World War II. A tracheostomy tube was inserted as a lifesaving measure, and the plastic splint was wired circumferentially to the remaining mandibular fragments to support the lower portion of the face. Because of bony instability, a plaster head cap was applied, and elastic support traction was provided to the left zygoma and mandibular symphysis. Fortunately, reasonable vision remained in one eye. This young man and many others like him came under the care of the Plastic Surgery Unit at the Valley Forge General Hospital, then under the supervision of Dr. James Barrett Brown and Dr. Bradford Cannon. Under their direction, six or eight different plastic surgeons operated on this patient over a period of approximately two and one-half years before he was finally rehabilitated and returned to his home. He is now, twenty years later, married and the proud father of attractive children. He supports his family and presents as a useful and effective citizen. The courageous example set by this man and many of his colleagues-at-arms should be an inspiration to all those interested in rehabilitation of the facially injured.

OTHER CERVICAL INJURIES

In addition to injuries of the larynx and trachea involving danger to the upper airway, injuries to the neck may involve other vital and important structures.

Not uncommonly, attempted suicides result in a transverse cut across the lower neck. The head is usually extended at time of injury, and, in most instances, the injury involves the external jugular veins and the sternomastoid muscles. Such patients have usually allowed bleeding from these veins to go uncontrolled until they are discovered by friends and incipient shock may be the greatest danger.

In children it is especially important to think of pneumothorax with injuries to the inferior neck. The apex of the pleura extends well up into the neck in young patients. If skin and soft tissues have been avulsed from the neck, it is important to provide a primary pedicle flap or a flap of sternomastoid or levator muscle to cover any ligated or repaired major vessels and nerves.

Cervical Vascular Injuries

The management of vascular injuries in the neck differs in a number of important ways from that of peripheral vascular injuries. In the extremities the control of hemorrhage and the management of possible distal ischemia are central issues. In the neck one must also be concerned with the development of late hematoma, airway obstruction secondary to bleeding, and the acute impairment of cerebral circulation which may be sudden, catastrophic and irreversible. Although young healthy adults or children may withstand complete interruption of the common or internal carotid arteries without major neurologic injury, older patients may develop permanent brain damage from cerebral ischemia of only a few minutes duration involving one internal carotid artery. In such patients a permanent hemiparesis, aphasisa or loss of memory may be tragically permanent.

It must be stressed that cerebral ischemia from division of a carotid artery is much more likely to be damaging if the patient should be in some degree of hemorrhagic shock from the associated injuries. It is important to prevent or correct ischemia in these patients before the clinical symptoms of neurologic damage have become established and irreversible. This is especially true in elderly patients with neck injuries who may have associated arteriosclerotic occlusive disease of the great vessels.

In spite of individual triumphs, the mortality of operations to restore carotid circulation after acute stroke within two to four weeks of the event is so high that overall results favor no operation at all. The selection of the favorable case for operation is extremely difficult. Patients having vascular injuries of the neck are certainly in a more favorable category than stroke victims, but it is important that circulation be restored as early as possible after great vessel injury.

TREATMENT PRINCIPLES WITH SUSPECTED VASCULAR INJURIES OF THE NECK

Penetrating neck injuries are best divided into three zones:

1. Injuries near the base of the neck (in the lower one-third). These injuries may involve not only cervical vessels, but also any vessels coming from the aortic arch. Exploratory incisions must be planned to extend into a median sternotomy and if necessary out through the third intercostal space to the right or to the left. If the patient is not massively hemorrhaging, angiography preoperatively is likely to be most helpful.

2. Midcervical region (central one-third). All penetrating injuries in this region should be explored. Angiography is usually necessary near the midline. Associated injuries to the larynx may indicate the need for thyroidotomy and in some instances intraluminal splinting of the laryngeal airway.

3. Upper one-third of neck (above angle of mandible). In this area of the neck arterial injuries to the carotid have the associated problem of making access to the vessel distal to injury quite difficult, and repair of the vessel in this region close to the base of the skull may be impossible. Ligation of the internal carotid artery is usually necessary. Angiography is very helpful for suspected vascular injury in this level of the neck, and surgical approach must be carried out quite carefully.

Thus, penetrating wounds of the neck should be routinely explored quite early. In most instances this requires the lighting, suction and equipment of a formal operating room. It should be carried out only by surgeons intimately familiar with the complex and important anatomy of the neck. The practice of attempting to control arterial bleeding in the neck by the application of hemastats or clamps deep into the neck is to be condemned. Further vessel damage and paralysis of the vegas nerve or nerves to the brachial plexus have occurred repeatedly with such efforts. Compression of the bleeding point until adequate exposure in the operating room is essential. With young patients, when the vessel has been exposed, the use of an internal shunt while carrying out repair is usually quite unnecessary. It is desirable to insert such a shunt when (1) neurological deficit is already present, (2) the patient is elderly or affected with occlusive vascular disease, or (3) when the nature of the repair will require a prolonged period of time.

Partial injuries to major arteries are best repaired by simple ligation with interrupted arterial silk. If this is not possible due to damage to the vessel wall, the alternative method of choice is the use of an autogenous vein graft. Since all of these wounds are to some degree contaminated one should avoid the use of prosthetic materials for grafting. Infection rate and late bleeding are extremely high in such cases.

At times exploration will reveal the vessel injury to be to one of the great veins. In such cases, it is wise to maintain the patient in Trendelenburg position to avoid air embolism. These veins may usually be repaired by simple suture, but if badly damaged, the internal jugular vein may be ligated with minimal danger. The vertebral arteries rarely require surgical intervention except for control of continued or late bleeding. Since the carotid arteries carry 90 per cent of the cerebral blood flow, colateral flow from the contralateral carotid artery through the Circle of Willis ordinarily provides protection against catastrophic brain injury. The technical methods of vascular reconstruction are described in Chapter 15 and identical to the principles used in the neck region. Hypercarbic, hypertensive anesthesia is of value to maintain cerebral circulation in most cases of arterial injury in the neck.

In addition to exploring the obviously damaged carotid artery, one should explore arteries in spasm and those with external signs of injury such as subadventitial petechiae or deeper intramural hemorrhage. The cervical hematoma, particularly when it extends into or from the area of the carotid-jugular sheath, should be approached warily on the assumption that it represents a communication hematoma or false aneurysm or an arteriovenous fistula. Proximal and distal control of the carotid-jugular vessels and availability of several sizes of plastic tubing (to serve as an internal shunt) are essential prerequisites for this venture It may be necessary to extend the preferred transverse cervical skin incision through the cervical fascia and along the anterior border of the sternocleidomastoid muscle and even into a sternal splitting incision. When explored early with this type of control and exposure, arteriovenous fistulas and false aneurysms are usually easily managed by primary repair of the vessels or by patch grafting after the poorly organized hematoma has been evacuated. Simple venous injuries may be repaired, but those more complicated should be treated by thrombectomy and double ligation, with special care being taken to avoid air embolism during these manipulations.

Penetrating wounds of the neck may often result from stab wounds made by knives or ice picks. The frequency of injury of important deep structures within the neck has been stressed repeatedly in recent years and in most instances such wounds should be explored in the operating room. In this way, holes in veins or major arteries may be identified and closed, thus reducing the danger of late hemorrhage or aneurysms. Attempts to clamp arterial bleeders in the depths of such wounds in the emergency room should be avoided as these clamps may result in damage to the vagus, hypoglossal, spinal accessory or brachial plexus nerve trunks. It is obviously essential that the neck explorations in such patients be carried out by surgeons who are intimately familiar with the detailed anatomy of the neck.

Although the common carotid artery can be ligated without the production of serious neurologic damage in the vast majority of young patients, it is usually unnecessary to do this when the wounds have not involved the esophagus or oral cavity. In such instances, irrigation, debridement and vessel repair or grafting are usually successful. The internal jugular vein, if injured, should usually be ligated without attempt at repair.

REFERENCES

1. Adams, W. M.: Internal wiring fixation of facial fractures. Surgery *12*:523, 1942.
2. Angle, E. H.: Classification on malocclusion. Dental Cosmos *41*:248, 1899.
3. Ashworth, C., et al.: Penetrating wounds of the neck. Re-emphasis of the need for prompt exploration. Am. J. Surg. *121*: 387, 1971.
4. Baudens, J. B.: Fracture de la machoire inférieure. Bull. Acad. de Méd., Paris 5:341, 1840.
5. Brown, J. B., Fryer, M. P., and McDowell, F.: Internal wire-pin fixation for fractures of upper jaw, orbit, zygoma, and severe facial crushes. Plast. Reconstr. Surg. 9:276, 1952.

6. Buck, G., Jr.: Fracture of the lower jaw, with displacement and interlocking of the fragments. Annalist, New York *1*: 245, 1846.
7. Cohen, C. A., et al.: Carotid artery injuries. An analysis of eighty-five cases. Am. J. Surg. *120*:210, 1970.
8. Dingman, R. O., and Natvig, P.: Surgery of Facial Fractures. Philadelphia, W. B. Saunders Co., 1964, p. 11.
9. Edgerton, M. T., and Hill, E.: Fractures of the mandible. Surgery *31*:933, 1952.
10. Fitchett, V. H., et al.: Penetrating wounds of the neck. A military and civilian experience. Arch. Surg. *99*:307, 1969.
11. Gerrie, J. W., and Lindsay, W. K.: Fracture of maxillary-zygomatic compound with atypical involvement of orbit. Plast. Reconstr. Surg. *11*:341, 1953.
12. Gillies, H. D., Kilner, T. P., and Stone, D.: Fractures of the malar-zygomatic compound, with a description of new x-ray position. Brit. J. Surg. *14*:651, 1927.
13. Hunt, T. K., et al.: Vascular injuries of the base of the neck. Arch. Surg. *98*:586, 1969.
14. Johnson, W. B.: New method for reduction of acute dislocation of the temporomandibular articulations. J. Oral Surg. *16*: 501, 1958.
15. Knight, J. S., and North, J. F.: Classification of malar fractures: An analysis of displacement as a guide to treatment. Brit. J. Plast. Surg. *13*:325, 1961.
16. Langer, C.: Zur Anatomie und Physiologie der Haut. Sitzungst. d. k. Acad. Wissensch. *45*:223, 1861.
17. LeFort, R.: Fractures de la machoire supérieure. Cong. internat. de méd. C. -r., Paris, 1900, Sect. de chir. gen., pp. 275–278.
18. McCoy, F. J., Chandler, R. A., Magnan, C. G., Jr., Moore, J. R., and Siemsen, G.: An analysis of facial fractures and their complications. Plast. Reconst. Surg. *29*:381, 1962.
19. Monson, D. O., et al.: Carotid vertebral trauma. J. Trauma *9*:987, 1969.
20. Robert, C. A.: Nouveau procede de traitement des fractures de la portion alveolaire de la machoire inférieure. Bull. Gen. de Therap. Méd. et Chirurg. *42*: 22, 1852.
21. Rubin, L. R.: Langer's lines and facial scars. Plast. Reconst. Surg. *3*:147, 1948.
22. Smith Papyrus: Translations by G. Kasten Tallmadge. *In* Dingman, R. D., and Natvig, P.: Surgery of Facial Fractures. Philadelphia, W. B. Saunders Co., 1964.
23. Swearingen, J. J.: Tolerances of the Human Face to Crash Impact. Report from the Office of Aviation Medicine, Federal Aviation Agency, July, 1965.
24. Wylie, E. J., and Ehrenfeld, W. K.: Extracranial Occlusive Cerebrovascular Disease: Diagnosis and Management. Philadelphia; W. B. Saunders Co., 1970.

chapter

9

TRACHEOSTOMY

Margaret M. Fletcher, M.D.

Tracheostomy is a procedure which has been done for more than two thousand years to relieve upper airway obstruction. In the past, it was performed as an unplanned terminal event in diseases such as diphtheria. Because the patients usually died from their primary disease, tracheostomies were seldom done. During the past thirty years, however, the management of the acutely ill patient has changed a great deal. One notes, as well, an attendant change in the indications and complications of tracheostomy.

The initial evaluation and treatment of the injured patient has been discussed in previous chapters. The importance of the airway cannot be overstressed. In the severely injured or acutely ill patient, inadequate ventilation and inadequate circulation rapidly lead to central nervous system anoxia. Three to five minutes of central nervous system anoxia lead to irreversible damage and death.

The purpose of this chapter is to provide guidelines on how to manage a patient with inadequate ventilation. Questions to be answered are:

1. Where is the ventilatory problem?
2. When is tracheostomy indicated and what is the technique which minimizes complications?
3. How does one do a tracheostomy?
4. What is adequate nursing care after tracheostomy has been done?

LOCATION AND MANAGEMENT OF VENTILATORY PROBLEMS

Head and Spinal Cord Injury

Seventy-one per cent of the victims of automobile accidents sustain injury to the head, midface or upper airway.[8] Sixty-four per cent of these patients die from intracranial and ventilation complications. Several mechanisms are responsible for ventilatory problems. First, cerebral edema seen with head trauma or direct damage to the respiratory center can decrease ventilatory rate and cause anoxia. Secondly, with unconsciousness, the tongue, pharynx and mandible become posteriorly displaced and obstruct the upper airway. Thirdly, the cough reflex is obliterated. Secretions, blood and foreign bodies can obstruct the airway and cause aspiration pneumonitis. Unconsciousness and/or brainstem involvement often result in copious, uncontrolled secretions of saliva and mucous which, when aspirated, cause severe and often irreversible pneumonitis. It is important to consider this problem early in patients with head trauma. Tracheostomy is done to maintain an airway, to maintain ventilation and to assist in the removal of tracheal secretions and aspirated materials. Once aspiration pneumonitis is established, it is difficult to treat. The mortality rate is approximately 70 per cent.[1, 3]

The diagnosis of head trauma is reviewed in Chapter 6. A brief check list when considering the airway would indicate the following:

1. Closely observe the patient's mental status and level of consciousness. The instant he becomes obtunded, an airway should be established.
2. Lacerations, contusions and palpated fractures of the skull may indicate possible central nervous system damage.
3. Cerebral spinal fluid otorrhea and rhinorrhea may indicate impending brainstem compromise.
4. Cranial nerve impairment may be shown by hoarseness (X), weak shoulder (XI), weak tongue muscle (XII). Other motor, sensory or cerebellar deficits indicate brainstem involvement.
5. Respirations are irregular and deep with coarse inspiratory stridor.

An airway can usually be established by proper position, oral airway and mouth-to-mouth respiration. An endotracheal tube is inserted to maintain the airway, to provide respiratory assistance, if necessary, and to assist in the clearance of secretions or blood from the pharynx. If the endotracheal tube must be in place for more than 48 hours, a tracheostomy is indicated to avoid complications of pneumonitis, laryngotracheal injury and stenosis.

Pharynx

The pharynx is the most common site of upper airway obstruction; it is also the easiest to manage. Unfortunately, it is often forgotten. If a patient has total airway obstruction, there will be no stridor—only paradoxical chest movements. These movements have often been mistaken for adequate ventilation, but auscultation of the chest and examination of the mouth reveal that no air is being exchanged. Many lives have been saved by pulling the jaw and tongue forward and by scooping gastric contents, blood, dentures, food and secretions out of the hypopharynx with one's fingers or with suction, if it is available.

The *diagnosis* of pharyngeal obstruction is made by evaluating the respirations and examination of the pharynx:

Respirations: Before complete obstruction, breath sounds are coarse with palatal and pharyngeal stridor, similar to exaggerated snoring. With complete obstruction, there is no movement of air.

Rate: Variable and labored.

Movements: Suprasternal and intercostal retractions with each attempted inspiration.

Color: Cyanosis is not present unless the patient has 5 gms./100 ml. of reduced hemoglobin circulating. It is not present if the patient has nasal oxygen being administered or if he is in shock and vasoconstricted.

Other traumatic causes of pharyngeal obstruction include displaced maxillary and mandibular fractures. These can sometimes be disimpacted by a constant pull against the muscles of mastication. If this is not readily accomplished, it is best to insert an oral airway or endotracheal tube or to proceed with a tracheostomy. Thermal burns of the head and trunk may also involve the mucosa of the oral cavity and pharynx. These are diagnosed by redness and edema of the palate and epiglottis, hoarseness, cough, pain and sometimes inspiratory stridor. Chemical burns are usually the result of caustic lye ingestion. Normal mucosa is replaced by a white fibrinous membrane, surrounded by redness and edema. Intubation often causes further damage. Tracheostomy is indicated early.

Hematomas of the retropharyngeal, parapharyngeal and visceral spaces occur as a result of cervical spine, carotid artery, internal jugular vein, thyroid, laryngeal and tracheal injury. Hematomas can cause severe airway obstruction and often extend deep into the mediastinum. Tracheostomy is often of little benefit in these instances, instead, it is important to intubate the patient, evaluate the hematoma and explore the injured sites for control.

Larynx

Vocal Cord Adduction. Incomplete laryngeal obstruction may have a characteristic high-pitched inspiratory crow. This is a result of air passing between two tightly opposed or edematous vocal cords. It is commonly associated with acute inflammation or extubation after anesthesia. Foreign bodies, mucus, blood and thermal burns in the larynx may also cause laryngospasm. Bilateral recurrent nerve paralysis and brainstem injury to the nucleus ambiguus bilaterally are less common causes of vocal cord adduction.

Laryngeal Fracture. Hoarseness, cough, hemoptysis, subcutaneous emphysema and neck contusions, when present with or without head injury, should indicate laryngeal fracture until proven otherwise.

The diagnosis can be confirmed by indirect examination. Complete airway obstruction may develop suddenly. Once a diagnosis of laryngeal fracture is made, tracheostomy is indicated. As soon as the patient's condition has stabilized, the laryngeal fracture should be reduced, mucosal lacerations repaired and an endotracheal stent inserted.

Tracheal, Pulmonary and Chest Wall Injuries

The diagnosis and management of these problems are covered in Chapter 10. Tracheostomy is important in a patient with multiple rib fractures or flail chest. It is done to assist ventilation and to remove bronchial secretions. Tracheostomy provides a means for ventilation in patients with lung contusions.

In the injured patient, the usual cause of ventilatory problems is a result of upper airway obstruction, loss of central nervous system control with head injury or a result of a chest injury. The diagnosis and immediate management of each of these problems have been discussed. In each instance a tracheostomy may be indicated, but only rarely is it used as the first line of defense of treatment. Instead, patient position, jaw and tongue position, clearing of secretions, foreign material, oral airway and mouth-to-mouth resuscitation are all that are indicated.

If ventilation cannot be maintained with the above maneuvers, then an endotracheal tube should be inserted. The technique of intubation is discussed in Chapter 4. Once an airway is established, one has gained control of the emergency situation with the patient and has converted it to a planned program based on logical priorities.

Endotracheal intubation causes a certain amount of injury in every patient. When compared with the lifesaving aspects of this procedure, the early injury is usually of no consequence and is acceptable. After thirty to forty hours of intubation, mucosal ulceration occurs on the laryngeal surface of the epiglottis, the arytenoids, glottis and subglottic space. Inflammation increases with time and after five days, 80 per cent of intubated patients demonstrate laryngeal cartilage necrosis.[5] If an endotracheal tube is necessary for more than 48 hours to maintain an airway or ventilation, then a tracheostomy is indicated.

TRACHEOSTOMY TECHNIQUE

Once the need for tracheostomy is established, an endotracheal tube or bronchoscope is inserted, after topical lidocaine 4 per cent. The airway can then be suctioned and ventilation begun.

Despite its apparent simplicity and frequency of performance, tracheostomy continues to be a hazardous procedure and should be performed in the operating room. Before proceeding one should take a few minutes to check on *four details*. This time will often save hours spent managing complications which otherwise occur.

1. Prepare for possible cardiac arrest and pneumothorax. These problems occur often in injured patients with ventilatory and circulatory compromise.

2. Prepare tracheostomy tube. (See Figure 9–1.)

   a. *Size.* Size of tracheostomy tube is the subject of controversy and confusion. Some authors advocate placing the largest tube possible, others the smallest. It is most important to insert a tube which is least traumatic to the trachea. Pressure necrosis at the cuff, stoma and tip should be avoided and the trachea should not be distended. The size of silver Jackson tubes corresponds to the patient's age up to size four and five. Number six is used in small women and number eight for the average male. The outer diameter of silastic (siliconized rubber) tubes corresponds with the Jackson standard. The silastic tube is thicker, therefore the inner diameter is less. Portex tubes are measured in the French system. (See Table 9–1.)

   b. *Cuff.* Check for leaks by inflating with 50 cc. of air slowly while immersed in hot water. This distension converts the cuff to a low-tension seal which is less traumatic to the trachea.

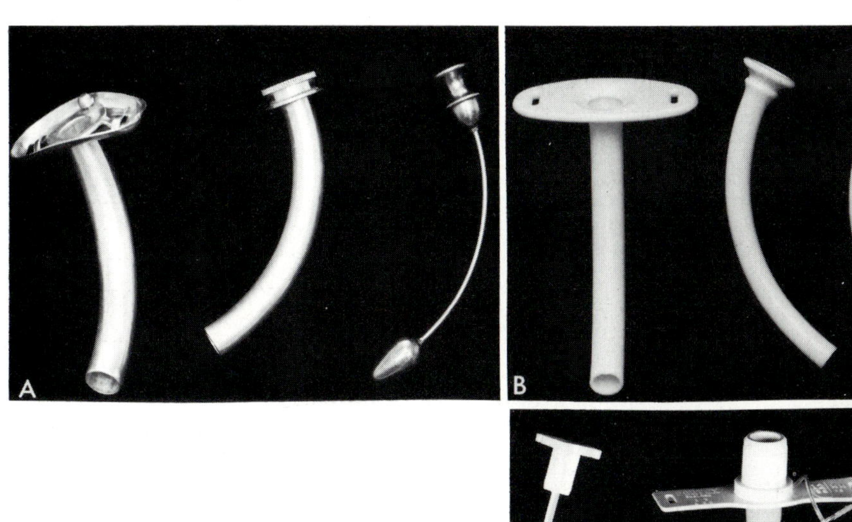

Figure 9–1 *A*, Tracheostomy tube, inner cannula and obturator. Jackson silver No. 7. *B*, Tracheostomy tube, inner cannula and obturator. Moore silastic No. 6. *C*, Tracheostomy tube and obturator. Portex No. 36.

TABLE 9–1

TRACHEAL DIAMETER	INFANTS TO 1 YEAR		1 TO 3 YEARS		4 TO 6 YEARS
Outer Diameter of Tube (mm.)	4.3	5	6	7	8
Jackson (Silver) Tube	00	1	2	3	4
Portex Tube (French System)	13	16	18	21	24
Silastic Tube		1		3	4.5

TRACHEAL DIAMETER'	ADOLESCENTS AND SMALL ADULTS		MOST ADULTS			
Outer Diameter of Tube (mm.)	9	10	11	12	13	14
Jackson (Silver) Tube	5	6	7	8	9	10
Portex Tube (French System)	27	30	33	36	39	42
Silastic tube		6				

Some tracheostomy tubes are available with low-tension cuffs on them.

c. *Material.* Silastic (siliconized rubber) tubes have been found to be superior to silver tubes, especially in pediatric patients.[9] They have less tendency to form inspissated plugs and granulation tissue and are also less traumatic. Portex or polyvinyl plastic tubes demonstrate similar advantages in adult patients. The tracheostomy tube must be checked and ready for insertion before the incision is made. This can prevent pneumomediastinum and pneumothorax in the following way. When the tracheal incision is made, the mucosa is irritated and the patient coughs, sometimes violently. If the tube is not ready, the assistant might lose control while retracting the trachea superiorly and anteriorly. When the trachea falls inferiorly, blasts of air are coughed into the mediastinum and thorax.

3. Prepare culture tube and suction. When the tracheostomy is performed, the cough reflex is often productive of a large amount of pus. Time and effort should not be wasted at this critical moment. A smear for gram stain and a culture are taken and excessive secretions are suctioned.

4. Recognize the importance of light and position. One can get into trouble if these simple details are ignored. A patient who is awake with an endotracheal tube in place experiences a great deal of pain with the neck in a hyperextended position. It is better to have the nurse place a bolster (pillow or rolled sheet) under the patient's shoulder after the surgeon has scrubbed and everything is ready to proceed.

The skin is prepped from the mandible to below the clavicle. Palpate midline structures to identify the hyoid bone, thyroid notch, cricoid cartilage and suprasternal notch. The skin and subcutaneous tissues are infiltrated with one per cent lidocaine in a transverse line halfway between the cricoid cartilage and suprasternal notch.

A transverse incision is made halfway between the cricoid cartilage and suprasternal notch (Fig. 9–2). It extends through the skin and subcutaneous tissue down to the superficial layer of deep cervical fascia. Small dermal vessels will be encountered and are easily controlled by pressure or clamping. The midline is then identified by palpating the cricoid cartilage and visualizing the linea alba seen between the bellies of the sternohyoid muscles. The cervical fascia is incised in the midline from the cricoid to one cm. above the sternal notch. The anterior jugular veins are located laterally and the anterior communicating veins are

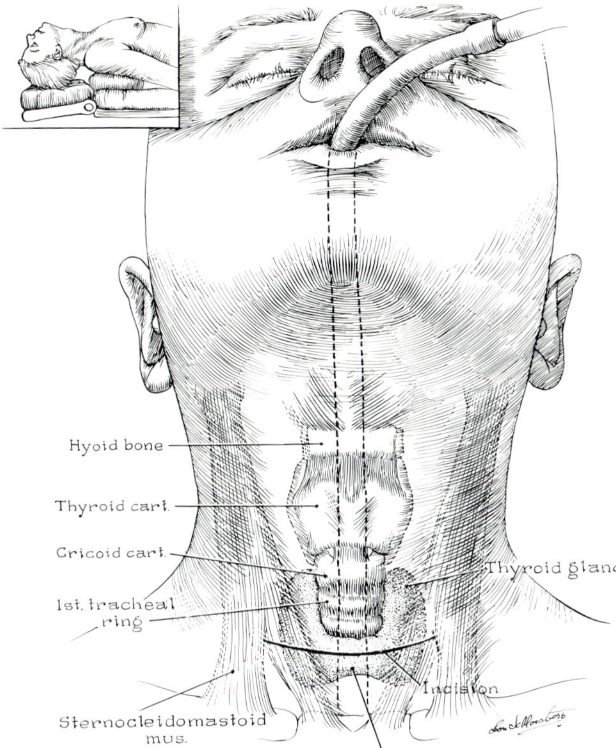

Figure 9–2 Illustration of position for tracheostomy, midline structures and incision.

located inferiorly. They should not be in the line of dissection. The strap muscles are retracted laterally with vein retractors exposing the thyroid gland and trachea. If the thyroid isthmus is freely moveable, it can be displaced superiorly or inferiorly with a vein retractor. In adults, the thyroid is often more fibrotic and firmly attached to pretracheal fascia. In these instances, it is preferable to clamp; divide and suture ligate the isthmus (Fig. 9–3). It is then bluntly dissected off the trachea. A tracheal hook is inserted beneath the first ring, and the trachea is retracted superiorly and anteriorly. The anesthetist is instructed to deflate the endotracheal tube cuff. One cc. of lidocaine is injected into the trachea. A cruciate incision (Fig. 9–4) is made between tracheal rings two and three. A window of cartilage is not removed because this is associated with an increased incidence of tracheal stenosis.[16] The endotracheal tube is removed, culture and smear taken and the trachea suctioned. The tracheostomy tube is inserted with its obturator in place. The obturator and the bolster are removed, head is flexed and tracheostomy ribbons are tied with a

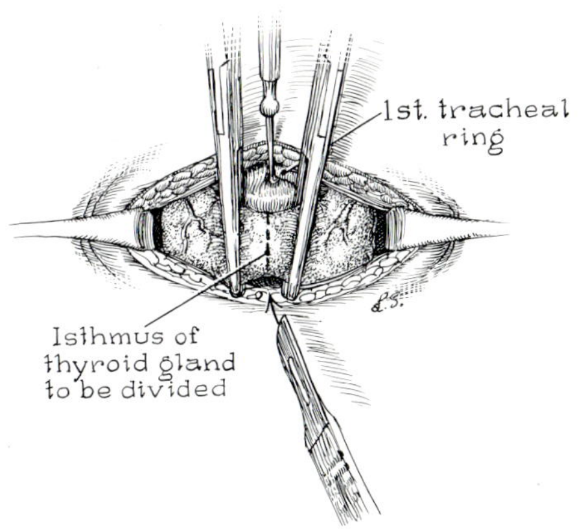

Figure 9–3 Transect thyroid isthmus.

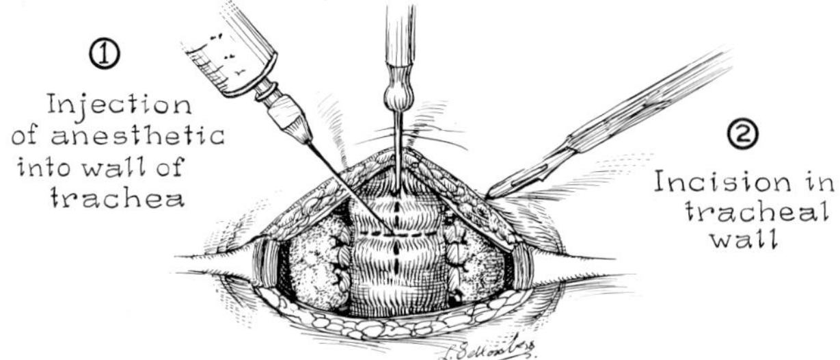

Figure 9–4 Incision between tracheal rings two and three after injecting with local anesthetic.

square knot. Wound sutures predispose to the development of subcutaneous emphysema (Fig. 9–5).

POSTOPERATIVE CARE AND COMPLICATIONS

The injured patient has a high mortality from airway obstruction. Because of complications such as laryngotracheal stenosis, pneumonitis and inadequate ventilation, endotracheal tubes cannot be used for long periods and tracheostomy is indicated. When tracheostomy is performed, one again must face the risk of high mortality and morbidity. Once the airway has been established, complications then arise from the operative procedure, inadequate nursing care and changed respiratory physiology.

Early Complications

Early complications associated with the surgical procedure and ways to avoid them have already been alluded to and are further discussed below.

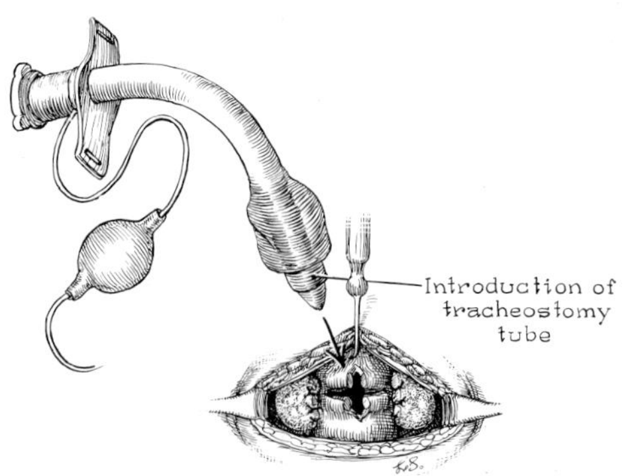

Figure 9–5 Insertion of tracheostomy tube.

Pneumomediastinum and Pneumothorax. Secure control of the trachea after making a tracheal incision with the tracheal hook in place. Suction the trachea and insert a tracheostomy tube without delay. Do not suture the wound, and do not ventilate the patient with high pressures which rupture alveoli. Lateral dissection in a struggling patient predisposes to cutting lung apices, though this is uncommon. Intubation preoperatively allows a less hurried operation with less struggle.

Air Embolism. This results from transecting anterior jugular veins or subclavian veins without control or recognition.

Hemorrhage. Early hemorrhage is due to improper suture ligation of thyroid isthmus, poor control of venous drainage, or inadvertent incision of the subclavian vein in the subclavian fossa. For purposes of management, identify source and secure hemostasis with suture or cautery.

Tracheoesophageal Fistula. Tracheoesophageal fistula is usually the result of using too much downward pressure with a large scalpel blade while making tracheostomy. The esophagus is often distended in a struggling patient. Immediate exploration of the neck is done with primary closure of the fistula.

Apnea. After tracheostomy has been performed, the patient is relieved of his airway obstruction and the hemoglobin is oxidized. He has lost his hypoxic drive and becomes apneic. Respirations should be assisted during this period with a respirator or manually with an Ambu bag.

Dislodged Tracheostomy Tube. If tracheostomy ribbons are tied while the neck is hyperextended, they are too loose when the bolster is removed. This allows the tracheostomy tube to be coughed out during suctioning. For the same reason, bulky dressings should be avoided on the tracheostomy wound. If the tracheostomy tube becomes dislodged within the first 24 hours, one again has an emergent obstructive problem to manage and the steps should follow a logical sequence.

Light, position, suction, tracheostomy tube, hook and retractors are all necessary tools to be used again for reinsertion. This was a critical moment in the operating room and is even more critical now. If the tube cannot be reinserted with direct visualization, it is important to reinsert an endotracheal tube. Valuable time is often lost by trying to thread a tracheostomy tube over a suction catheter, ostensibly in the trachea.

Late Complications

Inspissated Mucus. The most common cause of death from tracheostomy is obstruction due to inspissated mucous plugs. This can be avoided by efficient humidification to the tracheostomy by a "tracheal mask" or by the ventilatory apparatus. Suctioning is necessary almost every 30 minutes during the first 24 hours, then every one to two hours thereafter, more often if necessary. If secretions continue to be dry, one should be aware of the patient's general state of hydration, replacing known deficits. One to three cc. of sterile saline may be instilled within the trachea before suctioning.

Infection and Pneumonitis. After 48 hours, almost all tracheostomies have a positive culture for *Staphylococcus aureus*, *Pseudomonas aeruginosa*, *Proteus vulgaris* or *Escherichia coli*. The humidification and filtering systems of the nose and pharynx are bypassed along with the antibodies produced there. Dry, dirty air damages tracheal mucosa, causing a loss of cilia and its normal movement. The respiratory epithelium becomes atrophic and undergoes squamous metaplasia. With the normal physiology interrupted, bacterial infections are common. Tracheobronchitis due to tracheostomy usually does not require antibiotic therapy. The infection clears as soon as the tracheostomy tube is removed and the normal airway is established.

Twenty-five per cent of patients develop pneumonitis with fever, leucocytosis and radiographic changes. This is often associated with underlying pathology or aspiration of oral secretions. It can also result from contaminated sources in the environment..

Granulation Tissue. Granulation tissue develops after respiratory mucosa becomes ulcerated and the lamina propria is destroyed. This occurs as a result of pressure necrosis from the tracheostomy tube at the stoma, cuff or tip. Foreign body reaction from the tracheostomy tube also stimulates granulation tissue. When the tracheostomy tube is removed, granulation tissue can act like a ball valve obstruction. Hemorrhage is common. Granulation tissue can be excised and cauterized. Removing the tracheostomy tube (foreign body) is most helpful.

Tracheal Stenosis and Tracheomalacia. Further progression of tracheal injury from tracheostomy tubes, especially in patients on respirators, results in chondritis and cartilage necrosis. With loss of cartilage support, the trachea collapses when the rigid tube is removed. Obstruction occurs after decannulation. Acquired tracheomalacia is caused by using too-large tracheostomy tubes, trauma, infection, foreign body reaction and drag by respiratory tubing. The respirator tubing should be supported on the patient or his bed. Low-pressure cuffs should be used and deflated at hourly intervals.

Delayed Hemorrhage. Bright red blood that occurs in tracheal secretions three to five days after tracheostomy indicates ulceration of tracheal mucosa. This might be a superficial ulceration from traumatic suctioning, i.e., the catheter is too large and is used too often. It could also indicate deep erosion of the trachea, esophagus and/or innominate artery. Fifty per cent of cases of massive exsanguination are preceded by a small, bright, bloody ooze. When blood is obtained from the trachea, it should be a cause for alarm. The physician is obligated to identify its source by direct visualization and then to take necessary measures to stop it.

It is important to remove the tracheostomy tube and examine the stoma and trachea with a Jackson laryngoscope. Bronchoscopes are too long and narrow. The stoma, cuff site, and tip site should be carefully evaluated for types of secretion and depth of ulceration. AP and lateral chest x-rays are of some help.

Once the diagnosis has been made, then one can change suction catheters to size twelve French and re-examine the technique of suctioning. The length of the tracheostomy tube may be changed so that the cuff is at a higher or lower position.

Innominate Artery Erosion. This is a hazard which was seen more commonly with long, silver Jackson tubes but it still occurs. In reported cases,[12, 13, 14] most of the patients had neurological problems and were on respirators. Cough, retrosternal pain, pulsating tracheostomy tube and a bloody ooze often precede the final event by several hours. Rigid cuffed tubes, unusual pressure, drag of respirator tubes, tip erosion and infection predispose to innominate artery erosion. Inflation of a large cuff produces tamponade and allows a brief period to administer blood and perform a median sternotomy. Survival from innominate artery erosion is uncommon.

Tracheoesophageal Fistula. Tracheoesophageal fistula occurs after the seventh to tenth day and is a result of high-tension cuffs. It is more common in patients who are unconscious with nasogastric tubes. This complication is usually lethal. Patients cannot tolerate thoracotomy well in face of severe aspiration pneumonitis.

Tracheocutaneous Fistula. Most tracheostomies heal by secondary intention and are closed after 48 hours. If mucosa is continuous with skin, a fistula can be excised with a local anesthetic and the wound closed in mucosal, subcutaneous and skin layers.

Cosmetic Defects. Vertical midline incisions tend to heal with contractures. This is unappealing and requires a Z-plasty procedure for its correction.

Emergency Tracheostomy

Immediate tracheostomy is indicated with severe laryngeal injury, facial fractures and other instances when intubation cannot be performed. The midline structures of the neck are palpated. A vertical incision is made between the cricoid and one cm. above the suprasternal notch. Complications occur after most emergent tracheostomies. One must know what the complications are, how they are likely to occur and whether the complication itself is more life-threatening than the present patient status.

Coniotomy

A coniotomy is an incision made into the subglottic trachea through the skin, subcutaneous tissue and fascia in the cricothyroid interval. A small tracheostomy tube, number six (Jackson) or 32 (Portex) can be inserted to establish an airway if one doesn't have the time, skill, light or help to do a tracheostomy. A coniotomy is a lifesaving procedure done to provide an airway, to give the surgeon time to get the patient to an operating room and time to get appropriate equipment. It should not be left in place for more than six hours because the curved tracheostomy tube causes ulceration of both vocal cords and anterior commissure which are immediately above. When the ulceration heals, both vocal cords fuse, resulting in an absent airway and an aphonic laryngeal cripple. Coniotomy is rarely indicated.

POSTOPERATIVE ORDERS

Patients with tracheostomy should be transferred to an intensive care unit or have special duty nurses 24 hours each day. Nurses should be specially trained in aseptic technique to care for these patients. It is always the physician's responsibility to know whether or not the patient is getting adequate care. Casual observation by physicians is dangerous to the patient. Instead, he must personally suction the tracheostomy after the nurses, and he must observe the technique of cuff deflation, wound and tube care—not once, but on every shift and with every change of personnel. Postoperative procedures are briefly delineated as follows:

1. Transfer patient to intensive care unit or provide special duty nurses for every shift.
2. a. Suction tracheostomy every 30 minutes for the first six hours, then every hour or more often, as needed.
   b. Use number 12 French catheters for adults.
   c. Instill one to three cc. normal saline prior to suctioning if secretions are thick or dry.
   d. Suction trachea prior to and after deflation of tracheostomy tube cuff.
   e. Suction trachea prior to and after turning the patient.
   f. Suction trachea after each feeding.
   g. Suction oral cavity and anterior nares each hour—after tracheal suctioning and with number 16 French catheter.
3. Apply cold steam mask to tracheostomy at all times.
4. Provide bell at patient's side to notify nurse.
5. Provide magic slate and marker (or paper and pencil).
6. Be certain that number 36 (or appropriate size) tracheostomy tube, obturator, tracheal hook and dilator are at bedside or readily available.
7. Secure overhead light or gooseneck lamp.
8. Deflate cuff for five minutes every hour. Reinflate cuff slowly just to the point where no leak is heard in the oral cavity and nose. If more than three cc. are necessary, call physician immediately.
9. Observe for wheezing from tracheostomy tube (plugs), bleeding, unusual tracheal pulsations, subcutaneous emphysema, chest pain, gastric secretions or food in trachea. Notify physician if any of these occur.
10. Auscultate tracheostomy every 4-6 hours, noting absent or unusual breath sounds.
11. Make chest x-ray (portable) on arrival in room. Call physician when available.

REFERENCES

1. Awe, W. C., Fletcher, W. S., and Jacob, S. W.: The pathophysiology of aspiration pneumonitis. Surgery *60*: 232, 1966.
2. Belts, R. H.: Post tracheostomy aspiration. New Eng. J. Med. *273*:155, 1965.
3. Bigler, J. A., Holinger, P. H., and Johnston, K. C.: Tracheostomy in infancy. Pediatrics *13*:476, 1954.
4. Cameron, J. L., Anderson, R. P., and Zuidema, G. D.: Aspiration pneumonia: A clinical and experimental review. J. Surg. Res. *7*:44, 1967.
5. Carroll, D., and Dutton, R.: The management of respiratory problems in critically ill medical patients including indications for and results of tracheostomy. Johns Hopkins Med. J., *85*:(No. 3):163–176, 1969.
6. Cooper, J. D., and Grillo, H. C.: The evolution of tracheal injury due to ventilatory assistance through cuffed tubes: A pathologic study, Ann. Surg. *169*:334–348, 1969.
7. Flege, J. B.: Tracheoesophageal fistula caused by cuffed tracheostomy tubes. Ann. Surg. *166*:153–196, 1967.
8. Glas, W. W., and King, O. J., Complications

of tracheostomy. Arch. Surg. *85*:72, 1962.

9. Gosch, H. H., and Kindt, G. W.: Head injury—Some current concepts in management. Univ. Michigan Med. J. *37*:74, 1971.
10. Haller, J., and Talbert, J. L.: Clinical evaluation of a new silastic tracheostomy tube for respiratory support of infants and young children. Ann. Surg. *171*: 915, 1970.
11. James, A. E., MacMillan, A. S., et al.: Radiological considerations of granuloma and stenosis at tracheostomy site. Radiology. *96*:513–520, 1970.
12. Lowbury, E. J., Thom, B. T., et al.: Sources of infection with Pseudomonas aeruginosa in patients with tracheostomy. J. Med. Microbiol. *3*:39, 1970.
13. Lu, A. T., and Tamura, Y.: The pathology of laryngotrachial complications. Arch. Otol. *74*:323–332, 1961.
14. Mathog, R. H., and Hudson, W. R.: Delayed massive hemorrhage following tracheostomy. Laryngoscope *79*:107, May, 1969.
15. Meade, J. W.: Tracheostomy—Its complications and their management. New Eng. J. Med. *265*:519, 1961.
16. Neuman, M. M.: Tracheostomy, Surg. Clin. N. Amer. *49*:6, 1969.
17. Pearson, F. G., Goldberg, M., and Da Silva, A. J.: A prospective study of tracheal injury complicating tracheostomy with a cuffed tube. J. Laryng. Otol. Rhinol. *71*:867, 1968.
18. Rabuzzi, D. D., and Reed, G. F.: Intrathoracic complications following tracheostomy in children. J. Laryng. Otol. Rhinol. *85*:939, 1971.
19. Seed, R. F.: Traumatic injury to the larynx and trachea. Anesthesia *26*:55, 1971.
20. Silen, W., and Spieker, D.: Fatal hemorrhage from innominate artery after tracheostomy. Ann. Surg. *162*:1005, 1965.
21. Skaggs, J. A., and Cogbill, C. L.: Tracheostomy: Management, mortality, complications. Am. Surg. *36*:393, 1969.

chapter

10

THORACIC INJURIES

Robert B. Rutherford, M.D.

THE PROBLEM

Approximately 25 per cent of all civilian traumatic deaths in this country result primarily from chest injuries, and in another 25-50 per cent they contribute significantly to the lethal outcome; yet the relative contribution of chest injuries to mortality after trauma victims have reached the hospital ward is small. Although a significant number of these people die before reaching a medical facility and others, in spite of vigorous and well-directed attempts at resuscitation, expire shortly after arrival in the emergency room, the fate of many patients with chest injuries is determined by the responses of the physicians who first attend them.

It has also been shown that thoracotomy is required in only 10 per cent or less of cases of major thoracic trauma. Furthermore, most of the resuscitative procedures that suffice in the remainder should fall within the capabilities of the primary physicians who staff emergency departments: thoracentesis, intercostal nerve block, endotracheal intubation, tracheostomy, pericardiocentesis, blood transfusion, tube thoracostomy and nasotracheal suction. This is fortunate, because many of these injuries will occur in areas far removed from major medical centers served by thoracic surgeons; furthermore, the resuscitation of the critically injured patient with serious chest injuries usually cannot await his arrival.

This combination of therapeutic potential and necessity emphasizes the importance of the ability of "front-line" physicians to recognize and treat the various types of thoracic trauma. Van Waggoner[65] estimated, from an analysis of over 600 traumatic deaths occurring *after* arrival at the hospital, that one-sixth could have been prevented by prompt diagnosis and that an additional one-sixth could have been salvaged by institution of correct treatment. The best results are obtained by the physician who has a preconceived plan of action and the proper equipment with which to carry it out. In more severe cases, the three R's of trauma—recognition, resuscitation and repair—cannot be executed in orderly sequence punctuated by periods of contemplation. Therefore, before discussing in detail each of the different kinds of thoracic trauma, a general approach to the initial evaluation and management of chest injuries is presented, with emphasis on the critically injured. Later, the mechanisms and pathophysiology of the different types of thoracic trauma will be separately discussed.

Much of the basic equipment and the techniques used in the resuscitation of the injured patient are discussed in the chapters on "Initial Evaluation and Treatment," "Cardiopulmonary Resuscitation and Anesthesia in Trauma" and "The Treatment of Shock" and need not be enumerated here. Materials and methods peculiar to the resuscitation of chest trauma patients are described in conjunction with the condition to which they apply.

The Pathophysiology and Pathodynamics of Thoracic Trauma

Chest injuries are classically divided into two categories—penetrating and nonpenetrating. This separation has clinical importance beyond the simple consideration of the mechanisms of injury in that certain injuries fall almost entirely in one or the other group. For example, cardiac tamponade is encountered in an emergency room almost only after penetrating trauma, because myocardial rupture following blunt trauma is almost always immediately fatal and more minor pericardial bleeding usually either goes unnoticed or presents as a delayed pericardial effusion with or without tamponade as the red cells undergo lysis. By the same token, blunt trauma, as typified by a steering wheel injury, may be associated with sternal and rib fractures, flail chest, pulmonary or myocardial contusions, rupture of the thoracic aorta, diaphragm, or a major bronchus and other injuries rarely encountered following penetrating trauma. This type of knowledge contributes to the experienced physician's "index of suspicion."

Currently, blunt trauma causes the majority of serious (admitted) chest injuries with traffic accidents (55 per cent) and falls (15 per cent) contributing most heavily. However, in large urban medical centers, this ratio may be reversed. The mortality associated with blunt or non-penetrating thoracic trauma is greater only to the degree with which they are associated with multisystem injuries. The mortality of isolated chest injuries is in the range of 4–12 per cent, but increases to 13–15 per cent with another system involved and to 30–35 per cent with two or more systems involved.[6] The head, abdomen and extremities are affected in that order of frequency.

Stabbings account for almost three-fourths of penetrating chest injuries in most large civilian hospitals, but this is changing with an increasing preference for firearms among the criminal element. The mortality from stab wounds of the chest is lower (2–3 per cent) than from gunshot wounds, which approximates that of nonpenetrating chest trauma with involvement of another system (i.e., 14–20 per cent).[6] Nevertheless, hemothorax and hemopericardium caused by penetrating wounds still constitute the major indications for thoracotomy following chest trauma.

Understanding the effects of a penetrating injury may be as simple as tracing the trajectory of a knife or low-velocity missile through the structures in its path or as complicated as appreciating the degree of "blunt" trauma caused by temporary cavity formation perpendicular to the trajectory of a high-velocity missile.[8] Blunt trauma may be inflicted by a variety of direct and indirect forces, the latter being more important than the striking object. Classically, the extent of injury from a direct impact may be related to the magnitude and duration of the applied force, its velocity (rate of onset and decay) and duration and the area to which it is applied. Indirectly, within the thorax, these forces are translated into those of acceleration, torsion, compression and shear. Acceleration and deceleration themselves, over and above direct impact, may be responsible for serious intrathoracic trauma, as may be appreciated from Figure 10–1 *A* to *D*. By comparison a force of 20G may be associated with 40 mph impacts and 60G by 60 mph.[6] Shearing forces may result from differences in the degree of fixation or mobility of adjacent tissues, as in the site of predilection for disruption of the thoracic aorta near the ligamentum arteriosum, where there is a transition between mobile and fixed segments of the thoracic aorta. Compression and/or

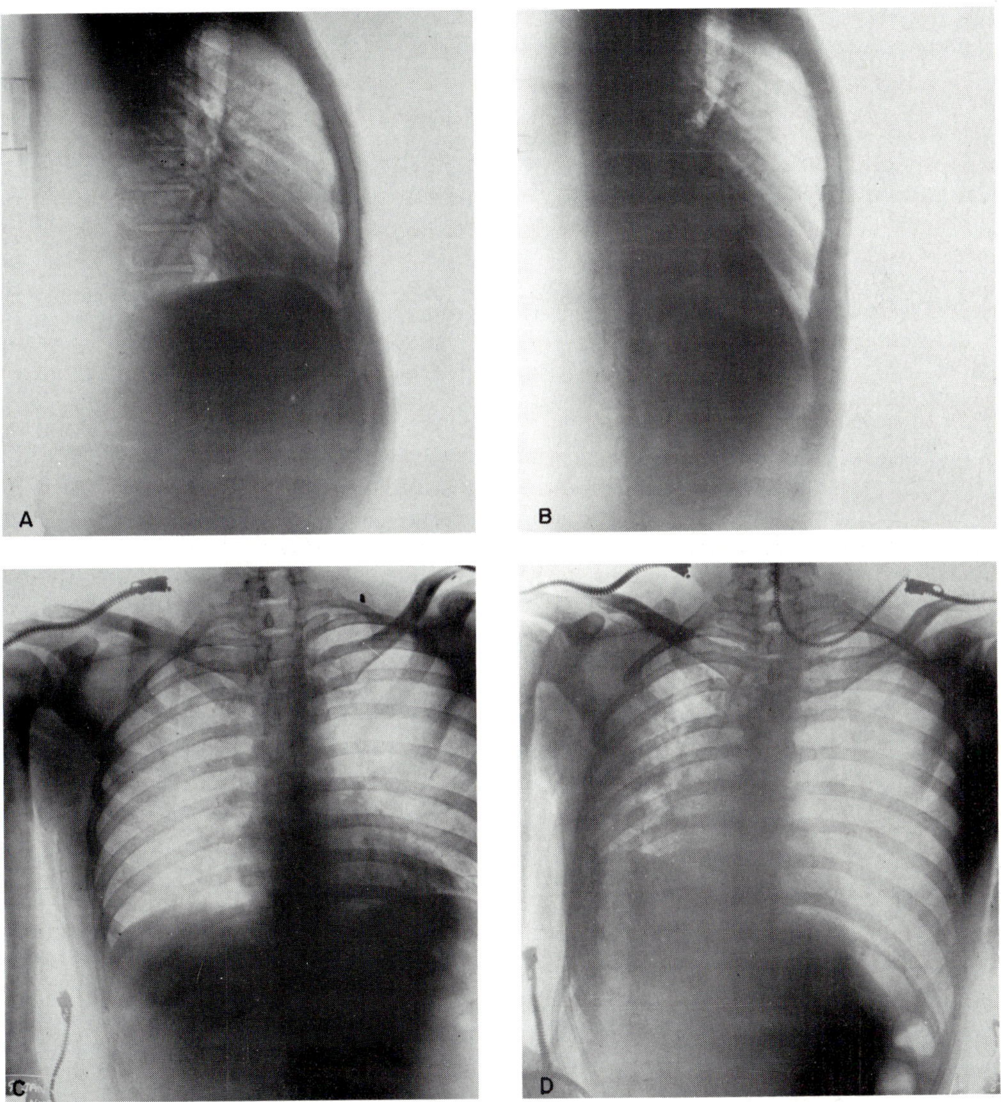

Figure 10–1 Displacement of the intrathoracic contents produced by a 5 G accelerating force in a forward (*A-B*) and lateral (*C-D*) direction. The distortion of the diaphragm, shift of the heart and mediastinum and change in the density of the pulmonary parenchyma in relation to the direction of acceleration (to the reader's right) can be seen in *B* and *D*. (Courtesy of Dr. Edward J. Hershgold: Aerospace Medicine *31*:213, 1960.)

decompression may play a major role in producing pulmonary contusions since the work of both Border[10] and Rutherford[58] and their coworkers suggest that a closed airway (glottis or experimentally an obstructed endotracheal tube) increases the likelihood and severity of pulmonary contusions.

AN APPROACH TO THE PATIENT WITH SERIOUS CHEST INJURY

Diagnosis. Fortunately, the different forms of thoracic trauma capable of causing *severe* cardiorespiratory embarrassment *soon* after injury are limited in number and are usually readily recognized if specifically sought. Thus, whenever ventilatory and/or circulatory insufficiency (shock) develop *soon* after chest trauma, initial examination should be quickly directed toward six conditions: open pneumothorax, airway obstruction, flail chest, tension pneumothorax, massive hemothorax and cardiac tamponade.

In addition, there are another half dozen potentially serious (lethal) conditions which may be causing only modest cardiorespiratory difficulties at the time of admission and which are usually not so readily diagnosed on the basis of physical findings. These include rupture or tear of the aorta, diaphragm, esophagus or tracheobronchial tree and pulmonary or myocardial contusion. The first five can often be diagnosed or at least strongly suspected, after viewing an upright chest film with these conditions specifically in mind. An EKG may provide the only clue to a myocardial contusion.

Beyond these "dirty dozen," the need for early diagnosis and treatment is less critical, for most of what remains are the "routine" problems of fractured ribs and lesser degrees of hemo- or pneumothorax. This is the basis for the advice to perform a brief but pointed chest examination, should inadequate ventilatory exchange or circulatory impairment be found, and to go ahead and obtain an upright chest film if they are not. While the x-ray is being developed, there is time for further examination. The remainder of this section will be devoted to elaborating on this initial approach.

The condition responsible for the patient's distress may be suspected immediately if one hears the characteristic sound of a sucking chest wound or the stridor or coarse rhonchi of airway obstruction. Knowledge of the wounding mechanism may suggest one condition above the others and alter the order of examination. For example, cardiac tamponade is considered in patients with precordial wounds; massive hemothorax with any penetrating wound; and flail chest, rupture of the aorta, bronchus, esophagus or diaphragm with steering wheel injuries.

Usually, gross assessment of the degree of ventilatory and circulatory impairment should come first. This may immediately orient the examiner toward certain lesions, since some produce mainly ventilatory insufficiency (e.g., airway obstruction, flail chest) and others mainly circulatory impairment (e.g., massive hemothorax, cardiac tamponade). If one places an ear close to the patient's mouth and nose, watches the movements of the bared chest and palpates the pulse at the wrist, much valuable information can be obtained (Fig. 10–2). With a little experience one can gauge the adequacy of ventilatory exchange by the force, duration and frequency with which the expired air strikes the ear. A strong blast of air would eliminate the possibility of significant interference with the ventilatory mechanism; and if such a patient was in shock, cardiac tamponade or massive hemothorax would be the primary considerations.

If the exchange is poor in spite of good effort, inspection of the chest may provide the answer. An open pneumothorax should be obvious, as should any paradoxical movement of the chest

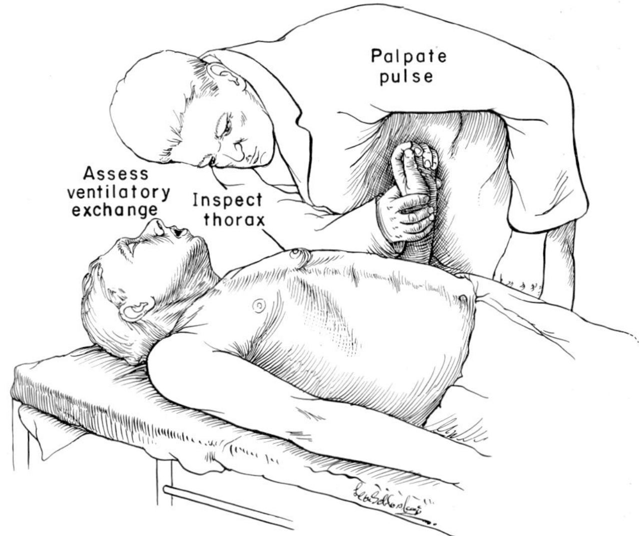

Figure 10–2 Initial evaluation for chest injuries. Assessment of the adequacy of ventilatory exchange, the integrity and movements of the thoracic cage, and the degree of circulatory impairment provide a quick orientation to the nature of the patient's problem.

wall severe enough to cause respiratory embarassment, particularly since the flail segment usually involves the anterior or lateral thorax. On the other hand, if the exchange is poor in spite of symmetrical and vigorous respiratory efforts, airway obstruction probably exists. This is not necessarily associated with stridor, crowing or audible, coarse rhonchi. However, if one hemithorax is *prominent* and does not move well with respiration, the problem is probably a large pneumo- or hemothorax, whereas the involved hemi-thorax is *diminished* in volume when poor excursions are the result of splinting against painful rib fractures or massive atelectasis. Before proceeding further with examination of the thorax, the neck should be examined to determine the relative position of the trachea, the presence of subcutaneous emphysema and fullness of the neck veins (independent of straining efforts). Both tension pneumothorax and a massive hemothorax may produce a prominent hemithorax with poor excursions, diminished breath sounds and a shift of the trachea to the opposite side. The former is more likely to be associated with subcutaneous emphysema and prominent neck veins, but a hyperresonant percussion note is of greater diagnostic significance. Massive hemothorax, on the other hand, is associated with a dull percussion note *posteriorly* and the neck veins are not full. Since two-thirds to three-fourths of patients with hemothorax also have some degree of pneumothorax, the percussion note anteriorly may be misleading.

Ventilation is not usually interfered with in cardiac tamponade and not until late in massive hemothorax. Therefore, if initial assessment discloses a diminished pulse but fairly adequate air exchange, consideration should first be given to these two conditions or to some extrathoracic cause of shock. The signs of hemothorax have already been mentioned. Cardiac tamponade should be suspected if there is a wound over or near the precordium. The diagnostic triad of low arterial pressure, elevated venous pressure and a small, quiet heart described by Beck[5] is not always present or readily apparent. A low arterial pressure is a common denominator in many traumatic conditions, and the struggling or straining of a patient may produce a misleading bulging of the neck veins. The muffling of heart sounds may be subtle and hard to ascertain in a noisy emergency room.

A tension pneumothorax on the left can easily be mistaken for cardiac tamponade. It may give bulging neck veins and, because of mediastinal shift, heart sounds over the normally precordial area may be absent or faint. Another "diagnostic" sign of cardiac tamponade, pulsus paradoxus, represents a fleeting stage in the development of cardiac tamponade and is elicited in only about one-third of such cases. The practice of using a central venous catheter in the management of patients in shock has particular value in this situation. If the central venous pressure is low, one can assume that there is low circulating volume and proceed with volume-expanding infusions. If, however, it is high in the face of shock or if it is normal and becomes quickly elevated with infusions, one should suspect cardiac tamponade and proceed with pericardiocentesis.

The above approach just outlined is admittedly oversimplified, but it is designed to detect only lesions of sufficient magnitude to cause early cardiac or respiratory embarrassment. Lesser degrees of these and other conditions may be missed while a search is made for the major threat to the patient's life. However, if this primary purpose is achieved, such lesser injuries can be detected when time allows a more painstaking examination and chest x-rays. The main failing of such an approach occurs in patients whose critical condition is the result of a summation of multiple injuries, none sufficient to be obvious on such a cursory examination. This is particularly true when multiple systems are involved. Such an examination, of course, represents only one part of the over-all evaluation of the critically injured patient.

Initial Resuscitation. The simplest effective resuscitative measures must be employed initially. Valuable time may be wasted waiting for the means to apply more involved methods, although they may be more effective. Consider again the six conditions just discussed. The simple covering of a sucking chest wound with a sterile towel or a gloved hand will transform it functionally into closed pneumothorax, which is reasonably well tolerated. With the major physiologic abnormality corrected, a definitive dressing can be prepared when assistance is available, following which a chest tube can be inserted.

An open airway should be established by the simplest effective means. Tracheostomy is employed too often and too early in combating the various forms of airway obstruction. In the unconscious patient simply clearing the pharynx and inserting an oropharyngeal airway may bring significant relief. If not, insertion of an endotracheal tube should be the next step. Emergency tracheostomy should be reserved for patients with mechanical obstruction or those in whom simpler measures bring only transient relief. Tracheostomy can be a risky and time-consuming procedure when carried out under the suboptimal conditions common in many emergency treatment rooms.

Similarly, placing the hands gently but firmly on a flail chest segment or laying the patient with the injured side down reduces the paradoxical movements that rob the thoracic bellows of its ability to move air. Later, multiple towel clips or pericostal sutures can be used to apply traction to this segment; or, as is more common in patients with a major degree of paradox, a tracheostomy may be performed and the patient be placed on a positive pressure respirator.

The quickest way to eliminate the lethal potential of a tension pneumothorax is to insert an intravenous needle through the chest wall into the involved pleural space, allowing it to equilibrate with atmospheric pressure. This maneuver converts the situation into that of an open pneumothorax, but with an opening so small that functionally it is little worse than a simple pneumothorax. The patient's condition is immediately improved, and there is then time to insert a chest tube and to apply suction to expand the lung.

In patients with massive hemothorax the first measure is to restore the blood volume. Only after this is underway (usually with *two* large-bore intravenous pathways established) *should the blood* be evacuated from the thorax through a posterolaterally placed chest tube. If large volumes are removed or the patient's response is not gratifying, immediate operation is indicated.

Pericardiocentesis relieves nearly all patients with cardiac tamponade *initially* and in a significant but selected number may be the only intervention necessary. Details of resuscitation in these and other conditions are included later in this chapter.

X-Ray. As previously mentioned, an upright chest film should be taken as soon as the initial evaluation and resuscitation have been accomplished. This does not mean that the patient should be "sent to x-ray." The attending physician's surveillance of the patient should not be interrupted by this examination. In the same vein, although one should take full advantage of the interpretation of the film by a radiologist, if he is in attendance, the treating physician should always bring his own index of suspicion to bear on this x-ray and interpret it independently before seeking consultation.

A widening of the mediastinal shadow may be the only clue to a temporarily contained rupture of the thoracic aorta. In a patient who has sustained severe blunt trauma to the thorax, such a finding, if unequivocal and associated with a left hemothorax, constitutes a valid indication for immediate thoracotomy. If the widening is equivocal, if there is no associated hemothorax and if the patient's condition is stable, the operating room should be alerted to stand by for emergency thoracotomy while a diagnostic aortogram is performed.

Rupture of the esophagus, though a rare complication of chest trauma, should be considered with any pneumomediastinum or left pneumothorax of traumatic origin, particularly if there are no fractured ribs or penetrating wounds on that side. In two-thirds of esophageal ruptures secondary to blunt trauma, an epigastric rather than a thoracic blow is responsible. Mediastinal widening is usually a late finding in this condition, but occasionally a stippling of air may be seen in the left cardiophrenic region. A swallow of contrast material (Hypaque) is a simple and harmless way to confirm this suspicion and may be lifesaving since failure to diagnose this condition is mainly responsible for the 80 per cent mortality rate (two-thirds of reported cases are discovered at autopsy).

Although a fully developed contusion pneumonitis or traumatic "wet lung" can usually be diagnosed by physical signs, an area of diffuse or fluffy opacification on the initial chest x-ray, signalling pulmonary contusion, may provide an early clue. Whenever marked changes such as this are already evident on a chest x-ray taken soon after injury, a severe degree of contusion pneumonitis can be anticipated. The importance of this early recognition is that the development of this "traumatic wet lung" can be suppressed by early tracheostomy and positive pressure ventilation.

Thoracoabdominal injuries, particularly rupture of the diaphragm, may be fatal unless diagnosed and treated early. Penetrating wounds of the diaphragm may be suspected from reconstruction of the course taken by the wounding agent and the victim's position at the time of impact. Operation is frequently dictated by penetration of the subjacent abdominal viscera with attendant bleeding or peritonitis. On the other hand, rupture of the diaphragm from blunt trauma is more likely to present acutely with herniation of abdominal viscera up into the thorax through the large defect. Herniation of air-containing viscera through a tear in the diaphragm may be misinterpreted as a "high stomach bubble." Similarly, an "elevation of the diaphragm" may be more apparent than real and should lead one to suspect diaphragmatic rupture.

Such suspicion can be confirmed by radio-contrast studies of the stomach or colon or by "diagnostic" pneumoperitoneum. An "elevated diaphragm" must also be distinguished from a subpulmonary collection of blood. Such subpulmonary "hematomas" will usually layer out in a lateral decubitus film. The rare herniation of the liver through a right leaf of the diaphragm is harder to diagnose but should be considered when the right leaf of the diaphragm is "elevated." Concomitant elevation of the lower border of the liver shadow strongly supports this suspicion.

The initial chest x-ray may also detect less obvious degrees of trauma that may have been missed in the initial examination. Even the lack of radiologic evidence of significant intrathoracic injury is valuable information and provides a baseline for later comparison. A preliminary chest x-ray will also facilitate the removal of foreign bodies at the time of thoracotomy. Finally, in extensive open wounds of the thorax, an accurate localization of the sites of fracture may be extremely valuable in planning reconstruction.

Reassessment. During the initial period of evaluation and resuscitation, the patient's cardiorespiratory function should be continually reassessed to determine whether his condition has deteriorated further or is responding satisfactorily.

Changes in the patient's condition with time, particularly his response to resuscitative measures, may be just as important as the type of injury sustained in determining the need for operative intervention. This requires more than merely checking the vital signs. In the past it was common to place almost sole reliance on the blood pressure in assessing the patient's hemodynamic state. However, it is well recognized that a 15 to 25 per cent loss in blood volume may be sustained before there is a significant decline in the blood pressure. During this period tachycardia, tachypnea and complaints of thirst may be the only warning signs of impending collapse but, unfortunately, these are nonspecific. In addition, not all hypotension following chest trauma is due to hypovolemia. Pericardial tamponade, severe acidosis, respiratory insufficiency and impaired venous return from the loss of negative intrathoracic pressure may be important contributing factors.

We have found the central venous pressure a valuable addition in monitoring such patients. A large bore plastic catheter inserted into the superior vena cava through the internal jugular or subclavian vein not only produces a major route for intravenous therapy but a reasonably sensitive index of the functional circulating volume. (See Chapter Three.) In addition to this, the rate of urine formation by the kidneys is a valuable guide to adequate tissue perfusion. Serial measurements of arterial and central venous pressures and urinary output are the most practical means of assessing the hemodynamic state of the injured patient.

The adequacy of the respiratory exchange may be grossly estimated by the patient's color, the respiratory excursions of the thorax, and the rate, force and volume of air exchange. However, it must be remembered that although cyanosis is a valuable diagnostic sign when present, its absence should not be reassuring. Recent experience has taught us that significant degrees of respiratory insufficiency may not be appreciated without arterial blood gas analysis (pH, pCO_2 and pO_2). This diagnostic capability is particularly desirable in evaluating the need for or the adequacy of artificial ventilation by a respirator.

If a chest catheter has been inserted, the chest drainage bottles should be carefully inspected since they may provide information about the size of the air leak, the pressure gradients being developed within the pleural space and the rate of bleeding into the chest.

The above guides supplemented with repeated physical and x-ray examinations are the keys to the continuing assessment of the patient with severe chest trauma. If the patient's condition continues to deteriorate or if the response to resuscitation has been only temporary, it may be necessary to proceed immediately with exploratory thoracotomy. Cases that demand such bold action almost invariably involve hemorrhage from the heart or great vessels. In most cases, however, the patient's condition will respond to the appropriate resuscitative measures.

Indications for Early Thoracotomy. These must be individualized for each patient and must take into account trauma to other systems as well as intercurrent diseases.

The following are *relative* indications for immediate or, at least, early thoracotomy: (1) massive or unrelenting intrapleural hemorrhage; (2) cardiac tamponade from gunshot wound or from stab wound if it recurs quickly or is ineffectively relieved by pericardiocentesis; (3) widened mediastinum with a left hemithorax or aortogram confirming aortic disruption; (4) ruptured esophagus; (5) open pneumothorax with major chest wall defect; (6) massive pleural air leak, subcutaneous emphysema, hemoptysis or complete unilateral atelectasis of a degree suggesting ruptured bronchus; (7) gross contamination of the pleural space with foreign bodies; (8) traumatic diaphragmatic hernia, usually requiring laparotomy; (9) valvular or septal cardiac injuries with acute heart failure. These indications will be further qualified along with less immediate indications in the discussion of the individual conditions which now follows.

THE THORACIC CAGE

Soft Tissue Injuries

The principles that apply to the management of soft tissue injuries in general apply equally to injuries of the musculocutaneous superstructure of the thorax and need not be reviewed at this point.

Subcutaneous Emphysema

Subcutaneous emphysema results when air is forced into the subcutaneous tissues from any source. There are three routes by which air can reach this plane of least resistance (Fig. 10–3): (1) through a major disruption of the pleura and intercostal muscles, e.g., a pneumothorax associated with rib fractures; (2) as an outward dissection of mediastinal emphysema, e.g., rupture of bronchus or esophagus, or pneumothorax with a break in the mediastinal pleura; or, rarely, (3) by direct connection with the external wound. Although the air is subcutaneous in many areas, the real planes of dissection are the various fascial planes of the neck and the loose areolar tissue plane between the chest wall proper and musculature of the shoulder girdle.

Though it is an important sign following chest trauma, subcutaneous emphysema itself is usually of little significance, amounting to no more than an annoyance to the patient. Occasionally, air dissecting the deeper fascial planes of the neck may lead to changes in phonation or even mild laryngeal obstruction, but the most annoying problem from the dissection of air in the subcutaneous plane is closure of the eyelids. Secondary infection of the involved tissues rarely occurs. The patient rarely complains once he is assured that the condition is innocuous.

Whenever the unmistakable crepitus in the skin is encountered, its extent and the area of maximal development should be noted. When

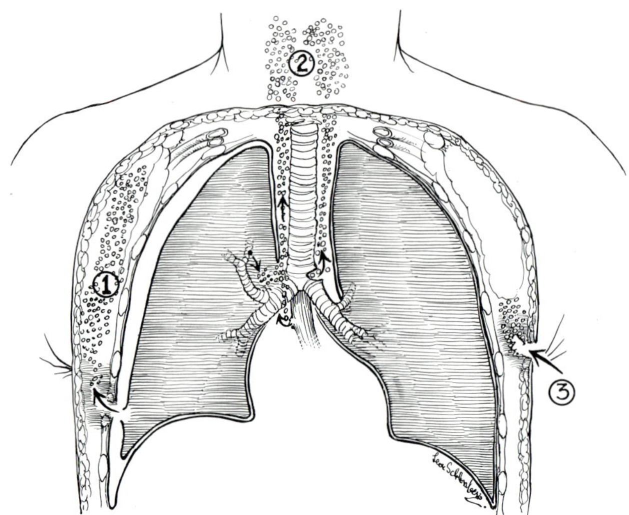

Figure 10–3 The three major sources of subcutaneous emphysema as described in the text.

associated with a traumatic pneumothorax it is maximal in the area of rib fractures. Occasionally it is detected in the area overlying rib fractures without an apparent pneumothorax. Although this is theoretically possible if there is underlying pleural symphysis, the more probable explanation is the failure to detect a small degree of pneumothorax which has almost completely evacuated itself along the lines of least resistance through a defect in the pleura and intercostal muscles. An an outward expression of mediastinal emphysema, subcutaneous air first appears in the neck and is maximal in its development there. This carries a more serious connotation. Whenever it is extensive and progressive, rupture of the esophagus or tracheobronchial tree should be considered. The subcutaneous emphysema associated with an external wound is usually limited in extent and not progressive.

Treatment. Subcutaneous emphysema will progress no further and will be resorbed gradually once its source has been controlled. Therefore, treatment should be directed toward the underlying cause rather than the emphysema itself. In this regard, a halt in the advancing perimeter of the subcutaneous emphysema or its retreat may serve as an important indication of the effectiveness of treatment. Patients with chest injuries not infrequently require tracheostomy. Subcutaneous emphysema may develop secondary to this procedure if the skin is closed too tightly around the tracheostomy. Conversely, subcutaneous emphysema in the neck may vent itself through an open tracheostomy incision. In addition, both tracheostomy and evacuation of a pneumothorax by tube thoracostomy and suction will arrest the progress of subcutaneous emphysema by eliminating or at least decreasing the pressure differentials that force air into the tissues. The breathing of pure oxygen will also help to speed the reabsorption of subcutaneous air by washing nitrogen out of the blood and improving its diffusion from the sequestered air into the circulation. Subcutaneous emphysema will usually yield to such measures. The use of cervical mediastinotomy, venting skin incisions and needle aspiration should be reserved for the uncommon instances in which the subcutaneous emphysema is massive and symptomatic.

Rib Fractures

A simple rib fracture is usually considered a trivial injury by the physician if not the patient. Even a simple rib fracture can lead to serious consequences if treated too lightly, however. This is particularly true in elderly patients whose more rigid, brittle thoracic skeleton can be fractured by relatively minor trauma. Such a patient, with limited cardiorespiratory reserve, fairs poorly if atelectasis or pneumonitis develops secondary to splinting from failure to control pain.

Rib fractures do not occur frequently until adult life and even then, during the third and fourth decades, require a well directed blow of considerable force. Such a forceful blow may result in other more subtle intrathoracic injuries which may not be apparent on initial evaluation. Nor will their subsequent development be anticipated unless the force of the trauma and the manner in which it was inflicted are considered. The number, position and type of rib fractures incurred can provide such information.

The upper ribs are somewhat protected anteriorly by the clavicle, posteriorly by the scapulae and laterally by the arms, as well as by the heavy musculature of the upper thorax and its appendages. For this reason fractures above the fifth rib imply that there has been considerable trauma, and they are not uncommonly associated with serious intrathoracic injuries. Fractures of at least one of the first three ribs were present in 91 per cent of all patients over the age of 30 with rupture of the tracheobronchial tree.[14] Posterior fractures of the upper ribs, especially the first rib, are not infrequent in deceleration accidents when the arms have been held stiffly in extension to brace against the impact, as in automobile and motorcycle collisions. The lower ribs are more mobile and are rarely fractured by indirect forces. However, the lower ribs may be fractured posteriorly by a direct blow and, in such cases, associated injury to the spleen or kidneys should be sought.

The middle ribs, the fifth through the ninth, sustain most blunt thoracic trauma and are the site of most rib fractures. Anteroposterior compression of the thorax causes a decrease in the radius of the rib curvature and results in an outward breaking in the midshaft. This "spring fracture" rarely results in damage to the underlying lung. A direct blow may fracture one or more ribs directly under the point of the impact. The more localized and severe the force, the greater the possibility that fractured rib ends are driven into and damage the underlying lung and pleura. A hemo- or pneumothorax are naturally more common with this type of injury. Severe but more diffusely applied blows, on the other hand, are more likely to fracture the ribs on either side of the point of impact. Fracture of a series of ribs in more than one plane may so destroy continuity with the rest of the thorax that the involved area may move paradoxically, responding to changes in the intrapleural pressure rather than to the muscles of respiration. This serious consequence, known as "flail chest," will be discussed separately later.

Diagnosis. The conscious patient with rib fractures will usually complain of localized chest pain which is aggravated by coughing, deep breathing or changes in position. Pressure on the area indicated by the patient usually elicits point tenderness, and occasionally subcutaneous and bone crepitus is felt. A grating sound may be heard by auscultation of this area as the patient breathes. On the other hand, the patient may not complain of specific discomfort in the period immediately following the trauma. Splinting of respirations on the involved side may be the only clue. Anteroposterior compression of the thorax during the examination will often elicit pain and localize an unsuspected rib fracture and is a useful maneuver in the examination of the injured. This reproduction of the patient's pain by pressure in an area away from the fracture site also helps to differentiate rib fracture from a "strained" or "pulled" intercostal muscle. Pain associated with rib fractures may result in marked splinting and so limit the respiratory excursions and transmission of breath sounds in the involved hemithorax that the presence of fluid or air in the pleural space is suspected.

X-ray examination is important in evaluating such patients. This is not because it is a much surer method of detecting rib fractures. On the contrary, even with special views, overpenetration and the grid technique, it is still difficult to demonstrate some fractures, particularly those located anteriorly and midlaterally. X-rays are superior to physical examination, however, in detecting rib fractures in the more protected parts of the thorax, especially in heavily muscled or obese patients. More important, x-ray films make it possible to diagnose associated intrathoracic injuries with more certainty, to demonstrate the presence of air or blood in the pleural space, and to localize accurately the position and displacement of the rib fractures. Even the x-ray documentation of a simple rib fracture has occasionally proved important in obviating operation for a "pseudotumor" of the rib some time after the original injury had been forgotten.

Treatment. The decision as to how and where to treat the patient must be individualized. Some of the considerations that govern the decision to admit the patient with rib fractures to the hospital are (1) advanced age, (2) underlying cardiorespiratory disease, (3) significant associated injuries, (4) inability to cooperate because of deficient intelligence or personality, (5) jagged rib fragments with marked inward displacement, (6) bleeding dyscrasia, (7) multiple fractures and (8) inability to control the pain with moderate analgesics. Most simple fractures sustained by young or middle-aged patients who are otherwise healthy can be managed on an outpatient basis, with the use of analgesics alone. In such cases one should assess the response to the proposed medication before allowing the patient to leave the hospital, noting particularly the patient's ability to breathe deeply after the analgesic has taken effect. Those not admitted should return within 24 to 48 hours for a follow-up examination and chest x-ray to rule out late complications (bloody effusion, atelectasis, etc.). They should be instructed to take their temperature twice a day and to cough and breathe deeply periodically, preferably at the time of maximal analgesic effect.

INTERCOSTAL NERVE AND EPIDURAL BLOCK. The best means of managing severer degrees of pain from rib fractures is by intercostal nerve block. Although a well-performed nerve block occasionally lasts much longer than the expected four to six hours, it is usually necessary to perform two or three blocks a day for the first few days. Such measures require hospital admission. Here again it is good practice to instruct the patient to breathe deeply and to cough following each block.

Intercostal block is only feasible if the rib fractures are reasonably discrete, since one or two spaces above and below the level of the rib fracture must be infiltrated. The technique is similar to local infiltration prior to thoracentesis except that the nerves are blocked in the paravertebral plane and the infiltrating needle is walked *under* the rib to reach the nerve rather than over it to avoid intercostal vessels (Fig. 10–4). A wheal is made over each of the interspaces proposed for block about three finger breadths lateral to the vertebral spine. A small amount of local anesthetic (1 per cent Xylocaine) is infiltrated as the needle is advanced toward the lower edge of the rib. The needle is walked underneath the lower edge of the rib and at this point, after aspiration to make sure a vessel has not been entered, approximately 3 cc. of the agent is infiltrated.

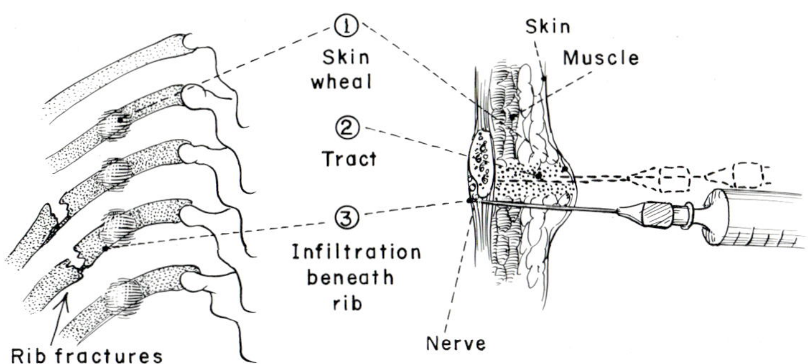

Figure 10–4 The technique of intercostal nerve block as described in the text. Note that the infiltrating needle is "walked" under the lower rilb margin, unlike the technique of thoracentesis.

If several rib fractures have been sustained, the patient may have difficulty localizing the pain well enough to determine the intercostal levels which need blocking. Here x-ray localization will be helpful. A technique for prolonged intercostal block using indwelling polyethylene catheters has been advocated and may prove worthwhile in some instances. Extensive intercostal blocking has the theoretic disadvantage of producing, by summation of intercostal nerve paralysis, almost as much interference with respiration as do narcotics. This fear has not been justified in our clinical experience. More recently, when multiple ribs have been involved, we have used an indwelling epidural catheter placed by an anesthesiologist. This has the advantage of allowing repeated injections and giving sensory without much motor paralysis if the range of the block is not too extensive. In practice, cases of multiple rib fractures requiring such extensive blocks often have "flail chest" and will be managed by tracheostomy and a respirator, in which case control of respirations allows the liberal use of narcotics.

Adhesive Strapping of the Chest. Controversy exists over the use of adhesive strapping of the chest to control the pain of rib fractures. Although this measure undoubtedly makes many patients more comfortable and may be employed without penalty in good risk patients with simple rib fractures, enthusiasm over its use is tempered by the following: (1) it limits the expansion of the thorax and therefore predisposes to atelectasis and secondary pneumonitis; (2) the wide expanse of adhesive tape interferes with examination of the chest; (3) it often leads to a blistering dermatitis, which can be more uncomfortable than the rib fracture itself; (4) it is often no more effective than moderate analgesics, particularly in obese patients and in women with large breasts, which make it difficult to get good splinting with the tape; and (5) it is most effective in controlling pain in patients with lower rib fractures, which constitute a decided minority. Antibiotics are not ordinarily administered, although they may be justified if there is associated cardiorespiratory disease, such as chronic bronchitis and emphysema.

Sternal Fractures

Fracture of the sternum occurs about once in every 20 instances of severe chest trauma, but it rarely requires operative reduction. Laustela,[40] in reporting 304 cases of major chest trauma noted 17 sternal fractures, only four of which required reduction. The mortality rate associated with sternal fractures, however, is high—ranging from 25 to 45 per cent. This, of course, is not the result of the sternal fracture itself, but of as-

sociated injuries. A blow severe enough to cause a sternal fracture will frequently cause serious damage within the thorax. This is attested by the *relatively* frequent association with sternal fractures of disruption of the thoracic aorta, tracheal or bronchial tears, ruptured diaphragm or esophagus, flail chest and contusion of the myocardium or lung. Head injuries are also a frequent accompaniment. It is reported that three-quarters of the sternal fractures resulting from steering wheel injury are associated with head trauma.[29] For these reasons, all patients with sternal fractures, even those with minimal displacement and discomfort, should be admitted to the hospital and observed closely.

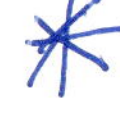

The diagnosis is usually suspected from the nature of the trauma and the patient's complaint of sternal pain aggravated by deep breathing. Localized tenderness, deformity, crepitus and/or false motion over the sternum at the site of fracture (commonly near the junction of the upper and middle thirds) are the physical signs, but there is usually no cause for vigorous attempts to demonstrate the latter two. Nevertheless, it is common for sternal fractures to be discovered hours or even days after the accident because the patient may have been distracted initially by other discomforts and may not complain of sternal pain. X-ray views of the sternum will usually confirm the diagnosis, although lateral films of excellent quality may be required to demonstrate undisplaced fractures.

Treatment in the form of reduction and fixation is usually required for completely displaced fractures and for partially displaced fractures with false motion. Some completely displaced sternal fractures are not exceedingly painful, but the deformity and restriction of thoracic movements usually warrant reduction. Pain from false motion justifies reducing some incompletely displaced fractures, but there is no indication for interfering with an impacted fracture or a partially displaced fracture that is not causing significant discomfort. The pain from most sternal fractures gradually subsides over the first two weeks even though a firm union may not occur for six to eight weeks.

It is neither necessary nor desirable to undertake reduction of the sternal fracture immediately since the threat of associated injuries takes precedence. The most commonly employed procedure is open reduction, with the use of heavy wire sutures to achieve fixation. Although closed reduction may occasionally be achieved by pressure over the more anterior of the two fragments with the patient's thorax at full inspiration and the arms extended over his head, this maneuver is usually too painful to be undertaken without general anesthesia, and once this step is taken it is better to assure both accurate reduction and proper fixation by operative means.

Flail Chest

One of the most serious consequences of blunt thoracic trauma is what has been variously called flail, floating, or crushed chest. With the increasing frequency of high-speed automobile accidents this condition is gaining an increasingly important position in the spectrum of chest trauma. It is relatively more frequent in older patients because their less resilient rib cages fracture more readily, and because their declining agility makes them prone to auto-pedestrian accidents and heavy falls.

When several ribs are fractured on both sides of the point of impact, the intervening rib segments may lose their firm continuity with the rest of the thorax so that this region responds to intrapleural pressure changes rather than to the pull of the muscles of respiration. As a result, the involved area moves in an opposite direction

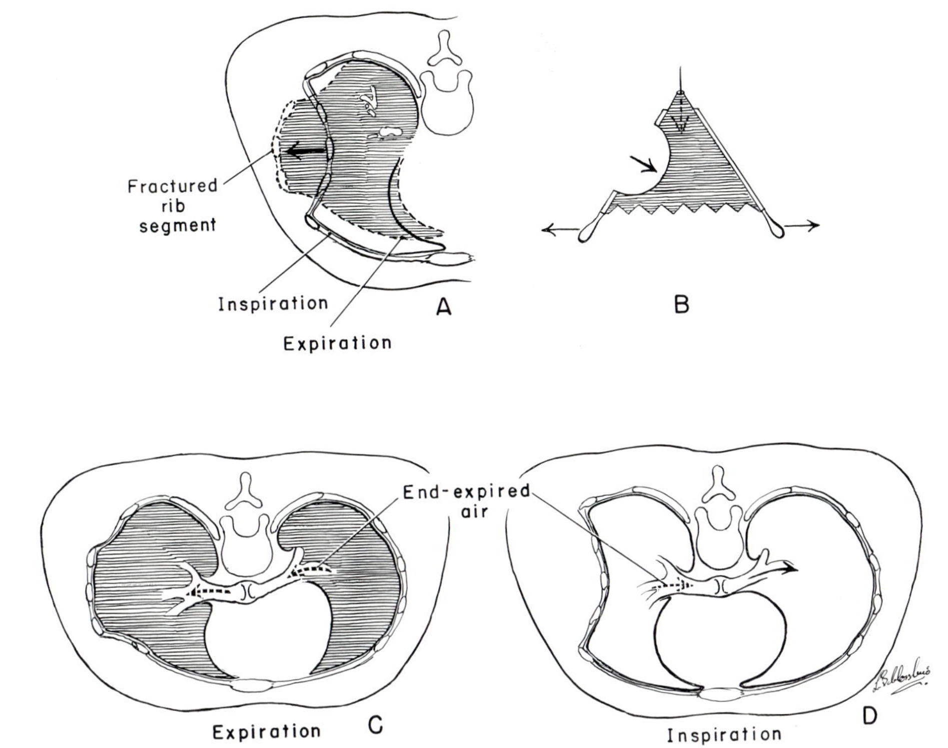

Figure 10–5 The pathophysiology of flail chest. *A*, Cross-sectional cut of the involved hemithorax showing (exaggerated) paradoxical motion. *B*, The mechanical interference with the function of the thoracic cage is likened to that of a bellows in which one of the rigid sides has been partly replaced by a semielastic membrane. *C* and *D*, Cross-sectional views in expiration and inspiration showing the to-and-fro movement of end-expired air across the carina between the two lungs during the respiratory cycle as suggested by the concept of "pendelluft."

to the rest of the thorax during the respiratory cycle (Figs. 10–5*A* and 10–6*A*); hence the term "paradoxical" chest movement.

Similar paradoxical movements occur after an extensive thoracoplasty. One of the first to appreciate the deleterious effects of this phenomenon was Brauer, the Marburg internist who guided the early development of thoracoplasty techniques in the late 19th century. As a result of his observations, Brauer suggested that thoracoplasty be done in stages. He also developed methods of dressing the chest after thoracoplasty to minimize the paradox, and these were later adopted in the treatment of traumatic flail chest.

Pathophysiology. The mechanisms advanced to explain the respiratory embarrassment associated with this condition are still unsettled. The German concept of "pendelluft," signifying a to-and-fro movement of useless end-expired air between the two lungs during the respiratory cycle is still popular in modern texts. Shown diagrammatically in Figure 10–5 *C* and *D*, it suggests that during inspiration end-expired air leaves the paradoxically collapsing ipsilateral lung and is drawn into the expanding contralateral lung. Conversely, during expiration, some of the end-expired air leaving the lung on the contralateral side is drawn into the ipsilateral lung which is paradoxically expanding. In essence, this to-and-fro movement of end-expired air results

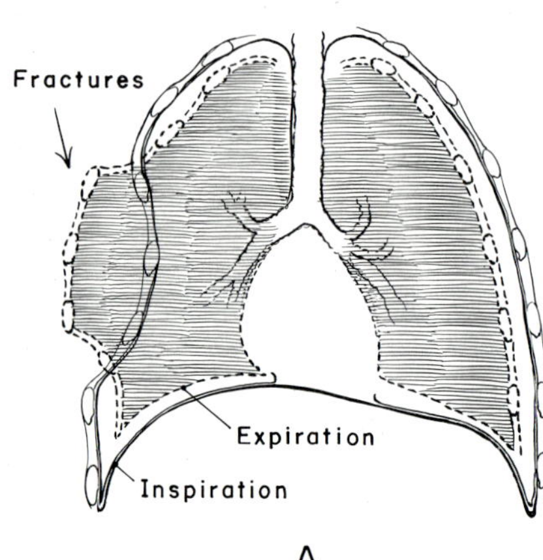

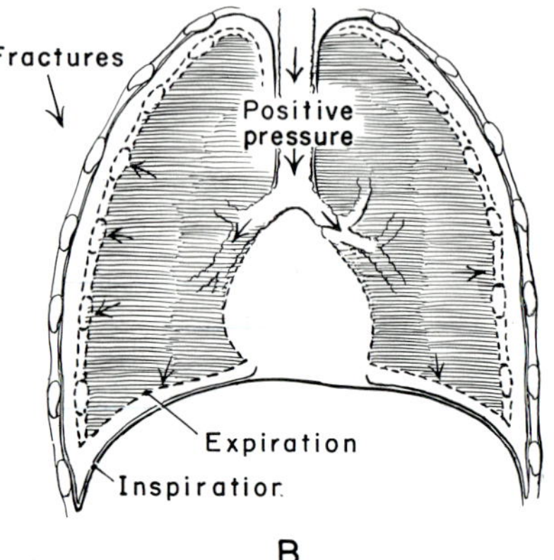

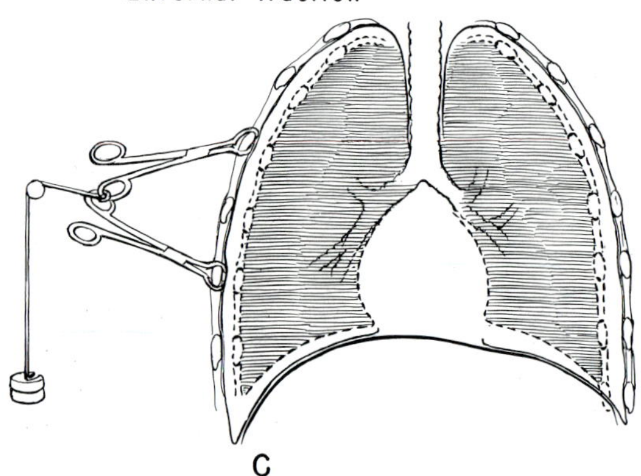

Figure 10–6 Stabilization of the flail chest. *A*, The paradoxical motion associated with active breathing. *B*, Stabilization of the fractured segment in the "out" position throughout the respiratory cycle by controlled positive pressure respiration. *C*, Stabilization of the fractured segment in the "out" position by external traction, using towel clips and orthopedic weight suspension.

in an increase in the dead space. This may be so great that the patient is unable to compensate for it by hyperventilation, particularly in the presence of painful rib fractures.

Only recently have doubts regarding the soundness of this theory been given experimental support. Maloney et al.[46] point out that such an explanation must assume that pressure differentials can exist between the two hemithoraces. They have shown that such differentials do not exist in a dog when flail chest is produced by a large extraperiosteal thoracoplasty. In their experiments the lungs acted as if suspended in a single chambered thorax. Moreover, their work suggests that during inspiration the lung on the side of the flail undergoes net expansion even though the lung subjacent to the flail segment sinks in. Finally, they were unable to detect any to-and-fro movement of end-expired air by continuous CO_2 measurements in each main bronchus. Since this experiment measured the effects of a standard-sized flail segment on an anesthetized animal known for its flimsy mediastinum, it is not possible to say with certainty that some degree of pendelluft does not occur in the unanesthetized human with large flail segments and a more rigid mediastinum.

In experiments with tension pneumothorax in goats and monkeys, animals which have a more substantial mediastinum, it has been shown that pressure gradients can exist across the mediastinum between the two pleural spaces.[57]

Nevertheless, logic favors the alternative view that the major difficulty in flail chest stems from the fact that pressure gradients developed by the thoracic bellows are dissipated by the paradoxically moving segment of chest wall so that the ability to exchange air against atmospheric pressure is greatly hampered (Fig. 10–5*B*). Air could be exchanged after the flail segment has completed its displacement, but the extra effort required for this would be limited by the pain of the rib fractures.

The clinical observation that supports this theory that the bellows function of the thorax is crippled by the flail segment is that patients who have a central flail segment from rib fractures on either side of the sternum have just as much ventilatory embarrassment as those with unilateral flail chest. Since this region straddles both hemithoraces, one could not incriminate a pendelluft mechanism.

Even with mild degrees of flail chest, a considerably greater respiratory effort is required to effect adequate ventilation. The pain of multiple rib fractures will discourage this extra effort, and even if such compensation is made initially, fatigue, central nervous system depression or accumulating tracheobronchial secretions usually tip the scales eventually against the patient.

Diagnosis. Paradoxical movement of the chest wall should be looked for in any patient who has sustained severe blunt chest trauma. The flail segment is usually anterior or lateral since the posterior thorax is not struck so commonly and is more protected by its heavier musculature and the shoulder girdle. The paradoxical movement is often obvious on inspection, but subtler degrees may not be apparent except by palpation, when the abnormal movement may be detected by comparison with the other hand placed on the normally moving side. This technique is particularly useful when the lighting is poor, in obese patients or in women with large breasts.

Treatment. The diagnosis having been made, there are several therapeutic alternatives. The most expedient of these is to stabilize the flail segment by firm but gentle manual pressure. Although this decreases the thoracic volume, it allows the work of the thoracic bellows to be more fully expended toward the exchange of air, and it is a useful temporizing maneuver. The same effect can be obtained by using sandbags. However, the weight and the restrictive dressings needed to hold them in place limit their usefulness. Another useful approach at the scene of the accident is to place the patient with the injured side down. Flail chest is said to be the only condition in which this commonly recommended position can be shown physiologically to be beneficial.[61]

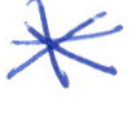

However, it is more desirable to stabilize the flail segment in the "out" position, and many ingenious methods have been devised for this. One of the simplest employs large towel clips passed percutaneously around each of several ribs in the flail segment. Traction is then applied to these towel clips by a cord to which are attached weights via an orthopedic suspension, as shown in miniature in Figure 10–6*C*.

This method has the advantage of being easily applied with equipment that is usually readily available. However, this traction system interferes with attempts to move the patient or to care for him in other ways. Particularly significant in extreme degrees of flail chest is the increased work the respiratory muscles must do in moving the thorax against the traction force applied to it. Nevertheless, there is much to be said for it as an initial procedure or in the definitive treatment of mild to moderate degrees of flail chest.

Operative fixation of multiple fractures is neither feasible nor necessary. The segment can be drawn out against an external strut, such as a Jacob's ladder, by passing heavy sutures around the ribs at several points, but this too has lost its popularity. *Tracheostomy* is beneficial in these patients,[10] although one must use a large cannula (No. 9 or No. 10) placed low in the cervical trachea. In this way, dead space may be decreased and airway resistance lessened so that air can be exchanged with less effort. This also facilitates removal of tracheobronchial secretions that accumulate because of the patient's ineffective cough. In fact, short of continuous positive pressure ventilation, tracheostomy is probably the simplest and most effective measure in that it both reduces the degree of flail and allows control of secretions.

At the present time, the "external" methods of stabilization referred to above have been largely superseded in the management of the patients with significant degrees of flail chest by what has been termed "internal pneumatic stabilization." This approach, first introduced in 1955 by Avery, Mörch and Benson,[3] employs controlled continuous positive pressure ventilation (C.P.P.V.), adjusted to just beyond the point of apnea. By this means the flail segment is "floated" out into a reduced position by the positive pressure from within; and since there are no active inspiratory efforts by these apneic patients, the flail segment is never drawn in (Fig. 10–6*B*). At the point of apnea there is a mild degree of alkalosis. This has a sedative effect and reduces the analgesic requirements, although with respiration controlled such agents may be given without fear of respiratory depression. The respirator not only assures an adequate exchange of air but eliminates the work of breathing. No surgery other than tracheostomy is required, and this is often indicated anyway for removal of blood and secretions from the trachea. The use of positive pressure has the added advantage of minimizing the outpouring of bronchial secretions and pulmonary transudates which are frequently associated in the form of "wet lung" or contusion pneumonitis.[56]

At the moment, few would disagree with the statement that C.P.P.V. is the most effective and definitive means of treating flail chest. But since no treatment, and certainly not respirator therapy, is without risk, the question remains—Do all patients with multiple rib fractures with some degree of paradoxical motion need it? One must remember that one is usually committing the patient to at least 10–14 days of respirator therapy—the usual time required for sufficient chest wall stabilization to allow C.P.P.V. to be discontinued—and that even by this time fixation is not complete, and a certain amount of the reduced or "out" position will be lost to the continuous inward pull of the negative intrapleural pressure. In patients with *lesser* degrees of flail, significant ventilatory impairment initially and a restrictive-type of pulmonary functional impairment eventually are *not* important considerations, and the major problems of control of pain and tracheal toilet can be handled by other means.

In general, the following can be considered as indications for respirator (C.P.P.V.) treatment of flail chest: (1) significant mechanical interference with ventilatory exchange; (2) significant associated pulmonary contusion; (3) uncooperative patient (e.g., comatose from head injury); (4) the need for general anesthetic and surgical intervention for associated trauma; (5) need for more than five to six L./min. O_2 to maintain reasonable arterial oxygen tension; (6) a need for voluminous I.V. fluid therapy for other injuries; (7) significant initial impairment of or deteriorating blood gases; (8) pre-existing underlying lung disease; (9) increasing respiratory distress, tachypnea, increased work of breathing and signs of fatigue; and (10) involvement of over five ribs in the flail segment.

Earlier problems with the respirator

treatment of flail chest have largely been overcome by the development of more efficient humidification and prophylactic bilateral chest tube drainage to avoid the threat of tension pneumothorax. A general controversy concerning pressure- versus volume-regulated respirators has also arisen in regard to treatment for this condition. Although both can be used effectively, the author feels that when contusion pneumonitis is an associated problem, volume-controlled respirators have the advantage of providing adequate ventilation without requiring adjustment for changes in compliance.

In summary, a flail chest associated with respiratory embarrassment should be immediately stabilized by the most expedient method, whether external compression or traction with towel clips. Then, as soon as feasible, a low cervical tracheostomy should be performed and a large diameter cannula inserted. If after this a significant degree of flail persists, or any of the above indications are met, one should place the patient on continuous positive pressure ventilation. Occasionally, with lesser degrees of flail, careful tracheostomy care, oxygen inhalation and control of pain by intercostal nerve block may suffice. Serial blood gas analyses are extremely helpful, if not essential, in determining the adequacy of therapy, particularly in regard to the use of a respirator.

Flail chest is associated with a high mortality rate, almost 40 per cent in the recent large series of Conn et al.[18] More universal application of recent advances in treatment should reduce this, but it must be recognized that many of these deaths are at least partly related to serious associated injuries.

Open Pneumothorax and Chest Wall Defects

Open pneumothorax is more likely to be encountered in combat casualties, but occasionally it is seen in civilian practice as a result of shotgun wounds at close range or bizarre accidents in which the patient is impaled or struck by a flying object.

However, this condition was the focal issue in the early development of the treatment of chest injuries. For six centuries interest in the treatment of chest injuries was kindled by the controversy between the "closed" versus the "open" treatment of the sucking chest wound. This controversy can be traced to 1267 when Theodoric advised closing such wounds so that "the natural heat would not escape or cold air enter the chest." This contradiction of accepted practice gained little immediate support. Even three centuries later Ambroise Paré, an authority in his time, insisted that although it was permissible to close small sucking chest wounds immediately if they were not associated with internal bleeding, it was best to allow the remainder to drain openly for two or three days before closure.

In 1767 William Hewson recorded his observations of a patient with marked respiratory distress from such a wound who was promptly relieved when the wound was covered. Forty years later Baron Larrey, Napoleon's surgeon, gave the concept of closed treatment its first authoritative backing after a similar personal observation. He had elected to cover the wound of a soldier near death from an open hemopneumothorax—ostensibly to hide it from the sight of other wounded men with whom the patient was quartered. To his surprise the patient not only responded but survived. Further bolstered by experiences during the Crimean War, this approach was given an extensive trial in the American Civil War, but the favorable initial response was so frequently followed by a fatal empyema that it was again abandoned.

Gradually, by the late nineteenth century, opinions exclusively favoring one or the other approach yielded to the realization that the problem lay between the immediate consequence of respiratory insufficiency from an open pneumothorax and the late complications of an undrained, contaminated hemopneumothorax if the wound were closed. Some selected one or the other approach, the decision depending on the size of the opening or the amount of bleeding and contamination. Others compromised by covering the wound with voluminous dressings in which a drain was incorporated. The eventual development of tube thoracostomy drainage made such compromises unnecessary.

PATHOPHYSIOLOGY. One of the most important outgrowths of this controversy was an aroused interest in the physiology of the open pneumothorax. In 1896 Paget, in the first major work devoted entirely to chest surgery, expressed the opinion that "vibration" of the mediastinum in open pneumothorax destroyed the piston action of the diaphragm. This same year Quénu and Lonquet brought the experimental method to bear on this problem. Their work suggested a method of sustaining expansion of the lung with the chest open by maintaining a positive differential between the intratracheal and intrapleural pressures. Frasier had suggested earlier that the thoracic wound competed with the natural airway; thus, whenever it was of greater diameter than the glottis, it offered less resistance to air flow so that the major portion of the air moved by the thoracic bellows passed through the open wound.

From the German literature came the concept of pendelluft, the to-and-fro motion of air, which was used to explain the ventilatory impairment associated not only with open pneumothorax, but with other forms of paradoxical respiration such as flail chest and paralyzed diaphragm. This concept has been described earlier in this chapter in relation to flail chest, and Figure 10–7 shows how it is thought to apply to open pneumothorax. Maloney et al. have cast doubt on its occurrence in flail chest,[46] and carbon dioxide analysis from the trachea and mainstem bronchi in experiments in the author's laboratory suggests that although it may occur to some degree it is not the major cause of ventilatory impairment in open pneumothorax.

A more logical explanation for the ventilatory embarrassment associated with open pneumothorax is that rapid equilibration of atmospheric pleural pressure occurs through the open defect. This limits the ability of the thoracic bellows to develop the necessary pressure gradient for air exchange (Fig. 10–7). Other factors undoubtedly contribute as well. The loss of intrathoracic negative pressure decreases the efficiency of venous return to the heart. Intermittent torsion of the caval-atrial junction by mediastinal shift or "flutter" may further impede this. Inability to build up pressure against a closed glottis, as required for effective coughing, may eventually lead to retention of bronchial secretions. The relative contributions of the several mechanisms mentioned above have not been determined.

DIAGNOSIS. There should be no problem in diagnosing an open pneumothorax. The sucking chest wound is usually obvious on inspection, and it makes a characteristic sound as air moves through it. No further examination should be carried out before covering the wound.

TREATMENT. Often the wound will already have been covered by the time the patient reaches the hospital, although the dressing used may not be adequate and may have to be replaced. Occasionally, in patients with pneumothorax secondary to a penetrating wound of the chest, the communication may be reopened by unnecessary manipulation of the wound at the time of examination. For this reason it is wise to dress all chest wounds definitively.

It is axiomatic that the sucking chest

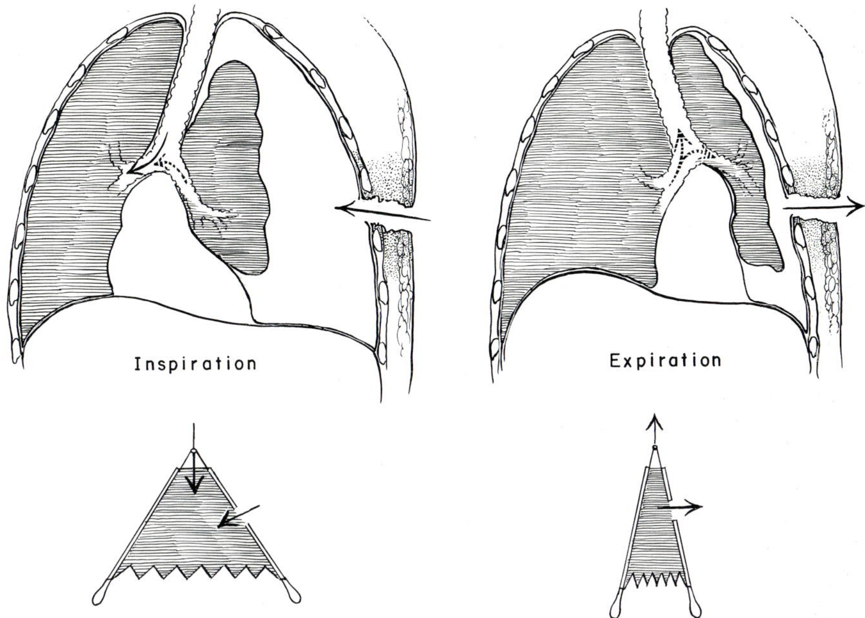

Figure 10–7 Open pneumothorax. The movements of the intrathoracic contents occurring with open pneumothorax are shown in the inspiratory and expiratory phases. The broken arrows in the upper diagrams denote the transcarinal movement of end-expired air suggested by the "pendelluft" concept. The mechanical interference with function of the thoracic "bellows" is depicted below.

should be covered immediately. This simple maneuver converts the condition to that of a closed pneumothorax and eliminates the major physiologic abnormality. Because time is required to prepare a definitive dressing, one should cover the wound first by the cleanest available means, preferably a sterile towel or sterile gloved hand. This coverage can then be maintained until a definitive dressing can be prepared. Such a dressing should consist of several layers of gauze, the innermost impregnated with petrolatum or some other means of rendering it impervious to air. It should be wide enough to extend two inches or more beyond the wound margin in all directions. It should be applied to the chest with several strips of adhesive. "In the field," no attempt should be made to completely seal the dressing to the chest wall with adhesive. In that way the dressing can not only prevent air from entering the chest on inspiration, but allow it to exit during expiration or at least whenever positive pressure builds up within the thorax. This could allow gradual expansion of the collapsed lung, but more importantly, it acts as a safety valve against the development of tension pneumothorax. These considerations are not usually important once the patient has reached the hospital, since a chest tube will be inserted shortly after application of the dressing and immediately connected to water-seal drainage or suction. Thus, in the most common situation—civilian emergency room practice—the dressing can and should be occlusive.

With evacuation of the pleural space and expansion of the lung, the resuscitative phase is completed. If operative debridement and repair of the chest wound are indicated because of the degree of contamination loss or devitalization of the chest wall tissues they can and should be delayed until the patient is thoroughly evaluated and resuscitated from other significant injuries. It is desirable to obtain chest x-rays at this point. In addition to the usual upright chest film, additional views of the ribs and soft tissues in the area of the wound should be made in anticipation of the problems of reconstruction that may present at the time of wound exploration. A lateral chest film should also be taken if there is an intrathoracic foreign body whose removal is planned at the time of surgery.

The Repair of Traumatic Defects in the Chest Wall. Not all thoracic wounds require formal exploration and debridement. In civilian practice, the majority can simply be covered with a dressing and allowed to heal by secondary intention. However, any large or grossly contaminated wound should be debrided. This is particularly true of the high-velocity gunshot or close-range shotgun wounds in which considerable tissue damage can be expected. Once debrided, the larger wounds may present reconstructive problems, since more than mere skin coverage may be required. Integrity of the chest wall must be restored so that it is not only airtight but also does not allow significant paradoxical movement. Often this can be satisfactorily achieved by mobilizing a flap of adjacent muscle into the defect.

In the case of larger defects in which much of the overlying muscle has been destroyed or removed by debridement, it may be impossible to accomplish this end by using the available surrounding muscle. Instead, it may be necessary to mobilize a rib from the upper or lower margins of the wound and swing it diagonally across the wound as a strut to stabilize this segment of the thoracic cage. Skin coverage is usually no problem since the surrounding skin can be readily mobilized or, if necessary, a large flap can be swung to fill the defect. Fortunately, the huge chest wall defects that tax the ingenuity of the surgeon dealing with cancer are rarely encountered with trauma; a discussion of the reconstructive procedures involved is beyond the scope of this chapter.

The techniques that have been developed to repair defects following the en bloc removal of invasive chest wall tumors involve the use not only of rib struts and large pedicle grafts but, occasionally, sheets of prosthetic material such as heavy Marlex mesh or tantalum wire. These techniques may not be applicable to traumatic defects because of damage to adjacent structures that might be used in reconstruction and because of the undesirability of using prosthetic material in the grossly contaminated wound.

With the advent of safer and more sophisticated respirators, we have not hesitated in recent years to maintain patients with the more complicated open chest wounds on a respirator after thorough debridement and simply dress the wound, exposed lung and all, until fixation occurs and granulation tissue can cover the defect. Skin grafting follows and definitive chest wall reconstruction, if functionally indicated, can be done later when one will be dealing with tissues which have healed and are no longer contaminated.

THE PLEURAL SPACE

Hemothorax

Hemothorax is one of the most common presenting problems following major chest trauma. In the companion studies of Gray et al.[31] and Harrison and associates[34] of penetrating and major nonpenetrating injuries to the chest from all causes, there was a 79 and 70 per cent incidence of hemothorax, respectively. In these reports the mortality associated with hemothorax was 4 per cent with penetrating injuries and 49 per cent with nonpenetrating injuries. The latter mortality rate is misleading because it is mainly a reflection of the severity of associated injuries. In fact, with the exception of traumatic disruption of the arch of the aorta, blunt trauma usually results in less severe degrees of hemothorax, whereas hemothorax resulting from penetration of the heart or great vessels provides one of the major indications for *immediate* thoracotomy.

At one extreme, the hemothorax may be so small that it is not detected initially. (A hemothorax of less than 300 ml. is often not demonstrable on an upright chest film.) At the other extreme, 30 to 40 per cent of the blood volume may be rapidly lost into one pleural space, with little resistance offered by the lung. Such major intrathoracic bleeding invariably stems from the heart, great vessels or a major systemic artery rather than the pulmonary parenchyma, which is perfused at low pressures, is rich in thromboplastins and tends to collapse around the bleeding site.

Diagnosis. A hemothorax of major proportions should rarely be missed. Shock will be the major feature and will precede and overshadow the ventilatory embarrassment that results from compression of the lung and the shift of the mediastinum.

Although only about 25 per cent of hemothoraces are large enough to produce shock, loss of blood into the pleural space is still the most common cause of shock following chest trauma. In Andersen and Halkier's large series of chest injuries,[1] shock developed in 48 patients, hemothorax being the cause in 31. The physical findings are diminished breath sounds and dullness to percussion posteriorly over the involved hemothorax, which may appear more prominent but move poorly with respirations. With major degrees of hemothorax, tracheal shift to the opposite side may be detected. In lesser degrees of hemothorax, these signs may be difficult to elicit, particularly when there is an associated pneumothorax. Fortunately, there is time for a chest x-ray in these cases. The importance of the *upright* chest film is underscored by the observation that almost a liter of blood may produce only a slight, diffuse increase in density over the involved hemothorax on a supine film. A missed hemothorax may present later as a pleural effusion and is a more common cause of delayed post-traumatic pleural effusion than the usual suspect, chylothorax. Aspiration of blood by thoracentesis establishes the diagnosis. This confirmation is not academic, for an esophageal rupture can produce shock and an x-ray picture not unlike pneumohemothorax.

Treatment. If shock is present, restoration of the blood volume should be the first therapeutic measure. The general principles of treating hypovolemic shock have already been discussed and will not be restated here.

It should be emphasized, however, that a central venous catheter is invaluable in treating shock from intrathoracic bleeding, not only as a major route and sensitive guide for massive volume replacement, but because the central venous pressure will allow detection of the other major cause of early shock after chest trauma, cardiac tamponade.

Once efforts at blood volume replacement are underway, a chest tube should be inserted through the 6th or 7th intercostal space posterolaterally and connected to constant gentle suction (−20 cm. water). This is designed to accomplish the following: (1) re-expand the collapsed lung, (2) remove the blood from the hemothorax, thus reducing the risk of fibrothorax from organizing blood clots and the risk of empyema by removing a source of bacterial nutrition, (3) reduce further bleeding by negative pressure coaption of the pleural surfaces, and (4) provide an accurate guide to the rate of continuing blood loss.

Today few would argue against the use of chest tube drainage in dealing with a major hemothorax. However, the choice between this approach and needle aspiration for evacuating moderate degrees of hemothorax is another matter. Such a debate is academic in many instances since a chest tube will be indicated for the pneumothorax that will coexist in at least half of the cases.

During World War I there was debate over the desirablility of evacuating the blood at all, those opposed arguing that the accumulating blood tamponaded the bleeding. This opposition gradually faded following the war, and by the time of World War II it was the method of evacuating the blood that had become controversial. It was not until the Korean conflict that advocates of chest tube drainage gained the upper hand. However, a recent review of civilian experiences suggests that this increasingly aggressive attitude may not be without some penalty. Three consecutive experiences with penetrating chest trauma reported from Grady Memorial Hospital for the years 1922 to 1935, 1936 to 1942, and 1948 to 1957[31] showed a drop in mortality from 13 to 6.4 to 3.8 per cent. However, they also document a rise in the incidence of empyema from 1.6 to 2.0 to 3.3 per cent. In their most recent series, four out of five cases of hemothorax were managed by a single aspiration with no instance of empyema. Multiple thoracenteses carried a 2.3 per cent incidence of empyema, and when chest tube drainage was employed, the incidence of empyema was 10 per cent. This is partially explained by the selection of chest tube drainage for the more complicated cases that are associated with a higher incidence of shock and multiple injuries.

In spite of this and other retrospective evidence that the vast majority of cases could be adequately handled by thoracentesis alone, the author still favors the chest tube in managing traumatic hemothorax in the majority of cases because this judgment is difficult to make prospectively, particularly soon after the injury, and because it represents a more decisive and practical approach to the problem in the emergency room setting. To state this in more specific terms, tube thoracotomy is indicated in the management of traumatic hemothorax (1) if it is already of major proportions shortly after injury and admission, e.g., causes shock, covers the dome of the diaphragm on x-ray and exceeds 500 ml. on thoracentesis; (2) if it is associated with pneumothorax; (3) if there are significant associated injuries and particularly if they will require operative treatment; and (4) if a significant hemothorax reoccurs shortly after initial treatment by thoracentesis. On the other hand, whenever more than an hour or two have passed since the injury, even a moderately large hemothorax can be reasonably managed by thoracentesis alone, if it is essentially an isolated injury. Minor degrees of residual hemothorax may be ignored since it is difficult to "tap the chest dry" and even moderate-sized hemothoraces, if they don't become secondarily infected, will usually resorb with surprisingly little residual evidence. This realization has caused us to be less aggressive with "clotted hemothorax" as an indication for early thoracotomy, preferring to wait at least six weeks to see if the degree of restrictive pulmonary dysfunction is significantly greater than that which may result from thoracotomy.

THORACOTOMY FOR MASSIVE HEMOTHORAX. Whenever a patient arrives at the hospital *in shock* from a hemothorax, the operating room should be alerted. Failure to respond fully to vigorous resuscitative measures or to maintain that response justifies immediate thoracotomy. Although this approach may seem bold, the benefit to those who could be saved only by immediate thoracotomy outweighs the cost to those who *might* have been controlled without such a step.

Even if a patient's response to volume replacement can be maintained, one may still be justified in proceeding with thoracotomy under the following circumstances: (1) bleeding that continues at a significant rate, arbitrarily set at greater than 500 ml. per eight hours after initial replacement, (2) a rate of bleeding that is steadily increasing rather than decreasing, (3) inability to empty the chest of large amounts of clotted blood, or (4) association of a widened mediastinum with a left hemothorax (i.e., suspected rupture of the thoracic aorta).

A lateral thoracotomy should be employed in the 5th interspace unless otherwise indicated by the trajectory of the penetrating agent, a widened mediastinum or other factors. In critical cases the chest is opened without the usual concern for chest wall hemostasis, the blood clots are evacuated, and the source of bleeding is sought first in the region of the heart and great vessels. If possible, the bleeding should be controlled with pressure, until the blood volume is replaced (usually 1 or 2 units beyond return to normotensive levels). It is foolish to attempt to repair the site of bleeding immediately if it can be controlled by pressure. This interval can be well spent gaining better exposure, controlling bleeding from the wound edges and obtaining proximal and distal control of the site of hemorrhage. Specific details in the operative management of bleeding from the heart and great vessels, which constitute the majority of cases of massive hemothorax, will be dealt with later in this chapter. Major sources of bleeding from lesser systemic vessels, usually either the intercostal or internal mammary arteries, can be managed by proximal and distal suture ligation while being controlled by finger pressure. Lacerations of the pulmonary parenchyma are rarely a source of major or uncontrolled hemorrhage and can usually be controlled by suture ligatures. Unless the parenchyma has been severely disrupted or the major hilar vessels have been torn, there is little reason to resort to resection to control hemorrhage.

Pneumothorax

Traumatic pneumothorax follows both penetrating and nonpenetrating chest injuries. In both instances, there is usually some degree of associated hemothorax. In the case of penetrating wounds, the wounding agent determines the frequency of this association. For example, icepick wounds frequently result in pneumothorax alone, whereas an associated hemothorax most frequently follows gunshot wounds. In nonpenetrating wounds, the pneumothorax will usually be associated with and often caused by rib fractures, which are present in 90 per cent of the adult cases of traumatic pneumothorax secondary to blunt trauma.

Pathophysiology. The respiratory embarrassment caused by a simple pneumothorax depends on the degree of collapse, but even when collapse is complete, the other lung is normally capable of carrying on adequate ventilation. Lesser degrees of pneumothorax are so easily compensated for that patients with *spontaneous* pneumothorax frequently experience little respiratory distress. Pneumonectomy could not be tolerated without this pulmonary reserve. However, this comparison can be carried further. Even patients in whom preoperative pulmonary function studies predict sufficient residual capacity for adequate ventilation after pneumonectomy may have difficulty getting through the immediate postoperative period to fulfill this prediction. The differences between the postoperative and the recovered state following pneumonectomy are not unlike those between the traumatic and spontaneous pneumothorax in that the ability of the remaining functional parenchyma to compensate may be interfered with by the complications of retained secretions and chest pain.

In addition to the simple loss of functioning lung tissue, blood circulating through the collapsed pulmonary parenchyma does not become fully saturated with oxygen. Fortunately, the degree of unsaturation resulting from this pulmonary arteriovenous shunting is somewhat reduced by increased resistance to flow through hypoventilated areas.

Diagnosis. The physical signs associated with significant degrees of pneumothorax are diminished breath sounds, hyperresonance to percussion and a prominent but poorly moving hemithorax. Each of these signs implies a comparison with the normal side. Such a comparison may not be entirely reliable in severely traumatized patients, especially if there are painful rib fractures. Tracheal deviation is an important sign when present, but it is not specific for pneumothorax since it occurs in other traumatic conditions such as hemothorax, mediastinal hematoma and pulmonary collapse distal to a totally severed bronchus. The sign that is most diagnostic, of course, is hyperresonance to percussion.

Although major degrees of pneumothorax can be diagnosed by physical examination, a chest x-ray is usually required to rule out a minor pneumothorax. Even this may not consistently demonstrate a pneumothorax of less than 10 per cent. *Expiratory* films of good quality may be required to reveal minor degrees of pneumothorax, and patients with chest pain may not be able to cooperate sufficiently for these. Even greater degrees of pneumothorax may be missed on emergency chest x-rays unless specifically sought. The appearance of a rib fracture or subcutaneous emphysema should alert the examiner to this possibility, and the lung markings should be followed to the periphery along the involved side to detect the separation of the parietal and visceral pleurae.

Treatment. Traumatic pneumothorax should be treated by tube thoracostomy through the use of either water-seal drainage or constant gentle suction. Needle aspiration and/or observation of "minor" degrees of traumatic pneumothorax are even less defensible than in spontaneous pneumothorax. This so-called conservative approach is associated with a much lower success rate than when used for spontaneous pneumothorax. In one series, it was successful in only 53 per cent of *selected* cases, which can be compared to a 97 per cent success rate obtained through use of a chest tube. In addition to being a surer and safer method of evacuating a pneumothorax, tube thoracostomy is less time-consuming in the long run, requires less frequent personal re-evaluation of the patient and results in earlier expansion of the lung.

The tube thoracostomy drainage system also provides important information regarding the persistence and relative magnitude of an air leak. For example, persistent large air leaks, which cause bubbling in the chest bottle during inspiration as well as expiration, signify a tear in a major radical of the tracheobronchial tree. Small leaks cease fairly promptly, if indeed they still persist by the time the chest tube is inserted. Failure of the chest tube to bubble when the patient coughs is a reliable sign that the air leak has closed, provided respiratory excursions of the fluid level in the drainage tube assure its patency. Such information allows this condition to be managed with a sureness and decisiveness which is gratifying to all concerned. Statistics do not justify the fear that infection may be introduced by tube thoracostomy (unlike the situation which may exist for hemothorax), nor is there any evidence that the use of *gentle* suction results in persistence of air leaks. An additional benefit from this method of management is shorter hospitalization for the patient.

Tension Pneumothorax

Except for patients in whom underlying disease limits cardiorespiratory reserve, total collapse of one lung, as occurs in simple pneumothorax, is well tolerated. However, in some cases the communication that permits air to enter the pleural space may act as a one-way valve, allowing air to enter during expiration but not exit during inspiration. As a result, there may be progressive accumulation of air under pressure in the pleural space, a situation that may prove fatal if not promptly detected and treated. This condition may develop in a number of ways. An oblique laceration in the pulmonary parenchyma may be so situated that a flap of tissue lies over a bronchial communication. If a rupture of the main bronchus communicates with the pleural space through a rent in the mediastinal pleura which does not lie directly over the bronchial tear, this pleural flap may similarly act as a one-way valve over the bronchial opening. Obliquely communicating chest wounds rarely may allow movement of air between the pleural space and the outside atmosphere in an inward direction only. Today, with tracheal intubation and artificial ventilation becoming so commonplace, a new and *relatively* frequent cause of tension pneumothorax is puncture of the lung by a fractured rib when positive pressure ventilation is being applied. It is the reason why all cases of flail chest treated by positive pressure ventilation should have prophylactic chest tubes inserted and why tension pneumothorax should be considered as the cause of unexplained deterioration in any patient with chest injuries being artificially ventilated.

Pathophysiology. As air builds up under pressure in the pleural space, the mediastinum is swung to the opposite side, with compression of the lung on that side. Progressive impairment of the venous return and ventilatory exchange occurs. It has been suggested that the venous return eventually becomes obstructed by distortion of the caval-atrial junction, secondary to mediastinal shift. Others feel that the obstruction is due to collapse of the intrathoracic venae cavae from positive pressure. Our experiments with goats and monkeys[57] suggest that impairment of venous return is related to the progressive increase in intrathoracic venous pressure in relation to that in the peripheral veins; in the final stages, resistance to blood flow through the compressed pulmonary parenchyma may further impede the right side of the circulation. Ventilatory impairment results not only from a loss of functioning pulmonary parenchyma, but also from the progressive difficulty of the thoracic bellows in achieving sufficient negative pressure gradients for adequate inspiration.

These experiments further suggest that the major lethal factor may be ventilatory rather than circulatory since blood pressure and cardiac output were maintained long after respirations ceased. Initially, the goats compensate with increased respiratory effort and rate, maintaining their minute volume, pCO_2 and pH close to normal. Yet from the outset progressive hypoxia occurs because of a marked degree of shunting through nonventilated pulmonary vascular channels. Finally, as hypoxia deepens, compensatory efforts gradually weaken until respirations cease. Although it is likely that the same mechanisms observed in goats are involved in the lethal outcome of tension pneumothorax in humans, their relative contributions may, of course, differ—particularly in children, in whom mediastinal shift is more marked and circulatory impairment appears to assume a more dominant role, as observed in young monkeys (Fig. 10–8 *A* and *B*).

Diagnosis. Both ventilatory and circulatory impairment may be grossly apparent in advanced stages of tension pneumothorax. The involved hemithorax may be prominent, move weak ly with respirations and transmit breath sounds poorly. There may be a shift of the trachea to the opposite side, with distention of the neck veins and subcutaneous emphysema. However, the most important sign is hyperresonance to percussion over the involved hemithorax. A tension pneumothorax of this degree of severity should be readily suspected on

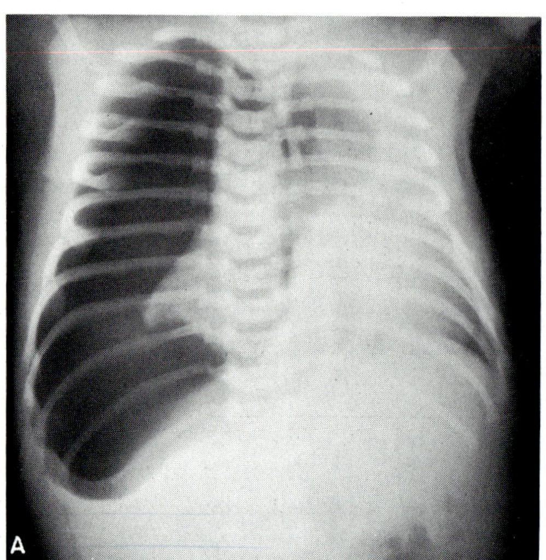

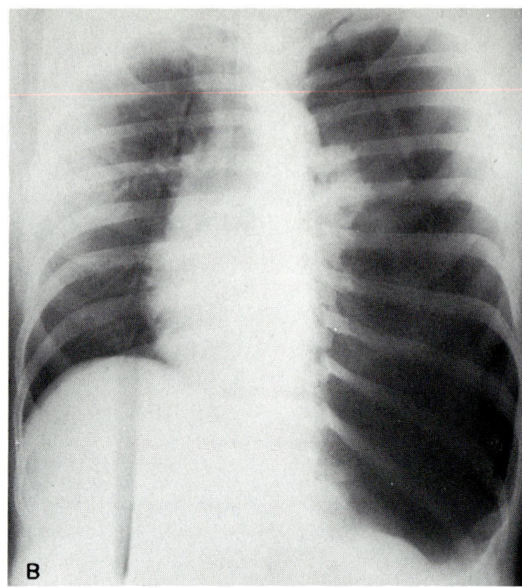

Figure 10–8 The x-ray appearance of the tension pneumothorax in a child (*A*) and an adult (*B*). In both instances there is a characteristic downward depression of the diaphragmatic contour. However, note the marked degree of the shift of the heart and mediastinum and the infringement upon the contralateral lung seen in the child.

the basis of physical examination alone and treatment instituted immediately without further diagnostic measures. Occasionally, however, it will not be realized, until a chest x-ray demonstrates a shift of the mediastinum, that what was thought to be a simple pneumothorax has already progressed to a tension pneumothorax (Fig. 10–8).

Treatment. The most expedient form of treatment for a tension pneumothorax involves equilibration of the pleural space with atmospheric pressure by percutaneous needle puncture of the involved hemithorax. This maneuver converts the condition into an open pneumothorax but with an opening so small that it is functionally little worse than a simple pneumothorax. If done early enough, the patient's condition will improve dramatically. There is then time to insert a chest tube and to expand the lung with suction. However, if the situation has progressed to a point at which the respiratory drive is failing, and before chest tube insertion, artificial ventilation with oxygen should be employed in addition to the venting of the pleural space.

The common association of tension pneumothorax with rupture of the bronchus should not be forgotten. Such a possibility should also be considered whenever there is evidence of a large and persistent air leak with almost constant bubbling in the chest drainage bottle and difficulty in expanding the lung.

Traumatic Chylothorax

Ordinarily, the problem of chylothorax does not arise early in the management of chest trauma. It rarely becomes clinically manifest until several days after the injury. Because thoracic duct flow is depressed while diet and activity are restricted, it takes time for a significant chylothorax to accumulate. Also, until diet is resumed and the thoracic lymph turns milky, it may be thought at first that one is dealing with a simple pleural effusion. The true incidence of traumatic chylothorax is probably greater than reports would indicate because many minor degrees of chylothorax go undetected and others "dry up" before the diagnosis is established. Only 90 instances of traumatic chylothorax had appeared in the literature at the time of Goorwitch's review in 1955.[30] However, subsequent reports have almost doubled this total.

Surgery and automobile accidents contribute the majority of the cases of traumatic chylothorax seen today. With the exception of the troublesome cases seen after cavopulmonary shunt, the problems presented by this condition are basically the same regardless of the original injury. Initially, chylothorax presents the problems of systemic loss of protein-rich fluid and the space-occupying effects of fluid accumulating in the pleural space. Eventually, persistent chylothorax may lead to fibrothorax, but secondary infection is rare, possibly because of the bacteriostatic properties of chyle.

Diagnosis. The diagnosis is usually not suspected until milky fluid is aspirated from the chest, and even then empyema is usually the first thought. The differentiation can be readily made because the chylous effusion is sterile on culture, contains predominantly lymphocytes rather than polymorphonuclear cells and will lose its milky color on shaking with ether. Refractile droplets may be seen under the microscope and can be demonstrated to take up lipophilic stains. Ingestion of vegetable dyes that are absorbed from the intestines will color the effusion and confirm the diagnosis in difficult cases.

Treatment. Until Lampson[39] first successfully controlled a case of traumatic chylothorax by thoracic duct ligation in 1948, the treatment had always been nonoperative, with the employment of multiple thoracenteses. Lampson's approach was further supported by Goorwitch's review, which pointed to the 10 per cent mortality from duct ligation as compared to 19 per cent in those treated nonoperatively. Transthoracic ligation of the thoracic duct just above the diaphragm was recommended if thoracenteses did not result in spontaneous closure of the fistula in two weeks.

It has been pointed out that the difference in mortality between the operative and the nonoperative approach reported by Goorwitch could be attributed to general advances in patient care, since all the cases treated by ligation had occurred in the six years prior to 1954, whereas the nonoperated cases dated back to 1695. More recent reports, particularly those of Maloney and Spencer[47] and Williams and Burford[68] have swung the pendulum back toward a more prolonged attempt at nonoperative management. Williams and Burford pointed out that almost any chylothorax will close in the absence of malignant obstruction or abnormal superior caval pressures.

At present, the following indications for surgical intervention are used: (1) a general deterioration of the patient because of large amounts of protein-rich fluid being lost, (2) inability to maintain expansion of the lung, with the threat of a "trapped" lung from fibrothorax, and (3) prolonged persistence of the chylothorax. One must consider the socioeconomic impact of indefinite hospitalization on the patient. In the majority of cases, spontaneous closure of the chylous fistula will occur in two to four weeks. Maloney and Spencer noted that the rate of reaccumulation has no prognostic significance since a sudden cessation of the drainage was more common than a gradual diminution. Attempts to accelerate spontaneous closure by restricting the patient's activity and diet have experimental backing but have the disadvantage of aggravating the nutritional drain resulting from the loss of protein-rich chyle and of conflicting with the goal of progressive mobilization of the patient.

Recently, it has been proposed[21] that chylothorax is better managed by chest tube drainage using continuous negative pressure. This is felt to help close the fistula by apposition of the pleural surfaces and to reduce the risk of infection and fibrothorax which may attend management by multiple thoracenteses. Although experience with this approach is still limited, it appears to have merit on theoretical grounds at least.

In the minority of patients in which operative intervention is indicated, ligation of the thoracic duct just above the diaphragm through a right lower thoracotomy will suffice. It is helpful to use dyes to aid in localizing the thoracic duct at surgery. The passage of a long tube into the upper small intestines preoperatively will allow one to instill a blue vegetable dye after the chest has been opened. Earlier instillation of the dye may stain the entire thorax by the time the chest has been opened. Williams suggests a simpler approach in which a small amount of cosmetic blue dye is injected into the wall of the lower esophagus at the time of thoracotomy. Lymphangiogram may occasionally be helpful in localizing the leak preoperatively.

In cases of longstanding chylothorax, concomitant decortication may be necessary. This possibility should be considered preoperatively in a left-sided chylothorax since the usual right-sided approach to the thoracic duct would have to be modified.

Procedures Employed in Evacuating the Pleural Spaces

The choice between thoracentesis and tube thoracostomy drainage in the management of pneumo- or hemothorax has been discussed in preceding sections of this chapter. The site chosen for evacuating the pleural space depends on whether one is dealing with a pneumothorax, a hemothorax or significant degrees of both. Since free air rises to the top of the pleural space, its evacuation is usually carried out through an upper interspace. With the patient in a semiupright position, the highest point in the pleural space is anterosuperior. For this reason, and because it is a reasonably avascular location in a wide interspace, the second intercostal space in the midclavicular line is usually selected for evacuation of air (Fig. 10–10*A*).

Conversely, if one wishes to evacuate blood or other fluid, a dependent location should be chosen. Because the moving diaphragm constantly changes the size and contour of the lower pleural recesses and is itself subject to injury during these procedures, the 6th or 7th interspace is preferred rather than a lower point in the thorax. For tube thoracostomy, insertion in the midaxillary line with tunneling posteriorly is chosen so that the patient will not lie upon and obstruct the chest catheter (Fig. 10–10 *B*).

It has been previously noted that variable degrees of hemothorax and pneumothorax frequently coexist following chest trauma. If there are significant degrees of both it is not always wise to try to evacuate them through a single chest catheter but rather to apply the method indicated for the treatment of each. Some blood may be evacuated through a superiorly placed chest tube, but this cannot be efficiently accomplished in the face of persistent large air leak, because only the air, which offers the least resistance to evacuation, will be obtained. Even the choice of a dependent site for tube thoracostomy in this situation may fail to completely evacuate the hemothorax.

If there is a major hemothorax and a pneumothorax without persistent air leak, one can insert a low posterolateral chest tube for the hemothorax and evacuate the pneumothorax by keeping the patient in the anterolateral supine position for a few minutes before returning him to the semiupright position. If, however, an air leak is still present, a second, high anterior chest tube should be inserted to deal with this. Generally, a pneumothorax should be evacuated through an anterosuperior chest tube and suction applied if an air leak persists. As previously stated, the indications for thoracentesis versus tube thoracostomy for hemothorax are subject to considerable differences of opinion. It is our practice to aspirate even minor hemothoraces initially, to confirm the diagnosis and to rule out chylothorax and particuarly, ruptured esophagus. In addition, a minor hemothorax may obscure the radiologic signs of ruptured diaphragm. For any major hemothorax, the authors prefer posterolateral tube thoracostomy with suction drainage. Lesser degrees of hemothorax may be aspirated or even watched as long as they produce only a blunting of the costo- or cardiophrenic angles. Whenever the fluid spans the width of the hemithorax, tube thoracotomy is justified.

Technique of Thoracentesis (Fig. 10–9). The patient should be seated or semierect. The interspace chosen is identified by counting ribs but in an emergency may have to be approximated. The second interspace anteriorly is broad and is level with the sternal prominence, the angle of Ludwig or Louis. To identify the 6th or 7th interspace posterolaterally it is easier to count backwards from the 12th rib. One should not rely on the fact that the 8th rib normally lies at the tip of the scapula since changes with shift in position may be misleading. The area is prepared with an antiseptic solution and draped with sterile towels. An intradermal wheal is raised with 1 per cent Xylocaine using a No. 25 needle. Then a No. 20 needle is advanced with gentle infiltration toward the upper border of the lower rib of the interspace. The needle is passed, or walked, over the upper border of this rib, at which point an additional 2 ml. is infiltrated before the pleural cavity is entered.

After aspiration of air or fluid establishes the proper depth of insertion, the needle is clamped at the skin level to mark the distance required for its entrance and then it is withdrawn. At this point, a change is made to a larger syringe (50 ml.) and needle (No. 18 or larger). The new needle is clamped at the same distance from the tip as the needle used to infiltrate, to serve as a constant guide to the correct depth of insertion, and attached to the syringe by a three-way stopcock. It is then introduced along the same tract into the pleural space. The three-way stopcock allows each 50 ml. aspirated to be discharged through a side arm without disconnecting or withdrawing the needle. The volume removed should always be measured. Aspiration is continued until no longer productive, or until over 500 ml. of blood or 1000 cc. of air have been removed, at which time the use of tube thoracostomy is usually indicated.

Closed Tube Thoracostomy. (Fig. 10–10). Small catheters (16 F) connected to water-seal drainage are used to evacuate modest air leaks. Larger leaks, indicating communication with

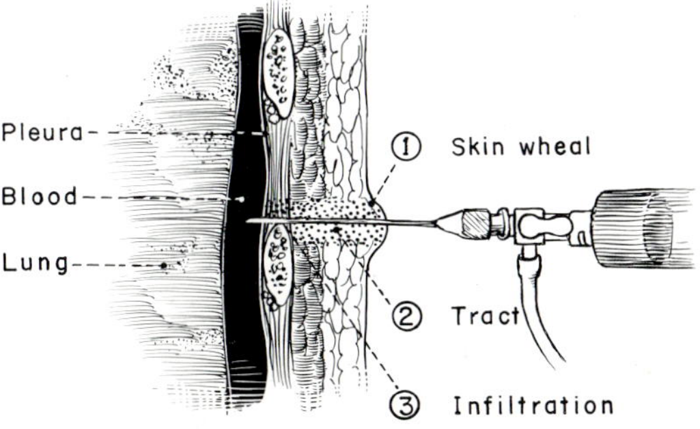

Figure 10–9 The technique of thoracentesis as described in the text.

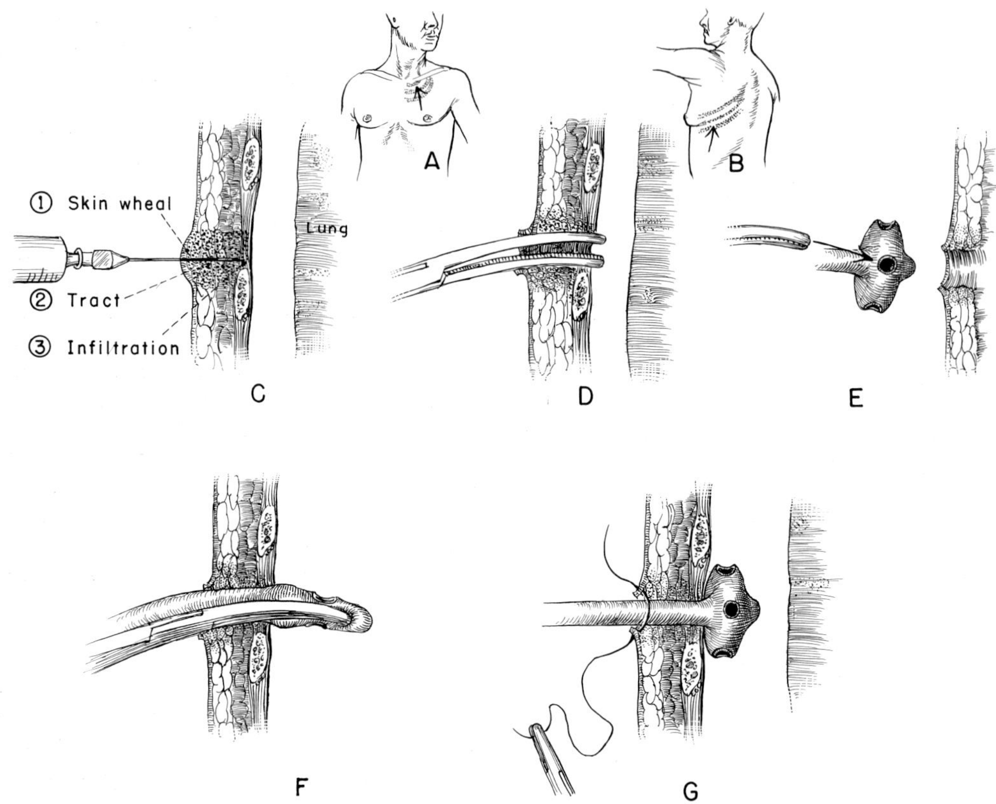

Figure 10–10 The technique of closed tube thoracostomy as described in the text. The second interspace in the midclavicular line (*A*) is selected for the removal of air and the 6th or 7th intercostal space in the posterior axillary line (*B*) for the removal of fluid.

a sizable bronchial radical, may require even more than one larger (24-28° F) catheter attached to suction. Larger catheters (32-36° F) are also used to evacuate a hemothorax. The initial technique is similar to that described for thoracentesis (Fig. 10–10 *C*). The chosen interspace is prepared and draped, and a tract into the interspace is infiltrated with 1 per cent Xylocaine but more widely than for thoracentesis. Specially designed trocars are available for inserting the catheter but are not widely used, because of the potential danger of damaging the underlying lung or diaphragm. We prefer to make a small incision and develop a tract through the underlying subcutaneous tissue and muscles down to the pleura by advancing a large Kelly clamp in increments and spreading it gently (Fig. 10–10*D*). The pleura is entered with a short quick thrust of the clamp. (The danger of damaging the underlying lung is minimal with this small instrument because it is separated from the parietal pleura by the accumulated air or fluid. There need be no fear of creating or increasing a pneumothorax since the pleural space will soon be completely evacuated.) Then a catheter of appropriate size, clamped at its distal end, is grasped by its forward tip and introduced into the pleura through this tract (Fig. 10–10 *E* and *F*). The skin is snugly closed around the catheter with a heavy silk or wire suture, which is then used to anchor the chest tube (Fig. 10–10*G*). "Mushroom-tip" or Malecot catheters have been popular since they can be pulled back until the flange abuts the parietal pleura, assuring the position of the tip of the catheter at the proper depth. However, clear plastic "Argyle" catheters with multiple holes near the end and a radiopaque marker to indicate position of the tube and its outermost hole on the chest x-ray are now the most popular type of chest tube. The clear plastic material allows ready visualization of the contents of the tubing and inhibits adherence of blood clots. An occlusive dressing may be applied around the tube, but this is usually not necessary if the suture is properly placed. The tube is unclamped after it has been securely connected (with adhesive tape) to the drainage system.

Pleural Drainage Systems. There are basically two types of pleural drainage systems. One employs a one-way water-trap mechanism, the other uses continuous suction. Their relative merits and indications are discussed in relation to the condition for which they are used.

The so-called water-trap or water-seal drainage achieves its purpose of allowing only the egress of pleural contents by the placement of the end of the drainage tube just under water some distance below the level of the patient's chest. The usual drainage bottle used for this purpose is illustrated in Figure 10–11 *left.* Pleural air or fluid will exit through the system whenever pleural pressure exceeds atmospheric pressure by more than the distance the drainage outlet is submerged below the water. This usually occurs during expiration, coughing or straining. During inspiration, however, the intrathoracic negative pressure must exceed the distance between the chest and the water level in the drainage bottle in order for fluid to rise up and enter the chest. Since this distance is usually 100 cm. or more, the system progressively evacuates the pleural contents with each expiration. If only fluid is involved, its egress will be further promoted by a siphon effect. Such a system is adequate for evacuating air and fluid accumulating at a modest rate and will prevent tension pneumothorax.

THE USE OF SUCTION SYSTEMS. The one-way drainage systems just described depend upon changes in intrapleural pressure to evacuate the pleural space. Their efficiency can be enhanced by having the patient cough, strain or breathe deeply, but if the rate of air leak or hemorrhage is rapid, this system will not keep the pleural space evacuated. This can be accomplished by applying negative pressure to the system. A number of devices, from complex pumps to simple faucet attachments, are used as the suction source, but the most important consideration is control of the

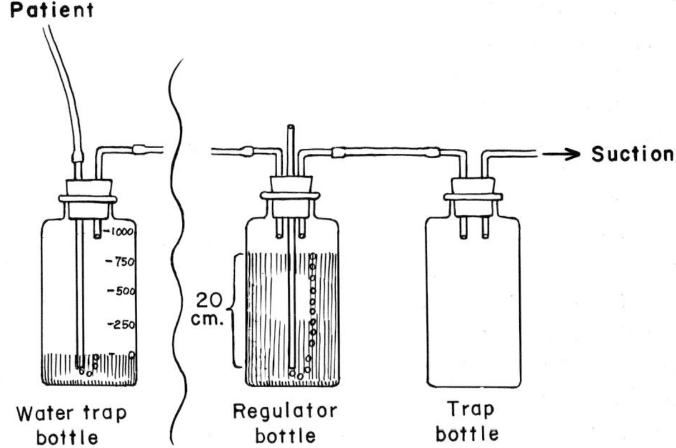

Figure 10–11 Pleural drainage systems. To the left is shown in the simple water trap bottle that utilizes respiratory excursions in intrapleural pressure to provide egress of the pleural contents. The suction drainage is provided by the addition of the two bottles on the right, the degree of suction being controlled by the depth of the middle tube below the water in the regulator bottle. See text for full description.

degree of negative pressure applied. A simple and effective means of achieving this employs a regulating bottle interposed between the suction source and the primary chest drainage bottle, as shown in Figure 10–11 *right*. In it a glass tube open to the atmosphere at one end and submerged below water at the other is used to limit the maximum degree of negative pressure that can be developed in the drainage system. When the negative pressure in the system begins to exceed the distance its tip is submerged below the water, outside air will be drawn in through the tube and will bring the pressure within the system back to this level again. Thus, by filling the regulator bottle to the desired level above the tip of this tube (usually between 5 and 20 cm.), one can limit the negative pressure applied, regardless of the amount of suction, and as long as bubbles are emerging from the tip of this tube, this level of negative pressure is assured. The system is usually completed by a third, or trap, bottle interposed between the regular bottle and the suction source to protect the latter against accidental spillover.

This "three bottle system" is the most common pleural suction apparatus used in this country. It has the advantage of being simple and inexpensive. There are more elaborate commercial systems available that are based on the same principles; their chief advantage lies in their capacity to remove large volumes rapidly at relatively low negative pressures. This is useful for large air leaks, from which air may accumulate more rapidly than the conventional three bottle system can remove it. It is also claimed that evacuating the pleural space at a lower pressure differential is less likely to delay the closure of air leaks. These features, though desirable, are a significant advantage in only a small minority of cases. In most instances the three bottle system is quite adequate.

Management of Chest Drainage Systems. Frequent checks should be made to see that all connections are secure and airtight and that the drainage tube has not become inadvertently occluded by the patient's sitting on it, by the inertia of fluid filling a bend in the tubing or by a fibrin or blood clot. These hazards can usually be avoided by seeing that the drainage tube has no excess length and by periodically "milking it down." Much practical information can be gained from careful periodic inspection of the chest bottles and tubing. Oscillations of the air-fluid level in the drainage tube in response to respirations, if greater than 1 to 2 cm., indicate that the system is patent. A persistent air leak is signalled by air intermittently bubbling out from the bottom of the drainage tube. This usually occurs only during expiration.

If bubbling occurs throughout the respiratory cycle in a water-seal drainage system, a large volume air leak is present and the presence of a ruptured bronchus should be considered. When suction is applied, the rate of air leak will be partly dependent on the degree of negative pressure applied as well as the size of the bronchopleural communication. The hourly rate of bleeding can be documented by marking a vertical strip of adhesive tape on the side of the bottle. The color of the blood may be helpful, but it must be kept in mind that if air is being evacuated through the tube with the blood, the latter can become oxygenated, misleading one as to its possible source.

Removal of Chest Tubes. Chest tubes are removed whenever they are no longer functioning or when blood or air has stopped accumulating. A petrolatum-impregnated gauze dressing, such as is used to cover an open pneumothorax, is prepared, and the anchoring suture is removed. The patient is instructed to hold a forced expiration for the period commanded and, after practice assures that this will be done, the tube is quickly withdrawn during the expiratory phase.

The communication is immediately occluded with the dressing, which is then firmly taped in place. Another alternative is to use a twisted wire to anchor the suture initially and to close the tract by tying this down at the time of removal of the chest tube.

THE LUNGS

Intrathoracic Foreign Bodies

The proper management of intrathoracic foreign bodies is a problem associated with penetrating thoracic injuries, particularly those resulting from military action. The problem is rarely urgent. However, after successful completion of the resuscitative phase, a decision should be made regarding the need for removal; if prophylactic removal is indicated, it is best done early. Factors influencing this decision are the nature of the foreign body, its size, shape and position, and the degree of contamination associated with its penetration of the thoracic cavity. Generally, foreign bodies in or near the tracheobronchial tree, the heart or great vessels warrant removal. One should also consider early removal of those that are large, (i.e., over 2.5 cm.), sharply contoured or associated with gross contamination. Objects that do not in themselves constitute an indication for surgical removal should nevertheless be removed when feasible during thoracotomy for other indications.

The removal of foreign bodies in or intimately associated with the heart and great vessels is dealt with later in this chapter. The majority of the remainder involve the lungs or pleura. In general, these are best left alone until they produce symptoms. Laustela[40] followed 502 Finnish casualties of World War II who had this complication and found that only 20 per cent developed complications requiring subsequent removal. Of the 104 presenting with late symptoms, 39 had chronic bronchitis; 31 developed lung abscess; 24 presented with empyema; 5 had bronchiectasis; and 5, bronchopleural fistula. Thus, the major problem was secondary infection.

The mortality from removal of intrathoracic foreign bodies in Korean War casualties was only 1 per cent when surgery was delayed until symptoms developed.[64] In 60 per cent of the cases the indication for operation was secondary infection. However, 85 per cent of the foreign bodies necessitating subsequent removal were shell fragments. In civilian practice the incidence of late complications would be even less. Indeed, in the Korean War experience, only 10 per cent of bullets lodged in the pulmonary parenchyma caused secondary infection. In spite of a few memorable exceptions, the generalization can be made that complications from foreign bodies develop relatively early, since many of the infections are related to the initial contamination and because it is rare for foreign bodies to migrate after the first few weeks unless they are closely related to hilar structures, are wholly intrapleural or are very sharp.

Primary Pulmonary Parenchymal Trauma

Trauma to the pulmonary parenchyma did not receive much attention in this country until widespread interest was aroused by the World War II experience with "wet lung."[12, 13] Just as there was a higher incidence of serious blast and blunt injuries to the thorax in that war, there has been a progressive increase in serious nonpenetrating thoracic injuries in civilian practice in the subsequent two decades. Penetrating injuries of the pulmonary parenchyma, excluding those from high velocity missiles, are relatively well tolerated. The reparative ability of the pulmonary parenchyma is remarkable. Unless hilar structures are damaged, the leakage of air and blood soon stops, and resections are rarely necessary for peripheral parenchymal damage. In the absence of a foreign body and gross contamination, infection is rare. On the other hand, although blunt trauma to the pulmonary parenchyma usually produces lesser degrees of local injury, it can result in far more serious, even life-threatening consequences by the summation of multiple lesions and secondary reflex changes.

The separation of various types of parenchymal damage is somewhat artificial since they so often occur in combination. In addition, with the exception of blast injuries, parenchymal lesions from nonpenetrating trauma are often associated with other intrathoracic damage.

Localized Pulmonary Contusion. This is a common sequel to thoracic injury. In its simplest form it represents suffusion of blood from disrupted vessels through air spaces into the surrounding parenchyma. As an isolated lesion it has little importance, although occasionally if there is bleeding into a main order bronchus, consolidation of the entire distal parenchymal segment may result. Nevertheless, when there is no significant disruption of the pulmonary parenchyma resorption will be prompt.

Parenchymal Laceration. Tearing of the pulmonary parenchyma may disrupt both blood vessels and air passages. Subsequent developments partially depend on whether the laceration connects with the pleura. If there is communication with the pleura, either a hemothorax, a pneumothorax or a pneumohemothorax will be produced. The latter is the most common occurrence with penetrating injuries. On the other hand, parenchymal disruptions resulting from blunt trauma are often localized in the region of the intermediary bronchus, so that the extravasated blood and air accumulate in the space created by the parenchymal laceration, resulting in either pulmonary hematoma or cystic cavities.

Pulmonary Hematoma. In contrast to the consolidation of pulmonary parenchyma with suffused blood occurring after contusion, pulmonary hematoma implies the accumulation of extravasated blood in a space created by parenchymal disruption. This is a much more common sequel to blunt chest trauma than generally appreciated. In a review of 124 cases of nonpenetrating injury to the thorax, Westermark[67] found radiologic parenchymal abnormalities in 94. In 14 of these, slightly over 10 per cent, lesions suggestive of single or multiple pulmonary hematomas were observed.

Errion et al.[26] reviewed 50 cases of pulmonary hematoma resulting from blunt thoracic trauma and made the following observations: When present, pain and hemoptysis were moderate in degree, usually disappearing in less than a week. Low grade fever and dyspnea were not uncommon, the latter being characteristically greater than expected from the radiologic appearance of the parenchymal lesion. Typically, these lesions appear fuzzy in outline on initial films but in a few days, as the surrounding suffusion of blood resorbs, the outline sharpens. This creates a parenchymal lesion which may be indistinguishable from other coin lesions without the benefit of earlier films. The hematomas are ordinarily 2 to 5 cm. in diameter and characteristically are located posteriorly in the lower lobes. In 18 of the 50 cases, a radiolucency developed later in the lesion. Resolution usually took place in two to four weeks.

Their characteristic location has suggested to some that pulmonary hematomas following blunt trauma result from a contrecoup mechanism in which shearing forces develop in the region of the intermediary bronchi. The main clinical problem created by such pulmonary hematomas results from failure to recognize their traumatic origin. This dilemma usually develops when there is no pretrauma x-ray available for comparison and the early evolution of these lesions is not observed. Thus, there may be no way to distinguish them from a pre-existing coin lesion. The problem may be resolved by progressive resolution of the lesion; but if this has not occurred in three weeks, the lesion should be excised to establish its identity.

Another problem that occasionally arises during exploration for other indications is whether something should be done about coexisting hemorrhagic parenchymal lesions. In view of the remarkable reparative properties of the pulmonary parenchyma, resection is recommended only for extensive parenchymal damage. Otherwise, bleeding and air leaks should be controlled by suture ligation, the laceration left open, and a chest tube placed near this area and connected to suction.

Traumatic Pulmonary Cavity. More rarely, the disruptive forces mentioned above will tear a small bronchiole without significant vascular damage, resulting in the formation of a pulmonary cavity. These usually resolve spontaneously without secondary infection but occasionally, if associated with disruption of a main order bronchus, they may fail to regress and actually enlarge. These exceptional cases require operative control of the bronchial communication, after which the opened cavity will collapse with catheter drainage and suction.

Contusion Pneumonitis or Wet Lung. Although a clear description of this entity was published many years ago by Morgagni and further elaborated in European—particularly French—literature, it was not until Brewer[11] and Burford[12] and their respective associates reported their experience with this condition during World War II that it became widely appreciated in this country. Brewer felt that "persistence of fluid in the pulmonary tree" resulted from increased production and decreased removal of this fluid—bronchial secretions, serum and blood. Drinker and Warren[23] elucidated some of the factors contributing to increased pulmonary fluid production, emphasizing anoxia, changes in tissue permeability, increased respiratory movements and tracheal obstruction. In addition, it was suggested that the extravasated blood produced a reflex bronchospasm.

Probably one of the most important factors limiting the patient's ability to clear these fluids from the air passages is the inability to cough because of uncontrolled chest pain. Similarly, any interference with effective coughing (e.g., flail chest, elevated diaphragm, central nervous system depression) will aggravate the situation. These factors initiate a vicious cycle that produces progressive ventilatory impairment.

What determines why one patient with blunt chest trauma ends up with only a localized pulmonary contusion and in another this process progresses to the diffuse secondary consolidative changes of "traumatic wet lung" is not clear. The severity of the trauma itself is one obvious factor, and the volume of intravenous fluids administered after the injury may be another. Rutherford and Valenta[59] have succeeded in producing pulmonary contusions in dogs which spontaneously progressed into a lethal "traumatic wet lung" by high-velocity, low-mass blunt trauma inflicted during tracheal obstruction, suggesting the importance of a closed glottis at the moment of impact. Histologically, the secondary areas of consolidation were indistinguishable from those of "shock lung" and other pulmonary parenchymal consolidative lesions of traumatic origins, adding to the conviction that the lung responds in a common manner to all forms of insult and injury. Hypoxia secondary to pulmonary vascular "shunting" through consolidated areas, decreased compliance and hyperventilation with hypocarbia were the main physiologic abnormalities observed.

DIAGNOSIS. After a variable period of delay, the patient usually develops an ineffective cough and progressive hyperpnea and dyspnea. Physical examination reveals scattered bronchial rales. These may be fine or "sticky" and do not completely clear on coughing. Local areas of wheezing are often a prominent finding. The overall picture resembles those of pulmonary edema associated with a degree of bronchospasm but is more variable in degree and distribution than seen on the initial x-ray.

The x-ray picture is characteristic but may not correspond temporally to the developing clinical picture. A few fluffy opacifications seen on the initial x-ray may quickly progress into a veritable "snowstorm" in which little functional parenchyma would appear to remain. Usually these lesions appear first on the side of impact, and the changes in this area will be more marked, even though scattered lesions may subsequently appear bilaterally. Blood gas analysis will usually show decreases in oxygen and carbon dioxide tension in the arterial blood.

TREATMENT. Treatment depends on the severity of the condition. If the contusion pneumonitis remains relatively localized, it may be weathered without specific therapy. However, one has no assurance when this localized process is first discovered that it will not progress into the severe, widespread form. The latent period between the development of symptoms and the rate of progression are only rough guides. Early vigorous therapy should not be delayed until serious symptoms develop. The patient should be placed in a semi-upright position in an oxygen-rich, humidified atmosphere. Chest pain must be controlled by analgesics or, if necessary, intercostal block. This alone may allow the patient to maintain a clear airway by coughing. Otherwise, nasotracheal suction should be used. Bronchodilators have proved helpful, particularly the use of small doses of aminophylline.

Although saline infusions have made experimental models of wet lung worse,[20] the inference that patients should be kept dehydrated does not appear justified. This may result in more viscid bronchial secretions that complicate tracheal toilet. However, one should assiduously avoid overhydration whenever intravenous fluids are being administered. Expectorants and mucolytic agents have been advocated, but their benefit has not been clearly shown. Antibiotics should be administered. In Westermark's series, 26 of the 28 patients who developed clinical bronchitis with purulent sputum after blunt chest trauma had x-ray evidence of contusion pneumonitis on earlier films.

Although a significant proportion of cases will respond satisfactorily to the above measures, it has become common practice in recent years to perform a tracheostomy and to place the more severely affected patients on positive pressure ventilation, using a respirator. The indication for tracheostomy here is inability to control secretions in spite of other measures. It has the additional benefit of decreasing airway resistance, respiratory dead space and the work of breathing. The benefit of positive pressure breathing has been implied from the report of Ransdell et al.[56] of a series of patients with traumatic flail chest treated with and without a respirator. Four of 17 treated without a respirator developed the wet lung syndrome, while none of the 16 placed in a respirator developed this complication. This agrees with earlier experience with the use of positive pressure oxygen therapy in the treatment of acute pulmonary edema.

In the previously mentioned experimental study,[59] the author showed that lethal outcome could be reduced from 70 per cent to 10 per cent by only an hour of positive pressure ventilation if it was applied soon after the injury. While the value of prophylactic or, at least early, respirator therapy seems clear, the practical problem of selection remains, since the majority of patients, those with mild, localized pulmonary contusions, will not need this form of treatment. Our experiments showed that pulmonary scans are much more sensitive than chest x-rays in predicting the severity of the parenchymal involvement, but this is not a practical diagnostic approach in most hospitals. Instead, we rely heavily on serial blood determinations. In general, the use of continuous positive pressure ventilation should be considered in the treatment of pulmonary contusions under the following circumstances: (1) multiple or large pulmonary contusions are evident on the admission x-ray, (2) the contusions are associated with multiple (more than 5) rib fractures or even minor degrees of flail chest, (3) surgery under general anesthesia will be necessary for associated injuries, (4) arterial blood gases are significantly depressed below normal, (5) voluminous intravenous fluid therapy is anticipated in the treatment of other injuries, (6) underlying dysfunctional lung disease exists (e.g., asthma, emphysema), (7) serial x-rays show progressive opacification, and (8) in the absence of other criteria, if rapid, labored respirations ensue.

Respirator Therapy of Chest Injuries. In addition to flail chest and contusion pneumonitis, there are a number of other "traumatic" forms of pulmonary parenchymal consolidation that may benefit from use of C.P.P.V. (e.g., shock lung, fat embolism, smoke inhalation, aspirative pneumonitis, "pump-oxygenator lung"). Serial arterial blood gas analyses usually provide the most objective guides for institution and discontinuation of respirator therapy. It is beyond the scope of this chapter to discuss respirator therapy in detail. The reader is referred to more comprehensive publications for this.[6, 53] However, several aspects are worth mention here. One is the controversy over the choice between pressure-cycled versus volume-cycled ventilators. In this particular setting, with changing degrees of parenchymal consolidation, the volume-cycled respirator is definitely superior. Pressure-cycled respirators cannot be relied upon to produce adequate ventilatory exchange in the face of increased and *changing* pulmonary compliance. Furthermore, most of them do not have a very high peak-pressure capacity or good control of inspired oxygen concentrations. Time-cycled devices, such as the Engstrom respirator, will deliver the required tidal volume with high pressure capacity but have the disadvantages of a fixed inspiratory:expiratory ratio and cannot be patient-cycled. The volume-cycled respirators deliver a metered amount of air at whatever delivery pressure is required. However, some of the newer respirators, like the Ohio 560 and Bennett MA-1 have such a variety of features that the above arguments become almost academic. Although they are basically volume-limited ventilators with range-controlled high-pressure capacity in which the inspired oxygen concentration can also be accurately controlled, they have a wide range of flow capacities, a spirometer to monitor each tidal volume, built-in warning devices, a sigh mechanism to protect against atelectasis, an ultrasonic nebulizer and the important capability of applying positive end expired pressure (P.E.E.P.) or the inflationary hold (I.H.).

While tidal volumes of 10 cc./kg. and a rate of 12-14 breaths per minute are sufficient in dealing with most forms of respiratory insufficiency, minute volumes of more than twice this level are commonly required in dealing with traumatic parenchymal problems. The resultant hypocarbia and alkalosis are then converted by adding one to three feet of dead-space tubing between the trachea and the expiratory valve. In an attempt to keep the inspired oxygen concentration below 40 per cent and avoid superimposing an oxygen toxicity lesion on an already damaged lung, one may have to accept slightly subnormal arterial oxygen tensions and, of course, supranormal levels are inexcusable in a properly functioning respiratory care unit.

Rather than increasing inspired

oxygen concentration for any extended period of time, it is worth trying other ancillary measures. One of the most popular of these is P.E.E.P., in which, by a special expiratory valve, 6 to 7 cm. of positive and expiratory pressure can be maintained. This maintains a larger functional residual capacity with which more alveoli may remain open and better ventilation:perfusion ratios may be achieved. Another occasionally useful technique is that of "inspiratory hold" in which peak inspiratory pressure is held for ½ to 1½ seconds to allow additional time for alveolar recruitment and more effective distribution of inspired air throughout the lungs. The fear that these maneuvers might interfere with venous return to the heart, as they can do in normal subjects, appears to be unfounded, as the noncompliant lungs dissipate these higher pressures so that they do not result in comparable rises in intrapleural pressure. In fact, these adverse hemodynamic effects occur in these patients only if the blood volume is diminished and their appearance is cause for volume restoration rather than discreditation of respiratory therapy.

The value of other measures, such as furosemide and concentrated salt-poor albumin to "dry-out" these "wet" lungs, is hard to prove, but it is the author's impression that they will usually produce worthwhile results in the early stages when interstitial and intra-alveolar edema are the dominant lesions and are readily reversible. Short-term, high-dose, Cortisone therapy also produces occasional dramatic results when there is a strong inflammatory component, as in fat embolism and aspiration pneumonitis.

The Tracheobronchial Tree. Although the tracheobronchial tree may be violated by a variety of penetrating objects, most tracheobronchial tears are the result of severe blunt trauma. There were 61 instances of this complication recorded in the medical literature in 100 years prior to 1948 and 94 in the decade that followed.[4] This fifteenfold increase in the reported incidence is attributable in part to increased frequency of severe blunt trauma and in part to the interest generated by successful surgical treatment, first achieved by Griffith in 1948.[32] Since that report, excellent results have been achieved in over 60 per cent of the operated cases reported.[49]

By far the majority of these injuries involve the mainstem bronchi. Only 18 of 98 cases reviewed by Hood and Sloan[36] were tracheal tears, and of the remaining 80, all but six were in the main bronchus. The distribution between right and left side was roughly equal. The mechanism involved has not been established, but shearing forces, compression of the trachea against the vertebral column, airway distention against a closed glottis and sudden vertical stretch of the tracheobronchial tree all have been suggested.[17] Whichever theory is true must explain the fact that over 90 per cent of the tears occur within an inch of the carina. The typical tear in the bronchus is circumferential and incomplete. The less frequent tracheal tears are usually vertical along the line of membranous-cartilaginous transition. Complete division of the trachea, however, is extremely uncommon.

DIAGNOSIS. The manner of presentation varies considerably (Fig. 10–12). The lesion may prove rapidly fatal or allow survival without surgical intervention. In more severe cases only prompt recognition and resuscitation will achieve survival. In Burke's series,[14] 52 per cent of the deaths occurred within one hour of injury and an additional 44 per cent within four days of injury. Fortunately, the majority of cases do not present in critical condition. In the same series, immediate operation was carried out in only 11 per cent, 21 per cent presented with a collaped lung which resisted attempts at re-expansion and were explored after bronchoscopic confirmation of the injury; and the

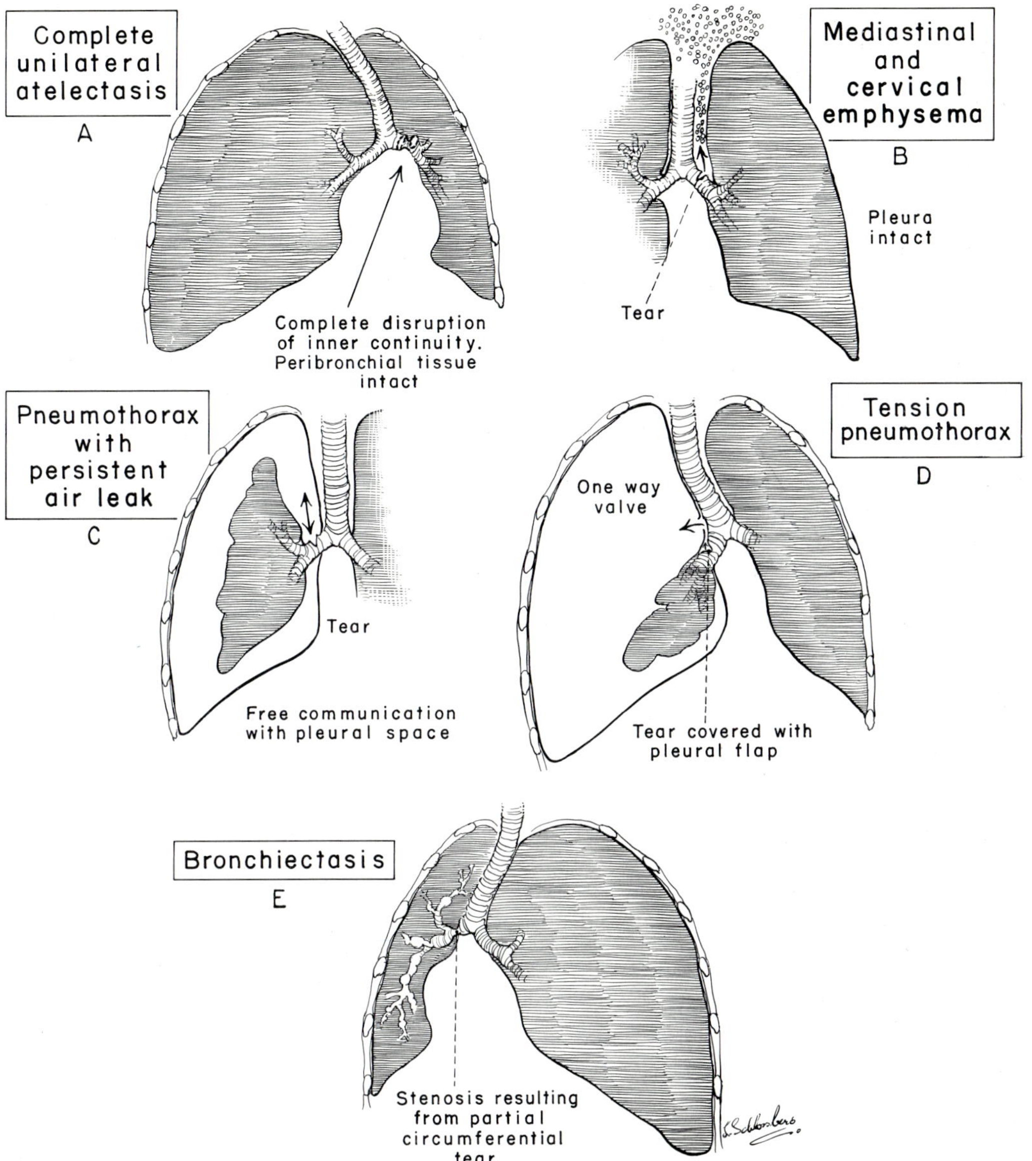

Figure 10–12 Common forms of presentation of tracheobronchial rupture as described in the text.

remaining 68 per cent presented later with bronchial stenosis. This is similar to the observation of Hood and Sloan that the diagnosis was made with 24 hours of injury in only a third of the cases.

Depending on the location and size of the tear and the involvement of bronchial vessels or the mediastinal pleura, these injuries may present with one or more of the following: massive hemoptysis, airway obstruction, progressive mediastinal and subcutaneous emphysema, tension pneumothorax, pneumothorax without tension but with persistent air leak, or massive collapse of one lung (Fig. 10–12). Although the patient with a ruptured bronchus is said to present characteristically with dyspnea and cyanosis, subcutaneous and mediastinal emphysema, fractured ribs, pneumothorax and hemoptysis, over two-thirds of the patients in Burke's series did not show this combination. In one of seven, the thoracic contents appeared normal on the initial chest x-ray.

Pneumothorax was found in only 55 of the 82 patients reported by Hood and Sloan and tension pneumothorax in only 21. Subcutaneous emphysema was present in just over one-half the cases and hemoptysis and thoracic skeletal fractures were demonstrated in only one-fourth. Furthermore, one cannot always depend upon other evidence of severe thoracic trauma to alert one's suspicions, for this injury may show remarkable selectivity. In 42 of the 80 bronchial tears reported by Hood and Sloan, this was the only major intrathoracic injury. Although one cannot expect to find all the "characteristic" features in any one patient, any one of them should arouse suspicion. This association of rib fractures is high *if* one considers only the age group in which rib fractures readily occur. Thus, 91 per cent of patients over 30 years of age had fractures involving one of the upper three ribs, and all had a fracture of at least one of the upper five ribs.[4] Similarly, mediastinal and cervical subcutaneous emphysema should raise the question of such an injury. This is likely to be prominent in tracheal tears or bronchial tears on which the mediastinal pleura remains intact. However, if the pleura is torn, a pneumothorax results. This usually presents either as a tension pneumothorax or a pneumothorax with persistent air leak. A tension pneumothorax often is produced because the tear in the mediastinal pleura occurs some distance from the point of airway rupture so that a valve-like mediastinal flap exists. However, tension pneumothorax is not so common an association as it once was thought to be.

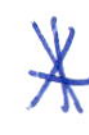

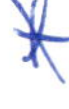

Another common variation is for the edges of a complete bronchial tear to be separated, yet for the surrounding tissues to remain intact so that pneumothorax does not occur. These cases may present early with complete unilateral atelectasis or late with bronchial stenosis. Most bronchial tears bleed, but hemoptysis may be absent because the bleeding may have stopped by the time the patient is seen or the blood may not have been coughed up. Nevertheless, there are cases in which the hemoptysis is massive, presenting a difficult problem in management. Significant hemoptysis following chest trauma is a symptom that should not be ignored and, even in the absence of other symptoms suggesting tracheobronchial rupture, it is an indication for bronchoscopy.

TREATMENT. Patients presenting with massive hemoptysis, airway obstruction or tension pneumothorax need immediate resuscitative measures. Emergency tracheostomy may be necessary to remove accumulating blood. It also helps to minimize the subcutaneous emphysema and to reduce the rate of air leak. The lethal potential of a tension pneumothorax can be eliminated by percutaneous needle puncture of the involved hemithorax. This should be followed by tube thoracostomy and evacuation of pleural air by suction. A large intercostal catheter and an efficient (low pressure–high volume) suction system may be required to evacuate the pleural space if there is a large air leak. In such cases, a point may be reached beyond which the rate or removal of pleural air prevents adequate intake of air into the lungs. Such an impasse, of course, demands immediate thoracotomy. Until this can be accomplished, it is better to settle for a pneumothorax without tension than to persist with more vigorous attempts to expand the lung.

Fortunately, such cases are not frequent. More commonly, these patients present with mediastinal and subcutaneous emphysema and a pneumothorax without marked tension. The initial treatment has often been simple water-seal drainage. It may be some time before the diagnosis is suggested by the fact that the air leak is unusually large and persistent or that the lung has failed to expand completely even though suction has been applied. Such clues will arouse the suspicion of the alert physician and will lead to bronchoscopic confirmation of the diagnosis. Not only are the bronchoscopic findings diagnostic but they may determine the need for definitive repair. For example, if there is only a fourth to a third circumferential tear, or a tear of less than one inch, tracheostomy alone may be tried since the majority of such tears will heal without stenosis. On the other hand, all large or irregular incomplete tears and all complete tears should be repaired.

Repair. If repair is indicated it should be done as early as feasible. Recent years have witnessed an increasing realization of this goal. Previously, most of the operations for tracheobronchial rupture followed the development of bronchial stenosis. Pulmonary resection was usually carried out, but this is now reserved for irreversible parenchymal damage secondary to infection. It has been shown that in the absence of superimposed infection, significant function may be restored by reanastomosing a lung that has been totally collapsed for years.[44] However, such remarkable instances of late functional restoration are exceptional and, in most cases, one can expect a progressive loss of recoverable function beginning between two to six months after bronchial occlusion. Fortunately, total bronchial occlusion almost never results in bronchiectasis or serious parenchymal infection. These complications are usually seen as a result of the incomplete obstruction that develops after a partial bronchial tear.

Immediately following injury, primary anastomosis can usually be accomplished after simple debridement of the edges of the tear. The exposure may be difficult on the left side because of the aortic arch. Except for smaller air leaks that can be controlled by intermittent finger pressure, it is preferable to have the anesthetist use a Carlens catheter (a bifid endotracheal tube with separate lumina for each stem bronchus) or advance an endotracheal tube into the opposite bronchus. Cardiopulmonary bypass has also been used to allow reconstruction of extensive tears. Delayed repair is technically more difficult because of inflammatory or scirrhous reaction in the surrounding tissues. These operative difficulties have prompted some to recommend dilatation for late bronchial stenosis, but this is rarely successful except for mild strictures. Resection of the stricture and reanastomosis is preferable to bronchoplastic techniques whenever possible. The latter are more applicable for the long, postinflammatory strictures for which they were originally devised.

Airway Obstruction

Patency of the airway and adequacy of the respiratory exchange should be among the first considerations in the evaluation and management of the injured patient. The stridor of laryngeal obstruction or the noisy rhonchi emanating from a trachea filled with retained secretions or blood demand immediate attention. More commonly, however, the airway obstruction associated with chest injuries is subtle in presentation. It may be completely absent on initial examination and vary in degree from moment to moment. The cause is often extrathoracic. Head injuries frequently accompany thoracic trauma, particularly when automobile collisions are involved. Depression of the state of consciousness from this, the effects of alcohol or indiscriminately administered narcotics are three common factors contributing to airway obstruction.

As noted, the adequacy of the ventilatory exchange can be grossly assessed by placing one's ear close to the patient's face and, at the same time, watching the respiratory movements of the thorax. By this maneuver one can evaluate not only the ventilatory exchange but the effort used to produce it. Initially, the patient may be able to compensate for minor degrees of obstruction with extra effort. Later, exhaustion, depression in the state of consciousness or accumulating tracheobronchial secretions may tip the scales against the patient.

Treatment. When the obstruction is positional, secondary to the relaxation of the muscular support of the tongue and mandible, manual repositioning of these structures will relieve the obstruction temporarily. This gain should be consolidated by an oropharyngeal airway or even an endotracheal tube. The latter may be left in for 24 to 48 hours, but if it is evident that the problem will continue beyond this time, a tracheostomy is indicated. Ordinarily, however, this should wait until other serious injuries have been dealt with and the patient's condition has stabilized.

In the conscious patient, on the other hand, airway obstruction usually develops because of retained secretions and blood. This is particularly true of patients with multiple rib fractures, flail chest or contusion pneumonitis, although it may be seen in any patient with chest trauma in whom pain is not properly controlled. There will often be a variable period of delay before this problem becomes manifest, a period during which its appearance may be prevented by control of pain by intercostal block, restoration of the integrity of the thorax, evacuation of the pleural space or attention to nasotracheal toilet. In severe cases, even these measures may not suffice and one must resort to tracheostomy.

Obviously, the methods used to maintain the airway free of blood and tracheobronchial secretions must be chosen to fit the individual case. A brief description of some of the techniques recommended above is included here. Others will be found in Chapters Four and Nine.

NASOTRACHEAL SUCTION. This maneuver, introduced by Haight in 1942, is a valuable means of providing adequate pulmonary toilet after thoracic trauma. The technique can be easily learned. If possible, the patient is seated in an upright position. He is instructed to project the mandible forward and protrude the tongue. The latter is grasped with a gauze pad and drawn gently forward. A sterile No. 14 to 18 French catheter is introduced into the posterior oropharynx through a nostril so that its tip lies pointed above the glottis. The depth of insertion can be guided initially by watching its passage down from the nasopharynx through the open mouth. Its arrival over the glottis is signaled by a "nearness" of the breath sounds heard through the proximal end of the tube. Once the catheter is in this position, the patient is induced to take a deep breath, at which moment the tube is quickly advanced through the open glottis. Even uncooperative patients will open their glottis after a cough or breath holding.

The successful introduction of the catheter into the trachea will result in vigorous coughing unless the patient has a depressed cough reflex. In such cases, the patient's inability to phonate or the forceful jet of air coming through the end of the nasotracheal catheter with each expiration will serve as a clue. At this point, the catheter is connected to a suction source by a Y-connector and intermittent tracheal aspiration is carried out with *brief* periods of suction, lasting no longer than ten seconds or the length of time this patient can hold his breath. More prolonged suctioning is contraindicated because much of the inspired air is being removed. Even when passage of the nasotracheal tube is not successful, the paroxysms of cough resulting from the attempts partly achieve the desired goal. This procedure must be repeated at four- to six-hour intervals. If much more frequent tracheal aspiration is indicated, a tracheostomy is usually warranted.

TRACHEOSTOMY. The technique and care of a tracheostomy are described elsewhere in this book (Chapter Nine). The following comments are directed toward its role in the treatment of thoracic trauma. For more than a century after Trousseau reported its use in 200 diphtheritic children in 1833, tracheostomy was employed only to relieve airway obstruction. In 1943 Galloway suggested its use in aspirating the tracheobronchial tree, and considerable experience with its use for this indication was obtained during poliomyelitis epidemics, particularly in Scandinavia in 1952 and 1953. At about this time, its potential in the treatment of chest injuries, particularly crushed chest, became more fully appreciated following reports of Carter and Giuseffi.[16] The progressive wave of enthusiasm that followed has only recently been tempered. Unfortunately, the procedure has become a "prophylactic" or "routine" measure in the hands of many. It has often been said that "the time to do a tracheostomy is when you first think about it." However, the need for following strict indications can be appreciated if one considers the risk this procedure carries in terms of serious complications.[38] Furthermore, this risk is trebled when tracheostomy is performed as an emergency procedure under suboptimal conditions. This is not to deny the value of this important resuscitative procedure but rather to stress the need for indications based on attainable objectives.

Mechanical obstruction to the upper air passage is an unchallenged indication and is one of the few indications for emergency tracheostomy. Fortunately, injuries resulting in true mechanical obstruction to the air passage proximal to the cervical trachea are not frequent. More often, it is the associated bleeding from such injuries that prompts tracheostomy.

As previously mentioned, position obstruction secondary to central nervous system depression is common, but this can be initially treated by insertion of an oropharyngeal airway or endotracheal tube, with tracheostomy performed later when the patient's condition has stabilized and the long-term need for tracheal intubation has been established.

Another relative indication for tracheostomy is the accumulation of tracheobronchial secretions. Maloney and MacDonald[45] have cautioned that most of the secretions removed from an established tracheostomy are aspirated saliva since it is known that some degree of laryngeal incompetence frequently follows tracheostomy. However, there remains a definite role for tracheostomy when simpler measures have failed to remove retained tracheobronchial secretions and blood.

It has been suggested that tracheostomy reduces dead space and resistance to air flow and in this way decreases the work of breathing. Indeed, the respiratory dead space can be reduced by tracheostomy although not by so much as once thought. Estimates based on anatomic studies assume that all the respiratory exchange passes through the tracheostomy cannula, a situation which is true only if cuffed tubes are used. The reduction in dead space that can be expected is therefore closer to one-third than the two-thirds formerly predicted. It should be also pointed out that resistance to airflow is reduced only when large diameter tracheostomy cannulas are used. It has been shown by Garzon et al.[28] that the work of breathing through a No. 7 or 8 cuffed tracheostomy tube is equal to that of mouth breathing. Only when a No. 9 or 10 tube is used can a significant reduction in resistance be expected. Thus, whenever relief of the work of breathing is the major goal, a respirator should usually also be employed.

By the same token, if one wishes to reduce the paradoxical movement of a flail chest by tracheostomy, it is necessary to use a large cannula placed low in the cervical trachea. This allows air to be exchanged at relatively lower pressure differentials and, in some cases, reduces the paradoxical movements of the flail segment enough so that use of a respirator is not necessary. However, need for prolonged artificial ventilatory support is the major indication for tracheostomy.

With the above qualifications, tracheostomy remains one of the most valuable resuscitative procedures available to the physican treating chest injuries. The indications for its use are summarized below:

1. True mechanical obstruction of the upper air passages.
2. Positional airway obstruction secondary to central nervous system depression, if prolonged over 24 hours.
3. Retention of tracheobronchial secretions and blood that cannot be controlled by simpler methods.
4. Use of a respirator.
5. Rarely, massive or progressive cervical subcutaneous emphysema.
6. Minor tears of the tracheobronchial tree (less than 1 cm. or one-third of the circumference).
7. Flail chest (use with or without a respirator).
8. Traumatic tracheo-esophageal fistulas.

THE ESOPHAGUS

Since caustic burns of and foreign bodies in the esophagus are primarily encountered in children, they are dealt with in Chapter Twenty. Essentially all other significant forms of esophageal injury involve disruption of its wall by one mechanism or another. The esophagus may be perforated from within by instrumentation or a swallowed foreign body, penetrated from without by a bullet or other missile or ruptured by blunt trauma to the abdomen or chest. Except for missile perforation, which may occur anywhere, these different mechanisms have characteristic sites of predilection. Perforation from instruments (esophagoscope, dilator or biopsy forceps) or by ingested foreign bodies almost invariably occurs at the site of esophageal narrowing, either at the three natural points of constriction (the pharnygo-esophageal junction, the level of the aortic arch and the cardia) or at the site of an inflammatory or neoplastic stricture. The esophagus usually ruptures from blunt trauma at the same site in the lower third of the esophagus above the cardia at which "spontaneous," or postemetic, ruptures occur. The relative weakness of this area has been clearly demonstrated by MacKenzie[41] and Mackler.[43] Rupture following a blast injury frequently occurs at this point too.

Diagnosis. Although these various mechanisms all result in disruption of the esophageal wall, the clinical picture may be quite variable, depending on the site of rupture and the degree of contamination. At one extreme is the relatively benign course that follows instrumental perforation at the pharyngo-esophageal junction when it is immediately recognized and the patient given nothing by mouth. At the other is the fulminant and often fatal condition that results when the gastric contents are ejected through a rent in the wall of the lower esophagus. In the former, discomfort may be minimal and noticed only with swallowing; with the latter, pain may be so excruciating that a coronary occlusion or some intra-abdominal catastrophe is suspected.

The indications of cervical esophageal perforation are painful dysphagia and subcutaneous emphysema. Later, there may be signs of local inflammation. Occasionally, this may spread downward inside the prevertebral fascia and result in serious mediastinitis. The development of such an infection is usually heralded by rising temperature and increasing pain.

Mediastinitis, of course, is more common after perforation of the thoracic esophagus. It characteristically occurs after internal perforations that do not violate the pleura. The dissection of air throughout the mediastinum may be detected on physical examination, if a "mediastinal crunch" is heard on auscultation, or if it reaches the neck so that the subcutaneous emphysema in the suprasternal area is noticed. The diagnosis may be confirmed, or even first suggested, by chest x-ray if stippling of the mediastinum with air is visible. Widening of the mediastinum is a late sign, and its absence should not delay the diagnosis.

Larger perforations, missile injuries and rupture of the lower esophagus secondary to blunt or blast injury are usually associated with a penumothorax. Depending on the degree of contamination of the pleural space, there will be a variable amount of reactive pleural effusion. When gastric contents have been ejected into the esophagus and out through the rent, the pleural space may contain more fluid than air. The fluid losses resulting from such contamination of the mediastinum and pleural space may be massive.[69]

Patients with esophageal rupture secondary to blunt or penetrating trauma may be thought at first to have a simple pneumothorax or hemopneumothorax. However, once a chest tube is inserted the diagnosis should become obvious from the appearance of the drainage. The diagnosis should be considered whenever there is a pneumothorax with a persistent air leak. Dyspnea, cyanosis and shock are common in severe cases. Hematemesis is a helpful but inconstant sign.

It is important to establish the diagnosis as early as possible. If esophageal rupture is even remotely possible, the patient should be made to swallow an absorbable contrast medium (not barium) and x-rays should be taken. This study is desirable even if the diagnosis is obvious, since it is important in planning the operative approach to know the site of the tear. However, this examination should not delay or take precedence over vigorous resuscitative efforts.

Treatment. Common to the treatment of all esophageal tears should be vigorous intravenous fluid administration, massive doses of antibiotics and restriction of oral intake. These are the mainstays of nonoperative treatment, an approach that should be limited to *selected* cases of cervical esophageal perforation. In most instances, these measures are intended only as support for definitive surgical intervention. In addition to these measures, the pleural space should be drained as early as possible by closed tube thoracostomy.

The earlier the exploration, the better the result. Operation should not be delayed indefinitely while awaiting optimal response to supportive measures. As soon as a reasonable initial response has been obtained, the patient should be explored with these supportive measures vigorously continued during surgery. The central venous pressure is a valuable means of determining the rate at which intravenous therapy should be administered. The work of Ware and Strieder,[66] showing no improvement in survival of animals given antibiotics and intravenous fluids alone, gave further impetus to the policy of early operative intervention. Also, early exploration allows definitive repair to be carried out before inflammatory changes in the tissues at the site of the tear have occurred. It should be emphasized, therefore, that severe debilitation, shock and moribund appearance are not contraindications to surgery, but indications for more aggressive supportive care before and during operation. Even in delayed cases in which primary closure of the tear cannot be expected to succeed, operative drainage of the site of rupture can be lifesaving.

The operative approach will be determined by the site of rupture. Generally, upper third perforations should be explored through the neck; middle third, through the right chest; and lower third, through a left thoracotomy. If possible, repair should be performed in two layers. A drainage tube should be placed with its tip near but not on the suture line and the pleura left open to avoid mediastinitis and abscess formation should the repair not hold.

It the tissues will not hold sutures, as may be the case if there has been considerable delay, one may have to rely on this drainage tube alone, accepting the fistula that will develop. If repair is possible, drainage of the suture line should be continued until it has been tested first by esophagogram and then by oral feedings. Concomitant gastrostomy should be performed to allow management of the patient during this period. Esophageal stricture not infrequently follows a difficult repair, particularly if a fistula forms. Unless a pseudodiverticulum develops, these can usually be managed by dilations.

Results. The outcome of esophageal rupture depends upon the mechanism of injury, the site of perforation, the degree of contamination and the delay in treatment. Instrumental perforations carry the best prognosis, and rupture secondary to blunt trauma the worst. The high mortality (80 per cent) in the latter situation is mainly the result of failure to make the diagnosis, which was not suspected until autopsy in two-thirds of the recorded cases.[70] That better results can be obtained is reflected by the statistics for postemetic rupture. Prior to 1951, only 13 of 100 reported cases had survived. However, the prognosis has steadily improved since then and in several recent series this mortality rate has almost reversed. This improvement stems as much from early diagnosis and operative repair as from a more aggressive supportive therapy.

Post-traumatic Tracheo-esophageal Fistula

As a consequence of blunt chest trauma, this condition stands somewhere between esophageal and tracheobronchial rupture, both in incidence and development. It most commonly occurs after automobile or auto-pedestrian accidents and rarely occurs in association with externally penetrating injuries. Up to 1965, 98 cases had appeared in the literature since Vinson's first report in 1836.[2] Like tracheobronchial rupture it is located near the carina, and the same mechanism is thought to be involved in the development of both conditions, with a fistula resulting when the adjacent esophagus is also damaged. Because of the late presentation of the majority of cases, it has been suggested that an abscess develops at the site of tracheal rupture and that this later breaks through the weakened esophageal wall.

Diagnosis. The initial symptoms are similar to those following a small localized bronchial or esophageal tear with localized mediastinitis. Later, the patient develops a paroxysmal cough aggravated by feeding. This pathognomonic feature should suggest the diagnosis, although it may be attributed erroneously to a degree of laryngeal incompetence associated with tracheostomy which has been performed. Confirmation may be obtained by an esophageal swallow using contrast material suitable for bronchography.

Treatment. The timing of the repair will be dictated largely by the patient's condition at the time of diagnosis. Although definitive repair would be preferable, delay in development or diagnosis usually prevents this, and commonly several months intervene between injury and definitive surgery. Once operation has been delayed, it is better to wait for local inflammatory changes to subside. During this period tracheostomy and feeding gastrostomy are used to avoid further complications. The dissection is frequently difficult, particularly in delayed cases. Small fistulas may be ligated and divided. Moderate-sized fistulas should be excised and the ends inverted. Excision of larger fistulas may result in defects of such magnitude that other tissues must be employed to bridge the gap. In such situations, the bronchoplastic techniques developed for postinflammatory strictures and the vascularized pericardial flap may be useful adjuncts.

Results. The mortality associated with post-traumatic tracheo-esophageal fistulas is much less than that of esophageal or bronchial rupture alone. Survival rates range between 70 and 85 per cent. This may be because the very nature of a fistula implies that the injury has been confirmed by surrounding tissues and that it develops relatively late when survival from other injuries has already been achieved.

THE DIAPHRAGM

The integrity of the diaphragm may be violated by either penetrating or nonpenetrating injury. Recent experiences[71] suggest that the incidence of diaphragmatic injuries has steadily increased since World War II, mainly as a result of the increase in automobile accidents. Today the majority of diaphragmatic disruptions are caused by blunt trauma rather than penetrating injuries. Automobile accidents are responsible for over 80 per cent of tears following blunt trauma, with falls from great heights and crushing injuries providing most of the remainder. Penetrating wounds, of course, are usually the result of a stabbing or shooting.

Blunt trauma results in larger diaphragmatic tears, a higher incidence of acute herniation, less external evidence of trauma and, because of the common association with other serious injuries, a higher mortality rate than is seen with penetrating wounds. The latter usually result in small defects which are either discovered early during exploration for other indications or present later with intestinal obstruction from an incarcerated or strangulated diaphragmatic hernia. Occasionally, the condition may be discovered on coincidental chest x-rays or when interval complaints of dyspepsia, discomfort in the left chest or shoulders, flatulence or postprandial fullness are being investigated.

Regardless of the type of injury, there is an overwhelming left-sided predominance in clinically manifest diaphragmatic tears, often as high as 90 per cent. This can be explained by the buttressing of the right diaphragm by the liver, the predominance of right-handed assailants, and the left-sided position of the usual intended target, the heart. Penetrating injuries may involve any area of the diaphragm, although knife wounds are characteristically anterolateral. Blunt trauma most commonly ruptures the diaphragm at the junction between the tendinous and posterior leaves, a weak point related to the fusion of two of the diaphragm's embryonic components. These tears are usually radial. They may extend to, but rarely through, the hiatus or may even involve the pericardium. Occasionally, the diaphragm will tear loose from its peripheral attachments. Distortion of the diaphragm by the changes in gravitational force that accompany decelerating accidents can be appreciated from inspection of Figure 10–1 *B* and *D*.

Larger tears usually result in acute herniation of the abdominal viscera into the chest. The stomach, spleen, left colon, small bowel and the left lobe of the liver may pass through the defect. Herniation of the liver through the right leaf of the diaphragm is rare but can occur with the large tears associated with blunt trauma. Progressive herniation through the larger defects may be encouraged by the increased pleuroperitoneal pressure differential caused by labored respirations. A progression of events similar to those occurring in patients with congenital diaphragmatic hernia may eventually lead to almost total collapse of one lung and infringement on the other as mediastinal displacement occurs.

Diagnosis. If acute herniation has

occurred, the earliest complaints are usually shortness of breath and left chest pain which may be referred to the shoulder. With small hernias the physical examination may reveal nothing abnormal or, at most, a small area of dullness and diminished breath sounds with limited excursion of the diaphragm. In the acutely injured patient, these signs are hard to elicit and even harder to interpret, particularly since the respirations on that side are usually splinted and some degree of hemothorax is commonly associated. One cannot expect the classic combination of diminished breath sounds and audible peristalsis over the lower hemithorax which greets the physician who examines such a patient in the interval following recovery.

With larger degrees of herniation, the examiner may be perplexed by a strange mixture of areas of dullness and tympany on percussing the chest. Peristalsis is usually suppressed initially, so that chances of auscultating bowel sounds over the thorax are slight. A shift of the mediastinal structures to the opposite side may occur with larger hernias, but by this time severe respiratory distress, cyanosis and shock have usually entered the picture and the finer points of physical diagnosis have been abandoned.

The diagnosis usually rests on proper interpretation of the chest x-ray. An associated hemothorax not uncommonly obscures both the physical and radiologic signs of herniated viscera, a good reason for repeating chest films after evacuating a hemothorax. The diagnosis should be suspected whenever the left diaphragm is high following injury to the chest or abdomen, or when radiolucent areas appear above the usual level of the diaphragm. Common misdiagnoses are loculated pneumothorax in the lower chest due to pleural adhesions or elevation of the diaphragm secondary to acute gastric dilatation. Passage of a nasogastric tube at this time may provide an important clue. If the stomach has herniated into the chest, distortion of the cardia may impede passage of the tube or, if it can be passed, it may be seen to deflect upward into the thorax. Upright films taken after induced pneumoperitoneum may result in the collection of air in the thorax. Finally contrast studies with barium in the stomach or the colon may be attempted if the patient's condition permits. Before one diagnoses traumatic herniation of the liver into the right chest on the basis of a high diaphragm, one should take lateral decubitus films to rule out the subpulmonary entrapment of a hemothorax. A further clue here is elevation of the x-ray shadow of the inferior border of the liver.

The small diaphragmatic tears resulting from penetrating injuries can result in acute herniation, but they are just as likely to be discovered incidentally during exploration for other indications. One might expect all such injuries to be discovered early because of the almost universal policy of exploring all penetrating wounds entering below the level of the nipple. However, small diaphragmatic wounds may be overlooked during exploration. Furthermore, the possibility of penetration of the diaphragm may not be entertained unless the physician is aware of the height to which the diaphragm may rise in the crouching or straining patient. Thus, the penetrating chest wound may be thought to involve only the thorax, and the associated pneumo- or hemothorax may be treated simply by chest tube drainage.

Initially, only a piece of omentum may herniate through the small defect. Sometime later, even years later in many cases, a sudden increase in intra-abdominal pressure may push the abdominal viscera through the defect in the diaphragm maintained by the omentum's "toe in the door." This mechanism was responsible for the long-held belief that diaphragmatic wounds do not heal well. Since these diaphragmatic defects are usually small, delayed cases commonly present with obstruction and even strangulation of the herniated viscera. The pain associated with this delayed presentation may be severe enough to suggest coronary occlusion. X-rays at this stage should be diagnostic, but because of a remote history of injury and overlooked small scar, they are frequently misinterpreted. Common misdiagnoses include multiple lung abscesses, cystic disease of the lung, multiloculated empyema or atypical pneumothorax secondary to pleural adhesions.

Treatment. When diagnosis is made in the acute period, operative reduction of the hernia and repair of the diaphragmatic tear should be undertaken as soon as feasible. A brief delay for further evaluation of significant associated injuries is permissible if the hernia is small and is causing little or no cardiorespiratory embarrassment. In any event, an attempt should be made to decompress the stomach by nasogastric tube as soon as possible.

There is some difference of opinion as to whether a thoracic or abdominal approach should be used. Because of the significant incidence of associated injury to abdominal viscera, the abdominal route is preferred by acutely presenting diaphragmatic tears secondary to a penetrating injury. However, because of adhesions that develop between the herniated viscera and intrathoracic structures, hernias with delayed presentation should be initially explored through the chest. This approach may also be selected for hernias secondary to blunt trauma, hernias in which there is a major hemothorax or evidence of other significant intrathoracic injury, or if previous abdominal operations are expected to interfere with the abdominal approach. Regardless of the initial incision, one should not hesitate to combine the abdominal and thoracic approaches in difficult cases, and the patient should be prepared and draped for such an eventuality. The repair should employ two layers of interrupted nonabsorbable suture and the chest should be drained.

THE HEART

Penetrating Injuries of the Heart

The management of penetrating injuries of the heart has challenged the judgment and technical skill of physicians for centuries. Even at the present time, surgeons in the medical centers with the greatest experience with this type of injury are unable to agree on its management.

In most reports of penetrating wounds of the heart, emanating as they do from urban medical centers, and reading back for many years, stab wounds outnumber gunshot wounds by a ratio of three or four to one. This not only reflects a preference for the knife or icepick rather than the gun in choice of weapons but also the fact that fewer victims shot in the heart survive to reach the hospital for treatment. Randall and Glass's[55] report in 1960 of 20 cases of cardiac gunshot wounds was the first sizeable experience with this type of injury reported from a civilian hospital.

Penetrating wounds of the heart may present in several different ways. Most commonly, the problem is one of hemopericardium with cardiac tamponade. However, if the pericardial wound communicates freely with the pleural space, exsanguinating intrathoracic hemorrhage may dominate the picture. Only rarely will traumatic hemopericardium lead to recurrent pericardial effusion or constrictive pericarditis. Penetrating wounds of the heart may occasionally result in rather selective injury to certain vulnerable parts of the heart's anatomy so that valvular or septal defects, infarction from injury to a coronary vessel or arrhythmias from damage to the conducting system may be encountered. A final point of consideration in such wounds is the problem of intracardiac foreign bodies.

Nonpenetrating Injuries to the Heart

At one time cardiac injury secondary to blunt thoracic trauma was thought exceedingly rare. This was partly because myocardial rupture, the greatest threat in such injuries, is almost invariably fatal and thus seen by the pathologist rather than the clinician. It was also due in part to the fact that cardiac contusion, the most common clinically presenting problem, was not fully appreciated until recent years when serial electrocardiograms and serum enzyme determinations were used to study chest trauma victims. Although nonpenetrating chest trauma can cause, with the exception of intracardiac foreign bodies, the same forms of injury mentioned in regard to penetrating trauma, these occur so rarely that only cardiac contusion warrants separate discussion.

In the following sections the management of cardiac wounds is discussed according to the type of problems they present clinically.

Cardiac Tamponade

In penetrating wounds of the heart, bleeding is usually significant enough to produce either cardiac tamponade or, if the penetrating agent has also produced a large enough pleuropericardial communication, massive hemothorax. Because many wounds penetrating the pericardium are located anteriorly where it is not in contact with the pleura and because, in many others, the traumatic pleuropericardial defects are not large enough to effectively vent the hemopericardium, the most common form of presentation is cardiac tamponade.

Diagnosis. With each systolic contraction, blood spurts from the myocardial laceration into the pericardial sac; and as it accumulates, it leaves less and less space for the heart to occupy in diastole. Therefore, diastolic filling and stroke volume progressively decline. Initially, cardiac output can be maintained by increasing rate, but eventually this can no longer compensate for impaired venous return and cardiac output falls. At this point there will be an elevation of venous pressure and decline in arterial pressure which, along with the muffling of heart sounds by the hemopericardium, constitute Beck's triad.[5]

Another feature of cardiac tamponade is an accentuation of the normal tendency for cardiac output to decrease during inspiration. This was originally observed as a weakening of the pulse during inspiration and still bears the name "pulsus paradoxus." A more objective criterion is a greater than 15 mm. Hg decrease in systolic pressure during normal inspiration. The underlying mechanism is still unsettled. One thought is that, although the decreased intrathoracic pressure during inspiration normally enhances venous return and compensates for concomitant expansion of the pulmonary vascular bed, this is prevented because tamponade impedes venous return. Another explanation is that tensing of the pericardium by diaphragmatic descent during inspiration increases the tamponading effect of the hemopericardium.

It might seem that the diagnosis of cardiac tamponade would be a simple matter of finding Beck's triad or pulsus paradoxus in a patient with a penetrating chest injury. However, as previously pointed out, hypotension is common to many forms of injury. The loudness of heart sounds may be difficult to assess in a noisy emergency room. Bulging neck veins may be absent if much blood has been lost, although they may occur in the absence of tamponade in a straining patient or in a patient with tension pneumothorax or compression of the superior vena cava by hemorrhage into the mediastinum. A left tension pneumothorax may superficially mimic cardiac tamponade, with bulging neck veins and inability to hear heart sounds clearly when auscultating the precordium.

If one considers the problem as that of a patient presenting with shock without significant ventilatory impairment after chest trauma, the diagnosis usually rests between exsanguinating hemorrhage and pericardial tamponade. If the differentiation is not readily apparent, a central venous catheter should be advanced into the superior vena cava through the external jugular or subclavian vein. (See Chapter Three.) If the central venous pressure is low, cardiac tamponade is unlikely and one can then use this catheter as a channel for vigorous blood volume expansion. If it is high or soon becomes elevated in response to intravenous infusion, the diagnosis of cardiac tamponade is virtually assured. The importance of serial determination of the central venous pressure in such a situation has been emphasized by two recent studies,[52, 72] which showed that one-third of patients developing tamponade after penetrating injury to the heart did not have a significant elevation of the venous pressure on the initial determination, but elevation occurred later when blood volume had been restored.

One of these reports also noted that pulsus paradoxus was detected in only one-third of the cases. This is because pulsus paradoxus represents a transient early stage in the development of acute tamponade. However, it is a valuable warning sign of the redevelopment of tamponade after pericardiocentesis.

X-RAY. Several authors have referred to the diagnostic significance of enlargement of the cardiac silhouette on chest x-ray. However, as Doubleday[22] has pointed out, patients can succumb with as little as 200 ml. of blood in the pericardium, yet 300 or more ml. can be present without a detectable increase in the cardiac silhouette. In addition, one rarely has an adequate enough chest x-ray to be sure of increased heart size without previous films for comparison. Some success has been reported using fluoroscopy to detect diminished pulsations of the cardiac silhouette, but this finding may be equivocal and lack of time and facilities limits this approach.

Treatment. There is little disagreement regarding the indication for immediate pericardiocentesis once the diagnosis of cardiac tamponade is made or even, in more desperate situations, strongly suspected. Sudden and dramatic relief may follow the removal of even 30 cc. of blood although as much blood should be aspirated as possible. The technique of pericardiocentesis is described later.

It is important to be sure that the blood obtained by this maneuver has been aspirated from the pericardium and has not been obtained by puncture of the heart through an empty pericardial space. Several considerations will help in making this distinction. First, blood aspirated from the pericardium should not clot in the syringe, having been defibrinated within the pericardial sac by the motion of the heart. Second, the removal of blood should be rewarded by hemodynamic improvement on the part of the patient. On the other hand, if the heart has been entered, pulsations transmitted to the needle and syringe will usually be felt and, since patients in the acute stages of shock become hypercoagulable, the blood obtained should rapidly clot in the syringe.

It is at the point at which the immediate threat of pericardial tamponade has been relieved by aspiration that a divergence of opinion concerning management exists. The history of the treatment of cardiac tamponade is interesting in this respect. In 1649 Riolanus first suggested the use of pericardiocentesis in the treatment of cardiac tamponade. The first successful outcome of such treatment was reported in 1829 by Larrey. However, in 1868 Fischer,[27] in a collective review of 425 cases, reported an 84 per cent mortality following use of pericardiocentesis and its popularity waned. It was not fully appreciated, however, that in most cases pericardiocentesis had been used in combination with venesection. Following Del Vecchio's experimental work in 1895, Rehn reported the first successful control of a bleeding heart wound by cardiorrhaphy. There followed a period of popularity for the direct surgical control of penetrating heart wounds. Not until the classic paper of Blalock and Ravitch[8] in 1943 reporting survival in 17 of 18 patients in whom pericardiocentesis was used did this approach become popular again.

In review of the experience at The Johns Hopkins Hospital by Isaacs[37] in 1960, 40 of the 60 patients reported were treated by a pericardiocentesis alone, with only one death. In the remaining 20 there was a 50 per cent mortality from surgery regardless of the employment of preliminary pericardiocentesis. This experience has been shared by some institutions[18, 25] but not others[11, 48] so that a divergence of opinion still exists between those recommending immediate operative intervention and those who feel that the percentage of patients who can be controlled by pericardiocentesis alone is significant enough to justify the attempt. This difference of opinion is in part related to the wounding agent predominating in the experience reported, since stab wounds of the heart are more likely to be manageable by pericardiocentesis than gunshot wounds.

Adopting a position at either extreme seems unwise. Experience indicates that certain patients are not likely to be successfully managed by pericardiocentesis alone. These are patients who are also bleeding into the chest through a pleural-pericardial laceration, patients with cardiac wounds from large knives or large caliber bullets, and patients with a partially clotted hemopericardium that yields only a small volume on aspiration so that continued bleeding will quickly lead to tamponade again. In such patients, or in any patient whose response to pericardiocentesis is weak or evanescent, immediate surgical intervention is indicated. Otherwise, the operating theater is maintained in readiness while the nearby patient is closely monitored for signs of recurrent tamponade.

Repeated pericardiocentesis may be required, and the rate of redevelopment of tamponade will soon determine if persistence with the nonoperative approach is justified. Although it has been argued that the mortality from unnecessary thoracotomy will be less than that from pericardiocentesis failures, it remains our impression that most deaths from penetrating heart wounds occur *in spite* of thoracotomy rather than *because* of attempts at pericardiocentesis and that both an unselected policy of routine thoracotomy and overpersistence with pericardiocentesis represent weakness in surgical judgment.

TECHNIQUE OF PERICARDIOCENTESIS. A long large bore needle (16 to 18 gauge) is attached to a 50 cc. syringe via a three-way stopcock. The needle is either passed to the left of the sternum in the fourth interspace or at a 45-degree angle inward and upward from a point just lateral to the xyphoid (Fig. 10–13). If time permits, as it often does with subsequent aspirations, a precordial electrocardiogram lead will signal contact with the heart and warn of overpenetration. Attaching the lead to the needle itself creates an electrical hazard which may manifest itself by ventricular fibrillation. A "popping" sensation will often be noted as the pericardium is penetrated and the withdrawal of nonclotting blood associated with the relief of the patient's distress will mark the successful pericardiocentesis. The needle should be withdrawn until aspiration stops and then reintroduced slowly until blood returns in the syringe. The proper depth of penetration can be maintained by placing a clamp on the needle flush with the skin. This prevents inadvertent overpenetration and provides a reference for future aspiration.

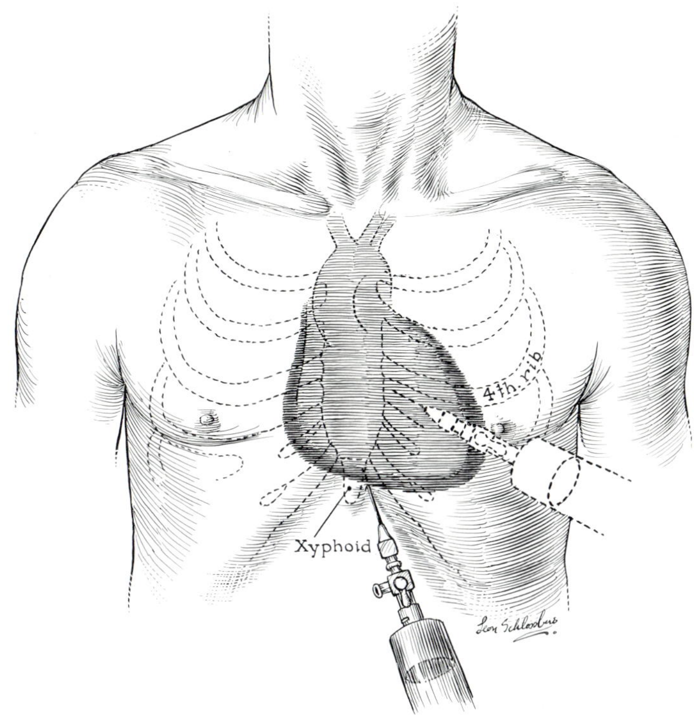

Figure 10–13 The technique of pericardiocentesis as described in the text.

THORACOTOMY FOR PENETRATING CARDIAC WOUNDS. Ordinarily, an anterior thoracotomy in the left fourth intercostal space will provide adequate exposure. This can be extended across the sternum with ligation of the internal mammary vessels if more exposure is needed. Division of the costal cartilages near their insertion into the sternum can be used to gain room in a cephalad or caudal direction. A sternal splitting incision provides even better exposure but is more time consuming.

The opening of pericardium is usually followed by a gushing of blood at a more rapid rate than anticipated as the countereffect of tamponade is broken and the cardiac wound bleeds unopposed. It was because of the difficulty of controlling bleeding from a writhing heart in a gushing pool of blood that Sauerbruch[60] first suggested gripping the heart with the fingers in the transverse sinus. Ordinarily, however, "Sauerbruch's grip" is not necessary. Bleeding can be controlled by finger pressure while 2-0 silk sutures are passed deeply through the myocardium in the underlying wound. By crossing and applying gentle traction to these sutures the bleeding usually can be controlled well enough to visualize their placement and to assure that no major coronary artery will be occluded if they are tied. However, even if the initial sutures are poorly placed they provide traction and hemostatis until definitive sutures are placed and tied. After satisfactory hemostasis is established, the pericardium is loosely reapproximated with interrupted sutures to allow free drainage of the pericardial space. The thoracotomy is then closed in layers after placement of a dependent or posterolateral thoracotomy drainage tube. The use of prophylactic antibiotics is indicated in this situation.

Myocardial Contusion

This condition should be considered in any patient who has received a severe blow to the chest, particularly a steering wheel injury. Estimates of its frequency have risen steadily with the more frequent use of the electrocardiogram and serum enzyme determinations in evaluating patients with such a history. The patient complaining of precordial discomfort after blunt trauma to the thorax may be thought to have a contusion of the chest wall, costochondral separation, or nondisplaced fracture of the anterior ribs or sternum. Patients whose pain arises from such chest wall injuries usually complain of aggravation or discomfort from breathing; the discomfort from myocardial contusion is more independent of respiratory movements. However, this differentiation is frequently complicated by the coexistence of such chest wall injuries. It is a reasonable approach to assume that any blow sufficient to have so injured the chest wall may also have resulted in myocardial contusion and to take steps to establish or eliminate this possibility.

Many of the signs and symptoms of myocardial contusion are similar to those of pericarditis with or without an effusion because such patients have a focal area of pericardial irritation. If there has been some bleeding from the contused pericardium, a secondary effusion may result. The electrocardiogram may show T-wave inversion or, in some instances, QRS changes or conduction disturbances. In older patients it may be hard to decide whether there has been a myocardial infarction precipitated by the stress of the accident or a myocardial contusion secondary to the chest trauma. This may not have immediate therapeutic significance since the initial treatment is similar, but from a prognostic and medical-legal standpoint, the differentiation may be quite important. The evolution of a classic infarction pattern on serial electrocardiograms or its failure to appear will usually settle this issue, but it should be remembered that a coronary artery can be damaged by a severe blow to the precordium, and that a severely contused area of myocardium may be virtually indistinguishable from the damage caused by regional coronary occlusion. Generally, however, the myocardial contusion produces milder, more variable electrocardiogram changes that do not fit the distribution patterns classically ascribed to occlusion of the coronary branches.

A myocardial contusion may be missed if serial electrocardiograms and enzyme studies are not done. An elevation of the serum glutamic oxalacetic transaminase (SGOT), creatinine phosphokinase (CPK), or lactic acid dehydrogenase (LDH) may confirm the suspicion of myocardial contusion in cases in which the electrocardiogram shows only fleeting or variable changes. These studies are also helpful in older patients when one does not know whether the EKG abnormalities existed prior to injury.

The outcome of a myocardial contusion depends to a large extent upon its severity and the association of conduction disturbances which may, as in the case of coronary occlusion, lead to fatal arrhythmias. The damage is rarely extensive enough to lead to delayed rupture or ventricular aneurysm, although isolated cases of this have been reported. When rupture does occur it usually results in immediate fatality and, as shown by Parmley and associates' review of the records from the Armed Forces Institute of Pathology,[50] this is the major cause of death from nonpenetrating injury to the heart. Although cardiogenic shock is rarely a problem after myocardial contusion, Pomerantz[54] has shown that acute reductions in cardiac output are not uncommon with this injury.

Treatment. The treatment of patients with myocardial contusion consists of restricted activity and continued observation. Patients with arrhythmias should be carefully monitored. Digitalis and antiarrhythmic drugs are given for the usual indications. The patient can be discharged after stabilization of the electrocardiogram and subsidence of symptoms, although restricted activity for a full six weeks is usually advisable.

Rarer Cardiac Injuries

Although the following cardiac injuries are encountered too infrequently to warrant detailed discussion, one must be aware of such possibilities. Valvular insufficiency may result from a ruptured cusp (usually aortic) or a torn attachment to a papillary muscle (usually mitral). Atrial or ventricular septal defects may be caused by penetrating wounds and, occasionally, the membranous ventricular septum may be torn after severe blunt trauma. Severe damage to the myocardium may result in ventricular aneurysm, but this is much less likely than myocardial rupture. Hemorrhage into the area of the major conduction pathways is seen in cases of severe hypoxia and shock but also has been reported after blunt trauma. The indications for surgical intervention follow those for similar conditions of a nontraumatic origin, with the exception that the acute hemodynamic derangements resulting from traumatic defects are often not so well tolerated as those acquired more gradually.

Foreign Bodies in the Heart. The management of missiles in the heart is a controversial subject which has been fanned by the flames of each of the great wars of this century. In World War I the bolder surgeons favored their removal. Delormé in France cited 13 operations (with three deaths), including the successful removement of fragments from the right ventricle. In 1918 LeFort reported the first successful removal of a missile from the left ventricle and recorded nine consecutive cardiotomies for removal of foreign bodies with only one death. By the advent of World War II, however, opinion was still divided. Decker reported that the mortality from expectant versus operative treatment were both about 20 per cent but suggested that many more unsuccessful surgical attempts had probably escaped publication. In 1914 Sauerbruch in Germany advised removal of all foreign bodies from the heart to forestall later complications and reported 105 cases, with an operative mortality of 8 per cent. At the same time, in England, Turner still cautioned that "it would seem a good rule to leave the foreign body alone unless the heart continues to rebel against its presence."

American opinions on this subject were expressed by Harken[33] and Swan et al.,[63] who noted that recurrent pericardial effusion and infection were the usual indications for surgical removal. Since that time the development of bolder cardiac operations has been fostered by the use of hypothermia and extracorporeal bypass. This has allowed a more confident approach to the intracardiac missile. However, the consensus still opposes searching for small, scattered foreign bodies that are causing no symptoms.

Bland and Beebe[9] recently reported an enlightening 20-year follow-up of 40 patients with missiles left in the heart after injury sustained in World War II. They noted that pericarditis was a common accompaniment and that an effusion of considerable degree (sometimes delayed) occurred in 25 per cent. Elective removal was later attempted in eight of these 40 patients. It was successful in only three and was abandoned in five, in two of whom the foreign body could not be found. In one the shell fragment lodged first in the left pulmonary artery, and later migrated into the right pulmonary artery where it eroded into and obstructed the bronchus. Although benign clinical courses have been recorded in the remainder of the cases, the psychic strain of living with a missile in the heart has been formidable. All these veterans are generally concerned about the threat of this condition, and five were totally incapacitated by an anxiety neurosis. This experience also suggested that once the foreign body is fixed in the myocardium, subsequent migration was unlikely; erosion or infection was not encountered during the 20-year follow-up period.

Considering the above facts and the availability of advanced techniques in open-heart surgery, the following approach is recommended. Barring other complications of the injury which have therapeutic precedence, all missiles of reasonable size in the heart should be carefully localized by fluoroscopic examination. If movement of the missile suggests that it is free in one of the chambers of the heart, immediate plans for its removal by open cardiotomy using cardiopulmonary bypass should be made. At operation these patients should be placed on a table with an x-ray cassette under the chest that will allow portable chest x-ray to be made at the commencement of the procedure and again later if the foreign body cannot be found. After caval drainage catheters are inserted, the aorta and pulmonary arteries should be cross-clamped at the beginning of inflow occlusion to prevent migration of the missile out of the heart. The initial attempt at removal of the missile should be through a wide atriotomy.

If fluoroscopy suggests that the missile is not moving with the contracting myocardium, one should also consider the possibility that it lies free in the pericardium. At the time of exploration the pericardium and great vessels should always be carefully explored before continuing with preparations for open removal.

Occasionally, one may be fortunate to be presented with a foreign body whose surface is visible in the myocardial wound. Unless easy extraction can be expected it is wise to cannulate the cavae and have a vascular clamp ready to close on the great vessels through the transverse sinus before extraction is attempted lest the attempt result either in the loss of the foreign body into the underlying heart chamber or uncontrollable massive bleeding on its removal.

The fact that a missile has penetrated the heart demands careful evaluation for traumatic septal or valve defects. Any murmurs should be thoroughly assessed by cardiac catheterization or angiography before surgical exploration. If the missile is not free in the chamber of the heart, its accurate localization by careful cinefluorometric study will greatly facilitate its localization and removal. All patients with this complication warrant heavy antibiotic coverage.

THE AORTA AND GREAT VESSELS

Penetrating Injuries

A laceration of the aorta or its major branches or the hilar pulmonary vessels is one of the most lethal forms of penetrating chest trauma. Depending on whether the site of vessel injury is intra- or extrapericardial, the trauma may result in cardiac tamponade or exsanguinating hemothorax. Occasionally, if the wounding agent is small, such as an icepick or small missile or if the vessel has been barely nicked, the rate of bleeding may not be very rapid or a false aneurysm may form. Equally rare is the formation of an arteriovenous fistula. In most cases, the patient expires before reaching the hospital and most of those who manage to reach the hospital present the attending physician with the problem of massive hemothorax or rapidly reforming cardiac tamponade. These patients may survive if a decision for immediate thoracotomy is quickly made.

The first successful outcome of such a penetrating wound of the aorta was recorded by the Russian Dshanelidze in 1922.[24] His patient had an 8 mm. laceration in the aorta 1 cm. above the heart. In 1932 Blalock reported the successful suture of an icepick wound of the intrapericardial ascending aorta. In a subsequent review, Blalock[7] noted that only 13 of 66 cases survived the immediate postinjury period. In a more recent report Beall[4] reported 23 cases; 10 of these survived operation and seven were long-term survivors. In 1958 Perkins and Elchos[52] reported the first successful early repair of a stab wound of the extra-pericardial aorta. They pointed out the reasons such wounds carry more serious prognosis than cardiac stab wounds: (1) high pressure is sustained in the aorta; (2) the thinner aortic wall does not seal so well as the myocardium; (3) the easily distensible medistinum offers less resistance to the egress of blood than the intact pericardium; (4) delayed rebleeding is common; and (5) if the patient survives the initial injury, later problems such as false aneurysm or arteriovenous fistulae remain.

Nonpenetrating Injuries

The most common cause of death among victims of traffic accidents who do not reach the hospital alive is rupture of the aorta (36 per cent). The most common site of rupture in decelerating injuries is near the aortic isthmus just below the origin of the subclavian artery. This is also the most frequent site for crushing injuries; but in falls from great heights, the tear may be near the root of the aorta, resulting in hemopericardium and cardiac tamponade. Although such injuries are usually immediately fatal, it has been pointed out that 15 per cent of these patients survive beyond one hour after reaching the hospital and 11 per cent live over six hours.[51] Those patients who survive this long do so because the tear has not traversed the full thickness of the aortic wall; instead, the outer layers of the aorta, mediastinum and pleura have contained the egress of blood and a false aneurysm has formed. This damming of the exsanguinating flood may be successful for minutes, hours or weeks. Occasionally, the aneurysm may remain intact indefinitely.

Cammack et al.[15] have estimated that the occupants of cars involved in a 60 mph head-on collison develop a sudden elevation in aortic pressure to about 1250 mm. Hg, or 250 mm. Hg more than required to rupture the aorta. However, Zehnder[73] has estimated that it requires 2000 mm. Hg to rupture the aorta. The frequency of the injury suggests that something more than simple elevation of the intraluminal pressure is involved. The frequent location of this tear at the aortic isthmus just below the origin of the subclavian artery provides the probable clue to the mechanism. This is the point of greatest fixation of the aorta to the chest wall, and it is thought that the sudden forward movement of the aorta above and below this fixed point produces a shearing force which, in combination with the increased intraluminal pressure, causes the injury. Maximum stress occurs at the inner surface of the vessel. The adventitia, having a higher elastic limit, withstands the stress best and occasionally by remaining intact allows the formation of a false aneurysm. A similar explanation has been postulated for the frequent location of aortic disruption at the root of the aorta following falls from great heights.

Diagnosis. At one extreme the patient may present with exsanguinating hemorrhage into the left chest or a rapidly reforming pericardial tamponade and, at the other, with an asymptomatic aneurysm of the distal arch of the aorta accidentally discovered by routine x-rays after the injury. It is the situation between these two extremes that offers the greatest therapeutic potential—a false aneurysm whose rupture has been temporarily delayed by the adventitia and surrounding tissues. The key to survival in these patients is the recognition of the possible significance of mediastinal widening on the initial chest x-ray (Fig. 10–14A). This feature should be specifically sought in any victim of severe blunt trauma to the chest. If such a finding is associated with significant bleeding into the left chest, immediate operation is justified. Otherwise, it is recommended that an aortogram be obtained while the

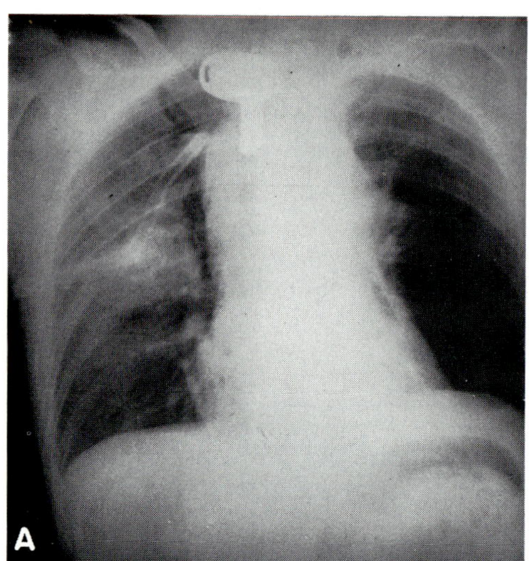

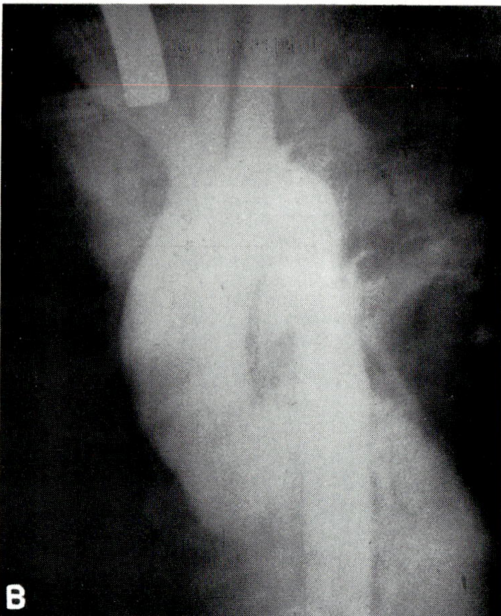

Figure 10–14 Traumatic rupture of the thoracic aorta. The condition was suspected from the initial anteroposterior chest film (*A*), which demonstrated a widened mediastinum with loss of definition about the aortic knob. Aortography (*B*) revealed complete intimal disruption in the descending aorta just distal to the level of the ligamentum arteriosum. An irregularity at the origin of the left subclavian artery suggests its avulsion. (From Blazek, J. V.: Acute traumatic rupture of the thoracic aorta demonstrated by retrograde aortography. Radiology *85*:253, 1965.)

operating theater stands by in readiness. The aortogram may be obtained by retrograde catheterization, but this may not be done without risk of rupturing the aneurysm. For this reason some have suggested the use of a "forward" aortogram, obtained by injecting a large bolus of dye through a central venous catheter whose tip lies near the heart. However, the brachial approach is probably the most commonly used.

MacKenzie et al.[42] have suggested that extravasation of blood into the anatomical spaces of the neck may be a valuable diagnostic sign of rupture of the great vessels of the thorax. They recommend the use of a minor supraclavicular incision to establish this fact. In an autopsy study of 38 accident victims, 16 of 17 patients with ruptured aorta showed blood within the carotid artery sheath. Blood was found within the sheath of the jugular vein in four patients with rupture of the superior vena cava. Four patients with rupture of the pulmonary arteries bled into the tracheal esophageal compartment in the neck; in 13 in whom there was no great vessel rupture, blood was not found in these cervical spaces. These autopsy observations were confirmed experimentally by the injection of varying amounts of blood around the intrathoracic vessels at the usual site of rupture. Significantly, it required 75 ml. of blood or less to stain the cervical vascular spaces but 400 or more ml. to cause a radiologically visible widening of the mediastinum. Further clinical experience is needed to fully assess the merit of this approach. The aortogram has the important advantage of localizing the site of injury and determining the appropriate thoracotomy exposure, but the use of a diagnostic supraclavicular incision may have merit when facilities for emergency aortography are not readily available.

Treatment. Intrapericardial injuries to the great vessels will present with hemopericardium, as discussed earlier in this chapter. Extrapericardial injuries usually produce massive bleeding into one hemithorax (usually the left). In such cases, it is hopeless to persist with efforts at transfusion and evacuation of the hemithorax; only prompt recourse to thoracotomy will lead to survival. Unless the location of the site of bleeding has been clearly suggested by the injury itself, a lateral thoracotomy in the 4th or 5th intercostal space should be performed. Bleeding points in a thoracotomy incision should be ignored initially. The hemothorax should be evacuated and the source of bleeding localized. No attempt should be made to control the bleeding directly by clamps; instead, pressure should be applied to control the bleeding site. If the bleeding can be controlled by pressure, the surgeon should gain adequate exposure, proximal and distal control of the bleeding vessel and wait for adequate blood volume replacement before renewing his attack.

Small stab wounds can usually be controlled by direct suture with or without the aid of partial occluding vascular clamps or brief cross-clamping. Patients with larger penetrating wounds are not likely to reach the operating room. The cases of nonpenetrating trauma present more challenging technical problems. Extensive mediastinal hemorrhage and false aneurysm formation make it difficult to evaluate the extent of damage to the aortic wall. There may be a small intimal tear or complete circumferential laceration with discontinuity (Fig. 10–14*B*). Intramural dissection or intramural hematoma may involve a variable segment of aorta adjacent to the tear. Such injuries must be opened to determine the extent of injury and to assure complete repair. To do this, the involved segment of aorta must be isolated and bypassed. The site of the injury determines whether a temporary shunt or left heart bypass is required. Occasionally, such injuries can be repaired with sutures alone; more often than not a segmental replacement is required. The risk of dissecting the false aneurysm and disrupted segment from the vital structures running through the surrounding mediastinal hematoma often dictates that the prosthesis replacement bypass the area or be laid in its bed after it has been opened and collateral bleeding controlled from within.

Most traumatic false aneurysms of the thoracic aorta rupture relatively early. However, it has been shown that if rupture has not occurred by two months it rarely does.[62] Because of the technical difficulties involved in excision of an organized false aneurysm and the danger of injury to surrounding structures such as the esophagus, recurrent laryngeal nerve and left stem bronchus, it has been suggested that patients presenting more than two months after injury be operated only because of signs of enlargement or other significant symptoms. However, many of these cases still require thoracotomy for these indications, and a common manner of the late presentation is compression of the left main bronchus. Because of more recent experiences using temporary nonthrombogenic plastic tube bypass (which avoid heparinization and partial cardiac bypass) and laying the graft inside the bed of the aneurysm, this conservative approach to the "older" aneurysms is losing its hold.

REFERENCES

1. Andersen, I., and Halkier, E.: Closed injuries of the thorax. Acta chir. scandinav. Suppl. *332*:32, 1964.
2. Anderson, R. P., and Sabiston, D. C., Jr.: Acquired bronchoesophageal fistula of benign origin. Surg. Gynec. Obstet. *121*:261, 1965.
3. Avery, E. E., Mörch, E. T., and Benson, D. W.: Critically crushed chests; new method of treatment and continuous mechanical hyperventilation to pro-

duce alkalotic apnea and internal pneumatic stabilization. J. Thorac. Surg. *32*:291, 1956.

4. Beall, A. C., Jr.: Penetrating wounds of the aorta. Am. J. Surg. *99*:770, 1960.
5. Beck, C. S.: Wounds of the heart. Arch. Surg. *13*:205, 1926.
6. Blair, E., Topuzlu, C., and Deane, R. S.: Major Blunt Chest Trauma in Current Problems in Surgery. Chicago, Year Book Medical Publishers, May, 1969.
7. Blalock, A.: Successful suture of a wound of the ascending aorta. J.A.M.A. *103*: 1617, 1934.
8. Blalock, A., and Ravitch, M. M.: Consideration of nonoperative treatment of cardiac tamponade resulting from wounds of the heart. Surgery *14*:157, 1943.
9. Bland, E. F., and Beebe, G. W.: Missiles in the heart: A twenty year follow-up report of World War II cases. U. S. Navy Medical News Letter, *48* (No. 3):3, August 12, 1966.
10. Border, J. R., Hopkinson, B. R., and Schenk, W. G., Jr.: Mechanisms of pulmonary trauma: an experimental study. J. Trauma *8*:47, 1968.
11. Boyd, T. F., and Strieder, J. W.: Immediate surgery for traumatic heart disease. J. Thorac. Surg. *50*:305, 1965.
12. Brewer, L. A., Burbank, B., Samson, P. C., and Schiff, C. A.: The wet lung in war casualties. Arch. Surg. *123*:343, 1946.
13. Burford, T. H., and Burbank, B.: Traumatic wet lung; observations on certain physiologic fundamentals of thoracic trauma. J. Thorac. Surg. *14*:415, 1945.
14. Burke, J. F.: Early diagnosis of traumatic rupture of the bronchus. J.A.M.A. *181*:682, 1962.
15. Cammack, K., Rapport, R. L., Paul, J., and Baird, W. C.: Deceleration injuries of the thoracic aorta. A.M.A. Arch. Surg. *79*:244, 1959.
16. Carter, B. N., and Giuseffi, J.: Tracheotomy: Useful procedure in thoracic surgery with particular reference to its employment in crushing injuries of the thorax. J. Thorac. Surg. *21*:495, 1951.
17. Carter, R., Warsham, E. E., and Brewer, L. A.: Rupture of the bronchus following closed chest trauma. Am. J. Surg. *104*:177, 1962.
18. Conn, J. H., Hardy, J. D., Fair, W. R., and Netterville, R. E.: Thoracic trauma: Analysis of 1022 cases. J. Trauma *3*: 22, 1963.
19. Cooley, D. A., Dunn, J. R., Brockman, H. L., and DeBakey, M. E.: Treatment of penetrating wounds of the heart: Experimental and clinical observations. Surgery *37*:882, 1955.
20. Daniels, R. A., Jr., and Cate, W. R., Jr.: Wet lung—an experimental study. Ann. Surg. *127*:836, 1948.
21. Decancq, J. G.: The treatment of chylothorax in children. Surg. Gynec. & Obst. *121*:509, 1965.
22. Doubleday, L. C.: Radiologic aspects of stab wounds of the heart. Radiology *74*:26, 1960.
23. Drinker, C. K., and Warren, M. F.: The genesis and resolution of pulmonary transudates and exudates. J.A.M.A. *122*:269, 1943.
24. Dshanelidze, I. I.: Manuskript Petrograd, 1922. Quoted by Lilienthal, H.: Thoracic Surgery. Philadelphia, W. B. Saunders Company, 1925, p. 489.
25. Elkins, D. C., and Campbell, R. E.: Cardiac tamponade: Treatment by aspiration. Ann. Surg. *133*:623, 1951.
26. Errion, A. R., Houk, V. N., and Kettering, D. L.: Pulmonary hematoma due to blunt, nonpenetrating thoracic trauma. Am. Rev. Resp. Dis. *88*:384, 1963.
27. Fischer, G.: Die Wunden des Herzens und des Herzbeutels. Arch. klin. Chirurgie *9*:571, 1868.
28. Garzon, A. A., Seltzer, B., Lichtenstein, S., and Karlson, K. E.: Influence of tracheostomy cannula size on work of breathing. Ann. Surg. *162*:315, 1965.
29. Gibson, L. D., Carter, R., and Hinshaw, D. B.: Surgical significance of sternal fracture. Surg. Gynec. Obstet. *114*: 443, 1962.
30. Goorwitch, J.: Traumatic chylothorax and thoracic duct ligation: Case report and review of literature. J. Thorac. Surg. *29*:467, 1955.
31. Gray, A. R., Harrison, W. H., Jr., Coures, C. M., and Howard, J. M.: Penetrating injuries to the chest. Am. J. Surg. *100*:709, 1960.
32. Griffith, J. L.: Traumatic fracture of the left main bronchus. Thorax *4*:105, 1949.
33. Harken, D. E.: Foreign bodies in, and in relation to, the thoracic blood vessels and heart. Surg. Gynec. & Obst. *83*:117, 1946.
34. Harrison, W. H., Jr., Gray, A. R., Coures, C. M., and Howard, J. M.: Severe nonpenetrating injuries to the chest. Am. J. Surg. *100*:715, 1960.
35. Hershgold, E. J.: Roentgenographic study of human subjects during transverse accelerations. Aerospace Med. *31*:213, 1960.
36. Hood, R. M., and Sloan, H. E.: Injuries of the trachea and major bronchi. J. Thorac. Cardiov. Surg. *38*:458, 1959.
37. Isaacs, J. P.: Sixty penetrating wounds of the heart. Surgery *45*:696, 1959.
38. King, O. J., Jr. and Glas, W. W.: Complications of tracheostomy. Rocky Mountain M. J., *57*:36, 1960.
39. Lampson, R. S.: Traumatic chylothorax. A

review of the literature and report of a case treated by mediastinal ligation of the thoracic duct. J. Thorac. Surg. *17*:778, 1948.

40. Laustela, E.: Thorax traumatology. Acta chir. scandinav. Suppl. *332*:17, 1964.

41. MacKenzie, M. A.: *A Manual of Diseases of the Throat and Nose.* II. Diseases of the Oesophagus, Nose and Nasopharynx. New York, William Wood & Co., 1884.

42. MacKenzie, J. R., Hackett, M., and Munro, D. D.: Diagnosis of ruptured great vessels of the thorax. A simple and reliable method. J. Trauma. (In press.)

43. Mackler, S. A.: Spontaneous rupture of the esophagus, an experimental and clinical study. Surg. Gynec. Obstet. *95*: 345, 1952.

44. Mahaffey, D. E., Creech, O., Jr., Boren, H. G., and DeBakey, M. E.: Traumatic rupture of the left main stem bronchus successfully repaired eleven years after injury. J. Thorac. Surg. *32*:312, 1956.

45. Maloney, J. V., Jr., and MacDonald, L.: The treatment of blunt trauma to the thorax. Am. J. Surg. *105*:404, 1963.

46. Maloney, J. V., Jr., Schmutzer, K. J., and Raschke, E.: Paradoxical respiration and "pendelluft." J. Thorac. Cardiov. Surg. *41*:291, 1961.

47. Maloney, J. V., and Spencer, F. C.: The nonoperative treatment of traumatic chylothorax. Surgery *40*:121, 1956.

48. Maynard, A., Avecilla, M. J., and Naclerio, E. A.: The management of wounds of the heart. Ann. Surg. *144*:1018, 1956.

49. Munnell, E. R.: Fracture of major airways. Am. J. Surg. *105*:511, 1963.

50. Parmley, L. F., Manion, W. C., and Mattingly, T. W.: Nonpenetrating traumatic injury of the heart. Circulation *18*: 371, 1958.

51. Parmley, L. F., Mattingly, T. W., Manion, W. C., and Jahnke, E. J.: Nonpenetrating traumatic injury of the aorta. Circulation *17*:1086, 1958.

52. Perkins, R., and Elchos, T.: Stab wound of the aortic arch. Ann. Surg. *147*:83, 1958.

53. Petty, T. L.: Intensive and Rehabilitative Respiratory Care. Philadelphia, Lea and Febiger, 1971.

54. Pomerantz, M. Personal communication. 1973.

55. Randall, H. T., and Glass, A.: Gunshot wounds of the heart. Am. J. Surg. *99*:788, 1960.

56. Ransdell, H. T., McPherson, R. C., Haller, J. A., Williams, D. J., and Conner, E. H.: Treatment of flail chest injuries with a piston respirator. Am. J. Surg. *104*:22, 1962.

57. Rutherford, R. B., Hurt, H. H., Jr., Brickman, R. D., and Tubb, J. M.: The pathophysiology and treatment of progressive tension pneumothorax. J. Trauma *8*:212, 1968.

58. Rutherford, R. B.: Personal communication.

59. Rutherford, R. B., and Valenta, J.: An experimental study of "traumatic wet lung." J. Trauma *11*:146, 1971.

60. Sauerbruch, F.: Die Verwendbarkeit des Unterdruchverfahrens bei der herz Chirurgie. Arch. klin. Chirurgie *83*: 537, 1907.

61. Schramel, R. J., Tyler, J., Kirkpatrick, J. L., Ziskind, M., and Creech, O.: Respiratory function after thoracic injuries. J. Trauma *3*:206, 1963.

62. Spencer, F. C.: Treatment of chest injuries. Curr. Prob. Surg. Jan., 1964.

63. Swan, H., Forsee, J. H., and Goyette, E. M.: Foreign bodies in the heart. Ann. Surg. *135*:314, 1952.

64. Valle, A. R.: An analysis of 2,811 chest casualties of the Korean conflict. Dis. Chest *26*:623, 1954.

65. Van Waggoner, F. H.: Died in hospital: A three-year study of deaths following trauma. J. Trauma *1*:401, 1961.

66. Ware, P. F., and Strieder, J. W.: Spontaneous perforation of the normal esophagus. Dis. Chest *16*:49, 1949.

67. Westermark, N.: A roentgenological investigation into traumatic lung changes arising through blunt violence to the thorax. Acta Radiol. (Stockholm) *22*:331, 1941.

68. Williams, K. R., and Burford, T. H.: The management of chylothorax related to trauma. J. Trauma *3*:317, 1963.

69. Worman, L. W.: Fluid Volume Deficits in the Mediastinum. Paper presented before the Society of University Surgeons, Milwaukee, Wisconsin, February 10, 1966.

70. Worman, L. W., Hurley, J. D., Pemberton, A. H., and Narodick, B. G. Rupture of the esophagus from external blunt trauma. Arch. Surg. *85*:333, 1962.

71. Wren, H. B., Texada, P. J., and Krementz, E. T.: Traumatic rupture of the diaphragm. J. Trauma *2*:117, 1962.

72. Yao, S. T., Carey, J. S., Shoemaker, W. C., Weinberg, M., and Freeark, R. J.: Hemodynamics and therapy of acute hemopericardium. J. Trauma. (In press.)

73. Zehnder, M. A.: Delayed posttraumatic rupture of the aorta in a young healthy individual after closed injury. Mechanical-etiologic considerations. Angiology *7*:252, 1956.

chapter

11

ABDOMINAL INJURIES

Charles B. Anderson, M.D.
and
Walter F. Ballinger, M.D.

INTRODUCTION

The management of abdominal injuries has been extensively discussed in the surgical literature, and problems of diagnosis and treatment are well defined. For those interested in the historical aspects of abdominal injuries, Loria's excellent contributions are recommended.[81, 82] Most of the ancient accounts concern penetrating injuries and their well-known mortality. Conservative management was usually adhered to from the time of the Egyptians to the early 1800s. Operative intervention was limited and of no great magnitude during this period. In 1836 Baudens published the results of his experiences in the French-Algerian war and suggested "bold operations" in some cases of gunshot wounds of the abdomen. On the basis of two cases operated on in 1830, one of which survived, he is probably the first to have performed laparotomy for gunshot wounds of the abdomen. Sims was the first in the United States to advocate surgical intervention; Walter, in 1859, and Kinlock, in 1863, were the first to perform abdominal operations in this country for blunt and gunshot injuries, respectively. In 1887, the American Surgical Association expressed a favorable opinion for operative intervention. Réclus, of France, strongly opposed surgical intervention and showed that 66 of 88 dogs with abdominal bullet wounds recovered without surgery. Controversy between the interventionists and the arch-conservatists continued throughout the nineteenth century. Because of the 75–85 per cent mortality associated with laparotomy, and since 25–75 per cent of penetrating wounds were not associated with visceral injuries, the general policy was to avoid surgical procedures. Nevertheless, the British, at the start of the Boer War in 1899, advocated surgical intervention for penetrating abdominal injuries. The mortality rate, however, was highest among patients treated by laparotomy, and thus the policy of conservatism again ruled until the early part of World War I. Because of the larger caliber missiles and higher velocity weapons used in World War I, the mortality associated with abdominal injuries was inordinately high. This led to the popularization of surgical intervention which reduced the mortality from 85 per cent to 56 per cent. Controversy in the management of abdominal wounds continues, however, especially with regard to stab wounds in which some advocate immediate surgical intervention in all cases and others postulate selective management.

Recent innovations in diagnostic methods have included peritoneal lavage, radioisotope scanning, arteriograms and sinograms. Enthusiastic supporters can be found for each of these modalities.

Improved methods of treating specific organ injuries, particularly those of the vascular system, liver and pancreas, and of managing infections, shock and respiratory insufficiency have significantly reduced the mortality from abdominal injuries. Loria's series of 478 abdominal wounds between 1927 and 1942 had an overall mortality rate of 55 per cent.[80] Today the mortality rate has decreased to somewhat less than 5 per cent for penetrating wounds of the abdomen.[121] As a comparison, the mortality rates during World War I (53.5 per cent), World War II (25 per cent) and the Korean War (12 per cent) are of interest.[121]

The main problem with all abdominal injuries lies in establishing the correct diagnosis soon enough to prevent death and limit morbidity. Two major life-threatening situations occur following either penetrating or blunt trauma to the abdomen: hemorrhage and hollow viscus perforation with associated chemical and bacterial peritonitis.

Much experience has been gained in time of war regarding the management of injuries to the abdomen. Military surgeons become civilian surgeons, and principles learned during wartime are then applied to the general public. The principle in treating any abdominal injury is operative control of hemorrhage and deterrence of peritoneal contamination and is applicable to the management of both civilian and military casualties. It is essential, however, that the difference between combat and civilian casualties be understood.[101] Abdominal wounds sustained during combat are more serious and had an associated 10 per cent mortality in the Vietnam war[59] as compared to a 3 per cent mortality rate associated with the usual civilian penetrating abdominal wound.[121] Military injuries are caused by missiles in 60 to 80 per cent of cases and are frequently multiple. The remaining one-third of cases are caused by bullets of the high-velocity type. Large areas of destruction necessitate wide debridement and healing of wounds by granulation and skin grafting.

Although civilian weaponry contributes considerably to the high incidence of abdominal wounds seen in large urban emergency treatment rooms, an ever-increasing number of nonpenetrating abdominal injuries result from automobile accidents caused by excessive speed on crowded highways. Diagnosis soon after arrival of the patient in the accident room is often difficult because of the high incidence of serious extra-abdominal injuries and the frequent association of shock. The penetrating wounds most often encountered in civilian life are knife and bullet wounds, and there is an inordinately high incidence of drunkenness among such patients with its attendant stupor and masking of abdominal signs. The soldier—young, healthy, sober and usually efficiently transported—presents no problem in diagnosis of a large shrapnel wound involving the anterior abdominal wall. Immediate therapeutic measures are undertaken with full knowledge of the nature of the injury. In contrast, an elderly man found semicomatose by the side of the road presents a serious problem in quick and efficient diagnosis. A high index of suspicion and repeated, painstaking examination are needed to point to the correct diagnosis.

CLASSIFICATION OF INJURIES

Methods of classifying abdominal injuries are, of necessity, artificial and arbitrary. Of major consideration in abdominal injury is the degree of urgency and the chance for survival. Thus, a patient is automatically classified according to the speed with which treatment is required. Some have injuries which are so severe that there is little chance for survival. Others have massive intra-abdominal hemorrhage and require immediate transfusion and laparotomy. Those who exhibit no evidence of severe internal hemorrhage but display signs of peritoneal irritation will require operative intervention on a less than immediate basis. Finally, some individuals have evidence of abdominal trauma but no indication that there has been visceral injury and consequently may be watched for further developments. In essence, then, individuals with evidence of hemorrhage require urgent treatment, and those with peritonitis may have operation delayed temporarily. Every patient is immediately classified by the physician according to the priority of treatment required. Classifications involving the delay before treatment, the number of organs injured, the association of extra-abdominal injuries, or the particular organ injured are not practical methods of diagnosing or treating abdominal injuries. A classification devised by Farrell[36] identifies abdominal injuries according to the principal manifestations: hemorrhage, peritonitis and injuries such as contusions to the abdominal wall, mesentery or diaphragm. However, *recognition of the two major groups of abdominal injuries—penetrating and nonpenetrating (or open and closed)—is of greater importance for prospective treatment* and has a direct relationship to accuracy and speed of diagnosis, mortality and morbidity. In Table 11–1 is an etiological classification of abdominal injuries which is useful in caring for individuals with abdominal trauma and facilitates discussion of this topic. In addition to the usual classifications of penetrating and nonpenetrating injuries, an iatrogenic classification is added because of the peculiar circumstances and effects associated with these latter injuries.

TABLE 11–1 ETIOLOGICAL CLASSIFICATION OF ABDOMINAL INJURIES

PENETRATING:
- Stab wounds
- Gunshot wounds (velocity)
- Shotgun wounds (range)
- Other (shrapnel, picket, stake, glass)

NONPENETRATING:
- Blunt injury
- Crush injury
- Blast injury
  - Air
  - Immersion
- Seat belt syndrome
- Ingestion
  - Corrosive agents
  - Foreign body

IATROGENIC:
- Endoscopy (biopsy)
- External cardiac massage
- Paracentesis and Thoracentesis
- Peritoneal dialysis
- Inhalation therapy (gastric rupture)
- Barium enema
- Peritoneoscopy
- Liver biopsy
- Radiation therapy
- Other

Penetrating Wounds

In recent years the hand gun has replaced the knife as the most common weapon used in assaults. Gunshot wounds of the abdomen are now more frequent than stab wounds in many major trauma centers.[64]

The incidence of organ injury in penetrating wounds of the abdomen is shown in Table 11–2. This represents a compilation of series in the literature which includes 3162 patients with 1623 positive laparotomies.[61, 69, 80, 93, 105, 106, 107, 118, 149] The percentages relate to those cases having sus-

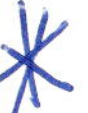

TABLE 11–2 FREQUENCY OF INJURY IN PENETRATING ABDOMINAL TRAUMA

VISCERA	PER CENT
Liver	37
Small Bowel	26
Stomach	19
Colon	16.5
Major Vascular and Retroperitoneal	11
Mesentery and Omentum	9.5
Spleen	7
Diaphragm	5.5
Kidney	5
Pancreas	3.5
Duodenum	2.5
Biliary System	1
Other (uterus, sciatic plexus, bladder, muscle, ovary, vagina, adrenal)	1
Injuries per patient	1.4

tained at least one intra-abdominal injury. For any individual case, such a list only provides a guide along with the location of the wound, indicating where to look first during exploratory laparotomy. In the selective treatment of abdominal stab wounds, the incidence of liver injuries will decrease because many liver wounds are trivial, require no surgical repair, and thus do not require laparotomy. Forty per cent of liver injuries are of no import when "routine" laparotomy is employed.[106] Although the small bowel is not the most frequent organ injured, there are, on the average, five and a half perforations per patient with bowel injury.[175]

The immediate mortality from penetrating abdominal wounds depends on the injury to major vascular structures and resultant intra-abdominal hemorrhage. Otherwise, mortality is directly correlated with the number of abdominal organs injured. Wilson and Sherman[175] reported the relative lethality associated with particular visceral injuries as follows:

vena cava	33%
biliary tract	33%
duodenum	26%
pancreas	20%
urinary bladder	17%
kidney	15%
vascular	12%
colon	12%
small intestine	11%
spleen	11%
stomach	9%
liver	7%

Penetrating wounds of the thorax can often traverse the diaphragm and result in intra-abdominal injury because of the variable position of the diaphragm during respiration—often reaching the level of the nipple or the fourth intercostal space during exhalation (Fig. 11–1). In high wounds like this, prophylactic insertion of a thoracostomy tube prior to laparotomy, despite the absence of a hemo- or pneumothorax, is a wise precaution against tension pneumothorax during positive-pressure anesthesia.

Stab Wounds. Knives, screw drivers, scissors, pencils, glass bottles, automobile radio antennae, bicycle spokes and numerous other articles are used to inflict stab wounds. The size, shape and length of the instrument is important in estimating the amount of damage which might have been caused. The skin and subcutaneous injury is usually not significant and requires no particular treatment.

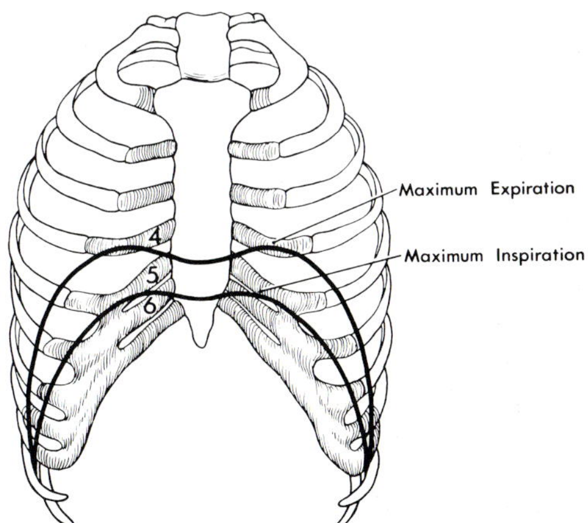

Figure 11–1 Because of the high position of the diaphragm on forced expiration, penetrating wounds of the lower chest frequently pierce the diaphragm and injure intra-abdominal structures.

Simple cleansing and primary closure may be performed. Frequently, a dressing alone suffices. The injury to intra-abdominal viscera is confined to the immediate area of penetration and only limited debridement is required. Multiple stab wounds occur in 20 per cent of cases and the thorax is penetrated in 10 per cent.[93] Whether selective management or mandatory laparotomy is the best method of treating stab wounds is heatedly debated in the literature and will be discussed below.

Gunshot Wounds. Gunshot wounds technically include shotgun injuries, but because of the particular characteristics of the latter they are discussed separately. Civilian gunshot wounds are usually caused by low-velocity pistols, whereas military bullet wounds are of the high-velocity type and result in extensive tissue destruction which requires wide and thorough debridement. The physical factors involve the kinetic energy imparted to the body by the missile. The kinetic energy of a missile is expressed by the formula: $E = mv^2/2g \times 7000$, where E equals kinetic energy in foot pounds, m equals mass of the missile in grains, v equals velocity in feet per second, g equals gravitational acceleration in feet per second and 7000 is a conversion factor. Kinetic energy is thus proportional to the mass of the object and the square of the velocity. Revolver muzzle velocities are in the range of 1000–1500 feet/sec., whereas military rifles have velocities of 2000–3250 feet/sec.[168] It follows that a threefold increase in velocity results in nine times the kinetic energy. The amount of energy imparted to the body is the difference between the kinetic energy of the missile entering minus that when leaving the body. This energy is dissipated by the movement of tissues in a perpendicular direction from the trajectory of the bullet. The definition of a high-velocity injury is arbitrarily one in which the wounding missile has a velocity over 2500 feet per second. In high-velocity injuries a large temporary cavity is formed which determines the extent of damage. After passage of the bullet, the tissues collapse and a relatively small tract is left which leads to underestimation of the injury. Low-velocity gunshot wounds require limited debridement because less kinetic energy is imparted to the tissues and consequently the amount of destruction is not as great.

Characteristics of the tissues determine the extent of destruction. Fascia, skin and lung reveal little devitalization when struck by high-velocity missiles, whereas solid tissue such as muscle, bone, liver and spleen are violently disorganized and devitalized.

With few exceptions[122, 149] all agree that gunshot wounds of the abdomen should be explored. Even tangential wounds which have not entered the peritoneal cavity can cause intra-abdominal visceral injury from the "blast effect." Occasionally, low-velocity .22 caliber tangential wounds confined to the right upper quadrant of the abdomen can be observed to determine the need for operative intervention.

Shotgun Wounds. The ballistics and characteristics of shotgun wounds have been described.[27, 91, 139] The term "shotgun wound" usually implies a pellet load, although slugs of rather heavy weight can be implicated. The amount of powder charge, size of pellets, choke of the gun, and distance to the target all determine the destructive effect. The pattern is the area over which the pellets are dispersed at any given distance. A close pattern concentrates more kinetic energy in a localized region and is thus more destructive than when pellets are widely spread. Usually when a major portion of the charge is concentrated within a wound of entry having a diameter of 15 cm. or less, one can assume that the velocity has been sufficiently high to produce a severe deep wound.[27] In addition, in shotgun blasts, the wad and plastic cups used to separate the powder charge from the shot very often penetrate deeply into the wound. Removal of wadding, clothing and other foreign materials is essential to prevent wound suppuration.

Innumerable combinations of shotgun gauge, shot size, powder load and barrel choke are possible. It is difficult, therefore, to categorize the damage likely at various distances. Usually a No. 6 shot or smaller is used, and a 12-gauge shotgun is the most frequent weapon employed. As an example, at ten yards approximately 95 per cent of No. 6 shot pellets will be within a skin wound nine inches in diameter if fired from a full-choke barrel, and within an 18-inch diameter if fired from a cylinder bore. At 20 yards wound diameters are doubled.[27] An initial muzzle velocity of 1300 feet/sec. will be reduced 25 per cent to 950 feet/sec. after traveling 20 yards. The unfavorable ballistic characteristics of the pellet (sphere) are responsible for the rapid fall-off of velocity and thus most serious human shotgun injuries occur within a short range. Distance is the most critical factor in determining seriousness of shotgun wound injuries. Sherman and Parrish[139] describe three types of injury. Type I injuries are sustained at long range (a distance of more than seven yards) and result in subcutaneous or deep fascia location of the pellets. Type II wounds are sustained at close range of three to seven yards, and structures beneath the deep fascia are perforated. In Type III massive wounds occur at point-blank range under three yards.

The treatment of shotgun injuries sustained at close range requires extensive debridement. Other injuries produce only a few scattered small wounds of minimal significance. A wide spectrum of injury exists between these two extremes and requires careful evaluation and management. An interesting observation by several authors involves the expectant treatment of multiple, widely scattered shotgun injuries that have penetrated the abdominal cavity.[15, 33, 91, 172] Perforations may be legion, thus making it impossible to locate all visceral wounds. Moreover, small holes in the intestine made by the pellets show no pouting of mucosa, no eversion of the wound edges and no significant leakage or soiling. When minimal leakage does occur, the holes usually close spontaneously and with appropriate antibiotic therapy the peritonitis will be limited and the patient will recover. Handling the bowel with innumerable perforations results in milking of the intestinal contents through the perforations and causes serious contamination. It is thus reasonable to treat certain selected shotgun wounds by the conservative method of careful observation.

Overall, shotgun wounds of the abdomen have twice the mortality of other gunshot injuries, and those involving the chest lead to ten times the mortality.[139]

Other Wounds. Fragmentation and secondary missiles from grenades, bombs and antipersonnel mines constitute the most frequent cause of injury in wartime. During the Vietnam conflict only 19 per cent of injuries were due to small-arms fire, whereas 65 per cent were attributed to fragmentation missiles.[62] Shrapnel wounds are usually large and result in extensive destruction of tissues. Impalement on stakes and picket fences occurs and requires innovations of treatment determined by the circumstances of the particular injury. Flying missiles from lawn mowers, explosions, storms and automobile accidents are only a few of the numerous and sundry causes of penetrating trauma to the abdomen.

Nonpenetrating Trauma

A comprehensive review of blunt abdominal trauma was published by Griswald and Collier[53] in 1961. Aristotle has been given credit for being the first to describe visceral injury from blunt abdominal trauma by noting that the intestine of the deer was so delicate that it might be ruptured by a slight external blow without injuring the skin. Today the incidence of blunt abdominal trauma is increasing primarily because of soaring automobile accident rates. The automobile is responsible for at least 50 per cent of nonpenetrating abdominal injuries. In a series of 518 cases of blunt abdominal trauma reported by DiVincenti and associates,[28] auto accidents and pedestrian accidents combined accounted for 74 per cent; blows to the abdomen, 14 per cent; falls, 9 per cent; and other causes, 3 per cent.

Although blunt abdominal trauma constitutes only 0.1 per cent of all hospital admissions and one per cent of all trauma admissions, it is associated with a 20- to 30-per cent mortality rate,[70] much of which is attributable to associated injuries of the head and chest, and fractures of the extremities. Di Vincenti's group noted the following:[28] Ten per cent of cases will die before treatment is instituted; 30 per cent will not be operated on, and 18 per cent of these will die—one-third because of other severe injuries and two-thirds from error in diagnosis. Diagnostic errors occur either because of distraction by associated injuries (fractures) or the absence of a history of trauma. Of the 70 per cent who are explored, 14 per cent will succumb.

The incidence of specific organ injuries is listed in Table 11–3. Griswald and Collier[53] derived these figures by reviewing numerous series in literature. A 50-per cent mortality occurs with liver injuries, ruptured diaphragms, kidney lacerations and retroperitoneal hematomas. A 25-per cent mortality is seen with ruptured spleens and urinary bladders, while pancreatic injuries and hollow viscus ruptures have a 15-per cent mortality. Naturally, much of this mortality was in association with other injuries.

TABLE 11–3 FREQUENCY OF INJURY IN BLUNT ABDOMINAL TRAUMA[53]

VISCERA	PER CENT
Spleen	26.2
Kidney	24.2
Intestine	16.2
Liver	15.6
Abdominal Wall	3.6
Retroperitoneal Hematoma	2.7
Mesentery	2.5
Pancreas	1.4
Diaphragm	1.1

Mechanisms of blunt visceral injury include crushing, shearing and bursting forces. The first is the crushing of an organ against the posterior abdominal wall, especially the anterior ridge in the midline produced by the vertebral bodies. Second, a sharp shearing force may suddenly be applied to both solid and hollow organs, resulting in tears with perforation or hemorrhage or both. Finally, an intra-abdominal hollow viscus can be burst open by a sudden increase in its intraluminal pressure.

A sudden application of pressure is more apt to rupture solid than hollow viscera, thus accounting for the greater incidence of solid organ injury. The more elastic tissues of the young tolerate trauma better than the less resilient tissues of the aged. A strong, firmly muscled abdominal wall constitutes a better barrier than the flaccid, relaxed abdomen of the old or intoxicated.

Blast Injuries. These can occur in air or under water (immersion). Gas-filled cavities such as the lung and intestines are primarily affected, and air blast injuries are not as severe as immersion blasts. Solid organs transmit blast waves better and are therefore less often injured. Indeed, Greaves and associates did not observe pathological changes in solid organ tissues that did not contain air or gas.[52] Observation and treatment are similar to that performed with blunt abdominal trauma.

Crush Injuries. These imply a diffuse and prolonged application of great force with all the attendant problems seen in the usual blunt trauma patient.

Seat Belt Injuries. Since Kulowski and Rost[74] in 1956 first attributed a case of intestinal obstruction to a previously incurred seat belt injury, numerous cases of the "seat belt syndrome"[49] have appeared in the literature. Williams and Kirkpatrick[171] collected 87 cases of lap belt injury. Intra-abdominal injuries occurred in 42 of these, and 39 had intestinal or mesenteric injuries. Thirty-seven were subjected to surgery with three deaths. Lumbar spine injuries occurred 51 times and in seven instances were associated with intra-abdominal injury as well. Twenty-four cases wearing a shoulder restrainer sustained predominantly skeletal injuries, although intra-abdominal trauma was also noted. Sixty-three individuals wearing the three-point shoulder-lap belt restrainers had primarily fractures of the ribs, clavicle or sternum but intra-abdominal injury was rare. This last device was the most effective in preventing injuries.

The method of injury to the bowel in this syndrome involves direct trauma which results in seromuscular tears and closed-loop obstructions which temporarily increase intraluminal pressure, resulting in intestinal rupture. Shearing and torsion forces are probably also active. Besides the intestines and mesentery, practically all abdominal structures, including the gravid uterus, have been injured by seat belts. The terminal ileum is the most common location for the intestinal injuries. A correctly worn seat belt rests low over the anterior iliac spines and should not result in intra-abdominal trauma. However, the seat belt is often worn improperly above the iliac crests or migrates there during the accident and thus predisposes to injury of the abdomen. Properly worn seat belts seldom cause serious injury and are definitely effective in reducing mortality and morbidity in automobile accidents.

The "seat belt sign" consists of a transverse band of contusion, abrasion or ecchymosis across the lower abdomen. It occurs in less than one-third of the cases of intra-abdominal injury but should always alert the examiner to the possibility that the accident victim may have incurred an abdominal visceral injury or fracture of the lumbar spine or pelvis.

Most seat belt injuries have had significant delays in diagnosis with increased morbidity and mortality. Deterioration is usually apparent by 12 hours,[171] but delays of up to 65 days are reported.[181] Diagnosis and treatment of these injuries have all the problems and pitfalls of managing other blunt abdominal trauma.

Corrosive Gastritis. Trauma to the abdominal viscera is not limited to blows and bullets. Corrosive gastritis is a form of abdominal injury which requires expert diagnostic and therapeutic acumen. Citron and associates[22] have thoroughly reviewed this problem.

The selective effects produced by acid and alkaline corrosives on different parts of the alimentary tract are well documented. Acids spare the esophagus and damage the stomach, whereas alkalis affect primarily the esophagus, causing gastric injury in only 20 per cent of the cases. These findings are attributable to the rapid passage of acid in an esophagus lined with acid-resistant squamous epithelium and to the neutralizing effect of the gastric content on ingested alkali. Concentrated acids produce a coagulative necrosis with subsequent eschar formation but little likelihood of perforation, whereas alkalis cause a liquifying necrosis with deep penetration and increased probability of perforation.

Hydrochloric, nitric, trichloracetic, sulfuric and carbolic acids are the most common causes of corrosive gastritis. The primary effect in the stomach is on the antrum because rapid passage along the lesser curvature "Magenstrasse" and pylorus spasm initiated by the acid causes the corrosive to accumulate in the distal stomach. An empty stomach is more likely to be diffusely involved.

Following ingestion the patient is seized with acute generalized abdominal pain which becomes more localized to the epigastric area. Retching, hematemesis and cardiovascular collapse may ensue. If the patient survives, pyloric outlet obstruction usually develops, requiring surgical intervention.

The emergency management of gastric corrosive injuries involves cautious passage of a large, soft rubber nasogastric tube, taking care to avoid further injury to the already damaged esophagus and stomach, followed by gastric lavage with antacids or specific antidotes. Supportive measures include sedation, antibiotics and appropriate intravenous fluid administration. Anticholinergic agents may be beneficial in relieving spasm.

After the acute period, signs and symptoms of peritonitis may develop. Steigmann[152] has stressed that emergency laparotomy should be avoided at this time because the process is a chemical burn–producing coagulative rather than liquifying necrosis and rarely perforates. Allen and associates,[2] however, recommended immediate laparotomy if signs of perforation or massive bleeding develop. They noted that a total gastrectomy with no anastomosis was the most common procedure performed. No doubt a spectrum of damage to the stomach exists with limited mucosal inflammation at one extreme and frank perforation at the other. Expert judgment is obviously required in deciding if surgery is indicated.

Following this initial period, healing and scarring occur and may result, months later, in pyloric outlet obstruction. Pyloroplasty, gastroenterostomy and subtotal gastrectomy are the usual procedures employed to rectify this problem.

Ingested Foreign Bodies. Swallowed foreign bodies that reach the stomach almost always pass completely through without causing obstruction or perforation. Only one per cent of 800 patients treated for ingested foreign bodies at Boston City Hospital had perforations.[60] An almost unending assortment of objects—sharp or dull, pointed or blunt, and large or small—have been treated by watchful waiting.

Perforations, when they do occur, commonly result from small objects becoming trapped in the appendix or Meckel's diverticulum. In addition, some pins probably perforate the bowel on their way to the rectum but heal spontaneously and cause no symptoms. If the object is radiopaque, serial x-rays taken twice a week will insure that the object is not being held up. If the object does become fixed, or if pain, fever, tenderness or signs of peritonitis develop, removal by celiotomy is indicated. Bulk diets are not indicated and cathartics should be avoided.

Iatrogenic Injuries

In Table 11–1 are listed some of the iatrogenic causes of abdominal injury. These represent an assortment of commonly performed diagnostic and therapeutic procedures which can, albeit infrequently, lead to injury of the intra-abdominal viscera.

Sigmoidoscopy, particularly in conjunction with biopsy, has been associated with perforations of the lower bowel. Extraperitoneal perforations are not nearly as serious as the intraperitoneal perforations. When the perforation occurs, a piece of fat or omentum may be seen plugging the newly made hole. However, perforation is often not diagnosed until signs of peritonitis develop. Immediate laparotomy with primary closure of the perforation is indicated. A diverting colostomy may not be necessary, particularly since most of these patients have had a lower bowel prep prior to the endoscopy and contamination is negligible.

The injuries which may be associated with external cardiac massage can be considerable and become significant if the resuscitation is successful. Fractures of the sternum and multiple ribs with hemopneumothorax, flail chest and rupture of the spleen or liver are the most frequent injuries. Often the critical status of the patient distracts the attending physician from recognizing these injuries.

Abdominal paracentesis, performed with a needle, rarely causes significant intra-abdominal injury even if the bowel is perforated. Needle puncture wounds of the intestine quickly seal without leakage, except in the presence of intestinal obstruction. However, laceration of the intestine can occur and will usually require operative repair. Trocar insertion can cause serious laceration or perforation of the bowel, particularly in areas where the bowel is fixed by adhesions. The withdrawal of intestinal contents during paracentesis is diagnostic of this complication. Avoidance of abdominal scars when selecting the site of trocar insertion is important. Trauma to the iliac vessels has also occurred from this maneuver and requires immediate exploration to prevent exsanguination and vascular thrombosis. Insertion of an abdominal catheter for peritoneal dialysis has the same potential for complications as the abdominal trocar paracentesis. Both thoracentesis and tube thoracostomy have been associated with injuries to the liver and spleen. Treatment is determined by the degree and type of injury.

Inadvertent insertion of a nasal oxygen line into the esophagus can cause gastric distention, rupture and even tension pneumoperitoneum with compression of the inferior vena cava and obstruction to venous return to the right heart. Immediate insertion of a large needle into the peritoneal cavity will relieve the pressure, after which laparotomy is indicated to repair the gastric rent.

Perforation of the colon during a barium enema examination introduces a potentially lethal combination of barium and feces into the peritoneal cavity. Biopsy of the rectosigmoid colon, done shortly prior to the barium enema, may at times be a predisposing factor by creating an area of weakness in the bowel wall. Celiotomy with closure of the perforation, a completely diverting proximal colostomy and thorough lavage of the abdominal cavity with large amounts of saline solution are no guarantee that the patient will recover.

The procedure of Fallopian tube interruption by peritoneoscopy has resulted in perforations of the small bowel during electrocoagulation of the tubes. Perforation is not necessarily immediate and symptoms may appear after several days as the necrotic area in the small bowel sloughs, resulting in leakage of intestinal contents.

Liver biopsies associated with significant hemorrhage or bile leak are not very common. On the other hand, liver biopsies or percutaneous cholangiograms performed in the presence of obstruction to the common bile duct will usually result in a bile leak. Therefore, if percutaneous cholangiography does demonstrate obstruction, abdominal exploration should be carried out immediately.

Radiation effects on the rectum or the small bowel fixed in the pelvis by adhesions during radiotherapy create problems of irradiation proctitis with bleeding and obstruction and stricture of the small intestine.[134] Symptomatology determines when operative intervention is necessary.

ASSOCIATED CONDITIONS

Other factors that may have an important bearing on the diagnosis, management and prognosis of abdominal injuries deserve comment.

Extra-abdominal Injuries. Such injuries are associated with a higher mortality in patients with abdominal trauma. Fitzgerald and associates[39] reported on 100 patients who arrived dead at the hospital following nonpenetrating abdominal trauma. Extra-abdominal injuries were present in 97 per cent of patients who were dead on arrival but in only 70 per cent of those arriving alive. Seventeen of the patients who arrived alive died before resuscitative measures could be instituted. Another three patients died because of failure to recognize intra-abdominal bleeding in the presence of other severe injuries. Of the remaining 80 patients, 50 had extra-abdominal injuries, 78 per cent of whom survived, whereas of the 30 patients with injuries limited to the abdomen 93 per cent survived. These figures emphasize the fact that mortality in abdominal injuries is low if the diagnosis is made early and if there are no extra-abdominal injuries.

Aside from affecting prognosis, associated injuries complicate and hamper the transportation and examination of the injured. A patient with a fractured cervical vertebra or femur with the appropriate splinting and traction devices in place is difficult to transport and almost impossible to position for proper abdominal x-rays.

London reported 58 deaths following laparotomy for abdominal injury, 45 of which occurred in patients with extra-abdominal injuries.[77] Wilson and coauthors[174] indicate that the presence of head injury in association with abdominal injury not only increases the mortality rate by a factor of four but also increases the likelihood of nonpenetrating abdominal trauma being undiagnosed. Only 22 per cent of their patients with combined injuries did not exhibit coma, shock or both (Fig. 11–2). In patients sufficiently reactive to respond to painful stimuli, the presence of abdominal rigidity and tenderness is an important finding and should not be discounted. These authors stress the importance of abdominal paracentesis in such patients and note a diagnostic accuracy of 95 per cent when the procedure yields free blood, bile and air. The most important lesson learned from this reported experience is that preoccupation with other injuries, misinterpretation of obvious clinical signs and avoidance of abdominal paracentesis are the chief factors leading to unnecessary deaths.

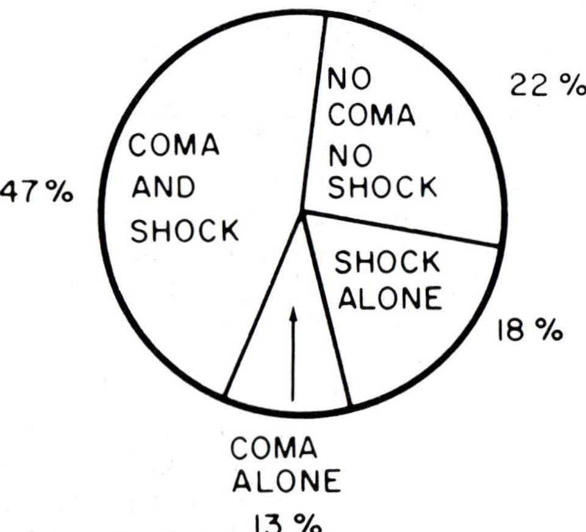

Figure 11–2 Incidence of coma and shock in 91 patients with combined head and abdominal injuries. (Reproduced with permission from Wilson, C. B., Vidrin, A., Jr., and Rives, J. D.: Unrecognized abdominal trauma in patients with head injuries. Ann. Surg. *161*:608, 1965.)

Alcohol. Hopson and coauthors[61] noted that 87 per cent of 297 patients with stab wounds of the abdomen had probably been drinking. Maynard and Orapeza,[93] in a series of 569 patients, noted that 35 per cent were obviously intoxicated. The obtunded reactions of inebriated patients make abdominal evaluation difficult. Also, the histories are less accurate, the chances of aspiration greater, and the likelihood of postoperative delirium tremens enhanced. The combative, obnoxious drunk must at times be restrained for his own as well as the attending personnel's protection. Poor judgment and physical defects complete the triumvirate of the most common causes of trauma and, particularly, automobile accidents.

Narcotics and Other Drug Abuses. The recent increase in the use of "hard drugs" has provided yet another set of complicating circumstances in the management of abdominal trauma. Obtunded sensation, lack of response to usual analgesic doses, postoperative withdrawal, the need to continue methadone maintenance therapy, the lack of veins for intravenous infusions because of drug-induced thrombophlebitis, and the higher incidence of hepatitis are a few of the added problems encountered. A 26-per cent incidence of narcotics addiction has been reported in one series of trauma.[69]

Treatment Delay. The delay between injury and definitive medical management has a very significant bearing on the outcome. In over 80 per cent of cases, admission to the hospital occurs within four hours of the accident. Injuries managed soon after the insult have less mortality and morbidity than when treatment is postponed.[79] Some authors have attempted to show that minor delays in performing laparotomy have no effect on morbidity.[16, 101, 175] Nance and Cohn, in a study on selective management of abdominal stab wounds, reported a 49-per cent complication rate in those operated on in less than six hours after injury and a 50-per cent complication rate in those with a delay exceeding six hours.[106] However, individuals with continued bleeding or peritonitis will succumb if corrective surgery is *not* performed. Deterioration is a continuous process and it seems unlikely that a definite time interval can be defined during which delay is not harmful.

Shock. That the mortality of patients admitted in shock is greater than those without hypotension is well established. The point which requires emphasis is that *shock in association with abdominal trauma is due to an abdominal injury until proven otherwise.* Other frequent etiologies of shock after trauma include spinal cord transection, cardiac tamponade, hemothorax, tension pneumothorax, obstructive airway, external blood loss, fractured pelvis, fractured femur and myocardial infarction. *Head injuries do not produce hypotension except in terminal stages.* The possibility of extra-abdominal injuries obviously complicates matters. A 25-year-old patient with hypotension and a single stab wound of the abdomen is certainly less of a diagnostic dilemma than a 60-year-old man who had an accident while driving his car and is admitted unconscious and hypotensive.

Psychosis. Psychotic individuals can be a formidable challenge to the trauma surgeon. Self-inflicted stab and gunshot wounds or ingestion of foreign objects are the most common forms of presentation. Repetitive attempts at self-destruction and an uncooperative attitude may be encountered. Large doses of thorazine in divided doses up to 400 mg. per day may be required to control such agitated individuals.

DIAGNOSIS

In acute abdominal trauma, the history, physical examination and treatment are integrated and concurrent aspects of total patient care. Of necessity, artificial divisions are employed to facilitate discussion.

History

In all cases of trauma it is important to obtain as accurate a history as possible. However, because of urgent requirements for therapy, it may be necessary to gather this information piecemeal. The history may be inaccurate or impossible to obtain. The emotional stress associated with trauma affects both patient and bystanders, especially relatives. Shock, semistupor and drunkenness all tend to prevent a clear recitation of the events leading to hospitalization. Furthermore, a history may be inaccurate because of legal or moral problems raised by the nature of the accident. Therefore, the examiner must always be alert to the possibility of distortion of the history in his evaluation of abdominal injuries.

Especially pertinent in trauma victims are the time and circumstances of the injury. Knowing the trajectory of the bullet or the direction of a knife thrust can be helpful. The coexistence of systemic diseases should always be sought. General comments which apply to all injured patients will not be discussed further here.

Physical Examination

The physical examination may be complicated by the presence of shock, coma, drunkenness or other conditions which prevent full cooperation on the part of the patient. Associated injuries may mask the presence of abdominal trauma.

The physical examination should be

modified to fit the needs of the particular situation. A patient with a gunshot wound of the midabdominal region who is in shock does not need a detailed examination of the abdomen in an attempt to document tenderness, guarding or hypoactive bowel sounds since immediate exploration is mandatory; with blunt abdominal trauma, a detailed baseline examination of the abdomen may be critical in making this decision. Repeated examinations by the same observer are often needed to correctly assess the situation. Initially, a quick cursory examination of the entire patient should be performed to detect any other life-threatening problems. Often, resuscitative measures must be carried out in conjunction with the physical examination. Once the immediate threat to life has been alleviated, a more detailed and methodical examination can be completed.

Location of Wound. In penetrating injuries the location of the wound is of diagnostic importance. Approximately three-quarters of all penetrating wounds occur in the upper abdomen.[105] The majority of these are in the left upper quadrant, reflecting the fact that when two assailants face each other, a right-handed opponent is most likely to inflict a left upper quadrant injury.[61, 93] Since many stab wounds are inflicted with relatively short-bladed knives, the location of the wound will help the surgeon to gain a rough idea preoperatively of the extent of the abdominal injury.

Penetrating missiles, such as bullets or bits of wire or stones thrown up from a rotary lawn mower, may travel in erratic paths through the abdomen, ricochetting from one of the lowermost ribs or vertebral bodies or the inner walls of the pelvis. Nevertheless, knowledge of the wound of entrance, the angle or trajectory of the missile and the wound of exit usually provides significant information as to its intraabdominal course. If the type of missile used in a shooting assault is known, the surgeon may also know whether to expect a greater or lesser degree of tissue damage. This depends upon whether a rifle, shotgun or pistol was used and whether or not the bullet was soft-tipped and likely to flatten out during tissue penetration.

The back, perineum, rectum and vagina should always be examined for wounds of entrance or exit. The location of the entrance wound, more than its size, may have significant bearing on the decision to perform laparotomy. A tiny puncture wound may have been inflicted by a long, stiletto-like weapon that caused considerable intraperitoneal injury. Patients with stab wounds usually present at the hospital within four hours of the time of injury, but a latent asymptomatic period may be present so that there are virtually no physical findings other than a small puncture wound accompanied by minimal tenderness and normal bowel sounds. This fact led to the dictum, practiced by surgeons for many years, that laparotomy is the single most important diagnostic tool in such situations since waiting for the physical signs of hemorrhage or perforation to develop results in higher mortality and morbidity. This concept, however, has been vigorously challenged over the past 12 years by those advocating selective management.

Signs and Symptoms. Physical examination of the abdomen of patients with nonpenetrating injuries presents much greater difficulties. A wide variation in signs and symptoms can occur. A patient may present following an automobile accident with an obvious history of severe blunt abdominal trauma but with virtually no physical findings. At the other extreme is the patient with extensive guarding, rebound tenderness and other strongly suggestive findings with no history of an abdominal blow. The state of consciousness or the presence of other painful injuries may make examination of the abdomen extremely difficult to perform and to evaluate. The presence of profound shock may produce a degree of unresponsiveness in which the injured patient may not complain even during thorough examination.

Discussions in the literature are often devoted to the physical signs resulting from injury to a specific organ. As Fitzgerald and associates[39] have pointed out, such descriptions are necessarily retrospective. When the examiner is confronted with a patient with blunt abdominal trauma, one or more of many organs may have been injured to a greater or lesser degree; the picture is rarely one of a single organ injury. Furthermore, they noted that many descriptions in standard works of reference use classic findings of physical diagnosis more applicable to less acute disease states than external trauma. The signs and symptoms of blunt abdominal trauma result from blood loss, bruising and tearing of solid organs and leaking of irritating juices from hollow abdominal viscera.

Thus, a patient with few or no physical findings may be safely observed or may require laparotomy based upon a high degree of probability of internal injury. Most patients with intra-abdominal injuries exhibit one or more positive signs which aid the examiner. Abdominal rigidity alone warrants exploration in most cases of blunt trauma, despite other known causes for rigidity such as fractured lower ribs or contusions. Rigidity is a variable sign but a dangerous one to ignore. Local infiltration about the fracture site of a broken rib relieves associated pain but does not abolish abdominal guarding or rigidity due to intra-abdominal injury. It may be quite difficult to differentiate intra-abdominal injury from the pain associated with severe contusion of the abdominal wall. Usually the patient with intraperitoneal injury will be able to sit up unassisted and with less abdominal wall pain than the patient with contusion of the subcutaneous tissues and musculofascial planes of the abdomen. When any doubt at all exists, however, it must be assumed that the guarding or rigidity is caused by intraperitoneal injury.

The presence of an abdominal hernia, particularly an umbilical hernia, affords an excellent opportunity to elicit peritoneal signs. We have noted excellent correlation between exquisitely tender umbilical hernias and visceral injuries or blood in the peritoneal cavity.

REFERRED PAIN. Sites of referred pain are frequently helpful in diagnosing intraperitoneal injury. A common site is the shoulder, especially the left shoulder (Kehr's sign) in patients bleeding from a ruptured spleen. Similarly, pain in the right shoulder can result from laceration of the liver. When attempting to elicit shoulder pain, it is useful to place the patient in Trendelenburg's position for a few minutes, thus permitting either blood or chemical irritants from the alimentary canal to collect beneath the diaphragm.

ABDOMINAL MASS. The presence of an abdominal mass following blunt abdominal trauma occurs late in the progression of the clinical picture, as do most physical signs. Such a mass most likely represents a semicontaining or subcapsular hematoma of the liver, spleen, mesentery or omentum. The presence of a mass may, however, be an important diagnostic aid in the evaluation of a patient with forgotten or only dimly remembered trauma of days or weeks past.

HEMORRHAGE. Massive intraperitoneal bleeding is associated with shock and demands immediate control. Signs of shifting dullness are indeed late manifestations of not much help. However, dissection of blood between the leaves of the mesentery or directly into the abdominal wall or retroperitoneal tissues and its eventual appearance in about three days as an ecchymosis is a valuable delayed sign. Since such dissection requires a certain period of time to develop, it is usually indicative of slow, steady bleeding or recurrence of bleeding following a period of stability.

AUSCULTATION. Classically, the injured abdomen has been described as silent upon auscultation, and Jarvis,[63] in a review of 128 patients, found no cases of free peritoneal bowel perforation in which peristaltic sounds were audible. Others have noted decreased or absent bowel sounds in 89 per cent of visceral injuries.[61] However, the *presence* of peristaltic sounds is not a reliable sign since it has been demonstrated that normal peristaltic sounds can be heard both in the presence of active intraperitoneal bleeding and following rupture of hollow abdominal organs. Thus, reliance upon the presence of peristalsis as assurance that no intra-abdominal injury exists is fallacious and dangerous. However, absence of peristaltic sounds, when carefully sought, should be given serious consideration. Abnormal location of peristaltic sounds has diagnostic importance. Peristaltic sounds heard in the chest in this setting are diagnostic of traumatic diaphragmatic hernia, as discussed in the chapter on chest injuries.

PALPATION. Subcutaneous emphysema of the abdominal wall is most likely the result of an intrathoracic injury. However, rupture of the retroperitoneal duodenum, rupture of any intestine along its mesenteric border or rupture of the distal colon and rectum may produce this finding.

RECTAL AND PELVIC EXAMINATION. Digital examination of the rectum should never be omitted in examining any patient who has sustained significant trauma. Although the presence of emphysema or gross bleeding is relatively rare, pelvic tenderness may be elicited or the presence of fluid in the pelvis detected. In women, vaginal and bimanual examination are of great aid in detecting the presence of pelvic bleeding or injuries to adjacent viscera following pelvic fracture. Culdocentesis can be helpful in documenting the presence of blood, bile or air in the peritoneal cavity. Other even less common signs of intraperitoneal injury include priapism, which may result from retroperitoneal injuries, especially those involving the spine, or the presence of testicular pain as a sign of retroperitoneal perforation.

INTUBATION. The nasogastric tube and the Foley catheter both serve as important diagnostic and therapeutic aids in the care of the severely traumatized patient. Insertion of a nasogastric tube, or at times a larger Ewald tube, permits decompression of the stomach, removal of gastric contents and prevention of further accumulation of gastrointestinal air or gas. Moreover, the aspirated contents can be checked for blood which, if present, provides a valuable diagnostic clue. The insertion of a Foley catheter into the urinary bladder will provide an immediate specimen of urine which can be examined for blood. A positive test would indicate the need for a cystogram and intravenous pyelography. Instillation of several hundred cubic centimeters of normal saline solution with no return on aspiration would confirm the suspicion of a major bladder rupture, probably in the dome and communicating with the peritoneal cavity. Following pelvic fractures and other perineal trauma, the urethra is often damaged and may be transected. Early insertion of a Foley catheter before the severed urethral ends are displaced will provide an adequate splint and often provide definitive care of this type of injury. Undue delay in inserting a Foley catheter may miss the period when the urethral ends are still in relatively close approximation. Surgical intervention will then be necessary to repair the transected urethra. Aside from its specific diagnostic value, the use of a Foley catheter enables hourly monitoring of urine output, which is essential in the management of severely injured patients.

Laboratory Studies

The most valuable laboratory tests in the evaluation of the patient with abdominal trauma include a hematocrit and leucocyte count, urinalysis and serum amylase. BUN, glucose and electrolyte determinations are usually obtained for baseline values. The diagnosis of massive hemorrhage is usually fairly obvious and the hematocrit merely confirmatory. Recent experience from Vietnam has indicated that massive hemorrhages of more than 20 per cent of blood volumes were associated with rapid plasma refill rates and consequently early decreases in the hematocrit level.[18] In cases of hidden massive intraperitoneal hemorrhage, a low hematocrit early in the treatment of the patient may, indeed, be quite significant.

Leukocytosis is commonly associated with trauma in general, and except for late evaluation in blunt trauma cases it has little significance. Fifteen thousand cells per cubic millimeter are commonly seen shortly after injury. Urinalysis will indicate the presence of bleeding in the genitourinary tract, the presence of diabetes mellitus, or severe underlying renal disease. The serum glucose and the BUN are also useful in discovering systemic disease.

Serum amylase values can be normal in the face of major pancreatic injury,[5, 66, 169, 179] but elevated values give important information. In the presence of blunt pancreatic trauma, the serum amylase values are elevated in from 48 to 91 per cent of patients. In the presence of penetrating trauma to the pancreas, the serum amylase is elevated in from 9 to 40 per cent of cases. Injuries to the head of the pancreas are more commonly associated with elevated serum amylases than when the tail of the pancreas is injured. Elevated serum amylase values usually return to normal within 48 hours after injury.[169] Elevated amylase values can also be associated with perforations of the gastrointestinal tract, particularly retroperitoneal ruptures of the duodenum.[9] Gamble and Mason [48] believe that the determination of the diastase in a two-hour urine collection is the most reliable index of pancreatic injury. Increased concentrations of amylase in the peritoneal fluid following pancreatic injury have been noted.[71, 118] A peritoneal amylase concentration in the lavage fluid greater than 100 Somogyi units per 100 ml. has been uniformly diagnostic of injuries to the pancreas or upper small bowel.[118]

Liver function studies are not usually carried out in patients requiring emergency procedures. However, the presence of subcapsular hematoma or hematobilia after injury may require a more sophisticated evaluation. These studies are discussed under liver injury.

Roentgenologic Studies

It is necessary to exercise judgment in the use of roentgenographic aids for the diagnosis and localization of intra-abdominal injury. In the presence of shock, resuscitative measures take precedence over x-ray studies. When laparotomy is clearly indicated, undue delay caused by unnecessary x-ray examinations is unwarranted. Nevertheless, when there is adequate time, proper utilization of x-rays adds much to the precision of diagnosis and planning of therapy.

The basic roentgenographic examination consists of an upright posterior-anterior chest roentgenogram, an anterior-posterior supine abdominal film and a left lateral decubitus abdominal film. If possible, an upright x-ray of the abdomen is performed, but this often is not feasible in the seriously injured patient. Careful radiographic technique is essential to provide the proper detail necessary for interpreting subtle findings. Amplification of these studies by the use of water-soluble opaque medium often provides important additional information. X-rays of the pelvis, spine and ribs are obtained as indicated.

A chest x-ray is considered an integral part of the abdominal examination because thoracic injuries are frequently associated with abdominal trauma. Even if no positive findings are demonstrated, the chest x-ray will have provided a valuable baseline study.

A standard approach should be followed in examining roentgenograms in cases of abdominal trauma. The following routine has been useful:

1. Examine the skeletal structures, looking for fractures of the vertebral bodies, transverse processes, pelvis and ribs. Fractures of the transverse process are often associated with retroperitoneal hematomas and left-sided rib fractures with splenic injury.

2. Note any foreign bodies and attempt to determine the trajectory of missiles by correlation with the wound of entrance. The absence of a missile when no exit wound is present connotes peripheral arterial embolization, proximal migration to the right heart and pulmonary artery via the venous system, or entrance into and passage through the gastrointestinal tract.

3. Inspect for free intraperitoneal air, indicative of a ruptured hollow viscus, which may be seen subdiaphragmatically beneath the lateral abdominal wall on a lateral decubitus film or as the "dome sign," "falciform ligament sign," or the "double wall sign" on a supine film. Both walls of the bowel (inner and outer) stand out sharply when there is air inside and outside of the bowel (Fig. 11–3). Stomach and colon perforations frequently give rise to free air, whereas small bowel perforations only occasionally do so. Positioning the patient for 10 to 15 minutes prior to taking the x-rays will improve the ability to identify free air.

4. Look for the classic "stippling" of retroperitoneal air, usually indicating rupture of the retroperitoneal portion of the duodenum or rectum.

5. Delineate the psoas shadows whose absence may indicate retroperitoneal bleeding.

6. Examine for separation of the gas-filled right or left colon from the properitoneal fat line, indicating intraperitoneal blood or fluid in the flanks. Also, flotation of the small bowel toward the center of the abdomen, increased space between loops of small bowel and a general ground glass appearance are all compatible with intraperitoneal accumulation of blood. With intraperitoneal bleeding the retroperitoneal structures will remain sharp.

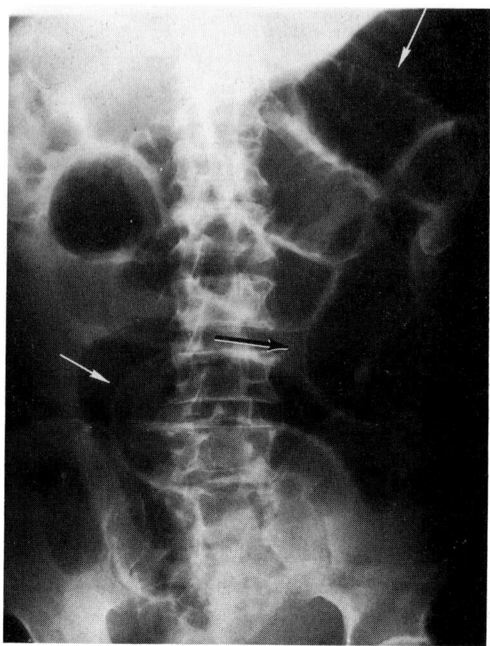

Figure 11–3 A supine roentgenogram of the abdomen demonstrating the double wall sign. The presence of free intraperitoneal air permits visualization of the small bowel outer wall (arrows).

7. Look for enlargement or distortion of the outlines of the spleen, kidneys or liver, indicating a subcapsular hematoma or a hemorrhage confined to that vicinity. A distinctive finding in splenic rupture is medial displacement of the stomach with indentations along its greater curvature caused by hemorrhage into the gastrosplenic ligament (Fig. 11–4).

Hypaque studies have proven useful in documenting injuries at first suspected on the "routine" films. This applies particularly to perforations of the duodenum. Cystograms and intravenous pyelograms are needed to assess injuries of the urinary tract. Detailed discussion of these tests is covered in the chapter on genitourinary trauma.

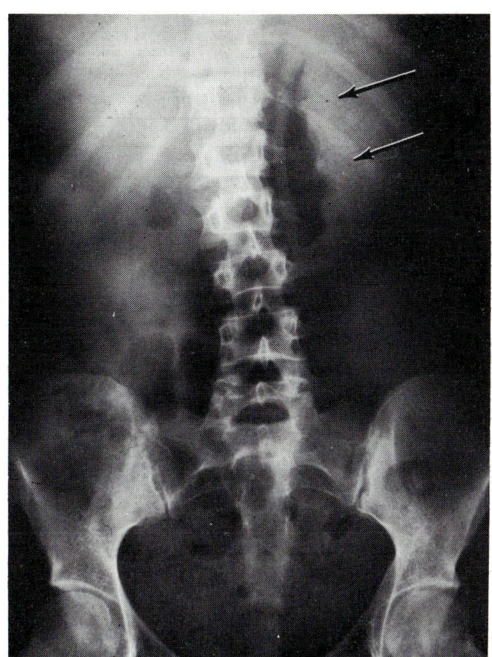

Figure 11–4 A supine roentgenogram of the abdomen in a patient with rupture of the spleen due to blunt trauma. The arrows indicate medial displacement of the stomach with indentations along the greater curvature due to hematoma in the gastrosplenic ligament.

Many experienced observers have noted that roentgenographic examinations provide useful information in less than one-third of patients with abdominal injuries. Nonetheless, any additional information is important particularly with blunt abdominal trauma where diagnosis is always a difficult challenge. For those interested in a more detailed discussion of diagnostic x-rays in blunt abdominal trauma, McCort's book has a succinct, well-illustrated, pertinent discussion.[98]

Angiography. Norell[110] was the first to use abdominal aortography in blunt abdominal trauma when he diagnosed a splenic rupture by this method in 1957. Since then numerous reports have appeared with Freeark[41, 44, 45] being the most enthusiastic supporter of this diagnostic approach, encouraging more frequent use of arteriography and emphasizing its usefulness pre-, intra- and postoperatively.

Both false positives and negatives occur with arteriography, and it has not been effective in the identification or management of injuries to the stomach, small and large intestines, or the more peripheral mesenteric vessels. Its primary benefit has been in the evaluation of injuries to the spleen, kidneys, liver, pancreas and duodenum. Selective arteriography provides better visualization and is preferable to midstream aortography.[76] Arteriography is indicated in blunt trauma to the abdomen when injuries to the spleen, liver, pancreas, duodenum or kidneys are suspected but the physical examination and the other common diagnostic studies are equivocal. The arteriographic findings are peculiar to each organ injured. For example, splenic injuries display extravasated contrast material (Fig. 11–5), radiolucent defects due to the hematoma (Fig. 11–6), and arteriovenous shunting manifested by splenic vein opacification one or two seconds after visualization of contrast material in the splenic artery.

Sinograms. Cornell, Ebert and Zuidema,[26] in 1965, described a method of injecting abdominal stab wounds with water-soluble contrast material in order to determine if the peritoneal cavity had been perforated. At last report, there was one false positive and three false negatives in 192 cases.[183] Sixty-eight demonstrated peritoneal perforation and underwent laparotomy, and 78 per cent of these had significant injuries. Steichen and associates[149] also had success in predicting peritoneal cavity perforation with only one false negative result in 95 patients studied. However, they found that selective management by clinical signs alone resulted in 7.3 per cent "unnecessary" laparotomies, whereas the radiographic technique led to 15.9 per cent laparotomies in which no significant visceral injury was found. Others have reported poor results with frequent false negative tests.[162] The pitfalls in interpreting the study have been discussed.[19] Pain in the area after injection makes it diffi-

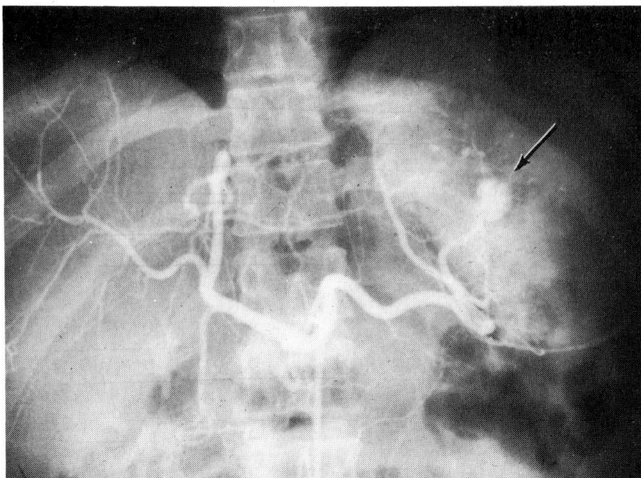

Figure 11–5 Selective celiac artery arteriogram in a patient with blunt rupture of the spleen demonstrating extravasation of contrast material (arrow).

cult to evaluate abdominal findings, but if the test can be performed with a high degree of accuracy, there is no need for close observation once nonperforation has been demonstrated. The method entails proper antiseptic preparation and draping of the area surrounding the penetrating wound, followed by instillation of a local anesthetic. A small (14F) catheter is inserted through the wound of entry, and the skin edges are tightly secured around the catheter with a purse-string suture. Sixty to 80 ml. of 50 per cent sodium diatrizoate (Hypaque) with one milliliter of methylene blue added is injected under moderate pressure through the catheter. Recumbent and lateral abdominal roentgenograms will then demonstrate whether the opaque material has passed into the peritoneal cavity (Fig. 11–7) or whether the wound itself was superficial and nonpenetrating. Failure to demonstrate contrast material in the peritoneal cavity is considered reliable evidence that the peritoneum has not been perforated (Fig. 11–8).

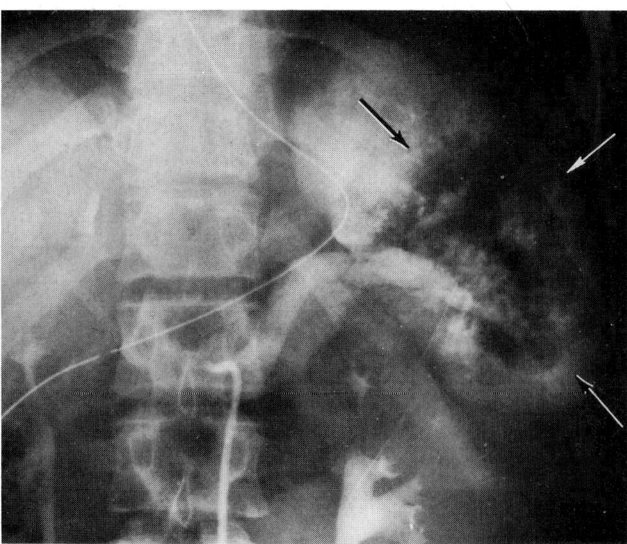

Figure 11–6 Late phase of a selective celiac arteriogram in a patient with blunt rupture of the spleen. Arrows indicate a filling defect caused by a large intrasplenic hematoma.

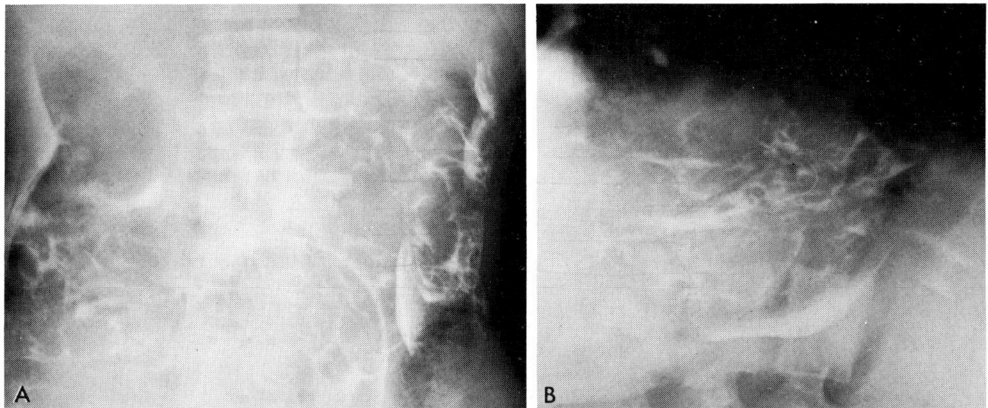

Figure 11–7 *A* and *B*, Injection of 60 ml. of sodium diatrizoate into a stab wound, followed by a roentgenogram in the anteroposterior and lateral positions, reveals penetration of the material into the peritoneal space, outlining the viscera.

Abdominal Paracentesis

A diagnostic study of considerable usefulness, especially in nonpenetrating abdominal injuries, is paracentesis. This examination has been utilized for many years and has proven an invaluable aid in many circumstances. Yurko and Williams[180] indicated that a diagnostic accuracy of 90 per cent can be obtained when needle aspiration of the peritoneal cavity is properly performed. Nonclotting blood withdrawn in the syringe is considered strong evidence of intraperitoneal injury, as is air or bile-stained fluid. In those patients in whom the abdominal paracentesis was positive, the delay between initial examination and operation was reduced and the need for blood transfusions lowered as compared to patients who did not have paracentesis performed. Others have confirmed these results.[99] All investigators experienced in the technique of abdominal paracentesis have emphasized that *a negative abdominal tap has no diagnostic*

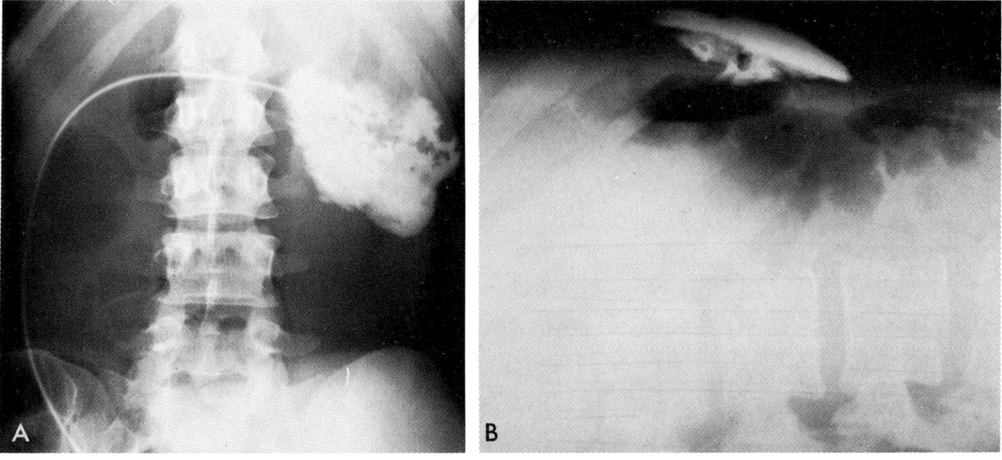

Figure 11–8 *A* and *B*, Injection of the radiopaque material into a stab wound of the left upper quadrant indicates extravasation into the subcutaneous extraperitoneal planes with no intraperitoneal extension.

significance, that is, one should act as though the study has never been performed.

Certainly, the most useful application of abdominal paracentesis is in patients with other serious injuries, especially craniocerebral ones. These patients, who may be in a coma and have severe respiratory difficulties from flail chest or extensive soft tissue and skeletal injuries, would obviously do better if they could be managed without the extra burden of a laparotomy to rule out intra-abdominal injury. It may be difficult, if not impossible, to determine whether shock is due to other injuries or to occult intraperitoneal bleeding. Paracentesis will usually help the surgeon in making his decision. In some situations abdominal paracentesis may provide the only opportunity to obtain a definitive indication for laparotomy. Wilson and associates[174] have not only emphasized this but have also urged that the paracentesis be repeated throughout the early hours of observation.

The technique for abdominal paracentesis is not difficult. A sterile syringe and a long 18- or 20-gauge spinal needle are the only essential instruments. It is preferable to have the patient void or to have the bladder emptied by catheterization before needle aspiration. The abdomen is inspected for scars of previous operations or injuries in order to predict and avoid areas where adhesions might be present. The study is contraindicated when the peritoneal space is suspected of being extensively involved with adhesions.

A four-quadrant approach, beginning with the left lower quadrant, is preferred. The sites of penetration are indicated in Figure 11–9. The needle should be introduced lateral to the rectus sheath in order to avoid a hematoma which may easily occur in this muscle because of its close association with the inferior epigastric vessels. Another technique employs aspiration along the lateral gutters to identify the presence of intraperitoneal bleeding.

An initial wheal is made in the skin with one per cent Xylocaine using a 25-gauge needle. It is wise to continue infiltration to the level of the peritoneum, including the fascia, if possible. Using a 10-ml. syringe, an 18- or 20-gauge spinal needle with a short bevel is gently inserted through the abdominal wall and peritoneum. It is usually an easy matter to determine whether the peritoneum has been

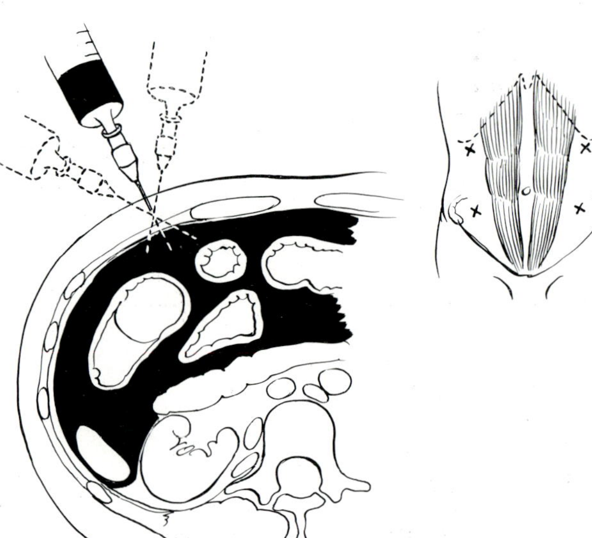

Figure 11–9 Diagnostic peritoneal tap.

penetrated since there is minimal resistance followed by a slight give to the needle as it enters. At this point, the operator applies gentle suction as the needle is slowly advanced in a lateral direction toward the gutters. Gentle repositioning of the needle within the peritoneal space may permit the withdrawal of a small quantity of fluid. As little as 0.1 ml. of nonclotting blood is sufficient evidence of intraperitoneal bleeding. Any nonbloody fluid obtained should be cultured and smeared immediately. The "tap" is repeated in the other quadrants if the first is negative. It is advisable to check the upper abdomen carefully for the presence of either splenomegaly or hepatomegaly prior to paracentesis, which in the upper quadrants should be directed downward to avoid these organs. The authors prefer to aspirate in the following order: left lower quadrant, right lower quadrant, left upper quadrant, right upper quadrant.

If the initial penetration with an 18-gauge needle is negative in the left lower quadrant, some observers prefer to thread a thin polyethylene catheter through the needle into the peritoneal space and then withdraw the needle over the tubing. This permits the catheter to lie either in the left gutter or in the pelvis, and repeated aspiration may be carried out over the subsequent minutes or hours. This has the advantage of permitting continued observation but the disadvantage of not allowing placement of the aspirating tip in different locations. We feel it is preferable to aspirate both in different locations and repeatedly, if necessary. The latter is particularly important in patients with multiple-system trauma.

A high degree of accuracy in abdominal paracentesis has not been the experience of all observers. Olsen and Hildreth,[112] in a prospective study comparing abdominal paracentesis versus peritoneal lavage on the same patients, showed that abdominal paracentesis was accurate in diagnosing significant hemoperitoneum in only 21 per cent of cases but that peritoneal lavage was accurate in 100 per cent of cases.

Peritoneal Lavage

Root first introduced diagnostic peritoneal lavage in 1964.[131, 132, 133] In a five-year experience with 304 patients there were three (one per cent) false positive tests and nine (three per cent) false negative tests. The technique involves insertion of a peritoneal dialysis catheter into the pelvis. Under local anesthesia a small lower midline incision is made just below the umbilicus and dissection is carried down to the peritoneum. After carefully securing hemostasis, the peritoneum is opened and the catheter inserted into the peritoneal cavity. If aspiration recovers gross blood, laparotomy is performed. If no blood is recovered, then one liter of normal saline solution is infused through the catheter, after which the fluid is siphoned back off into the bottle placed on the floor. In addition to grossly bloody lavage fluid, the following are indicative of a positive tap: more than 500 white blood cells per mm.^{3}, an amylase over 100 Somogyi units/100 ml., more than 100,000 red blood cells per mm.^{3}, or bile, bacterial or intestinal contents in the lavage fluid. These additional examinations of the fluid account for six per cent of the positive results.

Peritoneal lavage, like paracentesis, is of greatest value in those patients whose physical findings may be difficult to evaluate, when the patient cannot communicate and when there is unexplained hypotension.[118] Its advantages are that it can be quickly performed in bed with the patient in the supine position under local anesthesia with readily available equipment.

Thus, a variety of modalities is available to the examiner to determine whether an intra-abdominal injury is present. The most important tool to the examiner, however, is his awareness of the various injuries that may occur, their potential lethality, as well as the progression of signs and symptoms they produce. A physician suspicious of serious trauma, and prepared to operate if these suspicions are supported by physical examination and the studies described above, can at least reduce the consequences of diagnostic error to a minimum.

TREATMENT

Before discussing the treatment of specific individual injuries, a brief résumé of the prognosis of abdominal injuries and some principles of their initial care will be detailed. Throughout this text it has been repeatedly emphasized that injuries should never be treated as isolated entities, and it has been pointed out that patients with multiple injuries have a higher mortality than those with isolated injuries. Thus, a system of priorities of care should govern the actions of the surgeon who first takes charge of the injured patient in the emergency room. This priority of therapy need not be detailed extensively in this chapter: cardiorespiratory resuscitation always commands first priority, and relief of airway obstruction is an integral part of these maneuvers; next, control of major hemorrhage must be achieved; and restoration of the intravascular circulating volume follows. Further details are found elsewhere in this text.

Similarly, priority of care of certain types of wounds involving different organ systems is readily established. Aside from rapidly progressive craniocerebral injuries, such as an epidural hemorrhage, or similarly life-threatening situations within the thorax, such as massive continuing hemothorax, *abdominal injuries usually achieve highest priority.* There are two reasons for this. First, major hidden hemorrhage is commonly associated with both blunt and penetrating abdominal injury. Second, perforation of the alimentary tract results in peritoneal contamination with all its serious consequences. Confirmation of the degree of severity of the abdominal injury by prolonged observation can be disastrous, but unnecessary celiotomy can be equally calamitous and is never beneficial, especially in those individuals with associated injuries of a serious and complicated nature. Maturity in judgment, accuracy in diagnosis and therapeutic (surgical) skill are the essentials for successful management of abdominal trauma.

Treatment of Penetrating Abdominal Injuries

Gunshot Wounds. With few exceptions[122, 149] most authors agree that gunshot wounds of the abdomen should be explored. It is rare for a bullet to penetrate the peritoneal cavity and not cause visceral injury.[149] Tangential bullet wounds that apparently miss the peritoneal cavity should usually also be explored, as significant visceral disruption can result from the "blast effect." However, the authors have occasionally observed patients with tangential bullet wounds in the right upper quadrant caused by low-velocity .22 caliber "shorts" and have not had to perform delayed laparotomy. Shotgun injuries manifested by only a few subcutaneous pellets or a widely spread pattern (and probably only scattered single visceral perforations) may be managed conservatively in the absence of signs of bleeding or peritonitis. Otherwise, shotgun wounds are routinely explored.

Stab Wounds. The present controversy over treating abdominal stab wounds revolves about the "selective management" versus the "routine laparotomy" approach. The 25- to 75-per cent incidence of negative laparotomies has prompted clinicians to develop methods of trying to avoid surgery in those patients without significant injuries. Reports both from those in favor of mandatory exploration for all penetrating injuries[14, 61, 93, 105, 107] and from those proposing more selective management are prevalent in the literature.[25, 46, 92, 101, 106, 122, 127, 137, 145, 149, 150, 153, 160, 170]

Interpretation of the voluminous data available is difficult because different series of cases are often not comparable. Many authors do not distinguish significant from trivial injuries; stab and gunshot statistics are often combined; inclusion of morbidity rates depends on the whim of the investigator; and the incidence of associated injuries varies between series and contributes significantly to the final results. Table 11–4 lists the important points of contention between those advocating routine laparotomy and those proposing more selective methods of management.

Shaftan[137, 138] is credited with popularizing the selective approach to managing penetrating abdominal stab wounds by emphasizing meticulous clinical observation and defining the indications for exploratory laparotomy. Tenderness, rebound, guarding and absent bowel sounds were felt to be the prime indicators for surgical intervention. In his study of 535 patients, 90 per cent of whom had stab wounds, only 28 per cent underwent celiotomy with a mortality of 7.3 per cent. The nonoperative group had a mortality of 0.5 per cent and the overall mortality was 2.6 per cent. Morbidity of the operated group was 31 per cent versus only 3.3 per

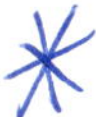

TABLE 11–4 POINTS OF CONTENTION IN THE MANAGEMENT OF ABDOMINAL STAB WOUNDS

IMMEDIATE LAPAROTOMY	SELECTIVE MANAGEMENT*
75 per cent have visceral injuries.	Only 25 per cent have *significant* visceral injuries.
Delay in treatment is significant.	Minor delays of more than 24 hrs. are probably inconsequential. Most injuries "declare" within 12 hrs.
Negative laparotomy carries a mortality of close to zero.	Negative laparotomy has been associated with a mortality up to 6 per cent.
Morbidity with negative laparotomy is 3 per cent.	Morbidity with negative laparotomy approaches 33 per cent.
Intoxication, drugs, and psychosis mask signs and symptoms.	Meticulous clinical evaluation and mature judgment are necessary. Increased risk with general anesthesia.
Lacerations of the diaphragm are often asymptomatic and may lead to herniation.	Late post-traumatic diaphragmatic hernias are not a frequent problem.
25 per cent of significant injuries initially lack signs of visceral trauma.	Only 5 per cent of those initially observed will require laparotomy.
Medicolegal implications—laparotomy is the accepted mode of therapy.	Minor assaults can become homicides if mortality is associated with negative laparotomy.
0–6 per cent overall mortality.	0–5 per cent overall mortality.

*Those proposing selective management claim that this method keeps the mortality rate the same but decreases the overall morbidity by 50 per cent because of avoiding unnecessary laparotomy.

cent for those avoiding operation. He concluded that no deaths could be attributed to delay or failure to recognize the need for abdominal exploration.

Several authors[92, 101, 106] have studied comparable series of "routine" exploration versus selective management, and all document reductions in overall morbidity with the same or improved mortality. Although this approach to managing abdominal stab wounds is a worthy one in terms of decreased morbidity and hospital time, definite risks exist for the 5 to 10 per cent of patients with serious abdominal injuries who initially do not present with abdominal findings. Frequent, usually hourly, observations are required. This method lends itself only to situations where full-time physician coverage is available to fulfill this responsibility. The surgeon in individual practice who only occasionally treats abdominal trauma will probably serve his patient best by following the approach of routine exploratory laparotomy.

Table 11–5 diagrams the options available in the management of abdominal stab wounds with outcome probabilities. The quoted percentages for the various approaches are approximations derived from numerous publications.

Mandatory indications for immediate laparotomy include:

1. Shock
2. Signs of peritonitis (rebound tenderness, muscle guarding, absent bowel sounds)
3. Gastrointestinal bleeding
4. Free air in the peritoneal cavity
5. Evisceration
6. Massive hematuria

These findings will be present in approximately 20 per cent of all stab wounds admitted to the emergency room. If none of these exists, five alternative avenues of management can be followed:

1. Close observation by the same examiner with laparotomy if evidence of bleeding or peritonitis occurs
2. Sinogram of the stab wound with laparotomy, if positive
3. Paracentesis, culdocentesis or peritoneal lavage followed by laparotomy, if positive

TABLE 11–5 MANAGEMENT OF ABDOMINAL STAB WOUNDS

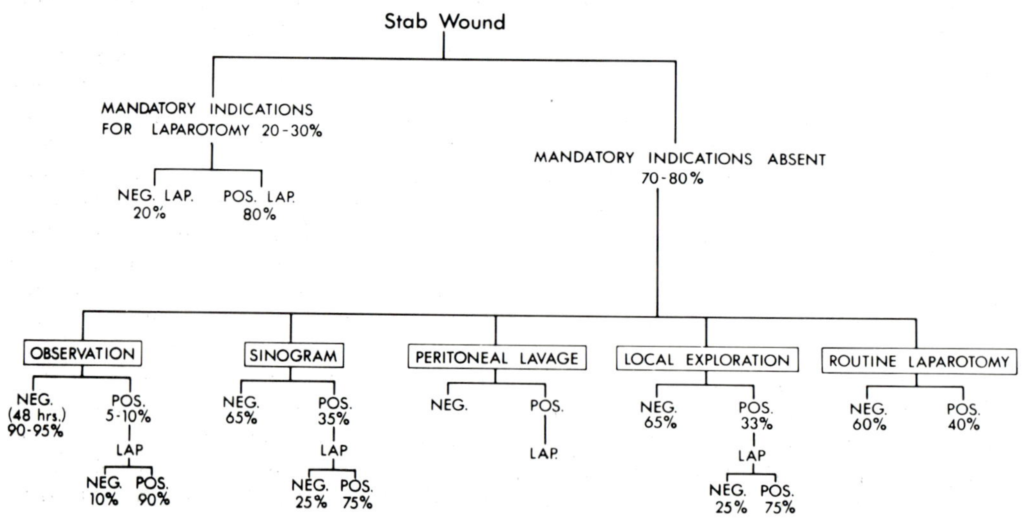

4. Exploration of the stab wound under local anesthesia proceeding to formal laparotomy, if penetration of the peritoneal cavity is documented
5. Immediate laparotomy

An inflexible approach to managing abdominal stab wounds can be impractical. Each patient will present with unique circumstances which must be considered before deciding on the most appropriate diagnostic and therapeutic procedures. A 25-year-old healthy male, who presents 24 hours after a single penknife wound of the abdomen and who is completely asymptomatic and has no abdominal findings, hardly seems suitable for anything other than continued observation. A busy trauma service in a large charity hospital may not have enough personnel either to explore every such patient or to examine each one hourly; thus, exploration of the wound under local anesthesia might be a reasonable compromise. The surgeon practicing without the support of house staff, who sees few stab wounds per year, would probably best manage the healthy young stabbing victim by routine exploratory laparotomy.

An approach to managing abdominal stab wounds that the authors have found useful is as follows:

1. Any patient with mandatory indications for celiotomy (as previously described) undergoes immediate operation.
2. Of the remaining patients:
   a. Those that present within six hours of stabbing have exploration of the wound under local anesthesia or a sinogram performed. If penetration into the peritoneal cavity is confirmed, laparotomy follows.
   b. Those presenting after six hours are observed. If questionable abdominal findings are present (a not uncommon circumstance), wound exploration is undertaken or sinogram studies done.
   c. Any patient who, for reasons of intoxication, narcotic addiction, psychosis or coma, cannot be properly evaluated or observed is also subjected to sinograms or local wound exploration.
   d. Patients with stab wounds inflicted through the lower rib cage which have probably penetrated the diaphragm are explored because of the risk of herniation through unrepaired diaphragmatic lacerations.
   e. *Multiple* stab wounds seen within the first 12 hours require laparotomy.
   f. Abdominal paracentesis may be done under any of the circumstances dictating local wound exploration or sinogram, but only positive "taps" are accorded any value.

Treatment of Nonpenetrating Abdominal Injuries

The approach to the management of nonpenetrating abdominal injuries is not surrounded with the controversy associated with stab wounds of the abdomen. Nevertheless, there is little question that the early diagnosis and treatment are much more difficult in nonpenetrating injuries. Frequent and repeated examinations of the patient by the same clinician are an absolute prerequisite for good management.

If the patient is not otherwise seriously injured and is alert and cooperative, the physical examination is usually quite reliable in evaluating patients for intra-abdominal trauma. The presence of generalized abdominal pain, rebound tenderness and rigidity usually reflect peritoneal irritation from blood or intestinal contents. These signs or symptoms, when localized to a particular part of the abdomen, indicate damage to subjacent organs. However, similar signs and symptoms may be due to contusions of the abdominal wall or fractured ribs. In blunt abdominal trauma rigidity alone probably warrants exploratory laparotomy. Shock and the suspicion of concealed hemorrhage are usually cause enough for laparotomy. Multiple considerations contribute to the final decision regarding operative intervention. The physical findings, the presence of associated injuries, the time of injury and the results of various diagnostic tests are all integrated into the final decision.

Much of the earlier discussion under diagnosis pertains to blunt abdominal trauma in particular. The discussion in that section of various physical findings and diagnostic procedures will not be detailed again. Although the management of each case must be individualized to fit the circumstances, it is desirable to have a general plan of approach. The basic decision, of course, is whether or not exploratory laparotomy is indicated. The following criteria are formulated to aid in making the decision:

1. Immediate laparotomy is indicated when:
   a. Signs of peritoneal irritation are unequivocal and persist.
   b. X-rays indicate free peritoneal air or rupture of the diaphragm.
   c. Hypotension persists in the absence of other likely causes or is unresponsive to or recurs after appropriate intravenous fluid therapy.
   d. Abdominal paracentesis is positive.
   e. Blood is present within the gastrointestinal tract.
2. Peritoneal lavage is indicated in those:
   a. With equivocal findings.
   b. Who cannot be accurately examined.
3. Scans and arteriograms are performed in those patients without indications for immediate laparotomy who have findings suggestive of a specific organ injury.
4. Intravenous pyelograms and cystograms are performed routinely in patients with hematuria or flank tenderness and in most patients in which exploration is planned.
5. All patients are closely followed for the development of new signs and symptoms until the need for operation has been clearly determined.

General Measures

Once the decision to operate has been made, the question of timing becomes important. Operations should be delayed as little as possible to prevent deterioration in the clinical situation and an increase in the operative risk. If not already present, a nasogastric tube and a Foley catheter are inserted. Typing and cross-matching of the patient's blood should have been performed by this time, and the responsible surgeon should ascertain that an adequate supply of properly matched blood is available.

If there are associated fractures, it may be necessary to use reasonable, temporary means to immobilize extremities so that the patient may be transported properly to the operating room. It may be necessary to perform a tracheostomy preoperatively in order to assure an adequate airway in patients with severe maxillofacial injuries. Usually, however, an endotracheal tube can be passed quickly, avoiding the necessity of tracheostomy. We prefer the use of antibiotics, especially penicillin and tetracycline, given intravenously in large doses beginning as early in the preoperative period as possible so that significant blood levels may be achieved during operation when hypotension and further disruption of protective mechanisms against the invasion of bacteria may occur. Fuller and associates[47] have recently documented the efficacy of penicillin and tetracycline, started preoperatively, in significantly decreasing the incidence of wound and deep infections after laparotomy for penetrating injuries to the abdomen. If shock ensues, large quantities of fluids are administered rapidly while the central venous pressure is monitored. Ethacrynic acid or furosemide are also given because of indications that it might prevent acute tubular necrosis.[154] Failure of the patient to respond to these resuscitative measures indicates the necessity for operation without delay. Usually, however, a significant response can be obtained. Patients respond better to the trauma of operation, and morbidity and mortality seem to be reduced if reasonable restoration of effective circulating volume can be accomplished preoperatively. One should not hesitate to continue these measures in the operating room in order that the procedure may begin as soon as blood volume replacement seems adequate. This is usually heralded by a rise in the previously subnormal central venous pressure toward normal.

Those patients in need of exploration who have a penetrating wound of the thorax should have a thoracostomy tube inserted, regardless of whether or not a hemo- or pneumothorax is present. "Prophylactic" insertion of a chest tube will prevent tension pneumothorax during positive pressure general anesthesia.

Operation

In general, endotracheal anesthesia is ideal for allowing as much muscular relaxation as required and permitting the patient to breathe a high percentage of oxygen. The patient is positioned supine with the right side elevated 20 degrees if a major liver resection is likely. Placement of a cassette under the patient to allow x-rays to be taken during the operation is worthwhile. While preping and draping, it is advised to widely expose the chest and groin as well as the abdomen.

Planning the incision and the operative maneuvers is important. Thoroughness, efficiency and controlled speed are the bywords of abdominal exploration for trauma. Patients do not fare well when unduly prolonged operative trauma is superimposed upon their original injuries. Nevertheless, it is important not to miss an intra-abdominal injury when more than one is present.

Midline incisions permit exploration of the entire intraperitoneal contents and management of whatever injuries may be encountered. Occasionally, extension of such an incision upward into the chest may be indicated for the management of injuries to the liver or, less frequently, the spleen. Rarely, a lateral limb to the left or right is needed to improve exposure. The midline incision also has the advantages of rapid execution and less bleeding.

Once the peritoneal space has been entered, one of two alternative situations usually presents itself. First, bleeding may be voluminous and continuing. Any hemorrhage noted to be coming from a specific area should be immediately controlled, but often the abdomen is filled with blood and its source is not obvious. Under these circumstances, immediate compression of the aorta as it passes through the diaphragm, either manually or with a sponge stick, can provide those few extra minutes of protection for volume restoration and definitive hemostasis. Otherwise, in the absence of significant hemorrhage, an orderly sequence of abdominal exploration, that varies little from patient to patient, can be performed so that no injury will remain undetected. It is usually advisable to repeat this exploration at the conclusion of the operative repairs.

The authors prefer to begin this exploration with the left lobe of the liver and the esophageal hiatus. The fundus of the stomach is examined next, followed by the spleen and the splenic flexure of the colon. The left kidney is palpated carefully, and the distal half of the pancreas examined. Next the descending colon, sigmoid colon and cul-de-sac are inspected, as is the mesentery of the sigmoid colon. In women the pelvic organs should be carefully examined. Following inspection of the cecum, ascending colon and hepatic flexure, a careful view of the right lobe of the liver over its dome and the diaphragmatic surface can be carried out. Attention is then directed to the gall bladder and biliary apparatus as well as the undersurface of the right lobe of the liver. The head of the pancreas, the lesser curvature of the stomach, pylorus and proximal duodenum are examined, as is the right kidney. If indicated, a Kocher maneuver is performed to fully examine the duodenum. The surgeon should provide enough exposure so that the foramen of Winslow can be seen. Blood may be seen escaping from the lesser sac into the peritoneal cavity. If this is true or if any doubt of its integrity exists, the lesser sac may be examined by dividing the gastrocolic omentum. There remain the transverse colon and the small intestine to inspect. It is most important to look at the base of the transverse mesocolon as well as the root of the mesentery of the small intestine for possible major vascular injuries. Also, at this junction, the aorta and inferior vena cava should be carefully examined for small hematomas which may signify partially contained areas of hemorrhage. If there are penetrating injuries of the intestines, the surgeon must assure himself that there is an even number of perforations, or prove that the injury to the intestine is tangential or that the penetrating missile is inside the bowel lumen. Otherwise, a small perforation may be missed. This is extremely important since a small perforation into the mesenteric surface of the small intestine may be easily overlooked. Filling the abdominal cavity with saline and compression of the small intestine can help identify bowel perforations. After careful inspection of the diaphragm for perforations, the exploration is completed.

Once the intra-abdominal portion of the operation has been concluded, the abdomen is closed. Some surgeons prefer to lavage the peritoneum with large quantities of sterile saline solution. The use of antibiotics, especially neomycin in large doses in the irrigating solutions, has resulted in rapid absorption and respiratory depression in some patients. Smaller doses of neomycin do not appear to cause this, but its usefulness in such situations may be questioned. Cephalothin instillation has not been effective.[124] Two double-blind, randomized clinical studies, one by Noon and associates[108] using kanamycin sulphate and bacitracin and another by Brockenbrough and Moylan[12] using kanamycin only, both show a 50 per cent decrease in infections with the use of these antibiotics. Although a categorical recommendation with regard to the use of antibiotics cannot be made at this time, thorough irrigation of the peritoneal cavity with copious amounts of isotonic saline solution is strongly advised.

The niceties of layer closure are of no advantage following exploration for abdominal trauma. The risk of infection is great, and these patients tend to become distended and to develop respiratory complications which necessitate forced coughing and often tracheal aspiration. Therefore, the linea alba and peritoneum should be closed with a single layer of interrupted figure-of-eight sutures of No. 28 wire. The ends of the cut wire should be turned into the fascia to prevent discomfort to the patient by their projection into the subcutaneous tissues. Retention sutures are used in very obese patients when massive contamination has occurred or when very rapid abdominal closure is necessary. The skin is left open and packed with saline-wetted fine-mesh gauze if contamination has occurred.

The use of drains has been much discussed in the surgical literature on trauma. Recent studies have shown that in 17 of 50 patients with prophylactic drains placed during laparotomy, there were definite skin contaminants on the insides of the drain ends.[109] In general, the authors prefer to drain the retroperitoneum when a hematoma has been evacuated or when significant quantities of nonviable tissue have been excised. This is especially true when such areas have been contaminated by spillage from the intestines.

However, drainage of the peritoneal space itself is usually not necessary or even advisable. However, drainage is necessary when significant wounds of the liver have required repair or resection. Draining of the left upper quadrant after splenectomy usually prevents the accumulation of serum or blood under the left hemidiaphragm, but whether there is a greater incidence of subphrenic abscess following drainage is an open question. Unless a significant accumulation is expected in this area, as from adhesions, the authors prefer not to insert drains following splenectomy. If the pancreas has been injured, drainage is mandatory. The use of soft rubber sump suction catheters for draining the liver or pancreas represents a distinct improvement. Drains should never be placed in contact with skeletal structures or intestinal suture lines. Separate stab incisions should be used to bring abdominal drains to the outside.

Bullets removed from individuals should be scored by the surgeon with his initials for later identification in court.

ABDOMINAL WALL

Hematoma

Injury to the abdominal wall alone occasionally produces clinical findings that suggest injury to intra-abdominal organs. Pain, anorexia, nausea, vomiting, tenderness, guarding and rigidity may all be associated with a hematoma of the abdominal wall. This hematoma is usually the result of hemorrhage inside the rectus sheath and may be caused by rupture of the rectus muscle or tears of the epigastric vessels. If the hematoma occurs below the line of Douglas, it may dissect through the extraperitoneal tissues of the pelvis and produce signs of pelvic peritoneal irritation.[67] Rarely, the extravasation of blood is sufficient to produce hypovolemia and shock. The fact that the hematoma is limited to the confines of the rectus sheath is of diagnostic help. Also, an abdominal mass that is palpable as the patient sits up and tenses his rectus muscle but which cannot be moved from side to side (Bouchacourt's sign) is more likely to be within the abdominal wall. Bluish discoloration of the skin over the abdominal mass suggests hematoma; however, the color change is usually not seen for several days after the bleeding, unless the anterior rectus sheath has been disrupted.

A patient may have severe intra-abdominal wounds in addition to an abdominal wall hematoma. In most instances it is safer to explore the peritoneal cavity, if the diagnosis is uncertain. If more serious injuries have been excluded and the hematoma is not large, the condition may be treated non-operatively by rest and heat applications. Since most patients with abdominal wall hematomas require laparotomy for diagnosis, it is usually preferable to evacuate the hematoma and ligate any bleeding points. The rectus sheath may then be repaired and drainage established if necessary.

Penetrating Injuries

Penetrating wounds of the abdominal wall itself are ordinarily relatively easy to manage. Following excision or debridement and thorough irrigation, they may be closed primarily, closed over a drain, or simply drained—depending upon the size and nature of the wound. Large defects of the abdominal wall, such as those which result from shotgun blasts at close range, must be adequately debrided and packed. Pedicle flaps of skin and subcutaneous tissue can be used to cover defects, but at times only packing of the defect with later skin grafting on the granulating bowel surface is feasible. If adequate primary closure is not possible without tension, Marlex mesh can be used to close large abdominal wall defects, even in the presence of infection. Once the bowel is fixed in position and covered, the Marlex is removed and skin grafts are applied.

DIAPHRAGM

Trauma to the diaphragm is discussed in the chapter on thoracic injuries. However, because diaphragmatic perforations are frequently associated with injuries to intra-abdominal viscera, it is the abdominal surgeon who sees the majority of these injuries.

All perforations require closure because of the potential for subsequent herniation and, in conjunction with liver injuries, the risk of a biliary-pleural fistula. Left hemidiaphragmatic injuries are usually easily identified. Right hemidiaphragm injuries, lying far posteriorly, are identified by palpation and exposure with difficulty. A method of facilitating exposure involves pulling the diaphragm forward by the sequential application of long clamps to the under-surface of the diaphragm (Fig. 11–10). Interrupted sutures of heavy silk are used for closure.

Low-velocity wounds located in the bare area of the liver are not usually explored or repaired. Spillage of intestinal contents through a laceration in the diaphragm requires thorough irrigation of the hemithorax before closure.

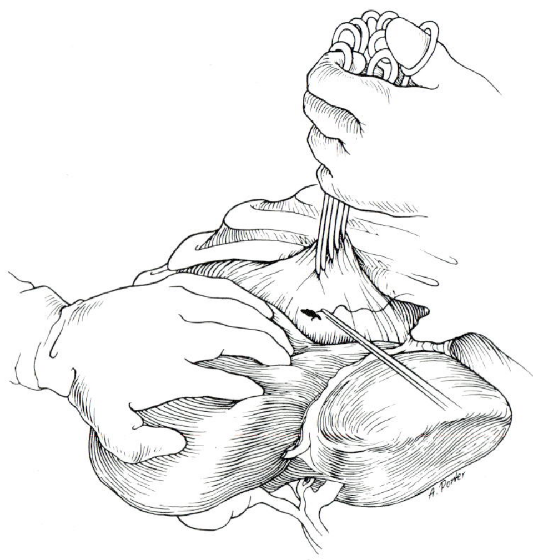

Figure 11–10 Exposure of the undersurface of the right hemidiaphragm is facilitated by the sequential application of long clamps which mobilize the diaphragm forward.

SPLEEN

The spleen is the intra-abdominal organ most frequently injured by blunt trauma (Fig. 11–11) and also is often lacerated by penetrating wounds of the left upper quadrant.[53] Massive intra-abdominal hemorrhage commonly occurs from injuries to this friable, vascular organ. The seriousness of splenic injury is adequately emphasized by the fact that the mortality rate is approximately 10 per cent; in the presence of multiple organ injury, the mortality increases to between 15 and 25 per cent.[6] In one series, isolated splenic injury occurred in only 20 per cent of patients.[118] Delayed diagnosis of a ruptured spleen contributes significantly to the mortality. The treatment of an injured spleen is nearly always splenectomy.

Signs and Symptoms

The signs and symptoms of ruptured spleen are, in general, those associated with intra-abdominal bleeding and vary according to the severity and rapidity of hemorrhage, the presence of other injuries and the time between injury and examination. The responsible injury may have been trivial and forgotten by the patient; this is especially true in children. Usually, however, the patient is seen because of and soon after a specific episode of trauma. Ordinarily, there is a generalized abdominal pain and nausea. The patient may have vomited. Pain localized to the left upper quadrant is noted in about 30 per cent of these patients. The reported incidence of pain at the tip of the left shoulder (Kehr's sign) has varied from 15 to 75 per cent. This sign can often be elicited

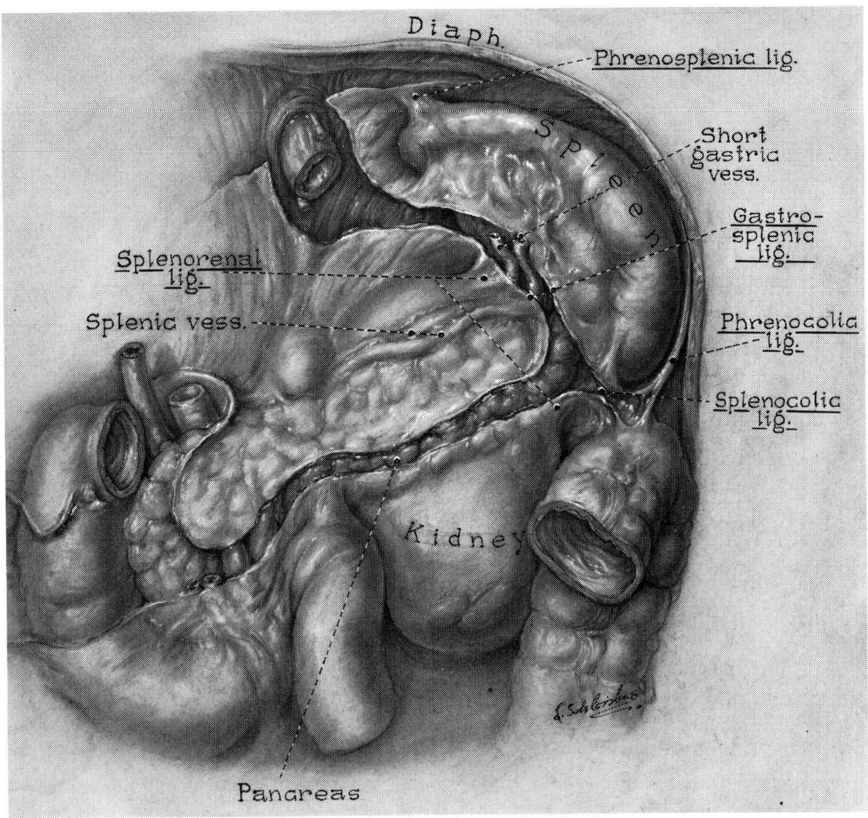

Figure 11–11 Tears of the friable, vascular spleen occur easily at the sites of ligamentous attachments, especially in the presence of splenomegaly. (From Ballinger, W. F., II, and Erslev, A. J.: Splenectomy. In *Current Problems in Surgery*, February, 1965. Used by permission of Year Book Medical Publishers.)

in patients with ruptured spleens if gentle, bimanual compression of the left upper quadrant is performed after the patient has been in the Trendelenburg position for several minutes. Tachycardia, hypotension, or both, may be present. Palpation of the abdomen usually reveals tenderness and muscle spasm, especially in the left upper quadrant. Rebound tenderness is often greater than direct tenderness in this area. Rarely, a tender mass can be palpated below the left costal margin, and occasionally, an area of fixed dullness in this region may be outlined by percussion (Ballance's sign) when a large extra or subcapsular hematoma or mass of adherent omentum is present.

The white blood cell count rises rapidly after splenic injury, and leukocytosis with white cell counts between 12,000 and 30,000 is the rule rather than the exception. The initial hematocrit level may not be helpful, but a progressive decrease should suggest intra-abdominal hemorrhage, even though the source of bleeding is not apparent. Many patients with ruptured spleens are first seen during the early period when examination may be relatively unrevealing. These patients may be dismissed, especially when there has been seemingly trivial blunt trauma, only to present later with serious hypovolemia. This error can usually be avoided if asymptomatic patients who have incurred nonpenetrating abdominal injury are observed for at least a period of four or more hours during which time careful examination is repeated frequently. Within this period, most patients with ruptured spleens will demonstrate one or more of the following:

1. tenderness to compression below the left costal margin
2. left shoulder pain while in the Trendelenburg position
3. tenderness or guarding in the left flank, and
4. some abdominal distention.

Any patient in whom one or more of these signs is elicited should be observed further and should have x-ray examinations and abdominal paracentesis. X-ray findings that suggest splenic injury include an increased splenic shadow, loss of the normal outline of the spleen, the left kidney or the left psoas muscle. The left half of the transverse colon may be depressed or the stomach shifted to the right. The greater curvature of the stomach may be serrated as a result of extravasation of blood into the gastrosplenic ligament (Fig. 11–4). Fractures of the lower left ribs, a bloody left pleural effusion, or hematuria should also arouse suspicion of a concomitant splenic injury.

Diagnosis

Despite precautions, the correct diagnosis is not made in a significant number of patients with this injury. It has been estimated that approximately 30 per cent of nonpenetrating splenic injuries result in delayed rupture.[143] About 75 per cent of these occur during the first two weeks following injury. Some of the patients with delayed rupture will have forgotten the responsible trauma.

Automobile-pedestrian accidents are the most common cause of nonpenetrating splenic injury; abdominal blows during fights and bicycle accidents are also common causes. Spontaneous rupture of the spleen is extremely rare, and even then, it usually occurs in an enlarged, diseased spleen. An apparently slight, forgotten injury almost surely precedes rupture of a normal spleen.

Splenic puncture is frequently used for measurement of portal pressures and for the injection of radiopaque material into the portal venous system. Occasionally, this results in laceration of the splenic capsule with continued bleeding. Few complications have been reported if the patient remains apneic during the procedures.

Splenic scintiscans[113, 167] (Fig. 11–12) and selective splenic artery angiograms[76] (Figs. 11–5 and 11–6) can provide useful information in a significant portion of individuals with obscure diagnostic features. False negative and false positive results can occur with both methods.

Treatment

If suspicion is high that the spleen has ruptured, operation should not be delayed. Blood and electrolytic solutions are administered intravenously during preparation for laparotomy. A left subcostal incision provides ideal exposure for splenectomy, but if injury to other intra-abdominal organs is suspected, a vertical midline incision is probably preferable (Fig. 11–13). The latter incision also permits more rapid entry into the peritoneal cavity and is therefore advantageous in the hypotensive patient. Once the peritoneal cavity has been entered, the left hand is placed over the diaphragmatic surface of the spleen, gently retracting it downward. If adhesions are present, this maneuver is not possible. The splenocolic ligament is brought anteriorly and divided. This ligament and the splenorenal and splenophrenic folds, which are divided next, are usually avascular and need not be clamped. If portal hypertension or congestive splenomegaly is present, numerous vessels that require ligation may pass through these folds.

When the ligaments have been

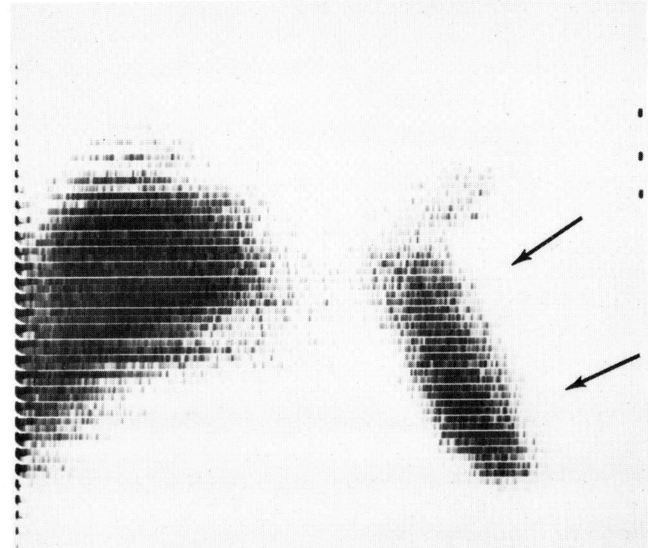

Figure 11–12 Radioisotope scan of a ruptured spleen demonstrating a large lateral filling defect (arrows) due to the formation of a hematoma.

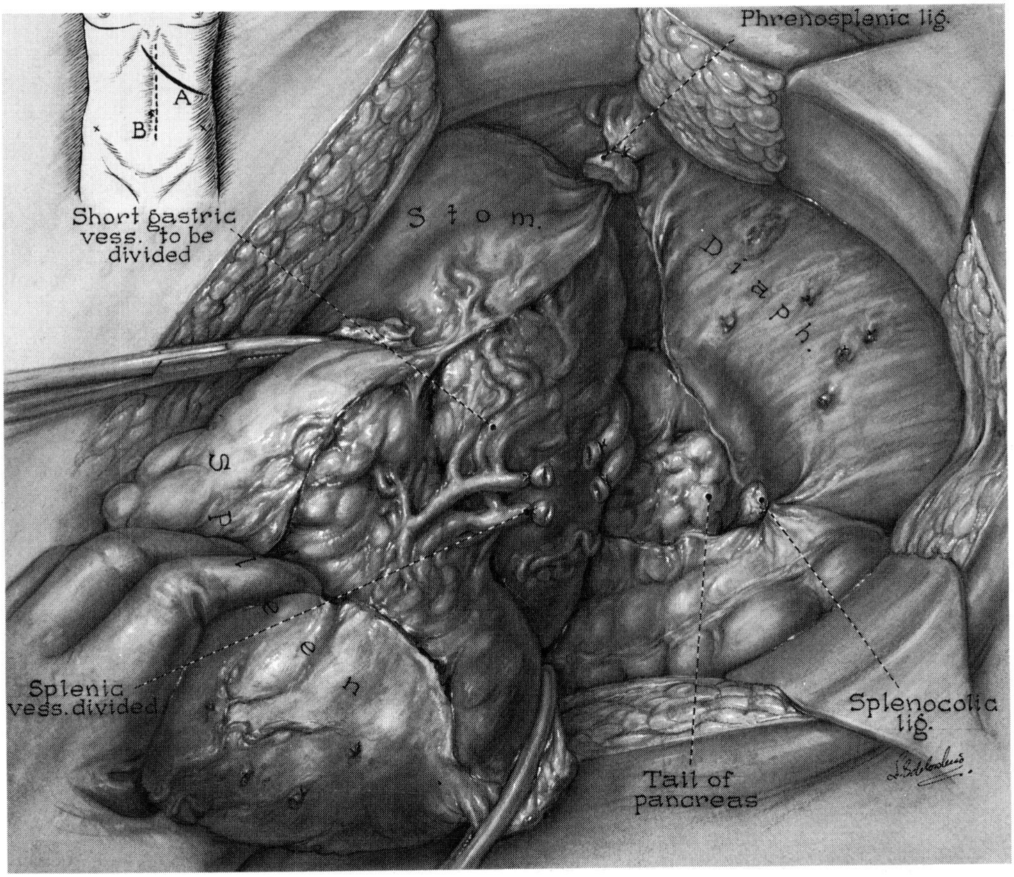

Figure 11–13 Technique of splenectomy. (From Ballinger, W. F., II, and Erslev, A. J.: Splenectomy. In *Current Problems in Surgery*, February, 1965. Used by permission of Year Book Medical Publishers.)

divided, the spleen is rotated forward and medially and delivered into the wound. In the presence of profuse bleeding from the spleen, the above maneuvers are performed rapidly and the vessels of the splenic hilum are controlled by finger compression. The short gastric vessels in the gastrosplenic omentum are divided between clamps and ligated.

The vessels in the hilum of the spleen may then be carefully isolated, clamped, divided and ligated without injury to the tail of the pancreas. The spleen is removed and the entire area inspected again for additional bleeding sites. In patients in whom the damaged spleen is solidly adherent to the diaphragm and the lateral abdominal wall, hemorrhage may be controlled by first compressing and then ligating the splenic artery at the celiac axis or on its course along the superior border of the pancreas. At these sites, the artery can be rapidly exposed by entering the lesser sac through the gastrocolic omentum. It is not necessary to ligate the splenic vein at this stage. The spleen is then mobilized deliberately by careful division of the diaphragmatic and abdominal wall adhesions. The splenic vessels are individually divided and ligated at the hilum after the spleen has been completely freed of its attachments. If there is considerable oozing from the diaphragm, a drain may be placed deep in the splenic fossa and brought out through an anterolateral stab wound. Frequently, sump suction catheters are used and removed in 48 hours if the drainage is negligible. Usually, however, drains are not necessary unless associated injuries, especially to the pancreas, are present.

Complications peculiar to splenectomy itself are few. Postoperative pancreatitis is not uncommon but usually subsides spontaneously. The potential of postoperative thrombocytosis leading to thrombosis has probably been overemphasized, but must not be ignored.[173] Temporary anticoagulation therapy should be considered if the platelet count rises to 1,000,000 or more. Splenic vein thrombosis with extension of the process into the portal vein is a rare complication today.

An interesting complication of splenic injury is "splenosis." This condition is characterized by the finding of numerous nodules of splenic tissue upon various peritoneal surfaces and is thought to represent autotransplantation of small pieces of a fractured spleen. In 1972, Trimble and Eason[163] were able to find 55 cases in the literature. Although splenosis is usually harmless, intestinal obstruction may occur if implants on adjacent loops of bowel become adherent.[50]

Increased susceptibility to infection or immunological disability has not been demonstrated in children having splenectomy *for trauma* after infancy.[35, 54, 114]

LIVER

Liver injuries encountered in civilian practice today vary from simple superficial lacerations to deep hepatic fractures with massive tissue disruption and destruction. In spite of the protection afforded by the lower ribs, the liver's size, weight, consistency, location and attachments make this organ particularly susceptible to injury from blunt trauma. Its size alone makes it the most frequent organ injured with penetrating injuries to the abdomen (Table 11–2).

In recent years, blunt trauma and gunshot wounds have been more common causes of liver injury than stab wounds. In large series of liver injuries, the mortality rate associated with knife wounds is three per cent, gunshot wounds, 18 per cent, and blunt trauma, 30 per cent.[84, 104] The patient's general condition, the number of associated injuries and the delay between injury and treatment influence the results of treatment.

A recent monograph by Madding and Kennedy is recommended for those interested in a complete and thorough review of the subject of liver injuries.[88] An understanding of the surgical anatomy of the liver is essential for surgeons contemplating major hepatic resections. Several authors have adequately described the details of liver anatomy as it applies to hepatic resection.[58, 104]

Treatment

The major goals in the management of liver trauma are control and prevention of bleeding and bile drainage, removal of all severely damaged and nonviable liver tissue, and adequate wound drainage. Ideally, the operative treatment of liver trauma includes one or a combination of the following: (1) suture, (2) drainage, (3) resection and (4) hepatic artery ligation.

Suture. Cleanly incised, superficial lacerations of the liver, similar to a hepatic biopsy wound, may be treated by suture only. All other hepatic injuries must be adequately drained. Madding[86] has stated that external drainage represents the most important step in the treatment of hepatic injury, and Sparkman and Fogelman[147] have emphasized that the size and appearance of a liver wound are not reliable indications of the probability of subsequent bile drainage. The possibility of preventing bile peritonitis or abscess by adequate drainage seems to make the omission of this simple procedure unwarranted. Lacerations with little surrounding devitalized tissue, such as stab wounds and small bullet wounds that are not bleeding, may be treated with external drainage alone. This can be accomplished with several soft rubber drains leading from the area of injury to the outside through a stab wound in the abdominal wall. Subsequent hemorrhage from simple hepatic wounds that are not bleeding at the time of exploration is unusual, and biliary drainage ordinarily stops after a few days. Suturing nonbleeding wounds is unnecessary and it may resume bleeding that is difficult to control. Also, the closure of the superficial portion of a deep wound may cause the accumulation of bile or liquified blood clots and necrotic tissue within the liver and lead to hepatic abscess or hemobilia.

Drainage. Hepatic wounds associated with bleeding that cannot be stopped by individual vessel ligature require either suture or resection in addition to drainage. The combination of suture and generous drainage provides adequate treatment for most liver wounds. When wounds are so situated that hemostasis and closure of raw surfaces can be accomplished by suture, this method is most satisfactory. If possible, bleeding vessels should be individually ligated before wound edges are approximated. Deep lacerations should be closed loosely around a soft rubber drain placed into the depths of the wound. This acts to prevent hematoma and dead space.[147]

The use of biliary decompression by T-tube drainage of the common bile duct, or occasionally cholecystostomy, is controversial. This method was advocated by Merendino et al.[103] for all but the most peripheral liver injuries. They contended that decompression of the common bile duct would decrease biliary fistula formation and intraperitoneal bile collection and prevent lysis of blood clots secondary to bile stasis. Moreover, it provides a method for checking bile leaks during surgery and permits cholangiograms in the postoperative period when abscess formation, hematobilia or jaundice occur. Recently, several authors[40, 83, 84, 117] have criticized routine common bile duct drainage. Lucas,[83] in a prospective randomized study of 107 patients with liver trauma, showed that in stab wounds larger than 1.5 cm. or in those requiring suture ligation for hemostasis of bullet wounds less than 3 cm. in diameter, the use of common bile duct drainage was associated with a significantly increased morbidity. The effect of common bile duct drainage in more extensive wounds could not be determined but is presently under study. The disadvantages of controlled extrahepatic biliary drainage includes the difficulty in inserting T-tubes in normal, small, common bile ducts and the possibility of later stricture formation, plus the increased incidence of stress ulcers as noted by Foster.[40] Our recommendation at this time is that common bile duct drainage be avoided for the minor injuries but that it be used where extensive debridement or resection is required, provided that the common bile duct diameter is larger than 5 mm.

The use of packing, except for temporary intraoperative control of bleeding, is generally condemned. The packing of liver wounds with nonabsorbable material leads to necrosis, prevents bile drainage, is followed by significant bleeding when the packs are removed, and is associated with increased mortality and morbidity. More recently, others have advised avoiding the use of hemostatic agents such as Gelfoam and Oxycel for packing liver defects.[97] These materials also act as foreign bodies and as such predispose to necrosis and infection. The cautious use of small amounts of hemostatic materials in conjunction with various suture techniques to control hemorrhage in difficult situations does not seem unreasonable and is probably more realistic than the absolute condemnation of such substances; also the gauze pack is valuable for the temporary control of bleeding during operation, although it must not be used as definitive treatment. Most hepatic wounds that would require large amounts of packing for control of hemorrhage are better resected or treated with hepatic artery ligation.

Intrahepatic hematomas are best treated by evacuation and adequate drainage. Likewise, it is advisable to explore, in most cases, subcapsular hematomas to locate and secure the site of bleeding. Formidable hemorrhage can occur in these situations, but it is better controlled at that time under direct vision rather than encountered days or weeks later when the abdomen is closed and rupture occurs.

Resection. Surgeons have recently advocated the more liberal use of hepatic resection because of the excessive morbidity and mortality following conservative suture and drainage of bursting liver wounds.[16, 96, 123] The techniques of hepatic resection are those outlined by the Quattlebaums,[123] Byrd and McAfee,[17] and McClelland and associates.[96] Exposure through a long vertical laparotomy incision is usually adequate. Depending upon the area of injury, the right or left triangular ligament is divided and the liver retracted inferiorly and medially. If this does not provide satisfactory access, the abdominal incision is extended obliquely into the right chest, usually through the eighth intercostal space. The diaphragm is then opened radially or around its perimeter to avoid injury to major branches of the phrenic nerve. Massive hepatic hemorrhage can be controlled in most instances by temporary packing and occlusion of the portal triad in the hepatoduodenal ligament with the fingers or a padded clamp (Pringle maneuver). The periods of occlusion probably should not exceed 15 minutes unless hepatic hypothermia has been instituted and not more than 5 to 10 minutes in the presence of shock.

If a total lobectomy is required, the porta hepatis is dissected next and the hepatic artery, portal vein and bile duct to the injured lobe are ligated and divided. Opening the common duct and inserting a probe into the appropriate hepatic duct is often helpful in the location and dissection of the lobar structures. Since the common duct will be drained at the end of the procedure, this step is not superfluous. When sublobar resection is to be performed, ligation of the vessels in the porta hepatis is omitted. The line of resection is then chosen, based on the more recent concepts of hepatic anatomy[58] (Fig. 11–14). A plane of resection passing through the falciform ligament should be avoided since branches of the left hepatic artery, portal vein and biliary ducts are especially profuse in this region (Fig. 11–15).

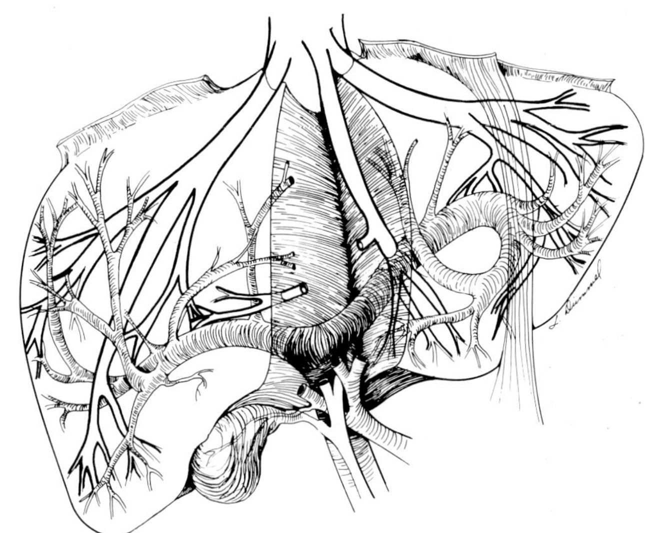

Figure 11–14 Intrahepatic anatomy. The liver is opened in the interlobar plane. The intrahepatic anatomy of the portal and hepatic venous systems is depicted. The middle hepatic vein lies in the interlobar plane and joins with the left hepatic vein proximal to the vena cava. The umbilical portion of the left portal vein is visualized in the plane of the falciform ligament. This plane is the division between medial and lateral segments of the left lobe. (From Donovan, A. J., Turrill, F. L., and Facey, F. L.: Hepatic Trauma. Surg. Clin. North Am. *48*:1313, 1968. Used by permission of W. B. Saunders Co.)

To resect the lateral segment of the left lobe, a line one to two cm. to the left of the falciform ligament is chosen (Fig. 11–16*a*). The entire left lobe may be removed by dividing the liver along a plane extending from the left gall bladder margin to a point just to the left of the vena cava (Fig. 11–16*b*). The plane for total right lobectomy crosses the liver from the right margin of the gall bladder to the right side of the vena cava (Fig. 11—16*c*). Use of these planes spares the middle hepatic vein in right and left lobectomies.

The so-called extended right lobectomy requires a line of division running from the left gall bladder margin to the right side of the vena cava. Here the middle hepatic vein, which courses in the hepatic tissue beneath the gall bladder fossa and above the vena cava, must be divided near its junction with the left hepatic vein, and great care must be taken to preserve the adjacent left hepatic vein. The vena cava usually receives three to five hepatic veins. The portions of these veins between the liver and vena cava are short and thin, and it is difficult to determine the area drained by each. It is therefore

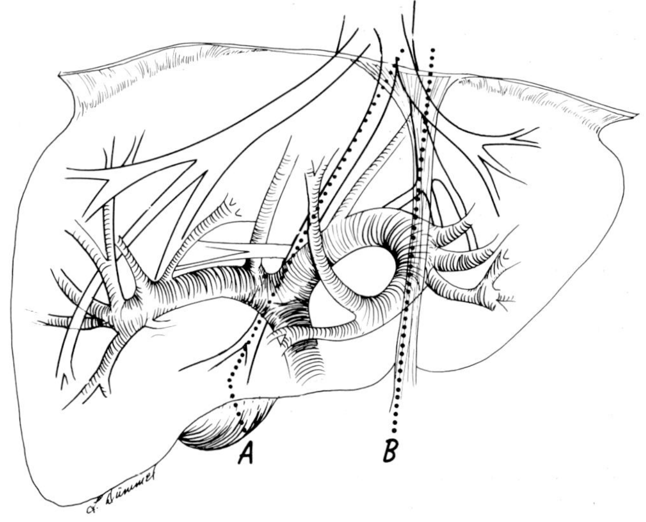

Figure 11–15 Interdicted planes for hepatic resection. The interlobar plane (*A*) should be avoided in either right or left hepatic lobectomy so as to avoid injury to the middle hepatic vein. The plane of the falciform ligament (*B*) should be avoided in extended right lobectomy or left lateral segmental resection so as to avoid injury to the umbilical portion of the left portal vein. (From Donovan, A. J., Turrill, F. L., and Facey, F. L.: Hepatic Trauma. Surg. Clin. North Am. *48*:1313, 1968. Used by permission of W. B. Saunders Co.)

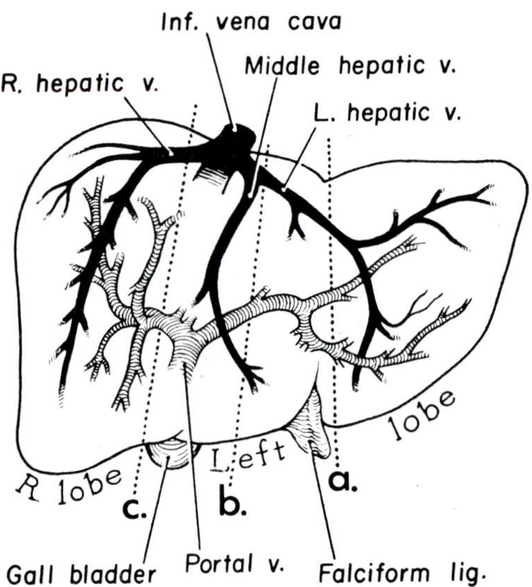

Figure 11–16 Diagram indicating major lobar and sublobar vascular divisions within the liver and the optimal planes for hepatic resection. *A, B* and *C* refer to lines of resection described in the text.

safer to divide the veins within the liver rather than at the cava. It is important when exposing the juncture of hepatic veins with the inferior vena cava that undue torsion not be applied for fear of occluding the inferior vena cava and acutely obliterating venous return from the lower portion of the body. After the line of resection has been chosen, long curved needles may be used to place rows of interlocking sutures of heavy chromic on either side of the intended line. Bluntly dissecting the tissues with a knife handle as suggested by the Quattlebaums[123] allows the blood vessels and bile ducts to be individually identified and ligated before division. This substantially reduces blood loss and bile drainage. When the liver has been divided to the depth of the first layer of sutures, a second tier is placed and blunt dissection is continued. These maneuvers are repeated until division is completed. Additional ligatures and sutures are then placed as needed. The raw area of liver can be covered with the falciform ligament or omentum to obliterate dead space. Rubber suction tubes and several soft rubber drains are placed in the bed of the resected liver and adjacent to the remaining raw surface and brought through the abdominal wall via a small subcostal incision. Drains are advanced slowly, beginning about the fifth postoperative day, and are usually out by the tenth day following operation. They are not removed if continued drainage is significant. In addition to anterior drains, McClelland et al.[96] place drains through the bed of the resected twelfth rib, thereby effecting a through-and-through drainage of the area. As mentioned, a T-tube or rubber catheter is placed in the common duct and exteriorized through a separate stab incision.

Smaller and easily accessible areas of devitalized tissue can be treated by resectional debridement.[120] The area of damage is excised between rows of tiers of interlocking catgut sutures, blunt dissection is used and, if possible, vessels are individually ligated before division. No attempt is made to close the defect and the area is well drained.

A word of caution is needed for those embarking on major liver resections. Despite favorable reports on its use, major hepatic resections are associated with significant risks and mortality and should be reserved for massive destruction or uncontrollable hemorrhage. Morton and associates[104] performed extensive resections in only three per cent of cases and noted an overall mortality rate similar to those who performed major resections three times as often. The niceties of an anatomical dissection as described by the Quattlebaums[123] or Madden and Brunschwig[85] are not always practical or feasible under some circumstances. Often simple hand compression of the liver by an assistant with the hepatic and portal blood supply occluded will permit a rapid resection followed by suture ligation of vessels and bile ducts.[38]

Hepatic Artery Ligation. Madding and Kennedy[89] have recently reviewed the use of hepatic artery ligation in hepatic trauma. Hepatic resection is certainly a formidable undertaking and the easier method of ligating the hepatic artery is often effective in controlling hemorrhage in many cases. The risk of hepatic necrosis is small, especially if the common hepatic artery is ligated proximal to the gastroduodenal or right gastric branches. Ligation of the right or left hepatic arteries probably carries more risk than ligation of the common hepatic artery but less than ligation of the proper hepatic artery. Mays[95] has demonstrated that lobar dearterialization is a safe and effective method of securing liver hemostasis. Rearterialization occurs in 7 to 10 days from the uninjured lobe via subcapsular arteries. During this period the patient is fasted and continuous glucose and albumin infusions are administered. Blood glucose and serum sodium levels as well as SGOT, SGPT and LDH values are monitored to detect evidence of liver necrosis. Hepatic arteriograms, cholangiograms and scintiscans are also useful in documenting necrosis. If in the postoperative period there is evidence of significant hepatocellular damage and necrosis, reexploration is indicated for resection of devitalized tissue.

Results of Treatment

Clinical and experimental studies indicate that survival is possible with only 20 per cent of normal hepatic tissue remaining, and the ability of liver to regenerate is remarkable. Liver function tests may be expected to be abnormal for days or weeks after major resection, but hepatic dysfunction rarely poses a serious problem if all devitalized tissue has been removed and drainage is adequate. The two most significant changes are decreases in the blood sugar and albumin. Continuous glucose infusions for several days with careful evaluation of blood sugars thereafter is necessary to prevent sudden, severe hypoglycemia episodes. The hypoproteinemia should be treated by the vigorous administration of serum albumin. The hypoalbuminemia, which may not be affected by the intravenous serum albumin, becomes most severe at one week and improves thereafter. Bleeding diathesis is not frequent, despite measurable decreases in multiple clotting factors, and when it occurs is probably due to multiple transfusions with subsequent thrombocytopenia, disseminated intravascular coagulation or pathologic fibrinolysis. Elevated bilirubin levels peak at two weeks and then gradually decrease over several weeks.

Pinkerton and associates[119] have stressed the malnutrition and gastrointestinal hemorrhage which follow major hepatic resection, and advocate parenteral hyperalimentation and early instillation of antacids into the stomach.

Abscess and hemorrhage require reoperation and must be watched for carefully. Hemobilia is easily detected if a catheter has been left in the common duct. If it has not, episodes of crampy abdominal pain and gastrointestinal bleeding with or without jaundice indicate the presence of this complication, which may occur from a few days to weeks after the injury. It is almost always associated with an intrahepatic abscess or cavity that has eroded blood vessels and biliary ducts. Hepatic scans[146] and arteriograms are helpful in locating the cavity, which must be resected or drained. Other significant complications include subphrenic abscess and bile peritonitis. Cholangiograms performed through the T-tube are helpful in diagnosing subphrenic and intrahepatic abscesses in the early postoperative period.[16]

Vena Cava and Hepatic Veins

Injuries to the juxtahepatic vena cava and hepatic vein tributaries are notoriously difficult to control and repair. Control of hemorrhage is at times unsuccessful and exsanguination results. Air embolus and, more rarely, hepatic tissue embolus are a danger.[119] Major injury to the liver may be associated with massive bleeding due to retrograde flow through injured hepatic veins which is not stopped by occlusion of the hepatic artery and portal vein.

Recently, several techniques have been suggested to solve this problem.[1,10,13,141,178] A variety of tubes, with and without balloons, for insertion into the vena cava both above and below the diaphragm, have been proposed. The main objective is to stop the bleeding yet permit the inferior vena cava blood to return to the right heart and thus avoid precipitous decreases in cardiac output. All methods include the Pringle maneuver to prevent inflow of portal vein and hepatic artery blood into the liver.

The fastest method to gain control, as demonstrated by Yellin and associates,[178] is to place four vascular clamps —one across the porta hepatis, one across the aorta above the celiac axis, another across the supradiaphragmatic inferior vena cava via a pericardiotomy incision, and the last above the renal veins. In those patients who cannot tolerate complete inferior vena cava occlusion, a shunt will have to be inserted.

Shunts inserted downward from above the diaphragm are secured by placing a purse-string suture around the right atrial appendage, excising the appendage and inserting either a No. 36 plastic chest tube or an endotracheal tube through the appendage into the inferior vena cava with the tip located at the level of the renal veins (Fig. 11–17). Side holes are cut at the appropriate level to permit the blood flowing up the tube to exit into the right atrium. A tourniquet is tightened around the intrapericardial inferior vena cava. When the endotracheal tube is used, the cuff is inflated as it lies above the renal veins. In the case of the chest tube, a second tourniquet must be placed and tightened around the suprarenal inferior vena cava. Along with the Pringle maneuver, this then effectively secures all blood flow to the juxtahepatic inferior vena cava.

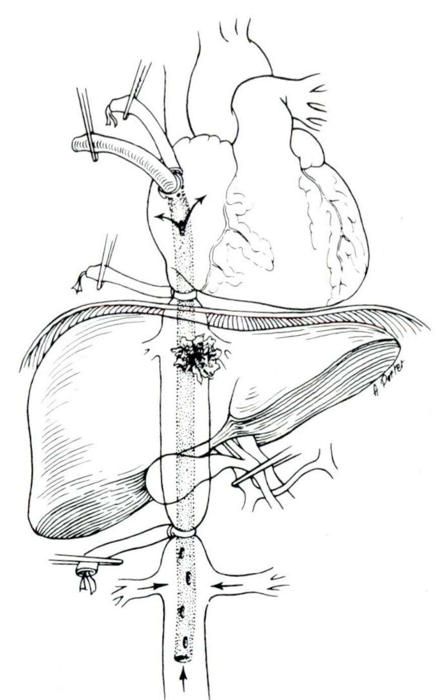

Figure 11–17 Diagram demonstrating a method of inserting a shunt via the right atrial appendage to bypass the retrohepatic inferior vena cava.

Shunts inserted upward from below the diaphragm have included Foley catheters and straight pieces of plastic tubing. Both are placed via an incision in the infrarenal inferior vena cava. The straight tube is completely inserted within the inferior vena cava with a suture secured to the caudal end for later removal. Tourniquets above and below the retrohepatic inferior vena cava are required. The Foley catheter is inserted with the balloon placed cephalad (Fig. 11–18). The side arm for inflating the balloon is brought out of the incision in the inferior vena cava. The balloon is inflated in the supradiaphragmatic inferior vena cava and a tourniquet placed around the inferior vena cava above the renal veins. Tubes with sausage-shaped balloons have been designed to eliminate the need for tourniquets and are inserted through the right atrium.[94] Despite these innovations, juxtahepatic inferior vena cava and hepatic vein injuries remain a formidable challenge.

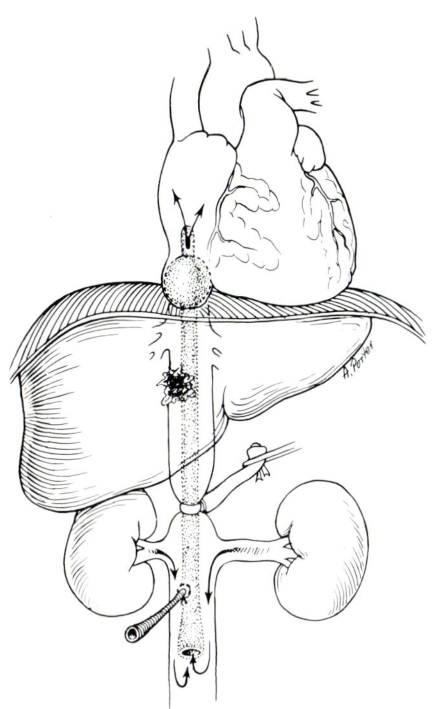

Figure 11–18 Diagram demonstrating a method of inserting a Foley catheter in the infrarenal inferior vena cava to bypass the retrohepatic vena cava.

Hepatoduodenal Ligament and Gall Bladder

Structures contained within the hepatoduodenal ligament are infrequently injured. The most common injuries are those sustained during biliary tract surgery.

Blood or bile found in the subhepatic space at laparotomy suggests injury to the structures in the hepatoduodenal ligament and requires thorough exploration of the hepatic artery, portal vein and extrahepatic bile duct. All clots should be removed, but this may restart substantial bleeding. Hemorrhage from wounds of the hepatic artery or portal vein can usually be controlled temporarily by digital compression of the hepatoduodenal ligament. Vascular or rubber-shod clamps may be applied for this purpose. Hepatic blood flow should not be completely interrupted more than 15 minutes at a time unless hepatic hypothermia is induced. The components of the portal triad are carefully dissected and exposed. Once the vascular injury has been located, it is isolated between vascular clamps and repaired by an appropriate technique of vascular surgery. Successful reconstruction of the common hepatic artery with an autogenous saphenous vein graft has been reported.[75] This technique warrants trial for hepatic artery and portal vein injuries that cannot be repaired directly.

If all attempts at repair of the hepatic artery or one of its branches fail, the artery must be ligated. Survival of patients with normal livers may be anticipated following hepatic artery ligation if the remaining hepatic inflow and oxygenation are not further reduced by shock, anoxia or high fever.[11, 89] The common hepatic artery can usually be safely ligated proximal to the gastroduodenal artery since the latter vessel will provide adequate collateral flow. Massive doses of antibiotics should probably be employed if hepatic artery ligation is required, although the efficacy of this has not been demonstrated in humans. Glucagon may be given at two mg. per hour intravenously for three to four days because of evidence that it increases portal venous flow.[87]

Portal vein injuries are usually fatal before repair can be accomplished. Hemorrhage during repair is significant and the application of vascular clamps difficult. Fogarty catheters inserted distally and proximally can be used to secure hemostasis. Primary repair or portacaval anastomosis may be used to rectify the injury. Often repair is not possible, in which case ligation is performed with the full expectation that a good result will be obtained. Child[20] has shown that acute portal vein occlusion in humans with normal livers is well tolerated.

Trauma to the extrahepatic biliary system is fortunately unusual but often leads to death if unrecognized. Although there was an 85-per cent mortality in a group of patients with bile peritonitis reported by Means,[102] the clinical course of patients with rupture of the bile duct is often surprisingly prolonged.[55] In isolated hepatic duct injuries, Zollinger et al.[182] reported an average delay of two weeks between injury and diagnosis. If hepatic duct injury was missed at the initial laparotomy, the delay was three weeks. Bile peritonitis resulting from a ruptured bile duct may manifest itself by jaundice, ascites, acholic stools and general deterioration in a patient who has suffered recent abdominal trauma. It can be particularly perplexing postoperatively if the biliary duct rupture was not recognized at laparotomy. During exploration for nonpenetrating abdominal wounds, the duodenum should be mobilized by a Kocher maneuver and the entire extrahepatic biliary system inspected. Bile straining without a demonstrable source is an indication for an operative cholangiogram.

Injuries of the gall bladder and cystic duct are best treated by cholecystectomy, although primary repair and cholecystostomy are effective when the wound is simple and may be preferred in patients with multiple other injuries or who are in shock.[144] Lacerations of the major bile duct should be carefully closed over one arm of the T-tube inserted into the common duct through an incision above or below the wound. When the common duct is completely transected, the distal end may retract behind the duodenum and be difficult to find. Duodenal mobilization, duodenotomy and retrograde probing of the common duct will facilitate the location of the distal end.[161] Using a catheter as a stent, end-to-end anastomosis with interrupted 4–0 silk sutures can then be performed. Necessary wound debridement of the injury itself may result in loss of tissue sufficient to prevent anastomosis, despite extensive duodenal mobilization. Cholecystoduodenostomy, cholecystojejunostomy, choledochoduodenostomy and choledochojejunostomy are all acceptable methods of bypass; the one preferable will depend upon individual considerations. However, the complication of anastomotic leak is more serious if the duodenum rather than the jejunum has been used to receive the bile. A very satisfactory procedure is the two-layer anastomosis of the common bile duct to a Roux-en-Y limb or simple loop of jejunum. The end of the Roux-en-Y limb should be closed and the bile duct implanted two to three cm. from this end. If the simple jejunal loop is used, an additional enteroenterostomy is advantageous in reducing reflux of intestinal contents into the biliary tract. In either instance, it is helpful to make the anastomosis over one arm of the T-tube placed through a separate incision in the common duct. The tube may be removed three to four weeks postoperatively.

PANCREAS

As surgeons throughout the country encounter an increasing number of patients with upper abdominal trauma, the treatment of pancreatic injuries has become a subject of considerable interest and controversy.[5, 32, 43, 65, 156, 158, 159] Recent reviews of the literature have clarified some of the details regarding pancreatic injuries and their management.[111, 157] Pancreatic injuries account for only one or two per cent of all abdominal trauma with penetrating trauma responsible for two-thirds of the injuries. The mortality rates (eight per cent for stab wounds, 25 per cent for gunshot wounds, and 50 per cent for shotgun wounds and blunt trauma) primarily reflect injuries to associated organs. Injuries to the head of the pancreas have twice the mortality of those to the body or tail.

The major complications of pancreatic injury are pancreatic fistulas (19 per cent), pseudocyst formation (12 per cent), pancreatic abscesses (5 per cent) and recurrent hemorrhage and pancreatitis (3 per cent). Pseudocyst and abscess formation are more common after blunt trauma and are probably indicative of inadequate drainage. A pancreatic fistula is not necessarily a complication but is the desired result in many cases of severe pancreatic injury.[111] Spontaneous closure of these fistulas is the rule and surgical intervention is rarely required. Even complicated pancreaticoduodenal fistulas have closed spontaneously with the aid of parenteral hyperalimentation.[34]

Diagnosis

Signs and symptoms are characteristically slow to appear following isolated blunt trauma to the pancreas. Some patients may be asymptomatic for years when a pseudocyst appears. At the other extreme, some injuries present with severe and persistent pain which suggests the need for immediate celiotomy. Ninety per cent of blunt pancreatic trauma cases may have an elevated amylase, but it might not be elevated initially due to transient secretory inhibition. Elevations seldom exceed 500 Somogyi units. Serial values are of prognostic importance because persistently elevated values beyond six days usually signal the development of a pseudocyst. A ruptured duodenum, among other causes, can account for an elevated amylase; therefore, if surgery is not planned but the amylase is elevated, hypaque duodenography is indicated.

The pancreas must be thoroughly examined in all patients operated on for trauma. The body and tail of the pancreas can be adequately exposed by dividing the greater omentum just below the greater curvature of the stomach and entering the lesser sac. Exposure of the head of the pancreas may be obtained by reflecting the right colon and mobilizing the duodenum. These maneuvers also allow inspection for injuries of the duodenum and the vena cava, aorta, renal and superior mesenteric vessels. Upper abdominal retroperitoneal hematomas should be considered presumptive evidence of pancreatic or other significant injury and therefore explored. Division of the ligament of Treitz will facilitate exposure of the third and fourth portions of the duodenum.

Treatment

The objectives in treating pancreatic injuries are control of hemorrhage, control of exocrine secretions and conservation of pancreatic function. The last consideration is the least important. In all the cases of pancreatic trauma reported in the literature, only two instances of exocrine and endocrine insufficiency are recorded.[111] Resections of traumatized pancreatic tissue can therefore be performed without fear of pancreatic insufficiency.

Control of hemorrhage, debridement of devitalized tissue, and adequate drainage constitute the basis for effective surgical treatment. Minor lacerations may be sutured superficially with silk, being careful to avoid the main pancreatic ducts. Sump drainage is more effective than Penrose drainage in preventing the complications of pancreatic trauma, six per cent versus 29 per cent, respectively.[5, 155] Soft rubber sump drains should be left in place for at least two weeks as drainage is frequently prolonged and may not become significant until after 7 to 10 days. Penrose drains should always be placed alongside the sump drains. The Penrose drains are slowly removed during the first two weeks, breaking up loculations.

Contusion of the pancreas with an intact capsule is best treated with drainage alone. Decompressive procedures on the biliary tract are not indicated. Lacerations without major ductal disruption should be sutured and well drained. Major ductal disruptions in the neck, body or tail are best managed by distal resection rather than intestinal pancreatic anastomosis[111, 156, 157] because: (1) exocrine or endocrine insufficiency is extremely rare, (2) resection is faster in critically ill patients, (3) bacterial contamination occurs with bowel anastomosis, (4) pancreatic enzymes are activated in the presence of bowel contents, (5) there is a 25-per cent incidence of fistulas with pancreatic intestinal anastomosis. If, however, major duct disruption is located in the head but is not complete, then an onlay Roux-en-Y limb can be sutured over the rent.[43] A complete transection should be treated by carefully closing the proximal end with nonabsorbable suture and anastomosing the distal end into a Roux-en-Y limb of jejunum.

Combined injuries to the pancreas and duodenum result in a much higher mortality rate than either injury alone. The morbidity is also increased with this injury and the treatment is much more difficult. Anderson and associates[3] claimed satisfactory management of this type injury with debridement, suture closure of the duodenum and pancreas and wide adequate drainage. Berne and associates[9] advocate antral exclusion by closing the duodenal perforation, drainage of the pancreas, antrectomy, gastrojejunostomy, vagotomy, biliary decompression and duodenal tube decompression. Pancreaticoduodenectomy is indicated when there is extensive injury to the duodenum and head of the pancreas or distal common bile duct. Sound surgical judgment is required in making a decision to perform a Whipple procedure for traumatic indications because of the significant risk involved in patients already seriously stressed by their original injuries. Thirty-four cases of pancreaticoduodenectomy have been reported with an overall mortality of 30 per cent.[3]

To summarize, blunt abdominal trauma and penetrating injuries in the vicinity of the pancreas require extensive mobilization and thorough examination of the extrahepatic bile ducts, pancreas, duodenum and other retroperitoneal structures in this area. Once hemostasis is obtained, the degree of pancreatic injury is assessed and the method of treatment is decided upon. Simple wounds may be sutured and drained externally. Distal pancreatectomy is used for extensive damage to the body and tail. Crushing injuries of the head of the pancreas are debrided and the open end of a jejunal Roux-en-Y limb sutured around the circumference of the injured area. Complex injuries of this area that involve the duodenum and common bile duct as well as the pancreatic head occasionally require pancreaticoduodenectomy, but usually more conservative measures suffice. If the patient's condition deteriorates rapidly during laparotomy, it may be necessary to confine treatment to achievement of hemostasis and establishment of external drainage. Such patients should be reoperated and definitive repair carried out as soon as their general condition permits. Regardless of the type of repair, all pancreatic injuries require external drainage, preferably with sump suction. Several Penrose drains in addition to the sump drain are placed in the area of the pancreas through a stab incision in the abdominal wall. The sump is connected to suction and the drains are not removed before the fourteenth postoperative day since drainage is frequently prolonged or becomes significant only after 7 to 10 days.

DUODENUM

Diagnosis

Duodenal wounds range from simple stab wounds to bursting or crushing injuries resulting from nonpenetrating trauma. The latter is frequently associated with complex wounds of the pancreas, liver and extrahepatic biliary systems. Such combined injuries in the right upper quadrant provide one of the major challenges for today's surgeon. The mortality and morbidity associated with complex wounds in this area remain high despite advances in resuscitation and surgical technique.[71, 165] Delay in treatment contributes to the high mortality. A delay of 24 hours before surgery is associated with a 65-per cent mortality. Those operated on in less than 24 hours from the time of injury have a 5-per cent mortality.[128]

Blunt duodenal injuries usually occur in the second and third portions and are often associated with fever, jaundice, signs of high intestinal obstruction and third-space fluid loss, especially when there is a prolonged delay between injury and examination. X-ray stippling of the retroperitoneal space, hyperamylasemia, hyperbilirubinemia and extravasation seen on intestinal roentgenographic contrast studies are all indicative of duodenal perforation.

Experience has shown that extensive duodenal mobilization, allowing adequate exposure and thorough examination of it and the adjacent organs, is essential when dealing with wounds of the pancreaticoduodenal area. Penetrating wounds in this region, bile staining of adjacent tissues, retroperitoneal hematoma and crepitation are all indications for painstaking examination of the entire pancreaticoduodenal area. The necessary exposure may be obtained by incising the peritoneum lateral to the right colon and retracting the right colon and the right half of the transverse colon to the left. This provides exposure of the retroperitoneal structures from the right side of the abdominal wall to the spine. The duodenum is then reflected to the left after incision of its lateral peritoneal reflection (Kocher maneuver). If necessary, the ligament of Treitz may be divided and the terminal duodenum retracted to the right beneath the mesentery and superior mesenteric vessels. A thorough examination of the duodenum, common bile duct, pancreas and the major vessels of the retroperitoneum may then be carried out.

Treatment

Several operative procedures have been proposed for the management of duodenal injuries.[23, 31, 158] Most authors agree that simple lacerations of the duodenum may be closed primarily, but severe duodenal wounds or combined pancreaticoduodenal injuries require procedures that provide duodenal defunctionalization in addition to repair. Cleveland and Waddell[23] listed a number of alternative procedures that may be used in the treatment of such injuries. Included in these was transection of the duodenum at the site of injury, closure of both duodenal ends and gastrojejunostomy or duodenojejunostomy. Thal and Wilson[158] have recommended pancreaticoduodenectomy, and recently Donovan and Hagen[31] have proposed wound closure combined with vagotomy, antrectomy, duodenostomy and gastrojejunostomy for pancreaticoduodenal or severe duodenal injury. Serosal patch repair has been recommended for closure of duodenal wounds in which primary repair would produce stenosis.[73, 100, 177] All these procedures have merit and are satisfactory in some instances but not in others. None is applicable in all situations, and the difference between a favorable and an unfavorable outcome often depends upon the surgeon's ability to decide which procedure is best suited for a particular situation.

It is helpful to consider not only the type and severity but also the location of the wound. Vagotomy, antrectomy and gastrojejunostomy are especially applicable in wounds of the first part of the duodenum where the injured portion of bowel may be resected along with the antrum. Tube duodenostomy is added if stump closure is difficult or insecure. Similarly, it may be possible to treat severe wounds of the fourth part of the duodenum by a resection of the distal duodenum and duodenojejunostomy of some type, end-to-end, end-to-side or side-to-side. The anastomosis must be made only to uninjured bowel. In conjunction with this, distal pancreatectomy and splenectomy may be employed for combined injuries of the body and tail of the pancreas. The major problem in the operative management of duodenal trauma arises in deciding what to do for severe injuries to the second and third part of the duodenum, particularly if combined with injury to the head of the pancreas. Primary closure of extensive wounds in these portions of the duodenum is frequently complicated by lateral duodenal fistula, postoperative hemorrhage and sepsis, which all too often lead to death of the patient.

Although it is relatively easy to transect the duodenum at the site of injury and perform a gastroenterostomy (preferably combined with a vagotomy), this leaves a long, blind, proximal duodenal loop that receives the bile and pancreatic juices. These secretions must move against the forces of peristalsis in order to decompress the proximal duodenum. Stasis and distention are therefore likely in the blind proximal duodenal limb and may contribute to the occurrence of a duodenal fistula. There is a distinct advantage in allowing the duodenum to drain in an isoperistaltic manner, and the recent report of Donovan and Hagen supports this concept.[31]

If a duodenal laceration can be approximated without tension following adequate debridement, and the associated injury to the head of the pancreas is not extensive, it may be closed with two layers of interrupted inverting silk sutures and antrectomy, vagotomy and gastrojejunostomy performed. The duodenal stump is closed over a sump-type drainage tube. If the duodenal wound is extensive and *cannot* be easily closed following adequate debridement, if the associated pancreatic damage is severe or if the common bile duct and pancreatic ducts have been avulsed from the duodenum, pancreaticoduodenectomy is the procedure of choice. By this means, all devitalized tissue can be resected and all anastomoses performed between tissues with good blood supply. If not severely damaged, the distal pancreas is preserved and the pancreatic capsule sutured to the circumference of the open end of the jejunal loop. The pancreas is further invaginated into the jejunum by additional layers of sutures placed between the pancreatic capsule and the jejunal serosa. Anastomoses are then made between the side of the jejunal loop and the common bile duct and stomach. The biliary anastomosis is made over a T-tube inserted into the bile duct through a separate incision above the anastomosis.

Regardless of the method of treatment, the area must be thoroughly drained to the outside and the gastrointestinal tract decompressed postoperatively. A sump drainage tube is laid along the pancreas and, in addition, several Penrose drains are placed in the area of injury and near, but not against, the anastomoses. Gastrointestinal decompression is achieved with nasogastric, gastrostomy or jejunostomy tubes, depending upon the surgeon's preference and the procedure performed. Combined decompressing and feeding jejunostomies are advantageous in these patients since they allow the patient to be fed distally while decompression is maintained proximally in the areas of injury and anastomoses. This approach is almost indispensable if a duodenal fistula or other regional complications occur and the patient cannot take food orally for perhaps several weeks.

The discussion of duodenal trauma must include some comment on two special forms of duodenal injury—retroperitoneal duodenal rupture and intramural hematoma.

Retroperitoneal Duodenal Rupture

This condition has been recently reviewed by Cocke and Meyer.[24] Retroperitoneal duodenal rupture usually follows some type of blunt abdominal trauma, commonly a blow to the body received during athletics, fights or falls. Cocke and Meyer postulate that the mechanism responsible for this injury is the rapid increase in the intraluminal pressure of a loop of duodenum closed between the pylorus and the ligament of Treitz. Under proper circumstances, a relatively minor force may produce a blowout injury of the duodenal wall. Since anatomic factors necessary to produce a closed loop in the duodenum exist in only a small number of people, retroperitoneal duodenal rupture differs from other types of duodenal wounds resulting from blunt abdominal trauma in that associated organ injuries are rare and the duodenal damage is usually not severe. Diagnosis is often difficult. The patient may give a vague history of trauma and have little pain and no significant physical, laboratory or x-ray findings; most patients, however, complain of pain in the epigastrium or right lower quadrant and give a definite history of trauma. Frequently, nausea, vomiting and even hematemesis have occurred. Signs range from mild epigastric or right-sided tenderness to those typical of a perforated viscus, including shock. Roentgenograms may be helpful but frequently are not. Intraperitoneal and retroperitoneal air and blurred psoas outlines should be sought; if the plain films are not diagnostic, administration of a water-soluble contrast material may demonstrate an intestinal perforation. When the diagnosis of retroperitoneal duodenal rupture has been made, laparotomy should be performed without delay. Ordinarily, simple two-layer closure of the duodenal tear is sufficient. The mortality and morbidity of this injury should be low, providing the diagnosis is made early and closure carried out promptly. Cocke and Meyer[24] point out that the duodenal rupture was not operated upon or recognized at laparotomy in 15 per cent of the reported cases, and among these patients the mortality was 71 per cent. They again emphasized the necessity for complete duodenal mobilization and examination in patients explored for abdominal trauma.

Intramural Hematoma

Traumatic intramural hematoma is another entity caused by nonpenetrating abdominal trauma; it is unusual but has been encountered more frequently in recent years.[4, 72] Patients exhibit clinical findings of upper gastrointestinal obstruction; occasionally the common bile and pancreatic ducts are also occluded. The diagnosis is frequently delayed but can often be made from a contrast study of the upper gastrointestinal tract which presents a typical appearance. Optimum treatment consists of laparotomy, complete assessment of the duodenal damage and a search for associated injuries. Since the bowel wall is intact in most instances, incision of the serosa over the hematoma and evacuation of all blood clots are sufficient in most of these patients. Duodenal decompression is maintained for several days. Gastrostomy and jejunostomy may be helpful during this period, but gastroenterostomy appears unnecessary in the management of intramural duodenal hematoma.

STOMACH

Gastric lacerations are encountered rather frequently in laparotomy for penetrating wounds of the upper abdomen and lower thorax. On the other hand, blunt abdominal trauma is seldom the cause of significant stomach injury; this is probably because of the protective location and the mobility of the organ. Bloody aspirate can usually be obtained from a nasogastric tube when the stomach has been injured. If a wound of the anterior wall is found or there is other reason to suspect gastric injury, the gastrocolic omentum must be divided and the posterior wall of the stomach thoroughly examined. In one-third of cases, both walls of the stomach are perforated. The stomach along the greater and lesser omental attachments should be carefully inspected since the fat in these areas hides wounds easily. All lacerations of the stomach should be closed with two layers of sutures; small perforations due to high-velocity missiles are excised and converted into linear closures; bleeding vessels are ligated. A continuous inverting 2–0 chromic catgut suture through the entire stomach wall is recommended for the first layer. This provides hemostasis in the highly vascular submucosa of the stomach. Interrupted Lambert sutures of 3–0 silk may then be used for the second layer of the closure. Purse-string sutures are not used because they are not as effective for the control of gastric wall bleeding. Resections of portions of the stomach should be carried out if necessary for debridement of devitalized tissue and, occasionally, partial gastrectomy is required for extensive injury. Removal of spilled gastric contents from the peritoneal cavity and copious lavage of the lesser sac and subhepatic spaces may decrease later abscess formation. As in the treatment of perforated peptic ulcer, the peritoneal cavity need not be drained if only the stomach has been injured.

MESENTERY AND SMALL INTESTINE

Injuries to the mesentery are often encountered in patients with abdominal trauma, and possible compromise of the intestinal blood supply makes correct appraisal and treatment of mesenteric damage necessary.

Blunt trauma to the intestine may be caused by shearing, crushing, tearing or compressive forces. Injuries to the proximal jejunum and distal ileum (points of relative fixation) are most common. Similarly, when adhesions are present, they may predispose to and localize intestinal tears. The mechanics of seat-belt injuries have been discussed previously. Penetrating injuries may occur anywhere and are commonly multiple, averaging five holes per injury.

The pH of the distal small bowel is often near neutral and produces less chemical irritation and thus an apparently milder, more delayed presentation is seen with lower ileal injuries when compared to those of the upper jejunum. The hazards of bacterial contamination are theoretically greater for more distal wounds in the small bowel because of the increasing bacterial flora in the caudal small intestine. Thus, it may be advantageous to close distal perforations first.

Methodical inspection of the small intestine, examining both sides including the mesentery, is essential. The ligament of Treitz is taken down and the large vessels at the root of the mesentery are inspected. Hematomas of the mesentery are evacuated, and bleeding vessels are identified and ligated. Hematomas on the mesenteric border of the intestine should be carefully inspected in case they represent perforation in this area. An even number of perforations should be found or a tangential wound identified.

Small contusions or perforations may be closed with interrupted silk. Linear lacerations should be closed in a transverse direction with a double layer of inverting sutures. High-velocity injuries require extensive debridement prior to closure, low-velocity injuries a little and knife wounds practically none. Adequate bleeding from the wound edges should be noted prior to closure.

Criteria for resection of bowel include:

1. injuries which cannot be closed without significantly narrowing the bowel lumen;
2. large or irregular wounds;
3. short segments containing multiple perforations;
4. areas that are infarcted or crushed;
5. bowel with injury in the leaves of the mesentery;
6. large hematomas at the mesenteric border;
7. large intramural hematomas;
8. avulsion of the mesentery;
9. large transverse tears of the mesentery;
10. long linear lacerations of the bowel.

In most cases where doubt as to viability exists, cover the area with warm packs and reinspect it later, prior to abdominal closure. End-to-end anastomoses are made only with bowel of unquestionable viability.

Injuries of the major mesenteric vessels are rare and usually require repair to prevent infarction. Ligation of large veins is better tolerated than that of arteries because of the more extensive collateral pathways. Intestines perfused by the injured vessels should be inspected prior to closure and resected if their circulation appears inadequate. When thrombosis of the superior mesenteric vessels occurs secondary to contusion, it usually involves the vein. Progression of the thrombus into the entire portal venous system may occur slowly over days or weeks with fatal results. There are probably many instances of minor mesenteric vessel thrombosis due to abdominal trauma which require no specific therapy and which resolve undetected. It has been suggested that some instances of idiopathic or spontaneous portal and superior mesenteric vein thrombosis are actually the result of previous unremembered abdominal trauma.[72] In any case, contusion of the superior mesenteric vessels may lead to bowel necrosis, which will require resection either initially or sometime following the responsible trauma.

COLON, RECTUM AND PERINEUM

The operative management of injuries of the large bowel may be outlined as follows:

1. primary closure;
2. resection and primary anastomosis;
3. primary closure with proximal colostomy;
4. resection with colostomy;
5. exteriorization.

During World War II the routine use of exteriorization of colon wounds by combat surgeons was associated with such a striking reduction in the mortality and morbidity that this procedure was used extensively in civilian practice following the war. The further reduction in complications attending the treatment of colon injuries observed during the Korean conflict appeared to confirm the efficacy of exteriorization in the treatment of colon injury.[135] However, several factors were responsible for the improved results. Among these were the decreased time between injury and definitive treatment, rapid replacement of blood loss, extensive use of antibiotics and intravenous fluid therapy, and the availability of well-trained anesthesia and surgical personnel. As war wounds are usually the result of fragmentation of high-velocity missiles, they differ significantly from the majority of wounds seen in civilian practice. It is now recognized that many civilian colon injuries can be treated definitively in one stage since these wounds often involve little tissue destruction and are encountered soon after injury.[8, 57, 129, 164, 177] Others have experienced excessive complication rates with primary repair.[21] Therefore, patients treated by primary closure or resection and anastomosis must be selected very carefully. An integral step in all methods of managing colon injuries involves thorough irrigation of the abdominal cavity with copious volumes of saline solution and the meticulous removal of all feculent material.

High-Velocity and Blunt Injuries

There is little disagreement that injuries to the colon from high-velocity missiles, shotgun blasts or blunt trauma should be treated by exteriorization or resection and colostomy. Right colon injuries under these circumstances are probably best treated by a matured ileostomy and mucous fistula.

Low-Velocity and Stab Injuries

If primary repair of the colon can be accomplished in selected patients without increased mortality or morbidity, those individuals are spared the time, risk and expense of a second hospitalization for closure of the colostomy. In deciding about primary repair, several factors must be considered. These include: the etiological agent, the location and extent of injury, the time since injury, the amount of peritoneal soiling, the number of associated injuries and the general condition of the patient. A young, healthy individual with a stab wound of the transverse colon measuring two cm., seen two hours after injury with no significant peritoneal soiling and no associated injuries, would be an exemplary candidate for primary closure.

Right Colon

Stab wounds of the cecum may be treated by converting it into a tube cecostomy. Other penetrating injuries may be treated by primary repair and may or may not need a venting cecostomy performed. More extensive injuries will require resection of the right colon and ileocolostomy. If there is significant soiling, contamination or multiple visceral injuries, exteriorizing colostomy or resection with a proximal ileostomy and distal mucous colonic fistula is advisable. The patient will be better able to cope with this temporary ileostomy than an anastomosis leak and abscess or fistula formation.

Transverse Colon

Primary repair, exteriorization, resection and primary anastomosis or resection with colostomy are all acceptable procedures, depending on the degree of injury. Exteriorization is reserved for injuries of the transverse and sigmoid colon in patients in whom primary repair or resection with anastomosis is considered unwise. The right and left colon are ordinarily difficult to exteriorize and are more easily managed by resection and colostomy. Exteriorization may be advantageous when the viability of a segment of colon and the necessity for resection are uncertain.

Left Colon

Exteriorization or the formation of a colostomy is difficult with this portion of the bowel. Therefore, in primary repair which is insecure, a completely diverting proximal colostomy is necessary. Those lesions with more destruction require resection and colostomy with mucous fistula formation. Rarely are resection and primary anastomosis advised.

Sigmoid Colon

If primary repair is not secure or if there is extensive destruction, then resection and colostomy with a mucous fistula should be done. There seems to be little reason to anastomose the colon primarily and then perform proximal colostomy. If primary anastomosis seems to be unwarranted following resection, the remaining bowel ends should be mobilized only enough to place them onto the abdominal wall as colostomies. The dissection required to bring the ends of colon together is better reserved for the second-stage operation when circumstances hopefully will be more favorable. The terminal colon may be too short to bring easily onto the abdominal wall following some resections of the distal large bowel; in these instances, it may be closed and left within the peritoneal cavity. The proximal colon is used for a colostomy.

Rectum

The treatment of injuries of the intraperitoneal rectum is the same as that for colon wounds. Damage to the rectum below the peritoneal reflection should be repaired primarily if possible and the retroperitoneal space adjacent to the wound drained. Access to the retroperitoneal space can be accomplished through an incision lateral to the coccyx or by coccygectomy. The latter gives the advantage of generous exposure of the distal rectum and thereby permits control of pelvic hemorrhage and repair of wounds which are otherwise inaccessible. If necessary, rectal resection with preservation of the anal sphincter can be performed through an abdominoperineal approach.[30] The repair of all but the smallest rectal wounds should be protected by a completely diverting proximal colostomy, preferably in the transverse colon, away from the area of damage where additional surgery may be required.[166] In all wounds of the anorectum, the anal sphincter muscles should be carefully repaired if at all possible and adequate drainage established. Perineal wounds must be widely debrided; if large and grossly contaminated, they are left open. Smaller wounds that have been well debrided may be closed with drainage. Extensive perineal injury requires a colostomy.

RETROPERITONEUM AND VASCULAR STRUCTURES

Retroperitoneal Hematoma

Retroperitoneal hematoma does not usually receive consideration as a primary diagnosis, except in the presence of pelvic fractures, but rather is a finding presenting at laparotomy for blunt or penetrating abdominal trauma. The retroperitoneal space can accommodate up to four liters of blood pushed into it under arterial pressure. It is possible, therefore, for hypotension to be secondary to a retroperitoneal hematoma alone. Abdominal pain, back pain, hypoactive bowel sounds (adynamic ileus), a tender abdominal or rectal mass and later bluish discoloration of the flanks are all possible symptoms and signs due to this entity. A falling hematocrit and obliteration of the psoas signs on abdominal x-ray are additional findings.

Blunt Trauma. When retroperitoneal hematoma is associated with blunt trauma, the most frequent source of bleeding is fractures of the pelvis or spine (50–60 per cent).[115] Less often, wounds of the kidney, bladder, pancreas and duodenum, and rarely injuries of the aorta or vena cava are responsible for the retroperitoneal bleeding. Evidence of major blood loss in the presence of pelvic fractures is due most often to a retroperitoneal hematoma. The bleeding will cease spontaneously in most circumstances, but in some situations over 20 units of blood may be given and the problem of stemming continued blood loss arises. The success of treatment by internal iliac artery ligation has been variable. Ravitch[125] has concluded that the mortality from operative intervention exceeds the risk of nonoperative management with continued blood replacement. Arteriography has been helpful in identifying major vascular injuries and in two cases selective injection of autologous clot into the anterior division of the internal iliac artery was successful in controlling bleeding from lacerated obturator arteries.[90] Continued need for blood replacement beyond ten units is probably a reasonable point at which to intervene surgically. At the time of surgery, the pelvic wall is explored with attention paid to the iliac vessels. If no definite source of bleeding is found, bilateral hypogastric artery ligation is performed.[136]

Other indications for operation with pelvic fractures are any findings compatible with intra-abdominal visceral injury, particularly a positive paracentesis or peritoneal lavage, or rupture of the bladder.

Retroperitoneal hematomas discovered at the time of laparotomy which are mainly situated in the pelvic area, associated with pelvic fractures and not expanding do not ordinarily need to be explored. However, rents in the peritoneum with continued blood loss or expanding hematomas and unstable vital signs after blood replacement may require exploration.

Upper abdominal retroperitoneal hematomas all require exploration because of the high incidence of injury to associated structures, particularly the kidney, pancreas and duodenum. Rupture of the aorta from blunt trauma with successful repair has been reported.[142]

Penetrating Trauma. Retroperitoneal hematomas caused by penetrating wounds must be explored to determine the source of bleeding. Some have advised leaving undisturbed those hematomas that are not actively bleeding.[116] However, the problems of rebleeding, false aneurysms, arteriovenous fistulas (Fig. 11–19) and possible injury to the main vessels, pancreas, duodenum or kidney dictate that exploration is the wiser choice after insuring that adequate preliminary precautions have been taken.[148] Large amounts of blood and a means for its rapid administration should be available. If possible, control of vessels proximal and distal to the hematoma should be obtained. When these preparations have been made, the hematoma may be opened and the retroperitoneal structures explored.

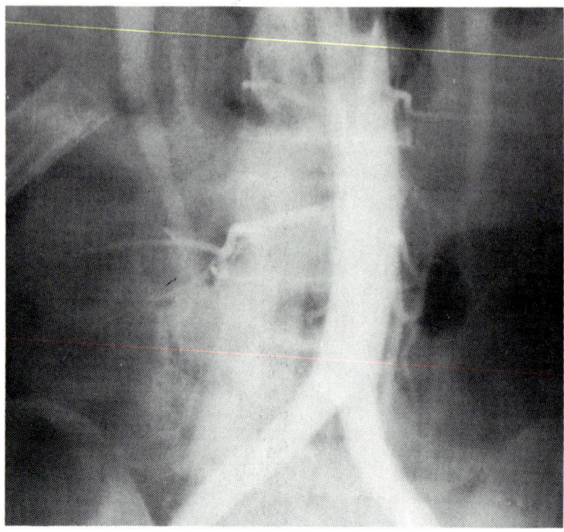

Figure 11–19 Arteriovenous fistula between lumbar artery and inferior vena cava caused by a gunshot wound. The right ureter was damaged and can be seen entering area of massive retroperitoneal hematoma. The aortogram reveals filling of the inferior vena cava via the right lumbar artery next to the bullet, which is embedded in the vertebral body.

Aorta and Inferior Vena Cava

Penetrating wounds account for the vast majority of injuries to the aorta and inferior vena cava. Patients with these injuries often arrive in the emergency room moribund and only immediate celiotomy and compression of the aorta at the diaphragmatic hiatus or direct pressure on the bleeding point will provide any chance for survival. The treatment of injuries to the juxtahepatic inferior vena cava has been previously covered in the section on liver injuries. Exposure of the aorta and inferior vena cava is provided by reflecting the right colon and the root of the small bowel mesentery superiorly and medially as well as mobil-

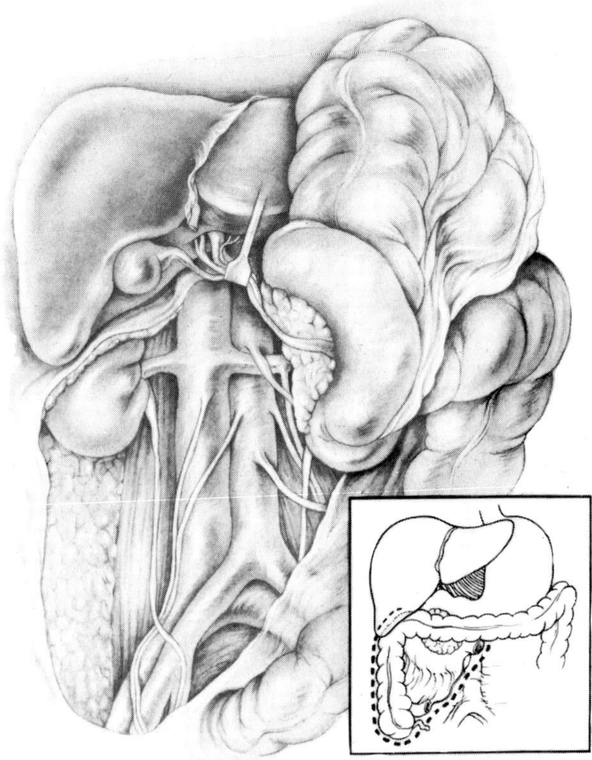

Figure 11–20 Exposure of the major retroperitoneal vascular structures by reflecting the right colon, root of the small bowel mesentery, duodenum and head of the pancreas superiorly and to the left.

izing the duodenum and head of the pancreas medially (Fig. 11–20).

Control of either the aorta or inferior vena cava will require not only proximal and distal clamps but pressure applied medially and laterally by sponge sticks or an assistant's fingers to control the lumbar vessels. Wounds are often through both the anterior and posterior walls, and at times transluminal repair of the posterior laceration will be required.[37] Most aortic injuries can be repaired by primary closure. Occasionally, a patch or circumferential graft is required. The use of prosthetics grafts should be avoided because of the high incidence of infection in these wounds. The experience in Vietnam demonstrated that a 75-per cent failure rate can be expected when prosthetic material is used in repair of the aorta or iliac vessels under these conditions.[126] A saphenous vein or an opposite internal iliac artery graft can be used in repairs of the iliac vessels when debridement and end-to-end suturing is not possible.

Inferior vena caval injuries are at best difficult and at times impossible to repair and in these circumstances the inferior vena cava may have to be ligated below the renal veins. Nevertheless, by doggedly gaining proximal and distal control and adequate exposure, repair of caval lacerations is usually possible, although occasionally only with the aid of massive blood transfusions. Iliac vein injuries may also require ligation and can be done with minimal morbidity. It is essential that suprarenal injuries be repaired.

Bullets not accounted for in vascular injuries must have appropriate x-rays to rule out peripheral or central embolism.[7] Combined arteriovenous injuries should be noted because of later fistula formation.

REFERENCES

1. Albo, D., Christensen, C., Rasmussen, B. L., and King, T. C.: Massive liver trauma involving the suprarenal vena cava. Am. J. Surg. *118*:960, 1969.
2. Allen, R. E., Morton, J., Thoskinsky, R., Stallone, J., and Hunt, T. K.: Corrosive injuries of the stomach. Arch. Surg. *100*:409, 1970.
3. Anderson, C. B., Weisz, D., Rodger, M. R., and Tucker, G. L.: Combined pancreaticoduodenal injury. Am. J. Surg. *125*: 530, 1973.
4. Bailey, W. C., and Akers, D. R.: Traumatic intramural hematoma of the duodenum in children. Am. J. Surg. *110*: 695, 1965.
5. Baker, R. J., Dippel, W. F., Freeark, R. J., and Strohl, E. L.: The surgical significance of trauma to the pancreas. Arch. Surg. *86*:1038, 1963.
6. Ballinger, W. F., II: Splenectomy. Curr. Probl. Surg., February, 1965.
7. Bartlett, H., Anderson, C. B., and Steinhoff, N. G.: Bullet embolism to the heart. J. Trauma *13*:476, 1973.
8. Beall, A. C., Jr., Crosthwait, R. W., and DeBakey, M. E.: Injuries of the colon including those incident to surgery upon the aorta. Surg. Clin. N. Amer. *45*:1273, 1965.
9. Berne, C. J., Donovan, A. J., and Hagen, W. E.: Combined duodenal pancreatic trauma. The role of end-to-side gastrojejunostomy. Arch. Surg. *96*:712, 1968.
10. Bricker, D. L., Morton, J. R., Okies, J. E., and Beall, A. C., Jr.: Surgical management of injuries to the vena cava: changing patterns of injury and newer techniques of repair. J. Trauma *11*:725, 1971.
11. Brittain, R. S., Marchioro, T. L., Germann, G., Waddell, W. R., and Starzl, T. E.: Accidental hepatic artery ligation in humans. Am. J. Surg. *107*:822, 1964.
12. Brockenbrough, E. C., and Moylan, J. A.: Treatment of contaminated surgical wounds with a topical antibiotic: a double blind study of 240 patients. Am. Surg. *35*:789, 1969.
13. Brown, R. S., Boyd, D. R., Matsuda, T., and Lowe, R. J.: Temporary internal vascular shunt for retrohepatic vena cava injury. J. Trauma *11*:736, 1971.
14. Bull, J. C., Jr., and Mathewson, C., Jr.: Exploratory laparotomy in patients with penetrating wounds of the abdomen. Am. J. Surg. *116*:223, 1968.
15. Bunch, G. H.: Shotgun wounds of the abdomen. Trans. South. Surg. Assoc. *41*:38, 1928.
16. Burne, R. V.: The surgical repair of major liver injuries. Surg. Gynec. Obstet. *119*:113, 1964.
17. Byrd, W. M., and McAfee, D. K.: Emergency hepatic lobectomy in massive injury of the liver. Surg. Gynec. Obstet. *113*:103, 1961.
18. Carey, L. C., Lowery, B. D., and Cloutier, C. T.: Hemorrhagic shock. Curr. Probl. Surg., January, 1971.
19. Carter, J. W., and Sawyers, J. L.: Pitfalls in diagnosis of abdominal stab wounds by the contrast media injection. Am. Surg. *35*:107, 1969.
20. Child, C. G., III: Liver and Portal Hypertension. Philadelphia, W. B. Saunders Co., 1964, p. 23.
21. Chilimindris, C., Boyd, D. R., Carlson, L. E., Folk, F. A., Baker, R. J., and Freeark, R. J.: A critical review of management of right colon injuries. J. Trauma *11*:651, 1971.
22. Citron, B. P., Pincos, I. J., Geokas, M. C., and Haverback, B. J.: Chemical trauma of the esophagus and stomach. Surg. Clin. N. Amer. *48*:1303, 1968.
23. Cleveland, A. C., and Waddell, W. R.: Retroperitoneal rupture of the duodenum due to nonpenetrating trauma. Surg. Clin. N. Amer. *43*:413, 1963.
24. Cocke, W. M., Jr., and Meyer, K. K.: Retroperitoneal duodenal rupture. Am. J. Surg. *108*:834, 1964.
25. Cornell, W. P., Ebert, P. A., Greenfield, L. J., and Zuidema, G. D.: A nonoperative technique for the diagnosis of penetrating injuries to the abdomen. J. Trauma *7*:307, 1967.
26. Cornell, W. P., Ebert, P. A., and Zuidema, G. D.: X-ray diagnosis of penetrating wounds of the abdomen. J. Surg. Res. *5*:142, 1965.
27. DeMuth, W. E., Jr.: The mechanism of shotgun wounds. J. Trauma *11*:219, 1971.
28. DiVincenti, F. C., Rives, J. D., LaBorde, E. J., Fleming, I. D., and Cohn, I., Jr.: Blunt abdominal trauma. J. Trauma *8*:1004, 1968.
29. Doersch, K. B., and Dozier, W. E.: The seat belt syndrome. The seat belt sign, intestinal and mesenteric injuries. Am. J. Surg. *116*:831, 1968.
30. Donaldson, G. A., Rodkey, G. V., and Behring, G. E.: Resection of the rectum with anal preservation. Surg. Gynec. Obstet. *123*:571, 1966.
31. Donovan, A. J., and Hagen, W. E.: Traumatic perforation of the duodenum. Am. J. Surg. *111*:341, 1966.
32. Doubilet, H., and Mulholland, J. H.: Some observations on the treatment of trauma to the pancreas. Am. J. Surg. *105*: 741, 1963.
33. Drye, J. C., and Schuster, G.: Shotgun wounds. Am. J. Surg. *85*:438, 1953.
34. Dudrick, S. J., Wilmore, D. W., Steiger, E., Mackie, J. A., and Fitts, W. T., Jr. Spontaneous closure of traumatic

pancreatoduodenal fistulas with total intravenous nutrition. J. Trauma *10*: 542, 1970.
35. Eraklis, A. J., Kevy, S. V., Diamond, L. K., and Gross, R. E.: Hazards of overwhelming infection after splenectomy in childhood. New Eng. J. Med. *276*: 1225, 1967.
36. Farrell, J. J.: Nonpenetrating abdominal trauma. J. Florida Med. Assoc. *43*:1104, 1957.
37. Field, S. B.: Transluminal repair of penetrating injury of the inferior vena cava. Ann. Surg. *31*:6, 1965.
38. Fischer, R. P., Stremple, J. F., McNamara, J. J., and Guernsey, J. M.: The rapid right hepatectomy. J. Trauma *11*:742, 1971.
39. Fitzgerald, J. B., Crawford, E. S., and DeBakey, M. E.: Surgical considerations of nonpenetrating abdominal injuries. Am. J. Surg. *100*:22, 1960.
40. Foster, J. H., Lawler, M. R., Jr., Welborn, M. B., Holcomb, G. W., Jr., and Sawyers, J. L.: Recent experience with major hepatic resection. Ann. Surg. *167*:651, 1968.
41. Freeark, R. J.: Role of angiography in the management of multiple injuries. Surg. Gynec. Obstet. *128*:761, 1969.
42. Freeark, R. J., Corley, R. D., Norcross, W. J., and Strohl, E. L.: Intramural hematoma of the duodenum. Arch. Surg. *92*:463, 1966.
43. Freeark, R. J., Kane, J. M., Folk, F. A., and Baker, R. J.: Traumatic disruption of the head of the pancreas. Arch. Surg. *91*:5, 1965.
44. Freeark, R. J., Love, L., and Baker, R. J.: The role of aortography in the management of blunt abdominal trauma. J. Trauma *8*:557, 1968.
45. Freeark, R. J., Shoemaker, W. C., and Baker, R. J.: Aortography in blunt abdominal trauma. Arch. Surg. *96*:705, 1968.
46. Friedmann, P.: Selective management of stab wounds of the abdomen. Arch. Surg. *96*:292, 1968.
47. Fullen, W. D., Hunt, J., and Altemeier, W. A.: Prophylactic antibiotics in penetrating wounds of the abdomen. J. Trauma *12*:282, 1972.
48. Gambill, E. E., and Mason, H. L.: One hour value for urinary amylase in 96 patients with pancreatitis. J.A.M.A. *186*:130, 1963.
49. Garrett, J. W., and Braunstein, P. W.: The seat belt syndrome. J. Trauma *2*:220, 1962.
50. German, J. D., and Davis, W. C.: Peritoneal splenosis following traumatic rupture of the spleen. Am. Surg. *32*:329, 1966.
51. Goldsmith, N. A., and Woodburne, R. T.: The surgical anatomy pertaining to liver resection. Surg. Gynec. Obstet. *105*:310, 1957.
52. Greaves, F. C., Draeger, R. H., Brines, O. A., Shaver, J. S., and Coreys, E. L.: Experimental study of underwater concussion. U.S. Nav. Med. Bull. *41*:33, 1943.
53. Griswold, R. A., and Collier, H. S.: Blunt abdominal trauma. Internatl. Abstr. Surg. *112*:309, 1961.
54. Haller, J. A., and Jones, E. L.: Effect of splenectomy on immunity and resistance to major infections in early childhood. Clinical and experimental study. Ann. Surg. *163*:902, 1966.
55. Hartman, S. W., and Greaney, E. M., Jr.: Traumatic injuries to the biliary system in children. Am. J. Surg. *108*:150, 1964.
56. Harvey, E. N., Korr, I. M., Oster, G., and McMillen, J. H.: Secondary damage in wounding due to pressure changes accompanying the passage of high velocity missiles. Surgery *21*:218, 1947.
57. Haynes, C. D., Gunn, C. H., and Martin, J. D., Jr.: Colon injuries. Arch. Surg. *96*:944, 1968.
58. Healey, J. E., Jr.: Clinical anatomic aspects of radical hepatic surgery. J. Internatl. Coll. Surg. *22*:542, 1954.
59. Heaton, L. D., Hughes, C. W., Rosegay, H., Fisher, G. W., and Feighny, R. E.: Military surgical practices of the United States Army in Vietnam. Curr. Probl. Surg., November, 1966.
60. Henderson, F. F., and Gaston, E. A.: Ingested foreign body in the intestinal tract. Arch. Surg. *36*:66, 1938.
61. Hopson, W. B., Sherman, R. T., and Sanders, J. W.: Stab wounds of the abdomen. Am. Surg. *32*:213, 1966.
62. Howard, J. M., and Brown, R. B.: Military Surgery, *In* Rhoads, J. E., Allen, J. G., Harkins, H. N., and Moyer, C. A., eds.: Surgery: Principles and Practice. 4th Ed. Philadelphia, J. B. Lippincott Co., 1970, p. 601.
63. Jarvis, F. J., Byers, W. L., and Platt, E. V.: Experiences in the management of the abdominal wounds of warfare. Surg. Gynec. Obstet. *82*:174, 1946.
64. Jett, H. H., Van Hoy, J. M., and Hamit, H. F.: Clinical socioeconomic aspects of 254 admissions for stab and gunshot wounds. J. Trauma *12*:577, 1972.
65. Jones, R. C., and Shires, G. T.: The management of pancreatic injuries. Arch. Surg. *90*:502, 1965.
66. Jones, R. C., and Shires, G. T.: Pancreatic trauma. Arch. Surg. *102*:424, 1971.
67. Jones, T. W., and Merendino, K. A.: The deep epigastric artery: rectus muscle syndrome. Am. J. Surg. *103*:159, 1962.
68. Jordan, J. S., and McAfee, D. K.: Wounds of the jejunum and ileum. Am. Surg. *29*: 630, 1963.
69. Kazarian, K. K., DiSpaltre, F. L., McKinnon, W. M. P., and Mersheimer, W. L.: Stab wounds of the abdomen: an analysis

of 500 patients. Arch. Surg. *102*:465, 1971.

70. Kennedy, R. H.: Presidential address: Problem areas in surgery of trauma. Am. J. Surg. *91*:457, 1956.
71. Kerry, R. L., and Glas, W. W.: Traumatic injuries of the pancreas and duodenum. Arch. Surg. *85*:813, 1962.
72. Killen, J. A.: Injury of the superior mesenteric vessels secondary to nonpenetrating abdominal trauma. Am. Surg. *30*:306, 1964.
73. Kobold, E. E., and Thal, A. P.: A simple method for the management of experimental wounds of the duodenum. Surg. Gynec. Obstet. *116*:340, 1963.
74. Kulowski, J., and Rost, W. B.: Intraabdominal injury from safety belts in auto accidents. Arch. Surg. *73*:970, 1956.
75. Lenyenwegen, F.: Hepatic artery reconstruction. Lancet *1*:21, 1965.
76. Lim, R. C., Jr., Glickman, M. G., and Hunt, T. K.: Angiography in patients with blunt trauma to the chest and abdomen. Surg. Clin. N. Amer. *52*:551, 1972.
77. London, P. S.: The management of persons with multiple injuries. *In* Rob, C., and Smith, R. (eds.): Operative Surgery. Philadelphia, F. A. Davis Co., 1964.
78. Longmire, W. P., Jr., and Cleveland, R. J.: Surgical anatomy and blunt trauma of the liver. Surg. Clin. N. Amer. *52*: 687, 1972.
79. Loria, F. L.: Prognostic factors in abdominal gunshot wounds. New Orleans Med. Surg. J. *83*:393, 1930.
80. Loria, F. L.: Abdomino-thoracic gunshot injuries. New Orleans Med. Surg. J. *95*:105, 1942.
81. Loria, F. L.: Collective Review—Historical aspects of penetrating wounds of the abdomen. Internatl. Abst. Surg. *87*: 521, 1948.
82. Loria, F. L.: Historical Aspects of Abdominal Injuries. Springfield, Ill., Charles C Thomas, 1968, Chap. XI, pp. 134–138.
83. Lucas, C. E.: Prospective clinical evaluation of biliary drainage in hepatic trauma: an interim report. Ann. Surg. *174*:830, 1971.
84. Lucas, C. E., and Walt, A. J.: Critical decisions in liver trauma. Arch. Surg. *101*:277, 1970.
85. Madden, J. L., and Brunschwig, A.: Right hepatic lobectomy. *In* Madden, J. L.: Atlas of Technics in Surgery, New York, Appleton-Century-Crofts, 1964, pp. 468–473.
86. Madding, G. F.: Wounds of the liver. Surg. Clin. N. Amer. *38*:1619, 1958.
87. Madding, G. F., and Kennedy, P. A.: The effects of glucagon on hepatic blood flow. J.A.M.A. *212*:482, 1970.
88. Madding, G. F., and Kennedy, P. A.: Trauma to the liver. *In* Dunphy, J. Englebert, ed.: Major Problems in Clinical Surgery. Vol. II, 2nd Ed. Philadelphia, W. B. Saunders Co., 1971.
89. Madding, G. F., and Kennedy, P. A.: Hepatic artery ligation. Surg. Clin. N. Amer. *52*:719, 1972.
90. Margolies, M. N., Ring, E. J., Waltman, A. C., Kerr, W. S., Jr., and Baum, S.: Arteriography in the management of hemorrhage from pelvic fractures. New Eng. J. Med. *287*:317, 1972.
91. Martin, J. B.: The management of shotgun wounds. J. Trauma *11*:522, 1971.
92. Mason, J. H.: The expectant management of abdominal stab wounds. J. Trauma *4*:210, 1964.
93. Maynard, A. de L., and Ordeza, G.: Mandatory operation for penetrating wounds of the abdomen. Am. J. Surg. *115*:307, 1968.
94. Mays, E. T.: Complex penetrating hepatic wounds. Ann. Surg. *173*:421, 1971.
95. Mays, E. T.: Lobar dearterialization for exsanguinating wounds of the liver. J. Trauma *12*:397, 1972.
96. McClelland, R., Shires, T., and Poulos, E.: Hepatic resection for massive trauma. J. Trauma *4*:282, 1964.
97. McClelland, R. N., and Shires, T.: Management of liver trauma in 259 consecutive patients. Ann. Surg. *161*:248, 1965.
98. McCort, J. J.: Radiographic Examination in Blunt Abdominal Trauma. Philadelphia, W. B. Saunders Co., 1966.
99. McCoy, J., and Wolma, F. J.: Abdominal tap: indication, technic and results. Am. J. Surg. *122*:693, 1971.
100. McKittrick, J. E.: Use of a serosal patch in repair of a duodenal fistula. Calif. Med. *103*:433, 1965.
101. McNabney, W. K., and McCanse, A.: Management of abdominal stab wounds. Am. J. Surg. *114*:726, 1967.
102. Means, R. L.: Bile peritonitis. Am. Surg. *30*:583, 1964.
103. Merendino, K. A., Dillard, D. A., and Cammock, E. E.: The concept of surgical biliary decompression in the management of liver trauma. Surg. Gynec. Obstet. *117*:285, 1963.
104. Morton, J. R., Roys, G. D., and Bricker, D. L.: The treatment of liver injuries. Surg. Gynec. Obstet. *134*:298, 1972.
105. Moss, L. K., Schmidt, F. E., and Creech, O.: Analysis of 550 stab wounds of the abdomen. Am. Surg. *28*:483, 1962.
106. Nance, F. C., and Cohn, I., Jr.: Surgical judgment in the management of stab wounds of the abdomen. Ann. Surg. *170*:569, 1969.
107. Netterville, R. E., and Hardy, J. D.: Pene-

trating wounds of the abdomen. Analysis of 55 cases with problems in management. Ann. Surg. *166*:232, 1967.
108. Noon, G. P., Beall, A. C., Jr., Jordan, G. L., Jr., Riggs, S., and DeBakey, M. E.: Clinical evaluation of peritoneal irrigation with antibiotic solution. Surgery *62*:73, 1967.
109. Nora, P. F., Vanecko, R. M., and Bransfield, J. J.: Prophylactic abdominal drains. Arch. Surg. *105*:173, 1972.
110. Norell, H. G.: Traumatic rupture of the spleen diagnosed by selective arteriography. Acta Radiol. *48*:449, 1957.
111. Northrup, W. R., III, and Simmons, R. L.: Pancreatic trauma: a review. Surgery *71*:27, 1972.
112. Olsen, W. R., and Hildreth, D. H.: Abdominal paracentesis and peritoneal lavage in blunt abdominal trauma. J. Trauma *11*:824, 1971.
113. O'Mara, R. E., Hall, R. C., and Dombroski, D. L.: Scintiscanning in the diagnosis of rupture of the spleen. Surg. Gynec. Obstet. *131*:1077, 1970.
114. Orlando, J. C., and Moore, T. C.: Splenectomy for trauma in childhood. Surg. Gynec. Obstet. *134*:94, 1972.
115. Orloff, M. J., and Charters, A. C.: Injuries of the small bowel and mesentery and retroperitoneal hematoma. Surg. Clin. N. Amer. *52*:729, 1972.
116. Ochsner, J. L., Crawford, E. S., and DeBakey, M. E.: Injuries of the vena cava caused by external trauma. Surgery *49*:397, 1961.
117. Payne, W. D., Terz, J. J., and Lawrence, W., Jr.: Major hepatic resection for trauma. Ann. Surg. *170*:929, 1969.
118. Perry, J. F., Jr.: Blunt and penetrating abdominal injuries. Curr. Probl. Surg. May, 1970.
119. Pinkerton, J. A., Sawyer, J. L., and Foster, J. H.: A study of the postoperative course after hepatic lobectomy. Ann. Surg. *173*:800, 1971.
120. Poulos, E.: Hepatic resection for massive liver injuries. Ann. Surg. *157*:525, 1963.
121. Pridgen, J. E., Herff, A. F., Jr., Watkins, H. O., Halbert, D. S., D'Avila, R., Crouch, D. M., and Prud'Homme, J. L.: Penetrating wounds of the abdomen: analysis of 776 operative cases. Ann. Surg. *165*:901, 1967.
122. Printen, K. J., Freeark, R. J., and Shoemaker, W. C.: Conservative management of penetrating abdominal wounds. Arch. Surg. *96*:899, 1968.
123. Quattlebaum, J. K., and Quattlebaum, J. K., Jr.: Technic of hepatic lobectomy. Ann. Surg. *149*:648, 1959.
124. Rambo, W. M.: Irrigation of the peritoneal cavity with cephalothin. Am. J. Surg. *123*:192, 1972.
125. Ravitch, M. M.: Hypogastric artery ligation in acute pelvic trauma. Surgery *56*: 601, 1964.
126. Rich, N. M., and Hughes, C. W.: The fate of prosthetic material used to repair vascular injuries in contaminated wounds. J. Trauma *12*:459, 1972.
127. Richter, R. M., and Zaki, M. H.: Selective conservative management of penetrating abdominal wounds. Ann. Surg. *166*:238, 1967.
128. Roman, E., Silva, Y. J., and Lucas, C.: Management of blunt duodenal injury. Surg. Gynec. Obstet. *132*:7, 1971.
129. Roof, W. R., Morris, G. C., Jr., and DeBakey, M. E.: Management of perforating injuries to the colon in civilian practice. Am. J. Surg. *99*:641, 1960.
130. Root, H. D.: When to explore the abdomen with penetrating wounds. *In* Pridgen, J. E., Aust, J. B., and Fisher, G. W., eds.: Penetrating Wounds of the Abdomen, Springfield, Ill., Charles C Thomas, 1970.
131. Root, H. D., Hauser, C. W., McKinley, C. R., LaFave, J. W., and Mendiola, R. P., Jr.: Diagnostic peritoneal lavage. Surgery *57*:633, 1965.
132. Root, H. D., Keizer, P. J., and Perry, J. F., Jr.: The clinical and experimental aspects of peritoneal response to injury. Arch. Surg. *95*:531, 1967.
133. Root, H. D., Keizer, P. J., and Perry, J. F., Jr.: Peritoneal trauma, experimental and clinical studies. Surgery *62*:679, 1967.
134. Roswit, B., Malsky, S. J., and Reid, C. B.: Severe radiation injuries of the stomach, small intestine, colon and rectum. Am. J. Roentgenol. Radium Ther. Nucl. Med. *114*:460, 1972.
135. Sanders, R. J.: The management of colon injuries. Surg. Clin. N. Amer. *43*:457, 1963.
136. Seavers, R., Lynch, J., Ballard, R., Jernigan, S., and Johnson, J.: Hypogastric artery ligation for uncontrollable hemorrhage in acute pelvic trauma. Surgery 55: 516, 1964.
137. Shaftan, G. W.: Indications for operation in abdominal trauma. Am. J. Surg. *99*:657, 1960.
138. Shaftan, G. W.: Selective conservatism in penetrating abdominal trauma. Surgery *59*:650, 1966.
139. Sherman, R. T., and Parrish, R. A.: Management of shotgun injuries. J. Trauma *3*:76, 1963.
140. Shirkey, A. L., Wukasch, D. C., Beall, A. C., Jr., Gordon, W. B., and DeBakey, M. E.: Surgical management of splenic injuries. Am. J. Surg. *108*:630, 1964.
141. Shrock, T., Blaisdell, F. W., and Mathewson, C.: Management of blunt trauma to the liver and hepatic veins. Arch. Surg. *96*:698, 1968.
142. Sinclair, T. L., and Stephenson, H. E., Jr.:

Survival following abdominal aortic rupture from blunt trauma. Missouri Med. *69*:271, 1972.
143. Sizer, J. S., Wayne, E. R., and Frederick, P. L.: Delayed rupture of the spleen. Arch. Surg. *92*:362, 1966.
144. Smith, S. W., and Hastings, T. N.: Traumatic rupture of the gallbladder. Ann. Surg. *139*:517, 1954.
145. Sorour, V. E., and Bijlsma, P. J.: Stab wounds of the abdomen. S. Afr. J. Surg. *4*:85, 1966.
146. Sparkman, P. S.: Massive hemobilia following traumatic rupture of the liver. Ann. Surg. *138*:899, 1953.
147. Sparkman, R. S., and Fogelman, M. J.: Wounds of the liver. Ann. Surg. *139*: 690, 1954.
148. Starzl, T. E., Kaupp, H. A., Beheler, Z. M., and Freeark, R. J.: Penetrating injuries of the inferior vena cava. Surg. Clin. N. Amer. *43*:87, 1963.
149. Steichen, F. M.: Penetrating wounds of the chest and the abdomen. Curr. Probl. Surg. August, 1967.
150. Steichen, F. M., Efron, G., Pearlman, D. M., and Weil, P. H.: Radiographic diagnosis versus selective management in penetrating wounds of the abdomen. Ann. Surg. *170*:978, 1969.
151. Steichen, F. M., Pearlman, D. M., Dargan, E. L., Prommas, D. C., and Weil, P. H.: Wounds of the abdomen: Radiographic diagnosis of intraperitoneal penetration. Ann. Surg. *165*:77, 1967.
152. Steigmann, F., and Doleheck, R. A.: Corrosive (acid) gastritis. New Eng. J. Med. *254*:981, 1956.
153. Stein, A., and Lissoos, I.: Selective management of penetrating wounds of the abdomen. J. Trauma *8*:1014, 1968.
154. Stone, A. M., and Stahl, W. M.: Effect of ethacrynic acid and furosemide on renal function in hypovolemia. Ann. Surg. *174*:1, 1971.
155. Stone, H. H., Stowers, K. B., and Shippey, S. H.: Injuries to the pancreas. Arch. Surg. *85*:525, 1962.
156. Sturim, H. S.: Surgical management of traumatic transection of the pancreas. Ann. Surg. *163*:399, 1966.
157. Sturim, H. S.: The surgical management of pancreatic injuries. Surg. Gynec. Obstet. *122*:133, 1966.
158. Thal, A. P., and Wilson, R. F.: A pattern of severe trauma to the region of the pancreas. Surg. Gynec. Obstet. *119*: 773, 1964.
159. Thompson, R. J., and Hinshaw, D. B.: Pancreatic trauma. Ann. Surg. *163*:153, 1966.
160. Tobias, S., DeClement, F. A., and Cleveland, J. C.: Management of abdominal stab wounds: Roentgenographic technique for diagnosis of peritoneal penetration. Arch. Surg. *95*:27, 1967.
161. Tolins, S. H.: Complete severance of the common bile duct due to blunt trauma. Ann. Surg. *140*:61, 1959.
162. Trimble, C.: Stab wound sinography. Surg. Clin. N. Amer. *49*:1217, 1969.
163. Trimble, C., and Eason, F. J.: A complication of splenosis. J. Trauma *12*:358, 1972.
164. Vannix, R. S., Carter, R., Hinshaw, D. B., and Joergenson, E. J.: Surgical management of colon trauma in civilian practice. Am. J. Surg. *106*:364, 1963.
165. Webb, H. W., Howard, J. M., Jordan, G. L., and Vowles, D. J.: Surgical experiences in the treatment of duodenal injuries. Internatl. Abstr. Surg. *106*:105, 1958.
166. Weckesser, E. C., and Putnam, T. C.: Perforating injuries of the rectum and sigmoid colon. J. Trauma *2*:474, 1962.
167. Werner, L.: Scintiscan diagnosis of splenic hematoma. Surg. Gynec. Obstet. *134*: 430, 1972.
168. Whelan, T. J., Burkhalter, W. E., and Gomez, A.: Management of war wounds. *In* Claude E. Welch, ed.: Advances in Surgery. Vol. 3. Chicago, Year Book Medical Publishers, 1968, pp. 227–350.
169. White, P. H., and Benfield, J. R.: Amylase in the management of pancreatic trauma. Arch. Surg. *105*:158, 1972.
170. Wilder, J. R., Habermann, E. T., and Schachner, S. J.: Selective surgical intervention for stab wounds of the abdomen. Surgery *61*:231, 1967.
171. Williams, J. S., and Kirkpatrick, J. R.: The nature of seat belt injuries. J. Trauma *11*:207, 1971.
172. Willis, B. C.: Shotgun wounds of the abdomen. Am. J. Surg. *28*:407, 1935.
173. Willox, G. L.: Nonpenetrating injuries of abdomen causing rupture of spleen. Arch. Surg. *90*:498, 1965.
174. Wilson, C. B., Vidrine, A., Jr., and Rives, J. D.: Unrecognized abdominal trauma in patients with head injuries. Ann. Surg. *161*:608, 1965.
175. Wilson, H., and Sherman, R.: Civilian penetrating wounds of the abdomen. I. Factors in mortality and differences from military wounds in 494 cases. Ann. Surg. *153*:639, 1961.
176. Wolfman, E. F., Jr., Trevino, G., Heaps, D. K., and Zuidema, G. D.: An operative technic for the management of acute and chronic lateral duodenal fistulas. Ann. Surg. *159*:563, 1964.
177. Wolma, F. J., and Williford, F., III: Treatment of injuries to the colon. Am. J. Surg. *110*:772, 1965.
178. Yellin, A. E., Chaffee, C. B., and Donovan, A. J.: Vascular isolation in treatment of juxtahepatic venous injuries. Arch. Surg. *102*:566, 1971.
179. Yellin, A. E., Vecchione, T. R., and Donovan, A. J.: Distal pancreatectomy in

trauma to the pancreas. Am. J. Surg. *124*:135, 1972.

180. Yurko, A. A., and Williams, R. D.: Needle paracentesis in blunt abdominal trauma: a critical analysis. J. Trauma *6*:194, 1966.
181. Zacheis, H. G., and Condon, R. E.: Seat belts and intraabdominal trauma: report of two unusual cases. J. Trauma *12*:85, 1972.
182. Zollinger, R. M., Keller, R. T., and Hubay, C. A.: Traumatic rupture of the right and left hepatic ducts. J. Trauma *12*: 563, 1972.
183. Zuidema, G. D.: In discussion of Nance, F. C., and Cohn, I.: Surgical judgment in the management of stab wounds of the abdomen: a retrospective and prospective analysis based on a study of 600 stabbed patients. Ann. Surg. *170*:569, 1969.

chapter

12

TRAUMA OF THE GENITOURINARY SYSTEM

Rainer M. E. Engel, M.D.

Motor vehicle accidents as etiologic factors of urinary tract injury by far outnumber others, such as industrial accidents, bullet wounds, stab wounds, the occasional iatrogenic trauma or the rare self-inflicted injury. The victims of such accidents usually sustain compound injuries that involve multiple organ systems in addition to the genitourinary tract, namely, skeletomuscular (e.g., fractures), gastrointestinal (e.g., perforated viscus) or vascular (e.g., hemorrhage) trauma. It is obvious that some of these injuries might be life-threatening, whereas others may not necessarily require immediate intervention. Thus, a rapid diagnostic evaluation to assess priorities in treatment is of utmost importance. Usually, genitourinary injury is of secondary importance. It is our strong conviction that, in the best interest of the severely injured patient, one individual, preferably a general surgeon, be charged with the overall care of the patient.

Team discussion and cooperation decide the priorities of treatment which has to be directed to life-threatening problems: restoration and maintenance of an adequate airway and pulmonary function, restoration of blood loss, control of hemorrhage, closure of perforations in various organ systems, and stabilization of fractures.

In injuries that are limited to the genitourinary tract, such intense teamwork is not necessary. Clinical evaluation in this group may be primarily directed toward the genitourinary tract, whereas in the patient with complex injuries, full urologic evaluation often has to wait until the overall condition of the patient has been stabilized or improved.

RENAL INJURIES

Injuries to a kidney can be classified by the causative factor into *penetrating* and *nonpenetrating* injuries, or, as we have found useful, on the basis of clinical symptomatology, into *minor, major* and *critical* injuries.

The adult kidney is extremely well protected by the rib cage posteriorly and posterolaterally and the abdominal viscera anteriorly. In addition, it is suspended in a fatpad confined by Gerota's fascia, which serves as a buffer. Renal injuries in the pediatric age group are somewhat more common since the kidney has not reached its protected position in the lower part of the rib cage, and because the para- and perirenal fatpad is not as well developed as in the adult. Thus, the renal parenchyma in children is somewhat more prone to contusions and lacerations. Also, the ureteropelvic junction has been seen to shear-off, probably also due to the lack of "buffering suspension" supporting the kidney.

It is worthwhile to remember that pre-existing renal disease may predispose to severe renal damage in even minor trauma. This is particularly true for hydronephrosis but also for cystic disease, chronic infection or malignant degeneration.[5, 46, 50]

Malpositioning of the kidney, particularly over bony prominences, such as the spine or sacrum, can also lead to significant damage with *minor* injuries.

Renal injuries account for approximately one-half of all injuries to the genitourinary tract. Waterhouse and Gross[57] found, in a series of 251 patients with genitourinary injuries, 116 renal injuries, 38 injuries to the bladder and 23 injuries to the urethra; the remainder were injuries to the external genitalia. The incidence of renal injuries in association with other trauma is difficult to assess from the literature as most authors do *not* state such figures. However, Scott et al.[49] report that in a total of 2525 patients with penetrating wounds of the abdomen, 7 per cent (181 patients) had associated renal injuries. This incidence was essentially equal for both gunshot wounds and stab wounds. Waterhouse[57] reports on 9660 patients who were admitted to the Trauma Service of King's County Hospital Center, of whom 251 patients (2.5 per cent) had injuries to the genitourinary tract. The incidence of renal injury is highest in the second and third decades and involves predominantly male patients.[12, 46, 57] (See also Table 12–1.)

Abdominal rigidity as a sign of renal trauma is often difficult to assess since

TABLE 12–1 RENAL INJURIES

		SCOTT (1)	SCOTT (2)	GLENN	SCHOLL	TOTALS Number	TOTALS Per Cent
No. of Patients		111	181	84	478	854	
Etiology							
	Gunshot Wounds		127	1	56	238	28 %
	Stab Wounds		54				
	Motor Vehicles	59 (52%)		34	264	357	42 %
	Falls	26 (24%)		27	88	141	16.5%
	Sports	26 (24%)		16	62	104	12 %
	Other			6	8	14	1.5%
Sex	Male			66	382	448/562	79.8%
	Female			18	96	114/562	21.2%
Flank or Abdominal	*Pain*	94 (85%)		74	359	567/673	78.3%
	Mass		170	11	88	269/743	36.2%
Hematuria	Gross	92 (83%)	140 (71%)	44	427	757/854	88.5%
	Micro	111 (100%)		35			
Associated Injury			> 80%	36	334	370/562	65.8%

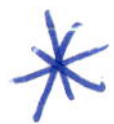

TABLE 12–2 ROUTINE FOR DETECTION OF UROLOGICAL TRAUMA IN THE PRESENCE OF OTHER INJURIES*

1. Transfer to Proper Stretcher.	6. Infusion Intravenous Pyelography.
2. Urological History.	7. Retrograde Cystourethrography.
3. Evaluation of Symptoms.	8. Retrograde Cystoscopy & Retrograde Pyelography.
4. Physical Examination.	9. Arteriography.
5. Initial X-ray Examination.	10. Catheter Drainage.

*Modified from Orkin.[38]

many of these patients have sustained other abdominal injuries; shock may be due to blood loss from renal causes due to extrarenal injuries.

The diagnosis of a renal injury may at times be difficult. We have adopted and, with modification, still adhere to the diagnostic outline presented over ten years ago by Orkin[38] for the diagnosis of trauma to the genitourinary tract (Table 12–2):

Proper Stretcher. Immediately upon arrival in the accident room, the patient is placed on a radiolucent stretcher. These stretchers are equipped with a Bucky and can be wheeled under a stationary x-ray machine. Films obtained in this manner are far superior to those obtained in bed with portable equipment. The stretcher allows not only rapid x-ray examination but also proper physical evaluation and emergency treatment.

Urological History. A careful urologic history is of utmost importance. The area of the greatest blow may direct attention to the injured organ in patients with blunt trauma. The patient will usually know the time of last micturition and whether or not the urine was bloody. A past history of urologic diseases, instrumentation and, particularly, surgery should be asked for. Some of this information may be gathered from relatives should the patient be unconscious. In particular, the preceding surgical removal of a kidney has to be ruled out.

Evaluation of Symptoms. The diagnosis of renal injury may at times be difficult. Hematuria, either gross or microscopic, is the most frequent finding of renal injury. However, we are at variance with Scott et al.,[48] who state, ". . . Indeed, microscopic hematuria was a required criterion of renal injury." It is evident from the literature that the absence of hematuria does *not* exclude even *major* renal injury since, in some injuries, occlusion or severance of the vascular pedicle or complete disruption of the ureter may prevent the passage of urine and blood into the lower urinary tract. Gross hematuria is seen in more than one-half of patients with renal injuries, and only 5–10 per cent do *not* exhibit microscopic hematuria. Hematuria may be transient and cease after a few hours or may continue for days. Gross hematuria usually clears within a matter of hours, but we have seen an occasional patient who has bled intermittently for weeks following renal trauma. It is important to point out that cessation of hematuria is *not* identical with healing of the injury since clots may obstruct the source of bleeding or the injured kidney may actually decrease its output and finally cease to function.

Localizing flank or abdominal pain is seen in 80–85 per cent of all patients. Since up to 80 per cent of patients with renal trauma have associated injuries, the symptomatology from the involvement of other organ systems may mask renal injury. The absence of flank mass does *not* exclude the possibility of even *major* renal trauma, as shown by Scott.[48, 49] Therefore, only a high degree of suspicion will lead to the early and correct diagnosis. Pain may be only slight but can be severe and agonizing. Typical renal colic can be seen with radiation from the flank into the groin, external genitalia and inner aspect of the thigh. Such colicky pains may be due to the passage of blood clots.

X-Ray Examination. A plain film of the abdomen is obtained. Fractures of the lower ribs or the dorsolumbar transverse processes are suggestive of associated renal trauma. Obliteration of the psoas shadow or the renal shadow may direct the attention of the attending physician toward renal trauma but is *not* reliable. Scott[48] reports 28 per cent of blunt *nonpenetrating* renal trauma to show such radiologic signs, but Glenn[12] found them in only 13 per cent of his patients. Thus, the absence of these findings is *inconclusive,* whereas their presence makes renal trauma highly suspicious.

Excretory urography is performed with *infusion pyelography.* There is significant discrepancy among the various authors concerning the percentage in which excretory urography is diagnostic of renal injury. Glenn[12] reports this figure as 50 per cent; Scott reports the incidence of diagnostic intravenous pyelograms as slightly over 60 per cent in patients with penetrating renal injuries[49] and slightly less than 40 per cent in patients with nonpenetrating renal injuries.[48] Rieser[44] reports this figure to be as low as 25 per cent of his cases. In patients who are in shock, renal perfusion is inadequate to permit adequate excretion of the dye and thus, insufficient visualization of the kidneys results.

The extent and exact localization of renal trauma is best visualized by other radiographic methods. The major value of excretory urography may well be in establishing the presence and adequate function of the contralateral kidney. *Retrograde pyelography,* in the absence of significant lower urinary tract trauma, may be performed to visualize the extent of the injury. Retrograde pyelography, however, continues to be a subject of controversy. It is diagnostic in approximately 20 per cent of cases.[12] Other radiographic methods may provide more accurate information. The possibility of introducing infection is frequently mentioned, but this risk is extremely small in our experience.

Nephrotomography has been advocated, but selective renal *angiography* by the percutaneous femoral route is preferable and has received wide acceptance in the study of renal trauma. Many centers are now equipped to perform excellent emergency renal arteriography. The renal arterial supply and its arborization within the parenchyma are concisely illustrated by the arterial phase of the angiogram as well as any thrombosis or rent with extravasation within the perfused area. Simultaneous injection of the celiac axis may help in delineating injuries to the spleen or liver.

As mentioned previously, renal injuries may be classified into *minor, major* and *critical* trauma, as illustrated in Figure 12–1. This classification has much practical value in determining the indications for an aggressive surgical approach as opposed to "watchful waiting."

Minor Trauma

Patients with minor trauma have suffered some damage to the renal parenchyma, which is contused. There is no rupture of the renal capsule or any tear into the collecting system. Unless other significant injury is

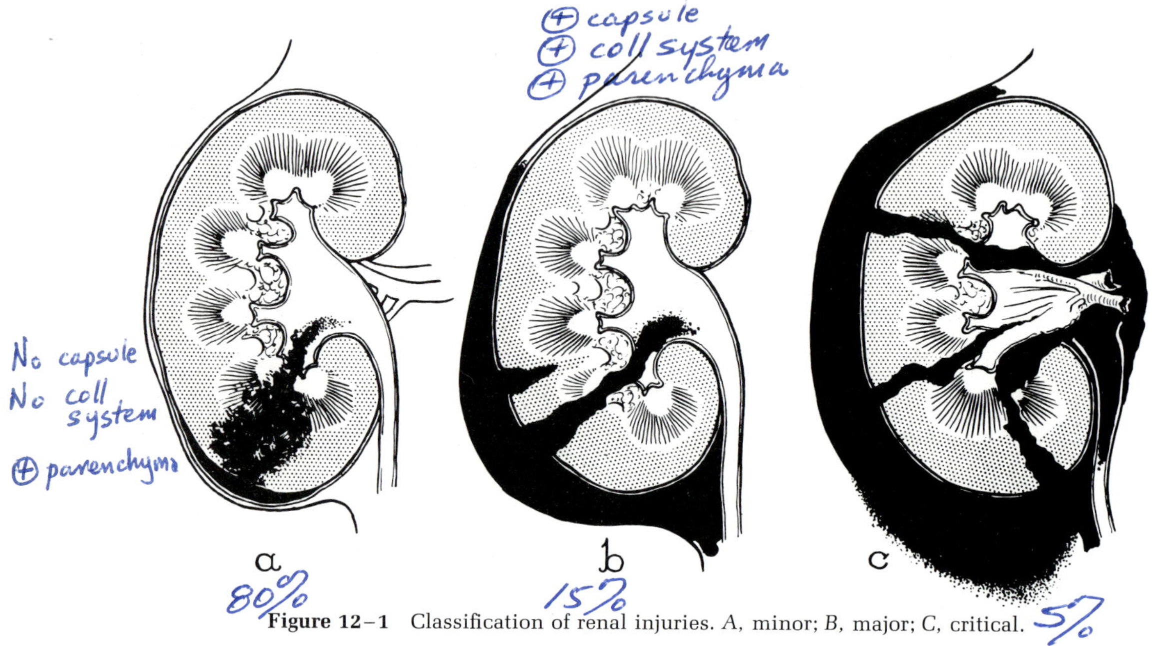

Figure 12–1 Classification of renal injuries. *A*, minor; *B*, major; *C*, critical.

present, such patients do *not* exhibit significant blood loss or shock. Hematuria may be gross initially but usually subsides rapidly. Pain and tenderness in the involved flank may be marked shortly after injury but also subside quickly. A flank mass is *not* palpable. Radiographically, no extravasation of dye can be demonstrated by intravenous pyelogram or retrograde urography. Excretion may be slightly decreased in such a kidney, and the nephrographic phase may show a subcapsular hematoma.

Fortunately, most renal injuries fall into this *minor* group. The incidence is cited by various authors as over 80 per cent of all renal injuries.[8, 12, 13, 17, 19, 21, 25, 46, 48, 49]

Treatment of this *minor trauma* type of renal injury consists of nothing but rest and observation. Full and uncomplicated recovery is almost always the case, and late complications of this type of renal injury have *not* been reported.

Repeated minor trauma may produce a distinctive lesion characterized by pericalyceal and peripelvic proliferations with distortions of the calyces. This is a very frequent finding in professional athletes (up to 50 per cent), producing microhematuria, pyuria, proteinuria and casts.[22] *Treatment* includes adequate rest, and stringent follow-up is necessary to prevent progressive renal deformity.

Major Injuries

The anatomic lesion in *major renal trauma* is, in addition to a marked degree of parenchymal laceration, a continuation of this laceration through the renal capsule and also into the pelvis. Although it is possible that a capsular and parenchymal tear may occur without extension of this laceration into the collecting system, this is rare. This laceration, extending from the collecting system through the parenchyma and through the renal capsule, allows free mixture of blood and urine not only within the collecting system but also in the space surrounding the kidney. Usually, this is confined by Gerota's fascia. This collection of blood and urine may present, on *physical examination*, as a palpable, either stable or expanding, flank mass.

Major injury may be caused by blunt trauma or by perforating or penetrating injuries. Approximately

15 per cent of all renal injuries fall into this group. Uncontrollable bleeding may also occur in 0.1 per cent of renal needle biopsies.[2, 47]

Physical findings may be misleading. Shock may exist initially, or it may develop later. Pain, tenderness and splinting may be due to the renal injury; however, the usually present concomitant injuries may very well mask the renal trauma initially. Hematuria, again, may not be proportional to the degree of trauma; however, symptoms and signs usually become worse with time, contrary to the gradual improvement seen in minor trauma.

Radiographic demonstration of extravasation of contrast medium is the diagnostic criterion for major renal trauma (Fig. 12–2). Intravenous pyelography, drip-infusion pyelography or retrograde pyelography may show this extravasation. Their advantages and disadvantages have been presented above, but it is important to stress that intravenous pyelography, even in penetrating renal trauma, may be normal in over 30 per cent of such patients.[49] The most reliable radiologic evaluation is performed with arteriography (Fig. 12–3), which, however, is *not* always possible in an acutely ill patient who may require urgent operation.

Severe blunt trauma may also lead to renal artery thrombosis, probably on the basis of intimal and intramural vascular damage. This lesion is well known in both pediatric[18] and adult[42] age groups. Hematuria is usually absent, but proteinuria may be present. Physical examination does *not* offer any significant findings. On excretory urography, the kidney shows no function, and retrograde pyelography will demonstrate a normal collecting system. Renal arteriography accurately demonstrates the site and nature of this lesion. Prompt thrombectomy is required to salvage renal function.

Treatment of major renal injuries depends largely on the extent of the renal injury. Most urologists will adopt an expectant policy as to the manage-

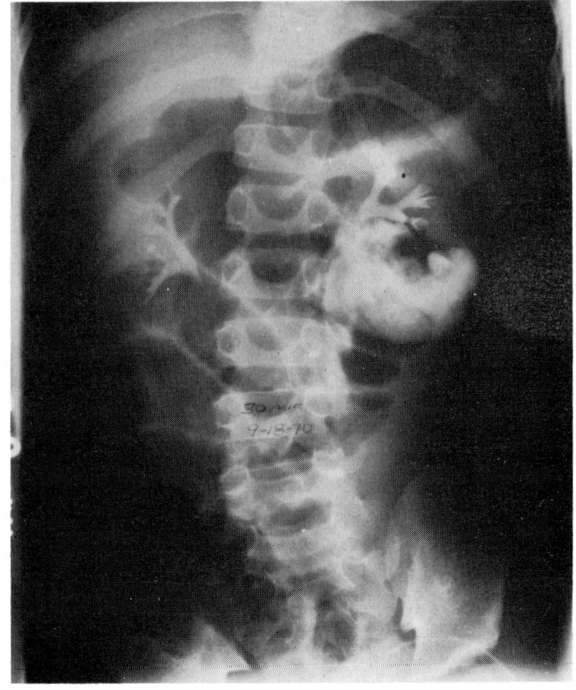

Figure 12–2 Eight-year-old boy was hit by a car. Back pain and persistent gross hematuria necessitated admission. On follow-up intravenous pyelogram three days later, marked extravasation of dye can be seen surrounding the lower pole and the upper ureter. At operation, complete transsection of the lower pole was found for which a heminephrectomy was performed.

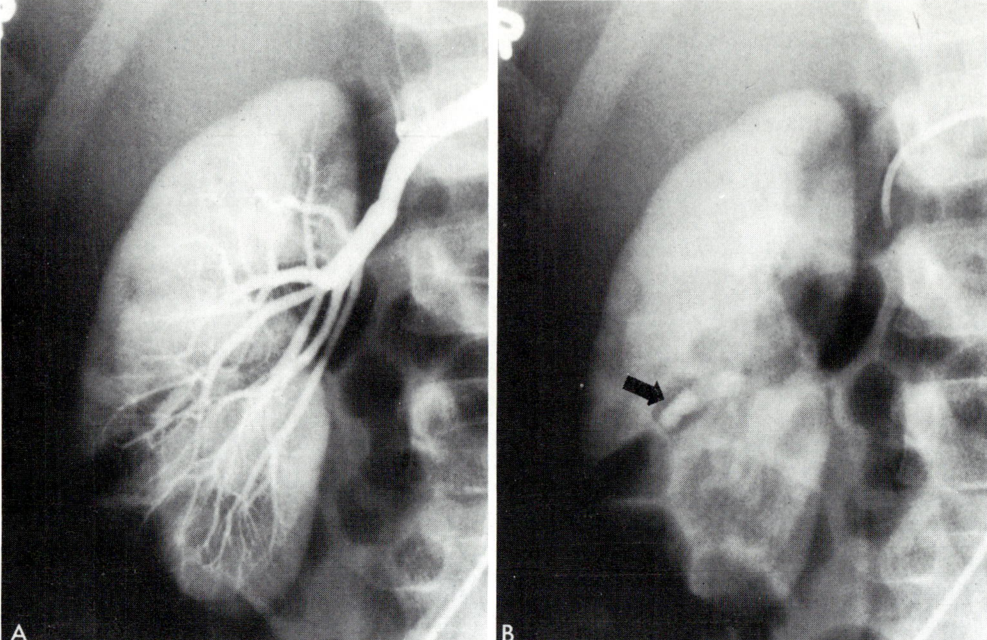

Figure 12–3 Young boy with intermittent gross total hematuria following a car accident injuring his right flank. *A*, Arteriogram shows collection of contrast material, outside the calyceal structures, which becomes more evident on (*B*) the delayed film (see arrow).

ment of such patients and will *not* intervene surgically as long as vital signs are stable, no significant blood loss occurs, and the flank mass is not expanding. Surgical intervention in the early post-trauma period has all too frequently resulted in nephrectomy for otherwise salvageable kidneys, simply because the extent of the perirenal hematoma and the continuous bleeding after release of the tamponade by opening of Gerota's fascia made it extremely difficult to identify and ligate any bleeding vessels. However, with the advent of angiography and, thus, the possibility of exact localization of bleeding vessels, it is possible to repair such kidneys during the acute phase of the trauma. In *nonpenetrating* renal injuries, surgical intervention is still limited to those patients with life-endangering hemorrhage. But with *penetrating* renal trauma, the following plan is proposed:[48]

1. Delineation of location and extent of injury
2. Control of renovascular pedicle prior to mobilization of kidney
3. Debridement of severely damaged parenchyma
4. Meticulous hemostasis
5. Primary approximation of the parenchymal margins
6. Extraperitoneal drainage of the renal fossa

With this approach, over 35 per cent of such kidneys may be saved.[25, 48, 49] Severe injuries in this category may require nephrectomy. Drainage only may be instituted in small lacerations. Debridement and primary closure are possible in those cases where vascular injury to the involved part of the kidney has *not* been so extensive as to devitalize this part of the parenchyma. Should a part of the kidney appear to be viable, then a partial nephrectomy may be the procedure of choice. This may be done sharply or with a Guillotine technique. (See Figures 12–4 and 12–5.)

Exploration of the injured kidney is best performed through an anterior

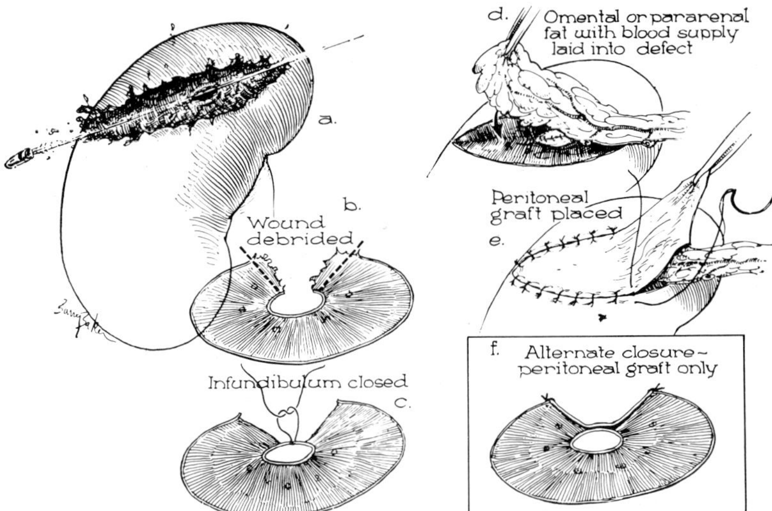

Figure 12–4 A transcapsular laceration. All larger vessels are suture-ligated. A watertight closure is used for the collecting system. The capsule is closed with running or interrupted sutures. Diverting pyelostomy is performed for clots in the renal pelvis. *A* and *B,* All devitalized renal tissue is debrided. *C,* Collecting system is then closed. *D, E* and *F,* It is desirable to place a patch of fat, omentum, or peritoneum over defect. (Reprinted by permission. From Scott, R., Jr., Carlton, C. E., and Goldman, M.: Penetrating injuries of the kidney: An analysis of 181 patients. *J. Urol. 101*:247–253, [March] 1969. © 1969, The Williams & Wilkins Co., Baltimore.)

transperitoneal approach, which yields quick access to the renal pedicle (Fig. 12–6). Non-crushing vascular clamps are applied to the pedicle as in surgery for renovascular hypertension. The kidney itself can then be approached through the paracolonic gutter after the colon has been reflected medially. The hematoma is evacuated and intermittent release of the pedicle clamp will allow accurate visualization of any bleeding vessels,

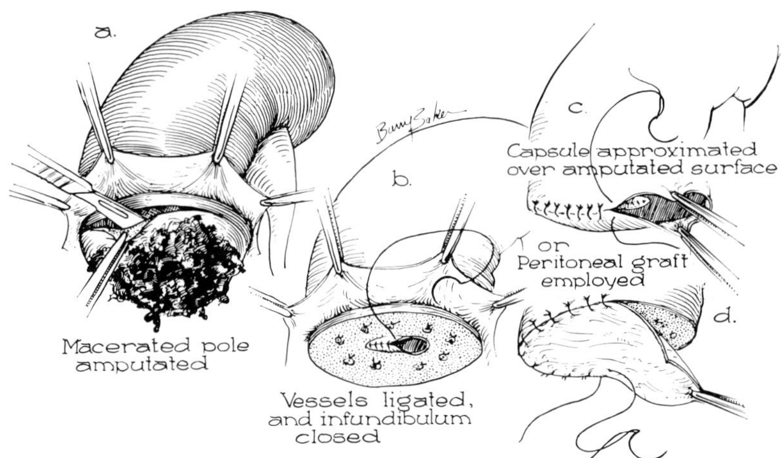

Figure 12–5 Partial nephrectomy for renal trauma. *A,* Amputation of injured renal parenchyma. *B,* Suture ligation of bleeding vessels is followed by watertight closure of the transsected calyces. *C* and *D,* A flap of renal capsule, which is seen reflected in (*A*), or a peritoneal graft, is used to cover the exposed renal surface. (Reprinted by permission. From Scott, R., Jr., Carlton, C. E., and Goldman, M.: Penetrating injuries of the kidney: An analysis of 181 patients. *J. Urol. 101*:247–253, [March] 1969. ©1969, The Williams & Wilkins Co., Baltimore.)

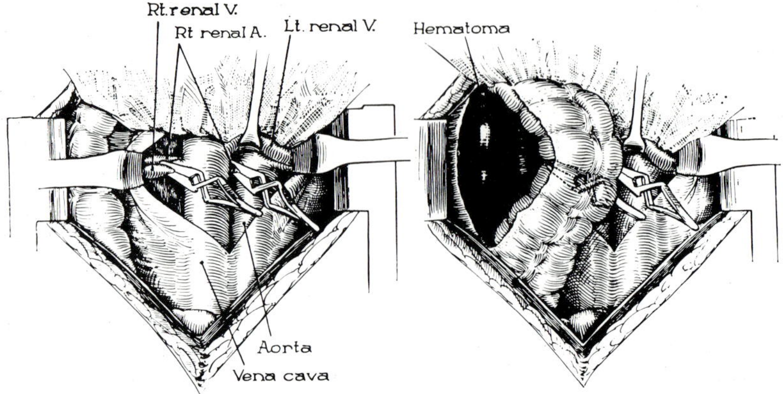

Figure 12–6 Vertical incision across the aorta at the renal hilum allows access to both renal pedicles. The renal artery of the injured kidney is clamped with noncrushing clamps before reflecting the colon and opening Gerota's fascia. (Reprinted by permission. From Scott, R., Jr., Carlton, C. E., and Goldman, M.: Penetrating injuries of the kidney: An analysis of 181 patients. *J. Urol. 101*:247–253, [March] 1969. ©1969, The Williams & Wilkins Co., Baltimore.)

which can be suture-ligated. Watertight closure of the torn pelviocalyceal system is important. This is followed by approximation of the renal parenchyma and closure of the renal capsule. Deep mattress sutures through the renal capsule, over a free fatpad or a peritoneal graft, may aid in covering a capsular defect. Should a heminephrectomy be required, it is advantageous to strip the renal capsule off the devitalized parenchyma prior to its removal. This capsule can then readily be used to oversew the amputated renal surface. (See Figures 12–4, 12–5 and 12–6.)

Critical Injuries

Fragmentation of the kidney or an extension of the injury into the renal pedicle places such a patient in the group of *critical renal trauma.* Renal pedicle trauma is more frequent in penetrating renal injuries (29 of 181) than in nonpenetrating injuries (7 in 111).[40, 48, 49] Blood loss in such injuries is apt to be severe and may be fatal in a short time.

A progressively expanding flank mass associated with early and profound shock as well as other evidence of massive hemorrhage readily point out the severity of this lesion. The primary value of the preoperative evaluation is to establish adequate function of the contralateral kidney. However, hemorrhagic shock with subsequent low renal perfusion may prevent adequate visualization of even a normal contralateral kidney.

Rapid intervention in such trauma is indicated to control hemorrhage and save the patient's life. In blunt trauma with destruction of the renal parenchyma and extension of the injury into the renal pedicle, ligation of the renal pedicle is the only possible treatment. However, in penetrating injuries with less damage to the parenchyma, and predominantly vascular pedicle injury, primary repair is possible in approximately 15 per cent.[49]

Mortality

Various authors have reported their mortalities from renal trauma.[12, 17, 25, 40, 45, 49]

It becomes apparent from the literature that most of these injuries are due to associated injuries. Rarely is the renal trauma itself the cause of death.

Early Complications

Early complications include those of persistent urinary drainage with the possibility of pararenal abscess formation. Gradual loss of function of the injured kidney, leading to "silent death," has been seen, but no data are available on the incidence of this complication. Organization of a large hematoma may lead to obstruction at the level of the ureter or ureteropelvic junction and, thus, predisposes to hydronephrosis. Persistent leakage of urine into the perirenal area may lead to the formation of a pararenal pseudocyst. These latter complications may have to be corrected surgically to prevent progressive renal attrition, infection and stone formation.

Late Complications

Patients with renal trauma should be followed routinely up to two years following their trauma to assess renal function and the possibility of renal hypertension. This is reported to occur in as many as 6 per cent of cases.[12, 60] Hypertension is felt to occur as a result of arterial constriction during the healing process with resultant ischemic renal tissue which produces a Goldblatt kidney. Heminephrectomy or nephrectomy is necessary to cure this complication.

URETERAL INJURIES

Incidence

The ureter is rarely the site of urinary tract injury. Throughout its entire course, the ureter is well protected from blunt external trauma by abdominal contents anteriorly and the ileopsoas muscle posteriorly. Approximately 2 per cent of all patients with genitourinary tract trauma sustain ureteral injury, and most of these are secondary to penetrating wounds of the abdomen.[7, 45, 51, 52, 56]

Surgical injury of the ureter, however, occurs more often than is apparent. The close relation of the ureter to rectosigmoid and female reproductive tract renders the ureter vulnerable during radical surgery on these organs.

Ureteral instrumentation with catheters, particularly with stylets or stone extraction baskets, has also produced a number of ureteral perforations. However, over the past decade, this type of trauma has drastically decreased in incidence.

Ureteral injury due to blunt trauma is frequently associated with fracture of one or more transverse processes of the lumbar vertebrae on the ipsilateral side.

Wertheim[58] reported an incidence of 10 per cent ureteral injuries in 500 radical hysterectomies. The incidence with this procedure today is still the same. With hysterectomies for benign diseases, the incidence is less than 0.5 per cent.[16, 45, 51]

The incidence for radical general surgical procedures is much lower and is quoted to be as low as 1 per cent in abdominal perineal resections.[16, 51] Ureteral injury during other intraperitoneal surgery is rare indeed, as is the occasional trauma to the ureter during spinal surgery. It may occur as a delayed complication following radiotherapy for carcinoma of the cervix.[1] (See Figure 12–7.) The high incidence of over 80 per cent in women is directly related to the risks of hysterectomy. Even with modern techniques, this risk has not been reduced. Important, however, is prompt repair. Higgins stated, "The venial sin is injury to the ureter, but the mortal sin is failure of recognition."[16] Parenthetically, it is a well-accepted surgical procedure to insert ureteral catheters into both ureters prior to radical pelvic surgery. This may well make identification of the ureters during such surgery much easier.

Symptoms and Signs

Localizing symptoms and signs of ureteral injury following surgical

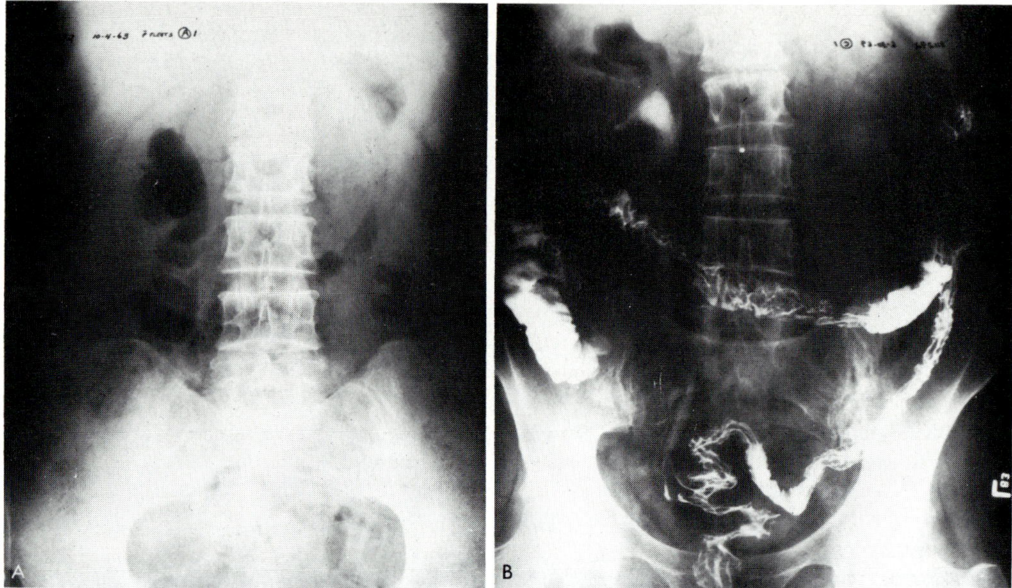

Figure 12–7 *A*, Flat plate of the abdomen shows a ureterosigmoid fistula following radium therapy for cervical carcinoma eight years previously. Right ureter and pelvis are filled with gas. *B*, Gastrografin enema demonstrates the ureterosigmoid fistula with reflux of the dye into the dilated upper tract.

trauma may initially be overlooked. Flank discomfort or fever of unknown origin in a patient who has undergone radical pelvic surgery should alert one to the possibility of ureteral injury. Hematuria may be absent in cases of complete transsection of the ureter; in partial transsection of the ureter, microhematuria is usually found. Complete or partial ligation by a suture or inadvertent application of hemostats, which compromises ureteral blood supply and may later result in necrosis and slough, is among the most frequent types of iatrogenic ureteral injury. In these patients, hematuria is usually *not* seen, but the signs of upper tract obstruction with flank discomfort, vague abdominal distress and possibly fever point toward the obstructed kidney. Unless relieved early, this kidney may succumb to a "silent death." Urinary sepsis can occur in approximately half of the patients whose upper tract has been obstructed through a surgical mishap. In patients with insufficient renal function of the contralateral side, or those with bilateral ureteral injury, azotemia and uremia may supervene. This makes it obvious that early and accurate diagnosis is important so that the necessary surgical treatment can be promptly instituted.

In patients with ureteral ligation, immediate release in the first 24 to 48 hours, or best at time of injury, is the proper course. Delayed release can make successful reconstruction of the ureteral continuity impossible, and nephrectomy may be necessary in 30 per cent of such patients.[15]

Urinary extravasation, if intraperitoneal, is dramatic. Acute peritoneal irritation and sepsis occur with marked urinary leakage, whereas mild spillage may simply lead to low-grade fever, leukocytosis and prolonged ileus. Extraperitoneal extravasation in patients with stab wounds will usually lead to a retroperitoneal urinoma which may be silent but can, not infrequently, be demonstrated on a flat film of the abdomen as a mass of "ground glass" appearance. Since the majority of ureteral injuries occur with radical gynecologic pelvic surgery, ureterovaginal fistulas are very common. Continuous dribbling of urine in patients who have an otherwise normal voiding pattern is characteristic for such a lesion.

Diagnosis

Excretory urography may be helpful in the diagnosis of ureteral trauma, but the most helpful diagnostic procedure is retrograde pyelography. In cases of disruption of the ureter, extravasation will pinpoint the exact location and extent of the ureteral injury. In patients with a ligated ureter, a varying degree of delayed function and hydronephrosis may be the result of this obstruction. This will be evident on excretory pyelography. Delayed films may be helpful in delineating the entire ureter down to the point of obstruction. Retrograde pyelography in conjunction with excretory urography will then visualize the lower segment of the ureter, and the nonvisualizing gap delineates the extent of obstruction.

Treatment

Much of the treatment of ureteral injuries is based on the concept of ureteral regeneration, which was pioneered by Davis.[6] Briefly, the ureter will regenerate its entire wall, epithelial lining and muscular coat along a narrow strip of ureteral wall bridging a gap. However, this regeneration does not occur across a transverse division unless the ends are directly approximated. The reasons for this extremely selective behavior of the ureter are still unknown.

The surgical procedure to be employed for repair of ureteral trauma depends in large measure on the extent of trauma. A simple transsection, if recognized early enough, can be primarily reanastomosed with an end-to-end anastomosis, preferably with spatulation of both ureteral ends. A urinary diversion with nephrostomy is usually *not* required in a primary repair but may be necessary in delayed repairs when the renal function has become impaired or the patient's general status has deteriorated owing to urinary sepsis and azotemia.

Gunshot wounds of the ureter may be deceiving since the tissue necrosis may frequently involve tissue that at first sight appears viable. Approximately a half-centimeter of healthy-appearing tissue on both ends of the ureter should be removed prior to reanastomosis. If end-to-end anastomosis is *not* possible, some other method of establishing ureteral continuity has to be employed.

In long strictures secondary to ureteral ligation, we have successfully utilized the Davis intubated ureterotomy, which is based on the principle of ureteral regeneration. In such ureters, the stricture is opened longitudinally and a catheter of inert material, such as silicone, and slightly smaller than the normal lumen of the ureter is used as a splint. This splint must be kept in place long enough to accomplish its purpose of allowing ureteral regeneration around its circumference, usually 4 to 6 weeks, at which time it can be withdrawn through the bladder. However, for the success of the Davis intubated ureterotomy, a continuous strip of mucosal surface bridging this gap is mandatory. Ureteral regeneration will *not* occur across a mucosal gap.

Fortunately, an obstructed ureter will usually dilate and elongate and thus make anastomosis possible even if several centimeters of the injured or obstructive segment cannot be utilized. A diverting nephrostomy is usually *not* necessary in patients where ureteral repair is performed immediately after injury but is advisable in cases of delayed surgical correction. An alternate method of diversion proximal to the site of injury is a ureterotomy.[14] The urine will drain along a Penrose drain placed at this ureterotomy. When normal peristalsis resumes across the suture line, this ureterotomy will close in a similar fashion to those after ureteral lithotomy. There is, however, some evidence[3] that urinary extravasation surrounding the ureter may lead to stricture formation. Carlton[3] describes a circular, watertight anastomosis associated with a much lower secondary complication rate than those of classical ureteral repairs. In patients with avulsion of the ureter at the renal pelvis, primary anastomosis may be successful; however, a pyeloplasty utilizing a pelvic flap is probably better. Patients with ureteral avulsion at the ureterovesical junction require a ureteral reimplantation,[53] for which the Politano-Leadbetter method probably gives the best results. An alternate surgical procedure has to be employed if primary anastomosis of the distal and proximal ureteral ends cannot be accomplished without stress on the suture line.[7, 10, 25, 45]

Prostheses of polyethylene, silicone or Teflon have *not* been successful. Homologous ureteral grafts, veins and arteries have also failed as ureteral substitutes.

A bladder tube flap, as described by Boari, can bridge a substantial ureteral defect. It is important that the anastomosis of ureter to this tube flap be performed with a submucosal tunnel technique to prevent the otherwise occurring reflux. In longer defects, substitution with segments of ileum has been described and used by us with good results. The use of intestine as substitute for portions of the urinary conduit is well known in urology. Transuretero-ureteral anastomosis employs the transfer of the remaining segment of one ureter into the intact ureter of the contralateral side. However, if the kidney on the injured side shows chronic pyelonephritic changes, one might have to expect possible damage and ascending pyelonephritis to the contralateral good kidney.

A promising new method[55] has been described recently which employs a posterior vesical flap with incorporation of the intact ureterovesical junction. This flap may permit advancement of the intact ureterovesical junction for about five centimeters, which will allow bridging of an equidistant deficit in the ureter without tension. Another method frees the bladder from its lateral and posterior attachments on the side of the ureteral defect. This also includes ligation of the superior vesical artery and vein. The bladder is then pulled up on this side and, with an anchoring suture, fixed to the psoas muscle. This procedure allows a significant superior advancement of the ureterovesical junction and thereby permits bridging a long ureteral gap without tension.

At times, urinary diversion is the only possible method of salvaging the upper tracts. If one deals with a solitary kidney and a dilated ureter, a ureterocutaneous anastomosis is the preferred method. Normal ureters have a high tendency to stricture if anastomosed to the skin. This complication is rarely seen in patients with dilated ureters. Diversions utilizing indwelling catheters should, if possible, be avoided unless they are temporary.

Indwelling catheters in the urinary tract carry with them the risk of chronic infection, ascending pyelonephritis and stone formation. Ureterosigmoidostomy has been utilized as urinary diversion in patients with significant injury to the ureters. We prefer the bilateral uretero-ileocutaneous urinary diversion, or ileal loop, as permanent urinary diversion. This procedure in our hands has given the best long-term results and has undoubtedly saved many a kidney that otherwise would have been doomed to chronic failure.

BLADDER TRAUMA

Bladder trauma is less frequent than injury to the upper urinary tract,[57] and is usually secondary to external force, either blunt or penetrating. By far, the majority are caused by blunt external trauma, usually motor accidents, which account for approximately 80 per cent of bladder trauma.[20, 36, 37, 57] Industrial crush accidents are less frequent today but still occur, particularly in the mining industry. Penetrating injuries by gunshot wounds or knives injuring the bladder are much less frequent than those afflicting the kidney. They usually are iatrogenic and are caused by instruments such as urethral sounds, wire catheter guides and resectoscopes.

Incidence

In a recent review by Clark and Prudencio,[4] tabulating about 2500 cases of pelvic fracture, the authors come to the conclusion that 14.5 per cent of pelvic trauma is associated with injury to the lower urinary tract. Of these, 32 per cent involve the bladder alone, 10 per cent bladder and urethra, and 58 per cent only the urethra.

Anatomy

Bladder perforation in pelvic trauma occurs usually with fractures involving the pubic arch. Fractures of the posterior aspect of the pelvic girdle rarely cause perforation of the bladder but may displace the bladder through hematoma formation. In its resting state, the bladder is fairly well-protected from direct injury (Fig. 12–8), but becomes more vulnerable with increased filling. Also, the severity of the injury increases with progressive distention. Most cases of intraperitoneal rupture of the bladder occur from a direct blow to the filled bladder.

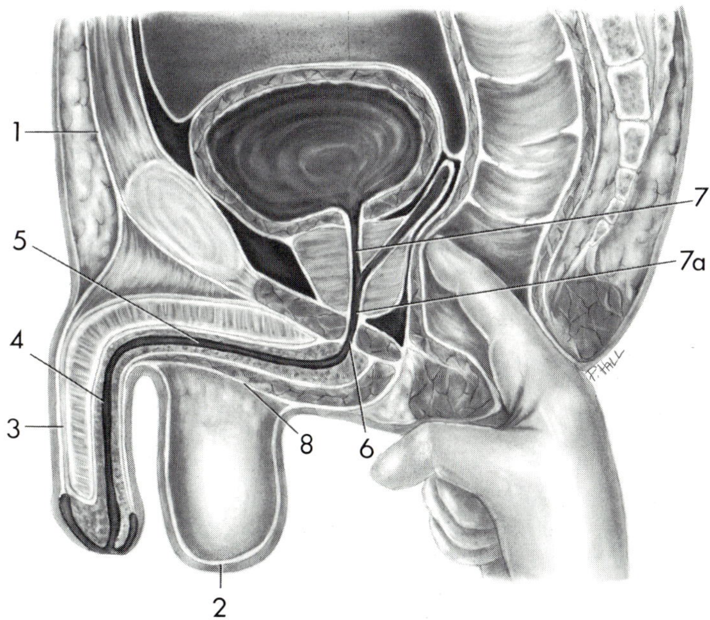

Figure 12–8 Sagittal section of the male lower urinary tract, demonstrating the relationship of the prostate to the rectum: (1) Scarpa's fascia, (2) dartos fascia, (3) Buck's fascia, (4) pendulous urethra, (5) bulbous urethra, (6) membranous urethra, (7) prostatic urethra, (7a) supramembranous urethra, and (8) Colles' fascia. (Reprinted by permission. From Clark, S. S., and Prudencio, R. F.: Lower urinary tract injuries associated with pelvic fractures: Diagnosis and management. Surg. *Clin. N. Amer.* 52[1]:183–201, [Feb.] 1972.)

Bladder Contusion

Up to one-third of patients with fractures of the pelvis, without demonstrable genitourinary trauma, may present with hematuria. This is felt to be due to a contusion of the bladder, in which minor damage has been sustained by the bladder wall. A number of these injuries can be caused by the snubbing action of the seat belt in car collisions.[11] The diagnosis is made by exclusion of penetrating injury to the urinary tract. No specific treatment is required.

Extraperitoneal Rupture

In their review of 1798 cases of pelvic fractures, Prather and Kaiser[41] report on 181 bladder ruptures, of which 82 per cent were of the extraperitoneal type. Extraperitoneal bladder rupture usually occurs with fractures of the pelvic girdle below the pelvic brim, particularly those of the pubic rami and symphysis. They are usually found, as Morehouse and MacKinnon[32] state, "on the anteriolateral wall rather close to the vesical neck." Urinary extravasation into the pre- and perivesical space occurs and may gradually, following fascial planes, ascend the anterior wall or, in the retroperitoneal space, may reach the kidneys. Extravasation can also extend via the inguinal canal into the scrotal compartment, through the obturator foramen to the thigh and through the greater sciatic notch into the buttocks. It may also spread under Colles' fascia, upward in the abdominal wall. (See Figure 12–9.)

Intraperitoneal Rupture

Intraperitoneal rupture usually occurs in direct trauma to a distended bladder. It involves not only complete penetration of the bladder wall but also a rupture of the visceral peri-

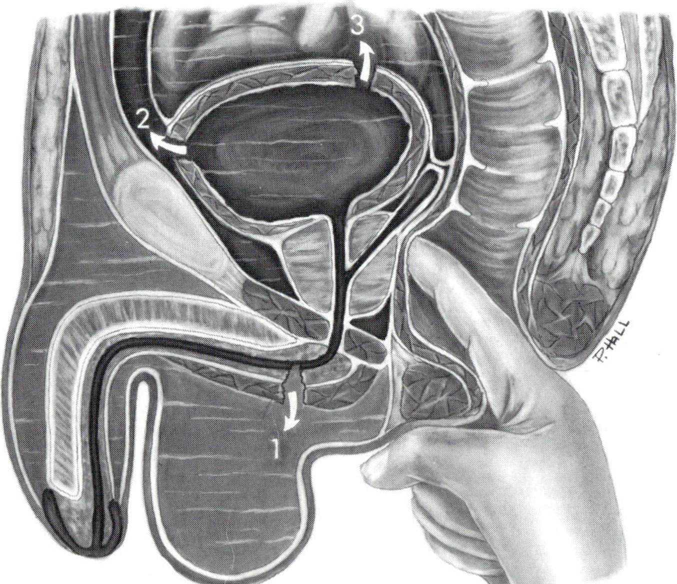

Figure 12–9 Routes of extravasation of urine and blood in (1) bulbomembranous urethral rupture with the hematoma appearing in the scrotum and beneath Scarpa's fascia, (2) extraperitoneal perforation with accumulation into the perivesical space, and (3) intraperitoneal perforation with extravasation into the peritoneal cavity. Rectal examination outlines the prostate in its usual position in any of these injuries. (Reprinted by permission. From Clark, S. S., and Prudencio, R. F.: Lower urinary tract injuries associated with pelvic fractures: Diagnosis and management. Surg. *Clin. N. Amer.* 52[1]: 183–201, [Feb.] 1972.)

toneum covering the dome of the bladder. Urinary extravasation will pool in the peritoneal cavity (Fig. 12–9). This type of injury occurs with somewhat higher frequency in children, whose bladders are still largely intraperitoneal and thus more vulnerable to this type of rupture.[9, 41]

Combined Intra- and Extraperitoneal Rupture

This condition is usually associated with severe crush injuries of the pelvis. It is also associated with a significantly higher number of injuries to adjacent organs, notably the rectum. The severity of the injury, plus the free mixture of blood, urine and contaminated feces, carries with it a very high mortality for this type of injury.

Crush trauma to the pelvis in a child will result in a different type of injury than in the adult patient group. The developing bony pelvis is less rigid than the mature pelvis. A crushing force applied to a child's pelvis may easily disrupt this at both symphysis pubis and the sacroiliac joints. "After the force has been removed, the pelvis springs back into a relatively normal position while the soft tissues, on the other hand, are compressed and rapidly decompressed resulting in total disruption of the rectum and urinary tract, with ensuing contamination of the pelvis with feces and urine."[4] Such a "sprung" or "exploded" pelvis may show remarkably few radiologic changes, whereas the damage to the lower urinary tract is enormous.

Diagnosis

Every pelvic fracture should lead one to suspect bladder trauma until proved otherwise. Examination should be done with the patient completely disrobed so that the suprapubic area and perineum as well as the external genitalia can be inspected and examined in detail.

Hematuria, microscopic or macroscopic, is usually present but may be absent in complete disruption of the urethra. Suprapubic tenderness and a "doughy" swelling may be palpated in patients with *extraperitoneal* bladder rupture and extravasation into the space of Retzius. Extravasation into scrotum, buttocks or perineum has to be sought. *Intraperitoneal* extravasation will rapidly lead to the classical signs of peritoneal irritation. Shock may accompany many pelvic fractures without bladder trauma. Blood loss in pelvic trauma can be severe, and 60 per cent of patients who succumb as a result of injury to the bony pelvis die of blood loss.[23, 26, 33] The iliac veins and the prostatic venous plexus of Santorini are the two most vulnerable vascular areas. In children, not only the major vessels but also the sciatic nerves in their courses overlying the sacroiliac joint are particularly vulnerable to trauma.[43] Absence of a femoral pulse and loss of sciatic nerve function is an ominous sign in this type of injury. Local tenderness is not a reliable sign in bladder rupture as the usually associated pelvic fracture masks any discomfort due to bladder trauma. In both *intra-* and *extraperitoneal* bladder rupture, the attempt to void will increase a patient's pain, and in *intraperitoneal* rupture in particular he may be unable to void.

The diagnosis in both intra- and extraperitoneal bladder rupture is made by a cystogram. An excretory urogram may show the typical "teardrop" deformity of the bladder, which is due to a mixture of blood and urine compressing and elevating the bladder. However, concentration of dye in the bladder on such a film is usually inadequate to visualize a small rent. Retrograde injection of *Renografin-60* into the bladder is the preferred diagnostic method. To avoid compounding a possible urethral injury, no catheter is used at this point; rather, the contrast material is injected into the urethra through a Brodney clamp or a Chetwood syringe. After obtaining adequate filling films of the bladder, an evacuation film is taken which will show the location and extent of extravasation. Not infrequently, a bladder perforation may be completely *missed* if a postevacuation film is *not* obtained. Also, oblique or lateral films may be helpful in establishing the diagnosis. With *intraperitoneal* rupture, the contrast medium may coat the intestinal loops and outline them, and it will pool in the most dependent portions of the abdominal cavity, usually the paracolic gutter (Fig. 12–10*A*). *Extraperitoneal* extravasation usually presents as an ill-defined, hazy, irregular contrast shadow which remains fixed with position changes of the patient (Fig. 12–10*B*).

Treatment

All *intraperitoneal bladder ruptures* require prompt surgical closure. The rent can usually be identified, the bladder wall closed, and the peritoneal tear closed in a separate layer. A number of surgeons prefer to drain such a bladder suprapubically.[23, 24, 36] Our preference is for urethral catheter drainage. The mortality rate with intraperitoneal rupture remains high.

Small extraperitoneal bladder perforations need not necessarily be closed. Transurethral catheter drainage for a week usually suffices in allowing adequate healing of small tears, particularly in patients who sustained such a tear from electroresection of a bladder tumor or false passage of a sound. However, if the prevesical extravasation is significant, and in all patients with infected urine,

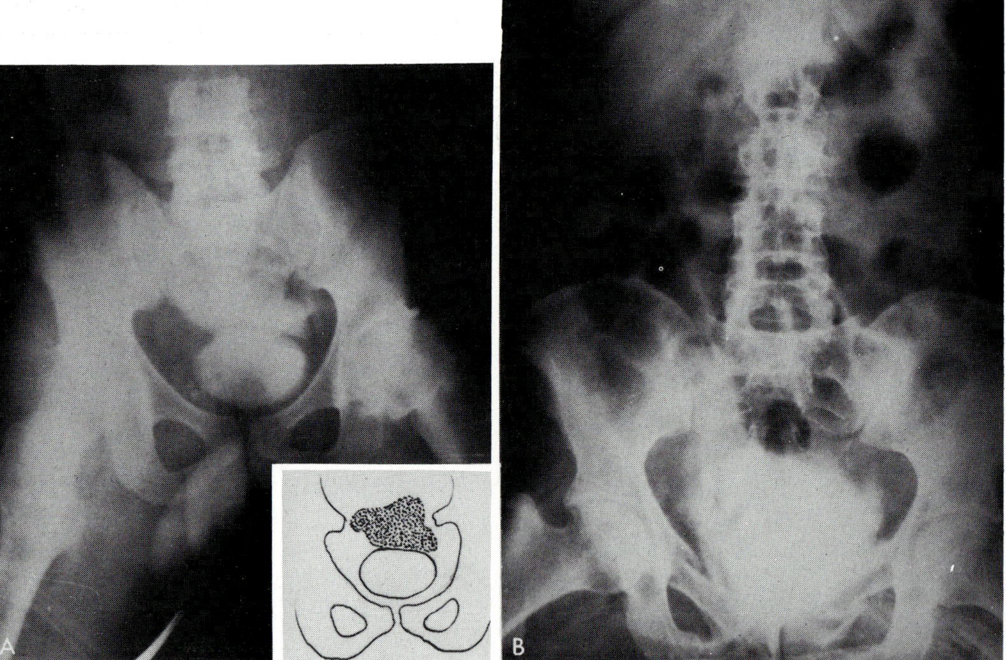

Figure 12–10 *A*, Retrograde cystogram and diagrammatic sketch illustrating intraperitoneal extravasation of dye from a bladder rupture. *B*, Retrograde cystogram shows extravasation of dye from an extraperitoneal bladder rupture.

it is advisable to approach the bladder through a suprapubic incision, close the bladder perforation anteriorly and place a suprapubic Penrose drain until a day after the catheter has been removed and the drainage from the Penrose drain site has ceased.

INJURIES OF THE URETHRA

As pointed out earlier, more than half of the injuries to the lower urinary tract involve the urethra, either alone (58.3 per cent) or in conjunction with bladder injuries (9.4 per cent).[41] Virtually all of these injuries occur in males. For the understanding of the mechanism of trauma to the urethra, a brief review of the *anatomy* is in order: The *prostatic urethra,* usually 2.5 to 3 cm. long in the adult, courses through the prostate along its longitudinal axis. Just below the apex of the prostate, the urethra traverses the urogenital diaphragm. This portion of the urethra is called the *membranous urethra* and is approximately 1.0 cm. long. It is firmly attached to the urogenital diaphragm and allows very little mobility. Following this begins the *bulbous urethra,* which lies within the superficial perineal space and extends in an S-shaped curve into the *scrotal* and *pendulous urethra* (see Fig. 12–8).

The membranous urethra allows little mobility, as pointed out above. The prostatic urethra, likewise, is fixed to the surrounding structures by the prostate which, in turn, is attached at its anterior surface, through the puboprostatic ligaments, to the posterior surface of the pubic symphysis. The prostatic base, joining the bladder at the bladder neck, is less restricted through its ligaments to the bony pelvis.

The *female urethra,* on the other hand, has no such firm and restricting attachments and, owing to its much greater mobility, almost always escapes trauma.

The cause of trauma to the urethra is usually a pelvic fracture, most often due to motor vehicle accidents. However, a significant number of such injuries are caused by industrial accidents. Falls resulting in straddle injuries, such as occur in the roofing or construction industries, are not infrequent. The compression of the perineum against the pubic arch may result in a crush injury of the urethra or an actual disruption of the urethra, usually at the urogenital diaphragm. Pelvic fractures which involve the pubic arch will traumatize the prostatic and bulbomembranous urethra in almost 70 per cent of such accidents.[32, 36, 41, 50] Not infrequently, fractures in this area also disrupt the periprostatic venous plexus, resulting in a large hematoma which may displace the prostate cephalad. Transsections of the urethra below the level of an intact external urinary sphincter usually do *not* result in extravasation of urine, and thus, the ensuing hematoma usually is *not* contaminated with urine. Disruption above the level of the sphincter leads to unrestricted urinary extravasation.

Diagnosis

Symptoms and signs of urethral trauma, again, may be masked by the accompanying pelvic fractures. A suprapubic mass may be the distended urinary bladder or a large hematoma resulting from injury above the urogenital diaphragm. Such a hematoma may extend underneath the inguinal ligament to the upper thigh.

A hematoma or urinary extravasation from trauma below the urogenital diaphragm will present itself as a swelling in the perineum, scrotum and penis (see Fig. 12–9). It may continue to extend underneath Colles' and Scarpa's fasciae and ascend on the anterior abdominal wall. If the urine is infected, cellulitis will rapidly supervene. This may lead to skin necrosis and gangrene of the genitalia.

Hematuria may be terminal or initial

in cases of urethral trauma, and if the injury occurs below the external sphincter, a constant dripping of bright red blood from the external meatus can frequently be observed. With disruption of the urethra, the patient will be unable to void spontaneously.

Rectal examination is an essential part of diagnosis. Frank blood per anum may well indicate a concomitant trauma to the rectosigmoid. In patients with urethral trauma above the urogenital diaphragm, such examination allows assessment of the expansion of a pelvic hematoma or the possible elevation of the prostate gland in complete disruption of the urethra. At times, the prostate may be displaced so high that it cannot be reached by the palpating finger; at other times, it can be freely ballotted (Fig. 12–11). Subsequent rectal examinations allow for follow-up of the resolution of the hematoma.

Following an excretory urogram (which preferably is done with an infusion drip after the blood pressure has been stabilized), further radiologic examinations are necessary. The excretory urogram is primarily indicated to assess function and integrity of the upper urinary tract. Films of the bladder, when filled and after evacuation, may be helpful in ascertaining the diagnosis of urethral injury in the posterior urethra since elevation of the bladder may be seen in complete transsection. However, we prefer retrograde cystourethrography as the diagnostic maneuver (Fig. 12–12). It is best *not* to insert a catheter for such a procedure since the necessary manipulation may convert an incomplete transsection of the urethra into a complete one. Twenty to thirty cc. of *Renografin-60* are injected with a Brodney clamp through the external meatus. A complete transsection of the urethra at any level will show extravasation and usually *no* filling of the urethra above the level of transsection. This study will show the site and degree of laceration, with one continuous wall in one projection, and filling above the level of trauma. In suspected trauma of the urethra, the catheter should be passed only by one who is best suited to do so, namely, a urologist.

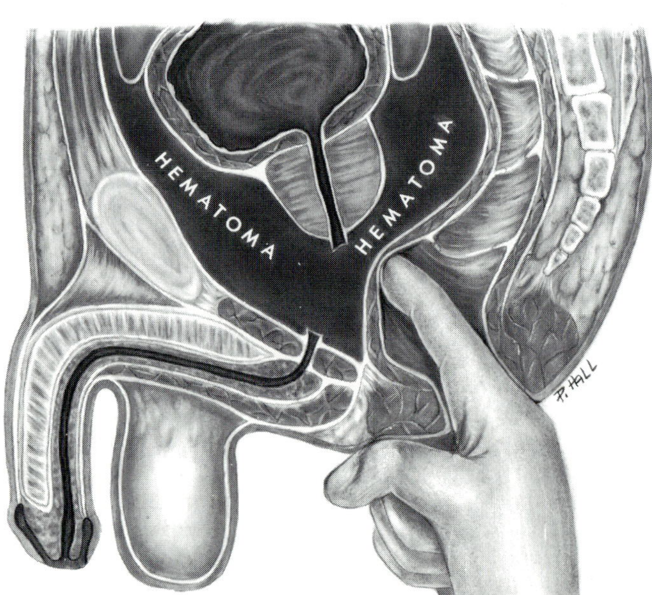

Figure 12–11 Transection of the posterior urethra with hematoma elevating the prostate and bladder. A finger in the rectum may not feel the prostate. (Reprinted by permission. From Clark, S. S., and Prudencio, R. F.: Lower urinary tract injuries associated with pelvic fractures: Diagnosis and management. *Surg. Clin. N. Amer.* 52[1]: 183–201, [Feb.] 1972.)

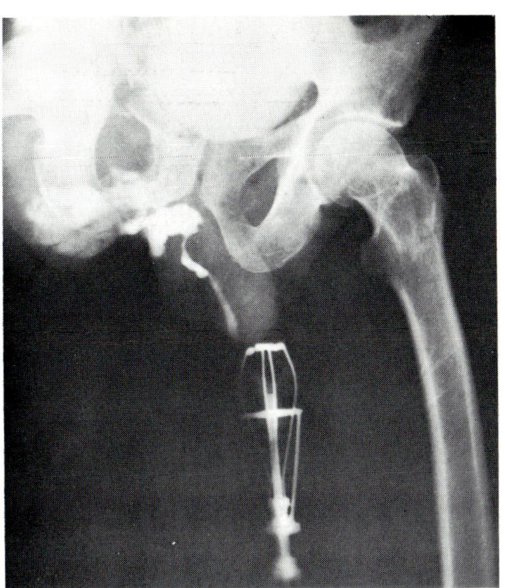

Figure 12–12 Retrograde cystourethrogram. Rupture of the posterior urethra is shown by the marked gap between the torn end of the urethra and the bladder base.

Treatment

Trauma to the posterior urethra may lead to significant long-term morbidity.[34, 39] Exact figures on the various complications are unknown, but incontinence, stricture formation and impotence are high. Recent authors[30, 31, 59] suggest that conventional management may actually increase the incidence of these complications.

Conventional management consists of reapproximating the transsected urethra via Davis interlocking sounds. These sounds are passed antegrade and retrograde until, with gentle manipulation, their tips meet and interlock. Rectal palpation by an assistant significantly aids in this maneuver. The sounds are then passed through the entire urethra, a catheter is tied to the tip of one of these sounds and then pulled into the bladder. After the balloon is inflated, traction is applied to the catheter to pull down the transsected segment of the urethra and approximate it to the distal end. Some authors[29, 34, 39, 59] have preferred to simultaneously evacuate the periurethral hematoma and perform a primary suture anastomosis of the transsected ends of the urethra through a perineal or retropubic approach. Clark and Prudencio[4] and Morehouse[30, 31, 32] strongly advocate simply diverting the urine suprapubically at the time of injury and leaving the hematoma and transsected posterior urethra undisturbed. Two to four months later, after the hematoma has been absorbed and the posterior urethra has returned to near normal position, a two-stage urethroplasty is performed to bridge the gap between proximal and distal segments. The methods of Johanson and of Turner-Warwick[54] are well suited for this purpose. Morehouse[32] reports on 11 patients who were managed this way. All 11 are voiding with good stream; they do *not* require dilation; all of them have normal urinary control, and nine have normal erection and ejaculation. While these reports are very promising, more experience with this method is needed before the procedure can be properly judged.

Trauma to the urethra below the urogenital diaphragm usually does *not* result in transsection, but rather laceration. Suprapubic urinary diversion may be performed. We prefer to let such a traumatized urethra heal over a medically inert silicone catheter. Extravasation of urine into the confines of Colles' and Scarpa's fasciae must be incised adequately to prevent necrotizing cellulitis.

INJURIES TO THE EXTERNAL GENITALIA

The external genitalia of the female are rarely involved in direct injury. In the male, the genitalia also usually escape trauma but are not infrequently involved in urinary extravasation secondary to lacerations or fistulas forming below the urogenital diaphragm. Trauma to the external genitalia accounted for roughly one-third of the trauma to the genitourinary tract in the series by Waterhouse and Gross,[57] but this incidence is significantly higher than the experience in other centers.[25, 50] They are secondary to motor vehicle accidents, industrial accidents, bullet or stab wounds, or self-inflicted trauma.

Abrasions, hematomas and minor lacerations constitute the bulk of genital injuries. These injuries will heal quite well with debridement and local treatment. Primary suture of lacerations is necessary. Small hematomas do well if left alone. Large hematomas will require incision and drainage, as do those that are complicated by infection.

Industrial accidents frequently are associated with significant skin loss which may require isolation of flaps from scrotum or thigh. Usually, penile skin deficits can be covered by temporarily burying the penile shaft under the scrotum or suprapubic skin. In a second-stage procedure, after complete wound healing, the penis is freed from its site of temporary implantation.

In deeper injuries that involve the penile shaft, as much of the penile body as possible should be preserved. If the urethra is involved in the injury, temporary urinary diversion with a perineal urethrostomy or suprapubic cystostomy is recommended. Strangulation with amputation in young boys who "dare each other," or self-amputation by psychiatric patients, has been reported.[27, 28] Treatment for these patients usually consists of oversewing the stump. Complete restoration to obtain anatomic and functional results is rarely possible. Prompt psychiatric treatment is important.

Testicular injuries can be divided into those that do *not* rupture the tunica albuginea and those that do. Testicular trauma is frequently characterized by severe pain which may radiate into the groin and flank, producing nausea, vomiting, and at times even shock. Blunt trauma which results in contusion or hematoma of the testis is best treated by analgesics, elevation of the scrotum, icepacks to reduce the swelling and discomfort, and rest. Surgical intervention is rarely indicated. A lacerated tunica albuginea, however, should be repaired. Testicular tissue outside the testis should be removed to prevent the formation of a sperm granuloma. As the testes are the site of androgen production, preservation of even the smallest amount of testicular tissue is worthwhile.

In patients with complete loss of their testes, replacement therapy with testosterone is required.

Herniorrhaphy in the young infant is associated with one to two per cent incidence of transsection of the vas deferens. At present, it is *not* known whether repair at a later age will allow transport of fertile sperm across the anastomosis into the ejaculate of such a patient.

Vasectomies, which are performed with increasing frequency today, also have a number of surgical complications. Hematomas of significant extent occur in less than one per cent. These should be surgically evacuated. The spermatic artery may accidentally be ligated. Should this occur bilaterally, testicular atrophy will occur, which again requires testosterone replacement therapy. As with all iatrogenic trauma, it is extremely important from a medicolegal standpoint to inform the patient of such incidents as ureteral transsection or ligation. Many legal problems can be prevented or ameliorated through complete honesty.

REFERENCES

1. Alfert, H. J., and Gillenwater, J. Y.: The consequences of ureteral irradiation with special reference to subsequent ureteral injury. J. Urol. *107*:369, 1972.
2. Cangiano, J. L., and Kest, L.: Use of a G-suit for uncontrollable bleeding after percutaneous renal biopsy. J. Urol. *107*: 360–361, 1972.
3. Carlton, C. E., Guthrie, A. G., and Scott,

R., Jr.: Surgical correction of ureteral injury. J. Trauma 9:457–464, 1969.

4. Clark, S. S., and Prudencio, R. F.: Lower urinary tract injuries associated with pelvic fractures. Surg. Clin. N. Amer. *52*:183–201, 1972.
5. Cohen, S. G., and Pearlman, C. K.: Spontaneous rupture of the kidney in pregnancy. J. Urol. *100*:365–369, 1968.
6. Davis, D. M.: The process of ureteral repair: Recapitulation of the splinting question. J. Urol. *79*:215–223, 1958.
7. Del Villar, R. G., Ireland, G. W., and Cass, A. S.: Ureteral injury owing to external trauma. J. Urol. *107*:29–30, 1972.
8. Del Villar, R. G., Ireland, G. W., and Cass, A. S.: Management of renal injury in conjunction with the immediate surgical treatment of the acute severe trauma patient. J. Urol. *107*:208–211, 1972.
9. Ezell, W. W., Smith, I. E., McCarthy, R. P., Thompson, I. M., and Habib, H. N.: Mechanical traumatic injury to the genital tract in children. J. Urol. *102*: 788–792, 1969.
10. Funkhouser, J. J., and Sacher, E. C.: The contiguous helix ureteral lengthening flap for repair of distal ureteral injury. J. Urol. *107*:567–571, 1972.
11. Garrett, J. W., and Braunstein, P. W.: The seat belt syndrome. J. Trauma *2*:220–238, 1962.
12. Glenn, J. F., and Harvard, B. M.: The injured kidney. J.A.M.A. *173*:1189, 1960.
13. Graham, W. H.: Injuries to the urogenital tract. Proc. Roy. Soc. Med. *61*:477–483, 1968.
14. Hamm, F. C., and Weinberg, S. R.: Management of the severed ureter. Trans. Am. Assoc. GU Surgeons *48*:130, 1956.
15. Herman, G., Guerrier, K., and Persky L.: Delayed ureteral deligation. J. Urol. *107*:723–728, 1972.
16. Higgins, C. C.: Ureteral injury during surgery. J.A.M.A. *199*:82–87, 1967.
17. Hodges, C. V., Gilbert, D. R., Scott, W. W.: Renal trauma: Study of 71 cases. J. Urol. *66*:627, 1951.
18. Jevtich, M. J., and Montero, G. G.: Injuries to renal vessels by blunt trauma in children. J. Urol. *102*:493–496, 1969.
19. Jones, R. F.: Surgical management of transcapsular rupture of the kidney: 24 cases. J. Urol. *74*:721, 1955.
20. Kaiser, J. H., and Farrow, F. C.: Injury of the bladder and prostatomembranous urethra associated with fracture of the bony pelvis. Surg. Gynec. Obstet. *120*: 99, 1965.
21. Kazmin, M. H., Brosman, S. A., and Cockett, A. T. K.: Diagnosis and early management of renal trauma: Study of 120 patients. J. Urol. *101*:783–785, 1969.
22. Khonsari, H., Morehouse, D. D., and MacKinnon, J. K.: Pararenal pseudocysts. Brit. J. Urol. *43*:164–169, 1971.
23. Levine, J. I., and Crampton, R. S.: Major abdominal injuries associated with pelvic fractures. Surg. Gynec. Obstet. *116*:223, 1963.
24. Lewis, L. G.: Treatment of wounds of the bladder and urethra. Surg. Clin. N. Amer. *24*:1402, 1944.
25. Lucey, D. T., Smith, M. J. V., and Koontz, W. W., Jr.: Modern trends in the management of urologic trauma. J. Urol. *107*:641–646, 1972.
26. McLaughlin, A. P., III, McCullough, D. L., Jerr, W. S., and Darling, R. C.: Use of external counterpressure (G-suit) in the management of traumatic retroperitoneal hemorrhage. J. Urol. *107*:940–944, 1972.
27. McRoberts, J. W., Chapman, W. H., and Ansell, J. S.: Primary anastomosis of the traumatically amputated penis: Case report and summary of the literature. J. Urol. *97*:105, 1967.
28. Mendez, R., Kiely, W. F., and Morrow, J. W.: Self-emasculation. J. Urol. *107*: 981–985, 1972.
29. Moore, C. A.: One-stage urethroplasty: a new one-stage anterior urethroplasty. J. Urol. *90*:203, 1963.
30. Morehouse, D. D.: Injuries to the bladder and urethra. Lawyer's Med. J. *7*:141–153, 1971.
31. Morehouse, D. D., Belitsky, P., and MacKinnon, K.: Rupture of the posterior urethra. J. Urol. *107*:255–258, 1972.
32. Morehouse, D. D., and MacKinnon, K. J.: Urological injuries associated with pelvic fractures. J. Trauma *9*:479–496, 1969.
33. Motsay, G. J., Manlove, C., and Perry, J. F.: Major venous injury with pelvic fracture. J. Trauma. *9*:343, 1969.
34. Myers, R. P., and DeWeerd, J. H.: Incidence of stricture following primary realignment of disrupted proximal urethra. J. Urol. *107*:265, 1972.
35. National Safety Council, Statistics Division: Accident Facts. Chicago, The National Safety Council, 1972.
36. Newland, D. E.: Genitourinary complications of pelvic fractures. J.A.M.A. *152*: 1515, 1953.
37. Ochsner, T. G., Busch, F. M., and Clarke, B. G.: Urogenital wounds in Vietnam. J. Urol. *101*:224, 1969.
38. Orkin, L. A.: Diagnosis of urologic trauma in the presence of other injuries. Surg. Clin. N. Amer. *33*:1473, 1953.
39. Pierce, J. M.: Management of dismemberment of the prostatic-membranous urethra and ensuing stricture disease. J. Urol. *107*:259–264, 1972.
40. Potempa, J., and Wenz, W.: Die Indikationsstellung zur konservativen und operativen Behandlung geschlossener Nierenverletzungen. Langenbeck's Arch. Klin. Chir. *321*:149–170, 1968.

41. Prather, G. C., and Kaiser, T. F.: The bladder in fracture of the bony pelvis; the significance of a "tear drop bladder" as shown by cystogram. J. Urol. *63*:1019–1030, 1950.
42. Prince, J. C., and Pearlman, C. K.: Thrombosis of the renal artery secondary to trauma. J. Urol. *102*:670–674, 1969.
43. Quinby, W. C., Jr.: Fractures of the pelvis and associated injuries in children. J. Pediat. Surg. *1*:353, 1966.
44. Rieser, C.: Diagnostic evaluation of suspected genitourinary tract injury. J.A.M.A. *199*:714, 1967.
45. Rusche, C., and Morriw, J. W.: Injury to the ureter. *In* Campbell, M. F., ed.: Urology. (2nd Ed.) Philadelphia, W. B. Saunders Co., 1963.
46. Scholl, A. J., and Nation, E. F.: Injuries of the kidney. *In* Campbell, M. F., and Harrison, J. H., eds.: Urology. (3rd Ed.) Philadelphia, W. B. Saunders Co., 1970.
47. Schreiner, G. E.: "The nephrotic syndrome." *In* Strauss, M. B., and Welt, L. G.: Diseases of the Kidney. Boston, Little, Brown & Co., 1963.
48. Scott, R., Jr., Carlton, C. E., Ashmore, A. J., and Duke, H. H.: Initial management of non-penetrating renal injuries: Clinical review of 111 cases. J. Urol. *90*:535, 1963.
49. Scott, R., Jr., Carlton, C. E., Jr., and Goldman, M.: Penetrating injuries of the kidney: Analysis of 181 patients. J. Urol. *101*:247, 1969.
50. Scott, W. W., and Engel, R. M.: Management of urinary tract trauma. Lawyer's Med. J. 2, Second Series (2):81–97, May, 1973.
51. Snyder, W. J., Jr.: The surgically traumatized ureter: Surgeon's viewpoint. Western Med. Surg. *3*:180, 1949.
52. Stone, H. H., and Jones, H. Q.: Penetrating and non-penetrating injuries to the ureter. Surg., Gynec. Obstet. *114*:52–56, 1962.
53. Thompson, I. M., Karow, W. F., and Ross, G., Jr.: Long-term results of ureteral reimplantation for trauma. J. Urol. *102*:308–315, 1969.
54. Turner-Warwick: The repair of urethral strictures in the region of the membranous urethra. J. Urol. *100*:303, 1968.
55. Vargas, A. D., and Silva, E. I.: Mobilization of the ureter by a posterior vesical flap in dogs: Preliminary report of a new technique. J. Urol. *107*:742–746, 1972.
56. Walker, J. A.: Injuries of the ureter due to external violence. J. Urol. *102*:410–413, 1969.
57. Waterhouse, K., and Gross, M.: Trauma to the genitourinary tract: A 5-year experience with 251 cases. J. Urol. *101*:241–246, 1969.
58. Wertheim, E.: Ein neuer Beitrag zur Frage der Radikaloperation beim Uletuskrebs. Arch. Gynäk. *65*:1–39, 1901.
59. Wiggishoff, C. C., and Kiefer, J. H.: Pull-through reconstruction of the posterior urethra. J. Urol. *93*:233, 1966.
60. Zimmerman, S. J., and Radding, R. S.: Hypertension due to trauma of the kidney. New Eng. J. Med. *264*:238, 1961.

chapter

13

OBSTETRICAL AND GYNECOLOGICAL INJURIES

James J. Delaney, M.D.

GENERAL CONSIDERATIONS

Women are subject to the same traumatic situations that men face. They spend as much time as men do behind the wheel of an automobile and, therefore, are at least as apt to be involved in automobile accidents as are men. They may be subject to beatings either by jealous mates or boyfriends or as the victims of sexual assault. As more women enter the labor market, they will become subject to more industrial accidents. The general principles involved in managing all these types of trauma are discussed elsewhere in this book. The purpose of this chapter is to discuss those traumatic injuries which are more or less specifically limited to the female pelvis and reproductive organs. This includes perineal trauma, trauma associated with sexual activity and assault, induced abortion and trauma resulting from automobile accidents, and blunt or penetrating injuries.

Anatomic Principles. The perineum is that area of the torso covering the pelvic outlet. It is well protected from most incidental traumatic injuries by its anatomical position. It becomes exposed only when the thighs are abducted. The anterior boundary is the symphysis pubis; the lateral boundaries are the ischial pubic rami, ischial tuberosities and the sacrosciatic ligaments; and the posterior boundary is the coccyx. The pelvic viscera include the urinary bladder and urethra, the vagina, uterus and tubes, ovaries and rectum. These organs are protected anteriorly, posteriorly and laterally by the bony pelvis and inferiorly by the pelvic diaphragm which is made up of a series of fascial and muscular planes. Figure 13–1 graphically demonstrates these relationships as well as shows the pelvic viscera and blood supply. There are eight planes and a knowledge of the limits of these planes will enable one to understand how hematomas and/or sepsis will be confined or the extent

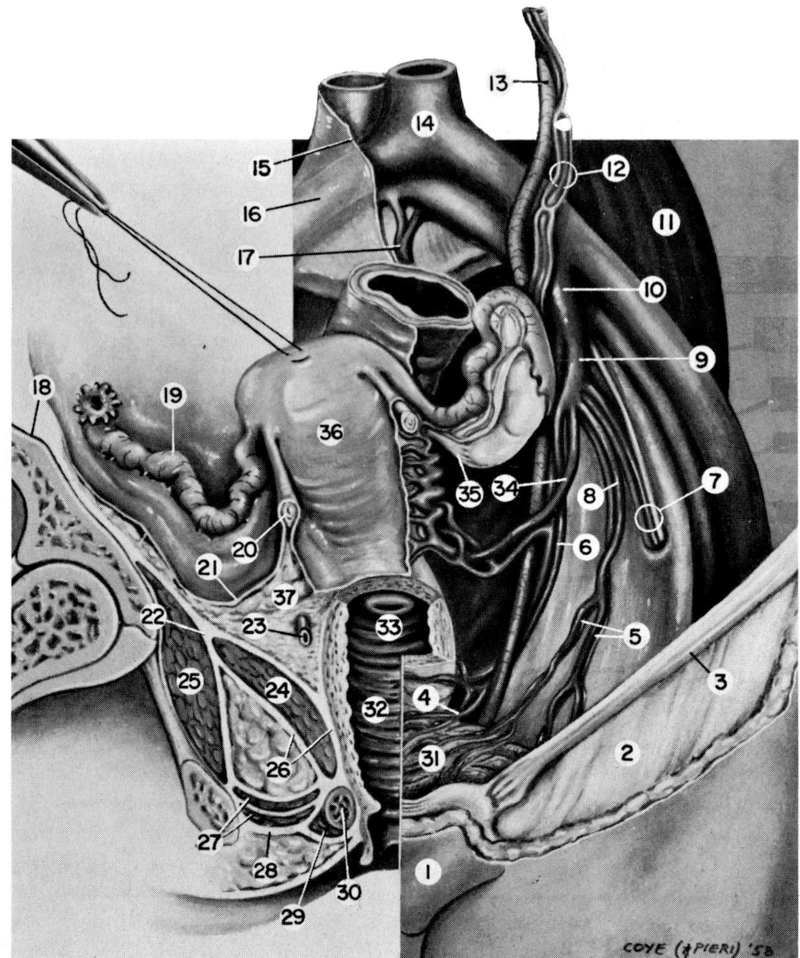

Figure 13–1 Composite illustration of main blood supply from anterior division of hypogastric artery: (1) labium majus; (2) fascia lata; (3) inguinal ligament; (4) inferior vesical artery; (5) superior and middle vesical arteries; (6) vaginal artery; (7) obturator vessels and nerve; (8) umbilical artery (superior vesical artery); (9) anterior divisions of hypogastric vessels; (10) hypogastric artery; (11) psoas muscle; (12) ovarian vessels; (13) ureter; (14) aorta; (15) cut edge of peritoneum; (16) common iliac artery; (17) middle sacral artery; (18) brim of true pelvis; (19) fallopian tube; (20) round ligament; (21) peritoneal edge; (22) superior levator fascia; (23) ureter; (24) levator ani muscle; (25) obturator internus muscle; (26) pelvic diaphragm; (27) urogenital diaphragm; (28) Colles' fascia; (29) bulbocavernosus muscle; (30) vestibular bulb; (31) bladder; (32) vagina; (33) cervix uteri; (34) uterine artery; (35) ovarian ligament; (36) uterus; (37) subperitoneal space. (From Pieri, R. J.: Obstet. Gynec. *12*:249, 1958.)

to which they may spread. Superiorly to inferiorly, the planes are as follows: The first plane consists of parietal peritoneum which is reflected over all the pelvic organs. The second plane consists of a layer of adipose tissue in which the blood vessels and nerves of the pelvis, lower extremities and the uterus are found. The clinical significance of this plane is that hematomata or infections arising in this plane may spread into the retroperitoneal space. This extension may occur posteriorly and superiorly to the diaphragm and laterally and anteriorly to the anterior abdominal wall. The third plane consists of the endopelvic or superior fascia of the levator ani muscles. The fourth plane consists of the levator ani musculature consisting of the iliococcygeus, pubococcygeus and coccygeus muscles. The fifth plane consists of the inferior fascia of the levator ani musculature. The sixth plane is divided into an anterior and posterior compartment by the superficial transverse perineal muscle. The anterior compartment is relatively small and bounded by the symphysis anteriorly and pubic rami laterally. This compartment contains the ischiocavernosus and bulbocavernosus muscles and the vestibular bulb made up of vascular erectile tissue. The posterior compartment is called the ischiorectal fossa and primarily contains adipose tissue. The lateral boundaries are the arcuate tendon of the levator musculature and the posterior boundary is the sacrum and coccyx. The clinical significance of the two compartments of this sixth plane is that a hematoma or infection in the anterior compartment will be localized in a small area. It cannot spread across the midline superiorly or posteriorly. On the other hand, an infection or hematoma in the posterior compartment will not spread anteriorly and can be at least five times as large as in the anterior compartment. The seventh plane consists of the superficial and deep (Colles') fascia. The eighth plane consists of the subcutaneous tissue and skin. This diaphragm is pierced by the rectum, vagina and urethra. Muscle fibers from the levator ani surround these orifices, forming sphincters of which the anal sphincter is most easily identified.

Trauma to the bony pelvis may spare the pelvic viscera. The female urethra is relatively short and much less apt to be transected than the male urethra. Pressure transmitted to the bladder from blunt trauma may cause the bladder to burst, but more often than not, such force will spontaneously empty the bladder without damage. This is probably due to the fact that the female urethra is relatively short. The diagnosis and treatment of urinary tract injuries are discussed in Chapter 12. In trauma-producing pelvic fractures, the femoral and obturator vessels and nerves are more apt to be damaged than are the pelvic organs, vessels or nerves. Extensive, concealed hemorrhage may occur in the retroperitoneal space as a result of a pelvic fracture.[6, 29]

Perineal and vaginal trauma is most commonly obstetrical in origin. The majority of perineal and pelvic lacerations and hematomas result from vaginal delivery. Such injuries may be associated with spontaneous deliveries, with forceps or with extraction deliveries. Most uterine ruptures are associated with obstetrical manipulation, although rupture may occasionally result from severe abdominal trauma.[5, 14, 20, 24, 26, 28] The reader is referred to standard textbooks on obstetrics for a discussion of trauma associated with obstetrical procedures.[12, 37]

Psychological Factors. Each and every part of the body has significant meaning to a patient and her family, but injuries involving the pelvis produce special anxiety. When it is apparent that the injury will not impair reproduction or sexual activity, the patient and/or her parents should be immediately reassured. In cases involving sexual assault, criminal abortion or pregnancy loss, extensive psychological support may be necessary, including psychiatric care. The physician must be careful not to make dogmatic statements regarding reproductive function or sexual activity in cases where either may be impaired. In doubtful cases, cautious optimism should be expressed. An unconcerned attitude or a rough or painful examination by the physician may seriously aggravate any associated emotional trauma.

Foreign Bodies. Occasionally a curious child, a sadistic attacker or a woman herself may place a foreign body in the urethra, vagina or rectum. Trauma may or may not result, depending on the type of object and the manner in which it is placed. Women will frequently consult a physician, claiming they have "lost" a tampon or diaphragm. In almost all such cases, the "lost" object has been lost in the toilet and the only treatment necessary is an inspection of the vagina and reassurance that the object is not present and has not been "lost" above the vagina. The problem of foreign bodies in small girls is usually one of infection rather than trauma, although perineal or vaginal lacerations may also have been produced. Because of the sensitivity of the vagina of a child, sedation or anesthesia may be necessary to adequately inspect the area and remove the foreign body.

Occasionally, severe trauma will be seen from a foreign body inserted into the vagina by a sexual pervert. Such an object may be driven through the cul-de-sac into the peritoneal cavity by a kick or other heavy blow. An exploratory laparotomy is indicated in such cases.

A woman or her sexual partner may place a foreign body in the vagina, urethra or rectum for the purpose of stimulating venereal pleasure. The trauma caused by such a practice will depend on the object used, where it is placed and what forces were used to place it. If the patient is unable to remove the object, the examining physician should have no trouble making the correct diagnosis. Treatment obviously consists of removing the object and repairing any lacerations that may be bleeding. The principles involved in managing trauma from foreign bodies include removing the object and then proceeding in a manner similar to that of managing trauma from other sources which will be discussed later.

PERINEAL INJURIES

Straddle Injuries. Very little is written in standard textbooks of obstetrics and gynecology regarding perineal injuries, especially straddle injuries. As the term suggests, such injuries are caused by falling on an object with the legs on either side of an object so that the perineum absorbs most of the impact. These injuries are most often seen in girls who fall while playing. With the increasing popularity of cycling and the preference by girls for the so-called boy's bike, we will undoubtedly see more straddle injuries.

Management. In this type of injury, the main concern of most girls and their parents is whether or not reproduction or sexual function will be impaired. In almost all cases, they can be reassured following a brief examination. Following initial inspection of the injury to determine its extent, treatment should begin by relieving any pain that may be present. This may require anything from oral analgesics to general anesthesia. It is usually impossible to perform an adequate vaginal examination on a prepubescent child without anesthesia. The extent of the examination will depend on the type of injury. Most straddle injuries produce blunt trauma and result in contusions or hematoma formation. Occasionally, the object may be sharp, resulting in lacerations or a puncture wound. Unless the injury is obviously minor, a digital vaginal or rectal examination should be done to determine the presence or absence of hematoma formation above the pelvic diaphragm. Hematomas can usually be treated nonoperatively. A hematoma should be evacuated only if it is growing or is excessively painful. If a hematoma is evacuated, usually no active site of bleeding will be found. If generalized bleeding is apparent, hemostatic sutures may be necessary using absorbable suture. If the bleeding is not brisk, a firm pack should be placed either in lieu of the sutures or in addition to the sutures. The pack should be removed in 24 hours. Prophylactic antibiotics should also be administered. Lacerations and puncture wounds should be treated the same as in any other area of the body. If there is a question of a rectal injury, the principles of managing bowel injuries, as described in Chapter 11, should be followed.

TRAUMA RESULTING FROM SEXUAL ACTIVITY

Trauma may result from either voluntary or involuntary sexual activity.[38] These injuries may be the result of normal heterosexual activity, homosexual activity, perverted activity or masturbation. The most common injury is a laceration and the most common presenting complaint is abnormal vaginal bleeding. Because of embarrassment, intoxication or fright, an accurate history may not be obtained, so trauma from sexual activity should always be considered in cases of acute onset of vaginal bleeding. Certain factors may render a woman susceptible to injury from sexual activity. These include a lack of estrogen effect (which normally produces a well-cornified vaginal epithelium and distensible vagina), pregnancy and recent vaginal surgery. The true incidence of such injuries is unknown, as most patients with these injuries probably do not seek care unless there is significant bleeding or pain. Wilson[38] reports only 37 cases of vaginal trauma from sexual activity over a 10-year period at the Harlem Hospital Center. Death has resulted from such trauma,[4] but is almost inexcusable with appropriate therapy.

Management. Careful inspection of the vagina should be carried out to make sure that there are no multiple lacerations. If a bivalve speculum is used, the speculum should be rotated laterally so that both the anterior and posterior walls of the vagina can be seen as well as the lateral walls. The presence of perineal lacerations should not prevent inspection of the vagina. A gentle bimanual rectovaginal examination should also be carried out to make sure there are no retroperitoneal hematomas developing as a result of the trauma. If the laceration is actively bleeding, fairly extensive or on the perineum, the best method of management is repair with absorbable suture. Packing should be utilized to control hemorrhage only when the trauma is too extensive to repair primarily. If a pack is placed, it should be soaked in Furacin or other antibiotic cream and packed tightly into the vagina. It should be removed in 12 to 24 hours. There are practically no residual complications from vaginal lacerations once the bleeding has been controlled. If the introitus has been injured, the repair may occasionally lead to a decrease in size of the introitus or it may result in some fibrous scar tissue which might make intercourse moderately painful in the future. However, this complication is only rarely seen and is more commonly associated with the repair of an episiotomy.

Assault and Molestation

Any female, regardless of age, may be the victim of an unprovoked sexual attack. The physician involved in caring for such patients must be cognizant of the individual needs of the patient as well as the potential legal ramifications of a particular case. Many physicians are reluctant to treat patients who have been the objects of assault because of the fear of getting involved with the legal aspects of the case. This reluctance to act is usually based on ignorance of what may be expected of the physician.

Legal Aspects. In most cases, the physician should have no fear of legal repercussions because he has cared for the victim of a sex crime. He should understand that state statutes regarding assault and molestation merely define what acts are illegal and prescribe a penalty for any individual convicted of having committed the defined offense. Rape is generally considered to have occurred if a woman is forced to submit to coitus without consent. Statutory rape is defined as coitus with a female below the age of consent. The age of consent varies from state to state, and it should be noted that consent is not a consideration in statutory rape. Sexual molestation is usually considered to have occurred if non-coital sexual contact has occurred in an individual below the age of consent.

The physician has three obligations in dealing with a patient who may have been the victim of criminal assault. His first obligation is to administer to the needs of the patient. His second obligation is to accurately record his observations and save any possible evidence that may be used in the case. His third obligation is to report the case to the appropriate law enforcement agency if he has reason to believe a crime may have been committed. The physician is neither competent nor required to make a judgment decision regarding whether a crime has been committed. By recording objective findings, he will not have to render a judgment as to whether or not the patient has been assaulted. Should such a case come to court, accurately recorded objective findings should be sufficient to provide the necessary evidence to determine whether a crime was committed. The physician should treat the patient the same, regardless of whether he is asked to examine the patient by a member of the local law enforcement agency or whether the patient comes to him herself or is brought in by her parents. The physician should record and document who is requesting the examination, especially if the individual is unconscious or below the age of consent. A "request for examination" form should be signed by the person making the request.

Management. In evaluating and treating the victim of an assault, the physician must consider the following priorities: First, he must give immediate care to physical injuries; second, he must treat the psychological trauma that always accompanies an assault; third, he must consider the prevention of pregnancy; and fourth, he must consider the prevention of venereal disease.

Institutions dealing with this problem on a fairly frequent basis, such as a large city or community hospital, would be well advised to have a standard operating procedure to which physicians could refer in such cases. The American College of Obstetricians and Gynecologists has a technical bulletin available covering most of the problems related to rape and suggests a procedure which should be followed.[1] Several articles have recently appeared in the literature which discuss the problems involved in dealing with cases of sexual assault.[15, 18, 19, 25, 31] The first thing to do is to obtain proper consent. If an examination is requested by a law enforcement officer, a form should be furnished for this purpose so that the signature of the requesting officer can be obtained and retained in the record. If the individual is a minor and a law enforcement officer is not requesting the examination, a parent or guardian should give consent. If the individual is over the age of consent and requesting the examination herself, this should so be stated in the record. An accurate history should then be obtained from the patient if she is capable of communicating in a rational manner. If the patient seems to be hysterical or there is any question about her mental status, notes should be made to this effect. Next an examination should be carried out and the initial examination should be done before the patient is disrobed. The appearance of the patient and her clothing should be described. It should be remembered that multiple injuries may be present and a complete physical examination should be carried out on all patients. Any evidence of trauma, including abrasions, contusions, lacerations, etc. should be recorded in terms of their location and their severity. If there is evidence that ejaculation has taken place, material should be obtained for the evaluation of the presence of acid phosphatase. Consideration should be given to combing the pubic hair and saving any loose hairs for possible evidence. The rationale behind this is that pubic hairs can be identified in a manner similar to finger prints as being that of a particular individual.

When the pelvic examination is done, three specimens should be obtained. A wet smear should be obtained and examined for the presence or absence of spermatozoa. It should be remembered that finding sperm does not necessarily mean that the patient has been raped, as the sperm may belong to her husband, and conversely, the absence of the sperm does not necessarily mean that she has not been raped. The findings of the wet smear should be recorded. A smear from the cervix and one from the upper vagina should be obtained and fixed in the usual manner for Papanicolaou smears. The slides should be labeled with a diamond-headed pen and either locked in a box or delivered personally to the pathologist so that there is no question regarding the origin of the slides should this information be subpoenaed in court. And finally, cultures should be taken for Neisseria gonorrhea organisms.

If the patient is a child, she should not be subjected to a pelvic examination without sedation, and serious consideration should be given to doing such an examination under anesthesia. Obviously, any severe trauma should be treated as soon as possible, but not before a complete examination has been performed.

Sedation may be necessary as a form of management but preferably should not be given prior to obtaining an accurate history. Hospitalization may or may not be required, depending upon the severity of injuries and the psychological state of the patient. Emotionally unstable patients should be kept in the hospital for observation. Psychiatric consultation may or may not be necessary, depending upon the psychological state of the patient. Victims of an assault may have been forced to submit to unnatural sexual activity as well as so-called natural activity, which may aggravate their anxiety. Some arrangements for follow-up should be made with the patient given a return appointment within a week.

Pregnancy Prevention. It is extremely unlikely that a pregnancy will result from criminal assault, but there is no excuse for not acting to prevent such a pregnancy in any woman who is in the first half of her menstrual cycle. As part of the history, the date of the last normal menstrual period should be obtained and information regarding contraceptive practices should also be included. If the patient is using oral contraceptives or an intrauterine device, it can be assumed that pregnancy will not result from the assault. This is likewise true of a woman who is past the menopause or of a prepubescent girl. If the woman is past midcycle and she has a cellular effect, as seen in her cervical mucus smear, it can be assumed that she has ovulated and will not be pregnant as a result of the assault. However, if the patient is in the first half of her cycle and has not been taking oral contraceptives, it is desirable to act to prevent a possible pregnancy. The use of relatively high doses of estrogen within 48 hours of the assault will prevent pregnancy.[23] The mechanism for action of this therapy is not known. The estrogen must somehow act by either preventing fertilization or implantation since an existing early pregnancy will not be terminated. One of the standard regimens in the past has been to give 25 mgm. of diethylstilbestrol daily for three days. However, because of the recent controversy over the delayed carcinogenic effect of diethylstilbestrol in the young female offspring of women who have been treated with stilbestrol, this drug is no longer used as often for the prevention of pregnancy. It would appear on the basis of current experience that conjugated estrogens may also be effective in preventing pregnancy. A regimen consisting of 40 mgm. of conjugated estrogen given intravenously following the examination followed by 5 mgm. orally three times a day for seven days will most likely prevent any pregnancy. Ten mgm. of Provera should be given during the last five days. The reason for giving estrogen and progesterone is to assure that there will be an adequate slough of the endometrium following hormonal therapy. Giving estrogen alone may lead to an incomplete slough of the endometrial lining and cause irregular bleeding. It should be stressed that there are currently no published data available documenting the effectiveness of conjugated estrogens in preventing pregnancy.

Venereal Disease Prophylaxis. Antibiotic therapy should probably be instituted to prevent the possible development of either gonorrhea or syphilis. Penicillin still is the drug of choice for treating these diseases; however, because of the recent controversies over the emergence of resistant strains of Neisseria gonorrhea, some consideration may be given to treating the patient with an alternative drug such as tetracycline.[32] It is important to see patients for follow-up evaluation to make sure they have not contracted either disease in spite of appropriate antibiotic therapy.

Children who are the victims of molestation should be evaluated in a manner similar to rape cases. However, the physician must be even more careful in dealing with a child to prevent unnecessary pain and psychic trauma.

ABORTION

Induced Abortion. Not too many years ago a woman who found herself unexpectedly pregnant had three alternatives. She could keep the child, give it up for adoption or seek a criminal abortion. If she chose the third option, more often than not, she would eventually end up in the hospital suffering from one or more of the potential complications of the procedure. Sepsis and/or bleeding were the most commonly seen complications and often existed simultaneously. The illegal abortionist would often prescribe or administer an antibiotic which was just effective enough to delay or mask some of the signs of sepsis, thus delaying an accurate diagnosis and the onset of appropriate treatment.

During the last few years, the change in public attitude has led to a change in our laws and consequently a change in physicians' attitudes toward induced abortion. An unknown number of "legal" abortions are now being performed by licensed physicians. This practice has led to a marked decrease in the number of criminal abortions performed but has not completely eliminated them. This in turn has led to a decrease in the number of complications resulting from illegal abortions. The type of complications seen have changed considerably and most of these complications are managed by the people performing the abortions. However, since many patients travel elsewhere to be aborted and because criminal abortions are still performed, it is important for physicians to understand how to manage these traumatic complications.

A viable pregnancy is relatively difficult to terminate. The cervix, especially in a nulligravida, is firm and tightly closed, rendering it subject to laceration upon forced dilatation. The trophoblastic tissue of the developing placenta burrows directly into the myometrium, exposing large blood vessels. This tissue is removed only with difficulty and when removed, results in considerable bleeding. The relatively thin wall of the uterus at the site of implantation may be perforated by a relatively sharp instrument. The uterine cavity with its vascular lining, the endometrium, may serve as a favored site for the proliferation of bacteria.

Methods of Inducing Abortion. At the present time there are essentially three methods of inducing abortion. The first and most commonly used method is the suction curettage. The development of this technique has made it possible to perform large numbers of abortions with relative safety and efficiency. The most difficult part of this procedure is to dilate the cervix. If the usual forcible dilatation is carried out using the standard dilators, the risk of cervical laceration is increased. The use of cervical laminaria and/or other methods, such as a Foley catheter, which seem to soften the cervix prior to performing the abortion, have decreased the risk of damaging the cervix. A cannula used for the suction portion of the curettage is usually plastic, disposable, approximately 1 cm. in diameter and blunted on the end to decrease the chances of perforating the uterus. Abortions may be performed utilizing this method until approximately 12 weeks as counted from the last normal menstrual period. Beyond this gestational age, the uterus and the products of conception are so large that the risk of perforation of the uterus and incomplete removal of the products of conception decreases the effectiveness of this method.

The second method of performing abortion is amniocentesis, utilizing some solution which will initiate the onset of labor and expel the products of conception. This method is generally performed during mid-trimester and is preferably done when the uterus is 16 weeks size or larger because it is technically easier than when the uterus is smaller. As much amniotic fluid as possible is removed and the solution to be used is injected into the amniotic sac. The most commonly used solution in the past has been 20 per cent sodium chloride. The mechanism of action in this type of abortion is not understood. The risk to the patient from this method of inducing abortion is considerably greater than with the suction curettage. If the hypertonic saline is absorbed rapidly into the vascular system, significant fluid and electrolyte imbalances may result. From 6 to 10 per cent of patients aborted in this manner have retained products of conception and require a uterine curettage to complete the abortion.[2,3,6]

The third most common way that abortions are performed is by hysterotomy or hysterectomy. Risks associated with these procedures are the same as those associated with any major surgical procedure.

Management. In the past, because of the criminal nature of these procedures, it was often difficult to obtain an adequate history from a patient. To some extent, this may continue to be the case because of the stigma that still attaches to abortion, but a woman may be much more apt to state that she has had an induced abortion and feels that her problem may be related to this procedure. It is important to obtain from the patient information regarding the method used to induce the abortion and the date of her last normal menstrual period so that an accurate gestational age can be calculated. In addition to a general physical examination with special attention to vital signs and abdominal signs, a careful pelvic examination should be carried out. At the time of pelvic examination, the amount of bleeding should be noted and the vagina should be inspected for the presence of lacerations. The cervix should be inspected and a bimanual examination should be done with special emphasis on determining the size of the uterus. If the uterus is compatible with the calculated gestational age or larger, it is probable that the abortion has not been completed and that products of conception most likely still remain in the uterus. Following the bimanual examination, either a sterile ring forceps or a Hegar dilator should be passed into the cervix to determine whether the internal cervical os is opened or closed. The presence or absence of fetal heart tones should also be determined, but this usually requires the use of a Doppler ultrasound instrument.

After a complete examination has been performed, appropriate treatment should be instituted. A complete blood count should be obtained. The hematocrit and hemaglobin values will serve as a reference for circulating blood volume. The white blood count can serve as a reference for the severity of infection. It should be remembered that every pregnant patient will have a slightly elevated white blood count and an elevated sedimentation rate. Therefore, a white blood count up to 14,000 cells per cc may be seen in the absence of infection. If there is minimal bleeding, if the uterus is eight weeks size or less and is firm and non-tender, and if the CBC is essentially normal and the cervix is either closed or open with no tissue present, the patient should be observed. If the uterus is larger than eight weeks size and fetal heart tones are present, the patient should also be observed. If the patient has signs of hypovolemia or frank shock, vigorous intravenous fluid therapy should be initiated to restore effective circulating volume. An indwelling Foley catheter should be used to accurately measure urine volume, and a central venous pressure catheter should be introduced to monitor the response to this therapy. The management of hypovolemic shock is discussed in further detail in Chapter 3. If there is evidence of infection, large doses of broad-spectrum antibiotics should be given intravenously.

The decision regarding surgical intervention should be made on the basis of whether residual products of conception are still present in the uterus or perhaps expelled into the pelvis from a uterine perforation. If fetal heart tones are present, the decision to intervene may be difficult to make. In spite of sepsis and excessive bleeding, it is well established that such pregnancies can continue to term with the delivery of a normal, healthy infant. In such cases, the blood volume has been replaced by transfusion and the sepsis eliminated by the use of antibiotics.

In most cases, surgical intervention should be delayed until appropriate supportive measures have been carried out. If there is no evidence of sepsis, which is rare, the patient may be taken to the operating room once effective circulating blood volume is sufficiently restored to allow the administration of anesthesia with safety. On rare occasions, bleeding may be so profuse that the maintenance of blood volume by transfusion may be impossible, in which cases early surgical intervention is indicated to control the hemorrhage. If sepsis is present, as it usually is, the patient should ideally be treated with antibiotics for six to 12 hours before any surgery is performed. In most cases, the only surgical procedure necessary is a curettage of the uterus. The cervix is usually already dilated and will readily admit a curette. The uterus should first be sounded with a dull probe to accurately determine its size and to rule out a possible perforation. The uterine cavity should then be gently curetted with either a sharp curette or a suction curette. Great care should be taken not to perforate the uterus during this procedure. The suction curette should not be used if a uterine perforation is thought to be present. However, a sharp curettage should be done to attempt to remove all the products of conception. An exploratory laparotomy should be performed if there is reason to believe that products of conception have been expelled into the abdominal cavity or if there is a probability that a bowel injury has occurred. Bowel may be sucked through a uterine perforation by the suction curette. When an exploratory laparotomy is performed and a uterine perforation is found, no attempt should be made to close the perforation. Any products of conception that are present should be removed, the bowel should be inspected for injury and the cul-de-sac should be drained either into the vagina or laterally in either lower quadrant. In most cases, the uterine perforation will heal and be of no concern if a subsequent pregnancy occurs. In cases of massive pelvic infection, a total abdominal hysterectomy and bilateral salpingo-oophorectomy may be necessary.

The complications arising from abortions induced by amniocentesis are usually so acute that the person performing the abortion is aware of the problem and must manage it. Probably all amniocentesis-induced abortions, regardless of the solution used, develop signs of intravascular coagulation. The reason for this is unknown, but one possibility is the release of placental thromboplastin into maternal circulation.[33] Fortunately, most cases are mild and require no treatment. As mentioned above, approximately 10 per cent of patients aborted by amniocentesis will require a uterine curettage for completion of the abortion. The same precautions mentioned earlier should be taken.

Miscellaneous Problems. For a variety of reasons, a woman may not seek legal termination of an unwanted pregnancy, preferring instead to seek some other avenue of terminating her pregnancy. She may take some form of medication. Quinine-containing drugs have frequently been used to this end. The side effects of excessive quinine may include nausea, vomiting, vertigo, tinnitus and diarrhea. Fortunately, these side effects are self-limiting. Other drugs may be ingested, so the physician must use common sense and consult a toxicology reference in managing any complications that arise.

A woman may also seek to terminate her pregnancy by introducing an irritating substance or foreign body into the vagina or uterus. Potassium permanganate tablets have been used for this purpose. These tablets react with the vaginal mucosa, resulting in ulceration and subsequent vaginal bleeding which may be extensive. Lye-containing substances have also been used with similar results. Treatment consists of vaginal irrigation, blood replacement when necessary, control of the bleeding with a vaginal pack saturated with a steroid cream and frequent follow-up to assure that healing occurs. Extensive burns may result in extensive scarring with vaginal stenosis. The use of a foreign body may produce vaginal or cervical lacerations and perforation of the cul-de-sac or uterus. Management of these complications was discussed previously in this chapter.

Spontaneous Abortion. Perhaps it is improper to discuss the management of spontaneous abortion in a book on trauma, but occasionally it is difficult to differentiate between a spontaneous abortion and an induced abortion, and the principles of management are similar. The subject is mentioned here only to remind the physician that spontaneous abortion may lead to excessive blood loss so that when the patient presents in the office or in the emergency room, general principles of management expressed in this book are applicable.

Summary. Any woman of childbearing age who presents with any of the symptoms of lower abdominal or pelvic pain, vaginal bleeding and/or infection should be evaluated for the possibility of the complications of abortion. At the time of the physical examination, special attention should be directed toward the presence or absence of lacerations of the vagina, lacerations of the cervix, the size of the uterus and the intactness of the uterine cavity. In most instances, supportive measures such as blood transfusions and antibiotics should be instituted before a patient is taken to the operating room. A curettage of the uterus should always be performed if there is any question of retained products of conception. Exception to this would be if fetal heart tones are detectible, the amount of bleeding is not significant and the evidence of excessive blood loss is not present. In such cases, even if an induced abortion has been attempted, the pregnancy may continue to viability.

A uterus that has been perforated should not be repaired. In the absence of massive infection, the perforation will heal spontaneously and will not jeopardize future childbearing. On the other hand, if widespread pelvic sepsis is present, the only treatment may be total hysterectomy and bilateral salpingo-oophorectomy.

TRAUMA IN PREGNANT WOMEN

In cases of trauma involving a pregnant patient, there are certain additional therapeutic considerations that the examining physician must be aware of. He must consider the well-being of the infant as well as that of the mother. He must also be aware of the potential late complications resulting from trauma and may often be asked in court whether or not termination of the pregnancy occurred as a result of the traumatic incident. Finally, the size of the pregnant uterus may actually serve as a protection to more severe trauma to a woman, especially in cases of penetrating trauma.

General Principles. For all practical purposes, the developing infant is extremely well protected within the confines of the uterine cavity. The amniotic fluid acts as an excellent shock absorber and it is extremely rare for a fetus to experience physical trauma as a result of anything but direct penetrating trauma. During the first trimester, the uterus is protected by the bony pelvis, while in the last two trimesters, the enlarging uterus distends the abdominal wall and at the same time displaces the bowel superiorly. Such an anatomical arrangement, although making the infant more susceptible to trauma during the last two trimesters, actually protects the major blood vessels and the intestines of the mother from damage from penetrating trauma, such as in the cases of knife wounds, bullet wounds or shrapnel wounds.

In cases of blunt trauma involving the abdomen, the major risk to the fetus is placental abruption. In such cases, the abruption may be either partial or total and vaginal bleeding may or may not be present. In cases of complete abruption, the infant will be dead at the time of the examination, but in cases of partial abruption, the infant may survive only to suffer intrauterine malnutrition from an incomplete placental circulation.

In evaluating injured women in the childbearing age, pregnancy should be considered possible until proved to be otherwise by examination. The risk to the mother and the prognosis of the pregnancy will vary, depending upon the type of trauma and the gestational age at the time the trauma occurred.[11, 16, 30] The physician must also consider the late sequelae of this trauma in regard to future pregnancy. A pelvic fracture may lead to a contracture, which will necessitate a cesarean section. It is also possible, but unlikely, that a traumatic incident may produce sterility.

The mechanism(s) that initiate labor are not known, but it has been observed that progesterone seems to inhibit uterine contractions. For this reason, many women are treated with progesterone to prevent the onset of premature labor. Whenever an exploratory laparotomy is performed or whenever a pregnant woman has been subjected to some form of trauma, it is probably a good idea to treat her with progesterone. The dosage is empirical. One-hundred mgm. of progesterone in oil should be given intramuscularly to give immediate elevated blood levels of progesterone. At the same time, 500 mgm. of hydroxyprogesterone caproate (Delalutin) should be given intramuscularly and repeated in two to three days. The longer-acting hydroxyprogesterone acetate (Depo-Provera) should not be administered because of the prolonged action and unpredictable effect on future menstrual normality. There are essentially no significant side effects from progesterone administered as recommended.

Deliberate termination of a pregnancy in a woman who has been subjected to trauma is indicated in only two instances. The first indication is excessive bleeding from the uterus, which is usually caused by a severe placental abruption, and the second is evidence of fetal distress (fetal heart rate less than 110) in a potentially salvageable pregnancy (30 weeks or more).

Non-traumatic Surgical Diseases. The pregnant patient may require surgery for the same reasons as the non-pregnant patient. The pregnancy should not be terminated in such cases and the prognosis for the pregnancy is excellent.[30] Progesterone may be used in the dosage recommended above.

Automobile Injuries. In the past there has been controversy over whether pregnant women should wear restraining harnesses or seat belts when traveling in automobiles. The reason for this concern had to do with the transmission of forces on impact from the restraints to the fetus. There now seems to be sufficient information to resolve this controversy.[8] Crosby and his co-workers have shown conclusively that the use of lap belts *with* or *without* shoulder harnesses has saved more fetal and maternal lives than has failure to use them.[9, 10] The leading cause of fetal mortality from automobile accidents is maternal mortality. In cases where the mother survives, the primary risk to the infant is from abruption of the placenta. This may occur at the time of the accident or may be delayed several days.

Management. Any woman involved in an automobile accident should undergo a thorough examination including a pelvic examination. Information regarding her last normal menstrual period should be recorded in the history, and all physical findings, including those found at the time of pelvic examination, should be accurately recorded. There are two reasons for this: (1) to determine whether a pregnancy is present so that its continuation can be closely monitored, and (2) because of the possible litigation which may occur if a pregnancy is lost as a result of the accident. If a pregnancy does exist, the management of the patient will depend in part on the gestational age of the fetus. The management of airway problems, hemorrhage, central nervous system injuries and fractures takes preference over the management of the pregnancy unless bleeding from an abrupted placenta or ruptured uterus is contributing to uncontrolled hemorrhage.

As mentioned earlier, the only indication for terminating a pregnancy is excessive uterine bleeding or evidence of fetal distress in a potentially salvageable pregnancy. If the gestational age is less than 20 weeks, usually no treatment is necessary. However, progesterone may be given in the dosage recommended above. If a spontaneous abortion subsequently occurs, the products of conception should be examined to attempt to determine the etiology of the abortion. If the fetus is well formed and the abortion resulted from the accident, placental hemorrhage should be evident. On the other hand, if an identifiable fetus is not present, the abortion could not possibly have been caused by the accident; it would have occurred spontaneously in spite of the accident. In more advanced pregnancies, especially those pregnancies beyond 25 weeks, the presence or absence of fetal heart tones should be determined as soon as practical. If fetal heart tones are absent, nothing can be done to salvage the pregnancy. The usual cause of this is complete abruption of the placenta. Management in such cases is to observe the patient for the development of shock or abnormal bleeding. If there is no sign of shock and no other evidence of serious injury, the patient may be observed and spontaneous labor will undoubtedly occur within a short period of time. Occasionally, a delay of several days may occur.

Sometimes the uterus is ruptured in a severe accident and the infant is expelled into the abdominal cavity. In such cases, the infant will have died from a lack of placental perfusion and the uterus will contract sufficiently to prevent continued hemorrhage. The diagnosis of a ruptured uterus may be difficult to make, but as long as the patient is not in shock or the shock can be prevented, the patient can be observed until a definitive diagnosis can be made. Once the diagnosis has been made, an exploratory laparotomy should be performed and the uterine defect repaired. A subsequent pregnancy should be terminated by cesarean section.

If fetal heart tones are present, these heart tones should be monitored, preferably with an external monitoring device for 24 to 48 hours. There are cases of partial abruption in which the infant does not die immediately, but there is insufficient placental circulation to maintain growth and development. This failure to grow can be documented by measuring the fundal height in centimeters. The height should equal the weeks of gestation between 20 and 32 weeks. Even if there are no significant physical injuries present in severe automobile accidents, it is advisable to hospitalize the patient and, if an external fetal monitor is available, to monitor fetal heart tones for a period of 24 to 48 hours. If a partial abruption of the placenta has occurred, evidence of fetal distress will eventually be noted and the pregnancy should then be terminated by cesarean section, as long as the patient is stable enough to tolerate this procedure.

The delayed complications of pregnancy resulting from automobile trauma are specifically related to pelvic fractures which may produce pelvic dystocia and result in the need for abdominal delivery. Figure 13–2 exhibits a typical pelvic contracture following pelvic fractures suffered in an automobile accident. It is extremely difficult to predict which patient will require abdominal delivery and which will be able to deliver vaginally on the basis of either clinical or x-ray pelvimetry. Any obstetrician who has had experience with patients with pelvic contractures realizes that the real proof of pelvic dystocia must await a trial of labor. As long as there is no complication of the pregnancy and no contraindication to allow a trial of labor (such as a previous cesarean section), every patient should be given an opportunity to deliver vaginally. However, no heroic efforts such as Pitocin stimulation should be carried out in an attempt to force an infant through a contracted pelvis. Dyer[11] and Spear[35] reported that four out of five patients who sustained pelvic fractures at the time of an automobile accident subsequently delivered vaginally without difficulty.

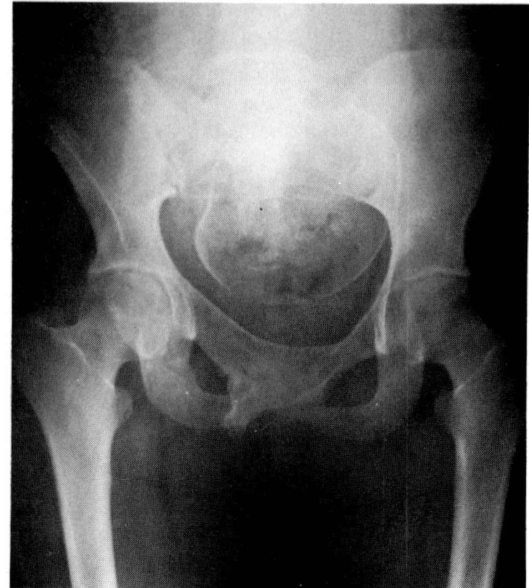

Figure 13–2 X-ray pelvimetry demonstrating a contracted pelvis following an auto accident.

MISCELLANEOUS TRAUMA

Penetrating Injuries. Penetrating abdominal or pelvic injuries in the non-pregnant woman should be managed as described elsewhere in this book, and penetrating injuries to the abdomen of pregnant women should be managed in a manner similar to that of non-pregnant women. Occasionally, if there is no evidence of shock, excessive blood loss or evidence of a ruptured hollow viscus, the patient may be observed closely in the hospital. The decision to do an exploratory laparotomy should be based upon the extent of trauma, the type of trauma involved and the condition of the patient at the time she is evaluated. As a general rule, all patients with penetrating abdominal wounds should be explored. If an exploratory laparotomy is performed, there is no justification for doing a cesarean section just to deliver the infant at that time. More often than not, these infants will die of the complications of prematurity, and the potential postoperative complications from the cesarean section may make management of the patient's other injuries more complicated than need be. Even if the fetus is dead, there is no indication for termination of the pregnancy.

In advanced pregnancy, the uterus will probably be entered by the penetrating trauma. Because of the muscular wall, damage to the uterus may be slight. The fetus may or may not be injured in such cases. There have been reports of a fetus surviving such trauma, including gunshot, stab and shrapnel injuries.[3, 13, 17, 21, 22] In such cases, the only indication for terminating the pregnancy is excessive bleeding or a large defect, in which case the infant will not have survived and may have been expelled through the defect. The uterine defect should be closed by suturing. Debridement, if necessary, should be done prior to the repair.

Blunt Trauma. Most blunt trauma sufficient to cause maternal injury or place the fetus in jeopardy results from automobile accidents. Occasionally, a woman may be subjected to a severe beating, fall from a considerable height or be crushed by a heavy object.[14, 16] The principles of management in these cases are the same as those discussed under automobile injuries.

One other problem that the physician should be aware of is the traumatic or spontaneous rupture of an epigastric vessel, which may simulate an acute abdomen or concealed placental abruption. The signs and symptoms usually are evidence of hidden blood loss, abdominal pain and uterine irritability. Treatment in such cases is blood transfusion and operation to ligate the ruptured vessel.

Spontaneous or traumatic rupture of the liver and spleen has been reported to occur in pregnancy.[7, 27, 34] The management of these problems is the same as it would be in the non-pregnant state. Termination of the pregnancy is no more indicated in such cases than it is in any of the other traumatic problems previously discussed.

SUMMARY

Some common principles regarding trauma to the external genitalia, pelvis and abdomen of women, both in the pregnant and non-pregnant state have been discussed. The principles involved in managing these cases are similar to those involved in managing any case of trauma. All of the patient's organ systems should be evaluated when appropriate and antibiotics used in the face of infection. Good common sense and reassurance are essential in managing these problems.

The treating physician should be cognizant of the potential litigation which may result from the traumatic episode, but the fear of having to testify in court regarding a particular case should not in any way prevent him from treating the patient in an appropriate manner. By recording objective findings, saving potential evidence and not recording subjective impressions, the physician should have no problem if litigation results from a case of trauma. There are two different potential legal problems. The most common situation is the one in which the victim of the trauma sues the instigator of the trauma or the instigator is prosecuted for a felonious act, such as rape. In these situations, the only information requested is an accurate description of the physical findings at the time the patient was treated. The second problem, the one most feared by physicians, is that the patient may have a bad result or be unhappy with the treatment she received from the physician and bring suit against him for malpractice. Most such cases can be avoided by following the principles described in this book and seeing that the patient has competent follow-up treatment. Hopefully, the fear of a malpractice suit will not prevent any physician from treating a patient who has been the victim of trauma.

REFERENCES

1. American College of Obstetricians and Gynecologists: Suspected rape. Am. Coll. Obstet. Gynec. Tech. Bull. No. 14, July 1970.
2. Ballard, C. A., and Ballard, F. E.: Four years experience with mid-trimester abortion amnio-infusion. Am. J. Obstet. Gynec. *114*:575–581, November 1, 1972.
3. Beattie, J. F., and Daly, F. R.: Gunshot wound of the pregnant uterus. Am. J. Obstet. Gynec. *80*:771–774, 1960.
4. Blair, R.: A fatal injury of the vagina. Brit. Med. J. *1*:828–829, 1925.
5. Bochner, K.: Traumatic perforation of the pregnant uterus. Obstet. Gynec. *17*:520–521, 1961.
6. Braunstein, P. W., Skudder, P. A., McCarroll, J. R., Musolino, A., and Wade, P. A.: Concealed hemorrhage due to pelvic fracture. J. Trauma *4*:832–835, 1964.
7. Cairns, J. D., Woods, J. M., and Sladen, J. G.: Traumatic rupture of the spleen with delayed intraperitoneal hemorrhage during pregnancy. J. Can. Med. Assoc. *90*:30–33, 1964.
8. Committee on Medical Aspects of Automobile Safety: Automobile safety belts during pregnancy. J.A.M.A. *221*:20–21, July 3, 1972.
9. Crosby, W. M., and Costilloe, J. P.: Safety of lap belt restraint for pregnant victims of automobile collisions. New Eng. J. Med. *284*:632–637, 1971.
10. Crosby, W. M., King, A. I., and Stout, A. C.: Fetal survival following impact: Improvement with shoulder harness restraint. Am. J. Obstet. Gynec. *112*:1101–1107, April 15, 1972.
11. Dyer, I., and Barclay, D. L.: Accidental trauma complicating pregnancy and delivery. Am. J. Obstet. Gynec. *83*:907–929, April 1962.
12. Eastman, J. J., and Hellman, L. M.: Williams Obstetrics (14th Ed.) New York, Appleton-Century-Crofts, 1971.
13. Eckerling, B., and Teaff, R.: Obstetrical approach to abdominal war wounds in late pregnancy. J. Obstet. Gynec. Brit. Emp. *57*:747–750, 1950.
14. Elias, M.: Rupture of the pregnant uterus by external violence. Lancet *2*:253, 1950.
15. Evrard, J. R.: Rape: The medical, social and legal implications. Am. J. Obstet. Gynec. *111*:197–199, 1971.
16. Fort, A. T., and Harlin, R. S.: Pregnancy outcome for noncatastrophic maternal trauma during pregnancy. Obstet. Gynec. *35*:912–915, June 1970.
17. Geggie, N. S.: Gunshot wound of the pregnant uterus with survival of the fetus. J. Can. Med. Assoc. *84*:489–491, 1961.
18. Hayman, C. R., and Lanza, C.: Sexual assault on women and girls. Am. J. Obstet. Gynec. *109*:480–487, February 1, 1971.
19. Hayman, C. R., Lanza, C., Fuentes, R., and Algor, K.: Rape in the District of Columbia. Am. J. Obstet. Gynec. *113*: 91–97, May 1, 1972.
20. Keifer, W. S.: Rupture of the uterus. Am. J. Obstet. Gynec. *89*:335–341, 1964.
21. Kobak, A. J., and Hurwitz, C. H.: Gunshot wounds of the pregnant uterus. Obstet. Gynec. *4*:383–391, 1954.
22. Kracke, A. D.: Congenital paraplegia from intrauterine injury. J. Pediat. *63*:1184–1185, 1963.
23. Kuchera, L. K.: Postcoital contraception with diethylstilbestrol. J.A.M.A. *218*: 28–29, 1971.
24. Lazard, E. M., and Kliman, F.E.: Traumatic rupture of the uterus in advanced pregnancy. Cal. West. Med. *45*:482–483, 1936.
25. Massey, J. B., Garcia, G. R., and Emich, J. P., Jr.: Management of sexually assaulted females. Obstet. Gynec. *38*:29–37, July 1971.
26. McClure, J. N., Jr.: Rupture of the pregnant uterus due to non-penetrating abdominal trauma. Surgery *35*:487–489, 1954.
27. O'Brien, S. E.: Spontaneous rupture of the spleen in pregnancy. J. Can. Med. Assoc. *89*:667–669, 1963.
28. O'Rourke, C. A.: Rupture of the pregnant uterus due to non-penetrating external trauma. Med. J. Australia *2*:496–498, 1963.
29. Quast, D. C., and Jordan, G. L., Jr.: Traumatic wounds of the female reproductive organs. J. Trauma *4*:839–841, 1964.
30. Radman, H. M.: Pregnancy complicated by nonobstetric surgical disease. Arch. Surg. *88*:279–282, 1964.
31. Robinson, H. A., Jr., Sherrod, D. B., and Malcarney, C.: Review of child molestation and alleged rape cases. Am. J. Obstet. Gynec. *110*:405–406, June 1971.

32. Schroeter, A. L., and Lucas, J. B.: Gonorrhea—Diagnosis and treatment. Obstet. Gynec. *39*:174–185, 1972.
33. Schwartz, R., Greston, W., and Kleiner, G. J.: Defibrination in saline abortion. Obstet. Gynec. *40*:728–737, 1972.
34. Sparkman, R. S.: Rupture of the spleen in pregnancy. Am. J. Obstet. Gynec. *76*: 587–589, 1958.
35. Speer, D. P., and Peltier, L. F.: Pelvic fractures and pregnancy. J. Trauma. *12*:474–480, June 1972.
36. Stewart, G. K., and Goldstein, P.: Medical and surgical complications of therapeutic abortions. Obstet. Gynec. *40*:539–550, October 1972.
37. Taylor, E. S.: Beck's Obstetrical Practice. (9th Ed.) Baltimore, Williams & Wilkins, 1971.
38. Wilson, F., and Swartz, D. P.: Coital injuries of the vagina. Obstet. Gynec. *39*:182–185, February 1972.
39. Wright, C. H., Posner, A. C., and Gilchrist, J.: Penetrating wounds of the gravid uterus. Am. J. Obstet. Gynec. *67*: 1085–1090, 1954.

chapter

14

SOFT TISSUE INJURIES OF THE EXTREMITIES

John E. Hoopes, M.D., and Michael E. Jabaley, M.D.

Statistics indicate that approximately three-fourths of all trauma involves the extremities. This information, coupled with the fact that extremity injuries produce significantly greater incapacity in terms of time lost from productive activities than trauma to other regions, provides some measure of the magnitude of the problem. The economic devastation attendant upon weeks and months of inability to work is literally inconceivable. The nature of permanent functional impairment frequently precludes return to the level of employment previously enjoyed.

The degree of functional recovery obtained directly reflects the attention to minute detail and basic surgical principles observed in initial management. Casual or misguided treatment adds insult to injury and assigns the patient permanently to the role of a relative cripple.

SURGICAL ANATOMY

A thorough knowledge of functional anatomy is essential in dealing with extremity injuries. Adequate diagnosis is based almost entirely on functional evaluation of the part distal to the site of injury. No attempt will be made to review morbid anatomy; rather, a concise guide to surgical anatomy is presented (Fig. 14–1).

Upper Arm. The upper arm is divided into anterior and posterior compartments by the lateral and medial intermuscular septa. The anterior compartment contains the coracobrachialis, biceps brachialis and brachioradialis muscles. The posterior compartment contains the triceps muscle. The brachial artery extends from the lower border of the teres major muscle to the antecubital fossa, at which point it bifurcates into the radial and ulnar arteries opposite the

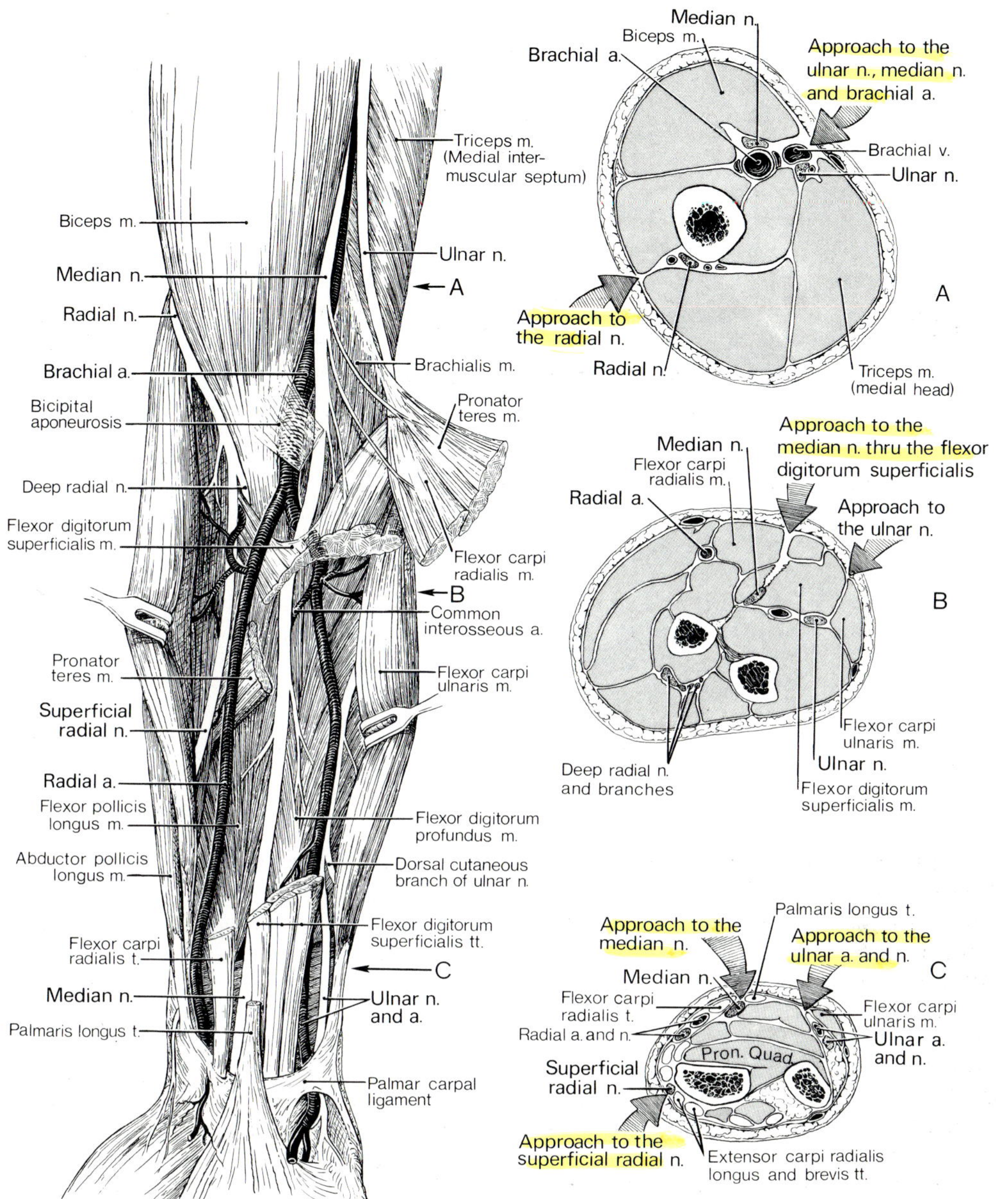

Figure 14–1 Soft tissue injuries of the extremities.

neck of the radius. The artery lies anterior to the medial intermuscular septum beneath the medial border of the biceps and enters the antecubital fossa beneath the lacertus fibrosis medial to the biceps tendon. The radial nerve progresses distally and laterally beneath the long head of the triceps muscle and, after supplying the triceps, penetrates the lateral intermuscular septum at the junction of the proximal and middle thirds of a line joining the deltoid insertion with the lateral epicondyle. The nerve divides into superficial (sensory) and posterior interosseus (motor) branches anterior to the lateral epicondyle. The musculocutaneous nerve diverges from the axillary artery to pass through the coracobrachialis and progress distally between the biceps and brachialis muscles; it supplies all the muscles of the anterior compartment. The median nerve accompanies the brachial artery, first on its lateral and then on its medial surface, crossing the brachial artery at the middle of the arm. The ulnar nerve accompanies the brachial artery on its medial surface in the proximal half of the arm and then penetrates the medial intermuscular septum to pass posterior to the medial epicondyle of the humerus.

FOREARM. The forearm musculature is divided into a volar-medial or flexor-pronator group and a dorsal-lateral or extensor-supinator group. The muscles of the flexor-pronator group all arise, at least in part, from the medial epicondyle of the humerus and are divided into superficial and deep layers. Progressing from lateral to medial, the superficial group consists of the pronator teres, flexor carpi radialis, palmaris longus, flexor digitorum superficialis and flexor carpi ulnaris muscles. The deep layer includes the flexor digitorum profundus, flexor pollicis longus and pronator quadratus muscles. All the muscles of the flexor-pronator group except the flexor carpi ulnaris and the flexor digitorum profundi of the ring and little fingers are supplied by the median nerve; these two exceptions are supplied by the ulnar nerve.

The musculature of the extensor-supinator group is divided into radial and dorsal divisions, the dorsal division being divided into superficial and deep groups. All the muscles of the radial and superficial portion of the dorsal group arise from the lateral epicondyle and are supplied by branches of the main trunk of the radial nerve. The deep muscles of the dorsal group arise from the dorsal surface of the radius and ulna and are supplied by the posterior interosseous branch of the radial nerve. The radial group of muscles includes the brachioradialis and the extensor carpi radialis longus and brevis.

The superficial division of the dorsal group contains the extensor digitorum communis, extensor digiti quinti proprius and extensor carpi ulnaris muscles; the deep division consists of the abductor pollicis longus, extensor pollicis brevis, extensor pollicis longus and extensor indicis proprius muscles.

The ulnar artery descends through the anterior surface of the proximal forearm on the surface of the flexor digitorum profundus between the flexor carpi ulnaris and flexor digitorum sublimis. In the distal half of the forearm it lies beneath the flexor carpi ulnaris and passes into the hand superficial to the transverse carpal ligament on the radial side of the pisiform bone.

The radial artery passes laterally on the surface of the supinator muscle beneath the brachioradialis and comes to lie between the brachioradialis and flexor carpi radialis in the distal half of the forearm. The distal third of the radial artery is subcutaneous and lies on the radius and the flexor pollicis longus muscle. The superficial branch of the radial nerve progresses distally beneath the brachioradialis on the lateral aspect of the radial artery; it pierces the deep fascia to become subcutaneous at the junction of the proximal and distal thirds of the forearm. The posterior interosseous branch of the radial nerve passes around the lateral aspect of the neck of the radius and through the supinator muscle to enter the interspace between the superficial and deep muscles of the dorsal group.

The median nerve passes between the superficial and deep heads of the pronator teres to lie between the flexor digitorum profundus and sublimis and progresses distally on the radial aspect of the palmaris longus. The ulnar nerve enters the forearm between the two heads of the flexor carpi ulnaris and descends on the ulnar surface of the flexor digitorum profundus beneath the flexor carpi ulnaris; it accompanies the ulnar artery into the hand on its radial deep surface.

Thigh. The musculature of the thigh is divided into three osteofibrous compartments: an anterior or extensor group consisting of the sartorius and quadriceps femoris muscles supplied by the femoral nerve; a posterior or flexor group including the biceps femoris, semimembranous and semitendinous muscles supplied by the sciatic nerve; and a medial or adductor group consisting of the adductor, pectineus and gracilis muscles supplied by the obturator nerve. The femoral artery enters the thigh beneath the inguinal ligament and is relatively superficial in the femoral triangle. It passes distally in the adductor canal beneath the sartorius to enter the popliteal fossa through a tendinous ring in the adductor magnus muscle. The profunda femoris branch leaves the common femoral artery approximately 4 cm. inferior to the inguinal ligament, passes lateral and posterior to the superficial femoral artery beneath the adductor longus muscle to gain the posterior surface of the shaft of the femur, and enters the popliteal fossa through the adductor magnus muscle. The femoral nerve enters the thigh beneath the inguinal ligament on the lateral aspect of the femoral artery and accompanies the superficial femoral artery in the adductor canal. The sciatic nerve descends between the greater trochanter of the femur and the tuberosity of the ischium beneath the long head of the biceps and terminates in the middle third of the thigh by dividing into the common peroneal and tibial nerves. The obturator nerve enters the thigh through the obturator canal and descends in two branches posterior to the pectineus muscle.

Lower Leg. The musculature of the leg is divided into anterior, lateral and posterior compartments. The anterior compartment contains the tibialis anterior, extensor digitorum longus, extensor hallucis longus and peroneus tertius muscles, all of which are supplied by the deep peroneal nerve. The tibialis anterior arises from the upper two-thirds of the lateral surface of the tibia and inserts into the medial aspect of the base of the first metatarsal. This muscle dorsiflexes and inverts the foot.

The lateral compartment consists of the peroneus longus and brevis muscles supplied by the superficial peroneal nerve. The tendons of both muscles pass posterior to the lateral malleolus. The brevis inserts into the lateral aspect of the base of the fifth metatarsal, and the longus crosses the sole of the foot to insert on the lateral aspect of the base of the first metatarsal. They permit plantar flexion, abduction and eversion of the foot.

The posterior compartment contains a superficial group of muscles consisting of the gastrocnemius, soleus and plantaris and a deep group consisting of the flexor digitorum longus, flexor hallucis longus and tibialis posterior muscles, all of which are supplied by the tibial nerve. The popliteal artery bifurcates into anterior and posterior tibial branches at the lower border of the popliteus muscle. The anterior tibial artery enters the anterior compartment through the upper part of the interosseous membrane. The posterior tibial artery descends in the interspace between the superficial and deep muscles of the posterior compartment to become subcutaneous between the medial malleolus and calcaneus. The peroneal artery is the largest branch of the posterior tibial; it progresses distally on the posterior surface of the fibula. The tibial nerve passes through the posterior compartment in close association with the posterior tibial artery. The common peroneal nerve divides into superficial and deep branches within the lateral compartment on the lateral aspect of the neck of the fibula. The superficial peroneal nerve descends immediately behind the anterior intermuscular septum between the fibula and peroneus longus. The deep peroneal nerve descends through the anterior compartment in association with the anterior tibial artery.

FIRST AID

The principles of the first aid management of injured extremities are as applicable in the large hospital emergency treatment room as at the scene of the accident. Preparation of injured patients for transportation to medical facilities demands that hemorrhage be controlled and fractures adequately splinted. This should be equally obvious at the time of initial evaluation in the emergency room, but all too commonly patients are referred for extensive radiologic evaluation or other diagnostic studies without due regard for protection from further injury. Hemorrhage is controlled by elevation and pressure, not by tourniquets and clamps. Improperly applied tourniquets readily produce peripheral nerve injuries; tourniquets properly applied but left unattended result in irreparable ischemia. Clamps applied directly to severed vessels preclude restoration of continuity; clamps indiscriminately plunged into the wound not infrequently incorporate vital structures. Adequate immobilization of fractures is imperative. Conversion of unsplinted closed fractures into compound fractures occurs readily, not to mention the tissue damage and blood loss associated with instability at the fracture site. Open wounds should be covered with sterile dressings. The physician may proceed with more leisurely evaluation only after assuring himself that his patient is comfortable, protected and free from danger.

INITIAL EVALUATION

All injured patients deserve a thorough physical examination before attention is focused on their outstanding injury. Complete, systematic evaluation is essential to the avoidance of catastrophe from some unsuspected injury. With thoughtfulness and a little practice, the physician quickly develops a routine that allows him to complete a truly thorough examination within a matter of minutes. The importance of developing such a routine cannot be overemphasized.

Preliminary preparations toward definitive operative management are made during or immediately following the initial physical examination. A route of intravenous fluid administration is secured as rapidly as possible in all severely injured patients and in all patients in whom it is anticipated that treatment will require the use of the operating room. Blood for baseline studies and for typing and crossmatching is obtained at the time intravenous fluids are begun. Occlusive sterile dressings are applied to open wounds. The nursing personnel are instructed to record the vital signs at appropriate intervals.

Having accomplished the above in a rapid and efficient manner, the physician is prepared to proceed with a more thorough evaluation of the total patient and his specific injury. A complete history is obtained, and emphasis is given to the specific circumstances of the injury. Minute details serve as valuable guides during the physical examination in pointing to the particular structures that might be injured. Victims of automobile accidents are questioned regarding loss of consciousness, chest and abdominal trauma, and so forth. Patients with injuries sustained at work are asked to describe in detail the machinery with which they were working and the exact nature of the accident. Patients with missile and sharp instrument injuries who have been victims of assault are questioned regarding the relative position of their assailant in an effort to determine the trajectory of the injuring agent. Knowledge of the time elapsed from injury to treatment is critical in evaluation of all wounds.

Facilities for the adequate evaluation of extremity injuries should be available in all receiving wards. Ideally, such facilities consist of the set-up usually found in a well-appointed minor surgery operating room; i.e., caps and masks, scrub sinks, operating room table with arm board, operating room light and sterile instruments and drapes. The facilities must permit a thorough, unhurried examination in peace and quiet.

Integument. As emphasized previously, the dressing of open wounds is an integral part of first aid treatment. Ordinarily, examination of the wound is deferred until completion of functional examination of the extremity distal to the site of injury. Aseptic technique is observed strictly. Examination of the wound is utilized as an opportunity to secure initial cleansing of the affected part. No solution other than sterile normal saline solution may be applied to the wound itself. The surrounding intact skin may be cleansed with a mild detergent such as Septisol or pHiso-Hex. Antiseptic solutions have no role in the management of open, traumatic wounds. Adequate shaving of the affected part is accomplished at this time. Gentle but thorough scrubbing with a surgical brush may be required to remove the accumulated dirt and grease from a working man's extremities and the imbedded foreign material associated with automobile accidents.

The major purposes of this portion of the initial evaluation are assessment of the soft tissue wound and determination of the forces involved in creating the injury. Assessment is made of the extent of soft tissue loss and of the viability of remaining tissue. Knowledge of topographical anatomy allows one to anticipate the subfascial structures involved on the basis of the location of the injury. Knowledge of the type of forces involved in producing the injury provides an index of the degree of soft tissue destruction and also of the possibility of subfascial injury, i.e., abrading, lacerating, avulsing, crushing and missile injuries. The deep structures are evaluated insofar as is possible without the benefit of dissection. Probing of wounds is of no value; suspicion of significant deep injury demands definitive surgical exploration. Following the examination, the wound is appropriately redressed if definitive repair is to be accomplished in the operating room.

Skeleton. Clinical suspicion of fractures is aroused by the usual signs of pain, swelling, crepitation, abnormal posture and abnormal motion. Confirmation is provided by radiologic evaluation. Fracture management is discussed in detail elsewhere. The presence of a compound injury is of considerable concern to the orthopedist and plastic surgeon alike in that adequate soft tissue coverage is absolutely essential to bony union. Initial evaluation must include deliberate consideration of means of securing reliable soft tissue coverage over a compound fracture.

Muscles and Tendons. Evaluation of dynamic function precedes direct inspection of the wound. Again, the importance of an all-encompassing routine of systematic examination cannot be stressed adequately. The location and appearance of the skin wound may be grossly misleading regarding the extent of subfascial injury. In addition, the presence of a severe skin wound does not exclude the possibility of injury proximal to this site. The full range of active and passive motion of all joints in a given extremity is elicited, following which the actions of specific muscle groups and tendons are tested. Differentiation between loss of function resulting from tendon injury and that resulting from nerve damage is not difficult.

The shoulder is tested for flexion, extension, abduction, adduction and circumduction. Point tenderness anteriorly and severe pain on all movements of the joint is indicative of a tear in the articular duff. Inability to initiate abduction but the ability to complete abduction if the initial 15 degrees of movement is assisted passively is pathognomonic of rupture of the supraspinatus tendon.

Flexion, extension, pronation and supination are evaluated at the elbow joint. Severe injury to the triceps prevents extension against gravity. Division or rupture of the biceps tendon prevents flexion with the forearm in supination and prevents supination with the elbow in flexion.

Simple observation of the attitude of the wrist and hand provides valuable information regarding possible tendon injury. In the normal hand at rest, the thumb is held in moderate opposition and flexion, and the fingers are held in progressively increasing flexion from the index to the little finger. Relative extension of one or more digits immediately suggests flexor tendon injury. Injury to the extensor tendons in the forearm results in increased flexion at the wrist and metacarpophalangeal joints.

In testing individual tendon function, it is exceedingly important that the effect of gravity be eliminated and that the part under examination be positioned so as to exclude substitution movements.

The flexor and extensors of the wrist are easily palpable when acting against resistance, making the diagnosis of division of these tendons relatively straightforward. It is well to remember that the palmaris longus tendon is absent in the hands of 10 per cent of people. Injury of the flexor carpi ulnaris tendon immediately raises suspicion of injury to the ulnar nerve. Laceration of the palmaris longus tendon renders imperative the exclusion of median nerve damage.

Accurate evaluation of injury to the long flexor and extensor tendons of the fingers is made somewhat difficult by the fact that discrete, dissociated movements of these structures disappear progressively at more proximal levels in the forearm. The flexor superficialis tendons are tested by mechanically blocking flexion at the distal interphalangeal joints of the other fingers and requesting that the proximal interphalangeal joints be flexed. The flexor profundus tendons are evaluated by mechanically blocking the proximal interphalangeal joints and requesting flexion at the distal interphalangeal joints. The long extensor tendons of the fingers act almost entirely at the metacarpophalangeal joints and are tested by requesting extension against resistance at this level. Injury significantly proximal to the extensor retinaculum of the wrist will usually include all extensor digitorum communis tendons. Injury to the superficialis tendon alone in the palm or the profundus tendon alone in the finger is seen commonly; forearm injuries involve either the superficialis alone or the superficialis and profundus. In evaluating tendon injuries, it is good practice to demonstrate clearly to the patient the action desired.

Tendon rupture is observed as a closed injury occurring "spontaneously" and attributed by the patient to a single, strenuous physical action. It is seen only rarely in association with other types of extremity trauma. The tendons most commonly ruptured in the upper extremity are the supraspinatus, biceps and extensor pollicis longus ("drummer's palsy"). In the lower extremity, Achilles and plantaris ("tennis leg") ruptures are seen. Tendons that rupture are usually abnormal and have been weakened by chronic trauma or disease.

Nerves. In evaluating motor and sensory loss, serious consideration must be given to the fact that the upper extremity represents an extension of the opposite cerebral cortex. Absence of motor function of cerebral etiology presents as a spastic paralysis without associated sensory disturbance. Cervical cord lesions produce a flaccid paralysis of structures innervated at the level of the lesion and a spastic paralysis below this level. Injury to the trunks of the brachial plexus results in functional impairment of segmental distribution; injury to the cords of the plexus exhibits a peripheral nerve-type distribution.

Subjective impressions of sensory changes usually are quite reliable guides in evaluating peripheral nerve injury. The majority of patients will remark somewhat quizzically that a certain area "feels peculiar" or is "dead." Almost invariably, such patients will prove at exploration to have a significant nerve injury. The same degree of reliability does not apply to motor function in that the majority of patients with peripheral nerve injuries are inexplicably unaware of their motor impairment. Motor function must be tested thoughtfully and specific defects carefully elicited.

Certain principles must be observed in evaluating peripheral nerve function. The ability to perceive light touch, as with a wisp of cotton, and pinprick are of very little value in the assessment of the relation between the degree of sensation and useful function, but are quite helpful in mapping out areas of sensory loss associated with acute injury. Caution must be exercised not to move the part being evaluated in that this will be interpreted as "touch" due to proprioception originating from tendons proximal to the site of injury. Areas tested must be unequivocal in their specificity because of the marked overlapping of peripheral nerve innervation, both motor and sensory. All degrees of hypesthesia are seen with peripheral nerve injuries; complete anesthesia is exceedingly limited in extent. The examiner performing sensory evaluation must appreciate subtle alterations.

RADIAL NERVE. Sensory evaluation is of little real value in the diagnosis of division of the radial nerve or its superficial branch because of the overlap provided by the median and ulnar nerves. At most, anesthesia is limited to a half-dollar-sized area overlying the proximal portion of the first dorsal interosseous muscle. Damage to the nerve proximal to the point at which it enters the supinator muscle results in wrist drop due to paralysis of all of the extensors of the wrist and fingers. The hand cannot be extended at the wrist and the fingers cannot be extended at the metacarpophalangeal joints. With support of the wrist and metacarpophalangeal joints in extension, the interphalangeal joints of the fingers can be extended by the intrinsic muscles of the hand. Division of the superficial branch produces no motor impairment and insignificant sensory loss; it is, however, the most common site of painful neuromata. Injury to the deep dorsal interosseous branch paralyzes the extensor pollicis brevis and longus and the abductor pollicis longus. The patient is unable to abduct or extend the thumb and holds the digit in a moderately adducted position.

MEDIAN NERVE. Sensory examination is essential to accurate diagnosis and reveals anesthesia of the radial two-thirds of the palm, the volar aspect of the thumb, index, long and radial half of the ring fingers, and the dorsum of the distal phalanges of the thumb, index and long fingers. The degree of peripheral nerve overlap varies considerably. Because of radial nerve overlap, the area of demonstrable anesthesia associated with median nerve division may be significantly smaller than that outlined. Diagnosis of median nerve injury on the basis of motor function is demonstrated by lack of opposition of the thumb: with the hand flat on a table palm up, the patient is unable to point the thumb directly toward the ceiling; classically, the patient is unable to bring the thumb into true opposition with the fingertips. In addition, division above the elbow results in inability to flex the index and long fingers: with the hand flat on a table palm down, the patient is unable to scratch the table top with the tip of the index finger.

ULNAR NERVE. Sensory examination reveals anesthesia of the ulnar third of the hand, the little finger and the ulnar half of the ring finger. Motor demonstration of ulnar nerve palsy consists of inability to adduct and abduct the fingers. In performing this test, it is important that the metacarpophalangeal and interphalangeal joints not be flexed; the fingers normally converge on flexion and are adducted by the long extensors. With injury to the ulnar nerve above the elbow, the patient is unable to scratch the table top with the tip of the little finger with the hand held palm down on the table. In attempting to produce a strong pinch between the thumb and index finger, the metacarpophalangeal joint of the thumb falls into hyperextension (Froment's sign). "Clawing" of the ring and little fingers, hyperextension at the metacarpophalangeal joints and flexion at the interphalangeal joints are most pronounced when the ulnar nerve is divided in the distal half of the forearm; paralysis of the intrinsics allows the long extensors to hyperextend the metacarpophalangeal joints, and the still-innervated profundus tendons pull the interphalangeal joints into flexion.

MEDIAN AND ULNAR NERVES. The sensory loss is that of the combined distribution of the two nerves. The attitude assumed by the hand is determined by the radial innervated musculature; i.e., the wrist is slightly extended and supinated, the metacarpophalangeal joints are hyperextended. The thumb is abducted and extended into the plane of the hand, and the longitudinal and transverse metacarpal arches are flattened. Injury distal to the innervation of the forearm muscles produces extreme "clawing."

SCIATIC NERVE. The sensory loss following division of the sciatic nerve encompasses the posterolateral aspect of the thigh, all the leg except a narrow area on its most medial aspect supplied by the saphenous nerve, and the entire foot. The hamstring muscles and all the muscles of the leg are paralyzed. Division of the tibial nerve produces paralysis of all the muscles of the posterior compartment of the leg with resultant inability to plantarflex the foot. Damage to the common peroneal nerve paralyzes the musculature of the lateral and anterior compartments and is manifested by inability to dorsiflex the foot.

Vasculature. The degree of vascular impairment is best judged on the basis of the color and temperature of the part. The rate of capillary filling in the nail beds, venous filling and rate of drainage are observed. Patency of the radial and ulnar arteries is established by the simple test of elevating the upper extremity, occluding both arteries, and then releasing them in turn. Immediate flushing on release of one artery with the other occluded demonstrates patency.

Special Diagnostic Methods. The logical step following a thorough physical evaluation is the consideration of diagnostic aids. It is assumed that the requisite basic laboratory data are obtained in all cases. The indications for radiography are self-evident. A baseline chest x-ray is obtained in all trauma victims who are to receive a general anesthetic.

Selective nerve blocks may be of value in resolving equivocal findings with respect to peripheral nerve injuries. Anesthetizing the ulnar nerve at the elbow or the median nerve at the wrist abolishes overlap and anomalous innervation, allowing clearer definition of the nerve injury in question. Electromyography and more sophisticated methods of testing are not utilized in the usual traumatic situation.

Angiography provides precise information regarding the status of the circulation and is indicated in highly specific complex situations. Usually, the nature, location and extent of vascular injury are grossly manifest and do not require refined techniques for elaboration.

INFECTION

Appropriate antibiotic therapy is instituted preoperatively in the management of all patients with extremity injuries. The drug of choice against gram-positive cocci should be instituted preoperatively and continued for a minimum period of five days.[2]

All patients receive tetanus prophylaxis: 0.5 cc. of tetanus toxoid if previously immunized or 4500 units of tetanus antitoxin in the absence of immunization. It must be emphasized that all patients receiving antitoxin also must receive a course of active immunization. Gas gangrene prophylaxis has been demonstrated to be of little or no value.

Clostridial cellulitis and myositis are the most dreaded complications, and massive debridement is indicated. Most patients will be salvaged only by amputation.[33]

OPERATIVE MANAGEMENT

A decision must be made whether the wound can be treated adequately in the emergency treatment room on an ambulatory basis or whether operating room repair and inpatient management are indicated. Treatment in the accident room is reserved for uncomplicated abrasions and lacerations involving only the skin and subcutaneous tissue. Penetration of the fascia is not in itself an indication for formal exploration; repair in the emergency unit is permissible provided the functional examination is unquestionably within normal limits. Small skin grafts may be applied in the emergency treatment room.

Complex injuries demand operating room repair by qualified surgeons. All tendon and nerve repairs, including isolated extensor tendon injury and digital nerve injury, are performed in the operating room. Crushing-type injuries, which invariably are followed by extensive hemorrhage and edema, demand hospitalization for purposes of observation if not for operative management.

All the usual adjuncts are employed in the operative management of extremity injuries. The pneumatic tourniquet is employed routinely except in cases exhibiting severe arterial insufficiency. In addition to its obvious benefits, the tourniquet provides an excellent method for assessing viability, i.e., the presence or absence of post-tourniquet hyperemia. The tourniquet is inflated to a pressure of 280 to 300 mm. of mercury on the upper extremity and 450 to 500 mm. of mercury on the lower extremity; it may be left inflated for a period not exceeding two hours, following which it must be released to permit adequate flushing of the extremity. Provided the tourniquet is released for at least 15 minutes during each two hours, tourniquet ischemia may be utilized for as long as is necessary. The pneumatic cuff must be applied sufficiently loosely to prevent it from acting as a venous tourniquet; prior to inflation, the extremity must be drained as completely as possible either by elevation or the application of an elastic bandage. The Boyes' hand table is utilized for all upper extremity repairs. No antiseptic solutions are used in preparation of the operative field. Intact skin is cleansed with detergent solutions; open wounds are prepared by irrigation with large volumes of saline solution. Regardless of the extent of injury the entire extremity is prepared and draped into the operative field. If there is any question regarding viability of skin and subcutaneous tissue, appropriate donor areas for either pedicle flaps or skin grafts are prepared and draped.

In order of priority, consideration is given to the repair of vascular injury threatening loss of viability, the integument, skeletal structures, muscles and tendons, and nerves. In the face of serious question regarding viability of the injured member, definitive repair of all structures is delayed for a period of 48 to 72 hours. Definitive repair of subfascial structures cannot be considered without provision for adequate soft tissue coverage. Consideration must be given to proper positioning and immobilization of fractures prior to embarking on tendon and nerve repair. Divided tendons retract and are, therefore, repaired in preference to nerves if a choice must be made. Delayed repair of nerve injuries is not only feasible but possibly desirable.

Conservation of all usable structures is the most basic of the surgical principles applicable to the management of extremity injuries. Structures which are in themselves irreparably damaged frequently prove of inestimable value in salvaging other structures. Injudicious sacrifice of tissue may effectively block subsequent reconstruction.

Amputation is considered only if the situation appears entirely hopeless in terms of restoration of function. Irreparable damage to any three of the five major structures comprising an extremity (skin and subcutaneous tissue, artery, bone, tendon and nerve) generally is indication for amputation. The concept of "sites of election" of amputation has become obsolete as a result of technical advances in the art of prosthesis manufacture.[13] As much length as possible is preserved in all cases.

Integument. Extremity skin and subcutaneous tissue will not tolerate tension. Wound closure of questionable integrity overlying a compound fracture courts osteomyelitis; exposed tendon and nerve repairs are doomed to failure. Wound margins are excised routinely to prevent traumatic tattooing and to provide nonbeveled, viable margins for suturing. Unlike the face, tissues of questionable viability in the extremities almost certainly will progress to frank necrosis. Debridement, therefore, must be adequate. Healthy tissue will successfully resist a significant degree of contamination; ischemic tissue almost invariably will become infected. Skin that has been avulsed completely but not severely traumatized is replaced as a full thickness graft after adequate defatting. Large, traumatic flaps are dealt with by removing all the subcutaneous tissue and replacing the skin as a full thickness graft, i.e., a combination pedicle-graft.

Definitive wound closure at the time of the primary procedure is highly desirable. Primary closure is preferable to other forms of securing coverage but may be utilized only if the wound margins are perfectly healthy and can be approximated without tension. The decision regarding pedicle flap versus free graft coverage is dependent upon the topography of the wound, the structures involved and the plan of repair. Free skin grafts provide the most expedient method of securing coverage and are utilized whenever possible. Pedicle flaps are indicated in securing closure over fractures lacking adequate muscle coverage, bone devoid of periosteum, exposed tendon, nerve and vascular repairs and in situations in which secondary reconstructive procedures will be required, i.e., tendon and nerve grafting (Fig. 14–2).

Donor areas to be considered for pedicle flaps are local tissues, the chest and abdomen and the opposite extremity. Local flaps are of limited value because of their exceedingly precarious blood supply. Such flaps are best designed as bipedicle advancement flaps. The disadvantage of

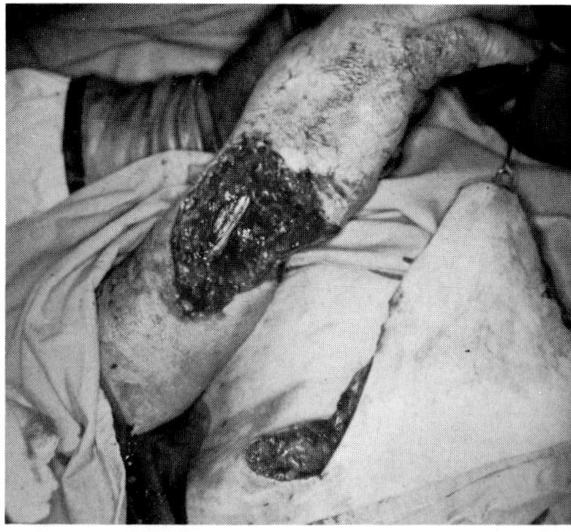

Figure 14–2 Soft tissue loss exposing the carpus and extensor tendons. Coverage was made immediately with an abdominal pedicle flap.

this method of repair is that of placing the suture line over the most critical portion of the wound. Rotation flaps must be planned generously and based proximally; they are utilized with extreme caution. Most commonly, the flap is obtained from the trunk. Pectoral flaps are preferred to abdominal flaps on the basis of the lesser quantity of subcutaneous tissue and the more acceptable position of the upper extremity from the standpoints of joint immobilization and ease of patient care. Flaps having a length to width ratio not exceeding 1:1 may be raised with impunity from any area on the chest or abdomen, may be based superiorly or inferiorly and may cross the midline. Oblique and transverse flaps are based laterally and must not cross the midline. If a long, relatively narrow flap is desired, it is based on the pattern of the classic thoracoepigastric tube pedicle flap extending from axilla to femoral triangle. The flap overlies the course of the thoracoepigastric vein and receives its arterial supply from the superior and lateral thoracic vessels above and the superficial inferior epigastric and circumflex iliac vessels below. One half of the thoracoepigastric flap, based either superiorly or inferiorly, can be raised without delay.

The only flap that will cover a large defect of the antecubital fossa is one based on the midaxillary line and extending transversely to the midline of the back. The major disadvantage of trunk flaps is the awkward position of the extremity and the imposed immobilization of the elbow and shoulder. Particularly with abdominal flaps, the wrist falls into flexion and the fingers into relative extension at the metacarpophalangeal joints. This position must be avoided by means of appropriate dressings. Cross-arm flaps are considered in dealing with exceedingly obese patients and in situations in which the defect requires local flap but less than is obtainable with a trunk flap. The disadvantages of cross-arm flaps are obvious; some thoughtfulness should disclose a better way to accomplish the desired result.

As always, the rule applies that the defect is adjusted to fit the flap and not the flap to fit the defect. Flap donor areas are covered immediately with split thickness skin grafts; care is taken to extend the graft over the exposed area of the pedicle. A completely closed wound allowing a reasonable degree of mobility of the extremity is achieved. All patients undergoing flap transfer to the extremities are instructed in active exercises to the extent permitted by the specific situation. Flap pedicles are left intact for a period of three weeks; ordinarily, a delay procedure need not precede division.

Muscles and Tendons. Determination of viability of traumatized muscle demands considerable judgment based on clinical experience. The color of frayed, contused, lacerated muscle is not a good index of viability, nor is the character of the bleeding from the cut edge. The "pinch test" is probably the most reliable guide: viable muscle fibers contract locally when stimulated by pinching. Adequate debridement is imperative for the avoidance of serious infection, particularly clostridial myositis. Uncertainty concerning muscle viability is an indication for delayed primary closure at a later date. Quite extensive sacrifice of muscle mass produces surprisingly little functional impairment.

Muscle fibers do not hold sutures, and repair is accomplished by meticulous approximation of the enveloping fascia. Division of multiple, discrete muscle groups requires anatomical approximation of all the intermuscular septa. Simple closure of the enveloping fascia of the extremity is adequate in most cases.

Successful tendon repair requires an understanding of tendon anatomy and healing. Tendon is composed of logitudinally oriented parallel bundles of collagen fibers with frequent cross-linking of adjacent bundles. Inactive fibrocytes, incapable of participating in the healing process, constitute the only cellular element. Blood supply is derived from three sources: muscular branches; vessels present in the periosteum of bone at the tendon insertion; and vessels in the surrounding connective tissue which enter the tendon through peritenon, mesotenon and vinculae. The vinculae provide the most important source of blood supply and have been likened to the vessels in the intestinal mesentery.[29]

The basic principle of "one wound—one scar" has been emphasized;[19] the difficulty of producing an anastomosis which possesses both tensile strength and gliding function accounts for the surgeon's dilemma in tendon surgery.

The initial cellular reaction phase of tendon healing entails fibroblast invasion of the anastomosis from surrounding tissues. The fibroblasts synthesize and discharge monomeric collagen and the various mucopolysaccharides necessary for scar synthesis. The monomeric subunits rapidly polymerize into discernible fibril and finally into dense scar. Remodeling of the scar along lines of tension is critical to the development of the thin, filmy adhesions which subsequently permit gliding ability. Short, thick adhesions doom the repair to functional failure if the anastomosis is allowed to remain motionless during the remodeling phase.

Fibroblasts appear in the wound as early as the third day, and collagen synthesis begins immediately. A dynamic process of synthesis and degradation achieves equilibrium on approximately the seventeenth day. A progressive increase in tensile strength allows initiation of active and passive motion shortly after this time.[14] Motion provides the dynamic stresses promoting reorientation of the collagen fibrils.

The blood supply to lacerated tendon ends is primarily through the mesotenon which is located on the deep surface of the tendon and must be protected. Trauma to the tendon by the careless use of instruments or sutures produces local wounds which will be invaded by fibroblasts and subsequently bound by adhesions.[20] Suture material must be non-inflammatory and securely placed to maintain union during the period when the fresh collagen has minimal tensile strength. Proper splint immobilization is all-important during this period. A careful program of guarded and progressive active and passive motion must be instituted during the proper phase of wound healing.

Tendon lacerations are repaired by means of the classic Bunnell buried crisscross suture of 4-0 synthetic material. Wire tends to cut into tendon, and the minute kinks at the points at which the suture changes direction tend to straighten out with time; both these factors contribute to separation of the anastomosis, with resultant elongation of the tendon and decrease in function. Division of a tendon at its site of origin from the muscle belly is repaired either with multiple, fine, interrupted sutures or by means of overlapping the muscle and its tendon and approximating the two with continuous longitudinal sutures separated by 180 degrees. Pull-out sutures are not indicated proximal to the wrist or ankle. Wire pull-out sutures-at-a distance are helpful in the lower extremity in relieving tension at the anastomosis.

Considerable local scarring inevitably follows tendon repair. The anastomosis should be surrounded insofar as possible with available soft tissue, either muscle or fat. This principle is particularly applicable when dealing with combined tendon and nerve injuries. Opinions differ regarding the wisdom of primary repair in the management of complex injuries. It can be argued that multiple tendon repairs jeopardize an associated major nerve anastomosis and produce scarring sufficient to compromise function in all tendons. On this basis, many surgeons would advocate repair of only the profundus tendons in dealing with a complex wound of the forearm. It is our feeling that total repair of all injured structures should be accomplished if at all possible, because this approach preserves the greatest number of motors for subsequent utilization as transfers.

Nerves. As clearly elucidated by Seddon,[25] there exist three discrete types of nerve injury which differ in etiology, pathophysiology, management and prognosis. Neurotmesis is defined as destruction of all the essential parts of a nerve, as is produced by complete division. Axonotmesis consists of interruption of the axons with preservation of all the supporting structures, as is seen most commonly in association with blunt trauma. Neurapraxia is defined as functional interruption of the nerve without loss of integrity; there is no axonal degeneration, but there may be localized degeneration of the myelin sheath. Neurapraxia usually is the result of a traction-type injury and is the nerve injury most commonly associated with displaced fractures. Spontaneous recovery of excellent function is to be anticipated with neurapraxia. Recovery of normal function probably never occurs following neurotmesis. Axonotmesis carries an intermediate prognosis.

The physiological processes involved in repair following nerve injury are well understood and adequately documented.[38] To review briefly, the stages which must be traversed sequentially for a successful outcome are: (1) closure of the gap between the severed nerve ends, mainly by the outgrowth of Schwann cells; (2) retrograde degeneration; (3) progression of axons across the scar; (4) disintegration of the axons and myelin in the distal segment and removal by macrophages; (5) multiplication of the nuclei and increase in the volume of the cytoplasm of Schwann cells to make Schwann bands which fill the old sheaths; (6) arrival of the growing axons at the end organs; and (7) increase in diameter and degree of myelination of the fibers. It is readily appreciated that the majority of factors influencing the ultimate result lie distal to the point of injury. The two critical areas are the anastomosis and the end organ. The final size reached by regenerating nerve fibers is directly dependent upon their connection with an end organ; proper connection results in an increase in size and a decrease in number of fibers in the distal segment.[1] The number of fibers available for connection with end organs is determined by the quality of the anastomosis.

A perfect anastomosis precisely approximates all the funiculi within the nerve and is probably not obtainable. Sunderland's[31] classic studies of intraneural topography demonstrate a constantly changing funicular pattern as one progresses peripherally in a nerve; cross-sectional areas separated by only a few millimeters exhibit grossly dissimilar patterns. In addition, the course of regneration following suture is greatly influenced by the size, number and composition of component funiculi and the total area occupied by the fibers of the individual branches within the nerve. A good result can be anticipated if the funiculi are large and few in number. If there are numerous small funiculi or if there are few large funiculi proximal to the anastomosis and multiple small funiculi distally, a poor result is to be expected.

Acceptable performance of a nerve anastomosis demands the utmost in technical ability. Consideration of the multiple factors determining success leads clearly to the conclusion that anything less than a perfect union is doomed to failure (Fig. 14–3). The technique to be described has proved most satisfactory. A proper anastomosis should always be performed with magnification, using either loupes or a microscope. A pneumatic tourniquet should be employed if at all possible; this may not be feasible with proximal injuries or in the presence of an arterial repair.

Any injury resulting in nerve divi-

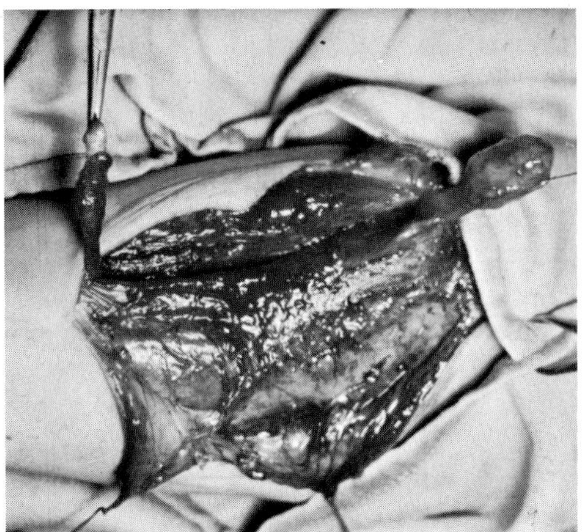

Figure 14–3 Median nerve neuroma—the inevitable consequence of a poor anastomosis.

sion, no matter how "clean," produces fraying of the severed ends. Preparation of the nerve for repair demands resection of the area of injury. The amount of nerve removed may amount to no more than a millimeter or so, but this is essential to precise anatomical approximation. The procedure is accomplished by supporting the nerve on a wet tongue depressor; resection is done with the sharpest instrument available, usually a fresh double-edged razor blade. Sufficient dissection of the nerve proximally and distally is carried out to permit a tension-free anastomosis. All possible guides to exact approximation are utilized; i.e., the position of the perineural vessels, the funicular pattern in the proximal and distal ends, and so forth. The slightest degree of relative rotation must be avoided. The finest suture material at hand, certainly not larger than size 7-0, is used for the anastomosis. Monofilament nylon is the usual material chosen because of its availability. Monofilament stainless steel wire may be employed but is difficult to obtain and requires considerable practice for adept usage. The sutures are placed through the perineurium only and must not penetrate the funiculi. Approximation is begun by placing two guide sutures separated by 180 degrees. The anastomosis is completed with multiple interrupted sutures; rotation of the nerve for exposure is performed with the initial guide sutures. The tissues are moistened repeatedly with Tis-U-Sol or normal saline solution throughout the procedure. Minimal manipulation of the nerve is observed. Forceps are never used to grasp any portion of the nerve; retraction and support are accomplished as needed by means of fine sutures through the perineurium. The level of injury and ability of the surgeon will determine the technique employed. Reports to date do not indicate a clear preference for interfascicular versus perineural sutures so long as precise technique is utilized.

A nerve that is partially severed is not completely divided and anastomosed; rather, the defect is approximated meticulously with as few sutures as possible. The incidence of neuroma-in-continuity and causalgia is greater than that following repair of a completely divided nerve, but the functional result is improved by not disturbing the intact fibers.

Microsurgical techniques have proved a valuable adjunct in the technical performance of nerve anastomosis. As pointed out by Edshage,[5] the intraneural topography following primary suture in the usual fashion is so bad that it is surprising that the results are not worse. Histological examination of nerves repaired by microsurgical technique has demonstrated less inflammatory reaction at the site of the anastomosis and a markedly improved funicular pattern distal to the anastomosis as compared with standard methods.[28] Microsurgical technique is advocated for all repairs.

Nonsuture anastomotic techniques enjoy recurrent periods of popularity but thus far have yielded variable results. Young and Medawar[39] achieved adherence with a clot of human plasma and chick embryo extract and demonstrated a markedly improved fiber pattern distal to the anastomosis over that obtained by nerve suture. More recent experience with synthetic adhesives and microporous tape[8] is encouraging, and this method deserves a careful clinical trial.

The value of "protecting" the anastomosis with a millipore-like wrapper is debatable. Decreased inflammatory reaction and improved distal fiber pattern have been reported using a variety of materials.[10] Further basic experimental evidence is needed before the technique can be advocated for routine clinical application.

Whether nerve suture performed at the time of injury (primarily) or several weeks later (secondarily) produces the better result cannot be answered. Experience clearly has substantiated the superiority of secondary suture in war wounds. Entirely satisfactory results have, however, been reported with primary suture in many series of civilian injuries. Unpublished data suggest that early secondary repair at 9–12 days may provide the optimal opportunity for regenerating axons to bridge the anastomosis. Considerable judgment is required in all cases, but it is felt that primary repair should be performed if at all feasible. Secondary suture is reserved for those cases in which an adequately trained surgeon is not available at the time of injury or in which the wound situation militates against definitive repair; i.e., delay in excess of six to eight hours following injury, crushing injury with questionable tissue viability, and so forth. In such instances, the nerve ends are tagged with suture material for ready identification at the time of the definitive procedure.

Direct approximation is far superior to other methods of restoring continuity. Rather appreciable gaps (3 to 4 in.) in the median and ulnar nerves can be overcome by a variety of techniques. Simple flexion of the wrist and elbow provides an additional 1 to 2 in. of relative length. Considerable length can be gained with the ulnar nerve by removing the nerve from the fibro-osseous tunnel posterior to the medial humeral epicondyle and transposing it to a subcutaneous position in the antecubital fossa (Fig. 14–4). The procedure is accomplished by splitting the two heads of origin of the flexor carpi ulnaris; detachment and replacement of the medial humeral condyle, as formerly practiced, is a crippling procedure. The ulnar nerve branches to the elbow joint are divided, but the motor branches to the flexor carpi ulnaris and flexor profundus muscles are preserved by carefully stripping them away from the main trunk with the back edge of a knife blade. The available length of the median nerve is increased by placing the nerve

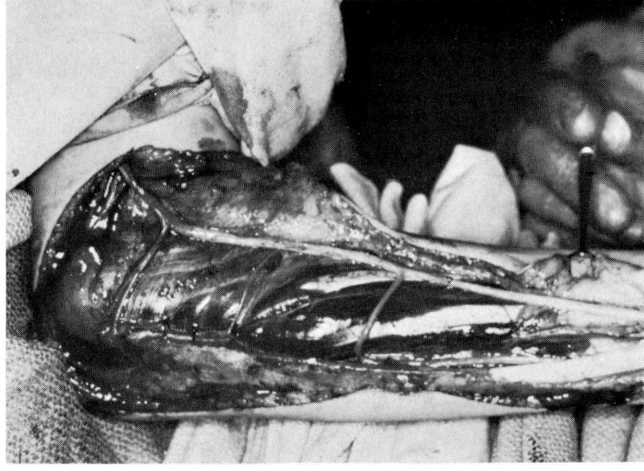

Figure 14–4 Ulnar nerve transposition at the elbow with preservation of all the motor branches; three and a half inches in length gained.

superficial to the antecubital fascia and the transverse carpal ligament. If lengthening procedures are required, the position of the extremity at the time of anastomosis is maintained for a period of approximately six weeks, following which the joints are progressively extended over a several week period. Loss of continuity over a distance exceeding 9 cm. precludes direct approximation.

Nerve grafting, pedicle nerve grafts and nerve transfer are reserved for elective reconstruction. Of the three methods, free nerve grafts give the best results. The sural and superficial radial nerves are chosen as donor nerves because of their accessibility and the absence of significant functional impairment imposed by their sacrifice. Obviously, two anastomoses instead of one are required, producing an expected decrease in the quality of the result. Pedicle nerve grafts are utilized only in very highly specific reconstructive situations; their advantages over free grafts have not been clearly demonstrated (Chapter 15). Nerve transference has limited application in clinical practice in that only crude sensation, at best, is achieved. In cases of irreparable damage, some useful restoration of function may be obtained by radial-median or radial-ulnar transfer.

Not uncommonly, one must deal with a nerve that is obviously traumatized but in continuity (axonotmesis). Resection of the involved segment is contraindicated as a primary procedure since a majority of such nerves spontaneously recover a satisfactory level of function. Neurolysis, either internal or external, is reserved for those few cases that fail to exhibit satisfactory recovery and is not considered for a minimum period of three to four months postinjury. Internal neurolysis is performed either by meticulous blunt teasing apart of the fascicles with the back edge of a knife blade or by mechanical separation of the fibers by means of distending the nerve with injection of saline solution through an extremely fine-gauge needle. The results obtainable with neurolysis recommend this procedure over excision and anastomosis.

Nerve palsies seen with blunt trauma, with or without associated fracture, almost invariably recover completely (neurapraxia). Operative intervention is indicated only if there is no evidence of recovery during an appropriate period of observation, usually not less than six months.

SPECIFIC INJURIES

Wringer Injuries. Washing machine wringers account for approximately 100,000 accidents per year in children under the age of 15 years; there are an equal number in adults.[21] The frequency with which these injuries are seen in the receiving ward of a large hospital leads to an attitude of relative complacency. Such injuries must be treated with utmost respect if catastrophe is to be avoided.

The injury produced is the result of a variety of forces, each of which must be given serious consideration in evaluating the extent of damage: compression, contusion, heat due to friction and avulsion.[6] The picture is one of a crushing injury with the usual anticipation of subsequent edema and hemorrhage.

Important features to be elicited in the history are the age of the machine and the status of the wringers, the level to which the extremity entered the wringer, the duration of exposure and the measures taken to extricate the extremity. Prolonged exposure results in deep burning of the skin and subcutaneous tissue and severe contusion of the underlying musculature. Strong countertraction produces avulsion and an increased incidence of peripheral nerve damage.

The most common sites of severe injury are the dorsum of the hand, the dorsum of the wrist, the flexor surface of the elbow and the medial aspect of the brachium at the axilla, represent-

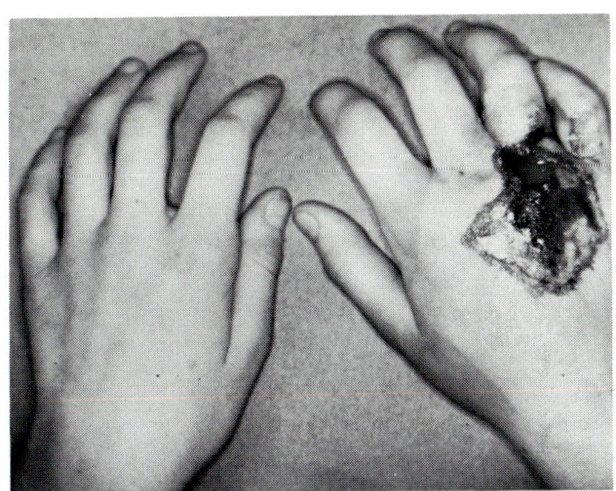

Figure 14–5 Full thickness loss over the dorsum of the hand secondary to a washing machine wringer injury. The true degree of soft tissue damage was initially indeterminate.

ing the areas at which the wringers are most likely to stop (Fig. 14–5). A tear in the web space at the base of the thumb is seen frequently. Separation of the skin and subcutaneous tissue from the underlying fascia results in large areas of hematoma accumulation. Severe pain on passive extension of the fingers indicates significant muscle damage and subfascial hematoma. Peripheral nerve damage usually is of the neurapraxia type, and spontaneous recovery can be anticipated. Fractures occur uncommonly (less than 5 per cent of patients) and usually involve the proximal phalanx or metacarpal of the thumb. Thorough radiologic evaluation is obtained routinely.

Whether to manage a given patient on an inpatient or ambulatory basis is a difficult decision and must be individualized. It is our strong feeling that the majority of patients should be hospitalized for a minimum 48-hour period of observation on the basis that delayed edema and swelling due to an expanding hematoma constitute the major threats. Wringer injuries are exceedingly deceptive, and accurate appraisal of the extent of damage may be impossible initially.

Initial management consists of thorough cleansing of the entire extremity with a mild detergent solution using aseptic technique. Obvious subcutaneous and subfascial hematomas are drained as an operating room procedure. Abraded areas and open wounds are dressed with Xeroform gauze. A bulky, immobilizing pressure dressing is applied from the fingertips to well above the most proximal extent of injury. Tetanus antitoxin is given, and antibiotic therapy is instituted. In the usual case, the patient is then admitted to the hospital, the extremity is elevated, and the nursing personnel are instructed to observe the fingertips frequently and to record the circulatory status. Definitive treatment of areas of full thickness loss is deferred until resolution of the swelling.

The dressing is changed and the extremity re-evaluated 48 hours postjury. At this time, preparations are made for grafting areas of full thickness loss; approximately 10 to 20 per cent of patients will require grafting.[6, 12] A careful search is made for undrained hematomas. These will produce diffuse fibrosis with resultant irretrievable loss of function if left untreated. In the absence of complications, the patient may be discharged at 48 hours with a well applied pressure dressing and a sling in place. Antibiotics are continued for at least five days. The dressing is changed at 48- to 72-hour intervals for a total period of ten days to two weeks postinjury, at which time the patient is allowed to gradually resume normal activity.

Missile. The gunshot and shotgun injuries encountered in civilian practice do not present the extensive soft tissue destruction seen with military wounds. Muzzle velocities of 850 ft./sec. (0.38 caliber) and 1150 ft./sec. (0.22 caliber long rifle) do not compare with the muzzle velocities in excess of 3500 ft./sec. produced by military weapons. The muzzle velocity of a shotgun is in the same range as that of a civilian pistol. Massive debridement is, therefore, not a consideration in the management of these wounds.

Gunshot wounds are not by definition "dirty" and are treated as clean wounds. All wounds are cleansed thoroughly with a mild detergent solution, the wound edges are debrided minimally, and a sterile dressing of Xeroform gauze is applied. A concerted effort is made to remove powder burns by means of scrubbing with a surgical brush to prevent permanent tattooing. The wounds are explored only on the basis of specific indications. Missiles that are easily palpable subcutaneously are commonly painful and subject to external trauma and are removed. Major vascular and peripheral nerve injury demand exploration and repair; no attempt is made to remove the missile if it is not easily accessible. All joint injuries are explored. Fractures are treated as closed injuries, with the usual indications for open reduction.

Shotgun wounds are responsible for a greater percentage of deaths than those from any other type of firearm. The single most important factor determining the magnitude of damage is the distance from which the injury was received.[27] Wounds received from greater than seven yards seldom demonstrate significant injury, whereas wounds inflicted at less than three yards exhibit massive tissue loss. Perforating injuries of subfascial structures are seen with injuries received from an intermediate range. The wounds are more "dirty" than other gunshot wounds because of the quantity of foreign material introduced in the form of wadding, bits of clothing, and so forth. Soft tissue destruction is due to direct damage by the injuring agent and not to a compression wave as is associated with high-velocity missiles.

Debridement consists of thorough irrigation with large volumes of saline solution, meticulous removal of all foreign material and resection of nonviable tissue. Contused muscle may be expected to survive. Inadequate debridement courts the ever-present threat of clostridial infection. Pellets are removed only if readily accessible within the wound. Major structures are repaired as indicated. Simple wounds of entry secondary to close range injury often may be closed primarily. Skin graft or pedicle flap coverage of larger wounds is secured at the primary procedure if at all possible. Definitive closure is delayed for a period of 48 to 72 hours in the face of massive muscle injury with questionable tissue viability. Multiple, small pellet wounds in the skin are dressed with Xeroform gauze. Adequate tetanus prophylaxis and antibiotic coverage are instituted preoperatively.

Impaling injuries are seen infrequently and are usually the result of industrial accidents. Necessary measures are taken to carefully dismantle the machinery and extricate the victim together with the impaling agent. First aid treatment is directed toward immobilizing the involved extremity and stabilizing the impaling agent. Removal of the impaling agent is accomplished as an operating room procedure with provision having been made for possible massive bleeding. Misguided efforts to shorten the impaling agent prior to removal result in increased soft tissue damage; it should be thoroughly cleaned and carefully withdrawn along the path of entry.[22] Repair is undertaken as indicated.

Massive Crush. Severe crushing injuries differ from other types of injuries in several basic respects: massive edema and interstitial hemorrhage, extensive damage to a multiplicity of structures and highly questionable tissue viability (Fig. 14–6). All these factors combine to render the true extent of injury initially indeterminate. The information obtainable by physical examination is only grossly reliable in determining the structures involved and the nature of their injury. Arterial insufficiency may be caused by vascular spasm, occlusion or division. Nerve deficits may represent neurotmesis, axonotmesis or neurapraxia. Loss of tendon function may be due to divi-

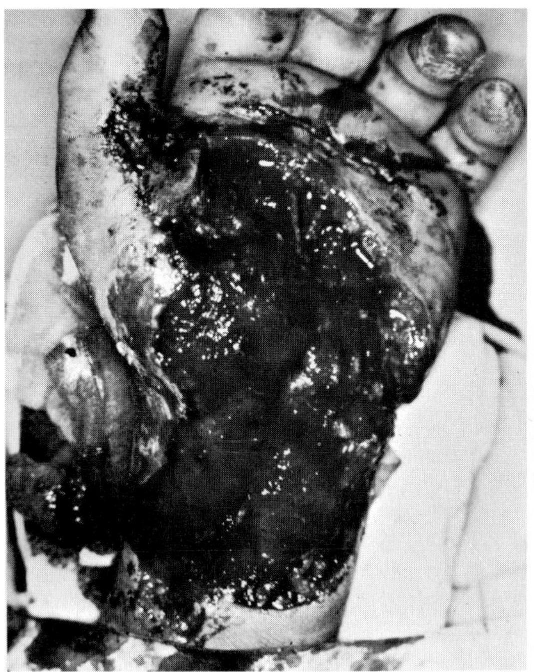
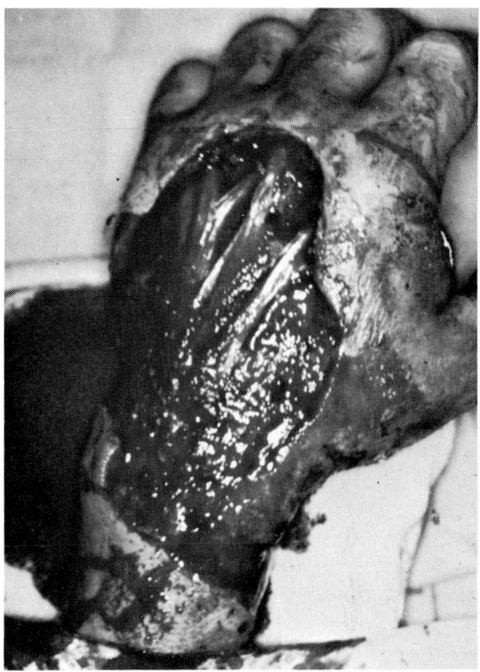

Figure 14–6 Massive crushing injury sustained in a printing press; soft tissue loss, multiple fractures, rupture of flexor tendons and division of the median, ulnar and multiple digital nerves. Reduction of edema and preservation of viability are the major postoperative considerations.

sion or rupture of the tendons or may be secondary to massive hematoma formation within their muscle bellies. Accurate assessment of soft tissue viability is impossible on the basis of simple inspection and is exceedingly difficult at best at the time of formal exploration. Radiographic evaluation is obtained routinely. Arteriograms and other diagnostic adjuncts are of little value.

Exploration is performed without benefit of tourniquet ischemia. The major goal is to restore adequate circulation, and the entire armamentarium of vascular techniques is used to accomplish this end: vascular anastomoses, flushing of occluded vessels with heparin-saline solution, periarterial sympathectomy, and so forth. All nonviable skin, subcutaneous tissue and muscles are resected, and a meticulous anatomical survey is made of the remaining structures. All too frequently, severe shredding and avulsion result in considerable loss of continuity of tendons and nerves. Anastomoses are performed only if normal tissue can be approximated without tension and covered with viable skin. Tendon and nerve ends that cannot be approximated are tagged with wire for easier identification at subsequent procedures.

Fasciotomy may be one of the most useful adjuncts in the care of such extremities and should be employed freely in the management of wounds resulting from crush, high-velocity missiles or ischemia. The fascia may be incised widely under direct vision in the presence of an open wound. Multiple small incisions should be employed in closed injuries. There must be no doubt regarding the adequacy of fasciotomy at the termination of the procedure. Fascial decompression should be considered for all wounds involving the regions of the intrinsic muscles, the volar carpal ligament, the forearm and upper arm, and the thigh and lower leg. It must be recalled that the anterior tibial compartment is anatomically discrete and receives no decompression from posterior or medial incisions.

It is doubtful whether these wounds should ever be closed at the time of the primary procedure: one can never be confident that the debridement was adequate; closure does not allow for the massive edema that inevitably follows these injuries. Skin flaps that are clearly viable at the time of closure may be compromised severely by subsequent swelling; edema within a closed compartment may reduce an already tenuous circulation to a critical level. Following debridement and repair of the deep structures to the extent possible, a bulky, immobilizing pressure dressing is applied. The patient is returned to the operating room for formal re-exploration and closure at the end of a 48- to 72-hour period.

Postoperative management is directed almost entirely at reduction of edema and preservation of viability. In the initial postoperative phase, elevation and pressure dressings are utilized. The Jobst pneumatic bandage provides an excellent method for both splinting and pressure. Stellate ganglion block, low molecular weight dextran, dimethyl-sulfoxide and local hypothermia, although not of proven clinical value, probably should be given a trial in cases demonstrating circulatory impairment threatening the limb. These measures must be instituted within four hours and probably are not beneficial beyond 24 hours. Interstitial precipitation of protein, brawny induration and diffuse fibrosis inexorably follow in the wake of persistent edema; the extremity literally becomes a coagulum.

All patients with severe crushing injuries require staged reconstructive procedures to a greater or lesser degree. Tendolyses and neurolyses are required to extricate these structures from a bed of dense scar. Complications in the form of indolent soft tissue wounds and chronic osteomyelitis are not uncommon. The economic devastation resulting from a two- to three-year period of unemployment is obvious.

Limb Replantation. The replacement of completely severed limbs has passed beyond a technical exercise in the laboratory to become a workable clinical reality.[36] A fair degree of success may be anticipated if the amputated member has not been excessively injured and can be retrieved within a reasonably short period of time. The member is placed under hypothermia as rapidly as possible and maintained at low temperatures while preparations are being made to flush the vasculature and maintain viability with the pump oxygenator. Bony approximation is accomplished by means of intramedullary fixation. Slight shortening of bone facilitates soft tissue closure and tension-free anastomosis. Vascular and nerve suture are performed in the usual fashion. Nerve regeneration is the major factor limiting success. Replantation of fingers is more difficult because of the small size of the vessels, but isolated successes have resulted from microvascular techniques.

LOWER EXTREMITY INJURY

The basic principles applicable to surgery of the lower extremity differ from those for other anatomical regions to such an extent that separate discussion is warranted. The primary reasons for this difference are: the somewhat unique vasculature of the lower extremity, and the essentially complete absence of "spare" skin.

The tissues of the lower extremity are relatively ischemic in comparison with the soft tissue of the face. Special features of the vasculature of the lower extremity include a primarily longitudinal orientation of blood vessels; blood vessel innervation by vasoconstrictor fibers only, resulting in a considerable degree of tone; and the superimposition of the hydrostatic pressure of a column of blood the length of the extremity.[23] Objective demonstration of the significance of this particular vascular pattern consists of a progressively decreasing skin temperature gradient below the knee. The skin derives its blood supply from a longitudinally oriented dermal plexus supplied by vessels perforating the fascia. Each perforating vessel nourishes an area of skin approximately 3 in. in diameter; very little overlap is provided by the dermal plexus.

Langer's lines are longitudinal in the lower extremity. The relationship between the deep fascia and the overlying soft tissue is such that no "spare" skin is available by undermining.

Surgeons assuming responsibility for lower extremity injuries must do so with these principles firmly in mind and must observe certain inviolate rules if primary healing and a stable scar are to be obtained: debridement must be stringent, wound closure must be absolutely tension-free, joints must be immobilized, and dependency and ambulation are prohibited. The rules are enforced rigidly for all but exceedingly minor injuries, i.e., small, clean lacerations involving only skin and subcutaneous tissue.

Soft Tissue Injuries. Longitudinal lacerations with minimal skin loss can be closed primarily. Even without skin loss transverse lacerations often demonstrate superficial necrosis along the distal margin of the suture line. Debridement in the lower extremity must not err on the side of conservatism. Wound margins are excised routinely. Tissue of questionable viability is sacrificed without hesitation, with the realization that necrosis on the basis of vascular insufficiency is a foregone conclusion. Wound closure is accomplished in two layers. Minute approximation of the skin margins is performed only if the tissues are unquestionably healthy. Continuous subcuticular pull-out sutures of nylon or wire give the best results. Skin sutures will produce necrosis of the wound margins in the presence of tension. In equivocal situations, meticulous skin closure is disregarded or accomplished by means of multiple adhesive straps applied transversely. The dressing incorporates a posterior plaster splint immobilizing the proximal and distal joints in functional positions, i.e., moderate flexion of the knee and neutral position of the ankle. Neither dependency of the extremity nor ambulation is permitted for three weeks. The period of immobilization may be varied within narrow limits in adaptation to specific situations.

Categorically, wounds distal to the knee exhibiting more than a minimal amount of skin loss require the introduction of additional tissue for adequate closure (Fig. 14–7).

The management of peripheral nerve injuries entails no specific features.

Tendon repairs in the leg and foot are immobilized for significantly longer periods than those in the upper extremities. The cast is left in place for six weeks; a walking heel may be applied at three to four weeks postinjury.

Plantar Injuries. The resurfacing of weight-bearing areas presents certain problems peculiar to their functional needs. The tissue utilized for cover must have protective sensibility and be able to withstand repeated trauma. Contrary to popular belief, free grafts prove surprisingly serviceable and in most instances are preferable to pedicle flap closure. As an extreme example, free grafts applied directly to the plantar surface of the calcaneus have been known to do well over long periods. The grafts develop protective sensibility; the wound becomes concave with healing, thereby offering some protection to the graft. Full thickness grafts obtained from the instep of the involved foot are utilized if possible. Local rotation flaps of generous proportions may be utilized to cover limited defects of the heel. Small defects in

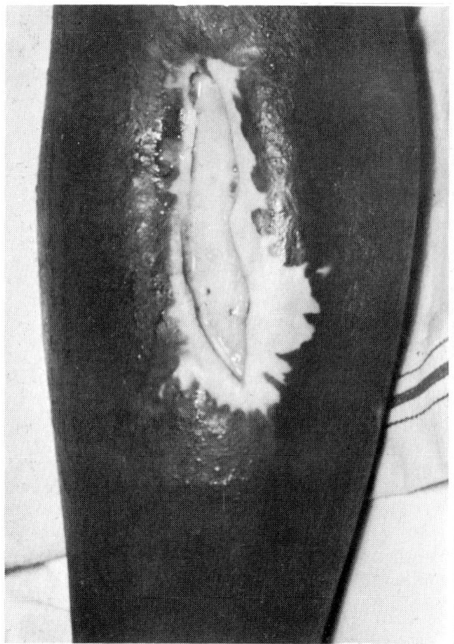

Figure 14–7

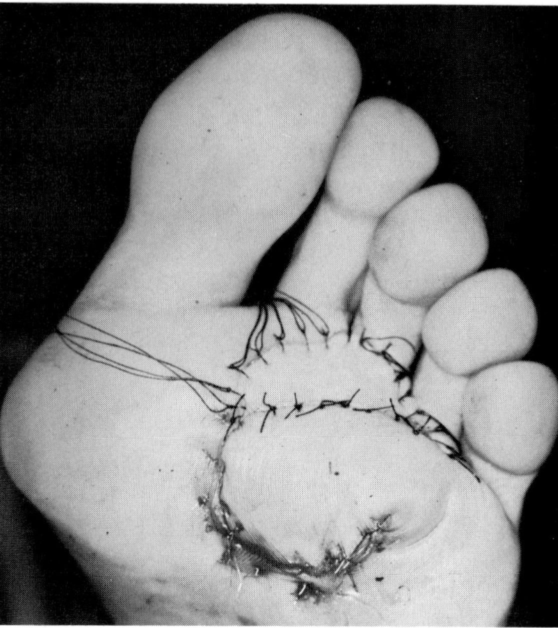

Figure 14–8

Figure 14–7 Soft tissue loss and osteomyelitis resulting from closure of a pretibial laceration with excessive tension.

Figure 14–8 Utilization of a local rotation flap for closure of a defect overlying the metatarsal heads. The skin graft is in a nonweight-bearing area.

the region of the metatarsal heads may be closed with a local flap taken from the area of the proximal flexion crease of the toes, thus transferring the skin graft to a nonweight-bearing position (Fig. 14–8). A filleted toe transferred on a neurovascular pedicle provides perfect cover for defects of intermediate size and will reach almost any area of the sole (Fig. 14–9). Distinct disadvantages are inherent in pedicle flaps from a distance: because of the quantity of subcutaneous fat, patients complain of instability of the flap which they graphically describe as "walking on a pillow"; there is complete lack of sensation.

Compound Fractures. A historical review of the treatment of compound fractures provides a fascinating chronicle of emergency war surgery in general.[4] The trend in therapy has been toward earlier definitive wound closure. Fortunately, we have progressed beyond the open wound, "closed plaster" method of Trueta,[32] beyond awaiting a clean, granulating wound, and partially beyond delayed primary closure on the fourth to sixth day postinjury. Adequate soft tissue debridement and provision for adequate skin cover are essential to bony union and prevention of osteomyelitis. Extreme conservatism is observed regarding sacrifice of bone. Obviously devitalized small fragments without periosteal attachment are discarded; all questionable bone is preserved. Closure is accomplished in accordance with the previously outlined principles. Adequate muscle closure allows utilization of a free graft. Massive soft tissue loss with exposed bone demands pedicle flap coverage. Failure of healing per primam is manged by conservative treatment designed to produce a granulating wound satisfactory for grafting; the graft is not considered definitive cover. Small areas of

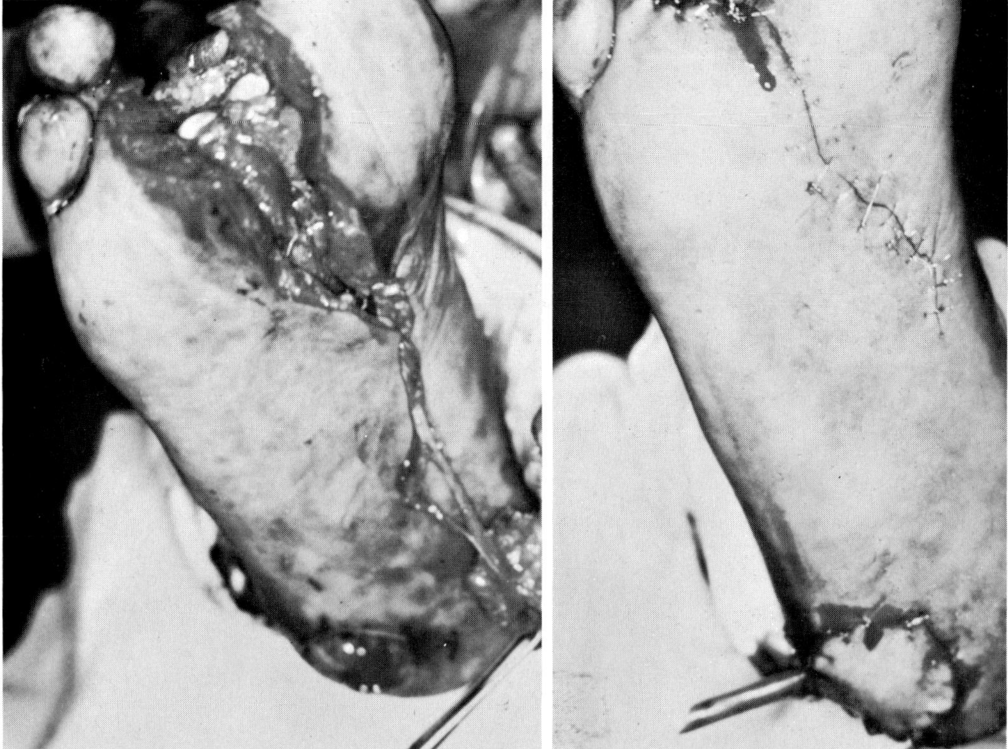

Figure 14–9 Utilization of a filleted toe transferred on an intact neurovascular pedicle to resurface a full thickness defect on the weight-bearing area of the heel.

exposed, nonviable bone may be disregarded during this phase of management. Definitive pedicle flap coverage is undertaken as an elective reconstructive procedure following wound healing. Nonunion responds dramatically to the introduction of healthy, blood-bearing tissue.

Free Grafts. Skin grafts provide the most expedient means of obtaining a clean, healed wound and on this basis are utilized whenever feasible at the time of the primary procedure. The graft can be applied directly to subcutaneous tissue, muscle and periosteum. Skin grafts do not survive well on cortical bone devoid of periosteum but may suffice on cancellous bone (Fig. 14–10). Failure of hemostasis and questionable viability are the only indications for delaying grafting 48 to 72 hours postinjury.

Elevation and immobilization of the extremity for three weeks is mandatory. A graft that appears to be healing satisfactorily at seven to ten days is readily lost by allowing the extremity to become dependent.

As noted previously, the graft may or may not be intended as definitive cover; its major function lies in securing a healed wound as rapidly as possible in situations in which pedicle flap coverage is unavailable or inappropriate. Perfect "take" of the graft is desirable but not essential. Small areas of exposed bone or tendon sequestrate with little or no local reaction.

Skin grafts around the ankle tend to be unstable. The technique of overgrafting[35] may provide a sufficient dermal layer to prevent recurrent ulceration; i.e., in multiple stages the epidermis is removed from previously applied skin grafts by means of derma-

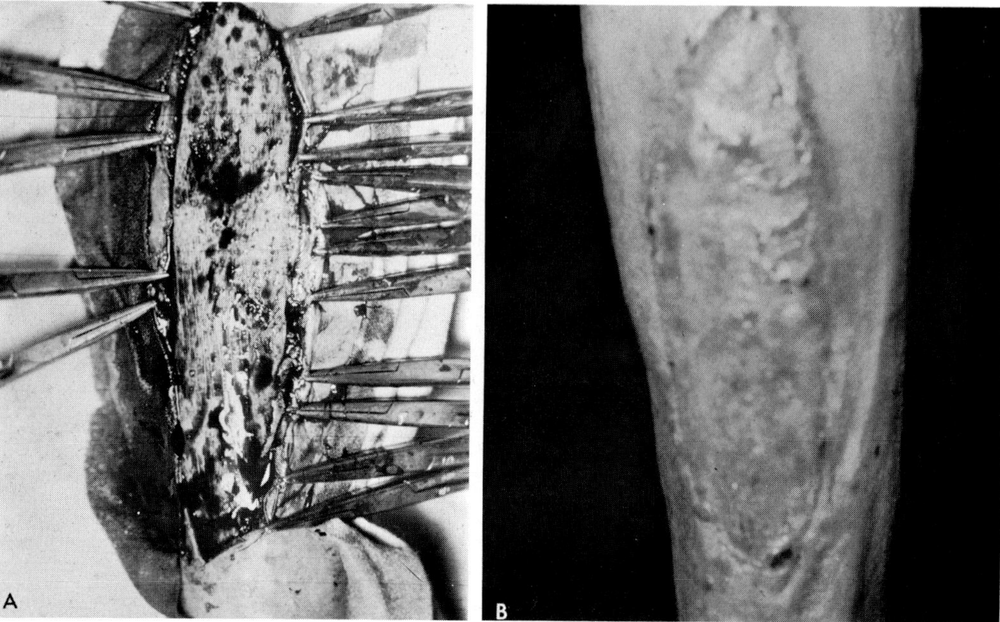

Figure 14–10 *A*, Decortication of the tibia for chronic osteomyelitis. *B*, The completely healed wound obtained by means of a skin graft applied immediately to bare bone.

brasion and new grafts are applied to the residual dermis. Pedicle flap coverage may be required.

Pedicle Flaps. Pedicle flap coverage may be utilized as a primary procedure, as a planned delayed procedure within the first week following injury or as a completely elective reconstructive procedure. The usual indications for pedicle flap coverage include exposure of important major structures such as bone, joints, tendons and nerves, and the necessity for subsequent reconstructive procedures on these structures. Adequate coverage of the acute wound may well determine whether deep structures survive or perish; if flap coverage is indicated, its accomplishment as a primary procedure is highly desirable. Pedicle flap coverage is performed as a planned delayed procedure when the superimposition of additional surgical trauma is inadvisable and when the wound is indeterminate in terms of tissue viability.

Possible donor areas for pedicle flaps are local tissues, tissues from the opposite lower extremity, and abdominal tissue in the form of a jump flap transported on an upper extremity.

The limited applicability of local rotation flaps because of their exceedingly precarious blood supply has been stressed previously.

Cross-extremity flaps may be based on the opposite leg, thigh or knee. The primary consideration is a purely mechanical one relating the defect to the opposite extremity in the most comfortable position for the patient. The cross-thigh flap is of limited value and is usually reserved for females who wish to avoid creation of a secondary deformity on the opposite leg. The geniculate circulation about the knee allows the designing of retrograde flaps (based distally) with considerable safety; such flaps serve admirably for limited defects involving the distal third of the leg. The cross-leg flap is most commonly used because of the frequency of compound fractures of the tibia and power mower injuries of the foot (Fig. 14–11). The cross-leg flap usually is based anteriorly and elevated from the posteromedial aspect of the calf. Provision is made for as broad a pedicle as possible; the length to width ratio of the flap preferably is maintained close to 1:1 and should not exceed 1.5:1.

Precise preoperative planning is absolutely essential to success and consists of substantial time spent in testing the relative position of the extremities, determining the dimensions of the flap and accurately mapping the location of the flap on the donor leg. Application of casts preoperatively hinders rather than helps the operative procedure. Properly designed cross-leg flaps are elevated and transferred without previous delay procedures. The pedicle is severed, usually without a delay procedure, at 21 days.

Abdominal jump flaps are reserved entirely for the elective resurfacing of extensive defects requiring more tissue than can be provided by cross-extremity transfers (Fig. 14–12). An initial procedure is required for the attachment of the abdominal flap to the upper extremity. Several delay procedures performed at seven- to ten-day intervals, beginning three weeks after the initial procedure, are required before the flap can be transferred.

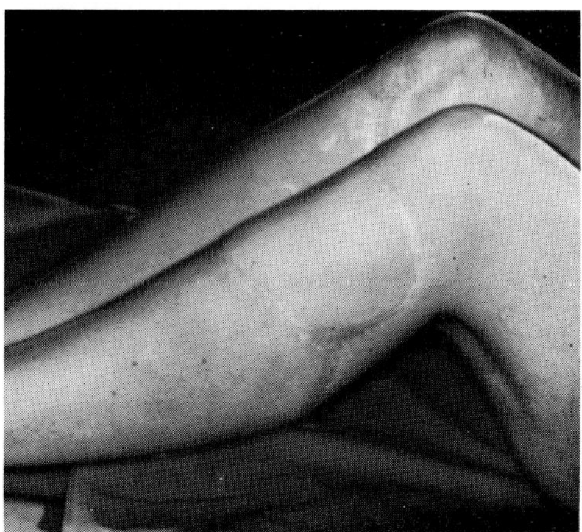

Figure 14–11 A cross-leg flap from the posteromedial aspect of the opposite calf utilized to secure closure of a chronic osteomyelitis of the tibia.

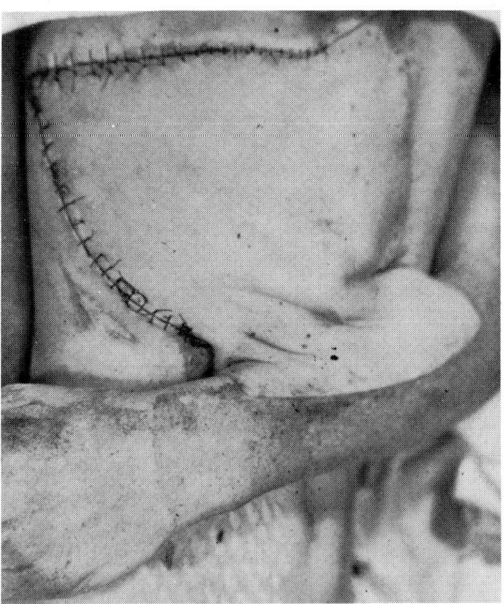

Figure 14–12 An abdominal jump flap to be utilized in resurfacing an extensive pretibial defect.

POSTOPERATIVE MANAGEMENT

The edema inevitably associated with extremity injuries is the major deterrent to recovery of normal function. Edematous tissues thicken and shorten and eventually become fixed in this position because of the deposition of protein and fibrin. Ligaments shorten, joints stiffen, muscles contract and tendons and nerves become encased in a dense fibrous sheath. Immobilization superimposed on edema and maintained for longer than absolutely necessary completes petrification of the extremity.

Attention during the immediate postoperative period is directed toward reduction of edema, preservation of viability and splinting of the wound. Almost without exception, extremity injuries are managed initially by means of elevation and pressure dressings. Elevation of the upper extremity is accomplished by means of an "arm bag" consisting of a canvas bag enclosing the entire upper extremity and suspended from an intravenous pole; the brachium and elbow rest horizontally on the bed, and the forearm and hand are suspended vertically. The lower extremity is elevated 15 degrees above the horizontal on pillows with care being taken not to exert pressure on the popliteal fossa. The extremities are not permitted to become either elevated or dependent in cases demonstrating severe arterial insufficiency.

Pressure dressings extend from the most distal part of the extremity to well above the area of injury; the toes and fingertips are exposed routinely for evaluation of circulation. Circumferential dressings applied to limited areas produce massive distal edema. Local hypothermia, low molecular weight dextran and stellate ganglion block are employed as therapeutic adjuncts in the face of severe vascular insufficiency. Institution of these measures as soon as feasible following trauma is essential; delay for more than four to six hours renders them useless. Elevation and complete immobilization of upper extremity injuries is maintained for a minimum period of 48 hours, following which ambulation with the extremity in a sling is allowed. Elevation and immobilization of severe lower extremity injuries is maintained for a minimum period of three weeks. Sutures are left intact and dressings continued for a period of two weeks.

Volkmann's ischemic contracture is a catastrophe that must be guarded against constantly, especially when dealing with casts and compression bandages. Although the etiology in the majority of cases is an unreduced supracondylar fracture of the elbow, the condition is seen with damage to the brachial or axillary artery and with massive subfascial hematoma secondary to crushing trauma of the forearm. Symptoms of impeding ischemia consist of constant pain exaggerated by forced extension of the fingers and hypesthesia and paresthesia of the hand, usually in the median nerve distribution. Examination reveals marked swelling of the hand and forearm, pale cyanosis, partial intrinsic paralysis and an absent radial pulse. Progression to this stage is prevented by repeated evaluation of the circulatory status of the toes and fingertips and repeated questioning of the patient. Damage occurs within six to 48 hours of trauma or the application of an excessively tight dressing. The presence of the above findings demands immediate removal of the dressings. Fasciotomy and sympathetic block are indicated if symptoms do not improve immediately. At exploration, the problem is found to be limited to the volar fascial space; findings consist of muscles that are either pale or blue-black from extravasation of blood, occlusion of all of the veins in the antecubital fossa, and rupture or thrombosis of the brachial artery.

Indolent wounds wreak havoc on the *entire* extremity by producing persistent edema and prolonging the period of inactivity. Postoperative management is not complete until a healed wound has been secured.

REHABILITATION

All except the most minor extremity injuries require organized effort directed specifically at restoration of normal function. Immobilization results in stiff joints that must be overcome by all means available. All surgeons assuming responsibility for extremity injuries must have a thorough working knowledge of static and dynamic splinting[18] and of the methods utilized in an organized program of physiotherapy.

All major peripheral nerve injuries require dynamic splinting until obviated by satisfactory recovery of motor function or the decision to proceed with muscle transfers, the goal being to prevent the creation of deformity by unopposed muscle groups. Dynamic splints are designed to provide the action of the paralyzed muscle groups, thereby offering resistance for the uninvolved muscles to work against. Construction of such splints by the surgeon caring for the patient serves two major purposes: the splint is custom designed to fit properly and to accomplish precisely the desired end; and the physician, of necessity, learns a great deal about the functional anatomy of the hand. One needs only the usual material required in applying a cast plus some ⅛ in. welding rods and leather working tools in order to construct a perfect dynamic splint. The splints are worn for increasingly longer periods as tolerated by the patient; night splints are utilized to overcome contraction of ligaments and tendons. Dynamic transfers are deferred until sufficient time has elapsed to judge the quality of the nerve repair.

The patient with a radial nerve palsy requires a static splint that maintains the wrist and metacarpophalangeal joints in extension; i.e., a volar thin plaster slab held in position by means of wrapping with an elastic bandage. A surprising degree of function is possible with the splint in place provided it does not extend beyond the proximal interphalangeal flexion crease. Such splints usually incorporate a dorsal outrigger with elastic traction producing extension of the thumb. The dynamic splint used in ulnar nerve palsy consists of a "knuckle-bender" component and a dorsal outrigger with elastic traction producing extension of the ring and little fingers (Fig. 14–13). The patient with a median nerve injury requires a splint designed to produce dynamic (elastic) opposition of the thumb. The need for dynamic splinting is increased markedly with median and ulnar nerve injuries distal to the site of innervation of the forearm musculature.

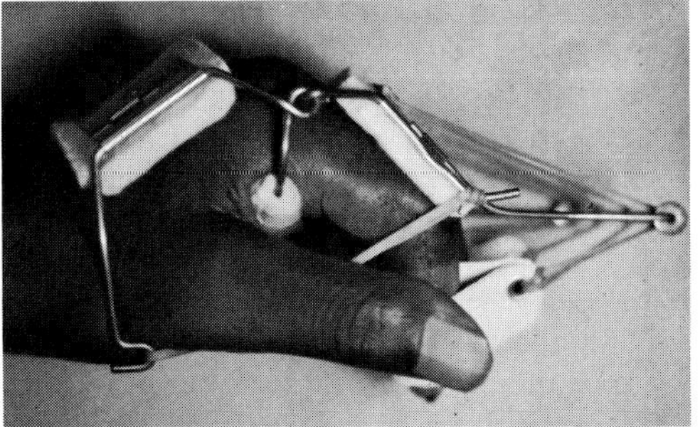

Figure 14–13 The proper "knuckle-bender" splint with extension outrigger to be utilized in the rehabilitation of median and ulnar nerve palsy.

The importance of precise follow-up records to the proper management of extremity injuries cannot be overemphasized. Treatment methods must be altered constantly to achieve maximal progress, and this is not possible if progress is not objectively measurable. Clinic notes such as "sensation improved" and "less flexion deformity" are totally worthless to the individual patient, and have no possible value in surveying the results of different methods of treatment. Measurements must be repeated sequentially and must be as objective as possible. Joint motion is recorded in degrees as measured with a protractor. The range of passive motion provides a good index of joint function, and the relation between this measurement and that of active motion gives valuable information in terms of tendon and muscle function. Sensory and motor return following peripheral nerve injury is best documented by the method of Nicholson and Seddon[17] (to be discussed later).

Sensory evaluation may be performed by a variety of methods, only a few of which are of real value. Coarse touch is the first sensation to return following peripheral nerve injury and is followed in order by perception of pinprick and light touch, the development of Tinel's sign and, finally, by stereognosis. Mohberg[16] and others[7] have demonstrated clearly the rather gross correlation between the usual tests of sensibility and the degree of functional usefulness of the hand. Response to pinprick and light touch is of no value in predicting the degree of *functional sensibility* of the hand. On this basis, the authors advocate utilization of the Weber two-point discrimination test,[34] the ninhydrin printing test and measurement of "tactile gnosis" by means of the Seddon coin test and the Mohberg pick-up test. Two-point discrimination of 12 mm. or less on the volar aspect of the distal phalanx represents a high degree of recovery; patients with this degree of recovery have little measurable functional impairment.

The ninhydrin printing test is based on Mohberg's excellent demonstration of correlation between sudomotor activity and functional sensibility. It consists of staining by ninhydrin of the amino acids normally present in sweat and is demonstrated by fingerprinting. The hand is applied to a sheet of glazed white paper which is then stained with a 1 per cent solution of ninhydrin in acetone acidified with five drops of glacial acetic acid per 10 cc. of solution. After a period of two to three days, the print is fixed in a 1 per cent solution of copper nitrate in 95 per cent methyl alcohol acidified with a few drops of nitric acid. Unstained areas have no functional sensibility.

An index of tactile gnosis is obtained by requesting the patient to manipulate a group of small and varied objects. As utilized by Seddon, this consists of asking the blindfolded patient to identify a variety of coins; Mohberg provides the patient with a variety of common small objects and requests that they be transferred from the table to a cup with and without the aid of vision.

Tinel's sign is of value primarily in judging the progress of recovery prior to reinnervation. Gentle tapping over the course of the nerve distal to the site of injury elicits paresthesia over the growing axons; this paresthesia is referred to the normal area of innervation of the nerve. In performing the test, it is important that vibration of the soft tissue proximal to the point of tapping be prevented. Tinel's sign is demonstrable four to six weeks following nerve suture and persists for a period of 18 to 24 months, i.e., until the regenerated axons have become myelinated.

Muscles return to function in the anatomical order of their innervation. A variable degree of irreversible atrophy may be anticipated and depends upon the time required for nerve regeneration.

Although nerve regeneration proceeds at a rate of approximately 1.5 mm. per day,[26] a considerably longer period of time than might be predicted on this basis is required for significant return of sensory and motor function. Beginning return of sensation may be appreciated within four to six weeks following nerve injury in the hand. Evidence of sensory return is not seen for a period of two to three months following nerve injury proximal to the level of the wrist, and motor return may not be appreciated for six to eight months. Function continues to improve slowly over a rather prolonged period of time in association with maturation of the regenerated nerve in terms of myelination and increase in fiber size. Recovery cannot be considered maximal for at least three years following major peripheral nerve injury.

The method of evaluation proposed by Nicholson and Seddon[17] should be used as a standard in recording results following peripheral nerve injury:

Sensory:

- (S:O) Absence of sensibility in the cutaneous zone supplied exclusively by the nerve concerned (autonomous zone).
- (1) Recovery of deep cutaneous pain.
- (2) Recovery of some degree of superficial pain and tactile sensibility.
- (2+) Return of tactile and pain sensibility throughout the autonomous zone but with persistent overreaction.
- (3) Return of superficial pain and tactile sensibility throughout the

autonomous zone with the disappearance of overreaction.

(3+) Return of superficial pain and tactile sensibility throughout the autonomous zone with the disappearance of overreaction, and good localization of stimuli with some return to two-point discrimination.

(4) Complete recovery.

Motor:

(M:O) No contraction.

(1) Return of perceptible contraction in the forearm muscles.

(1+) Median: Forearm muscles able to contract against gravity but paralysis of the thenar muscles.

Ulnar: Forearm muscles able to contract against gravity but paralysis of the ulnar intrinsic muscles of the hand.

(2) Median: Forearm muscles able to contract against gravity and weak action in the thenar muscles.

Ulnar: Forearm muscles able to contract against gravity and some power in the hypothenars but little or none in the interossei.

(2+) Ulnar: Forearm and hand muscles all active but the first dorsal interosseous muscle unable to contract against resistance.

(3) Median: Forearm and thenar muscles able to contract against resistance.

Ulnar: Forearm, hypothenars and first dorsal interosseous muscles able to contract against resistance.

(4) Median: All muscles able to contract against strong resistance with some independent action.

Ulnar: All muscles able to contract against resistance with some independent lateral movement of fingers.

(5) Full recovery in all muscles.

Patients with return of function to the S:3, M:3 level are classified as having a good result; those with return to the S:4, M:4 or 5 level are classified as having an excellent result. Combined data indicate that not more than 50 or 60 per cent of patients achieve a good or excellent result and that few, if any, patients regain completely normal function.[3, 11, 24, 30, 37] Results with mixed nerve injuries are poorer than those with injuries just to sensory or motor nerves; digital and radial nerve repairs are almost uniformly successful; ulnar repairs provide the least satisfactory results; and median nerve repairs are intermediate in results. Children uniformly obtain a better result than adults and often demonstrate relatively normal sensation after a two-year period.[11, 24, 30]

Electromyograph and nerve conduction velocity studies provide a more sophisticated measure of the extent of recovery following peripheral nerve damage. Multiple studies[9, 15] indicate that the conduction velocity never returns to normal following nerve suture; in the usual case, it probably does not exceed 60 to 70 per cent of normal. The electromyogram may be of considerable prognostic value.

The results presently being obtained leave much to be desired. Intensive effort must be directed toward the improvement of repair techniques.

RECONSTRUCTION

It is not our purpose to elaborate upon the complex techniques utilized in restoring function to a badly crippled extremity. It is sufficient to say that the hand is totally dependent on a finely balanced mechanism for functional integrity, and all possible efforts must be directed toward restoring this balance.

REFERENCES

1. Aitken, J. T., Scharman, M., and Young, J. Z.: Maturation of regenerating nerve fibers with various peripheral connections. J. Anat. *81*:1, 1947.
2. Altemeier, W. A., and Alexander, J. W.: Surgical infections and choice of antibiotics. *In* Sabiston, D. C. (ed.): Textbook of Surgery. Philadelphia, W. B. Saunders Co., 1972.
3. Benvenuto, R.: Peripheral nerves. Int. Abstr. Surg. *115*:528, 1962.
4. Brown, R. F.: The management of traumatic tissue loss in the lower extremity, especially when complicated by skeletal injury. Brit. J. Plast. Surg. *18*:26, 1965.
5. Edshage, S.: Peripheral nerve suture, a technique for improved intraneural topography. Evaluation of some suture materials. Acta. Chir. Scand. (Suppl.) *331*:1, 1964.
6. Entin, M. A.: Roller and wringer injuries: clinical and experimental studies. Plast. Reconstr. Surg. *15*:290, 1955.
7. Flynn, J. E., and Flynn, W. F.: Median and ulnar nerve injuries. Ann. Surg. *156*:1002, 1962.
8. Freeman, B. S.: Adhesive neuroanastomosis. Plast. Reconstr. Surg. *35*:167, 1965.
9. Hodes, R., Larrabee, M. G., and German, W.: The human electromyogram in response to nerve stimulation and the conduction velocity of motor axons. Studies on normal and injured peripheral nerves. Arch. Neurol. Psychiat. *60*:340, 1948.
10. Kline, D. G.: The use of a resorbable wrapper for peripheral nerve repair, experimental studies in chimpanzees. J. Neurosurg. *21*:737, 1964.
11. Lindsay, W. K.: Traumatic peripheral nerve injuries in children; results of repair. Plast. Reconstr. Surg. *30*:462, 1962.
12. Lindsay, W. K., Thomson, H. S., and Farmer, A. W.: The wringer injury. Can. J. Surg. *1*:189, 1957.
13. Marmor, L., and Sollars, R. E.: Amputation levels in severely traumatized extremities, with appropriate prostheses. J. Trauma *2*:585, 1962.
14. Mason, M. L., and Allen, H. S.: The rate of healing of tendons: an experimental study of tensile strength. Ann. Surg. *113*:424, 1941.
15. Mayer, R. F.: Nerve regeneration in replanted canine limbs. Am. J. Physiol. *206*:1415, 1964.
16. Mohberg, G. E.: Objective methods for determining the functional value of sensibility in the hand. J. Bone Joint Surg. *40B*:454, 1958.
17. Nicholson, O. R., and Seddon, H. J.: Nerve repair in civil practice. Brit. Med. J. *2*: 1065, 1957.
18. Peacock, E. A.: Dynamic splinting for the prevention and correction of hand deformities. J. Bone Joint Surg. *34A*:789, 1952.
19. Peacock, E. E., and Van Winkle, W. W., Jr.: Surgery and Biology of Wound Repair. Philadelphia, W. B. Saunders Co., 1970.
20. Potenza, A. D.: Tendon healing within the flexor digital sheath in the dog. J. Bone Joint Surg. *44A*:49, 1962.
21. Press, E.: Wringer washing machine injuries. Am. J. Pub. Health *54*:812, 1964.
22. Roberts, G. R.: Impaling and transfixion injuries to the limbs. Brit. J. Surg. *51*: 135, 1964.
23. Rozner, L.: Anatomical and physiological factors in below-knee wounds. Lancet *1*:1362, 1965.
24. Sakellarides, H.: A follow-up study of 172 peripheral nerve injuries in the upper extremity in civilians. J. Bone Joint Surg. *44A*:410, 1962.
25. Seddon, H. J.: Three types of nerve injury. Brain *66*:238, 1943.
26. Seddon, H. J., Medawar, P. B., and Smith, H.: Rate of regeneration of peripheral nerves in man. J. Physiol. London *102*: 191, 1943.
27. Sherman, R. T., and Parrish, R. A.: Management of shotgun injuries; a review of 152 cases. J. Trauma *3*:76, 1963.
28. Smith, J. W.: Microsurgery of peripheral nerves. Plast. Reconstr. Surg. *33*:317, 1964.
29. Smith, J. W.: Blood supply of tendons. Am. J. Surg. *109*:272, 1965.
30. Stromberg, W. B.: Injury of the median and ulnar nerve. J. Bone Joint Surg. *43A*: 717, 1961.
31. Sunderland, S.: The intraneural topography of the radial, median, and ulnar nerves. Brain *68*:243, 1946.
32. Trueta, J.: Treatment of War Wounds and Fractures. London, Hamish Hamilton, 1939.
33. Wagle, M. B.: Gas gangrene—conservative management. Brit. J. Plast. Surg. *16*:391, 1963.
34. Weber, E. H.: Cutaneous sensation. *In* Schafer, E. A. (ed.): Textbook of Physiology. New York, The MacMillan Co., 1900, p. 928.
35. Webster, G. V., Peterson, R. A., and Stein, H. L.: Dermal overgrafting of the leg. J. Bone Joint Surg. *40A*:796, 1958.
36. Williams, G. R.: Replantation of the extremities. *In* Sabiston, D. C. (ed.): Textbook of Surgery. Philadelphia, W. B. Saunders Co., 1972.
37. Woodhall, B., and Beebe, G. W.: Peripheral Nerve Regeneration. Washington, D. C., V. A. Medical Monograph, 1956.
38. Young, J. Z.: The functional repair of nervous tissue. Physiol. Rev. *22*:318, 1942.
39. Young, J. Z., and Medawar, P. B.: Fibrin

suture of peripheral nerves. Lancet 2: 126, 1940.

General

Committee on Trauma, American College of Surgeons: Early Care of Acute Soft Tissue Injuries. Philadelphia, W. B. Saunders Co., 1961.
Ellis, M.: The Casualty Officer's Handbook. London, Butterworth & Co., Ltd., 1962.
Emergency War Surgery. NATO Handbook. Washington, D. C., Department of Defense, U.S. Government Printing Office, 1958.
Flint, T., Jr.: Emergency Treatment of Management. Philadelphia, W. B. Saunders Co., 1964.
Kirkaldy-Willis, W. H., and Wood, A. M.: Treatment of Trauma. Baltimore, The Williams & Wilkins Co., 1962.
Schrire, T.: Emergencies. Springfield, Ill., Charles C Thomas, 1962.

chapter

15

PERIPHERAL VASCULAR INJURIES

Robert B. Rutherford, M.D.

The first crude vascular repair was performed by Hallowell over two centuries ago,[24] and the basic suture techniques, as we know them today, including the use of autografts and homografts, were well worked out by the end of the first decade of this century and summarized in the classic works of Carrel[3] and Guthrie.[9] By 1910, over 100 lateral repairs and 46 end-to-end anastomoses or segmental vein grafts had been performed clinically.[19] The stage was set for the application of these techniques to vascular injuries by the outbreak of World War I, and yet it was not until the Korean conflict was well under way over 35 years later that this came to pass. The development and use of high-velocity missiles and high explosives during World War I, the treatment priorities imposed by mass casualty situations, and the inordinately long evacuation times from embattled trench to operative theatre combined to perpetuate a discouragingly high failure rate and established the attitude that there was no place for primary vascular repair in military surgery. The emphasis shifted to the management of the delayed complications of vascular injury, arteriovenous fistulas and false aneurysms. Even under the more optimal conditions of civilian practice, treatment rarely went much beyond hemostasis, and not only was the injured artery ligated at the expense of patency but so was the accompanying vein. For inexplicable reason, this attitude was perpetuated through World War II, as indicated by DeBakey and Simeone's review[5] which revealed that direct repair was attempted in only slightly over 3 per cent of 2,471 arterial injuries with end-to-end anastomosis being performed in only eight instances. The overall amputation rate was 49 per cent.

The Korean War shared a period of very rapid advancement with cardiovascular surgery when bold innovative approaches seemed commonplace. Rapid evacuation, ample blood replacement, antibiotics, new vascular instruments and a more stable fighting front with trained surgeons at forward

(M.A.S.H.) hospitals set the stage for a complete reversal of the previously conservative military approach to vascular injuries. Immediate repair was attempted in 88 percent of arterial injuries.[11] In these cases, the amputation rate was only 13 per cent compared to 51 per cent for those in whom ligation of the injured vessel was carried out. The present-day (aggressive) approach to vascular injuries can be said to stem from this experience, although important additional refinements have been added by subsequent experiences in civilian practice and in the Vietnam conflict, as will be brought out later. However, it should be realized that today's relatively optimistic outlook toward peripheral vascular injuries is not due solely to adopting a policy of immediate operative repair. Rapid transportation, availability of blood and antibiotics, abandonment of mass tourniquet techniques, a better appreciation of the true nature of certain forms of arterial injury (high-velocity and blunt trauma), the increased use of arteriography, recognition of the importance of fracture stabilization, thorough debridement (including the traumatized arterial segment), fasciotomy, repair of concomitant venous injuries and the success of vein grafts in bridging major vascular defects in the face of major contamination and tissue destruction, heparin anticoagulation, Fogarty balloon catheters and improved suture material and instruments all have contributed greatly to this advance.

ARTERIAL INJURIES

A wide spectrum of arterial injuries may be encountered, depending on the mechanism of injury. Examples of these are shown in Figure 15–1. Penetrating wounds may take the form of a small puncture, a lateral or through-and-through (knife) laceration or a gaping (low-velocity) bullet hole. An artery will be cleanly transected if directly hit by a high-velocity bullet or, on a near miss, it may be literally torn apart by the explosive energy released in the temporary cavity which develops in the bullet's wake.[1] Blunt trauma may result in contusion and segmental spasm of the artery or, more commonly, its occlusion by intramural hematomata and segmental thrombosis, flap-like intimal tears or circumferential intimal disruption. Arteriovenous fistulas and false aneurysms are the most common late complications.

In the majority of instances, the arterial injury is not an isolated consideration. Associated injuries to the accompanying vein and nerves, concomitant fractures or dislocations, varying degrees of muscle and other soft tissue destruction and contamination of the wound with bacteria and foreign material frequently compound the problem. Other factors that play a role in the end result are the level of injury, the collateral circulation and, occasionally in civilian practice, underlying occlusive arterial disease. A good example of the significance of the level of injury is the popliteal artery, which may be injured by displaced fractures above or below the knee joint or dislocation of the joint itself in addition to penetrating trauma. It is the only major artery traversing this section of the lower extremity and most of its collaterals, i.e., the geniculate arteries, depart from it over a relatively short segment so that they may be involved primarily by the injury itself or secondarily by a relatively short segmental occlusion of the popliteal artery. The high amputation rate associated with ligation of an injured popliteal artery was documented early by Makins,[17] and even today it carries approximately a 30 per cent amputation rate in Vietnam, almost twice that of the next most serious site of peripheral arterial injury, the common femoral.[22] It should be understood that higher amputation rates are to be expected in the natural course of an acute traumatic occlusion than with acute thrombotic occlusion of an already arteriosclerotic vessel, in which

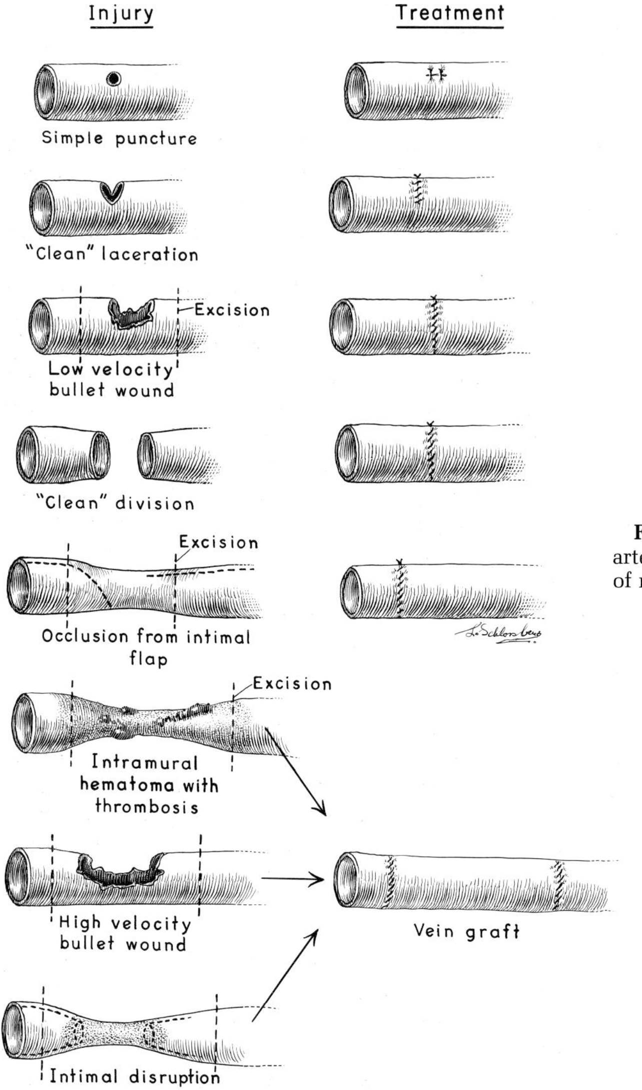

Figure 15–1 Common forms of arterial injury with the likely method of repair.

there has been time for the development of collateral channels.

DIAGNOSIS

The possibility of an arterial injury should be entertained whenever a penetrating wound is found along the course of a major vessel, particularly if there is excessive bleeding from the wound or a rapidly expanding hematoma. However, if the artery has been completely severed and its ends have contracted and become occluded by thrombus, the wound itself may not arouse suspicion. Non-penetrating injuries are a less obvious and therefore more treacherous cause of arterial injury. The existence of a displaced fracture, dislocation or extensive soft tissue injury in particular should lead to the consideration of concomitant arterial injury. Of course, the state of the extremity distal to the wound is usually more telling in this regard by absent arterial pulsations and coolness and pallor or mottled cyanosis of the skin. However, even this may be misleading, particularly following blunt trauma. In 271 civilian arterial injuries reported by Shires et al.,[25] distal pulsations were palpable in 69 and were normal in 40. In a later review,[21] the incidence of normal distal pulses in association with arterial injuries was approximately 10 per cent. Capillary filling should be noted, not only as an aid to diagnosis, but as an indication of viability, to help establish priority of treatment when other significant injuries are present.

Difficulty may arise in examining extremities in the presence of shock. This may not only mask the aforementioned signs but, in association with subclinical degrees of arteriosclerosis, may lead to confusing differences between compared extremities. In a similar regard, it may be difficult to decide in older patients if absent peripheral pulsations are due to the extremity injury or to pre-existing disease. A history of claudication or the presence of trophic skin changes or absent hair growth on the foot being examined should be sought to clarify this situation. Repeated examinations of the extremity for evidences of arterial injury are important in detecting delayed occlusion, the pulsating hematoma of a false aneurysm or the bruit of an arteriovenous fistula.

Finally, the value of arteriography in evaluating arterial injuries cannot be overemphasized.[27] It is particularly useful in dissociating arterial spasm from actual occlusion, in providing earlier diagnosis in cases in which clinical evidence is not decisive, in identifying the level of occlusion for more precise exploration, in assessing the condition of collateral circulation and in detecting incomplete occlusions, false aneurysms and arteriovenous fistulas. It is unnecessary only in penetrating wounds when the existence and location of the arterial injury are obvious.

TREATMENT

Once an arterial injury has been diagnosed, its relative priority in the overall management of the injuries to the patient must be established. Such a decision depends greatly upon the significance of the associated injuries as well as the immediate threat presented by the arterial injury itself. Although it is axiomatic that repair should be performed as soon as possible, it is equally true that once the possibility of exsanguinating hemorrhage has been controlled, there may be no immediate threat of loss of life or limb from this injury, and trauma to other vital areas may deserve prior or at least concomitant attention.

Nevertheless, the consequence of delay in restoring arterial circulation to the extremity must be recognized in making such decisions. Although it is recognized that the often quoted six- to 12-hour "golden period" is only relative, the results of treatments do correlate well with this concept. Edwards and Lyons[6] noted that gangrene was rare following successful repairs undertaken within six hours of injury but occurred in over 50 per cent beyond 12 hours. In Jahnke's experience[12] with 77 consecutive arterial repairs during the Korean conflict, no amputations were required when the delay was 12 hours or less but were required in 29 per cent after this lapse of time. Makin et al.,[16] reporting results with arterial injuries associated with fractures or dislocation, found the late amputation rate to be 16 per cent when delay was less than 12 hours and 80 per cent beyond that, with the remaining 20 per cent suffering permanent disability.

The degree of urgency for repair is often decided by the apparent viability of the skin. However, it should be recognized that outward appearances may be deceiving because the relative viability of ischemic nerves and muscle is much more limited than that of skin. The work of Malan and Tattoni[18] indicates that myelin degeneration and axon retraction begin after four to six hours of ischemia and that discoid degeneration with progressive loss of contractility may affect 90 per cent of the muscle fibers by 12 hours, beyond which time only partial recovery is possible. Failure to recognize this may lead to serious late disability from nerve deficits or ischemic muscle contractures. Areas of skin anesthesia and digital paralysis or foot drop should be considered *late* warning signs of serious limb ischemia. In this regard, Lavenson et al.[15] have shown a good correlation between viability and audible flow through nonpalpable distal vessels (e.g., the posterior tibial artery at the ankle) using an ultrasound flow detector.

In addition, before electing not to repair immediately a peripheral arterial injury in which there is no threat to viability of the extremity, consideration must be given to the possible dire consequences which distal propagation of thrombus with occlusion of additional collaterals might bring to the marginally viable extremity. If there is good reason to favor delayed reconstruction, one must still continue close observation and be prepared to reverse this decision at the first sign of deteriorization. As Eiseman[2] has pointed out, the error at the other extreme of repairing minor or noncritical arteries needs to be guarded against. It was emphasized that, particularly in the young, it is ordinarily not essential to limb survival to repair the brachial artery between the profunda and elbow collaterals, the ulnar or radial artery alone at any level, the profunda femoris artery, the superficial femoral artery proximal to the geniculate collaterals and the anterior tibial, posterior tibial or perineal artery alone at any level. By the same token, vascular repair in the face of serious neuromuscular or skeletal injuries which preclude the return of useful limb function must be decried. However, in a more favorable environment and particularly when not restricted by priorities dictated by other injuries, it is probably wise to at least explore all potential injuries to "name" vessels regardless of how inconsequential they may seen, for even if viability is not at issue, late aneurysms and arteriovenous fistulas may be avoided and those successfully repaired may serve an unexpected later purpose.

The most pressing indication for treatment following arterial injury is, of course, exsanguinating hemorrhage. This should be controlled initially with direct application of pressure over the site of injury or the course of the artery proximal to this. The use of a tourniquet is condemmed except under the most trying circumstances since this technique occludes collateral circulation as well as the injured vessel. In addition, improper application of the tourniquet frequently succeeds only in stemming venous outflow. In large wounds over superficial arteries, hemostasis may be achieved by direct clamping. However, blind clamping into the depths of a bleeding wound only allows additional blood loss at a time when it can be least well tolerated. Unless vascular clamps are available, the artery injury may be compounded by this practice, necessitating a more extensive debridement and possibly the need for a graft.

Once control of hemorrhage has been established, it should be maintained until circulating blood volume has been restored and additional blood is on hand to support definitive exploration. Tetanus prophylaxis should be administered and, in most cases, broad-spectrum antibiotic coverage should be provided for the indications of shock, tissue ischemia or gross contamination.

The actual technique of surgical exploration and repair of arterial injuries must be individualized, but certain principles should be considered. Ordinarily, general anesthesia can be used, but such considerations as an associated head injury, alcoholic intoxication or the desire to continue observation for suspected thoracic or abdominal trauma may dictate the use of regional anesthesia. Many actually prefer the latter because of the theoretical benefit of vasodilatation, and continuous epidural anesthesia is gaining popularity for elective vascular procedures in the lower extremity. The entire extremity and adjacent areas of the trunk as well as the area over the upper saphenous vein in an uninvolved extremity should be prepared and draped. Provision should *always* be made for intraoperative arteriography where available.

One of the first steps should be to gain proximal control of the injured artery. Often this is better done by use of a small, separate incision through which umbilical tapes may be passed around the vessel and occlusion achieved when desired by a noose tourniquet or vascular clamp. This provides a relatively bloodless field in which the injured vessel and surrounding tissues can be adequately exposed. In penetrating injuries one should not explore through wounds of entry or exit or modify one's incision to accommodate them; rather one should use the same incision that would be selected electively to obtain optimum exposure of this part of the arterial tree.

Although it is not necessary in early operations on simple peripheral arterial injuries, consideration should be given in other cases, as soon as control of hemostasis has been established, to inserting a temporary arterial shunt, using a length of thromboresistant plastic tubing to bridge the defect. This technique, as recommended by Eger et al.,[7] provides several advantages: early restoration of flow and prevention of further ischemia during the course of the operation; the ability to perfuse the distal vascular bed with heparin solutions (under pressure if necessary to overcome high critical closing pressures); allowance of more accurate debridement of nonviable tissues, repair of damaged veins *before* arterial repair and fixation of concomitant fractures prior to the vascular repair as well as the performance of most of the vascular reconstruction without interruption of flow. An important additional technical suggestion, to be carried out prior to the above and again just prior to the completion of the final anastomosis, is the removal of thrombus from the distal arterial tree using Fogarty balloon catheters. The presence of back bleeding cannot be considered reliable evidence of distal patency. Systemic heparinization is not without its dangers in the face of other injuries or prior to wound debridement. In such cases, brief intermittent release of the controlling clamps, with or without installation of a small dose of heparin (30 mg.) or a heparin-saline solution into the distal artery, may provide a reasonable alternative. Of course, this so-called "distal" or "regional" heparinization is only possible while circulatory interruption is maintained. In less complicated situations, systemic heparinization (1 mg./kg. every two to three hours) may be carried out as in elective arterial surgery.

Accurate assessment of the true nature and extent of the arterial injury is of utmost importance. One common mistake is to assume that an intact but narrowed arterial segment represents spasm alone when, in fact, mechanical obstruction exists from intimal disruption or dissection or from intramural hematomata and segmental thrombosis. In general, it is wiser to assume that arterial spasm is associated with some significant intramural injury and to explore the vessel than to persist with external efforts to relieve it or to close the wound with the expectation that the "spasm" will eventually abate.

However, if either exploration or a good arteriogram has ruled out mechanical intraluminal problems, a number of maneuvers may be attempted to relieve the arterial spasm (see Fig. 15–2). Segmental periarterial neurectomy, by excision of the adventitial layer, is worthwhile. In addition to this, the topical application of warm saline solutions of Xylocaine, sodium nitrite, pabaverine or Priscoline has been recommended, either by infiltration of the arterial wall or application of a gauze sponge soaked in these solutions. However, neither of these is as effective as mechanical dilation in overcoming simple segmental spasm. If the vessel has been opened, this may be achieved by spreading a clamp within the lumen

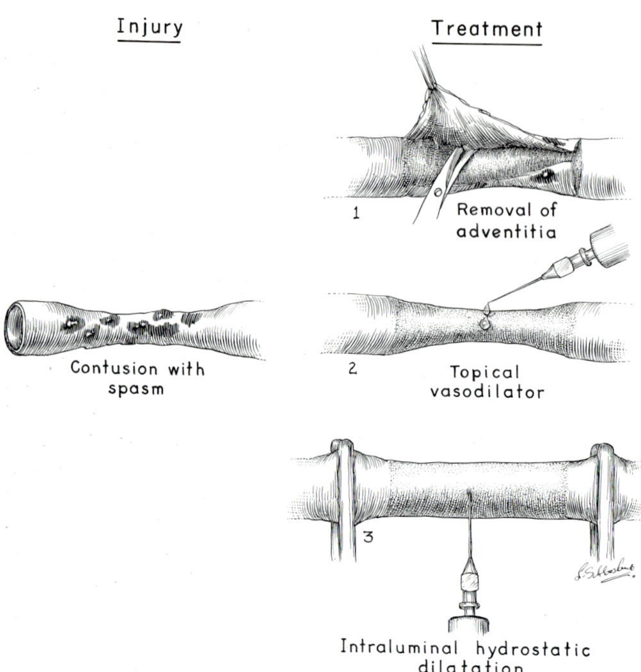

Figure 15–2 Local measures commonly used to relieve segmental arterial spasm.

of the segment or drawing an inflated balloon catheter through it. In the closed vessel, injection of saline into the lumen of the segment isolated between two vascular clamps may achieve the same effect. Although secondary diffuse spasm may respond to regional sympathetic block or intra-arterial injections of vasodilators, the segmental spasm more frequently encountered in arterial injuries appears to result from local, myogenic reflexes that are usually refractory to these latter measures. Finally, if all local measures fail to relieve segmental spasm, it is usually wiser to resect the involved segment and replace it with a vein graft. Careful examination of such segments will usually reveal evidences of more extensive intramural damage than suspected.

Another common mistake is to underestimate the *extent* of the injury to the arterial wall beyond the gross limits of the penetrating wound itself. This has proved particularly important in Vietnam, where high-velocity missile wounds are common. In such situations, histologic studies have shown microscopic damage for more than a centimeter beyond the limits of grossly visible injury. However, Rich[23] no longer recommends the arbitrary resection of two to three cm. margins, the policy which was initially suggested following these studies.

The method of reconstruction will depend on the extent of injury to the arterial wall. Figure 15–1 illustrates the usual repairs employed for the most common forms of arterial injury. Basically, they include reapproximation of cleanly incised wounds, wedge excision of small penetrating wounds with primary closure or saphenous vein patch graft, and segmental excision with reanastomosis or interposition of a hydrostatically dilated reversed segment of saphenous vein. The actual suture techniques have not changed greatly from the principles layed down by Carrel in 1907.[3] The adventitia should be cleared from the margins of repair. The suture should traverse the full thickness of the arterial wall; repeated inspection is necessary to insure inclusion of the intima. The size of the suture material, its pattern of placement and the choice of interrupted or continuous technique must be individualized. In general, finer interrupted technique is used in smaller arteries, and simple through-and-through sutures are preferred to everting mattress sutures. The newer synthetic suture materials are preferable to silk.

End-to-end anastomosis may be possible after mobilization of the proximal and distal ends of the artery, but suture line tension and narrowing must be carefully avoided. To this end, the use of autogenous vein for patch or circumferential grafting has been invaluable. The preference for an autogenous vein over a prosthetic graft is particularly valid for peripheral arteries and in the presence of gross contamination or significant tissue damage. An acceptable alternative to the saphenous vein and still preferable to the use of a prosthesis in this situation is provided by the cephalic or even the basilic veins in the arm. Any injury that is extensive enough to warrant the use of a graft is likely to be associated with injury to the accompanying vein or to require prolonged immobilization. To avoid an additional threat to the venous system in such an injured extremity, it is recommended that the saphenous vein graft be obtained from the uninvolved side wherever possible. Otherwise, the technique of saphenous vein grafting does not differ from that normally employed. The segment must be reversed to maintain normal orientation to flow. This is preferable to leaving it in its original orientation to the extremity and avulsing or excising its valves. Its lumen should be distended to physiologic pressures with saline, and, ideally, its distended diameter should be almost equal to or slightly exceed that of the artery it is to replace.

There are frequently other problems requiring attention, although the repair of the arterial injury usually takes precedence. One common exception to this involves the management of concomitant fractures, the stable reduction of which must be coordinated with the arterial repair. In such a circumstance, certain questions arise, the answers to which determine the sequence to be followed. How will reduction and stabilization best be achieved? How urgent is restoration of flow? Will subsequent reduction and stabilization of the fracture imperil the repaired artery or be interfered with by it? Will the final position of fixation cause tension on or kink the repaired vessel? Will skeletal shortening accompanying the reduction influence the length of the arterial segment of interposed graft to be anastomosed? Ordinarily, in civilian practice, the repair can follow reduction and fixation of the fracture and, in instances in which there is urgency to restore flow, a temporary internal shunt may be employed as suggested previously. The Vietnam experience has shown, however, that rigid adherence to this preferred sequence is not necessary and individualization should be allowed. In fact, the current trend is toward vascular repair first with *external* fixation being carefully applied at the end of the procedure to avoid introducing foreign material into the wound. In such cases, further support is provided by incorporating Steinman pins or Kirschner wires into the cast and immediately bivalving it to avoid constriction and allow frequent inspection.

Concomitant injuries to the accompanying nerves and veins are frequent, and their management in this setting bears comment. Distal motor and sensory function will have been assessed prior to operation, but the weakness and numbness that accompany ischemia may be misleading. Delayed repair of injuries to peripheral nerves is the usual rule in complicated, high-velocity or seriously contaminated wounds, but even in these situations, the operator can facilitate the subsequent repair by carefully assessing the appearance of the nerves at time of exploration and tagging their ends in line with the perineural vessels for future orientation. Although there is still considerable disagreement over immediate versus delayed (3 weeks to 3 months) repair, most now recommend concomitant nerve repair under less complicated circumstances than those described above, provided a surgeon experienced with these injuries is available. The decision to repair concomitant venous injuries will be dealt with later in this chapter, but in general is recommended.

Thorough irrigation and debridement of damaged muscles and other soft tissues should follow the principles outlined in the previous chapter. Skin coverage can normally be achieved by mobilization of surrounding skin, but if a flap is necessary, the defect it produces can be filled by a split thickness graft. It is undesirable to have a repaired artery covered only by skin, not only because it will be exposed if the skin closure breaks down, but because it will be more susceptible to trauma in the future. In addition, delayed skin closure may be dictated by the degree of contamination of the wound. This goal cannot always be easily achieved because of injury to surrounding muscle, but a muscle flap can usually be mobilized to cover the site of repair. In the femoral triangle, for example, the sartorius is usually available and can be used in the manner employed in radical groin dissections.

When there has been early and adequate repair of a discrete arterial injury, little more need be done to achieve excellent results. In other instances, ancillary measures bear consideration, particularly fasciotomy. The rationale for fasciotomy is that ischemia, particularly if associated with some degree of venous obstruction, will lead to swelling of muscles within the fascial compartments of the calf or forearm with eventual impairment of capillary flow to the muscles and, finally, necrosis and fibrosis. Although it has been debated that swelling alone cannot be responsible for this consequence (since the extravascular pressure it creates can hardly exceed the intravascular pressure that generates it), those who have seen the tense, pale muscle expand through fasciotomy incisions and become pink again feel that this argument is academic and cite venous gangrene of distended, obstructed gut and swollen pedicle flaps as a precedent.

Patman and Shires[20] have advocated fasciotomy under the following circumstances: undue delay, prolonged shock, extensive soft tissue damage, damage to venae comitantes and preoperative swelling of the limb. Their low amputation rate (3.8 per cent) has been partly attributed by them to the liberal use of these criteria. Theoretically, most vascular surgeons support the use of fasciotomy in most of these circumstances but, in practice, few employ it quite so liberally for "prophylactic" indications. The proponents of prophylactic fasciotomy argue that it can be carried out through small skin incisions with little additional time and risk and that it is only effective if carried out early, before irreversible changes in the muscle have taken place. The standard technique (Fig. 15–3) calls for three small vertical linear skin incisions in the mid-calf over each of the anterior, lateral and posterior muscle compartments through which the overlying fascia can be slit for most of its length by sliding the cutting edges of the partly opened scissors against the superior and inferior ends of the fascial defect. Skin closure may defeat the purpose of fasciotomy and may not even be possible without undue tension once the swollen muscle compartment expands. Some feel that the fasciotomy skin incision should be as long as the fascial incision, but most feel that should be done only if, after fascial incision, the skin can be seen to be providing a constricting effect. Finally, there has been increasing sentiment in favor of the more

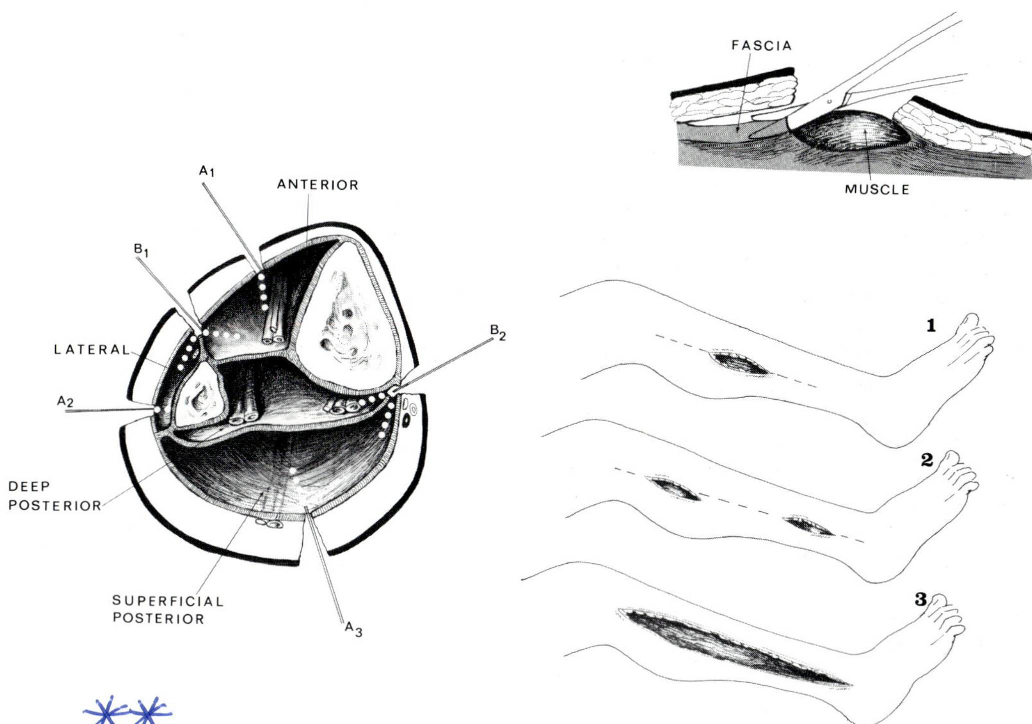

Figure 15–3 The "standard" fasciotomy approach involving three linear incisions (A_1, A_2 and A_3) through the outer fascia of the anterior, lateral and superficial posterior muscle compartments of the calf. This may be accomplished by one or two short skin incisions (1 and 2) through which the scissors may be passed and slid along the cut edge of the fascia (insert) or by a long incision (3) which may be loosely closed or left open for secondary closure or grafting. This approach does not decompress the deep posterior compartment. All four compartments can be opened through two incisions (B_1 and B_2) but full-length incisions (3) must be made.

radical fibulectomy-fasciotomy, as originally advocated by Kelly.[13] Its proponents claim that the standard fasciotomy does not decompress the important *deep* posterior muscle compartment and advocate removal of the middle three-fifths of the fibula through a single lateral incision which allows all four compartments to be decompressed (Fig. 15–4). Although removal of this portion of the fibula causes little or no functional disability, it leaves a major open wound to contend with. For this reason, most surgeons reserve this fibulectomy-fasciotomy for the more advanced situations and use the standard approach in early or prophylactic situations.

Sympathectomy is another adjuvant measure, but one of debatable effectiveness. Although the relief of arterial spasm is its usual justification, local rather than peripheral nervous factors appear to be more important in the spasm associated with direct arterial trauma,[14] and the local measures outlined previously seem to be more effective than sympathetic blockade. However, sympathectomy has been shown to acutely increase resting nutrient flow to muscle, skin and bone, particularly in the more distal part of the extremity.[24] This occurs even in the face of proximal arterial occlusion, but the flow increases are not as great as flowmeter studies would suggest since much of the increase in flow passes through opened arteriovenous shunts and does not nourish the tissues. Nevertheless, this non-nutrient flow may help in keeping grafts patent during the early days. Nonetheless, it

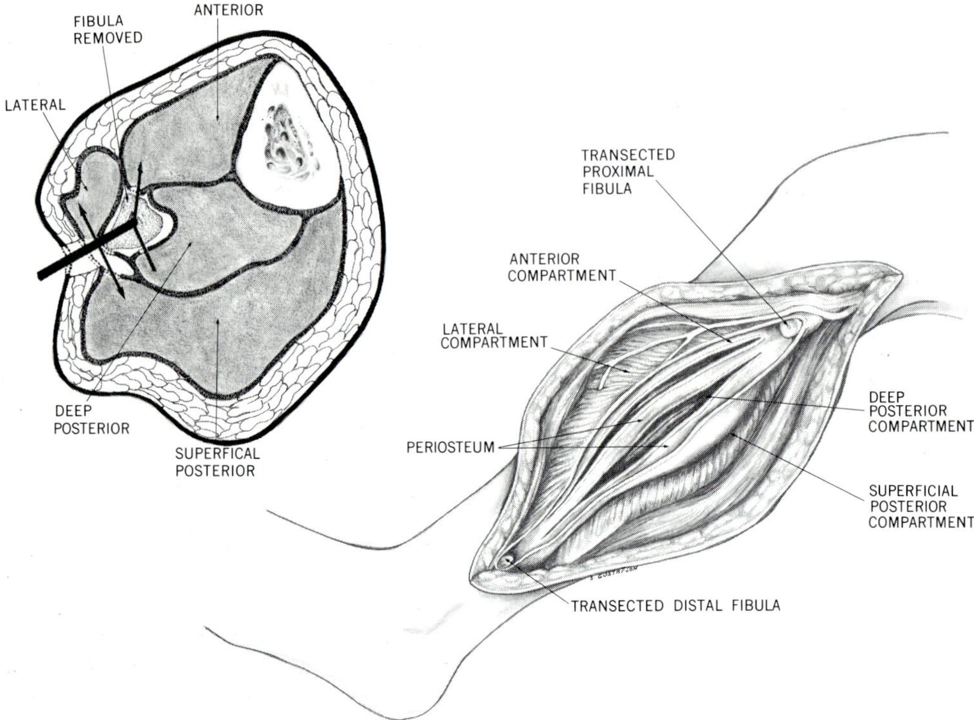

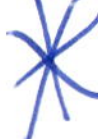

Figure 15–4 The "radical" fasciotomy or fibulectomy fasciotomy in which all four muscle compartments of the calf are exposed, incised and decompressed through the bed of a subperiosteal fibulectomy.

is the author's opinion that it will rarely spell the difference between success or failure in arterial injury repair, and obviously it will not cover up for technical inadequacies. During that short initial postoperative period where sympathetic denervation may be useful, intermittent lidocaine infusion through an indwelling epidural catheter can usually achieve this effect and avoid the necessity of adding an additional operative procedure.

The previously discussed, and other, measures are commonly resorted to when satisfactory return of circulation has not been achieved or when there is subsequent deteriorization from the level of circulation initially achieved by surgery. Before attributing this state of affairs to arterial spasm or compartmental swelling, technical failure at the site of repair must be ruled out by arteriography or re-exploration. The latter possibility is particularly likely whenever there is an abrupt deteriorization in the peripheral pulses, skin temperature or capillary filling. This underscores the importance of frequent monitoring of the state of the circulation of the injured limb in the early postoperative period. Routine intraoperative arteriography after the reconstruction has been completed and before closure will do much to uncover these problems before they become manifest, and provides welcome assurance to the surgeon during those early hand-wringing hours that nothing important has been overlooked in providing the best possible chance for restoration of limb viability and function.

VENOUS INJURIES

Venous injuries of significance may be isolated but more commonly occur in association with injury to the accompanying artery. They will be discovered if sought at the time of arterial exploration, but even a major deep venous occlusion will frequently be missed if it is an independent injury. It should be suspected whenever early swelling or cyanosis occurs distal to the injury.

Simple, clean lacerations of major veins should be repaired primarily after removal of secondary thrombus formation. Repair of more extensive injury rarely results in permanent patency and is more likely to lead to thromboembolic complications. However, in the Vietnam experience, where repair of the concomitant venous injury has been accomplished in approximately one-third of the cases, the threat of pulmonary embolism did not become manifest. Even though it is realized that eventual thrombosis of the venous repair is likely to occur in the majority of cases, repair of major venous injuries is currently being advised because it is felt that the success of the arterial repair is jeopardized when major venous outflow obstruction exists, and if this can be avoided by even a few days of patency of the venous reconstruction, it will be worthwhile. Fortunately, the situation in which the injury is severe enough to involve the major venous collaterals and dictate repair of the major vein also favors the patency of the repair because of the high rate of obligatory flow which must pass through the anastomosis. If the vein is not the major portal of venous return or is too badly damaged to repair, double ligation is recommended with the proximal ligature placed just distal to the next large tributary whenever feasible. Significant disability following such ligation is usually temporary if a careful postoperative regimen, similar to that employed following thrombophlebitis, is adhered to and additional venous thrombosis avoided. However, unlike the postphlebitic limb in which recanulization with valvular incompetence occurs and leads to permanent disability, elastic support and intermittent elevation may not be necessary indefinitely following uncomplicated ligation, and the tendency to dependent edema often subsides with the development of adequate collateral tributaries.

Amputation

Amputation may be indicated from the outset if the damage to the tissues of the extremity, and particularly the nerves, is so extensive that successful vascular repair and reconstruction of the remaining structures would not provide a useful appendage. In marginal cases, this decision requires experienced judgment and, unless the situation is clearly hopeless, it is better to proceed with reconstruction. Amputation may be necessary later on if the arterial reconstruction fails and the causes of this failure cannot be overcome. Unless the threat of systemic toxic effects from crushed, infected or gangrenous tissues becomes manifest, delayed amputation is preferred if for no other reason than that its unquestionable need will become clearly apparent to and better accepted by the patient. Even in this situation, the so-called "debridement amputation" has great merit as a preliminary procedure to control infection and allow the definitive amputation to be carried out with a higher degree of success in primary healing. Furthermore, the additional time allows for the development of collateral circulation and potentially a lower level of amputation. Immediate fitting of prostheses is important in the elderly to avoid unretrievable loss of walking skills and in the young for morale purposes. The details of definitive amputations are beyond the scope of this chapter.

LATE SEQUELAE AND RESULTS

The results of failure to achieve adequate arterial repair have already been mentioned. The degree of success achieved may not be apparent until the adequacy of circulation has been tested by normal use. Even then, the late results of arterial repair, particularly when grafts are used, may be hard to document and evaluate since these procedures are ordinarily performed for occlusive arterial disease of later life. Whether the repaired vessels of younger patients will be the site of predilection for arteriosclerosis and other degenerative changes will only be answered in time, but these considerations do not invalidate the procedures presently employed.

The most common late sequelae of arterial injury are false aneurysms and arteriovenous fistulas. The impression that these are delayed complications of arterial injuries is probably not justified. Rather it is their recognition that is delayed, a carry-over from the time when wounds not presenting an immediate threat to limb survival were not explored. Early exploration and definitive treatment of suspected arterial injuries, as practiced in the past 15 years, should continue to reduce the incidence of these sequelae.

The early recognition of an arteriovenous fistula usually depends upon the auscultation of a bruit in the region of a recent penetrating wound. Later, attention may be attracted by symptoms of decreased arterial circulation distal to the fistula, increased venous collaterals and, eventually, even varicosities in the vicinity of the fistula or, finally (in large, proximal fistulas), the signs and symptoms of high-output cardiac failure. The hemodynamic alterations associated with arteriovenous fistulas and their therapeutic implications have been thoroughly documented by the work of Holman[10] and Elkin.[8]

In general, an arteriovenous fistula should either be attacked early when it is little more than a poorly organized communicating hematoma and before major venous collaterals have had time to develop, or operated on six weeks to three months later when the acute inflammatory reaction has subsided. When done within the first day or two, fistulas are technically not much more difficult than any other acute arterial injury. The procedure of choice is repair of both artery and vein or at least repair of the artery and double ligation of the vein. If for some reason both artery and vein have to be sacrificed, the rationale for quadruple ligation (artery and vein proximal and distal to the fistula) as well worked out by Holman,[10] should be heeded.

Traumatic false aneurysms are usually allowed to develop because the possible significance of an innocuous-appearing wound over the course of a major artery is not considered. One should be particularly suspicious of excessive bleeding or hematoma formation following such wounds. The expansile or pulsatile nature of such hematomata may not be apparent until later. The same preference for very early or delayed operation that has been expressed in regard to arteriovenous fistulas applies to false aneurysm. At the time of operation, proximal and distal control of the involved vessel is necessary before approaching the aneurysm itself. It is frequently necessary to use a partial or circumferential graft to repair the vessel after excision of the aneurysm, although success has been reported in the use of endaneurysmorrhaphy, in which the communication is closed through the opened aneurysmal sac.

REFERENCES

1. Amato, J. J., Rich, Norman M., Billy, Lawrence J., Grubner, Ronald P., and Lawson, Noel S.: High-velocity arterial injury. J. Trauma *11*:412, 1971.
2. Brisbin, R. L., Geib, P. O., and Eiseman, B.: Secondary disruption of vascular repair following war wounds. Arch. Surg. *120*:522, 1970.
3. Carrel, A.: The surgery of blood vessels. Johns Hopkins Bull., *18*:18, 1907.

4. Carrel, A.: Heterotransplantation of blood vessels preserved in cold storage. J. Exp. Med. *9*:226, 1907.
5. DeBakey, M. E., and Simeone, F. A.: Battle injuries of the arteries in World War II. Ann. Surg. *123*:534, 1946.
6. Edwards, W. S., and Lyons, C.: Traumatic arterial spasm and thrombosis. Ann. Surg. *140*:318, 1954.
7. Eger, M., Gokman, L., Goldstein, A., and Hirsch, M.: The use of a temporary shunt in the management of arterial vascular injuries. Surg. Gynec. Obstet. *13*:67, 1971.
8. Elkin, D. C.: The treatment of aneurysms and arteriovenous fistulas. Bull. N. Y. Acad. Med. *22*:81, 1946.
9. Guthrie, G. C.: Heterotransplantation of blood vessels. Am. J. Physiol. *19*:482, 1907.
10. Holman, E.: Arteriovenous aneurysm. Abnormal Communications Between the Arterial and Venous Circulations. New York, The MacMillan Co., 1937.
11. Hughes, C. W.: Arterial repair during the Korean War. Ann. Surg. *147*:555, 1958.
12. Jahnke, E. J., Jr., and Seeley, S. F.: Acute vascular injuries in the Korean War: An analysis of 77 consecutive cases. Ann. Surg. *138*:158, 1953.
13. Kelley, R. P., and Whitesides, T. E., Jr.: Transfibular route for fasciotomy of the leg. J. Bone Joint Surg. *50B*:482, 1968.
14. Kinmouth, J. B.: The physiology and relief of traumatic arterial spasm. Brit. Med. J. *47*:59, 1952.
15. Lavenson, G. S., Rich, N. M., and Baugh, J. H.: Value of ultrasonic flow detector in the management of peripheral vascular disease. Am. J. Surg. *120*:522, 1970.
16. Makin, G. S., Howard, J. M., and Green, R. L.: Arterial injuries complicating fractures or dislocations: The necessity for a more aggressive approach. Surgery *59*:203, 1966.
17. Makins, G. W.: Gunshot Injuries to the Blood Vessels. Bristol, England, John Wright & Sons, Ltd., 1919.
18. Malan, E., and Tattoni, G.: Physio- and anato-pathology of acute ischemia of the extremities. J. Cardiovasc. Surg. *4*:2, 1963.
19. Nolan, B.: Vascular injuries. J. Royal Coll. Surg. *13*:72, 1968.
20. Patman, R. D., Poulos, E., and Shires, G. T.: The management of civilian arterial injuries. Surg. Gynec. Obstet. *118*:725, 1964.
21. Perry, M. O., Thal, E. R., and Shires, G. T.: Management of arterial injuries. Ann. Surg. *173*:403, 1971.
22. Rich, N. R., et al.: Popliteal artery injuries in Vietnam. Am. J. Surg. *118*:531, 1969.
23. Rich, N. R.: Vascular trauma in Vietnam. J. Cardiovasc. Surg., *11*:368, 1970.
24. Rutherford, R. B., and Valenta, J.: Extremity blood flow and distribution. The effects of arterial occlusion, Sympathectomy and Exercise. Surgery *69*:332, 1971.
25. Shires, G. T., and Patman, R. D.: Vascular injuries in the care of the trauma patient. New York, McGraw-Hill Book Co., Inc., 1966.
26. Schumacker, H. B., Jr.: Arterial suture techniques and grafts: Past, present and future. Surgery *66*:419, 1969.
27. Sinkler, W. H., and Spencer, A. D.: The value of peripheral arteriography in assessing acute vascular injuries. Arch. Surg. *80*:300, 1960.

chapter

16

INJURIES OF THE HAND

Raymond M. Curtis, M.D., John E. Hoopes, M.D., and Michael E. Jabaley, M.D.

The strength and flexibility of the human hand are unequaled by any other part of the human body. The hand is also an organ of expression, exposing the secrets of the heart and soul. This fact, coupled with concern regarding economic loss and inability to contribute to society, readily explains the psychological disturbances associated with crippling hand injuries.

Dr. Sterling Bunnell's[14] dictum that the *early* treatment of the acutely injured hand determines whether the hand is "doomed to disability" or "will regain usable function" cannot be emphasized sufficiently.

BASIC PRINCIPLES

A procedure of management so formalized that it may be followed by the emergency treatment room nurse as well as the intern, resident or staff doctor should be available in the emergency department of every hospital. The following is suggested as an optimal routine.

History. Information pertinent to the injury must be as detailed as possible. Specific attention should be paid to the time of occurrence, the mechanism of injury and the position of the hand when injured. The degree of contamination should be determined as well as the nature of first-aid administered.

Assessment of the Injury. Evaluation of total hand function is imperative. The examination must include a careful search for vascular injury, evaluation of flexor and extensor tendon function (Figs. 16–1, 16–2 and 16–3), an appraisal of sensation (Fig. 16–4), an assessment of all the small muscle functions of the hand (Figs. 16–5 and 16–6) and a roentgenogram if bone injury is suspected.

Initial Wound Management. The wound is covered with a small sterile gauze dressing, following which the injured extremity is shaved properly and cleansed thoroughly with soap and water. This cleansing must be done carefully so that none of the solution enters the wound. The wound is irrigated with copious quantities of nor-

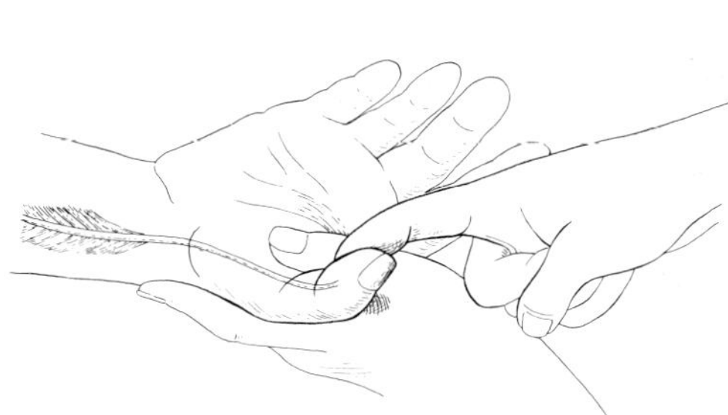

Figure 16–1 Illustrates testing for the function of the flexor pollicis longus to the terminal phalanx of the thumb.

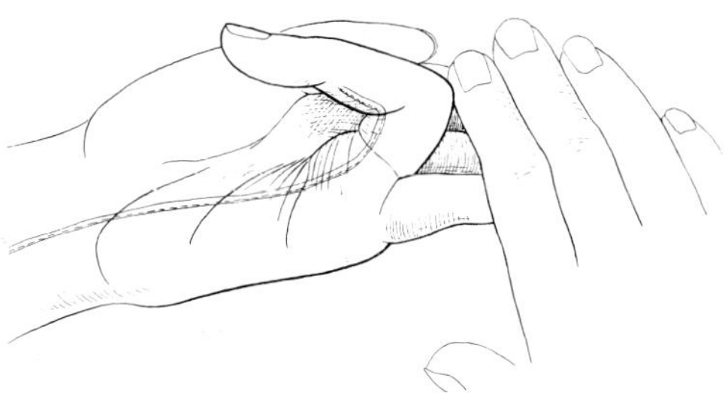

Figure 16–2 Illustrates testing for the function of the flexor superficialis in ring finger by blocking the action of the flexor profundus tendon by holding the middle and ring fingers in extension.

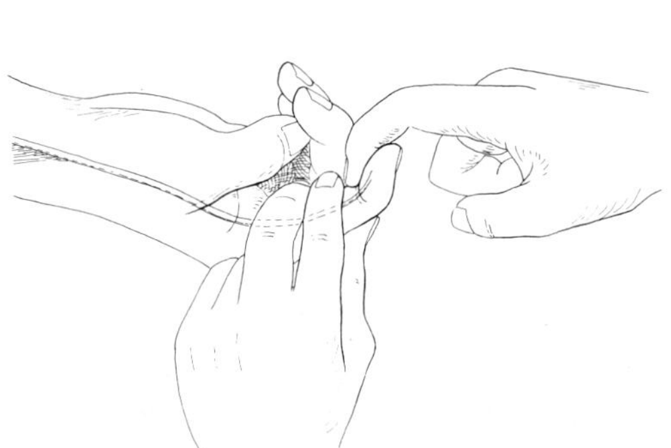

Figure 16–3 Illustrates method of holding finger to block flexion of the proximal interphalangeal joint so as to test for flexor profundus function in the terminal phalanx.

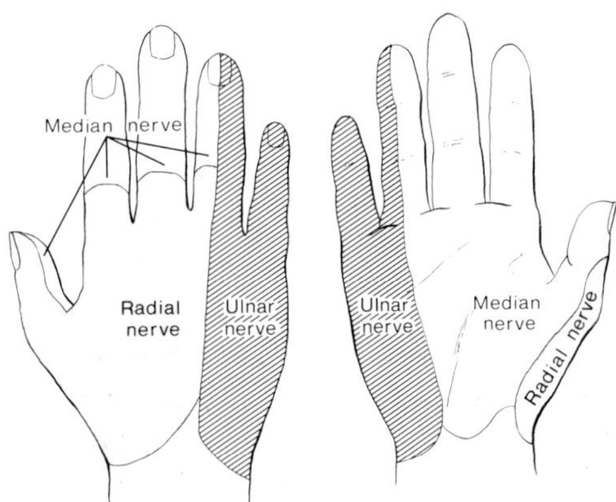

Figure 16–4 Diagram illustrates sensory distribution of median, ulnar and radial nerves to hand.

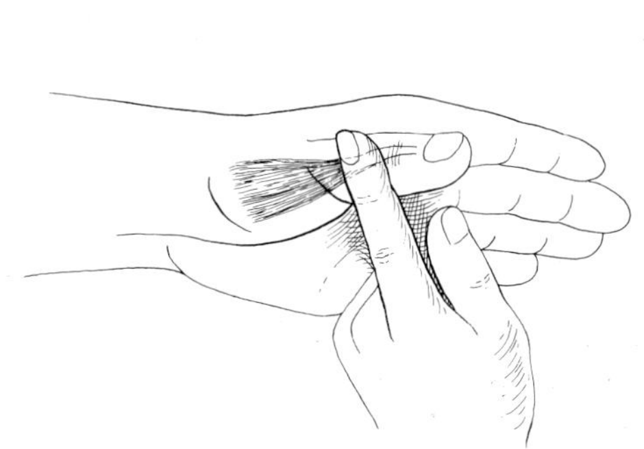

Figure 16–5 Diagram illustrates method of testing for function of the short abductor muscle of the thumb which is innervated by the median nerve.

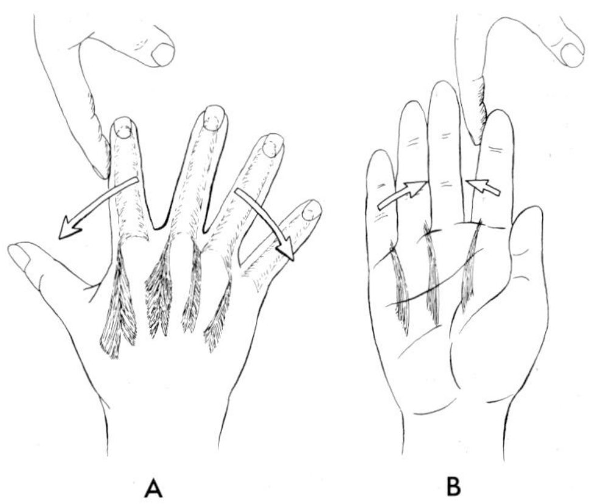

Figure 16–6 Diagrams illustrate method of testing for function of the dorsal interossei (*A*) and the palmar interossei (*B*) which are innervated by the ulnar nerve.

mal saline solution or, preferably, a buffered electrolyte such as Tis-u-sol,* since experimental work has demonstrated that normal saline solution alters wound pH. Following completion of irrigation, the wound is again covered with a sterile dressing; and the hand and forearm are prepared with an antiseptic solution and placed on a sterile arm board for examination.

Definitive Treatment. Suturing of hand lacerations in the accident room is permissible only if the examiner can be certain that there has been no tendon or nerve damage. The repair of injury to deep structures demands the following conditions:

1. A well-equipped operating room.
2. Adequate hand instruments.
3. A sufficient number of assistants.
4. Complete anesthesia.
5. A realization of the importance of the procedure.
6. A bloodless operating field provided by a pneumatic tourniquet.
7. Meticulous atraumatic surgical technique.

It is both impossible and dangerous to explore a hand and perform the necessary repair without the aid of a bloodless operative field provided by a tourniquet. Even in those instances in which suturing of a minor laceration is accomplished under local anesthesia in the accident room, the patient will tolerate a tourniquet for 25 to 30 minutes. The bloodless field allows visualization of the depth of the wound, and injuries not suspected clinically may be detected.

General anesthesia is employed uniformly when there are no contraindications so that unlimited operative time with complete tolerance of the tourniquet is provided. Other forms of anesthesia may be used for less severe injuries.

LOCAL ANESTHESIA. Lidocaine (Xylocaine), 1 per cent, locally infiltrated into the wound is useful for small lacerations. Epinephrine must not be used with the local anesthetic for fear of producing digital gangrene secondary to vasoconstriction. Adequate preoperative sedation of the patient and supplementation with intravenous Demerol, if necessary, greatly facilitate the use of local and nerve block anesthesia.

NERVE BLOCK ANESTHESIA. Block of the median nerve at the wrist, the ulnar nerve at the elbow and the radial sensory nerve in the distal third of the forearm can be used for local procedures on the hand. The patient will not tolerate a tourniquet for more than 30 to 45 minutes.

AXILLARY BLOCK ANESTHESIA. It is well to supplement the axillary block with local infiltration of lidocaine in a circular fashion about the upper arm in order to increase tourniquet tolerance time.

BRACHIAL PLEXUS BLOCK ANESTHESIA. Brachial plexus block with lidocaine, 2 per cent, with epinephrine 1:100,000, provides excellent anesthesia for hand surgery. It is particularly valuable for a patient who is not a suitable candidate for general anesthesia because of the recent intake of food.

The special arm board, the use of which was first described by Boyes[4] (Fig. 16–7), allows the operator to sit in the oval area and rest his elbows on the table for much of this work. This is of particular value for the more meticulous type of work and eliminates much of the fatigue associated with this fine surgery. A sphygmomanometer cuff of the wrap-around type is placed over a layer of glazed cotton applied to the arm, and a layer of gauze bandage is applied over the cuff to prevent ballooning on inflation. Some of the newer types of pneumatic cuffs are easier to use as arm tourniquets. Elevation of the arm

*Travenol Laboratories, Inc. Morton Grove, Illinois.

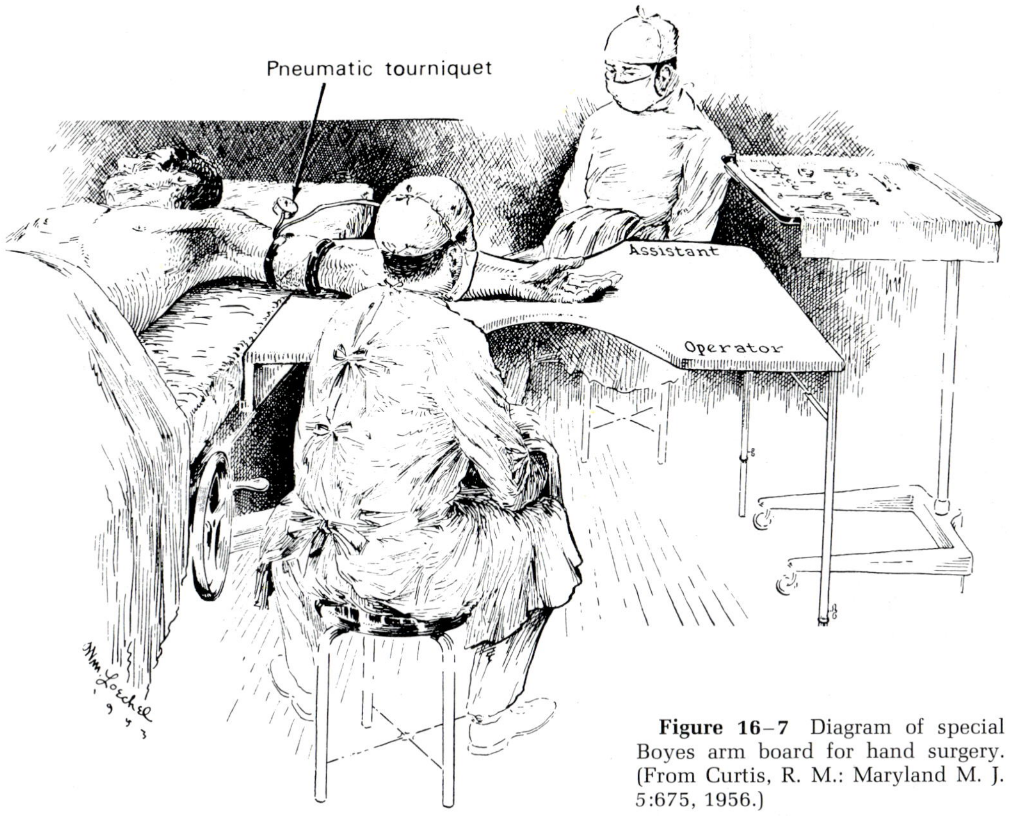

Figure 16–7 Diagram of special Boyes arm board for hand surgery. (From Curtis, R. M.: Maryland M. J. 5:675, 1956.)

for five minutes followed by inflation of the cuff will prevent bleeding during preparation of the extremity with antiseptic solution. Following the application of sterile drapes, the tourniquet is released, the extremity is wrapped firmly with a sterile Ace bandage from the fingertips to within one inch of the tourniquet to completely empty the extremity of blood, and the tourniquet is reinflated. A pressure of 300 mm. of mercury is utilized in adults. Children under 12 years of age require 260 mm. pressure; 150 mm. pressure provides adequate ischemia in infants.

The tourniquet may remain inflated for one and a half hours. If the operation has not been completed at the end of this period of time, a light pressure dressing is applied to the wound and the tourniquet is released for 15 minutes. The tourniquet is reinflated after the arm has once more been wrapped with an elastic bandage. If the wound is infected, the extremity is emptied of blood by means of elevation rather than utilizing an elastic bandage.

In many civilian hospitals a busy operative schedule may impose a delay of several hours in the definitive treatment of an acute hand injury. In these circumstances, a sterile dressing is applied to the forearm and hand after initial wound management in the accident room, and this dressing remains in place until the patient reaches the operating room. Administration of antibiotics is initiated preoperatively.

SKIN

The provision of adequate soft tissue coverage will determine, in many instances, the final result achieved in the management of a serious hand injury.

Primary closure can be secured at the time of initial management in the majority of acute injuries by strict observation of the surgical principles of thorough wound cleansing and debridement and by careful selection of the method of closure best suited to the situation. Delayed primary closure[1] is preferred for wounds which are severely contused, heavily contaminated, or which present for treatment after an unduly long interval following injury. Such wounds are thoroughly cleansed, surgically debrided and irrigated with copious quantities of a buffered electrolyte solution. The hand is dressed with a single layer of fine mesh gauze, padding, and a plaster splint and elevated continuously until the patient is returned to the operating room for wound closure. This should ordinarily be accomplished in 3 to 5 days in order to avoid the development of granulation tissue and excessive deep scar, and to permit active and passive motion of the joints and tendons.

There is no excess tissue on the hand. For this reason, closure of areas of skin loss simply by undermining and suturing the wound margins is doomed to failure. Tissue of questionable viability is far better excised primarily than allowed to become necrotic and secondarily infected. Accurate determination of viability is a decision of major importance. Observation of the return of circulation to the questionable tissue following release of the tourniquet can be of considerable value in making this judgment. Circulation within the skin margin may be assessed by small incisions into the dermis after the tourniquet has been deflated for 10 to 15 minutes.

Simultaneous repair of deep structures and provision for adequate soft tissue coverage comprise optimal management. It must be emphasized that the type of skin coverage provided is determined by the specific wound situation. The following plastic procedures are useful in providing the necessary coverage:

1. Partial thickness skin graft.
2. Full thickness skin graft.
3. Local pedicle flap.
4. Distant pedicle flap.

Partial Thickness Skin Graft

Utilization of a partial thickness skin graft is determined by the characteristics of the bed on which the graft is to be placed. In general, exposed tendons and compound fractures require pedicle flap coverage. An excellent clinical result can be obtained with a partial thickness graft if the paratenon and epitenon overlying the extensor tendons are intact (Fig. 16–8). A partial thickness skin graft may provide suitable coverage for the palm if the flexor tendons are within their sheaths. Pedicle flap

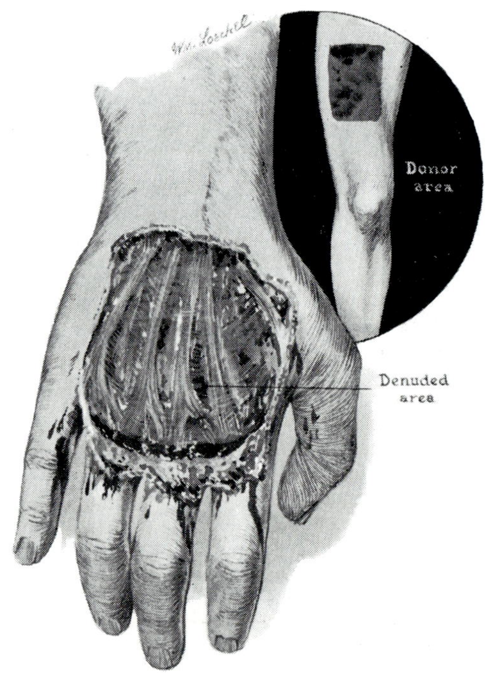

Figure 16–8 Drawing illustrates extensive avulsion of dorsum of hand and use of thigh as donor area for dermatome skin graft. (From Curtis, R. M.: Maryland M. J. 5:675, 1956.)

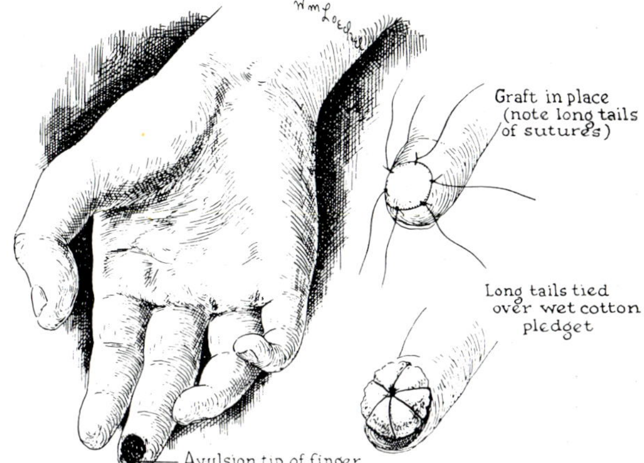

Figure 16–9 Drawing shows use of the split thickness skin graft for coverage of minor avulsions at the tip of the finger. (From Curtis, R. M.: Maryland M. J. 5:675, 1956.)

coverage is required if the tendon sheaths have been denuded and the flexor tendons lie exposed in the wound. The partial thickness graft is useful for the coverage of minor fingertip avulsions in which a good bed of subcutaneous tissue remains (Fig. 16–9). An alternative method for securing grafts employs steri-strips instead of sutures and allows the graft to conform better to the convex surface of the fingertip. Contraction of the graft with time will advance the normal skin of the finger distally so that at the end of one year there will be little evidence of the original injury and good sensation will be present over the tip of the finger.

In specific instances, the partial thickness graft may be utilized to secure early temporary wound closure with the realization that pedicle flap replacement of the skin graft at a later date will be necessary to allow further reconstructive procedures. The approach is particularly suitable for battle casualties.

A thick graft, approximately 0.018 in., provides good permanent skin coverage. The graft is obtained with the Reese Dermatome. Perfect hemostasis, adequate pressure and strict immobilization are essential for a proper "take" of the graft. One should select a donor site which is hidden or leaves a cosmetically acceptable scar. This is especially true in female patients and pigmented races.

Full Thickness Skin Graft

Full thickness grafts are valuable for the repair of small defects, particularly in those instances in which it is important that there be no subsequent shrinkage of the graft (Fig. 16–10). Full thickness grafts are preferred by some for fingertip avulsion.

The antecubital fossa and the flexion crease of the wrist are preferred donor areas since closure of the defect is accomplished more easily than in the central, volar aspect of the forearm. A perfect pattern of the defect should be outlined on the donor area of the full thickness graft to ensure suturing the graft into position with no more than normal skin tension (Fig. 16–10). All subcutaneous fat is removed from the graft either at the time of excision or by stretching the graft over the operator's finger and trimming away the fat with fine scissors. Full thickness grafts demand meticulous attention to every detail if survival is to be achieved. A partial thickness graft is preferred if there exists any question regarding the suitability of the recipient area.

The skin avulsed by a severe injury may occasionally be defatted and

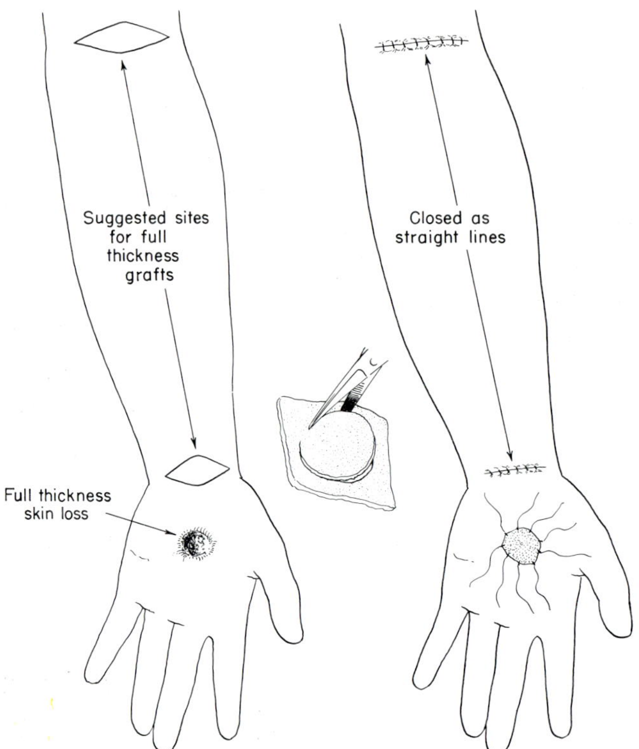

Figure 16–10 Drawing illustrates the use of the full thickness skin graft for replacement of skin loss. Note how sutures are left long to be tied over pressure dressing on graft and how graft is patterned to fit the defect perfectly.

replaced as a full thickness graft. Severely contused skin is not suitable for this purpose.

Pedicle Flaps

Blood-bearing skin and subcutaneous tissue often are needed to provide cover for exposed tendon and bone. The surgeon dealing with acute hand injuries must be in a position to apply such coverage at the time of primary treatment or soon thereafter.

Local Flaps. ROTATION FLAP. A local rotation flap is particularly suitable for wounds on the dorsum of the hand and can be raised from the dorsal or lateral aspects of the fingers as well. Skin flaps are difficult to rotate on the palm because of the fascial attachments to the underlying structures.

CROSS-FINGER FLAP. The cross-finger flap is indicated in the management of fingertip injuries in which the loss of both skin and subcutaneous tissue exposes tendon and bone. A satisfactory result cannot be expected with a partial thickness skin graft applied over a denuded flexor tendon. The cross-finger flap is of particular value for surfacing defects on the flexor surface of the finger and the fingertip.

Utilization of pedicle flap tissue from an adjacent finger offers many advantages: Vascular complications within the flap are unusual because of the abundant circulation. Only two adjacent fingers need be immobilized, and the flap can be divided safely under local anesthesia 10 to 14 days postoperatively. The functional and cosmetic result is superior, and the recovery of sensation is frequently faster than with other methods. The major disadvantage consists of imposing scarring and possible stiffness on a normal finger.

The cross-finger flap may be based distally, proximally or laterally depending upon how it can best be rotated to fill the defect (Fig. 16–11).

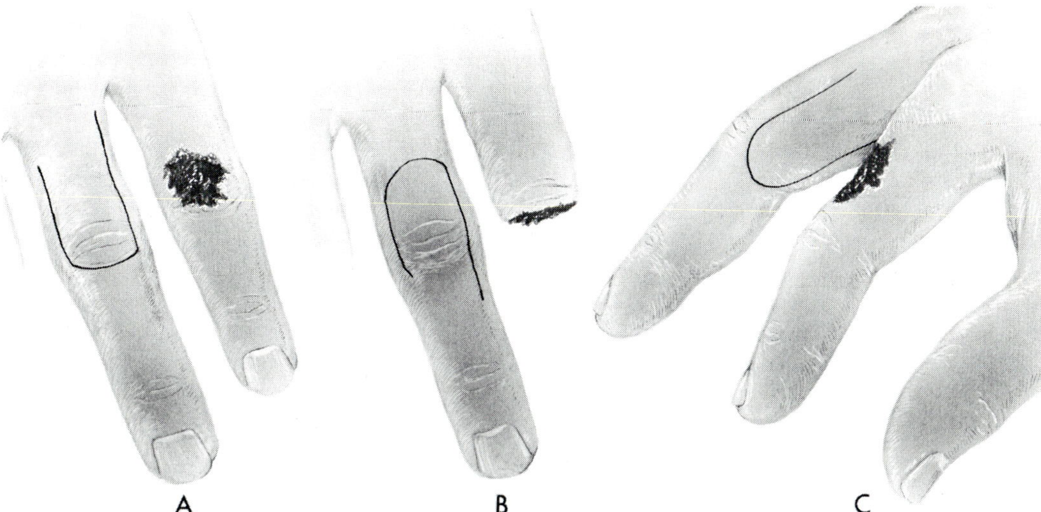

Figure 16–11 Diagram illustrates fact that pedicle flap may be based distally, proximally or laterally. (From Curtis, R. M.: Maryland M. J. 5:675, 1956.)

The flap should always be designed larger than the defect. The incision for creation of the laterally based flap should be carried to the midlateral position to minimize the danger of residual scarring and stiffness (Fig. 16–12). As the dissection reaches the lateral margin of the finger, it is necessary to separate a layer of oblique fascia (Cleland's ligament) joining the skin on the lateral aspect of the finger to the extensor mechanism and phalangeal periosteum. Release of these fascial bands adds approximately 0.25 in. to the length of the flap (Fig. 16–13). The flap is handled with meticulous atraumatic technique and sutured with fine nylon. The donor area is covered with a partial thickness graft 0.015 to 0.018 in. in thickness. Care is taken to line the raw area of the pedicle flap completely with the

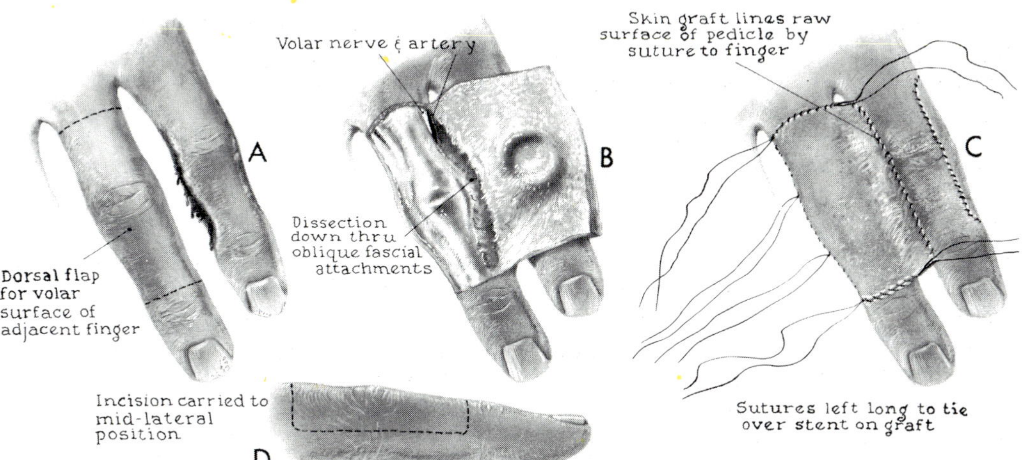

Figure 16–12 Technique of preparation of cross-finger pedicle flap for large volar defect and partial thickness graft to donor area. (From Curtis, R. M.: Ann. Surg. *145*:650, 1957.)

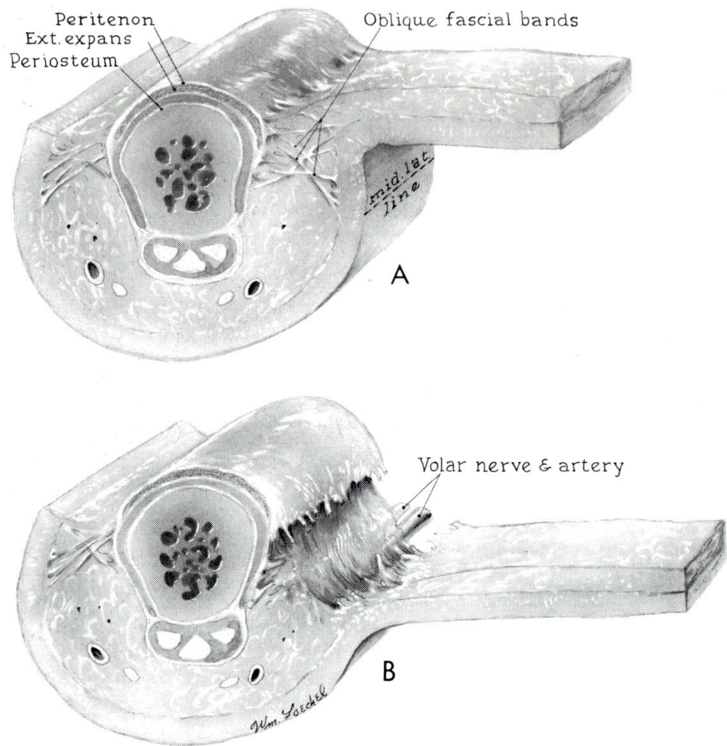

Figure 16–13 *A*, Cross section of finger through proximal phalanx, showing oblique fascial bands which fit skin to extensor tendon mechanisms and periosteum of phalanges. *B*, Release of skin obtained by dividing the oblique fascial fibers. (From Curtis, R. M.: Ann. Surg. *145*:650, 1957.)

skin graft (Fig. 16–12). A stent dressing is tied over the graft, and wet cotton is packed lightly between the two fingers. Care is taken not to jeopardize the circulation of the flap. The pedicle is divided in 10 to 14 days, and the margin of the pedicle on the donor finger is trimmed to lie in the midlateral position.

Cross-finger flaps may be required in late reconstructive procedures. Resurfacing of the volar aspect of a finger may be necessary prior to tendon grafting, and this is best accomplished with a cross-finger flap. In dealing with a severe flexion contracture requiring tenolysis, excision of tendon sheath and volar capsulectomy, the best results are obtained by Kirschner wire immobilization of the finger in moderate extension and immediate application of a cross-finger flap, if inadequate skin and subcutaneous tissue exist.

THENAR FLAP. The thenar flap[2] is of value in severe avulsions or amputations of the fingertips. The flap is elevated well posterior from the thenar area to avoid hyperflexion of the proximal interphalangeal joint; considerable care must be taken in resurfacing the donor site to prevent persistent discomfort in the resultant scar. Permanent stiffness of the proximal interphalangeal joint may follow immobilization of longer than 10 to 14 days, especially in older patients.

Distant Flaps. ABDOMINAL FLAP. An abdominal pedicle flap, elevated and sutured to the defect primarily, frequently is the procedure of choice for coverage of a large defect of the hand or forearm (Fig. 16–14). Complex and severely contaminated wounds are managed best by either immediate or delayed partial thickness grafting or delayed application of a pedicle flap.

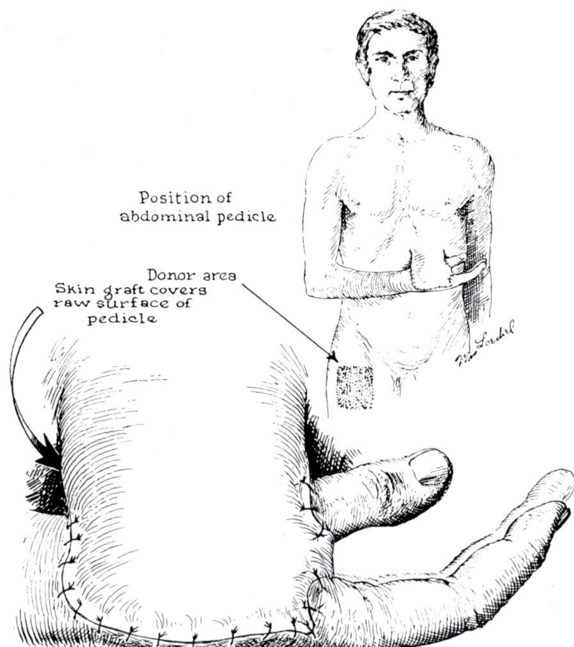

Figure 16–14 Drawing illustrates use of abdominal pedicle flap for coverage of extensive defect of wrist and hand. Note that abdominal donor site is covered primarily with dermatome skin graft. This graft also lines the raw surface of the pedicle. (From Curtis, R. M.: Maryland M. J. 5:675, 1956.)

Preparation of the flap is of utmost importance. The base should be broad and flaring, and the length-to-width ratio should not exceed two to one. The flap may be based above or below the umbilicus; those above the umbilicus are pedicled superiorly, and those below are pedicled inferiorly. Flaps, particularly if tubed, are raised in a plane parallel to the rib over the anterolateral aspect of the chest and abdomen, since thoracic vessels descend slightly obliquely. The flap should be precisely designed[2] by a pattern of the wound and elevated at a level to include a minimum amount of fat. This technique reduces the amount of "parasitic fat" which detracts from the blood supply and frequently avoids subsequent defatting procedures. A flap delay procedure may be utilized if a healed wound is being resurfaced; the flap is outlined as described, incised to the appropriate level and then the wound edges resutured. The flap is elevated and transferred to the defect two weeks later. Abdominal flaps may be partially defatted, if necessary, at the time of application. An open pedicle flap is never used on the hand because of the inevitable secondary infection and excessive scarring at the attachment of the pedicle. All pedicles are closed either by grafting of the raw surface or by tubing the base of the pedicle.

CROSS-ARM FLAP. The cross-arm flap is limited in the amount of tissue available but offers the advantage of being less bulky than an abdominal flap. The decision to employ a cross-arm flap, as opposed to an abdominal or infraclavicular flap, is based on its suitability in terms of thickness and availability.

TENDONS

Principles of Tendon Repair

The achievement of satisfactory results following tendon repair is dependent upon an understanding of the physiology of tendon healing. The experimental work of Skoog and Persson,[45] Potenza,[40] and others has demonstrated the peritenon to be the main source of the vascular bud which grows into the area of tendon injury.

Potenza[40] found in an experimental study of the healing process in the canine flexor digital tendons that the vascular bud was the source of fibroblasts from which collagen bundles develop. Fibroblastic activity was demonstrable within ten days postinjury. Initially, the collagen fibers are oriented in a plane perpendicular to the long axis of the tendon; they are realigned in the direction of the tendon fibers by approximately the 112th day[40].

Tensile strength studies indicate the anastomosis to be weakest on the third day following repair, coincident with maximal edema of the tendon ends. The degree of healing at the anastomosis will allow some active motion at three weeks, but it may be six weeks before the tendon can be considered strong.

Tendon repair demands sharp and meticulous dissection with a minimum of surgical trauma. The following principles of strictly atraumatic technique must be observed:

1. The tendon is handled when possible with the wet, gloved finger.
2. Traumatized tendon ends are removed sharply.
3. Stainless steel suture material on atraumatic needles is used.
4. The operative field is kept moist by frequent irrigation with a buffered electrolyte solution.
5. Sharp dissection is utilized exclusively; identification of dissection planes is enhanced by using a two- to three-power magnifying loupe.
6. Blood supply is preserved, and hematoma is prevented.

The tendon anastomosis should be placed in tissue that has not been traumatized by the original injury or surgery. Severe, crushing or mangling injuries may contraindicate primary tendon repair. All scar must be removed at the time of secondary repair in order that the tendon anastomosis will lie in good tissue.

The character of the wound, the mechanism of injury, the degree of contamination and the elapsed time between injury and definitive treatment determine whether primary or delayed tendon repair is performed. A maximum elapsed time limit of six hours, during which definitive treatment may be undertaken, is generally satisfactory. The time limit may be extended slightly when dealing with sharply incised wounds which have been cleansed and dressed within one hour of injury. When these requirements cannot be met, it is better judgment to defer tendon repair for two to four days. In crushing or mangling injuries in which there has been gross contamination, the tendon repair may be deferred for four to six weeks or until the wound is soft and pliable. Boyes[4] has stated: "It is difficult to prove that primary repair is superior to that done later, all other factors being equal. Unless the wound can be treated, unless healing can be obtained by primary intention, reactionless in type, the tendon and nerve repair probably should be delayed. We must approach the fundamental problem by graded steps and stages."

Suture materials should be inert, as fine as possible and swaged on atraumatic needles—stainless steel is preferred, but other synthetics, such as dacron (mersilene), are also employed. 5–0 size is used in the flexor tendon and 4–0 is used with the pull-out wire technique. The tendon being sutured should not be handled with forceps but rather with the moistened, gloved hand or with a transfixion needle. Utilizing the method of Bunnell, the tendon end that is held with clamp or forceps is trimmed away after the suture is inserted. Potenza[40] emphasizes that an adhesion is produced at each point of trauma. The Bunnell figure-of-eight buried suture (Fig. 16–15*B*) or the

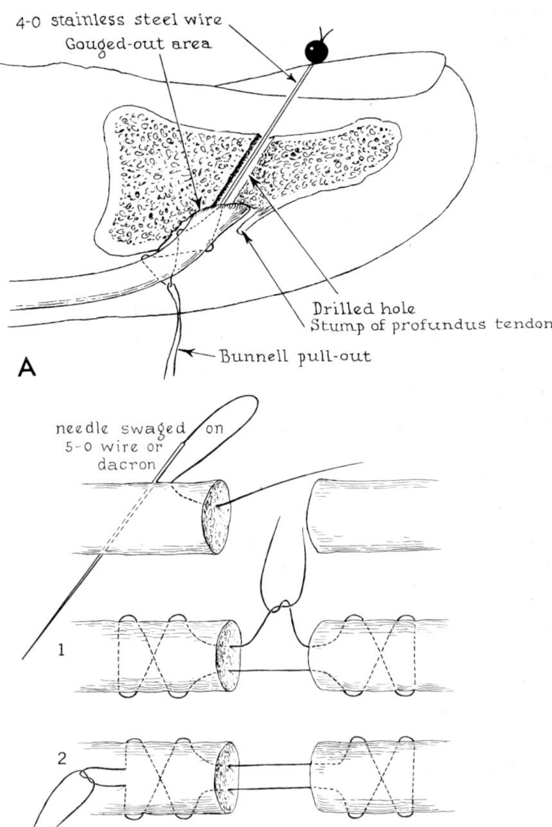

Figure 16–15 Diagram illustrates technique of tendon repair. *A*, Bunnell pull-out technique using 4-0 or No. 34 wire. *B*(2), Bunnell figure-of-eight tendon suture using 5-0 wire or dacron. *B*(1), Technique modified to allow knot to be tied within the anastomosis.

Bunnell pull-out wire technique (Fig. 16–15*A*) may be utilized. The latter is preferable for suturing of the flexor tendon to the terminal phalanx and for the repair of extensor tendon injuries on the dorsum of the hand. Interrupted sutures, 5–0 or 6–0, have been recommended for tendon repair by Verdan[51] and Mason[32] and are the method of choice for repairing extensor tendons over the metacarpophalangeal and interphalangeal joints, since wire sutures in these locations irritate the skin and may require removal.

Flexor Tendon Injuries

Distal Third of the Forearm and Wrist. The flexor profundus tendons, the flexor carpi radialis and the flexor carpi ulnaris are repaired with a figure-of-eight 5–0 wire suture. A fold of synovium is interposed between the flexor profundus and superficialis tendons if possible. The flexor superficialis tendons are repaired with interrupted sutures of 6–0 wire in order to produce a minimum of scarring between the superficialis and profundus tendons. Verdan[51] and others have suggested not repairing the flexor superficialis tendons at this level; certainly repair is not recommended in the badly contused or contaminated wound.

Carpal Canal. Lacerations through the transverse carpal ligament usually produce extensive damage. Division of all of the flexor tendons and the median nerve is not uncommon. Adequate exploration and repair demands excellent exposure which usually requires extension of the wound into the forearm and palm (Fig. 15–11*B*). The flexor profundus tendons to the fingers and the long thumb flexor are repaired with figure-of-eight 5–0 wire sutures. Repair of the flexor superficialis tendons should not be performed if the flexor profundus tendons are intact. Opinion differs as to whether the flexor superficialis tendons should be repaired in the presence of divided flexor profundus tendons. Repair of the flexor superficialis tendons, if undertaken, should be accomplished with interrupted sutures of 6–0 wire.

Long Thumb Flexor in the Thenar Area. Testing sensation and opposition and abduction is essential since lacerations in the thenar area frequently divide the volar digital nerves to the thumb and the motor branch of the median nerve. Primary repair of the tendon injury is accomplished if not contraindicated by wound considerations. Retraction of the proximal tendon above the wrist and difficulty in exposing the point of tendon injury are the major problems. The transverse carpal ligament may be divided and the area of division exposed after identification of the median nerve (Figs. 16–16*B* and 16–17*B*); or a midlateral thumb incision carried across the palm, allowing retraction of the superficial head of the short thumb flexor, may be utilized (Fig. 16–17*A*). The latter incision is used for secondary tendon repair and tendon grafting in the thumb and, in most instances, eliminates the need for dividing the transverse carpal ligament. The tendon is repaired with a figure-of-eight suture of 5–0 wire. An alternate technique is to use a 4–0 pull-out wire suture placed proximal to the laceration and several 6–0 wire sutures to approximate the tendon ends.

Long Thumb Flexor within the Flexor Tendon Sheath. The results of primary repair of the long thumb flexor within the tendon sheath warrant this procedure. The repair is accomplished with interrupted fine wire sutures, and that portion of the sheath overlying the anastomosis is excised. A pulley mechanism must be retained either over the proximal phalanx or over the metacarpophalangeal joint. The tendon advancement technique is the procedure of choice for lacerations near the insertion of the long thumb flexor and yields good results if no more than a half inch shortening of the tendon is required.

Flexor Superficialis Tendon Alone. Careful exploration is required to rule out injury to the profundus tendon. The flexor superficialis tendon is not repaired except in certain skilled artisans who require function of both the superficialis and profundus tendons. The best functional result is achieved by carefully controlled early motion.

Flexor Profundus Alone. Primary

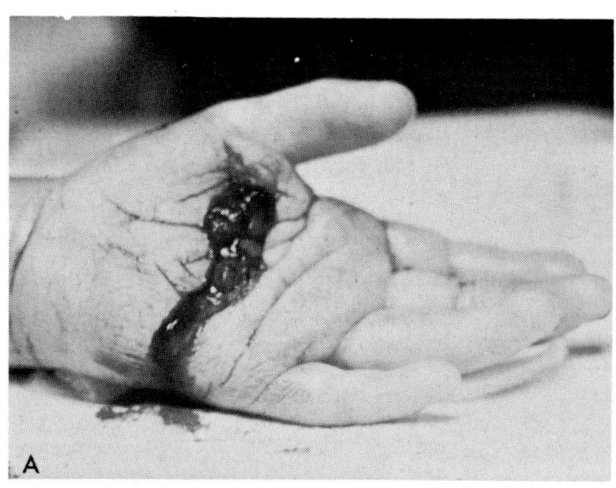

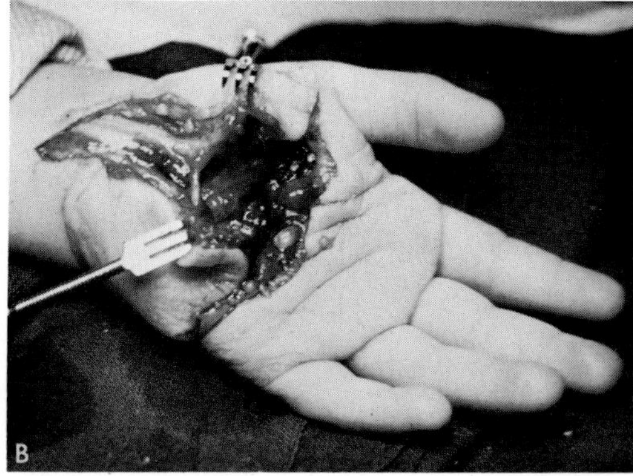

Figure 16–16 *A*, Photograph illustrates laceration of palm of the hand. *B*, Method of extending the laceration proximally with division of transverse carpal ligament in order to expose the divided flexor tendons and the median nerve.

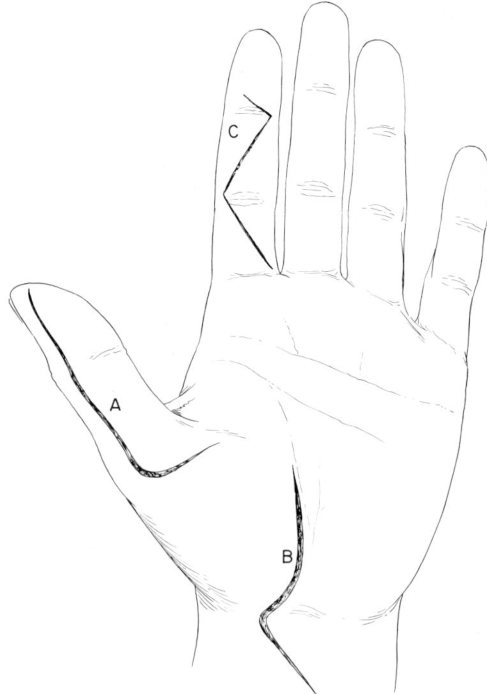

Figure 16–17 *A,* Diagram illustrates incision for exposure of the flexor pollicis longus tendon within the thumb. *B,* Incision for exposure of flexor tendons and median nerve within carpal canal. *C,* Bruner zig-zag incision for exposure of flexor tendons within the finger.

repair of flexor profundus tendon lacerations yields good results in the presence of an intact flexor superficialis tendon, provided the wound is ideal. The Bruner zig-zag incision[12] (Fig. 15–17C) may be used as an alternative to the standard midaxial approach in order to incorporate the wound into the incision. The advancement technique (Fig. 16–18), using the Bunnell pullout wire to anchor the tendon to the terminal phalanx, gives better results than tendon anastomosis but may be employed only if the distal stump of the profundus is short, i.e., 0.5 in. in the index finger, and 0.25 in. in the middle, ring and little fingers. Slight active motion may be initiated as early as 12 days following tendon advancement. Excision of an intact flexor superficialis tendon should never be done in an ideal wound. Secondary tendon grafting is the procedure of choice when the wound is less than ideal if a good passive range of motion persists in the distal interphalangeal joint.

Flexor Profundus and Flexor Superficialis Tendons within the Flexor Tendon Sheath of the Finger. The area of the flexor tendon sheath of the finger called "no man's land" by Bunnell, "the critical zone" by Littler and "the area of the expert" by Verdan, represents the most difficult area in which to achieve a satisfactory end result following the division of both tendons. Primary repair may be attempted with reasonable anticipation of success in children under the age of 12. At the other end of the chronological spectrum, Boyes reports results with tendon grafting in patients over 50 years to be no better than with primary repair.[5] Thus, the area of contention involves the group between children and the over-fifty. Two schools of thought exist regarding definitive treatment of these patients: whether to perform primary repair or close the wound and tendon graft the profundus in four to six weeks. In either case, the superficialis is usually not repaired. Likewise, all authorities agree that simple wound closure is the treatment of choice when dealing with a less than ideal wound.

The best results of primary repair have been reported by Verdan[51] and Kleinert.[29] Both emphasize that the technique should be performed only by the skilled hand surgeon, under ideal circumstances, and employing meticulous technique. Kleinert[29] excises only enough sheath to permit the anastomosis to glide freely (Fig. 16–19) and performs the suture with a modified Bunnell criss-cross combined with a running 6–0 dacron to the tendon edges. When circumstances preclude primary repair in an otherwise ideal situation, Madsen[31] has recommended wound cleansing and dressing, followed by delayed primary repair within a period of seven days, pro-

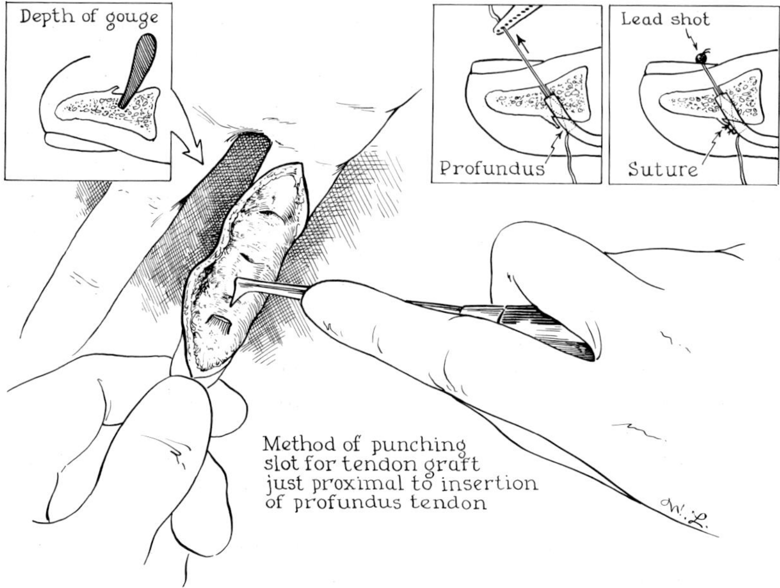

Figure 16–18 Diagram illustrates Bunnell pull-out wire suture for advancement of flexor profundus tendon or for attaching a tendon graft to the terminal phalanx.

vided the wound remains clean without drainage or infection.

Wakefield[52] doubts that conditions are ever ideal for primary repair in "no man's land," except possibly in children four to six years old, and states: "Some surgeons are endeavoring to perfect a technique which will permit successful primary repair within 'No Man's Land.' Although prospects seem to offer some promise, the method is not of general application. Tendon grafting in this situation gives vastly superior results in most surgeons' hands." Verdan[51] reports that 50 per cent of his primary repairs and approximately 50 per cent of his tendon grafts in "no man's land" flex to within 3 cm. of the distal palmar crease; one-third of the primarily repaired tendons required tenolysis. Boyes[7] reported the results of primary

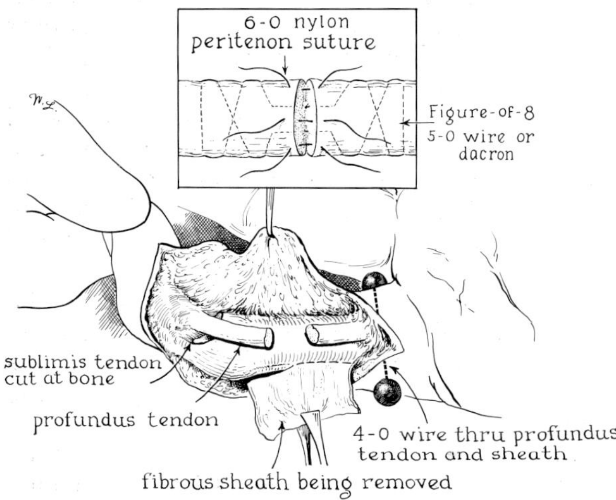

Figure 16–19 Method for primary repair of the flexor profundus tendon. Modified after techniques of Verdan and Kleinert. Nylon or 6-0 wire may be used for peritendinous suture and also mercilene as figure-8 suture.

repair in a selected series of ideal injuries in 12 patients. Forty-three per cent of these flexed to within 1.5 in. of the distal palmar crease; whereas, in a group of patients with secondary tendon grafts done under ideal conditions, all flexed to within 1 in. of the distal palmar crease.[9] Dupont and Crikelair[21] reviewed the cases done by resident surgeons on the Surgical Service of the Presbyterian Hospital: of 33 primary repairs in "no man's land," three patients obtained a good result; of 23 tendon grafts, 21 patients obtained a good result. Van't Hof and Heiple[50] reviewed the current literature on this subject and reported that, of primarily repaired tendons, 38 per cent flexed to 1 in. of the palm and 57 per cent flexed to within 1.5 in. of the distal palmar crease.

Tendon Grafting

The major criterion determining the suitable time for tendon grafting is the softness and pliability of the wound. With proper wound care, the tissues may be satisfactory within the four to six weeks of the initial injury. On the other hand, massage, passive stretching and soaking of the hand may be required for a significantly longer period of time before the tissues become soft and pliable.

The sources of a tendon graft are listed preferentially as follows:

1. Palmaris longus.
2. Plantaris.
3. Extensor digitorum communis of index.
4. Extensor indicis proprius.
5. Common extensors of the second, third and fourth toes.

The palmaris longus is absent in 14 per cent and the plantaris in 7 per cent of the population. Considerable dissection is required in removing the common toe extensors, particularly if a long graft is needed. The common toe extensors fuse at the ankle, and sharp dissection is necessary to isolate a single tendon. The muscle belly of the extensor indicis proprius frequently extends to the wrist. For these reasons, the common extensor of the index finger is preferred in the absence of a palmaris longus. The extensor digitorum communis of the index finger is readily available; it provides a long graft; and no disability results from its sacrifice since the extensor indicis proprius provides full extension of the index finger. Sharp dissection is required to section the juncture tendinum.

A midlateral incision on the radial side of the index finger or on the ulnar aspect of the middle, ring and little fingers together with a separate incision in the palm are utilized for tendon grafting. An associated digital nerve injury may determine whether the radial or ulnar aspect of the finger is explored. Better exposure is achieved by a continuous incision along the midlateral line of the finger and across the palm if the laceration is in the region of the metacarpophalangeal joint or the base of the proximal phalanx. In this area, sharp dissection is required to excise the tendon sheath and remove the stumps of the divided tendons. Adequate removal of scar is essential to a good result. In some instances, scarring may be so severe that the surgeon must content himself with excision of the fibro-osseous canal, all the flexor tendon remnants and no reconstruction. In such instances, four to six months are allowed for complete healing, following which the flexor profundus tendon and new pulleys are provided by tendon grafts. An alternative approach to the badly scarred finger involves the insertion of a silastic tendon prosthesis at the time of scar and tendon excision.[24] The formation of a synovium-lined sheath about the prosthesis greatly simplifies the second stage of the reconstruction and appears to significantly improve the functional result.

The flexor superficialis tendon stump is not removed if it has healed smoothly, as is so often the case with division of the tendon immediately proximal to the vincula. The flexor superficialis tendon must be excised to within a few millimeters of its insertion in the presence of dense scar for it may be limiting flexion of the proximal interphalangeal joint.

The amount of tendon sheath excised is determined by the degree of scarring within the sheath. In those instances in which the flexor superficialis tendon is intact and the graft is being inserted for flexor profundus action, the sheath usually is beautifully intact; and only that amount necessary to allow removal of the distal flexor profundus stump and exposure of the proximal stump for anastomosis need be resected. The sheath is subjected to minimal surgical trauma by passing the tendon graft blindly with a small probe or ureteral catheter. The sheath must be reduced to a two pulley system, one at the base of the proximal phalanx and one over the middle phalanx, when dealing with a severely scarred or completely collapsed sheath.

Passive excursion of the flexor profundus tendon is tested prior to performing the proximal anastomosis. A passive excursion of 35 mm. in the adult with the tourniquet elevated (measured by grasping the relaxed proximal cut tendon end and stretching distally, the wrist in neutral position) is equivalent to an active excursion of 55 to 60 mm. with the tourniquet released and is within the normal range (demonstrated by repair under local anesthesia; tendon stretched to maximum length with the wrist in neutral position; patient asked to flex the finger).[19]

The proximal anastomosis is performed with a figure-of-eight suture of 4–0 or 5–0 wire. The figure-of-eight suture technique allows the anastomosis to lie at the point of origin of the lumbrical muscle from the profundus tendon and to recede proximally into an area not traumatized by dissection. The lumbrical muscle is excised if badly scarred. The graft is passed through an area of normal synovial tissue within the carpal canal and the anastomosis performed proximal to the wrist if a good range of passive motion cannot be obtained by moderate dissection in the proximal palm.

The proper tension for the tendon graft is determined by placing the palm flat on the table with the wrist in neutral position and the fingers extended, stretching the graft distally as tautly as possible, and marking the point on the graft corresponding to the insertion of the flexor profundus tendon into the distal phalanx. If 35 mm. of passive excursion have been demonstrated in the profundus muscle-tendon unit, the graft tension is adjusted so that the finger rests in a normal position of function. With less than 35 mm. of passive excursion, the graft tension is increased correspondingly so that the finger rests in more than normal flexion; in this instance, complete extension may not be obtained.

The distal anastomosis of the tendon graft is performed by anchoring the graft to a slot in the terminal phalanx beneath the stump of the flexor profundus tendon with a figure-of-eight pull-out suture of 4–0 wire (Fig. 16–18). A sharpened dental root extractor provides an excellent instrument for creating the slot in the terminal phalanx. Injury to the volar plate of the distal interphalangeal joint in dissecting up the stump of the flexor profundus tendon must be avoided to prevent adherence of the graft at this point, with subsequent lack of flexion of the distal phalanx. A single knot is tied over the button on the terminal phalanx and the position of the finger tested before excising any excess graft. The stump of the flexor profundus is sutured to the graft with interrupted sutures of 6–0 nylon. The pull-out wire is brought out through a single skin opening near the tendon insertion. This distal position of the pull-out wire minimizes irritation and allows for better motion of the graft within the sheath than if the wire lies along the graft and exits over the middle phalanx.

Flexor tendon repairs and tendon grafts are immobilized with the wrist and fingers in slight flexion for three weeks. The hand is examined frequently to be certain that adjacent fingers are not becoming stiff. Slight passive extension of the proximal interphalangeal joint of the injured finger with the metacarpophalangeal joint held in flexion can be performed at the end of the second week. Protected active motion within the splint is begun at two and a half weeks, and graded active motion without the splint is allowed at three weeks. The suture is removed at the fourth week.

The minimum age at which tendon grafting may be performed successfully is debatable. A minimum age of five years has been suggested by some; however, it must be realized that a finger lacking flexor tendon function does not grow normally, and operation at a younger age may be desirable. The senior author has performed tendon grafting successfully in a 13 month old child.

Pulvertaft[41] reports a successful case of tendon grafting performed 17 years following the initial injury. In long-standing cases it may be necessary to use an adjacent flexor superficialis as the motor. The flexor profundus motor may be used if the tendon has been adherent within the finger and acting as a flexor of the metacarpophalangeal joint. In such instances, the tendon sheath must be reduced to a two pulley system because of the absence of synovium within the sheath.

Extensor Tendon Injuries

The Bunnell pull-out wire technique, augmented by a few interrupted 6–0 sutures at the anastomosis, is the method of choice for the repair of extensor tendon injuries on the dorsum of the hand. Repair of the extensor mechanism over the metacarpophalangeal or interphalangeal joints is accomplished with 6–0 silk or mersalene to avoid possible skin irritation by wire sutures. Splinting protects the sutured tendon.

Extensor tendon injuries distal to the wrist are immobilized for three weeks, with the wrist and metacarpophalangeal joints in moderate extension and the proximal interphalangeal joints in slight flexion. Extension of the wrist is maintained for four weeks following repair of the wrist extensors.

Mallet Finger. Mallet finger is produced by three types of closed injury (Fig. 16–20) in addition to open laceration of the extensor tendon inserting at the base of the terminal phalanx. Lacerations should be repaired by suturing of the tendon and immobilization of the distal interphalangeal joint in extension, either by splinting or Kirschner wire fixation.

1. Rupture of the extensor tendon or laceration of the distal interphalangeal joint.
2. Avulsion of a small fragment of bone with the extensor tendon.

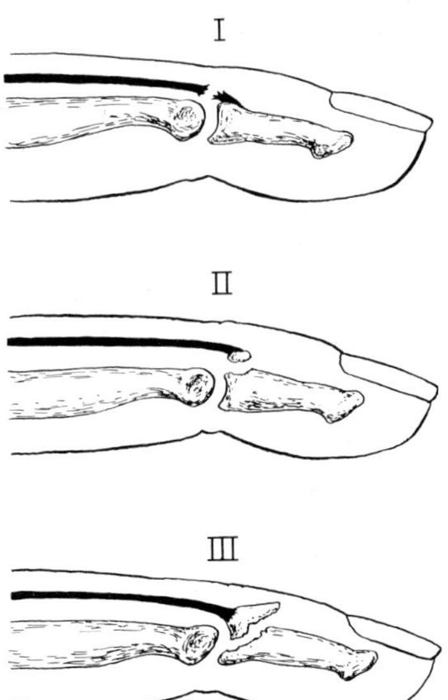

Figure 16–20 Diagram illustrates the three types of closed injury to the extensor tendon and its insertion to the terminal phalanx which produces the mallet finger deformity.

3. Avulsion of a large segment of the articular surface with the extensor tendon.

Rupture of the extensor tendon (Type I) only and avulsion of a small fragment of bone with the extensor tendon (Type II) are treated by aluminum splint immobilization of the distal interphalangeal joint in slight hyperextension for six to eight weeks (Milford[35]) (Fig. 16–21). The proximal interphalangeal joint is not immobilized. Patients lacking extension at the distal interphalangeal joint after a two-to-four-week period of improper splinting usually will achieve a good result following eight weeks of splinting with progressively increased hypertension of the distal interphalangeal joint. Some patients will respond to this course of treatment as long as three months after injury, provided slight active extension of the distal interphalangeal joint can be demonstrated prior to splinting.

Avulsion of a large segment of the articular surface (Type III) is managed by open reduction and Kirschner wire fixation (Fig. 16–22).

Tenolysis. Tenolysis is a very useful and rewarding procedure for dealing with tendon injuries in which a good functional result has not been achieved following primary repair, physiotherapy, dynamic splinting and active usage.

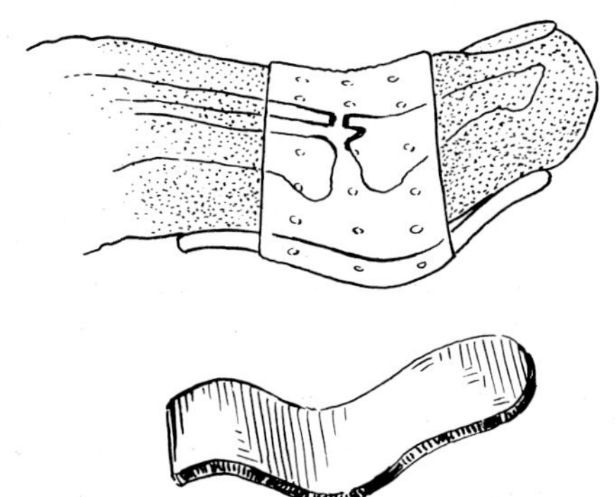

Figure 16–21 Mallet finger with rupture of extensor tendon treated on a biconcave aluminum splint with a band-aid immobilizing only the distal interphalangeal joint. (Redrawn after Milford, L.: Campbell's Operative Orthopaedics. 4th ed. St. Louis, The C. V. Mosby Co., 1963.)

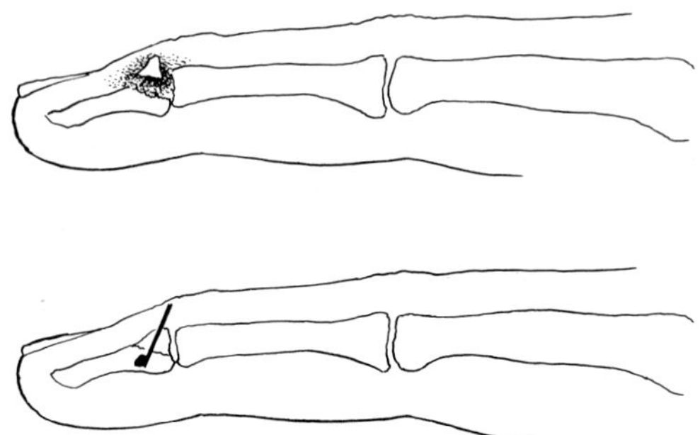

Figure 16–22 Diagram illustrates reduction and Kirschner wire fixation of a large bone fragment avulsed from the base of the distal phalanx.

The procedure demands meticulous removal of all scar tissue and precise hemostasis. Active and passive motion is initiated within 72 hours postoperatively and consists of placing the finger through a full range of motion once daily. The finger is splinted between these brief periods of exercise in order to prevent a recurrence of adhesions secondary to the reaction produced by the tendon moving through a fresh wound. Rubber band traction may be utilized to stretch a finger into extension following tenolysis; the traction is removed and the finger placed actively and passively through a full range of motion once daily. Active exercise is gradually increased.

PERIPHERAL NERVES

Primary repair of peripheral nerve injuries is preferred to secondary repair when there is a clean, sharp laceration (Onné)[38]. Lack of retraction of the nerve and the absence of a neuroma proximally and a glioma distally significantly reduce the amount of gap to be overcome. Secondary nerve suture is reserved for crushing and mangling injuries and situations in which a skilled surgeon is not available to perform the neurorrhaphy. If primary repair cannot be accomplished, the nerve is united with a single suture in the perineurium to prevent retraction. Repair should be performed as soon as the wound will allow—if at all possible, no later than six months after injury. Considerable care must be observed in serially sectioning the nerve proximally and distally until an area of minimal intraneural scarring is encountered, and equal care must be observed in properly aligning the fascicles at the time of suturing. Sunderland[34] has pointed out that the fascicular pattern is constant for only 5 mm. in the median nerve. Onné[38] noted no difference in the results when comparing primary repair with secondary suture performed within six months of the injury. Seddon[43] strongly advocated secondary suture on the basis of electively choosing the incision for exposure, ease of determining the amount of damaged nerve and ease of suturing provided by the thickened nerve sheath. Certainly this is the procedure of choice in treating battle casualties, but most civilian injuries can be repaired primarily.

A gap of 1 to 1.5 in. in the median and ulnar nerves at the wrist can be overcome simply by immobilizing the wrist in flexion. A gap of 4 in. in the ulnar nerve can be overcome by mobilization of the motor branches and transplantation of the nerve anterior to the elbow joint. A gap of 3 in. in the median nerve can be overcome by mobilization of the motor branches and transplantation of the nerve anterior to the pronator teres; flexion of the elbow will relax the tension on the suture line at the wrist. A nerve graft must be employed if the gap is greater than 4 in. in the ulnar nerve or 3 in. in the median nerve. Zachary[53] has emphasized that a successful outcome is unlikely following resection of a 5 cm. segment of nerve. The superior results reported by Millesi[34] will undoubtedly encourage surgeons to graft nerve gaps of smaller distances than these figures. The critical aspects of his technique are high magnification, topographical mapping of the nerve ends, resection of the epineurium, a minimum of fine sutures carefully placed and the absolute absence of tension. The suture material utilized for neurorrhaphy must be as fine and unreactive as possible. Most specialists now recommend size 8–0 or 9–0 nylon for perineural and interfascicular suturing. Precise placement of such material requires good quality magnifying loupes at the very least. Many authors advocate the operating microscope.

The suture material utilized for neurorrhaphy must be as fine and unreactive as possible. The technical difficulties encountered in using very fine wire lead most specialists to recommend nylon or silk, sizes 6-0 or 7-0. The sutures are placed only in the nerve sheath (Fig. 16–23).

The wrist is splinted in flexion for a minimum of four weeks following nerve repair. Abnormal tension on the suture line during the subsequent four-week period is prevented by weekly application of a new dorsal plaster splint, and the amount of dorsiflexion at the wrist is progressively increased until full dorsiflexion is attained.

Repair of the digital nerve is mandatory and, if possible, should be accomplished primarily. Secondary suture of digital nerves divided in the palm frequently is impossible because of retraction of the nerve ends and the resection imposed by the neuroma and glioma. Repair of digital nerve injuries as far distally as the distal interphalangeal joint is possible.

Nicholson and Seddon[37] reviewed 305 nerve repairs in 277 patients in civilian practice. When the injury was at the wrist level, two out of three sutures of the median nerve were followed by useful motor recovery and four out of five times there was a good sensory recovery. The results of ulnar nerve suture at the wrist were slightly better, with four out of five making useful sensory and motor recovery;

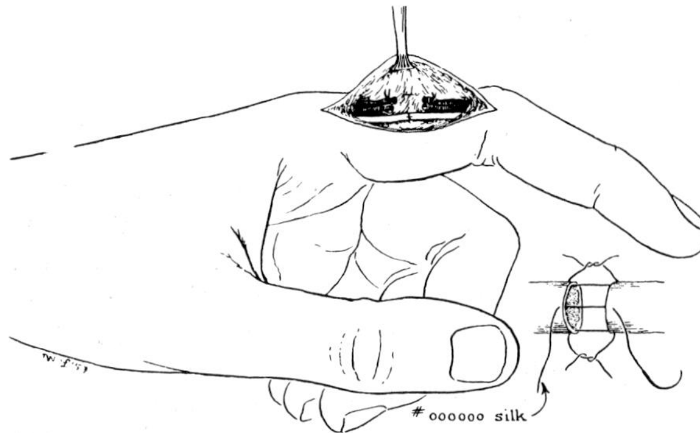

Figure 16–23 Drawing illustrates technique of peripheral nerve repair, using perineurial suture of 6-0 silk. (From Curtis, R. M.: Maryland M. J. 5: 675, 1956.)

in one case out of three some degree of lateral movement of the fingers was regained.

The causes for failure to achieve a satisfactory result following nerve repair may be summarized as follows:

1. Excessive elapsed time between injury and repair. (Zachary and Holmes[54] reported 15 months to be the maximum interval compatible with a satisfactory result.)
2. Excessive nerve gap to be overcome. (Zachary[54] reported that a gap of more than 7 cm. yields a poor result.)
3. Excessive mobilization of the nerve being repaired. (Nicholson and Seddon[37] indicated that local mobilization with flexion of the wrist and elbow yields better results than transposition.)
4. Failure to adequately resect the neuroma and glioma.
5. Failure to properly align the motor and sensory fibers.
6. Postoperative suture line separation.

Nerve Grafts

Bunnell[13] described successful digital nerve grafts, and Bunnell and Boyes extended the technique to larger nerves. They also demonstrated experimentally that small cable grafts survive whereas large nerve grafts, the size of the median and ulnar nerves, undergo fibrosis before the growing axons reach the distal anastomosis. The sural nerve serves beautifully as a graft for the digital nerve or provides two long strands of nerve of the proper caliber for construction of a cable graft. Seddon[44] reported a 50 per cent success rate (69 per cent, if the partial successes are counted) in a series of 107 nerve grafts. The successful results compared favorably with the best results following direct suture; the partially successful results provided return of useful sensory and motor function; and the failures exhibited no functional benefit from the procedure. Millesi[34] reported his series of 33 median and 32 ulnar nerves in 1972 using the technique described earlier. His results indicate better quality of sensory and motor return in a greater number of patients than has heretofore been reported by any other method.

Nerve Pedicle Grafts. The technique of pedicle nerve grafting was performed by Barnes and colleagues in 1945, according to Seddon,[44] and was subsequently described independently by Strange.[48] By the technique an otherwise useless median or ulnar nerve may be used for grafting. It should be emphasized that this procedure is applicable only when both nerves are injured and are not reparable by the usual means, such as grafting. Seddon[44] reports eight successful and five partially successful nerve pedicle grafts.

Nerve Compression Syndromes

Acute compression syndromes involving the median nerve in its course through the carpal canal or the ulnar nerve beneath the fibro-osseous tunnel adjacent to the pisiform bone give rise to numbness, muscle atrophy and early sympathetic dystrophy manifested by severe causalgia, swelling and stiffness of the hand. The syndrome may follow Colles' fracture or severe contusion of the hand. Failure to recognize and treat the syndrome may result in a hand permanently disabled by causalgia, with persistent swelling and stiffness. Treatment consists of release of the constricted area combined with internal neurolysis if there is definite scarring in the epineural tissues. The senior author has encountered two patients in whom acute carpal tunnel syndrome secondary to wrist fracture failed to improve following release of the transverse carpal ligament but who improved rapidly following subsequent internal neurolysis by blunt dissection of the fascicles.

BONES AND JOINTS

Principles of Fracture Management

The optimum treatment of fractures involving the metacarpals and phalanges achieves correct alignment and allows early movement, thereby preventing joint stiffness and adherence of tendons.

Correct alignment usually may be achieved only at the time of the initial manipulation. Closed manipulation, whenever possible, is preferable to open reduction. The reduction is maintained by a molded plaster splint, the hand splint suggested by Bohler[2] (Fig. 16–24) or, if necessary, by traction or Kirschner wire fixation. A Kirschner wire may be inserted blindly or at the time of open reduction under direct vision.

Malalignment produces malfunction. Rotation at the fracture site in the metacarpal or phalanx may cause scissoring of the fingers and malposition of a fractured phalanx is a frequent cause of adherent flexor and extensor

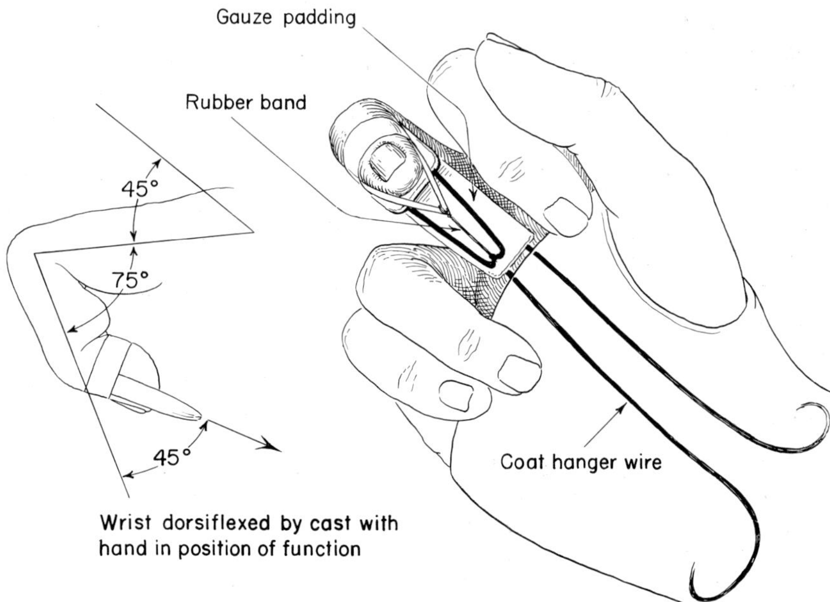

Figure 16–24 Drawing illustrates technique of using rubber band traction for fracture of phalanges and metacarpals. Insert shows angles which metacarpophalangeal and interphalangeal joints should assume during traction. Note that coat hanger wire is molded to fit finger. The traction should immobilize only and not distract the fracture site.

tendons. Pre- and postreduction radiographs are essential but do not replace functional evaluation. Rotation at the fracture site may not be detected on the x-rays but becomes immediately apparent on the basis of scissoring of the flexed fingers.

The wrist and fingers are splinted in the position of function. Motion, if only once daily, is initiated in the fractured finger as soon as possible.

Metacarpal. SIMPLE FRACTURE WITHOUT DISPLACEMENT. In the absence of instability at the fracture site, treatment consists of a volar plaster splint to the level of the metacarpophalangeal joint. Active motion of the fingers is allowed, but activity is limited until the pain and swelling have disappeared.

BASE OF THE THUMB METACARPAL (BENNETT'S FRACTURE). Closed reduction is obtained by forcing the thumb metacarpal into opposition and abduction. It is rarely possible to maintain the reduction with the thumb in this position. James[25] transfixes the thumb and index metacarpals with a Kirschner wire maintaining the reduction by thumb opposition (Fig. 16–25). Traction has been suggested by others. Open reduction with Kirschner wire fixation is indicated if reduction and fixation cannot be achieved by closed manipulation (Fig. 16–25).

OBLIQUE FRACTURES OF THE SHAFT. Closed reduction is preferred. Immobilization is by means of a plaster splint to the palm if the fracture is stable and without rotation or by Kirschner wire fixation (Fig. 16–26). Instability, rotatory deformity or inability to maintain length requires correction by closed or open reduction.

TRANSVERSE FRACTURE OF THE SHAFT. Closed reduction and immobilization occasionally may be accomplished. Open reduction and Kirschner wire fixation are frequently required as a result of the instability of the fracture. In testing the functional result following reduction, it is important to recall that all fingers point to the tubercle of the scaphoid when forced into full flexion at the metacarpophalangeal and proximal interphalangeal joints (Fig. 16–27). Axial rotation also is evaluated by examining the plane of the fingernails.

FRACTURE OF THE HEAD. Fractures of the distal metacarpal near the head usually are impacted. Volar angulation of as much as 30 degrees at the fracture site in the fourth and

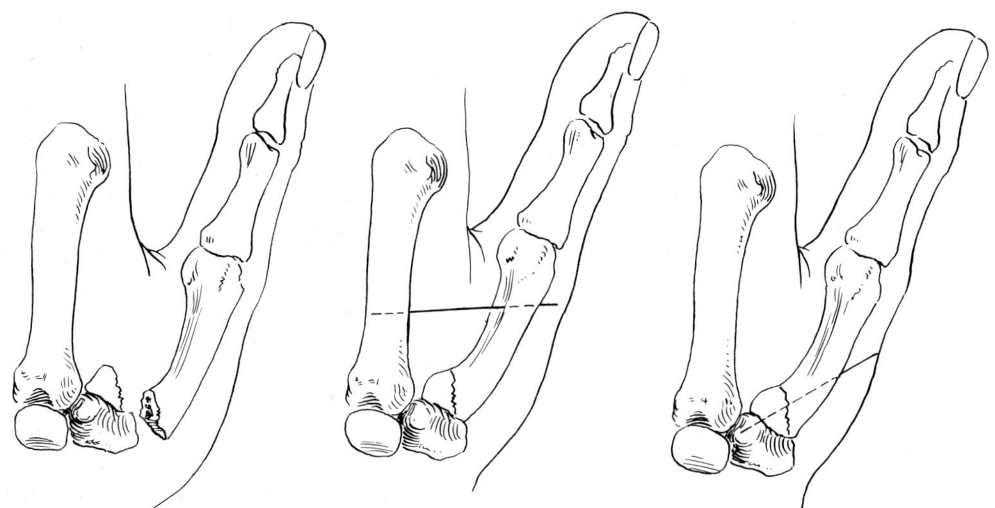

Figure 16–25 Alternate techniques of immobilization of Bennett's fracture of first metacarpal. Kirschner wire fixation can be used with closed reduction or open reduction.

fifth metacarpals is compatible with an excellent functional result because of the mobility of these metacarpals, and treatment consists of immobilization in a volar plaster splint to prevent excessive use of the hand until the pain and swelling have disappeared. Lack of full flexion at the fourth and fifth metacarpophalangeal joints indicates excessive angulation at the fracture site and requires closed or open reduction. The index and middle fingers tolerate less angulation at the fracture site and require open reduction with Kirschner wire fixation if proper alignment cannot be achieved by closed manipulation (Fig. 16–28).

Proximal Phalanx. BASE. The proximal third of the proximal phalanx frequently is the site of a compression fracture, with a dorsal concavity resulting from angulation at the fracture site (Fig. 16–29). The adequacy of closed reduction is evaluated on the basis of active extension of the fingers: failure of full extension at the proximal interphalangeal joint indicates an unsatisfactory reduction. Open reduction with Kirschner wire fixation usually is required and is accomplished through a dorsal incision with splitting of the extensor tendon in the midline. A slight amount of dorsal concavity as a result of improper reduction prevents full extension because of a tendon imbalance in the extensor mechanism. Fractures through this cancellous area usually heal within three to four weeks.

SHAFT. A linear fracture may be treated by taping the injured finger to an adjacent finger. Open reduction is required for spiral fractures with rotation and for transverse fractures with displacement at the fracture site. Open reduction and internal fixation with

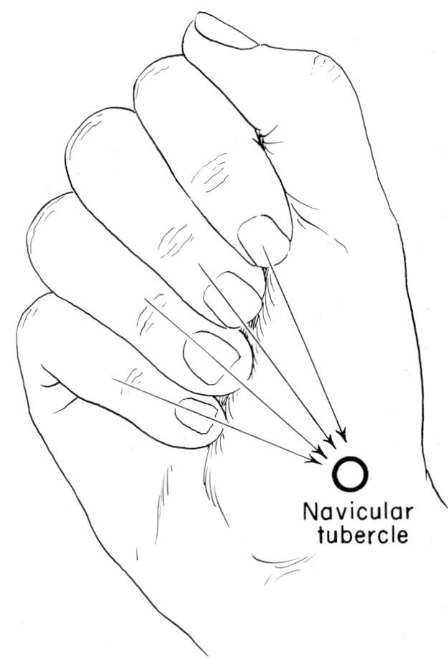

Figure 16–27 Diagram illustrates that when fingers are fully flexed at metacarpophalangeal and proximal interphalangeal joints all fingers point to tubercle of navicular. Axial rotation at fracture site is detected by the horizontal plane of fingernail.

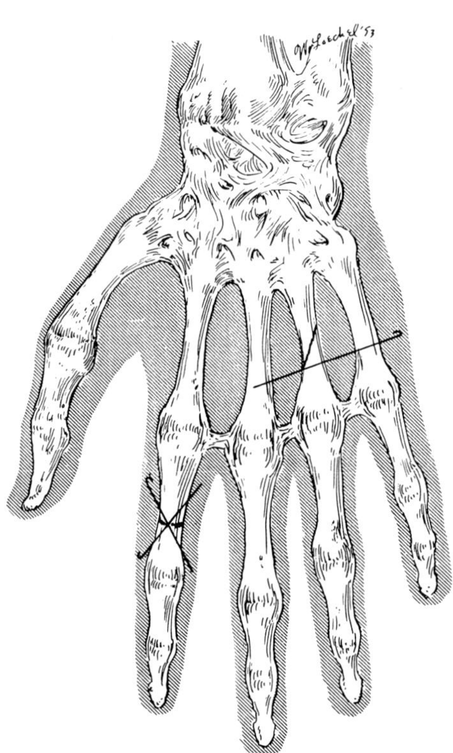

Figure 16–26 Drawing illustrates use of fine Kirschner wires for immobilization of fracture of phalanx and metacarpal. If possible, wires should be inserted so as to allow joint motion while fracture is being immobilized. Crisscross technique is also useful in metacarpal fracture. (From Curtis, R. M.: Maryland M. J. 5:675, 1956.)

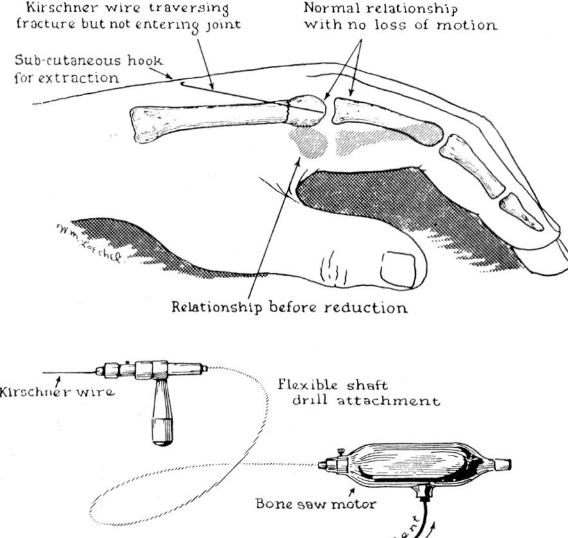

Figure 16–28 Drawing illustrates method of inserting Kirschner wires for fixation of fracture of head of 1st metacarpal. Note use of electric motor to facilitate insertion of fine wire. (From Curtis, R. M.: Maryland M. J. 5:675, 1956.)

Kirschner wires is accomplished through a doral incision and exposure of the fracture site by splitting the extensor tendon in the midline. Early motion in flexion and extension is allowed. Healing may be complete within five to seven weeks.

DISTAL. Open reduction is necessary to properly position the fracture fragments when there has been a fracture of one or both condyles (Fig. 16–30). Open reduction is accomplished through a midlateral incision with division of the retinacular ligament. Exposure of the lateral aspect of the joint and condyle is accomplished by removal of a portion of the capsular ligament (Fig. 16–31). Anchoring of the fracture fragment with Kirschner wire is performed under direct visualization of the joint surface. Repair of the collateral ligament may not be possible, but the retinacular ligament is always repaired.

Middle Phalanx. BASE. Subluxation of the proximal interphalangeal joint and injury to the lateral and volar capsules usually occur with fractures

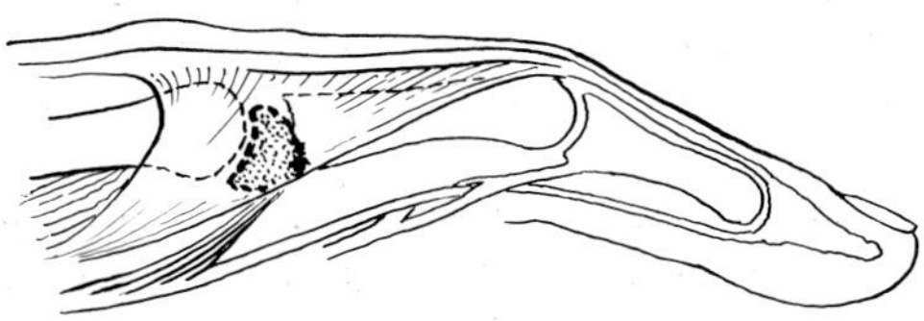

Figure 16–29 Deformity with impacted fracture of base of proximal phalanx. Dorsal concavity produces imbalance preventing full active extension at proximal interphalangeal joint.

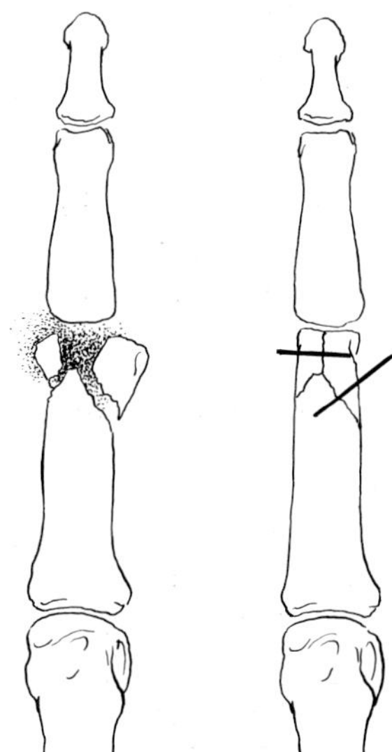

Figure 16–30 Kirschner wire fixation following open reduction of T-type fracture of the condyles of the proximal phalanx.

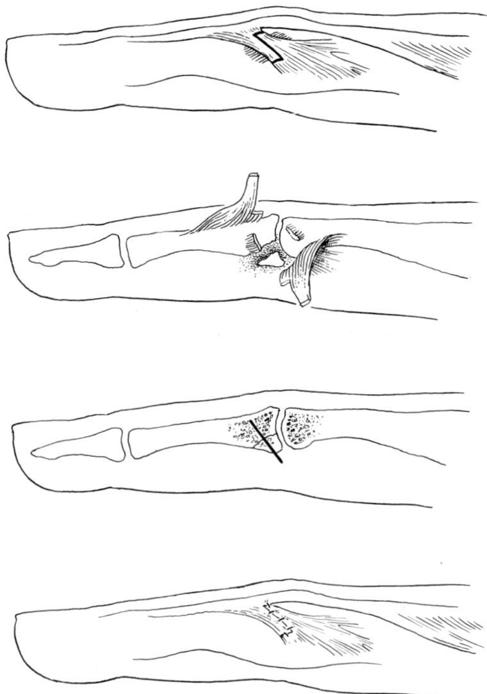

Figure 16–31 Diagram illustrates technique of step cutting the retinacular ligament and removal of the lateral capsular ligament for exposure of the proximal interphalangeal joint and fracture fragment, with Kirschner wire fixation of fracture.

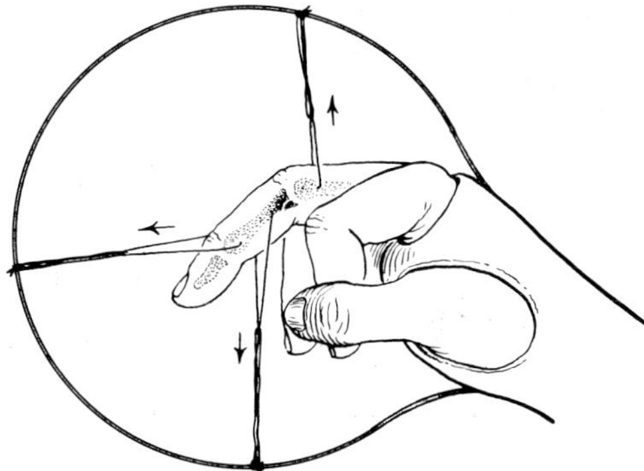

Figure 16–32 Method of Robertson, Cawley and Faris for treatment of acute fracture-dislocation of the proximal interphalangeal joint, with traction from Kirschner wire in proximal and middle phalanges. (Curtis, R. M.: Joints of the hand. *In* Flynn, J. E. (ed.): Hand Surgery. Baltimore, The Williams & Wilkins Co., 1966.)

of the base of the middle phalanx. The capsular injury produces considerable swelling of the proximal interphalangeal joint. Severe disability due to joint stiffness results from improper treatment. Closed manipulation is attempted by placing the proximal interphalangeal joint in 70 to 80 degrees of flexion. The traction technique described by Robertson et al.[45] is the method of choice for treating markedly comminuted fractures (Fig. 16–32). Open reduction is accomplished through a midlateral incision, with division of the retinacular ligament and resection of the lateral capsular ligament to gain exposure of the proximal interphalangeal joint (Fig. 16–31). The reduction is maintained by Kirschner wire fixation (Fig. 16–33); lateral stability of the joint is provided by repair of the retinacular ligament. An additional Kirschner wire may be utilized to hold the proximal interphalangeal joint in slight flexion for four to six days (Fig. 15–26). Protected active motion is initiated within five to seven days. Chronic fracture-dislocations in this area require capsulectomy to achieve reduction of the fragment and flexion of the proximal interphalangeal joint.[20]

SHAFT. Open reduction and Kirschner wire fixation (Fig. 16–26) are frequently required because of the severe displacement produced by the pull of the flexor superficialis on the proximal fragment. Linear, nondisplaced fractures and fractures proximal to the insertion of the flexor superficialis may be treated simply by using an adjacent finger as a splint.

DISTAL. The fracture usually is T-type with separation of one or both condyles from the middle phalanx. Open reduction with Kirschner wire fixation is accomplished through either a midlateral or dorsal incision. The Kirschner wire should be inserted in a manner that will permit early motion.

Distal Phalanx. BASE. Fractures producing large fragments involving a third or a half of the articular surface demand open reduction and Kirschner wire fixation (Fig. 16–22). Avulsion of a bone fragment volarly with the flexor profundus tendon requires immediate

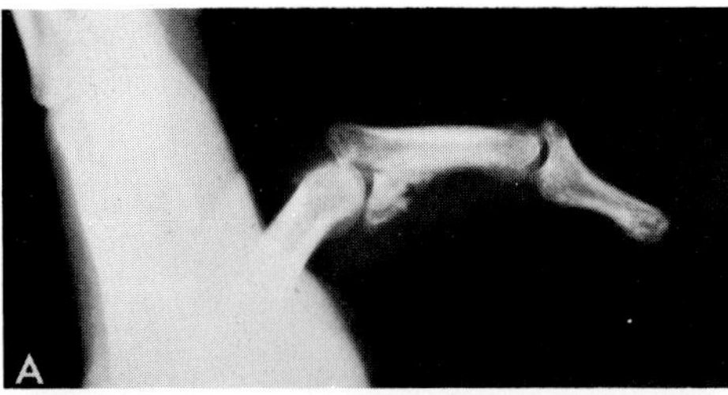

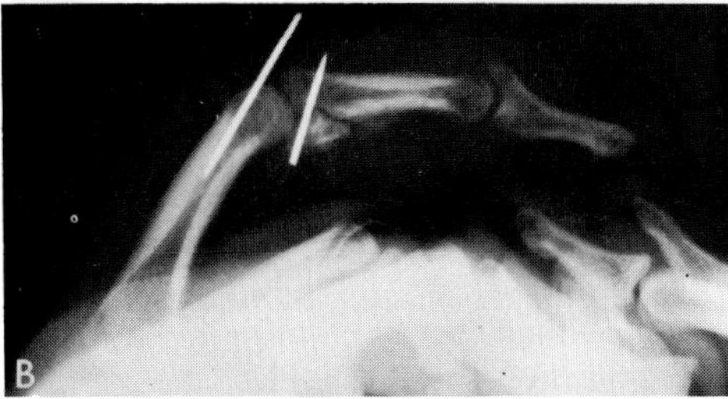

Figure 16–33 *A*, Fracture-dislocation of proximal interphalangeal joint. *B*, Open reduction and Kirschner wire fixation of fracture with temporary Kirschner wire to prevent recurrence of subluxation. (Curtis, R. M.: Joints of the hand. *In* Flynn, J. E. (ed.): Hand Surgery. Baltimore, The Williams & Wilkins Co., 1966.)

surgery consisting of fixation of the fragment with a Bunnell pull-out suture of 4-0 wire. T-type fractures of the base of the distal phalanx are managed by closed or open reduction; proper alignment of the articular surface is essential to a satisfactory result.

SHAFT AND TUFT. Fractures in this area are treated by means of simple splinting of the distal interphalangeal joint for three to four weeks. Radiographic evaluation frequently suggests nonunion although clinically the fracture is stable.

Dislocation

Carpometacarpal Joints. Closed manipulation rarely is successful in treating this severely disabling injury. Inadequate reduction of the metacarpal bases as seen on a lateral x-ray is indication for immediate open reduction with Kirschner wire fixation. Severe muscle and tendon imbalance with inability to flex the metacarpophalangeal joint follows improper treatment (Fig. 16–34).

Metacarpophalangeal Joint. FINGERS. Closed recduction should be attempted but infrequently is prevented by interposition of either joint capsule, natatory ligament or tendon (Kaplan[27]). Open reduction is indicated if there is any question whether a satisfactory reduction has been achieved.

THUMB. Closed manipulation should be attempted but should be followed by open management if the reduction is not entirely satisfactory. Exposure of the joint through a dorsal incision is accomplished by splitting the extensor tendon and retracting the extensor pollicis brevis. The reduction may be maintained with Kirschner wire fixation, if necessary.

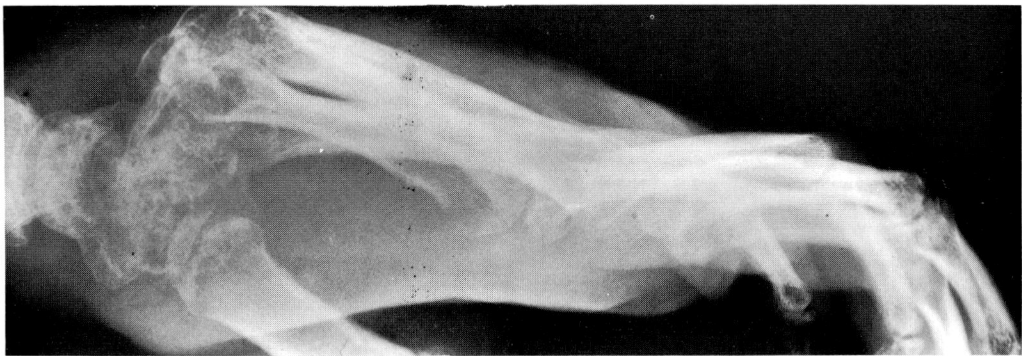

Figure 16–34 Carpometacarpal dislocation. Radiograph shows bases of middle, ring and little finger metacarpals dislocated on the carpus. Muscle and tendon imbalance produce hyperextension of proximal phalanx on metacarpal head and flexion at proximal interphalangeal joints. (Curtis, R. M.: Joints of the hand. *In* Flynn, J. E. (ed.): Hand Surgery. Baltimore, The Williams & Wilkins Co., 1966.)

Rupture of the ulnar collateral ligament of the metacarpophalangeal joint of the thumb requires open reduction (Stener[46]).

Sprain

Finger sprains represent partial tears of the capsular ligament secondary to overangulation of the joint. Early treatment consists of splinting the finger in the position of function for three weeks; the patient removes the splint once daily after the first week and performs slight, active extension and flexion. Aspiration of the joint for hemarthrosis may be indicated early. Injuries seen late exhibit stiffness secondary to thickening of the collateral ligament; pain may be a prominent complaint. Relief of pain in chronic cases may be provided by the injection into the joint of 2 ml. of Triamcinolone Acetonide (Kenalog*).

AMPUTATIONS

The two major problems encountered in dealing with amputations are: adequate closure of the stump and management of the volar digital nerves. Closure of the amputation stump may be accomplished by a variety of procedures (Figs. 16–35 and 16–36).

1. Primary closure with or without resection of bone.
2. A combination of volar and dorsal flaps created by midlateral incisions.
3. A lateral or dorsal flap rotation with skin grafting of the donor area (Fig. 16–36).
4. A local or distant pedicle flap.
5. Combination of two triangular flaps raised laterally from either side of the finger (Kutler method)[22] or a single volar flap on a subcutaneous pedicle.[1]

Partial thickness skin grafts do not provide adequate coverage over bone. Pedicle flaps from adjacent fingers are preferred to thick abdominal flaps. Divided volar digital nerves are placed in a drill hole in the phalanx to reduce the risk of disability from neuroma formation. Simple resection of the nerve, allowing the nerve end to retract proximally, may lead to disability due to compression of the neuroma between bone and objects coming in contact with the hand.

Thumb. Preservation of maximal length by all reconstructive techniques available is mandatory.

*E. R. Squibb & Sons, Inc. New York, N.Y.

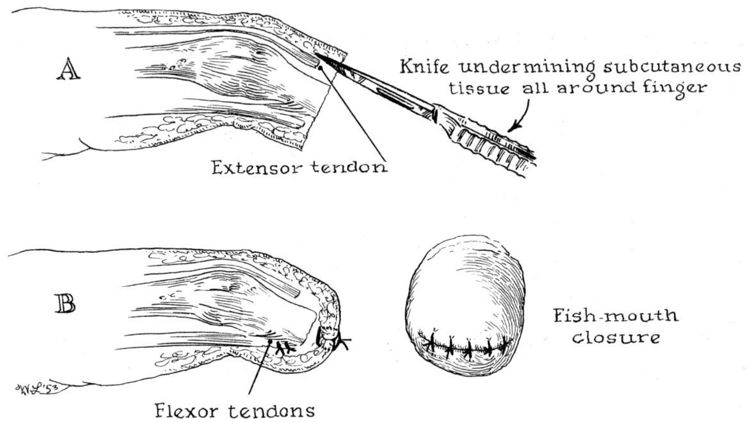

Figure 16 35 Closure amputation of finger by freeing dorsal and volar skin flaps. Lacerated flexor superficialis tendon sutured to tendon sheath.

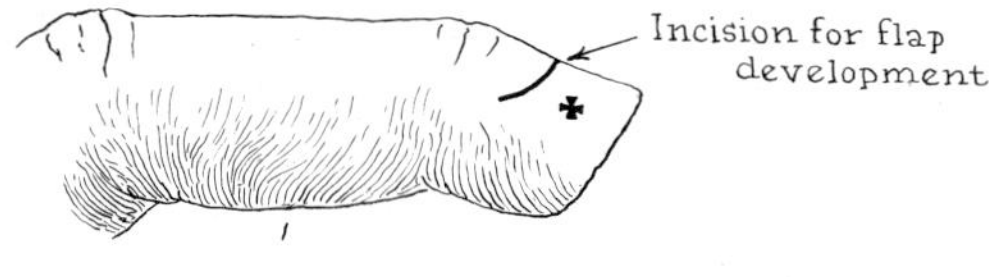

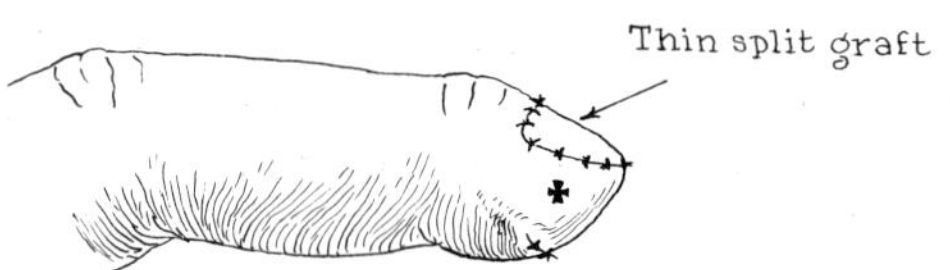

Figure 16–36 Local rotation flap from dorsum of finger for closure of amputation.

Fingers. Decisions regarding treatment must be based on considerations of the occupation and specific needs of the individual. The choice between primary closure following resection of bone and complex reconstructive technique must be made carefully in every patient. Useful function may be retained if proper coverage can be provided with traumatic amputations through the terminal phalanx distal to the flexor and extensor tendon insertions. Amputations through the middle phalanx are best managed by shortening the phalanx and closing the wound with available skin. Care in handling the profundus tendon is necessary to avoid paradoxical extension of the proximal interphalangeal joint due to the "lumbrical plus" syndrome.[39] Maximal length is preserved with amputations through the proximal phalanx, particularly in the little finger. Retention of the proximal phalanx of the index finger may prove a hindrance and require resection through the metacarpal.

INFECTION

Chemotherapy and an appreciation of the importance of hand infections have contributed equally to a decreased incidence and improved management. An attitude of complacency can lead only to disaster in the form of life-threatening systemic infection and permanent crippling of the hand.

Principles of Management

All hand infections of more than minor proportions require hospitalization. The most common organisms are staphylococcus, streptococcus, gram-negative and combination staphylococcus and gram-negative organisms. Antibiotic coverage with a bactericidal drug should be instituted at once on their presumed presence and adjusted when cultures and sensitivities become available.[23] Heat in the form of continuous warm, moist dressings, elevation and immobilization by plaster splint in the position of function are essential. Sedation is frequently necessary in that most serious hand infections are excruciatingly painful. Seriously ill patients require bedrest and parenteral fluid therapy.

The choice between conservative and surgical management demands exceedingly fine judgment. Space infections and localized soft tissue infections require immediate drainage. Premature surgical treatment is to be strictly avoided in the process of cellulitis and progressing lymphangitis. Therapy must be aggressive, whether conservative or surgical.

Operative management of hand infections demands adherence to the same principles employed in elective hand surgery. Virtually all hand infections require general or brachial block anesthesia for adequate drainage. Local infiltration anesthesia is hazardous, and digital gangrene is produced readily by finger block anesthesia. A bloodless field is essential. Incisions and dissection must be anatomically accurate so that important structures are not damaged and uninvolved areas are not contaminated. If there is a wound of entry, it should be explored and drained first before proceeding to other areas. The dictum, "go where the pus is," is appropriate. Through-and-through drainage is to be avoided. Drains, when utilized, are either soft rubber or grease gauze wicks. Proper postoperative management is of utmost importance and consists of sterile dressing technique, continuous moist dressings and physiotherapy as early as possible to prevent joint stiffness. Frequent examination during the postoperative period is essential. The persistence of pain and tenderness is most often due to undrained infection, and a second exploration may be indicated. When doubt exists as to the presence of pus, exploration is advised, especially in children. A negative exploration is much preferred to an overlooked infection. Lastly, the surgeon who overrelies on antibiotics courts disaster; the ideal treatment of closed space infection is still surgical incision and dependent drainage.

Anatomy

Hand infections may be classified into those involving primarily soft tissue and those involving the various potential spaces within the hand. A sound knowledge of anatomy is essential to proper diagnosis and treatment.

Tendon Sheaths. The tendon sheaths of the thumb and little finger extend from the terminal phalanx to a point 2 to 3 cm. proximal to the proximal flexion crease of the wrist. A septum occasionally separates the proximal and distal halves of the sheaths. The proximal halves of the thumb and little finger sheaths are referred to as the radial and ulnar bursae, respectively. The radial and ulnar bursae communicate proximal to the transverse carpal ligament. The tendon sheaths of the index, middle and ring fingers extend from the terminal phalanges to a line joining the radial extremity of the proximal palmar crease with the ulnar extremity of the distal palmar crease. The proximal extremity of the index finger sheath overlies the thenar space. The proximal extremities of the middle and ring finger sheaths overlie the midpalmar space. The tendon sheaths of the index, middle and ring fingers rarely communiate with the ulnar bursa.

Thenar Space. The thenar space is separated from the midpalmar space by a fibrous septum extending from the palmar aponeurosis to the third metacarpal (Fig. 16–37). The thenar space extends from the third metacarpal to the thenar eminence and from the transverse carpal ligament to within 1 cm. of the proximal flexion crease of the index finger. It lies between the flexor tendons and lumbrical muscle of the index finger and the adductor pollicis and extends radially between the deep aspect of the adductor pollicis and the palmar aspect of the first dorsal interosseous muscle.

Midpalmar Space. The midpalmar space (Fig. 16–37) extends from the third metacarpal to the hypothenar eminence; it reaches slightly more proximally than the thenar space. The roof of the midpalmar space is formed by the sheaths of the lubrical muscles to the middle, ring and little fingers.

Parona's Space. Parona's space is a potential space lying between the flexor pollicis longus and flexor digitorum profundus tendons and the pronator quadratus muscle.

It must be emphasized that infections confined initially to a given space may subsequently involve adjacent spaces. The firm attachment of the palmar aponeurosis to the thenar and hypothenar muscles prevents the

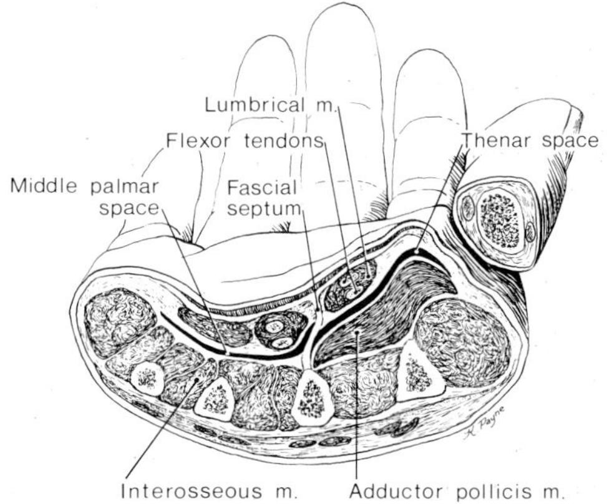

Figure 16–37 Diagram illustrates the midpalmar space and the thenar space and related anatomatical structures in cross section of hand approximately 3 cm. proximal to the metacarpophalangeal joints.

formation of a space in which pus may accumulate. The dorsal subaponeurotic space is not often infected because of the barrier provided by the metacarpals and interosseous muscles.

Lymphatic Drainage. The lymphatics of the fingers, web areas, distal palm, and thenar and hypothenar eminences drain to the lymphatic lakes within the loose areolar tissue on the dorsum of the hand; and the lymphatic trunks from the dorsum accompany the cephalic and basilic veins. The cephalic vein lymphatics drain directly into the nodes of the deltopectoral triangle, whereas the lymphatics accompanying the basilic vein pass through the epitrochlear and axillary nodes. The lymphatics of the central and proximal palm accompany the superficial and deep venous arches to the lymphatics associated with the radial and ulnar arteries. Tremendous edema of the dorsum of the hand is commonly associated with hand infection and, too frequently, is interpreted as localized infection in this area.

Soft Tissue Infections

Folliculitis. A low-grade infection involving the hair follicles occurs most commonly on the dorsum of the proximal phalanx. The process usually clears rapidly with placing the hand at rest and employing continuous warm soaks.

Furuncle. Subcutaneous abscesses usually occur on the dorsum of the proximal phalanx. General or proximal nerve block anesthesia is required for adequate drainage.

Carbuncle. Carbuncles are relatively uncommon but may occasionally be seen on the ulnar aspect of the dorsum of the hand. General or proximal nerve block anesthesia is required for adequate drainage; a linear rather than cruciate incision is utilized.

Collar Button Abscess (Web Space Infection). The thickness of the palmar skin permits formation of a localized abscess immediately beneath the cuticular layer (subcuticular abscess). A collar button abscess which has perforated the dermis to form a deeper abscess or which, in the palmar web area, has perforated the palmar aponeurosis to reach the dorsum of the web. Web space infections may extend proximally within the lumbrical sheaths to enter the thenar or midpalmar spaces.

Paronychia (Run Around). Localized infection between the nail and the cuticle constitutes a paronychia. Pain is a prominent symptom; the cuticle appears erythematous and tense. Early cases are treated simply by elevation of the cuticle; incisions proximally on the dorsum are not necessary. When the nail has become undermined, it acts as a foreign body, and the proximal third of the nail must be excised. Chronic cases exhibit exuberant granulation tissue beneath the cuticle; the granulation tissue and the proximal nail must be removed.

Felon. The multiple fibrous septa attaching the skin to the terminal phalanx form expansionless closed spaces. Infection and only slight swelling within these closed spaces readily produce thrombosis of the terminal branches of the digital arteries with resultant necrosis of the tuft of the terminal phalanx. Severe pain is an outstanding feature of a felon. The distal phalanx is tense, ischemic, hard and exquisitely tender. Drainage is accomplished through a midlateral incision paralleling the volar surface of the distal phalanx (Fig. 16–38*H*). The knife must extend to, but not through, the skin of the opposite side of the finger and must divide all the fibrous septa. Persistent drainage and the presence of exuberant granulation tissue within the incision or a sinus tract indicate osteomyelitis of the terminal phalanx. The bone is not attached surgically; adequate drainage is provided and sequestration allowed.

Human Bite. Wounds produced by human teeth contain virulent anaerobic organisms and spirochetes as well as streptococci and staphylococci

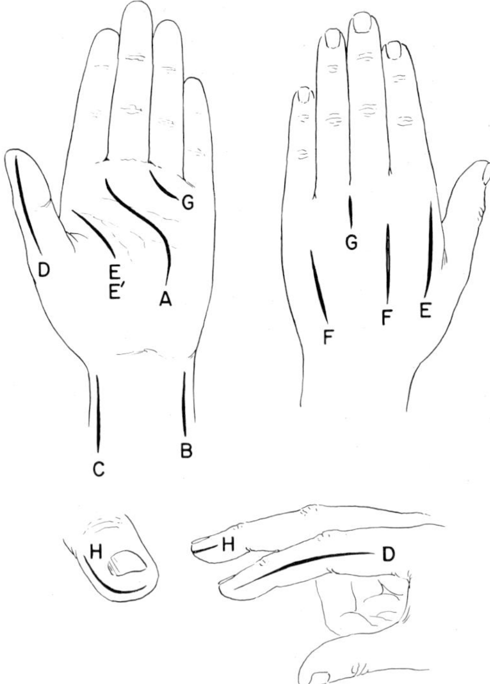

Figure 16–38 Indication of sites for incisions for drainage. *A*, For midpalmar space and palmar portion ulnar bursae. *B*, For ulnar bursae above wrist. *C*, For radial bursae above wrist. *D*, For tenosynovitis of flexor tendon. *E*, For thenar space abscess. *E'*, For palmar portion radial bursae. *F*, For subaponeurotic space. *G*, For collar button abscess palm and dorsum of hand. *H*, For felon. (Redrawn from Boyes, J. H.: Bunnell's Surgery of the Hand. 4th ed. Philadelphia, J. B. Lippincott Co., 1964.)

and can result in truly devastating hand infections. The wound usually overlies a metacarpophalangeal joint, and there is injury of the extensor tendon mechanism and direct contamination of the joint. Extension of infection to the palm occurs via the lumbrical sheaths. The wound is sometimes sustained with fist clenched; later, when the hand opens, the tissues slide back and seal the wound. Under no circumstances are wounds secondary to human bites sutured. Treatment consists of thorough cleansing, irrigation, debridement, adequate drainage, antibiotic therapy, splinting and elevation. Bone sequestration is allowed to separate spontaneously. Reconstructive procedures are deferred until wound healing is complete and the tissues are soft and pliable.

Herpetic Whitlow. Infection of the subcuticular layer of the skin by herpes simplex virus begins as an area of irritation and shortly becomes intensely painful.[47] Deep vesicles appear and spread. This may be resistant to all forms of treatment. Sudden improvement usually occurs within about ten days. The herpetic lesion may become secondarily infected with staphylococci and necessitate drainage.

Space Infections

Tendon Sheath. Suppurative tenosynovitis usually is secondary to a puncture wound over the volar aspect of the distal interphalangeal or proximal interphalangeal joints. Rapid extension of infection within the closed space provided by the tendon sheath leads to early necrosis of the flexor tendon secondary to pressure obstruction of the vincula and may produce systemic symptoms out of proportion to the wound. Severe pain is the outstanding symptom. The diagnosis is established readily on the basis of Kanavel's[26] four cardinal points:

1. The finger is held in flexion.
2. There is uniform swelling over the entire course of the tendon sheath, as opposed to the localized swelling seen with soft tissue infection.
3. There is discrete tenderness over the entire course of the sheath.
4. Passive extension of the finger produces intense pain.

Treatment must be prompt and efficient and consists of early, adequate drainage of the tendon sheath. Delayed treatment results in destruction and loss of function of the flexor tendons; the entire hand may be incapacitated by exudate. Drainage is accomplished through an incision extending from the base of the distal phalanx to the proximal flexion crease of the digit. Finger incisions are placed on the ulnar aspect of the index finger and the radial aspect of the little finger. The sheath is opened throughout its length. The proximal cul-de-sac of the sheath is drained through a transverse incision in the palm immediately distal to the proximal palmar crease. Incisions utilized for draining the tendon sheath of the thumb must extend no further than the midpoint of the first metacarpal in order to avoid injury to the motor branch of the median nerve. Anatomical landmarks may be entirely absent as a result of swelling, and if care is not taken the incision may be found to lie in the volar midline following resolution of the edema. The dorsal ends of the finger flexion creases provide the most accurate guides to placement of the incision (Fig. 16–38*D*).

Radial Bursa. Extension of infection to the radial bursa is manifested by tenderness from the distal phalanx of the thumb to above the carpal ligament. Draining is accomplished through an incision paralleling the thenar eminence and extending from the proximal flexion crease of the thumb to within 2 cm. of the transverse carpal ligament. It must be emphasized that the sensory rami of the median nerve, as well as the motor branch, cross the tendon sheath.

Ulnar Bursa. The earliest sign of infection within the ulnar bursa is an area of maximal tenderness at the point at which the distal palmar crease crosses the hypothenar eminence. Drainage is accomplished through an incision paralleling the hypothenar eminence and extending from the proximal palmar crease to the transverse carpal ligament (Fig. 16–38*A*).

Adequate drainage of the proximal extremities of the radial and ulnar bursae requires an incision in the midulnar line of the wrist immediately proximal to the transverse carpal ligament (Fig. 16–38*B*). The radial and ulnar bursae almost always communicate, and an infection in one is followed by infection in the other. A "horseshoe abscess" involves the tendon sheaths of the thumb and little finger together with the radial and ulnar bursae.

Parona's Space. Infection within Parona's space is secondary to infection of the radial or ulnar bursae or to infection within the midpalmar space. The diagnosis is based on localized swelling and tenderness on the volar aspect of the wrist immediately proximal to the transverse carpal ligament. Drainage is accomplished through an incision in the midulnar line of the wrist (Fig. 16–38*B*).

Thenar Space. Thenar space infections are secondary to direct puncture wounds or suppurative tenosynovitis of the index finger. The typical appearance of the hand consists of massive swelling of the soft tissues between the thumb and index metacarpals, with the thumb pushed away from the hand. Tenderness is maximal in the first interosseous space. Drainage is accomplished through an incision on the dorsal aspect of the thumb-index web paralleling the web margin and extending between the heads of the thumb and index metacarpals (Fig. 16–38 *E* & *E'*).

Midpalmar Space. Infections within the midpalmar space are secondary to direct puncture wounds or suppurative tenosynovitis of the middle or ring fingers. Severe pain and marked systemic toxicity are characteristic. The normal palmar concavity is lost, and the palm is flat and extremely tense. Tenderness is maximal in the center of the palm. Drainage is accomplished through a transverse incision immediately proximal to the distal palmar crease (Fig. 16–38*A*).

CHEMICAL INJURIES

Injection Injuries

Popularly known as "grease gun" injuries, a variety of devices in modern America are capable of injections, foreign and frequently caustic substances such as plastic and paint, into the hand at pressures varying from 1000 to 15,000 lbs./sq. in.[33] They may appear deceptively innocuous initially but rapidly progress to ischemia and gangrene if unrecognized and untreated. The clues to diagnosis are the history, a small puncture wound and mild discomfort which rapidly changes to exquisite pain. Initial redness about the wound becomes ashen gray, hard and tender. Treatment is wide surgical incision and exploration of all suspicious areas. Involved tissue must be debrided, removing as much of the offending agent as possible and employing open treatment. The postoperative course is often indolent and further debridement may be necessary. Many such cases eventually result in amputation.

Drug Related Injuries

The incidence of complaints related to various drug injections has paralleled their increased usage by the population. Three separate problems may occur, although they frequently are seen together.[36]

If infection is present, it must be recognized and treated as previously described. Many patients present with histories of "skin-popping" and inflammatory processes secondary to chemical irritation. Although many of the drugs employed are not themselves noxious, the diluents, notably sucrose, quinine and the like, are hypertonic and highly irritating.

The distinction between such inflammatory processes and outright infection is often difficult or impossible to make, but the former responds to bed rest, elevation, warm soaks and antibiotics.

Occasionally, injection is inadvertently made intra-arterially, resulting in spasm, thrombosis and distal ischemia. A variety of methods of treatment involving anticoagulants, antivasospastic agents, early fasciotomy and early arterial exploration have been only partially successful. The ultimate outcome of this injury is frequently amputation.

The accompanying problems of drug users, such as hepatitis, addiction and profound psychiatric disturbance, all combine to make this group of patients especially pathetic and difficult to treat. Their unreliability, uncooperative nature and unwillingness to return for follow-up visits pose a challenge to the hand surgeon unlike any other with which he must deal.

REFERENCES

1. Atasoy, E., Ioakimidis, E., Kasdan, M. L., Kutz, J. E., and Kleinert, H. E.: Reconstruction of the amputated fingertip with a triangular volar flap. J. Bone Joint Surg. *52A*:921, 1970.
2. Beasley, R. W.: Reconstruction of amputated fingertips. Plast. Reconstr. Surg. *44*:349, 1969.
3. Bohler, L.: Treatment of Fractures. 4th ed. Baltimore, William Wood & Co., 1935.
4. Boyes, J. H.: A philosophy of care of the injured hand. Bull. Am. Coll. Surg. *50*:341, 1965.
5. Boyes, J. H.: Bunnell's Surgery of the Hand. 4th ed. Philadelphia, J. B. Lippincott Co., 1964.
6. Boyes, J. H.: Demonstration of Arm Board for Hand Surgery. American Academy of Orthopaedic Surgeons, 1950.
7. Boyes, J. H.: Discussion of paper by Van't Hof, A., and Heiple, K. G.: Flexor tendon injuries. J. Bone Joint Surg. *40A*:262, 1958.
8. Boyes, J. H.: *In* Cramer, L. M., and Chase, Robert A. (eds.): Symposium on the Hand. St. Louis, C. V. Mosby Co., 1971, p. 191.
9. Boyes, J. H.: Evaluation of digital flexor tendon grafts. Am. J. Surg., *89*:1116, 1955.
10. Bruner, J. M.: Safety factors in the use of the pneumatic tourniquet for hemostasis in surgery of the hand. J. Bone Joint Surg. *33*:221, 1951.
11. Bruner, J. M.: The zig-zag volar-digital incision for flexor-tendon surgery. Plast. Reconst. Surg. *40*:571, 1967.
12. Bunnell, S.: Surgery of nerves of the hand. Surg. Gynec. Obstet. *44*:145, 1927.
13. Bunnell, S.: The early treatment of hand injuries. J. Bone Joint Surg., *33*:807, 1951.
14. Bunnel, S., and Boyes, J. H.: Nerve grafts. Am. J. Surg. *44*:64, 1939.
15. Burkhalter, W. E., Butler, B., Metz, W., and Omer, G.: Experiences with delayed primary closure of war wounds of the hand in Viet Nam. J. Bone Joint Surg. *50A*:945, 1968.
16. Curtis, R. M.: Reconstruction of the acutely injured hand. Maryland Med. J., *5*: 675, 1956.

17. Curtis, R. M.: Cross-finger pedicle flap in hand surgery. Ann. Surg. *145*:650, 1957.
18. Curtis, R. M.: Joints of the hand. *In* Flynn, J. E. (ed.): Hand Surgery. Baltimore, The Williams & Wilkins Co., 1966.
19. Curtis, R. M.: Lecture, Repair of Flexor Tendon Injuries. Emory University Hospital, April 1, 1966.
20. Curtis, R. M.: Capsulectomy of the interphalangeal joints of the fingers. J. Bone Joint Surg. *36A*:1219, 1954.
21. Dupont, C. G., and Crikelair, G. F.: A review of 135 cases of tendon lacerations in the hand and wrist. J. Bone Joint Surg. *42A*:913, 1960.
22. Fisher, R. H.: The Kutler method of repair of finger tip amputations. Proceedings Am. Soc. Surg. Hand. J. Bone Joint Surg. *48*:606, 1966.
23. Friedberg, A., and Waddell, J. P.: Proceedings of the American Society for Surgery of the Hand. J. Bone Joint Surg. *54A*:896, 1972.
24. Hunter, J. M., and Salisbury, R. E.: Flexor-tendon reconstruction in severely damaged hand. J. Bone Joint Surg. *53A*:829, 1971.
25. James, J. I. P.: Fractures of the phalanges and metacarpals. Proceedings of meeting British Hand Club for Surgery of the Hand, May 14, 1965.
26. Kanavel, A. C.: Infections of the Hand. (7th Ed.) Philadelphia, Lea & Febiger, 1939.
27. Kaplan, E. B.: Dorsal dislocation of the metacarpophalangeal joint of the index finger. J. Bone Joint Surg. *41A*:1081, 1959.
28. Kelleher, J. C., Sullivan, J. G., Baibak, G. J., and Dean, R. K.: The Distant Pedicle Flap in Surgery of the Hand. Orth. Clin. N. Amer. *1*:227, 1970.
29. Kleinert, H. E.: Presented at Society of Plastic and Reconstructive Surgeons, Los Angeles, California, October 6, 1970.
30. Littler, J. W.: The severed flexor tendon. Surg. Clin. N. Amer.. *39*:435, 1959.
31. Madsen, E.: Delayed primary suture of flexor tendons cut in the digital sheath. J. Bone Joint Surg. *52B*:264, 1970.
32. Mason, M. L.: Fifty years of progress in hand surgery. Surg. Gynec. Obstet. (Int. Abst. Surg.) *101*(6):541, 1955.
33. Meagher, S. W.: Special Wounds. *In* Flynn, J. E. (ed.): Hand Surgery. Baltimore, The Williams & Wilkins Co., 1966.
34. Milford, L.: The hand. *In* Crenshaw, A. H. (ed.): Campbell's Operative Orthopedics. (4th Ed.) St. Louis, C. V. Mosby Co., 1963, vol. 1.
35. Millesi, H., Meissl, G., and Berger, A.: The interfascicular nerve-grafting of the median and ulnar nerves. J. Bone Joint Surg. *54A*:727, 1972.
36. Neviaser, R. J., Butterfield, W. C., and Wieche, D. R.: The puffy hand of drug addiction. J. Bone Joint Surg. *54A*: 629, 1972.
37. Nicholson, O. R., and Seddon, H. J.: Nerve repair in civil practice. Brit. Med. J. *2*:1065, 1957.
38. Onné, L.: Recovery of sensibility and sudomotor activity in the hand after nerve suture. Acta. Chir. Scand. (Suppl. 300), 1962.
39. Parkes, A.: The "lumbrical plus" finger. The Hand *2*:164, 1970.
40. Potenza, A. D.: Tendon healing within the flexor digital sheath in the dog. J. Bone Joint Surg. *44A*:49, 1962.
41. Pulvertaft, R. G.: Tendon grafts for flexor tendon injuries in fingers and thumb; study of technique and results. J. Bone Joint Surg. *38B*:175, 1956.
42. Robertson, R. C., Cawley, J. J., Jr., and Faris, A. M.: Treatment of fracture, dislocation of the interphalangeal joints of the hand. J. Bone Joint Surg. *28*:68, 1946.
43. Seddon, H. J. (ed.): Peripheral Nerve Injuries. Medical Research Council Special Series No. 282. London, Her Majesty's Stationery Office, 1954.
44. Seddon, H. J.: Nerve grafting. J. Bone Joint Surg. *45B*:447, 1963.
45. Skoog, T., and Persson, B. H.: An experimental study of the early healing of tendons. Plast. Reconstr. Surg. *13*:384, 1954.
46. Stener, B.: Displacement of the ruptured ulnar collateral ligament of the metacarpophalangeal joint of the thumb. A clinical anatomical study. J. Bone Joint Surg. *44B*:869, 1962.
47. Stern, H., Elek, S. D., Millar, D. M., and Anderson, H. F.: Herpetic whitlow. Lancet *2*:871, 1959.
48. Strange, F. G. St. C.: An operation for nerve pedicle grafting. Preliminary communication. Brit. J. Surg. *34*:423, 1947.
49. Sunderland, S.: The intraneural topography of the radial, median, and ulnar nerves. Brain *68*:243, 1945.
50. Van't Hof, A., and Heiple, K. G.: Flexor tendon injuries of the fingers and thumb. J. Bone Joint Surg. *40A*:256, 1958.
51. Verdan, C.: Practical considerations for primary and secondary repair in flexor tendon injuries. Surg. Clin. N. Amer. *44*:951, 1964.
52. Wakefield, A. R.: Management of flexor tendon injuries. Surg. Clin. N. Amer. *40*:267, 1960.
53. Zachary, R. B.: Results of nerve suture in peripheral nerve injuries. *In* Seddon, H. J. (ed.): Peripheral Nerve Injuries. Medical Research Council Special Report Series No. 282, London, Her Majesty's Stationery Office, 1954, pp. 354–388.
54. Zachary, R. B., and Holmes, W.: Primary suture of nerves. Surg. Gynec. Obstet. *82*:622, 1946.

chapter

17

INITIAL MANAGEMENT OF FRACTURES AND JOINT INJURIES: THORACIC AND LUMBAR SPINE, PELVIS AND HIP

James L. Hughes, M.D.

The physician in the accident room setting, by his expertise in the diagnosis and initial management of an injured patient, can play a major role in how rapidly the patient may return to normal activity. Many long-term problems can be prevented by the appropriate initial management. This chapter will be limited to the general principles of initial diagnosis and treatment so as to guide a house officer or generalist prior to a consultation with the appropriate specialist. Where applicable, an outline of definitive care will be given.

Each physician responsible for the initial care of an accident victim must recognize that each injury requires a rapid diagnosis coupled with steps to prevent deterioration. Nowhere is this more true than in fractures of the spine and the pelvis. It must be remembered that these fractures are frequently associated with other injuries. It is good practice to alert the patient and his family, if possible, that other injuries may remain undisclosed for several days while attention is directed toward obvious life-threatening problems.

THORACOLUMBAR SPINE

Spinal injuries range from a paravertebral muscle contusion with little or no effect on the patient, to a dislocation of the thoracolumbar vertebrae with paraplegia. In all cases of trauma, damage to the spine must be considered and ruled out by appropriate examinations. It is estimated that approximately 7000 new cases of permanent injury to the spinal cord occur each year. Improper care in the emergency room may contribute to permanent damage, and it is this fact that governs the protocol for emergency care.

Evidence of Injury. Every accident victim should be quickly examined for weakness or paralysis, sensory impairment and pain or tenderness along the spine. A thorough neurological examination should not be done at the time the patient is first seen, but should be performed later when all parameters are stable. Until confirmation of stability is made via specific examinations, all spinal injuries are to be considered unstable.

Initial treatment should actually begin at the scene of the accident by a well-trained ambulance crew. If the patient arrives in the emergency room in a position other than a prone or supine one, this should be accomplished immediately. An emergency stretcher, such as that manufactured by the Stryker Corp. (Fig. 17–1), is useful in maintaining the proper position. Upon arrival into the accident room, all clothing is removed without altering the position of the patient. If a neurological deficit is present, great care is taken to prevent the patient from lying on any objects that may begin pressure necrosis of the skin (Decubitus ulcer).

Documentation should be made immediately as to the adequacy of the airway, the presence or absence of shock and the level of consciousness. Neurological injuries may cause a distortion of physical findings. Injuries to the abdomen may be masked by spinal cord injury. Loss of the normal pain sensation may cause a ruptured viscus to go unrecognized. With flaccid paralysis the abdomen may remain soft when the presence of blood, intestinal contents or urine in the peritoneal cavity would normally cause board-like rigidity. The opposite may also occur, in that with partial cord transection, rigidity of the abdomen may occur where no intra-abdominal pathology is present.

Spinal shock is a state that may immediately follow spinal trauma in which the cord is transected. Transection may occur either as a result of a complete laceration of the cord or by temporary loss of the blood supply, a physiological transection. In spinal shock all muscles below the level of the lesion are completely paralyzed, tone is lost and reflexes are initially abolished. When the lesion is above the thoracolumbar area, there is a

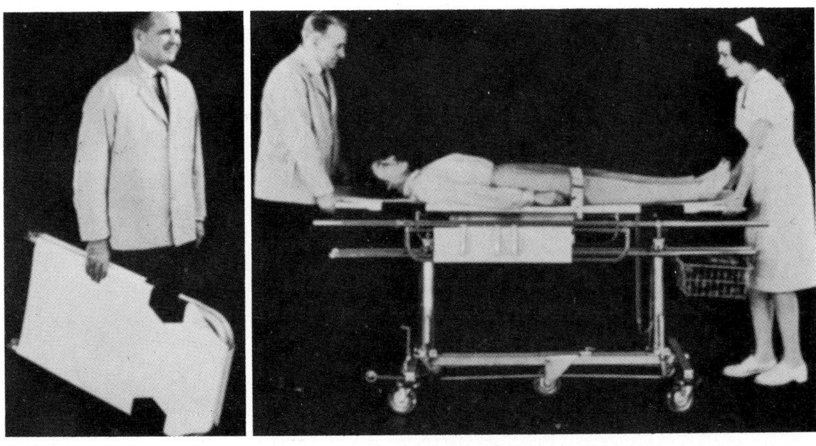

Figure 17–1 Emergency stretcher (used by permission Stryker Corporation).

temporary drop in blood pressure due to peripheral pooling of blood. In spinal shock the decrease in blood pressure is usually not accompanied by tachycardia. When one finds tachycardia and a falling hematocrit, attention should be turned toward the extremities, chest or abdomen in an attempt to find a source for hemorrhage.

A careful examination should be made of the lower extremities. In paraplegia the normal "pain signal" will be absent and a fracture or major vascular injury may be easily overlooked. A thorough manual examination should be made of all major joints and long bones and the distal pulses checked.

Approximately 30 per cent of patients having thoracic or lumbar spine injuries have concomitant lesions with the majority being craniocerebral in nature. A comatose or stuporous patient presents a difficult evaluation problem. Attention should be paid to any movement the patient makes in order to analyze the presence or absence of muscular activity. Only in profound coma will the normal withdrawal to painful stimulus be absent, provided the cord is intact. Usually, if one foot is raised and dropped directly over the other, the descending heel will not strike the resting foot unless paralysis is present in the falling limb. Care must be taken to control the comatose patient on the stretcher. Straps over the lower extremities should be separated from the skin by soft pliable material.

Preliminary Management. An adequate airway is the first priority. The standard procedures for maintaining an adequate airway have been covered elsewhere and may be applied here.

Circulatory support is next in order and this is accomplished by an intravenous infusion through a number 18 needle. When the I.V. is being started, blood should be drawn for type and cross-match, hematocrit, white blood count and differential, and electrolytes.

Attention should be paid next to the urinary tract. A number 14 or 16 French foley catheter should be utilized under strict aseptic technique. The amount of urine obtained should be carefully recorded. The catheter should then be placed to straight drainage.

Definitive Diagnosis and Management. Once emergency care has been rendered and the patient is stable and under control, a careful and thorough examination can be undertaken.

If the patient is conscious, a history should be obtained as to how the injury occurred and, if paraplegia is present, whether the onset was acute or gradual. In addition to this brief but important history, the patient should be asked to pin-point any area of pain or tenderness. Directions should be given to move the lower extremities and the presence or absence of movement recorded.

A detailed neurological examination should now be undertaken covering every dermatome of the trunk and lower extremity. It is helpful to have a chart, showing the dermatome distribution, on the wall of the accident room. Movement, sensation, tone and reflex changes should be recorded. This initial record is critical, for without an accurate and thorough recording of this examination, future changes in the neurological picture cannot be appreciated. Table 17–1 shows the common findings in injuries to the thoracic and lumbar vertebrae with cord damage.

An examination of the back should next be undertaken without moving the patient. If the patient is supine, the examining hand may be slipped gently beneath the patient. Prominence of spinous processes, local tenderness, palpable or visible deformities and the presence of muscle spasm help to delineate the area of injury. Abrasions should be noted about the abdomen, for this may lead one to suspect a seat-belt injury.

If a thorough physical examination of the extremities, abdomen, chest and head were not accomplished initially, it should now be done.

Special Diagnostic Procedures. After the physical examination determines the probable level of injury,

TABLE 17–1 TYPICAL FINDINGS WITH INJURY TO THE THORACIC OR LUMBAR SPINAL CORD

1. Injury of T–1 to T–12
   a. paraplegia
   b. Initial absent deep tendon reflexes in lower extremities, absent cremasteric and plantar reflexes; upper abdominal reflexes may be preserved in low thoracic lesions.
   c. Anesthesia below the dermatome level on the trunk corresponding with level of cord damage.
   d. Bladder and bowel retention; priapism in male.
2. Injury of L–1 to L–5
   a. Partial flaccid paraplegia, the extent depending on which roots of the cauda equina are involved.
   b. Above L-2 knee and ankle jerks and plantar reflexes are absent; cremasteric reflexes present. Below L-2 knee jerks are present.
   c. Anesthesia of perineum, sacral area, and lower extremities may be spotty and asymmetrical.
   d. Bladder and bowel retention at least temporarily but perhaps with some retention of sensation.

AP and lateral radiographs are made without moving the patient. This study should include at least four vertebral bodies above and below the suspected level of injury. These roentgenograms are examined for the contour and alignment of the vertebral bodies and the presence or absence of bone fragments protruding into the spinal canal. The most common area of injury, in which the cord is damaged, is at the junction of the mobile lumbar spine, and the less mobile thoracic spine. Special attention should be paid to this area, looking for a slice fragment of the upper border of the body of the lower vertebrae (see Fig. 17–3*B* and *C*). If found, this represents the most unstable of all the injuries to the thoracolumbar spine. It must be kept in mind that all fractures of the spine will appear stable in the supine or prone position. If any questions arise as to the presence or absence of stability after the initial x-rays, tomograms should be taken.

Spinal taps should not be done as a routine procedure on these patients. This procedure should only be done in conjunction with a myelogram. There is a great difference of opinion as to when these procedures should be carried out. Consideration should be given to doing them if one suspects a block in a fracture dislocation or if protrusion into the cord by a fragment of bone or an intervertebral disc is suspected. Normal manometric studies in the spinal tap are more significant than an abnormal study, for tears in the dura or cord edema may prevent a rise in pressure on jugular compression.

Early Definitive Therapy. Open injuries of the vertebral column and spinal cord are extremely rare. When present, surgical repair is carried out as in any other soft tissue injury. A laminectomy is indicated if there is a persistent spinal fluid leak, indicating a laceration of the dura either by bone or a foreign body. All tears of the dura should be closed, utilizing fascial graft if necessary. Antibiotic coverage intravenously is indicated in conjunction with copious and frequent irrigation during surgery in an attempt to abort meningitis. Many of these injuries will be secondary to a puncture wound with the point of entry away from the midline.

Paravertebral Muscle Tear. A paravertebral muscle tear will reveal acute spasm and a list toward the injured area. X-ray examination will be within normal limits save for perhaps a scoliosis secondary to muscle spasm. Treatment is directed toward ablation of pain by the appropriate analgesics, bed rest and warm compresses.

Intervertebral Disc Injury. Protrusion of an intervertebral disc may be diagnosed by the history and physical findings that include a positive straight-leg-raising test in association with reflex and sensory changes. Positive identification is made by a myelogram. Conservative care of an acute disc should be undertaken initially just as was recommended for the paravertebral muscle tear.

Wedge or Compression Fractures. Wedge or compression fractures (Fig. 17–2A) are the most common fractures of the thoracic-lumbar spine in persons under fifty years of age. These occur most commonly as a result of a fall from a height in which the patient lands on his feet, transmitting acute flexion forces to the spine. The injury may well be coupled with a fracture of the os calcis. Occasionally, falling objects may strike the patient's shoulder, causing acute flexion of the spine and a compression fracture of the thoracic spine. In persons over fifty years of age certain pathologic conditions such as multiple myeloma, metastatic tumors, or osteoporosis may predispose the patient to a fracture of the vertebral bodies with a minimum of external force. Occasionally, coughing, sneezing or just getting out of a chair may be the only history obtained.

X-rays will show a diminution in the anterior height of the vertebral body. This diminution in height may be from 10 to 90 per cent of the vertebral body. Neurologic deficit rarely occurs with this fracture, for the posterior elements remain intact.

Early treatment in the younger age group can be outlined as follows. The patient must at all times remain supine, having been given enough sedation to overcome the severe discomfort. It must be kept in mind that adynamic ileus may occur secondary to the paravertebral hematoma accompanying this fracture. If ileus occurs, I.V. fluids along with a nasogastric tube must be utilized. If the collapse of the

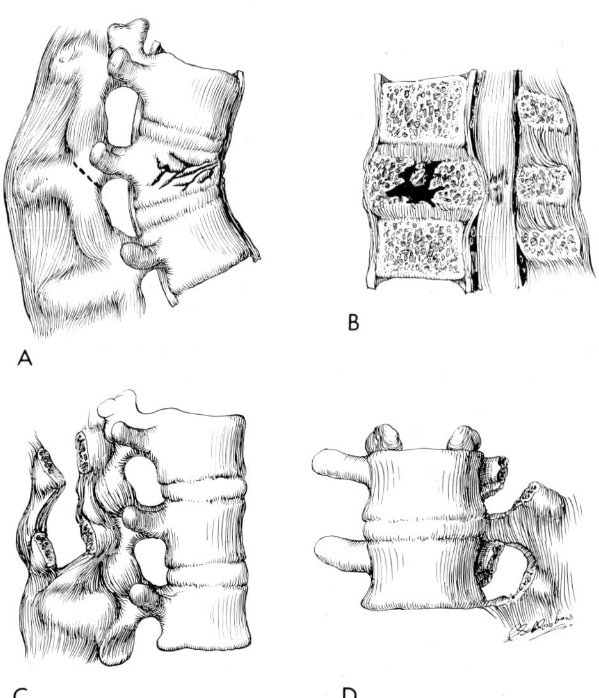

Figure 17–2 Stable thoracolumbar spine fractures.

vertebral body is over 30 per cent of the total height of the body, the patient should be carefully placed with his head at the foot of a hospital bed in order that the knee-gatch can be utilized to obtain hyperextension of the fractured area. A hinged fracture board is placed between the mattress and springs. The knee-gatch is then gradually elevated at approximately one turn of the crank per hour until it is believed that sufficient extension has been accomplished to reduce the fracture. This method should obtain some reduction by tension on the anterior longitudinal ligament. A lateral x-ray should be taken to confirm the amount of reduction obtained. When the patient stabilizes, he should be transferred to a Goldthwait frame for application of a hyperextension plaster jacket. Care must be taken in applying this plaster jacket to obtain pressure over three important bony prominences: the upper sternum and anterior chest, the iliac crests and the spine directly overlying the level of the fractured vertebra. Care must be taken to cover the iliac crest, rib margins, pubic and upper sternum with felt pads. Hyperextension exercises should be initiated very early after the injury, for maintenance of an adequate paravertebral musculature is of prime importance in lowering the morbidity of this fracture. If the collapse is less than 30 per cent of the total height of the body, rest followed by hyperextension exercises will be sufficient treatment for a good result. In persons over fifty years of age or in persons who have sustained minimum trauma, complete bed rest with the patient flat in bed coupled with the early use of hyperextension exercises will be adequate early treatment. Early mobilization of the patient can be accomplished by the use of the Taylor back brace. Appropriate attention should be paid to any pre-existing pathology which predisposed to the fracture.

"Burst" Fracture. "Burst" fractures (Fig. 17–2*B*) are similar to compression injuries except that in this instance the line of force is almost perpendicular to the vertebral column. As the forces are transmitted down the column, the affected vertebral body appears to explode. Due to the projection of fragments posteriorly, there may occasionally be a neurological deficit. This deficit is usually transitory in nature but if not, a myelogram should be done. If a block is demonstrated, appropriate surgical decompression should be accomplished.

If decompression is not necessary, treatment consists of bed rest in neutral position. The hyperextended position should be avoided. When the patient stabilizes, a plaster jacket should be applied in neutral position, or an appropriate spinal brace may be used. Owing to the multiplicity of fragments coupled with intact ligamentous structures surrounding these fragments, the fracture will heal very rapidly.

Transverse Process Fractures. Transverse process fractures (Fig. 17–2*D*) occur occasionally in the lumbar spine as an avulsion injury secondary to violent, sudden muscle contraction. The injury may also occur from a direct blow. Radiographic evidence of this fracture may be obtained on the AP view. The jagged line found at the fracture, along with the findings of tenderness and spasm, will separate this entity from a congenital separation. Treatment for this fracture should be directed toward making the patient comfortable. Bed rest for several days along with the appropriate analgesic is all that is necessary. Care should be taken to explain to the patient that he has no chance for neurological damage. Avoidance of over-treatment is strongly encouraged.

Spinous Processes. The spinous processes (Fig. 17–2*C*) may be fractured by direct trauma, as with an object falling from a height and striking the patient's flexed spine, or indirect trauma, such as the violent muscle pull associated with "clay-shoveler's" fracture. This latter fracture occurs primarily at the T–1 level. Diagnosis is made on physical examination and by lateral x-ray. No attempt at reduction should be undertaken and the patient should be treated symptomatically. No neurological deficit is found with this injury.

Unstable Fractures. All patients with acute traumatic injury to the spine should be treated as unstable until proved otherwise. Any degree of malalignment, however small, in either AP or lateral view of the spine should make the physician suspect instability. A "slice wedge" fracture of the upper part of the lower vertebra, when seen on both the AP and lateral x-rays, is indicative of a fracture-dislocation and denotes a very unstable situation (Fig. 17–3 *B* and *C*). Almost all of the fractures that are unstable will be found in the T–2, L–1 area. Even with severe trauma the thoracic spine remains stable owing to the rib attachments. L-1, L-2, and L-3 are most commonly involved in seat-belt injuries (Fig. 17–4*A* and *B*). Almost all of these fractures have either a complete or partial neurological deficit. Regardless of whether the neurological deficit is partial or complete, extreme caution must be maintained in the movement and care of these patients, for there may be the possibility of some neurological return. Any motor power or sensation present below the level of cord damage indicates a partial lesion of the cord. Total loss of sensation below the cord lesion is an indication of cord transection, especially if reflexes controlled by the segments below the lesion are present. Holdsworth feels that if complete loss of motor power and sensation persist longer than 24 hours irreparable damage to the cord is certain.[1]

Fractures of the posterior elements (Fig. 17–3A) may occur as a result of direct trauma or from hyperextension.

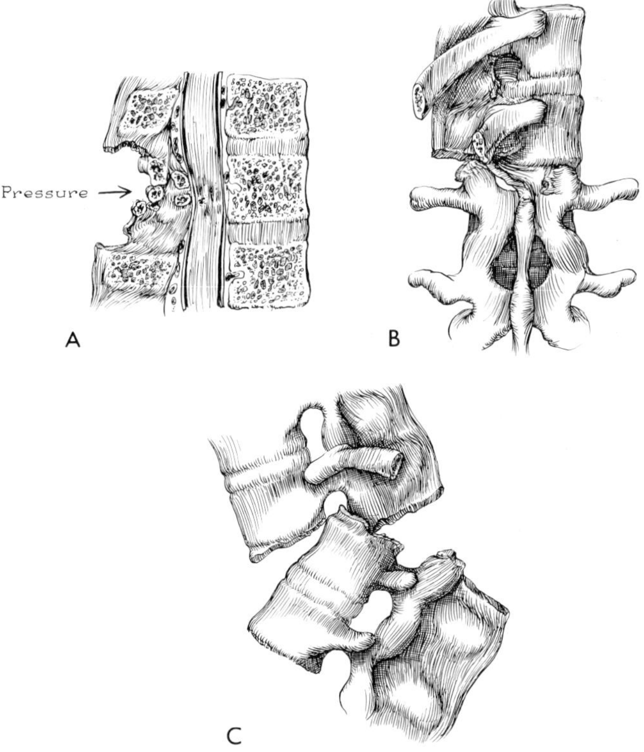

Figure 17–3 Unstable thoracolumbar spine fractures.

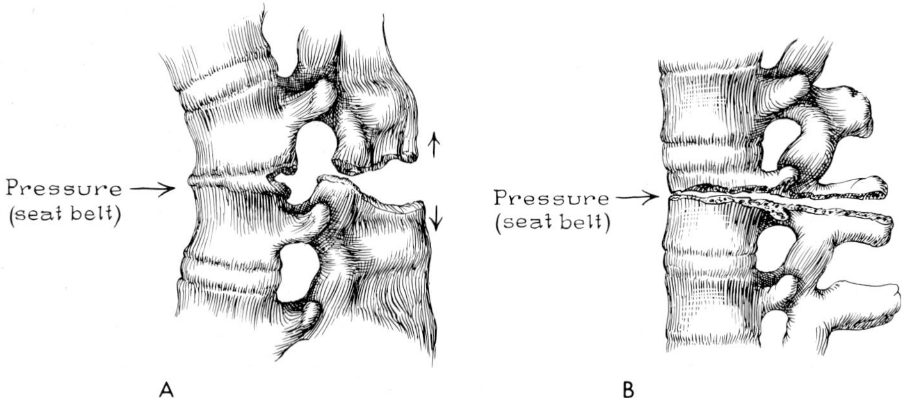

Figure 17–4 Unstable thoracolumbar spine fractures.

These are rare injuries but may be associated with injury to the spinal cord and should be considered unstable.

When the diagnosis of instability is made, appropriate nursing care is begun. The patient should be turned every two hours on a Foster Frame or a CircOlectric bed. An orthopedist and neurosurgeon should be consulted in order that a decision for definitive therapy may be made.

FRACTURES OF THE PELVIS

The pelvic ring is composed of the ilium, ischium, pubic and sacral bones, providing multiple functions. A number of early and late complications are associated with fractures of the pelvis. Because one of the early complications, hemorrhage, may lead to death, it is important to consider and diagnose fractures of the pelvis early. In combining all types of pelvic fractures, there is an average blood loss of two units. Other complications found in a high percentage of cases include rupture of the bladder, urethra or intestine. Any combination of these may be found in any patient.

These fractures are produced primarily by falls from a height, automobile crashes and crushing trauma. Less severe fractures are produced in the elderly by a simple fall and in the young by an avulsion of a muscle attachment.

Evidence of Injury. Evidence of a pelvic girdle fracture, which should be searched for on any accident victim, includes mobility of the symphysis pubis, lower limb paresis or hypesthesia, hematuria and perineal ecchymosis.

In order to adequately examine the patient, all clothing should be carefully removed. At all times the patient should remain in a supine position on a stretcher. Examination of the pelvic ring may be carried out in the following manner. The examining hands should be placed on the anterior-superior iliac spines and outward pressure gently applied. If the ring is broken, there will be an opening of the fracture and the patient will experience discomfort. Pressure over the symphysis pubis will demonstrate tenderness in a fracture of the pubic rami. Leg length discrepancy can be noted visually and documented by measuring the distance from the anterior-superior iliac spines to the medial malleoli. Attention should be directed toward the perineum, for swelling or discoloration in this area may indicate extravasation of urine or blood. Prior to any treatment of the fractures it is necessary that the patient's condition be stable. The blood pressure is monitored and recorded every five minutes or more frequently if shock is present. A number 18 needle or larger is utilized for transmission of I.V. fluids. A blood sample is sent promptly for typing and cross-matching; a minimum of five units of whole blood is set up. The monitoring of central venous pressure, urine output and hematocrit is a useful guide to fluid replacement. The presence of profound shock may necessitate utilizing a plasma expander such as dextran. If blood replacement is not keeping up with the loss, consideration is given to an abdominal exploration, looking for a tear of the iliolumbar or internal pudendal arteries or the iliac veins. If a retroperitoneal hematoma is found, it should not be opened, for more bleeding will occur, and this complication is not easily controlled. Ligation of the internal iliac artery is not helpful because of the rich collateral circulation. No manipulation of the fracture should occur prior to control of the bleeding, for this will only increase the blood loss. The degree of blood loss is proportional to the number of fractures of the pelvis. Bleeding from the fracture sites can be controlled by reduction and stabilization of the fractures.

Injury to the genitourinary tract, especially to the bladder, may complicate even the most minor injury to the pelvis. The integrity of the urinary tract should be confirmed in every pelvic injury regardless of how insignificant the injury may appear. A distended bladder is extremely vulnerable to any trauma about the pelvis. The bladder rupture may produce intraperitoneal extravasation of urine, resulting in acute peritonitis, or more commonly the rupture may be extraperitoneal, thus permitting urine to escape into the regional tissue spaces. Urethral injuries occur primarily in the male, usually in association with fractures involving the pubic rami and symphysis. The urethra is usually torn at the apex of the prostate and in most cases the tear is complete. If a urethral tear is present, the prostate may be freely moveable on rectal examination. If spontaneous voiding is not possible, a catheter is passed utilizing sterile technique. Bleeding from the urethral meatus or difficulty in passing the catheter should alert one to a probable urethral tear. The diagnosis of a tear is confirmed by retrograde urethrogram. With a catheter in place, urine is obtained and examined for hematuria. The presence of hematuria is not by itself significant, for this may occur simply from contusion to the bladder. Tears of the bladder are confirmed by the injection of radiopaque contrast material into the catheter followed by a roentgenogram. Extravasation of the contrast material may be noted, or the bladder may simply be pushed aside by a pelvic hematoma. An intravenous pyelogram may reveal a laceration of the renal parenchyma. In profound shock this latter study is not indicated, as the kidneys will not visualize.

Actual laceration or entrapment of the bowel may occur in the more severe fractures. Other known associated injuries include laceration of the vagina, rectum and diaphragm.[2]

Diagnostic Confirmation. An anterior-posterior x-ray of the pelvis is sufficient to permit classification of a fracture into the stable (Fig. 17–5) or unstable (Fig. 17–6) variety. Occasionally, a lateral x-ray is indicated to document displacement of a sacral fracture.

Specific Fractures. The pelvic skeleton is anchorage for powerful locomotor muscles. In youth sudden contraction of a muscle against resistance, such as in a hurdler or sprinter, may avulse the anterior superior iliac spine or the ischial tuberosity (Fig. 17–5). In the ischial tuberosity avulsion by the hamstring muscles the buttock is found to be tender, swollen and painful. The thigh cannot be flexed and the knee extended without pain in the buttock area. Maximum displacement occurs at the time of injury and does not usually exceed 2 cm. Bed rest and control of pain should be provided until ambulation with crutches is tolerated. Operative repair is contraindicated.

Avulsion of the anterior iliac spine occurs as a result of a sudden pull from either the sartorius or rectus femoris. Displacement is usually limited to 3 cm. or less by the surround-

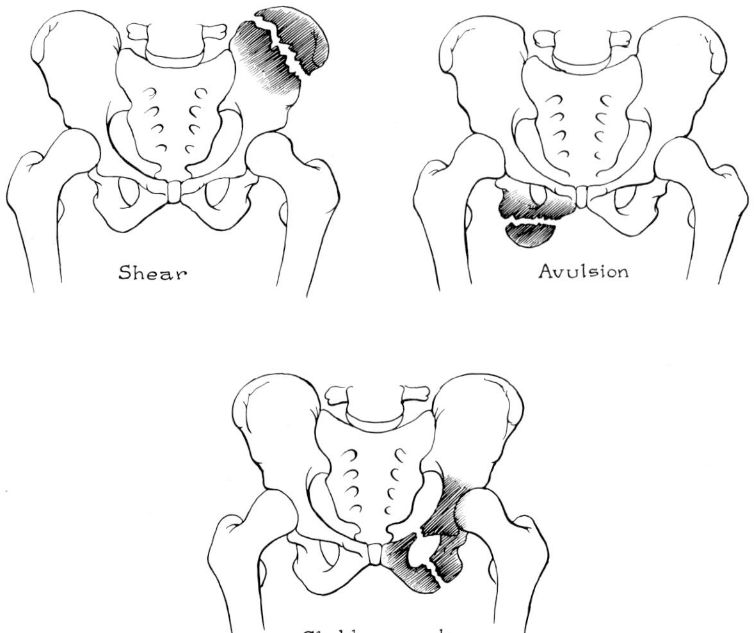

Figure 17–5 Stable pelvic fractures.

ing fascial connections. Treatment consists of bed rest with the thighs flexed for one or two weeks in conjunction with mild analgesics. Operative treatment is not indicated.

A shear fracture of the ilium occurs almost exclusively in a motorcyclist who, at the point of impact, is thrown forward, catching his iliac crest on the handlebar. Occasionally, this fracture will be associated with an open abdominal wound with or without rupture of a viscus. Attention is directed toward surgical cleansing of the wound followed by the appropriate repair of the viscus if necessary. The shattered ilium is treated as follows. If there is not other pathology present, bed rest followed by gradual ambulation will give an excellent result. If an open wound complicates the fracture, the broken fragments may be removed, reduced or left undisturbed as the local circumstances dictate.

Isolated fractures of the pubic rami in which the ring of the pelvis is not significantly altered may be treated symptomatically by early ambulation if no other injuries are present (Fig. 17–5). With fractures about the obturator ring the patient may be more comfortable on bed rest for a few days with a pillow beneath the knees. Before releasing these patients from the emergency area, one must make sure that the patient is stable, has a patent urinary tract and a normal abdominal examination. Even the most benign-appearing injury may produce pathology in the systems just mentioned.

Stable fractures of the pelvic ring also include diastasis of the symphysis in association with "spraining" of the sacroiliac joints. Depending on the severity of the separation, treatment may range from bed rest for several days to application of a pelvic band to provide support and relief of pain. Surgery is not indicated as early treatment.

Stress fractures may occur in the pubic rami as a result of excessive physical activity in an otherwise sedate individual. These should not be confused with bone tumors which may arise in this area. Treatment is rendered only as symptoms dictate.

Fractures involving the sacrum are

difficult to diagnose by x-rays and are usually found when the patient continues to complain of discomfort or when sacral nerve hypesthesia is seen in the perineal or posterior femoral cutaneous nerve areas. If displacement is noted, an attempt should be made to reduce the fracture by placement of the finger into the rectum and gentle manipulation of the fracture. Follow-up treatment consists of bed rest until the patient can ambulate normally.

Unstable fractures in which there are breaks in the anterior-posterior segments of the pelvic ring are treated only after the patient is stabilized, for these are the fractures in which blood loss may lead to severe shock and death. In addition the bladder, bowel or urethra may be involved.

"Straddle" injuries (Fig. 17–6) occur as a result of direct trauma to the pubis or perineum, producing grossly unstable fractures limited to the anterior segment of the pelvic girdle. Rupture of the urethra is common with this injury. After stabilization of associated injuries, the patient should be treated in a semi-sitting position in an effort to neutralize the various muscle pulls in the fracture fragments. A supine position may produce gross displacement of the fragments.

A Malgaigne fracture is one in which fracture lines are present through one set of pubic rami and through the region of the sacroiliac joint (Fig. 17–6). The fracture posteriorly may be on either the ipsilateral or contralateral side of the pubic fracture and may involve either the ilium or the lateral mass of the sacrum. On physical examination the affected lower extremity lies in external rotation and appears shortened. A palpable, tender hematoma is noted frequently over the separated fracture anteriorly. Shock and urinary extravasation are frequently found. Reduction should be accomplished as soon as possible, for no other special care can be undertaken until this is done. Small separations are

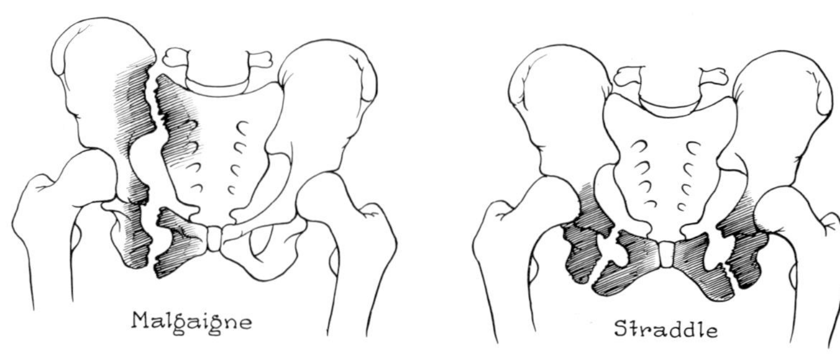

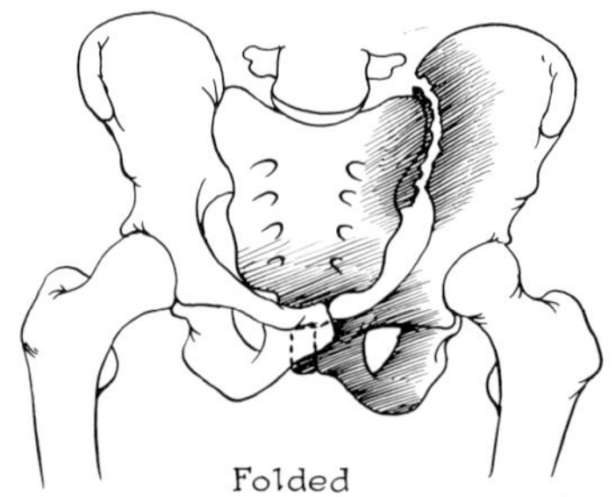

Figure 17–6 Unstable pelvic fractures.

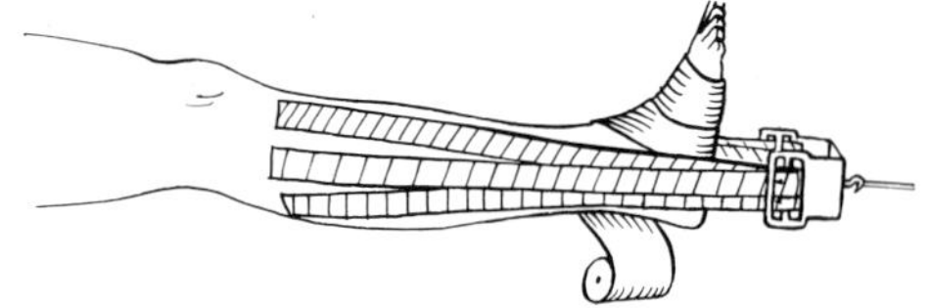

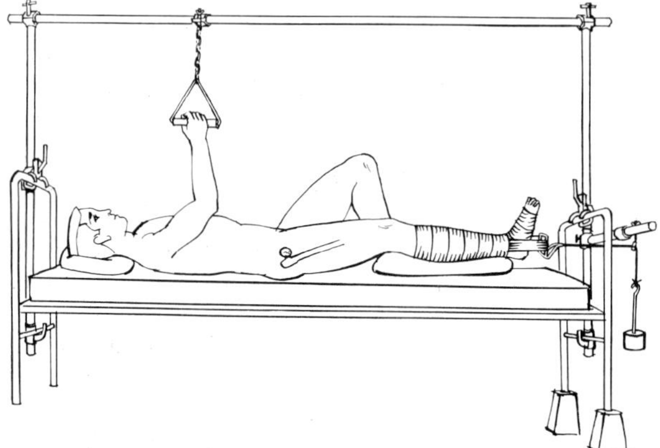

Figure 17–7 Buck's traction.

reduced simply by placing the patient in a lateral position with the normal side up and allowing the body weight to reduce the two pelvic fragments. Reduction is maintained by a canvas sling placed beneath the buttocks with weight and pulley systems attached to the sling elevating the pelvis till it is barely touching the bed. Buck's traction (Fig. 17–7) should be applied to the affected lower extremity in order to prevent cephalad displacement of the unstable fragment. This traction should be maintained until fibrous union occurs after several weeks. After stability is obtained, a plaster spica can be used in place of the suspension hammock.

In the case of an "infolding" or "telescoping" fracture of the pelvis (Fig. 17–6), the hip on the affected side is flexed and inwardly rotated in association with elevation of the thigh and buttock from the examining table. Urethral or bladder injuries occur as a result of overlapping of the pubes. The displaced pelvic bone may be either anterior or posterior to its mate. Reduction is relatively easy if the displacement is anterior, for simple pressure on the iliac crests with the patient supine will usually reduce the dislocation. If reduction is not accomplished easily or if the dislocation is posterior, it is necessary to place the uninvolved lower extremity in flexion, lateral rotation and abduction, and have an assistant hold this position while the affected extremity is likewise flexed, internally rotated and hyperabducted. The fracture dislocation will then be stable when reduced and the patient can be nursed while supine. A suspension hammock is not necessary in this injury. Bed rest is utilized for six to eight weeks with the affected lower extremity held in Buck's traction to prevent proximal migration of the unstable pelvic segment.

Crush injuries in children usually show multiple fractures of the "immature" pelvic bones with no joint disruption. Healing occurs rapidly as displacement of the fractures is not marked. When the integrity of the abdominal contents is confirmed, the child may be treated on bed rest in a supine position until healing occurs.

FRACTURES OF THE ACETABULUM AND DISLOCATIONS OF THE HIP

A normal hip maintains stability by the proper relationship of the femoral head to the acetabulum, the muscular framework surrounding the hip joint, and the hip capsule reinforced by accessory ligaments. When the thigh is flexed and abducted, a powerful force along the longitudinal axis of the limb forces the femoral head through the capsule posteriorly. This occurs most often in automobile accidents when the knee strikes the dash, and is described as a "dashboard" dislocation. If the force along the longitudinal axis of the femur is applied with the thigh crossed and abducted, there results a classical posterior dislocation. With less abduction of the thigh a dislocation of the proximal femur occurs in association with a fracture of the acetabular rim. If the thigh is abducted, either a simple fracture of the acetabulum with or without a central protrusion of the head or a fracture of the femoral neck occurs. In any dislocation of the hip or fracture of the acetabulum, the knee on the ipsilateral side should be investigated by physical examination and x-ray in that a great percentage will demonstrate fractures of the patella.

In describing fractures of the acetabulum, it is useful to divide the acetabulum into three components.[3] The ischium comprises the posterior pillar; the pubic ramus, the anterior pillar; and the ilium, the superior pillar. While a central fracture dislocation of the hip into the acetabulum may disrupt all three pillars, one should try to ascertain on x-ray exactly what has happened to each of the three individual pillars. In doing this, it is possible many times to outline a plan of reconstruction. The most important pillar of the acetabulum in relation to hip stability is the posterior pillar. The most important to weight-bearing is the superior pillar.

Consideration of a dislocated hip should be given to any patient who has multiple injuries or who has a fracture of the pelvis or femur. A routine AP x-ray of the pelvis may show one of the femoral heads to be smaller or larger than the opposite side and would lead one to suspect a dislocation. A stereoscopic AP or a tube lateral x-ray will confirm the dislocation. Other x-rays should be taken on any fracture of the acetabulum, or if there has been a dislocation. If a dislocation is present, these x-rays are taken only after reduction is accomplished. The first x-ray should be taken with the patient tilted 45 degrees on his sound side and the x-ray tube placed directly over the injured acetabulum. By this method the posterior acetabular rim will be shown in detail. By tilting the patient 45 degrees with the injured side down and the x-ray tube directly over the injured side, an excellent view of the anterior acetabular rim may be obtained.

An acetabular fracture with central dislocation of the hip occurs as a result of a blow to the knee with the extremity in abduction or as a result of a direct blow on the greater trochanter. The latter mechanism occurs most frequently when a pedestrian is struck by a car. This is a severe injury and attention must be given initially to replacement of the blood volume. Blood loss may be massive with this fracture and steps should be taken to insure that adequate blood is available for replacement. At least five units of blood should be set up for replacement as necessary. The abdominal viscera and the GU tract should be considered and their integrity proved. Shortening of the involved extremity may be present with this injury; otherwise a normal attitude exists. Any attempt to move the extremity will be extremely painful.

When the patient is stabilized, traction is applied in the lateral and longitudinal directions under general anesthesia. One person stands along the injured side and applies traction with a sheet placed on the inner aspect of the proximal thigh. When another person applies longitudinal traction, the resultant force should reduce the dislocation. After this is accomplished, x-rays should be taken, and if the superior weight-bearing portion of the acetabulum is intact, the extremity may be treated with skeletal traction through a distal femoral pin and balanced suspension for several weeks with 25 to 30 pounds initially, with later reduction to 10 to 15 pounds. Other techniques for reduction have been used such as placing a large wood screw or crossed Steinman pins in the greater trochanter for lateral traction; however, this is to be discouraged as initial management. On rare occasions it may be necessary to open the hip in order to reestablish a satisfactory weight-bearing surface.

Anterior Dislocation of the Hip. Anterior dislocation of the hip occurs most commonly as a result of a fall from a height with the blow being administered on the posterior aspect of an abducted, externally rotated thigh. The deformity of the leg is diagnostic (Fig. 17–8) and consists of a flexed, abducted, externally rotated extremity and may appear longer than the uninjured limb. The femoral head usually comes to rest in the obturator foramen.

Reduction is usually accomplished rather easily, often without anesthesia, by applying traction to the hip in the direction of the deformity. After the musculature surrounding the hip has been relaxed, the extremity is gently internally rotated and abducted. Post-reduction films are then made to determine reduction and also to check for any loose fragments of bone that may be in the joint. If loose fragments are found, they should be removed through an anterior approach to the hip. If no fragments are found, Buck's traction, using five to seven pounds, is then applied to the injured extremity. Bed rest in a semi-flexed position is maintained until soft tissue healing is present at about three weeks.

Posterior Dislocation. This is the most common dislocation and is often associated with injury to the sciatic nerve. It may or may not be in association with a fracture of the posterior pillar of the acetabulum. The typical deformity shows the hip to be slightly flexed, abducted and internally rotated (Fig. 17–8). There is also a shortening of the involved extremity. This dislocation should be considered an emergency, and manipulative reduction takes precedence over most other injuries. The late complication of aseptic necrosis of the femoral head is directly related to how long the head was dislocated.

Reduction cannot be accomplished in a posterior dislocation without satisfactory anesthesia. Several methods have been advocated for relocation of the hip. In Bigelow's circumduction method the patient is anesthetized on the x-ray table and the physician accomplishing the reduction removes his shoes and takes a position standing over the patient on the x-ray table. The adducted thigh and leg each are fully flexed over the abdomen. As traction is applied to the thigh, lateral circumduction followed by external rotation and abduction may effect reduction. This maneuver should not be carried out with force, especially in an elderly patient, for a fracture of the femoral neck may ensue. Another effective and safe method of reduction utilizes strong traction in the axis of the flexed and slightly abducted thigh in association with gentle maneuvering of the thigh toward external rotation and mild abduction. Stemson's method of reduction is an excellent one for elderly people. The patient is anesthetized in a prone position and the affected extremity is flexed at 90 degrees over the end of the table. With the knee flexed 90 degrees, pressure is gently applied to the calf. After the muscle spasm has been overcome, the hip will easily reduce. This method takes longer than the previously described procedures but it is probably the safest.

After reduction another series of x-rays should be obtained in order to check the reduction as well as the integrity of the acetabulum. If there has been an associated posterior pillar fracture with this dislocation, an x-ray utilizing the technique previously described will show whether or not this fragment has been reduced. Indications for opening a posterior dislocation include posterior instability of the hip, significant displacement of the acetabular fracture fragment, loose bone fragments in the joint and persistent or increasing signs of sciatic nerve injury. At all times, both pre- and post-reduction, the status of the sciatic nerve should be ascertained. After

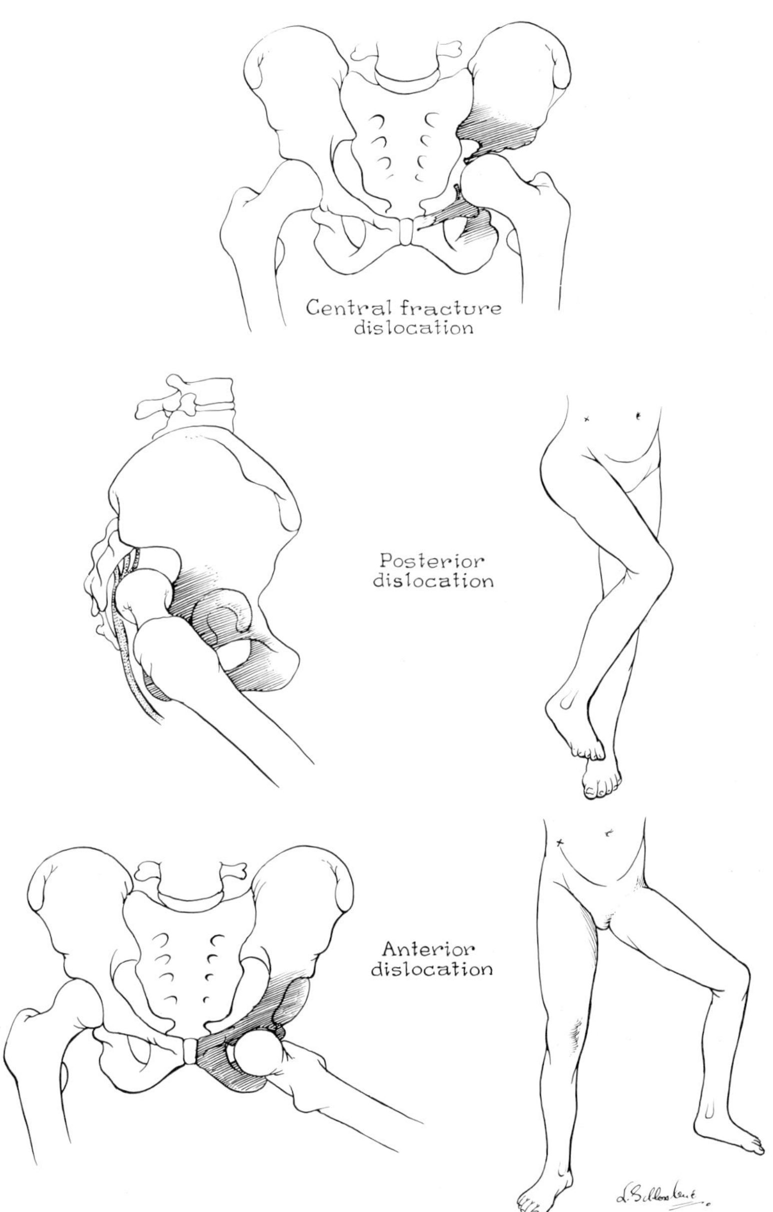

Figure 17–8 Basic types of hip dislocation.

reduction is accomplished, Buck's traction, using five to seven, is applied with the hip in a neutral position.

INJURIES OF THE HIP

The hip joint, functioning as the cornerstone of ambulation, is subjected to trauma throughout life. Most injuries, however, occur at the two extremes of life, either in the young prior to the closure of the epiphysis or in the later years when the bone has undergone degenerative changes. In the middle years of life when the proximal femur is strong, the most common injury is dislocation of the femoral head. In any injury about the hip, efficient and precise early management is essential, for complications of delayed management are frequent and severe.

In children, due to the presence of epiphyses, various injuries may occur. Prior to closure of the proximal femoral epiphysis, the femoral head and the femoral neck have separate blood supplies. The blood supply to the femoral head enters via the femoral neck; thus any injury to the neck may cause disruption of the blood supply. This is the reason for the frequent complication of asceptic necrosis of the femoral head after an injury to the hip in childhood.

The capital femoral epiphysis is the major site of injury in childhood. Displacement of the femoral epiphysis may occur following acute trauma as an "acute" slip or it may gradually slip over a period of several months. The slip takes place through the zone of hypertrophied cartilage, occurring more commonly in boys between the ages of 10 and 16. The body habitus of these youngsters is either of the obese "Fröhlich" type or of the rapidly growing, "Beanpole" type.

In an acute slip there is usually a history of a severe injury coupled with acute pain. On entrance into the emergency room the child will appear to be in severe pain and the lower involved extremity will be shortened and externally rotated. Any movement of the involved lower extremity will precipitate increased pain in the hip. A gradual slip will not be associated with any history of acute trauma, and the patient usually complains of pain in the knee region, fatigue and a limp. Physical examination here reveals a limitation of internal rotation. If the slip is quite severe when the leg is brought into flexion, the limb will rotate externally and move into abduction.

If one suspects an acute slip the involved extremity should be immobilized in a Thomas splint prior to any radiographic examination. Immobilization will reduce pain and minimize any damage that may occur to the remaining vascular attachment. X-rays taken by the AP and tube lateral techniques will reveal the true pathology. In an acute slip there will be a fracture through the epiphyseal line with the head lying inferior and posterior to the neck. There will be no evidence of new bone formation. If a gradual slip has occurred, there will be widening of the femoral neck and a tilting posteriorly and inferiorly of the femoral head. This tilting may be minimum or severe. It must be remembered that an acute slip may occur superimposed upon a chronic slip.

A patient with chronic slip should be placed on bed rest or on non-weightbearing with crutches until a decision can be made by the appropriate specialist as to the type of treatment needed. An acute slip, however, should be treated as a fracture following all the general principles of immobilization. Buck's traction should be utilized with five pounds and plans outlined for early reduction. This reduction may be closed or open. A gentle closed reduction may be attempted under an image intensifier, taking care not to injure any remaining blood supply. If this is accomplished easily, a spica cast may be applied. Open reduction is recommended by many authors utilizing atraumatic surgical technique with internal fixation being accomplished at the time of surgery.

Fractures of the hip in children are the result of severe trauma. These are uncommon injuries and are associated with a very high incidence of complications. The classification most commonly used divides the type of fractures into transepiphyseal, transcervical, cervical trochanteric (base of neck) and intertrochanteric fractures of the hip.[4] The most common fracture in a child is the base of neck type.

Because of the severe trauma that is necessary to reduce these fractures, the child must be examined carefully for other injuries. The most common complicating injury found on examination will be that of cerebral trauma. A consideration of the battered child syndrome should be entertained if no significant history of trauma is present or if no underlying disease such as osteogenesis imperfecta is present.

Examination of the involved extremity will usually reveal the limb to be shortened and externally rotated. Rarely, the limb may be normal in appearance if the fracture is impacted. When one suspects a fracture about the hip, a Thomas splint should be applied immediately. Only after this is accomplished should an AP and tube lateral x-ray be taken. A Frog Leg lateral should not be taken as this may further injure the blood supply of the hip.

After documentation of the type of fracture present, several avenues of therapy are open to the physician, depending on his skill and experience. Gentle, closed reduction coupled with a spica cast may be utilized, or open reduction attempted with atraumatic surgical technique and internal fixation by several pins. A nail should not be used in these fractures. Neither of these two methods of treatment has yet proved superior to the other. The complication of aseptic necrosis remains quite high in either treatment. It is very important, however, to carry out one or the other method of initial management early, if possible within the first six to eight hours after injury, for in this manner the high complication rate may be reduced.

Occasionally, the lesser trochanter is avulsed by the iliopsoas, or the greater trochanter by the abductor muscles. These avulsion injuries do not require operation and may be treated by non-weight-bearing with crutches for several weeks or until the pain subsides.

Fractures of the femoral neck (intracapsular) and of the trochanteric region (extracapsular) of the femur are primarily injuries of the elderly. Eighty per cent of these fractures occur in people over 60 years of age. Because of osteoporosis, a longer life expectancy, and a natural tendency toward coxa vara, women with this injury outnumber men about 3 or 4 to 1. The mortality rate of 15 to 35 per cent is a result not of the fractures themselves but of their complications. Pneumonia, pulmonary embolism and cardiovascular complications are responsible for the high death rate.

The mechanism of injury responsible for these fractures is usually a fall onto the injured side. Occasionally, however, the patient will actually fracture the bone before the fall as a result of a misstep or a twisting motion.

The chief complaint on admission is usually severe pain in the hip area with radiation into the knee. The injured extremity will usually appear to be shortened and externally rotated. These two findings are not always present, for the fracture may be impacted.

Roentgenograms in two planes are necessary to confirm and identify the type of fracture. In addition to an AP x-ray of the hip, a tube lateral should be taken. A Frog Leg lateral should never be taken of the hip in the accident room setting.

Throughout all examinations the injured extremity should not be moved about. As soon as possible, Buck's traction with a pillow under the knee should be applied.

In considering future management of these patients, several considerations are in order. As detailed a history as possible is obtained from the patient or the patient's family in an effort to determine the status of the patient's ambulation prior to the injury. A patient that was bedridden or confined to a wheelchair, or one in whom there was a history of previous malignant disease or other major medical problems, may best be treated by conservative means. If none of these is present, then the treatment of choice is operative intervention. After obtaining an EKG, chest x-ray and other studies appropriate to a geriatric workup, the patient should be scheduled in preparation for early operation. Usually the patient is in the best physiological condition at the time of the accident, and any lengthy delay will predispose the patient to thrombophlebitis, cystitis, decubitus ulcers or pneumonia. Delays in operation are only justified in an attempt to correct diabetic acidosis, cardiac failure and arrhythmia, acute myocardial infarction, cerebral hemorrhage, or dehydration secondary to the fracture occurring over 24 hours prior to the admission of the patient to the hospital. Treatment of any of these problems should be accomplished in association with an internist in an attempt to prepare the patient for early surgery. By operating early and mobilizing the patient quickly after surgery, postoperative complications of surgery in the elderly are diminished.

Intracapsular fractures can be classified according to the angle of inclination of the fracture as described by Pauwel. Type I fractures show an angulation of 30 degrees to the horizontal, type II 50 degrees and type III 70 degrees (Fig. 17–9). Because these fractures are intracapsular, they are not associated with significant hemorrhage.

A type I intracapsular fracture occurs most commonly from a fall causing a direct blow on the involved hip. These fractures may be considered stable if there is no posterior tilt on the tube lateral x-ray, the

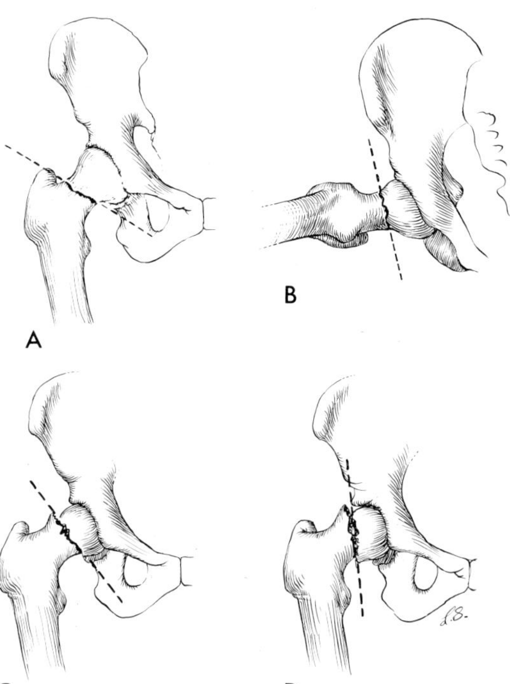

Figure 17–9 Femoral neck fractures.

head on the AP x-ray is in slight valgus and on physical examination the involved leg can be moved slowly without pain. If these factors are all present, the patient may be treated on bed rest with Buck's traction for several weeks followed by non-weight-bearing ambulation until healing takes place. If there is any question of instability, then the fracture may be fixed in situ by use of three Knowles pins.

Treatment of the unstable types II and III is best accomplished either by open reduction and internal fixation or by replacement of the head with an endoprosthesis. The use of an endoprosthetic replacement in fresh fractures should be considered in any patient over 70 years of age if his general condition would not permit possible secondary surgery if the nailing of the femoral head failed; if Parkinson's disease, spastic hemiplegia or severe arthritis of the hip is present; or if the patient is subject to pathological fractures. If the patient comes in late with a displaced fracture of the femoral neck, he should be considered for primary prosthetic replacement.

In the operative treatment of these fractures, great care must be taken to achieve adequate reduction, proper fixation of the fragments and atraumatic handling of all tissues.

Intertrochanteric fractures of the hip occur outside the hip capsule and therefore have an adequate blood supply, which allows for satisfactory union if the fracture is properly immobilized. Closed methods may be accomplished by means of traction and plaster immobilization, but the associated mortality rate is quite high. The type I or non-displaced intertrochanteric fracture can be treated by a nail and plate, thus enabling the patient to resume early non-weight-bearing ambulation. If the patient's general condition does not permit surgery, he may be managed on bed rest with frequent careful turning. The healing time is shorter here than in any other hip fracture.

In a type II intertrochanteric fracture there will be some displacement, but an intact medial calcar will allow good surgical results. These fractures are reduced at operation on the fracture table under Biplane x-ray control, and then internally fixed by use of a nail and side plate.

In a type III intertrochanteric fracture there is comminution of the medial calcar, which predisposes to instability and late varus deformity. These fractures are treated by medialization of the femur and implantation of the medial femoral calcar into the distal intramedullary cavity in association with internal fixation by a nail and side plate. Prior to transferring the patient from the operating table, Biplane x-rays should be taken. Technical errors include too long or too short a nail, too long or too short a plate, or an inadequate reduction of the fracture. Postoperatively, the patient is gotten out of bed and transferred to a chair within 24 hours after the operation. It is not necessary after an adequate reduction and internal fixation to immobilize these patients for any period of time in bed or in a cast. Metastatic disease causing a fracture of the femoral neck is best treated by an endoprosthesis. If the bone destruction results in an extracapsular fracture, internal fixation may be accomplished by a nail and plate enabling the patient to be nursed in a more comfortable manner.

REFERENCES

1. Holdsworth, F. W.: Early orthopaedic treatment of patients with spinal injury. *In* Spinal Injuries, Proceedings of a Symposium (P. Harris, ed.) London, Morrison & Gibb, Ltd., 1963, pp. 93–100.
2. McLaughlin, H. L.: Trauma, Philadelphia, W. B. Saunders Company, 1959.
3. Müller, M. E., Alligower, M., and Willenegger, H.: Manual of Internal Fixation, New York, Springer-Verlag, 1970.
4. American College of Surgeons: Fractures and dislocations of the lower extremity. *In* Early Care of the Injured Patient. 1972, pp. 263–276. Philadelphia, W. B. Saunders Company.

chapter

18

INITIAL MANAGEMENT OF FRACTURES AND JOINT INJURIES: UPPER LIMB

Gerhard Schmeisser, M.D. and Melvin Friedman, M.D.

Bone and joint injuries are among the commonest results of trauma and probably result in more lost man-hours of work time than any other type of injury. Because of the variation in these injuries and the significance of numerous details, large multiple-volume textbooks have been written dealing primarily with skeletal trauma. In contrast, this textbook is oriented primarily toward early management, and emphasis is placed on practical identification and initial management of the skeletal lesions discussed. Principles rather than details of definitive care are mentioned.

To facilitate rapid reference, the material in this chapter is organized regionally. The more proximal regions are considered first and the more distal ones last.

THE SHOULDER GIRDLE

Physical Diagnosis. In the unconscious patient, injury to the shoulder girdle must be suspected and localized by detection and analysis of deformity, whether it is visible or merely palpable. In the oriented patient, deficient function or the presence and nature of pain are of additional help. If the patient is able to supply intelligent cooperation, his examination is greatly facilitated. The ease and precision of establishing a presumptive diagnosis will vary greatly. Fortunately, a portion of the bones and joints of the shoulder girdle lie so close beneath the skin that they can be carefully palpated.

Sternoclavicular Joint Dislocation

The first area to be inspected and palpated for injury should be the sternoclavicular joints. Comparison with its opposite member is essential, both from the front and side of the chest wall. The clavicle may be dislocated either anterior or posterior to the sternum. Subluxations and dislocations of the joint are usually the result of trauma laterally while the opposite shoulder is fixed, i.e., against a car door or lying on the ground, although cases of direct trauma have been noted in the retrosternal type of dislocation. Retrosternal dislocations, which are exceedingly rare, can cause life-endangering problems due to the important structures behind the sternoclavicular joint. Carotid pulsations and subclavian pulsations must be appreciated as well as any airway obstruction from tracheal compression. Special oblique x-rays may be needed to verify this injury, as x-rays of this joint are often exceedingly difficult to interpret. Tomography is very useful whenever there is doubt in the examiner's mind.

Clavicular Fracture

The next structure to be palpated is the clavicle itself. The clavicle can be felt throughout its length and normally presents to the examining fingers a smooth gentle curve with no sharp angulations or tender spots. This bone is broken in children more frequently than any other bone with the possible exception of the radius. It is usually injured in a fall when the child extends his arms to soften his impact. As the clavicle is the only upper limb bone articulating directly with the skeleton of the trunk, it is subjected to severe axial compression forces when the arm is used as a shock absorber. When the examiner is attempting to detect an obscure fracture, it is useful to ask the patient to lift his arm. Full elevation of the upper limb rolls the bone and places it under a certain amount of stress from the weight of the raised limb. The patient with a fractured clavicle will avoid this motion and will localize the pain to the injured area. A fracture of the clavicle may occur just as easily as a result of a fall on the tip of the shoulder or a blow directly on the front of the bone. Fractures of this type are the most common fractures seen in newborn infants and may be caused by lateral compression in the birth canal.

Whenever a fracture is apparent, it is well to remember the proximity of the apex of the lung and the axillary neurovascular structures and to evaluate their function carefully. Pneumothorax from perforation by a sharp clavicular fragment is always a possible complication, particularly in the adult when the sharp fragments tend to displace more widely than in the child. Any standard shoulder x-ray views are usually adequate for identification and management of the fracture itself (Fig. 18–1). The management of pneumothorax is considered elsewhere in this text.

Acromioclavicular Subluxation and Dislocation

The third structure to be observed and palpated is the acromioclavicular joint. This connection between scapula and clavicle may be torn apart if the limb is suddenly forced caudally, such

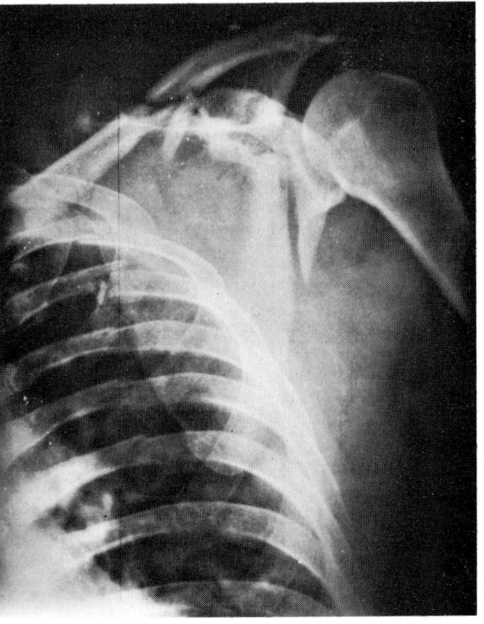

Figure 18–1 Fractures of both the clavicle and scapula.

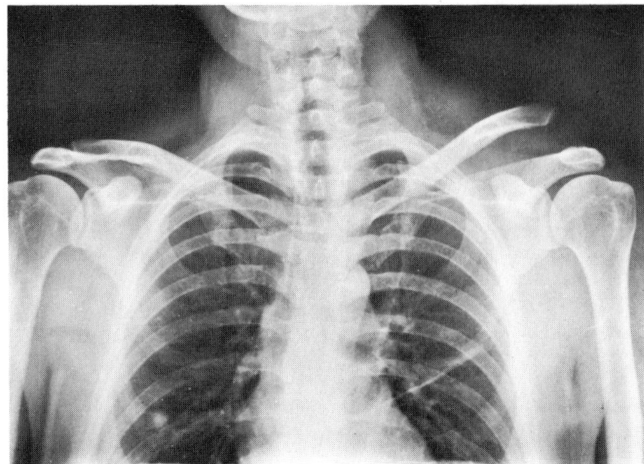

Figure 18–2 Left acromioclavicular joint dislocation.

as by a downward blow on the tip of the shoulder, particularly if this occurs at the precise moment the clavicle is fixed in elevation by the sternocleidomastoid muscle. The displacement of these bones may be both visible and palpable, provided no attempt is made by the patient to shrug his elbow, thereby reducing the dislocation. If there is doubt, the x-rays should be taken with both shoulders shown on the same film and with both arms pulled gently caudally (Fig. 18–2). The spaces of the acromioclavicular joints can then be carefully compared. Severe injuries of these joints are frequently self-evident without resort to such manipulation.

Scapular Fracture

The acromion is a prolongation of the spine of the scapula curving around the top of the shoulder. It can be palpated readily. The body, neck and glenoid, however, are parts not accessible to palpation; thus, pain is the only early evidence of fracture. The neck and body of the scapula followed by the acromion and the coracoid process are the areas fractured in order of decreasing frequency. The neck of the scapula, including the glenoid fossa, and the acromion are usually injured when the humeral head is driven into them, while fractures of the body are usually caused by direct violence. X-rays for fractures of the rest of the scapula should include one or more tangential views. When examining the films, the common error of mistaking the nutrient foramen and vascular canal on the axillary edge as a fracture should be avoided.

Scapulohumeral Joint Dislocation

Dislocation of the scapulohumeral joint, like an acromioclavicular dislocation, presents a specific deformity that can be almost diagnostic to the alert examiner (Fig. 18–3). Dislocations wherein the head of the humerus is displaced anterior or inferior to the glenoidal sockets are a common complication of hyperabduction injuries or falls on the outstretched arm. This injury classically occurs when the high school football player is brought down roughly with his arm out to the side while trying to pass the ball, or when the snowbound motorist pushing on a rear fender falls and slips beside a rear wheel while the fender pushes his arm backwards. This injury is usually seen initially in the younger individual as the weaker anterior capsule tears rather than the strong bone.

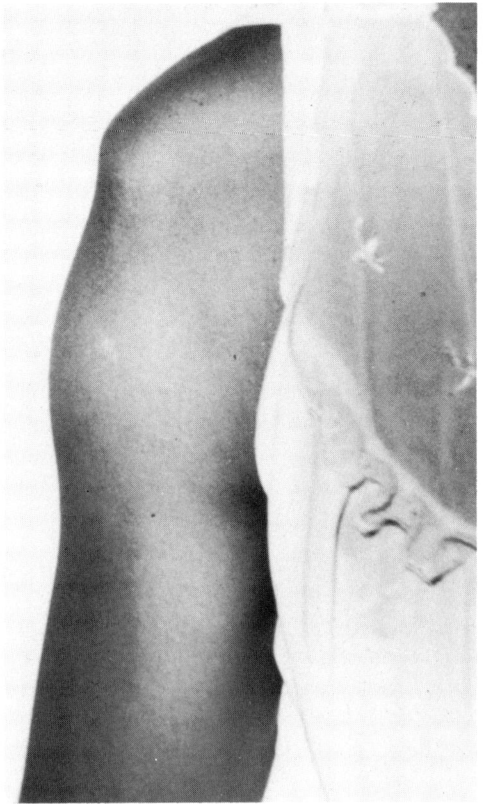

Figure 18–3 Anterior-inferior scapulohumeral dislocation. Note flattening of lateral deltoid bulge and prominence of the acromion.

In the older individual, the capsule is stronger than the bone and thus the bone fractures.

With the humeral head displaced anteriorly and medially from its socket, the astute examiner notices that the normal lateral bulge of the deltoid is flattened (Fig. 18–3). The greater tuberosity of the humerus is no longer palpable in its normal location. Instead, the humeral head may be felt as a firm fullness high in the axilla or anterior in the deltopectoral groove.

Since the humeral head is displaced somewhat inferior as well as anterior in most dislocations, the distance between the acromion and the olecranon is increased on the injured side. The elbow may be held out from the side of the body, and the patient, if this is his first dislocation, is in excruciating pain. Subsequent dislocations are progressively less painful until a veteran may be either blasé about his problem or may even relocate the joint himself without seeking special attention. An axillary x-ray must be taken as well as an anteroposterior or posteroanterior view in order to be certain of the location of the humeral head.

Proximal Humerus Fractures

In contrast to the shoulder dislocation, fractures of the head, neck or upper shaft of the humerus exhibit a full or accentuated deltoid bulge rather than a flattened one. As long as the humeral head remains in the glenoidal socket, a rounded deltoid curve will persist. In the presence of a fracture, hemorrhage will gradually occur, further accentuating the deltoid bulge. The proximal end of the shaft fragment frequently displaces upward, almost never downward; therefore, the distance from the acromion to the olecranon is decreased in contrast to the situation with a dislocation. Frequently, when the shaft fragment displaces upward, its sharp end may be felt beneath the deltoid or high in the deltopectoral groove. If this fragment has been pulled medially by the pectoralis major, a depression in the lateral contour of the arm appears below the level of the shoulder and humeral head.

The mechanism of injury and age distribution of fractures of the upper humerus is also different from those of dislocations of the scapulohumeral joint. Whereas the latter are usually due to hyperabduction and occur predominantly in younger adults, the former usually result from using the limb as a shock absorber when falling, and occur more frequently in older people.

It is most important to note fractures of the tuberosities of the humerus and realize their severity. Since these are the attachments of the major muscles of the shoulder, they should not be regarded as only a "chip." Also, displacement of these fractures is important to note as proper treatment is dependent upon the realization of such displacement. These fractures are often associated with anterior humeral dislocations, a problem which must not be overlooked.

The most useful x-rays for management of these fractures are an anteroposterior or posteroanterior and a transthoracic view with the injured shoulder against the cassette. An axillary view is frequently very helpful to ascertain extent and direction of displacement.

Acute Calcific Tendonitis

Occasionally, the physician sees in his practice a young to middle-aged patient with severe disabling shoulder pain. The pain at times is described as being unbearable and paroxysms of muscle spasm occur. A history of trauma may or may not be elicited. The pain may awaken the patient from his sleep or may be of several days duration, gradually building in intensity.

The patient presents with an extremely guarded extremity and indeed resists any motion of the arm, especially abduction. The pain can be well localized by palpation and the shoulder itself may be swollen and warm to touch. H. F. Moseley has said, "Any adult who, in the course of two or three days, has developed acute pain in the area of the humeral head, of such intensity that sleep is impossible and pain unbearable without analgesics, has a calcified deposit in the rotator cuff until proven otherwise by x-ray or operation."[1]

The diagnosis is often made by the clinical picture alone and confirmed by x-ray. One should always ask for an anteroposterior view of the humeral head in both internal and external rotation and with the x-ray tube angled 15 degrees caudally so that the joint space can be well visualized without superimposition of the acromion. An axillary view can also be quite helpful but may be exceedingly difficult to obtain due to the inordinate pain. A bicipital groove view may show calcification in the long head of the tendon. One must be certain not to mistake the opacity of the calcific deposit for a fracture fragment. Usually the deposit is located in the supraspinatus tendon, but it can occur in the biceps tendon, infraspinatus, teres minor and subscapularis tendons. It is possible to see this syndrome without observing the calcific deposit by x-ray, and the physician should be alert to this possibility.

Ruptured Rotator Cuffs

"Any patient, fifty years of age or over, who has a forcible strain or fall injuring the shoulder, and who suffers severe pain with inability to abduct the arm, and whose x-ray is negative for fracture, dislocation or calcium deposits, has almost certainly a rupture of the rotator cuff."[1]

The patient presents to the physician with severe pain in the shoulder after a strain such as lifting or after a fall. All too often when the x-ray is negative, the patient is sent home in a sling with a "sprain of the shoulder." Only by a keen awareness of this entity is it possible to make a correct diagnosis. An understanding of the anatomy and physiology is paramount if one is to be aware of this syndrome.

The rotator cuff is composed of four muscles: the supraspinatus, the infraspinatus, the teres minor and subscapularis. Ruptures generally involve the supraspinatus and the subscapularis and are usually due to degenerative changes and attrition of the tendons as they pass under the acromial arch. The traumatic episode is usually only the final event that causes the actual rupture.

The function of the rotator cuff musculature is grossly to abduct, internally rotate and externally rotate the shoulder. Thus, disruption of one of the muscles will produce a clinical picture dependent upon which muscle

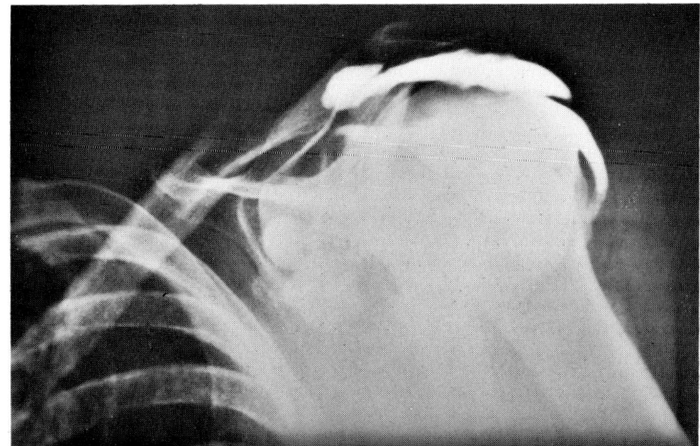

Figure 18–4 Shoulder arthrogram showing extra-articular extravasation of contrast media into the subacromial bursa.

is ruptured. Since it is usually the supraspinatus and subscapularis muscles that rupture, the classical picture is of a person who cannot abduct the shoulder.

Many people present for emergency treatment who are unable to abduct the shoulder. Often this is due to pain and if this can be eliminated, shoulder function approximates normal. If, after the arthrocentesis and injection of a local anesthetic, the patient is able to abduct the shoulder, the diagnosis is *not* a massive rupture of the rotator cuff. If, however, the patient has a positive drop-arm test, then the diagnosis is certain. This test is performed by passively abducting the arm and then having the patient hold the arm in abduction. If this fails, the patient is said to have a positive drop-arm test. Conclusive diagnosis is made by shoulder arthrography (Fig. 18–4), specifically by observing the extravasation of the contrast media outside the normal confines of the shoulder joint into the subacromial bursa. The importance of early diagnosis is evident when one notes the excellent results of early operative intervention.

Ruptures of the Long Head of the Biceps Tendon

This lesion presents acutely in healthy middle-aged men with no previous history of shoulder difficulty and is caused by a very strong contraction against a maximal load. The etiology is similar to that of ruptured rotator cuffs, i.e., degenerative changes. These occur due to friction of the tendon as it passes over the humeral head and under the transverse humeral ligament in the biceps groove of the humerus.

Ruptures of the long head of the biceps tendon occur either at the supraglenoid ridge or at the musculotendinous junction. Diagnosis is made by clinical signs, e.g., increased swelling of the muscle belly of the biceps tendon with a contraction of the muscle. Pain may or may not be the predominant symptom. One must also be alert for concomitant ruptures of the rotator cuff.

Initial Immobilization of the Injured Shoulder

Prior to x-ray evaluation, and at the time of initial examination, an injured shoulder, just like any other injured skeletal structure, should be immobilized. Because of the uncertainty of diagnosis on clinical grounds alone, a standard technique should be used that is harmful to none of the various injuries that might be present and helpful to as many as possible. If shock is not a factor and the sensorium is clear, the backrest of the stretcher may be elevated, a position which the patient is likely to prefer and one which facilitates immobilization of the shoulder. Any measure or posture that promotes angulation or overriding of fracture fragments should be avoided. A sling should be used to retard motion of the limb, but particular care should be taken to apply it so that it supports the wrist but does not lift the elbow. This is insured if the sling encircles only the patient's neck and wrist, i.e., a collar-and-cuff or necktie type of sling. In this way, it can also be applied with less disturbance to the patient, an additional advantage.

Sternoclavicular Dislocations

Subsequent Management. The anterior type is managed closed when seen early and simply requires backward and upward pressure with pressure exerted over the medial end of the clavicle. Immobilization is required for four to six weeks. Retrosternal dislocations must be reduced and it is best to have operating room facilities readily available. The medial clavicle can be grasped with a towel clamp and the dislocation reduced with traction anteriorly, laterally and superiorly. If the reduction is stable, then figure-of-eight bracing will suffice. For unstable situations, resection of the medial end of the clavicle is recommended, although some authors prefer fascial repair.

Clavicular Fracture

Fortunately, definitive management of most shoulder injuries by nonoperative technique is possible. Frequently, no reduction maneuver is necessary with a child's fractured clavicle. If the x-rays do show that some correction is desirable, all that is necessary is to have the child sit up very straight and draw his shoulders back. This distraction force may help to straighten the angulation, or it can be corrected by digital pressure. Unless the deformity is extreme, strenuous measures are unjustified. For strapping or bandaging around both shoulders, the figure-of-eight dressing, like knapsack straps that are crossed over the interscapular space and pulled tight enough to draw the shoulders back, is a standard and satisfactory treatment technique. This method works well probably because the injury is benign rather than because of any particular benefit in this type of dressing. Effort should be made to keep the straps adjusted to pull on the lateral ends of the clavicles, rather than to press on the center; pressure on the center increases the deforming force rather than relieving it. Binding the limb to the side (as with a Velpeau dressing) or lifting the elbow (as with a conventional sling) tends to compress the clavicle, causing angulation or overriding, deformities which should be avoided if possible. Immobilization should be for a period of three weeks for children and six or more weeks for adults. A lump over the fracture site is to be expected and the patients should be forewarned. In a majority of cases, this will regress with time.

In certain persons, clavicular fractures must be treated more aggressively. In athletes, open reduction is sometimes indicated so that the patient will have a more anatomical and, supposedly, a more functional result. In women, also, the lump of callus can be objectionable. Certainly, substituting a scar for a lump is a poor bargain. These people may prefer bed rest or traction. These methods avoid motion at the fracture site and reduce the quantity of periosteal callus. Patients who require more aggressive management are those with neurovascular compromise, and in these people, traction and/or surgery may be indicated.

Acromioclavicular Dislocation

Good x-rays tend to reveal acromioclavicular joint dislocations of two different degrees of severity: those with slight displacement that have torn the acromioclavicular joint ligaments, and are actually classified as subluxations, and others with total displacement that have also torn the coracoclavicular ligaments (conoid and trapezoid). Operative reconstruction is usually necessary in the latter and may ultimately be indicated in the former. However, with the milder injuries, a trial of strapping the limb in such a manner as to support the elbow while pulling down the clavicle is usually justified. One technique is simply to apply a conventional triangular sling rather tightly. To prevent discomfort, the neck and clavicle must be well padded where the sling presses on these areas.

Another technique is to apply a collar and cuff or necktie-type sling from neck to wrist (Fig. 18–5). Broad strips of adhesive tape are then applied under tension from the shoulder to the olecranon. The ends of the tape should extend around the olecranon and over the proximal part of the shoulder in order to lift the arm toward the clavicle. There is a well-padded acromioclavicular strap, commercially available, that accomplishes the same thing.

Operative intervention in which the joint is reconstructed, while best done early, can be done up to six months after the injury. After this time, resection of the outer end of the clavicle is the procedure of choice. Many operations have been described for the early repair. While some advocate repair of the coracoclavicular ligament, this has been found unnecessary when a good ligament reconstruction has been performed, such as in the repair described by Dr. J. Neviaser.[2] The articular disc of the A-C joint must always be examined and is usually excised.

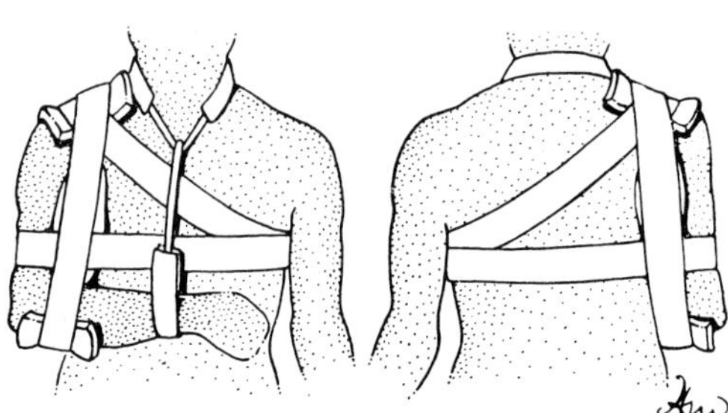

Figure 18–5 One type of bandaging for acute dislocation of acromioclavicular joint. (Courtesy of Moseley, H. F.: Athletic injuries to the shoulder region. Am. J. Surg. 98:401–422, 1959.)

Scapular Fracture

Fractures of the acromion or remainder of the scapula may be adequately immobilized by immobilizing the whole upper limb, as by bandaging the arm to the trunk in a sling and swathe or Velpeau dressing (Fig. 18–6). Fortunately, reduction is seldom necessary unless the glenoid is grossly disrupted. Even in this circumstance an adequate result can frequently be achieved with closed treatment since the shoulder, unlike the hip joint, is not subjected to weight-bearing forces.

Scapulohumeral Joint Dislocations

If x-rays confirm that the injury is a scapulohumeral dislocation, the precise location of the humeral head is of relatively little significance in executing reduction. It is very rare indeed that closed reduction cannot be done if complete relaxation is obtained. Complete relaxation not only facilitates reduction but also minimizes additional trauma to the rim of the socket or the surface of the head. This is particularly true if the patient is a muscular young man suffering from his first such injury. If good relaxation cannot be obtained with medication, then general anesthesia is necessary. The objective is to draw the head away from the rim, lifting it over the edge and allowing it to drop back into the socket.

The hyperabduction method of reduction is the safest, fastest and least

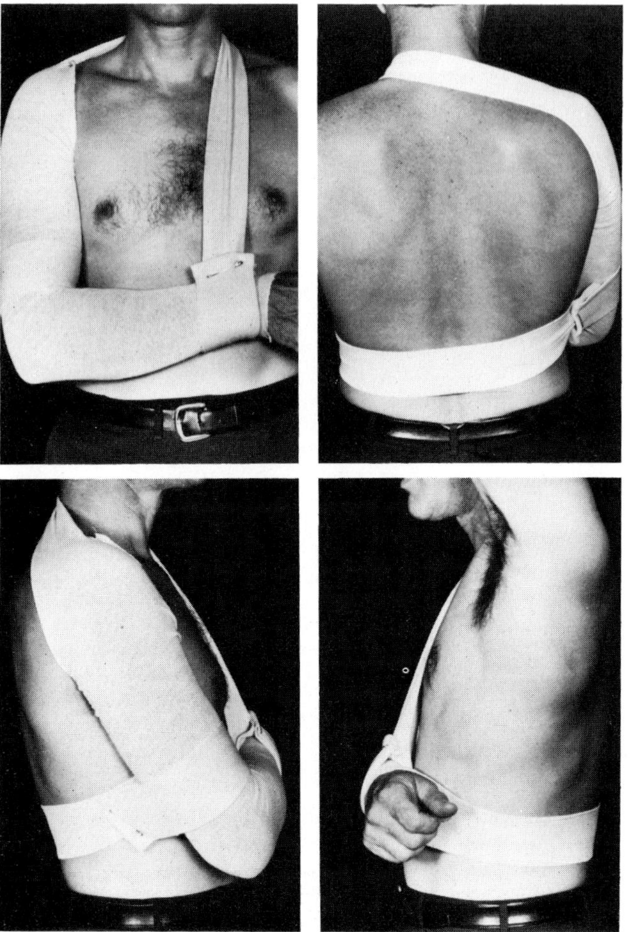

Figure 18–6 Stockinette velpeau dressing for lightweight immobilization of the shoulder. A long piece of stockinette tubing is slit in two places to allow insertion of the arm and emergence of the hand. The two ends are pinned or tied around the limb after encircling the neck and waist.

traumatizing. The patient is placed supine with an assistant holding him securely across the chest. The hand is grasped with the arm in external rotation and the elbow either flexed or extended. The physician then leans back with all of his weight in the opposite direction from the patient. After 30 to 45 seconds of prolonged traction, he takes a step cranially, still maintaining traction. This is repeated until the arm is fully hyperabducted. Usually the shoulder will reduce before getting this far and the arm is then quickly brought down to the side and the patient's hand placed across his abdomen with instructions to grasp his belt buckle. In those that don't reduce until full hyperabduction is achieved, one can palpate the humeral head and apply direct pressure while bringing the arm down to achieve reduction. Reduction is then secured and maintained by bringing the arm against the body, with the shoulder internally rotated enough for the forearm to lie across the patient's waist. Any dressing that will hold the limb in this position will maintain reduction. A collar and cuff sling with a swathe about the arm and chest is adequate. A stockinette velpeau is very comfortable in a trustworthy patient (Fig. 18–6). It is both unnecessary and uncomfortable to strap the limb in front of the chest with the hand positioned at the opposite shoulder.

Proximal Humerus Fractures

If the x-rays confirm that the injury is a fracture through the upper end of the humerus, the position of the fragments should be evaluated carefully and treatment selected with special consideration of the patient's age and activities. In the child, because of remodeling potential, considerable angulation and displacement are compatible with a good functional and cosmetic result. This is less true of an adult. Also, the functional demands of heavy labor may require more precise reduction than for more sedentary activities. In any group, attempt at reduction by closed manipulation beginning with manual traction in a caudal direction is justified by the probability of obtaining an adequate position. After reduction has been achieved by merely pulling down on the arm, it can sometimes be maintained with an arm-trunk binding such as a modified Velpeau dressing. On other occasions when reduction can be achieved only in abduction, a shoulder spica cast holding the limb in some degree of elevation or abduction is necessary.

If judgment or experience indicates that in the adult an adequate position cannot be secured, open reduction and internal fixation with screw or pin is appropriate. Early motion can usually be obtained in nonoperated cases despite the suboptimal position. Nonunions are rare complications of injuries of the proximal humerus as compared with those of the midhumerus.

Fractures of the tuberosities may be treated by a modified Velpeau dressing if they are not displaced. Fractures with displacement must be treated with open reduction and internal fixation. Too often, the inexperienced surgeon accepts a poor position, using the excuse that the shoulder is a non-weight-bearing joint. One must strive for an excellent result with these fractures.

Acute Calcific Tendonitis

Since the pain of acute calcific tendonitis is so severe and disabling, conservative management is not indicated. Immediate relief can often be obtained by injecting the area with a local anesthetic and steroid combination after an attempted aspiration. One should always puncture the deposit at several points in order to facilitate decompression. Operative intervention is indicated if the deposit recurs or fails to respond to non-operative treatments. This procedure, while not difficult, should be done by a surgeon experienced in shoulder surgery as the lesion is often difficult to extirpate. X-ray treatment is mentioned only to be condemned.

Ruptured Rotator Cuffs

Once the diagnosis of a massive rupture of the rotator cuff is made, then only operative intervention at the earliest time possible will suffice. It should be done under a general anesthetic with the patient in a semi-sitting position. A saber approach is made and an acromioplasty is performed. The coraco-acromial ligament is transected. Unabsorbable suture material is used for fixation. The technique of repair, of course, depends upon the pathology found at the time of exploration. Again, only a surgeon well acquainted with shoulder problems should attempt it. Even in the best of hands, results may leave some permanent disability. However, the operative results are far superior to simple immobilization or no treatment at all.

Ruptures of the Long Head of the Biceps Tendon

The treatment of this lesion is colored by many factors. Young, active men presenting acutely should be operated upon immediately. In the aged and sedentary, however, conservative management is often warranted. Physical therapy will help to relieve the pain. Functional disability will be minimal. Patients with lesions one month or older must be evaluated carefully due to secondary contractures of the muscle present. Surgical intervention at this stage may be difficult and may yield a poor result. If surgical intervention is performed, one must also explore the rotator cuff to rule out tears.

THE MIDHUMERUS

Fractures of the shaft of the humerus are usually self-evident. Like the thigh, the upper arm is a one-bone segment, and therefore a fracture of that one bone generally produces total instability. An exception occurs in the small child, in whom an incomplete, greenstick fracture may occur. Because of the relatively small muscle bulk around the upper arm compared with the thigh, the fracture deformity is visible and palpable as soon as any attempt is made to lift the limb. Because of the close association of important neurovascular structures to the humeral shaft, damage, particularly to the radial nerve, is not uncommon. Oblique fractures at the junction of the middle and distal thirds of the humerus are more frequently associated with radial nerve injury than other types. Certainly, with humeral fractures particular attention should be given to routine evaluation of peripheral neurovascular function.

Most methods of splinting these fractures are somewhat unsatisfactory and some techniques are truly hazardous. Among these, mentioned only to be condemned, is the upper limb traction splint, a modification of the lower limb Thomas splint. The padded ring is placed in the axilla and against the chest wall. For counter-traction, a hitch is placed about the wrist, fastened to the other end of the splint, and tightened for traction. Neither the wrist nor the axilla tolerates these forces as well as the ankle and the ischium. Furthermore, rotation, angulation and displacement of the fracture fragments can seldom be prevented as long as the elbow is extended. A long, inflatable plastic splint, extending the entire length of the limb to press in the axilla, is less hazardous than a traction splint, but it is equally ineffective in immobilization of the fracture.

The authors prefer to shorten the lever arm on the distal fragment by gently flexing the elbow. This also allows control of rotation of the distal fragment. The limb is then held in this position by a collar-and-cuff sling. If the condition of the patient permits, the backrest of the stretcher is raised to a partial sitting position to allow the elbow to drop downward, thereby reducing overriding of the fragments. A thin, padded wood splint, about ten inches long, may then be placed in the axilla. It is applied to the medial aspect of the arm and wrapped to it in order to minimize angulation. An additional splint of similar dimensions may be applied to the lateral aspect if desired. A roll of knitted gauze is much more effective in holding these splints than short strips of muslin. Throughout the splinting procedure, gentle manual downward traction the elbow is effective in maintaining or improving position safely.

A stockinette tube dressing, known as the "military velpeau," has recently become popular for either temporary or definitive immobilization (Fig. 18–6). A piece of stockinette tubing, wide enough for the upper arm and as long as one and a half times the height of the patient, is used. A longitudinal slit several inches long is made in the tube beginning at a point one-quarter of the length from one end. The middle portion is then slipped over the limb until it is entirely covered. The short end is passed around the back of the patient's neck and down in front of the chest to encircle his wrist at his waist. The tube is pinned or tied snugly around the wrist. The other end is passed around the patient's back at the level of his waist and tied or pinned around the supracondylar portion of the arm. The tube is slit open at the wrist to allow freedom of the hand. Splints can be added just as with the collar-and-cuff sling.

Once splinting has been accomplished, x-rays may be obtained. The easiest views to obtain are transthoracic and one in which the cassette is placed behind the upper arm with the x-ray tube positioned anteriorly. In the position of immobilization of the humerus which has just been described, oblique rather than true lateral and anteroposterior views are obtained. However, these views are in planes at right angles to each other and are easily reproduced later when the limb has been bound up in a postreduction dressing; therefore, they are more useful in fracture management than the conventional views. Occasionally, the bulk of the patient or the limitations of the x-ray equipment will prevent an adequate transthoracic view. In this case, a true lateral and a true anteroposterior view of the humerus should be obtained.

After the x-rays have been examined and the details of the fracture anatomy determined, it may be possible to achieve and maintain adequate position merely by refinement of the immobilization already applied. The padded wood splints can be removed without disturbing the collar-and-cuff or stockinette sling. In place of the wood splints a padded plaster "sugar tong" is applied with one-third of the splint placed up along the medial aspect of the upper arm into the axilla. The center of the splint is lapped around the elbow and the other end is placed up along the lateral aspect of the upper arm to the acromion. This sugar tong can be secured in place as it sets by circumferential wrapping with knitted gauze. Soft drainage dressings can be inserted between the arm and the chest wall to maintain the proper amount of shoulder abduction, which controls angulation in one plane while alteration of the length of the collar-and-cuff sling controls angulation in the other plane. Circumferential gauze wrappings about the trunk and limb keep everything in place.

It is important that care be taken not to telescope the elbow toward the shoulder with any of these wrappings; rather, an attempt should be made to keep the elbow pulled down. This is the principle of the "hanging cast," in which a circumferential above-elbow cast is applied with the elbow flexed and also with a collar-and-cuff sling. While the patient is in a vertical position, the weight of the cast tends to hang, drawing out and aligning the fragments of the humerus. In practice, unfortunately, this technique has been overexploited.

Occasionally, a shoulder spica cast is a superior method of immobilization of a humeral shaft fracture, permitting as it does placement of the arm in more abduction or flexion. Proper application requires technical skill and good patient cooperation. A good spica cast may obviate the need for open reduction and internal fixation, whereas a bad one may necessitate it.

Particularly if a patient has multiple coincidental serious injuries requiring prolonged recumbency and if access to the chest for auscultation or other measures is necessary, pulley and weight traction may be appropriate for a fractured humerus. Open reduction and internal fixation are wisely used when the patient's condition best tolerates the procedure and when adequate position cannot be obtained or secured by nonoperative techniques. It is particularly appropriate if the fractured humerus is explored for a related radial nerve palsy. Exact reduction with truly rigid fixation is important. For this purpose strong intramedullary rods or compression plates are indicated.

THE REGION OF THE ELBOW

Initial Management. A deformed, distorted or swollen elbow may represent any of a variety of dislocations or fractures. Distinction between them on the basis of physical examination alone is too inaccurate to justify the attempt. X-rays are far more revealing and should not be delayed. Therefore, the logical routine is to check for integrity of the skin and the neurovascular status, splint the limb and obtain anteroposterior and lateral views of the elbow.

Splinting. Splinting of an injured elbow is not to be undertaken lightly. Neurovascular compression or laceration by the fracture fragments leading to severe disability is perhaps more common following injuries to the elbow than anywhere else in the body. The first step in preventing these complications is immobilization of the fragments without disturbing the position in which the arm is first seen. In most other areas of the limbs, such as the lower leg or forearm, one can be assured that straightening the limb by gentle manual traction will not aggravate and may relieve a compression problem. In certain supracondylar fractures in children, straightening the elbow by gentle manual traction or any other technique can elevate the sharp distal end of the proximal fragment so that it presses directly on the artery in the antecubital space. The elbow, when first seen, is usually flexed about 45 degrees. Alteration of the degree of flexion in the process of splinting is most unwise and, therefore, despite common practice to the contrary, a straight inflatable plastic splint should not be applied. A splint must be modified to fit the deformity rather than the deformity distorted to conform to the splint.

In practice, a simple technique is to place in the axilla a light wood splint that extends to the hand (Fig. 18–7). The space between the straight splint and the bent elbow is then filled with drainage dressings or other paddings. One or more rolls of knitted gauze should be wrapped gently around the entire limb and splint without any attempt to straighten the limb. The patient is kept recumbent on the stretcher and the limb elevated on a pillow. A sling should definitely be avoided since it forcibly flexes the elbow, which may be just as deleterious as extending it. Particularly with elbow fractures, x-rays should be taken by moving the tube and cassette around the limb rather than by turning the limb between the tube and cassette.

Diagnosis and Subsequent Management. Among the most serious and common elbow injuries in childhood is the supracondylar fracture with angulation anteriorly and displacement of the distal fragment posteriorly. Most commonly occurring between the ages of four and 10 years, this fracture is usually not due to a hyperextension or longitudinal force occurring as a result of a fall on hand with the elbow extended; instead, it usually results from a fall in the face down position

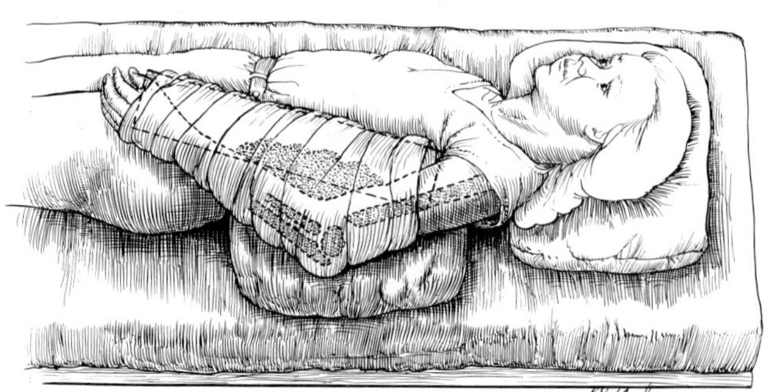

Figure 18–7 The injured elbow should be splinted to maintain the existing position. It should not be flexed or extended. A wood splint, properly wrapped to the limb with knitted gauze, is therefore preferable to an air splint.

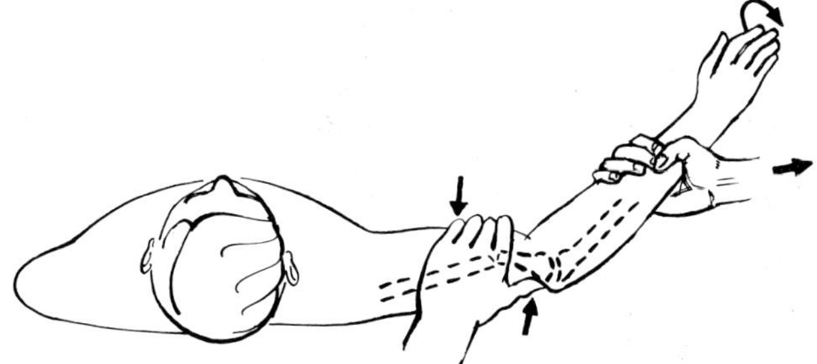

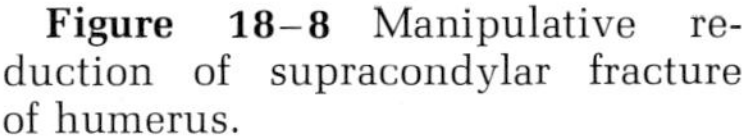

Figure 18–8 Manipulative reduction of supracondylar fracture of humerus.

with the upper limbs functioning as shock absorbers. The humeral condyles are driven back off the rest of the humerus by the force transmitted through the forearm bones at a moment when the elbows have flexed under the force of cushioning the impact. This is an important fact since, if the elbow is fractured by a force delivered when the elbow is in flexion rather than in extension, there is no logical reason for extending the joint in the course of manipulative or traction reduction. Furthermore, the threat to the antecubital neurovascular structures is an important reason for not doing so.

The reduction maneuver may be more safely performed by applying manual traction on the forearm while maintaining some elbow flexion (Fig. 18–8). Then, without relaxing the traction force, the olecranon should be forced forward while the distal end of the humerus is pulled backward. Finally, if it is felt that reduction has been achieved, and if the radial pulse remains intact, the elbow may be flexed while retaining the upward traction. A position of better than 90 degrees of flexion must be obtained to maintain reduction. But attempts to achieve it must be done carefully and with constant attention to the position of bony landmarks and the state of the pulse. If these physical aspects seem satisfactory, a plaster splint or cast with collar-and-cuff sling may be applied and the position checked by x-ray.

If a well-executed reduction maneuver has failed to achieve and maintain an excellent reduction, the safest course is to abandon further attempts and to apply Dunlop's traction (Fig. 18–9). In cases of severe displacement, manipulative reduction should probably not be attempted initially but instead Dunlop's traction should be applied and a reduction maneuver executed with the arm in traction. Locking the reduction by flexion is then unnecessary since it can be maintained by the traction force. If at any time good circulation in the hand cannot be restored quickly, prompt open reduction with arterial release or repair is imperative if severe disability in the form of Volkmann's ischemic contracture of the forearm muscles is to be avoided. Surgery is rarely necessary if these injuries are initially splinted and managed with the care they deserve.

The supracondylar fracture in the adult is usually more comminuted than in the child. Displacement may be im-

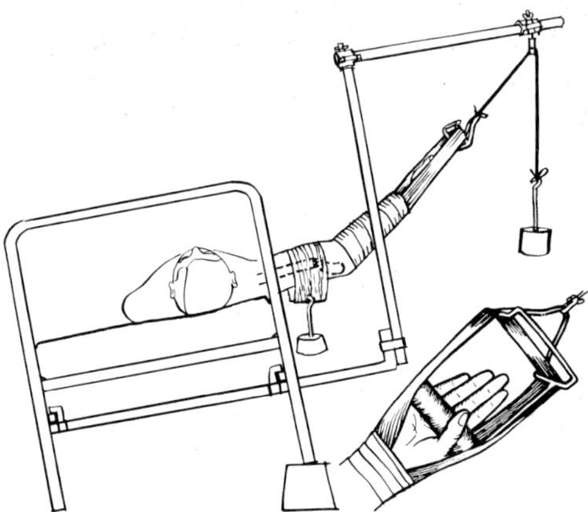

Figure 18–9 Dunlop's traction. (Schmeisser, G., Jr.: A Clinical Manual of Orthopedic Traction Techniques, 1963.)

possible to correct by manipulation or traction, and stiffness will result from prolonged immobilization. Open reduction with internal fixation and early motion may yield the best result.

Similarly, fractures of single condyles such as the capitellum may require internal fixation. Although open reduction of a closed fracture is almost never necessary in a child, the displaced capitellum of the humerus, like the displaced head of the femur, is a genuine exception to the rule.

Fractures of the olecranon are similar to those of the patella in that, if displacement is present, full, active extension of the joint may be lost unless surgical repair is performed. On the other hand, if displacement is absent and if full active extension is present, six weeks protection in a long cast in slight flexion is usually adequate treatment.

Fractures of the head or neck of the radius may, like those of the capitellum of the humerus, be due to force transmitted longitudinally up the radius or to an abduction force at the elbow, or both. Both these forces can result from a fall. The presenting complaint may be pain in the region of the radial head, but is almost as likely to be pain in the wrist. Tenderness, however, will be found on palpating the lateral aspect of the radial head. Pronation and supination of the forearm will produce pain at the elbow, whereas flexion and extension of the elbow are sometimes almost pain-free. The latter signs need not be elicited, as radial head tenderness alone justifies lateral x-rays, which will be diagnostic. If the patient's discomfort is minimal and the examination does not suggest a more serious injury, the immediate splinting recommended above for the deformed elbow is not necessary.

Fractures of the radial head and neck are not uncommonly associated with an elbow dislocation. They may be overlooked on both clinical and x-ray examination unless careful inspection of the head-neck junction is carried out. Generally, a loose fragment in the joint requires excision or reattachment. Most surgeons feel that the entire head should be removed if more than 30 per cent of the articular surface is destroyed. When the neck is angulated more than 20 or 30 degrees and this angulation cannot be corrected by digital pressure, either surgical reduction or excision is indicated in the adult. Since a growth plate is involved, excision of the radial head is contraindicated in the young as long as any growth potential remains in the forearm. Finally, immobilization requires a long arm cast or splint that prevents forearm rotation as well as elbow motion. In the adult, immobilization beyond a few weeks may result in prolonged elbow stiffness.

The distortion of an elbow dislocation may be very similar to a supracondylar fracture. Careful evaluation of the position of the epicondyles with respect to the tip of the olecranon may differentiate these injuries, but the need for an x-ray makes this painful exercise in physical diagnosis unnecessary. Prompt splinting in the position of deformity and anteroposterior and lateral x-ray studies are indicated on the basis of elbow deformity alone. Surprisingly, elbow dislocations are sometimes overlooked, particularly if certain radiologic details are not appreciated. First, slight displacement of the trochlea of the humerus from the sigmoid fossa of olecranon is not normal; second, the central longitudinal axis of the radius should pass through the center of the capitellum regardless of the x-ray view obtained. Dislocation of either or both of these components of the elbow may occur, and reduction of one component may be achieved without reduction of the other.

Reduction of the ulnotrochlear dislocation can be achieved by a maneuver identical to that executed in supracondylar fractures. Good anesthesia is imperative if additional damage to the articular surfaces is to be avoided. Reduction of radiocapitellar dislocation may be achieved by thumb pressure on the radial head while rotating the wrist back and forth with slight traction. The concept of subluxation is a dangerous one. A joint is either in proper position or it is not. After reduction, a splint or cast should be applied to hold the elbow in 90 degrees of flexion. At this point, the maintenance of exact reduction should be verified radiologically. If there has been radiocapitellar dislocation, the cast must maintain the position of forearm rotation that is found, on pronation and supination, to be most stable.

With a radiocapitellar dislocation as one of its components, the Monteggia fracture-dislocation is a composite injury that also includes a fracture of the ulna. This injury is caused by a blow on the ulnar aspect of the forearm when the elbow is flexed 90 degrees. It is usually sustained when the individual throws up his forearm to protect himself against a blow. After breaking and angulating the ulna, the remaining force drives the radius away from the capitellum. When there is significant displacement, deformity of the elbow is recognizable, and splinting should be performed as described for any elbow injury. This combination of injuries is so common that whenever x-rays reveal either a radiocapitellar dislocation without an ulnotrochlear dislocation or an ulnar fracture without a radial fracture, diligent search should be made for the other component.

When possible, closed reduction should be attempted by careful application of force to the forearm in the opposite direction to that of the injury. A useful technique is for the surgeon to place his own forearm across the front of the patient's elbow. With his other hand, he then flexes the patient's elbow over his forearm like a nutcracker over a nut. In this case, however, the object is to "straighten the nutcracker, not crack the nut." Post-manipulation films must show exact reduction; otherwise, further displacement will surely occur. If, as commonly happens, exact reduction cannot be achieved by closed methods, open reduction and internal fixation must be performed. A compression plate or intramedullary rod is used to secure the ulna; the orbicular ligament or a fascial substitute is resutured about the radial neck.

THE FOREARM BONES

Even if no visible deformity is present, fractures of forearm bones are easily detected. The ulna can be easily palpated throughout its length for any irregularity or point of tenderness. The distal half of the radius is concealed under the flexor muscles of the forearm, but fractures in this area produce pain on rotation of the wrist. Inflatable plastic splints are ideal for immobilization of forearm or wrist fractures. Only long splints extending above the elbow should be used. They may spontaneously straighten some of the deformity, which is desirable in fractures in this area. If such a splint is used, a sling is unnecessary since the elbow is held straight. Instead, the patient is kept recumbent on a stretcher with the limb elevated. Anteroposterior and lateral x-rays should be taken through the splint, rotating the tube and film about the limb rather than rotating the limb. Reduction should be attempted by manual traction on the hand, while manual countertraction is applied to the upper arm with the elbow flexed 90 degrees. One can achieve the same effect with the patient supine on a stretcher by suspending the arm from the ceiling by the thumb and one or more fingers and with the elbow flexed 90 degrees. A weight is then suspended from a band about the upper arm. Finger traps and other devices to secure traction to the thumb and fingers can be damaging and must be used with caution. Once the arm has been suspended, any residual angulation and displacement can be corrected by pressing the fragments into place and by rotating the wrist. The long arm cast can then be applied while the limb is still suspended and the reduction forces molded into the cast as it sets.

Deliberately increasing the initial deformity to "loosen the fragments" or to "break up the impaction" is a hazardous technique to be shunned by the novice or anyone unprepared to explore the arm to repair the damage that may occur. In a child, forearm fractures will unite quickly, even if barely touching, if adequate immobilization is provided. Remodeling can be relied upon to correct considerable deformity so that an adequate position can virtually always be obtained by close techniques. In the adult, the situation is different. Minimum standards for acceptance of reduction in the adult are 50 per cent end-on apposition of fragments with less than 15 degrees angulation on any x-ray view. Unless these standards are met, exact reduction with rigid internal fixation is indicated.

A particularly common fracture is that of the distal end of the radius, usually occurring in an adult as a result of a fall. The contour of the deformity was originally described by Abraham Colles as resembling an upside-down dinner fork when viewed from the side (Fig. 18–10). X-rays of the wrist will reveal that the distal fragment is tilted and impacted on the end of the proximal one. A small tip of the ulna may be avulsed. The long axis of the hand is tilted radially as well as dorsally. The apex of the angulation may impinge upon the median nerve as it enters the carpal tunnel.

Manipulative reduction is achieved by applying forces in reverse to those which caused the deformity. The fracture is disimpacted by manual traction. Residual angulation is then corrected by bending the wrist in a volar and ulnar direction while traction is retained. It is generally felt that the forearm should be fully pronated. The cast is applied and molded to maintain these forces. In the difficult case, an above-elbow cast gives greater assurance of maintaining pronation and some traction.

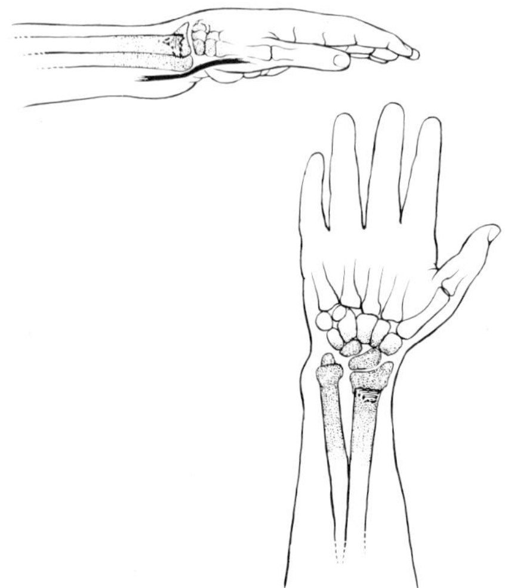

Figure 18–10 Colles' fracture.

As with other forearm bone fractures, swelling may be a serious problem. Elevation above the heart should be insisted upon. The patient is instructed to remain in bed for this purpose for at least 48 hours. Ideally, the arm should be suspended over the bed. If the patient is not hospitalized, an unplugged floor-standing lamp can be used for suspension. The next choice is to support the arm above heart level on pillows. Obviously, sitting up in bed or using a sling fails to provide sufficient elevation in the early period. Once the patient does get out of bed, he should rest his wrist on top of his head as much as possible and in a sling the rest of the time. If uncomfortable swelling does occur, decompression is imperative and is achieved by splitting and releasing both the cast and the cast padding. For this reason, inspection should be made routinely about 24 hours after application. The patient should be instructed to present himself sooner if pain, swelling or dysfunction of the fingers occurs.

THE WRIST (CARPUS)

Most carpal fractures and some dislocations can be detected only if the patient localizes pain in this area. Deformity is absent except in severe cases until after swelling has developed. X-rays should include oblique as well as anteroposterior and lateral views. A high index of suspicion should be used in reading the x-rays, and in doubtful cases, matching views should be obtained of the uninjured wrist. The most commonly overlooked injuries are a fracture through the navicular (Fig. 18–11) or a dislocated lunate. The former deserves a cast extending at least from the elbow to the distal phalanx of the thumb and designed to hold the thumb in abduction and apposition. The lunate injury requires prompt reduction and casting. The standard technique for reduction (by manual traction in dorsiflexion and "thumbing" the bone into place) is frequently unsuccessful, in which case open reduction is indicated.

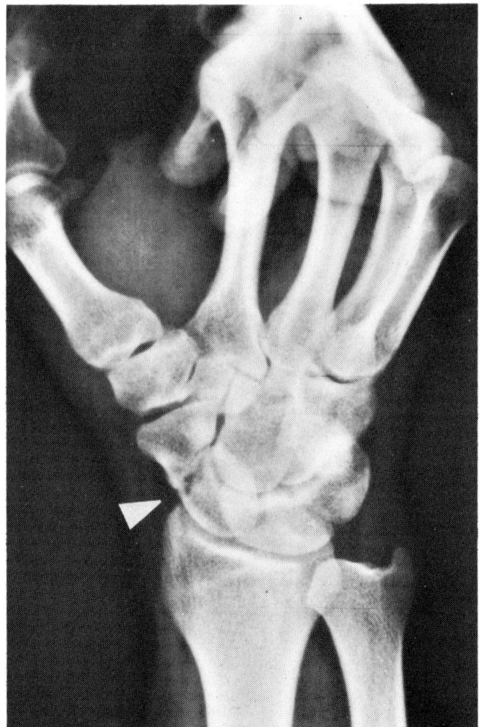

Figure 18–11 Oblique fracture, carpal navicular bone.

Ischemic necrosis of the lunate or of a fragment of the navicular is a frequent complication of these injuries. Various other types of carpal bone derangements do occur, some of which are more complex. Most of these can be identified by the same x-ray studies just recommended; however, a carpal tunnel view is sometimes helpful. The management of these more complex injuries is beyond the scope of this text.

THE HAND

Fractures or dislocations of hand bones are of major concern. The brief treatment that these injuries receive in this chapter is not a reflection of their importance; it is intended that additional information be sought elsewhere in this text and from textbooks devoted solely to this subject. In severe open injuries, tendons, nerves and other critical soft parts are generally involved as well as bones. The composite management of these is complex enough to support specialty interest, and such experienced help should be sought. Space is devoted in this chapter only to the management of specific isolated skeletal injuries.

Carpometacarpal Joint Injuries

Fracture dislocations of the first metacarpomultangular joint are commonly, but not exclusively, found among persons who have struck some other person or object with a fist. The force that drives the thumb metacarpal proximally may cause the anterior lip on the concave articular surface to break off on the palmar side while the major portion of the metacarpal dislocated proximally on the opposite side of the multangular bone. This is sometimes called a Bennett fracture. Pain and swelling occur just distal to the anatomical snuff-box, with slight shortening and marked limitation of abduction of the thumb. Emergency splinting is usually superfluous, as it is with most closed-hand fractures.

Traction is not so popular in the management of this injury as it was formerly. It may be possible to reduce the dislocation and fracture by pulling on the thumb and abducting it. These forces may be maintained by inserting a traction wire across the thumb and attaching it by rubber band to an "outrigger" extension from a gauntlet plaster cast. Unfortunately, such an arrangement is bulky, uncomfortable and frequently results in stiffness. For these reasons, open reduction with internal wire fixation, closed reduction with internal wire fixation or closed reduction with percutaneous Kirschner wire fixation is usually preferred. Accuracy of reduction is vital if the ability to fully abduct the thumb is to be retained and persistent pain in this important joint avoided. If malunion does occur, corrective osteotomy may improve the situation, but significant permanent physical impairment is still likely.

Dislocations of other carpometacarpal joints are very uncommon. The proximal end of one or more metacarpals may displace proximally and either volarly or dorsally over the wrist. A deformity in this area should be readily appreciated, but occasionally it is missed. A straight lateral x-ray of the hand is the most important view for detecting these injuries. Reduction may be accomplished by manual traction on the involved fingers while pressing the bones back into place. A well-molded cast may maintain reduction but if difficulty is encountered in either performing or maintaining reduction, surgical exploration and Kirschner wire fixation should be performed.

Metacarpal and Phalangeal Fractures

Fractures of metacarpals and phalanges are similar in many aspects. Fractures should be suspected in the presence of pain deformity or disability and oblique lateral and anteroposterior x-rays obtained. If precise reduction is already present or can be achieved by closed reduction and maintained by simple splinting in flexion, this is preferred. If not, open reduction and internal fixation, usually by oblique Kirschner wires, are indicated. Skeletal, fingernail or pulp traction seldom, if ever, provides proper immobilization of hand injuries. After reduction, residual malrotation may easily be overlooked. It must be specifically sought by ascertaining whether each finger, when *individually* flexed, points as it should to the tubercle of the navicular. Fingernail alignment provides a good guide to proper rotation of the digits. Parallel flexion of the fingers should be avoided as they are then forced into a strained position which may angulate or twist an unstable fracture.

Swelling must be prevented as much as possible by adequate elevation, as described in the management of the Colles' fracture. Dressings or casts must be decompressed if swelling does occur. No constriction or pressure points can be tolerated. In this regard, strapping a finger to an aluminum splint can be quite dangerous since it may cause swelling distal to the adhesive tape. Full immobilization for more than three to four weeks may result in intolerable stiffness.

When a man fractures his hand in a fist fight, examination usually reveals a depressed knuckle. Most frequently, the knuckle of the little finger is involved. The metacarpal is usually unduly prominent on the volar aspect of the hand and less prominent on the dorsal, although swelling may obscure the depression in dorsal contour. A very careful search should be made of the skin over the knuckle for a small cut that might indicate puncture by one of the teeth of the individual assaulted. In view of the virulence of infections caused by bacteria from the human mouth, it is most important that such an injury receive the same care as any compound fracture. If the deformity is due to a fracture through the neck of the fifth metacarpal, routine anteroposterior and oblique x-rays of the hand are adequate to determine the degree of tilt of the distal fragment toward the palm. On the other hand, if the second, third or fourth metacarpal is involved, the transverse arch of the normal hand necessitates a full lateral rather than an oblique view to evaluate angulation. A little tilt of the more mobile second or fifth metacarpal is less annoying than of the third or fourth. In the latter cases, a man who works with heavy hand tools may feel his displaced metacarpal head pressing uncomfortably against the palm whenever he grips an object tightly. Furthermore, the muscle balance of the finger may be disturbed by the angulation.

In managing these injuries, the metacarpal head must be pressed back up and a splint applied with the finger in moderate flexion to maintain reduction. Ninety-degree flexion of the metacarpophalangeal and interphalangeal joints should be avoided since the necrosis of the skin in the flexor creases may occur as a result of swelling and maceration. As with fractures of other bones in the hand, the hand should be explored if adequate reduction is not obtained and stable reduction assured, if necessary, with Kirschner wire fixation.

Finger Joint Injuries

A finger that is unstable, deformed or angulated at a joint may represent any of the following injuries: a fracture extending into the joint, a tendon avulsion or tear, a ligament tear or a frank dislocation. If a fracture is present, the fragments must be replaced and secured as accurately as possible if stiffness is to be minimized. If a collateral ligament is torn, the joint will be unstable in the coronal plane. Careful splinting for three or four weeks may be adequate to restore stability. If the tear is of the ulnar collateral ligament of the metacarpophalangeal joint of the thumb, conservative management by splinting is less likely to be effective. In this injury, sometimes called a "gamekeeper's thumb," surgical reconstruction of the ligament may be necessary. If an avulsed tendon insertion does not heal properly, weakness and loss of muscle balance will occur.

In certain cases, surgical reattachment is indicated; in others, simple splinting to facilitate spontaneous reattachment may be adequate. An example of this is the "baseball finger." In this condition the most distal extensor tendon insertion may be torn loose as the ball strikes the tip of the extended finger, causing sudden forceful flexion of the distal, interphalangeal joint. Clinically, there is pain and swelling centered about the distal interphalangeal joint with inability to straighten the tip independently. X-ray may show avulsion of a tiny fleck of bone from the dorsal lip of the distal phalanx. If the fragment is large enough to permit subluxation of this joint, open reduction and wire fixation are indicated.

If a finger cannot be extended at the proximal interphalangeal joint and the distal interphalangeal joint will not flex, avulsion of the extensor tendon from its insertion into the dorsal lip of the middle phalanx or a longitudinal tear of the extensor hood may have occurred. These two injuries allow the lateral bands to drop into an abnormally volar position, thus upsetting the muscular balance of the finger and producing the observed deformity known as a "boutonniere" deformity; it may require meticulous surgical repair.

A deformity of the thumb consisting

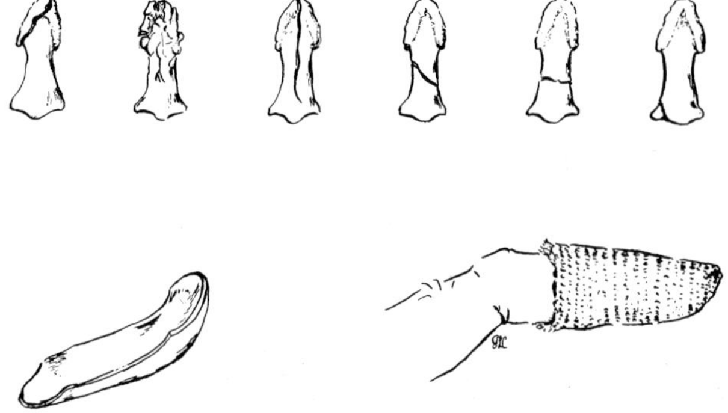

Figure 18–12 Crush injuries of the distal phalanges and their management. (Courtesy of Dr. Gaylord Clark.)

of a hard prominence at its base on the volar aspect and an outward angulation of the distal portion of the thumb in a radial direction is probably a metacarpophalangeal dislocation. It commonly results from forced hyperextension. The proximal end of the phalanx is displaced above the metacarpal head. It cannot usually be reduced by direct manual traction, but hyperextending the phalanx and then pushing it distally may be successful. If this maneuver fails, open reduction will probably be required since the metacarpal head may be trapped between the dual tendon insertions of the flexor pollicis brevis. Following reduction, immobilization in mild flexion should be maintained for three weeks.

Interphalangeal joints may be similarly displaced from forced hyperextension. Reduction should be performed in the same fashion as above and is usually more easily obtained. Again, immobilization in mild flexion is indicated for not more than three weeks; otherwise, severe stiffness may result. Dislocation of metacarpophalangeal joints other than that of the thumb is very uncommon.

The Crushed Distal Phalanx

Crush injuries of the distal phalanx, particularly from being caught in car doors, are important because of their frequency (Fig. 18–12). The fingernail, if still reasonably well attached, should be left in place to serve as a splint during early convalescence. The pain from blood collecting beneath the nail may be partially relieved by the creation of a small hole through its base by drilling, shaving with a razor blade or burning with a hot needle. A very light, small splint of aluminum, collodion-soaked tube gauze or plaster extending back to the proximal interphalangeal joint will add to the patient's comfort if not too tightly applied. It is important that the dressing not be bulky. No padding is necessary. Constant high elevation will minimize throbbing, as will an ice pack during the first few hours. If the skin is broken, thorough cleaning is just as important as with larger injuries. If a partial amputation has occurred and the distal piece is viable and contains a single, relatively large bone fragment, axial wire fixation may be indicated. An adequate supply of an analgesic should be provided and arrangements made for close follow-up care so that proper steps may be taken if any sign of infection occurs.

The proper care of the injured hand requires attention to detail with all the zeal and skill that are appropriate for any other part of the musculoskeletal system.

REFERENCES

1. Moseley, H. F.: Shoulder Lesions. London, E. & S. Livingstone, Ltd., 1969.
2. Neviaser, J. S.: Acromioclavicular dislocations treated by transference of the coracoacromial ligament. Clin. Orthop. 58:57, 1968.

chapter

19

FRACTURES OF THE LOWER EXTREMITIES

Virginia M. Badger, M.D.
Marshall B. Conrad, M.D.
Fred C. Reynolds, M.D.
Ronald E. Rosenthal, M.D.
and
Arthur H. Stein, Jr., M.D.

FRACTURES OF THE SHAFT OF THE FEMUR

Closed fractures of the distal two-thirds of the femur are frequently seen in the preschool child as a result of torsional force on the femur or a direct blow against the shaft. These fractures generally are not associated with other injuries and should be treated by closed conservative means consisting of Russell's traction[31] or balanced skeletal traction (Fig. 19–1) with a pin through the proximal tibia away from the tibial tuberosity to control and/or regain length and alignment and to control rotational deformities for a period of two to four weeks or until callus is visible by x-ray. The patient can then be immobilized in a plaster spica and treated at home until the fracture is united (Fig. 19–2). Mobilization of the joints occurs rapidly without the need of extensive supervised physical therapy.

Similar fractures in people over sixty are more prone to occur in patients with stiffness in the hip or knee and usually are the result of torsional forces, frequently with the knee extended. These fractures are rarely open or associated with arterial injury or extensive soft tissue injury.[20] They do, however, unite slowly and are often associated with considerable residual stiffness in the knee. Because of associated osteoporosis, these patients are poor candidates for internal fixation but they may occasionally be treated with dual-plate fixation. More often they have to be treated with skeletal traction followed by plaster immobilization. Although this form of treatment precludes wound infection,

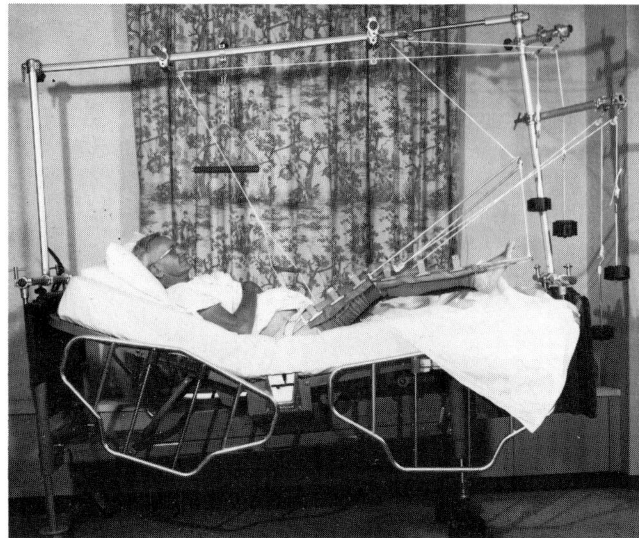

Figure 19–1 This is an adult patient in balanced suspension and skeletal traction. This is a common method of management for fractures of the shaft of the femur.

it adds considerably to the risk of thromboembolic disease, hypostatic pneumonia, severe nursing problems and slow recovery. At times the better part of valor is to ignore the position of the fracture and get the patient out of bed when dealing with an old, debilitated individual.

More extensive fractures of the distal two-thirds of the femur are often associated with multiple injuries resulting from deceleration accidents (Figs. 19–3 and 19–4). Most of these patients are young adults, although these injuries may occur at any age. These patients are frequently in shock even with a closed fracture due to sequestration of blood and serum about the fracture. Initial emergency management is to establish and maintain an airway, control hemorrhage and combat shock. Definitive treatment of closed fractures not associated with circulatory impairment is not an urgent matter once splinted, and should be delayed until associated life-threatening injuries are under control. In fact, there is substantial evidence that delay of one or two weeks before either open or closed reduction decreases the incidence of delayed or non-union.[39] Early treatment then is to prevent deformity and undue shortening by cast or traction until the time of reduction.

The aim of the physician in treatment of fractures is to restore the injured part or parts to normal function at the earliest possible time with the least risk to the patient. In open fractures, he should convert them to closed fractures as early as possible, again with the least risk to the patient. Treatment of an open fracture, therefore, is treatment of the wound. It matters not how beautifully the fracture may be reduced and maintained if the wound becomes infected as a result of inadequate care. For then the result, at best, is destruction of bone, loss of position and delayed or non-union of the fracture; at worst, it is loss of limb or life.

Care of an open fracture or fractures cannot be separated from care of the patient. The condition of the patient either from disease or associated injuries may force alteration in fracture management but rarely in wound therapy.

The immediate problem is resuscitation and maintenance of vital functions. Once an airway is functioning, hemorrhage is controlled and shock is being combated, sterile dressing should be applied to the wounds and

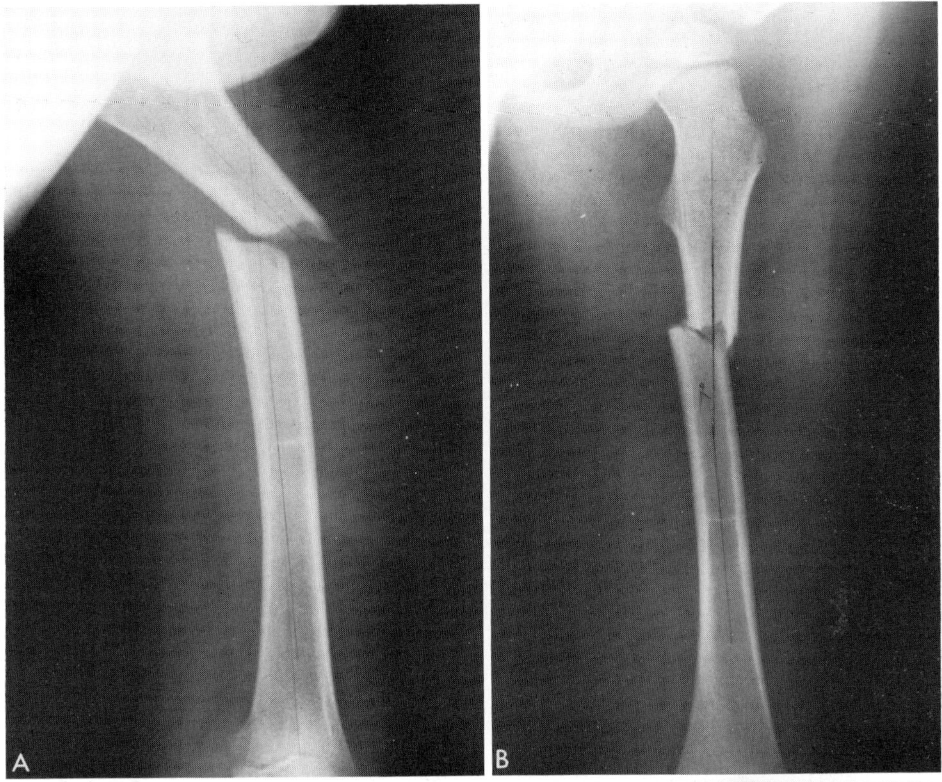

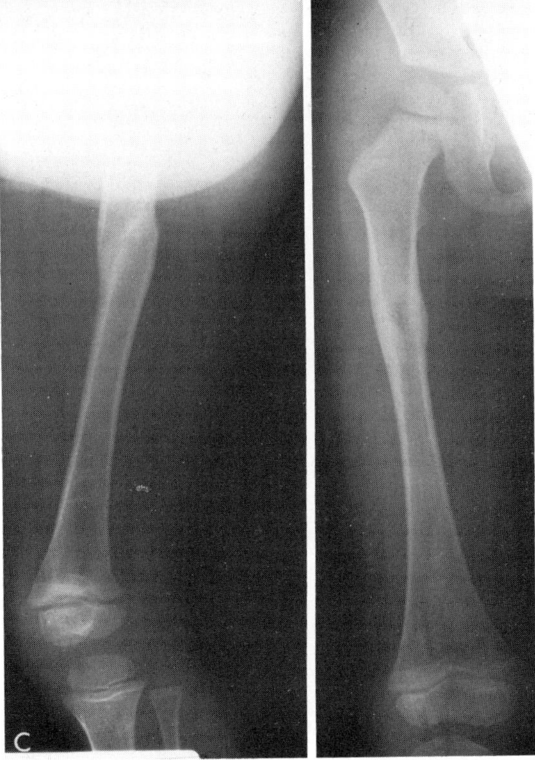

Figure 19–2 *A* and *B*, These are anteroposterior and lateral x-rays of a fracture at the junction of the proximal and middle thirds of the femur in a 5-year-old child. *C*, This fracture was maintained by means of skeletal traction through the proximal tibia for four weeks followed by eight weeks in a plaster spica cast. The film above shows the fracture six months after the injury with solid bony union and good early remodeling at the fracture site.

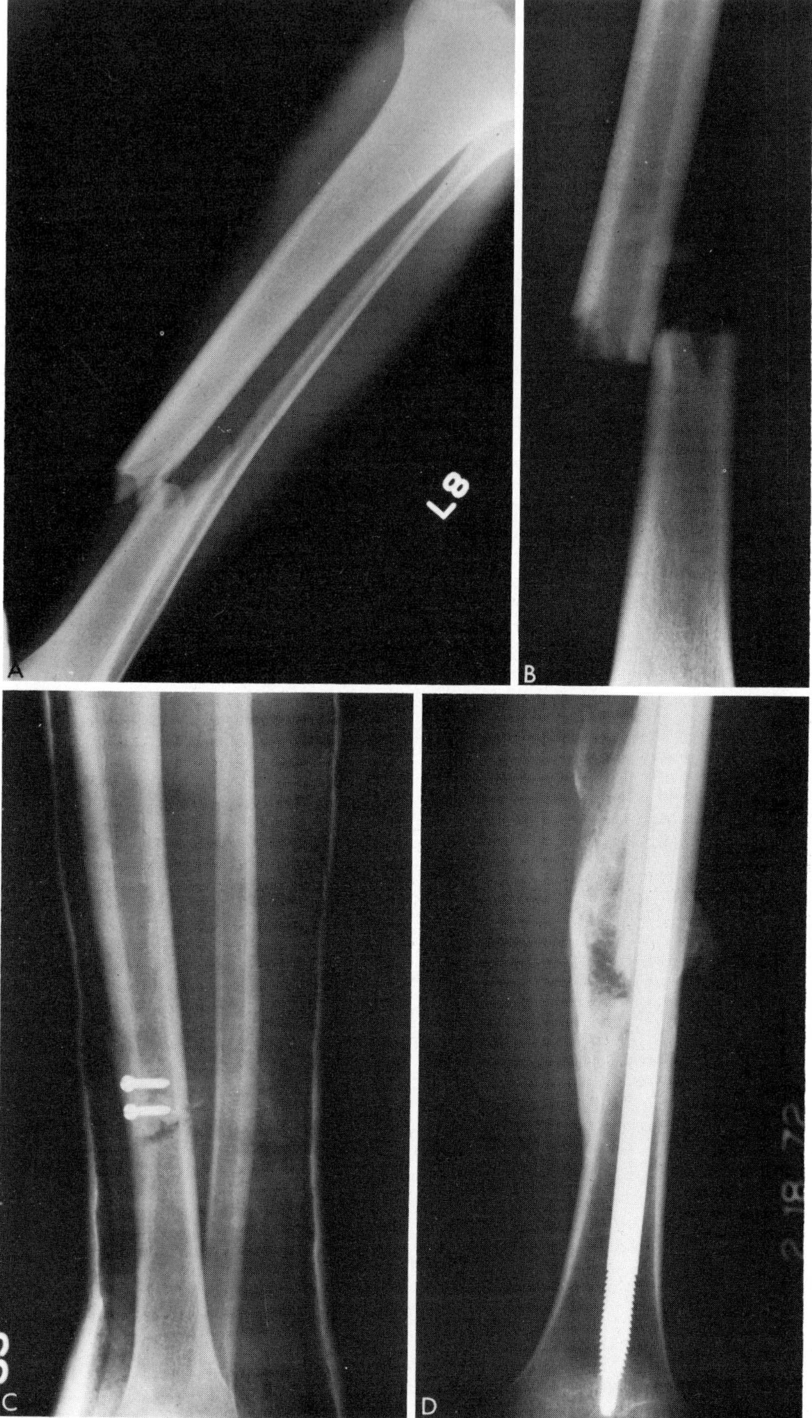

Figure 19–3 This is a 16-year-old male who was involved in an automobile accident and received fractures of the left tibia (*A*) and the left femur (*B*). Stabilization of the fracture of the left tibia was necessitated due to the inability to achieve a satisfactory closed reduction. The fracture of the femur was electively stabilized by intramedullary rod fixation. This allowed early ambulation and a minimal stay in the hospital for this combination of injuries. *C* shows the tibia immobilized with a long leg plaster cast. *D* shows the degree of bony union approximately one year after the injury.

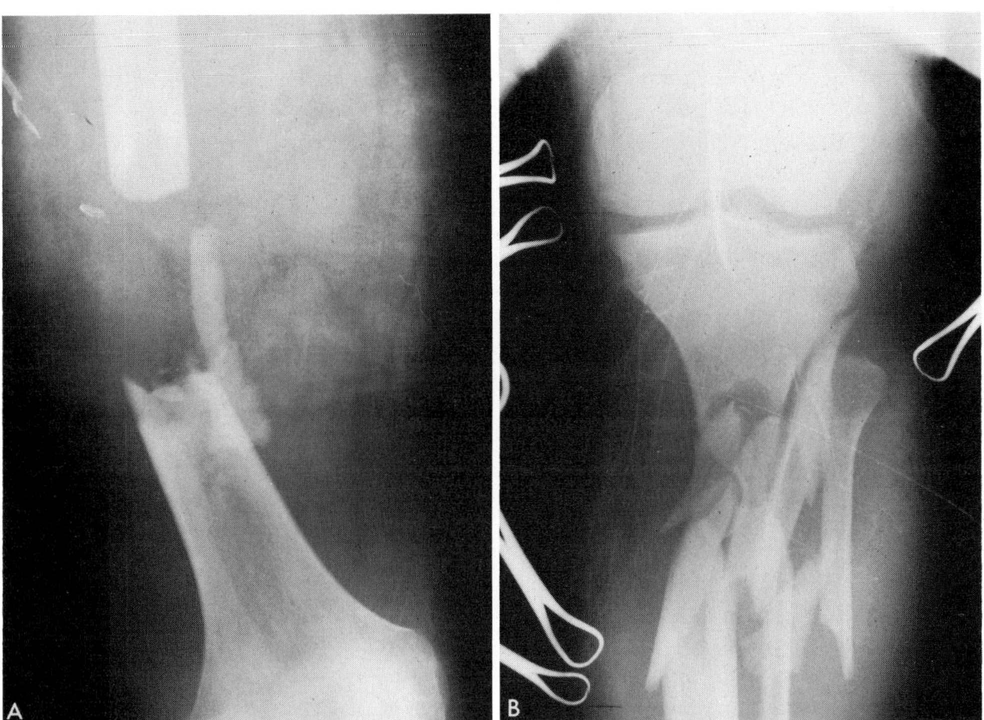

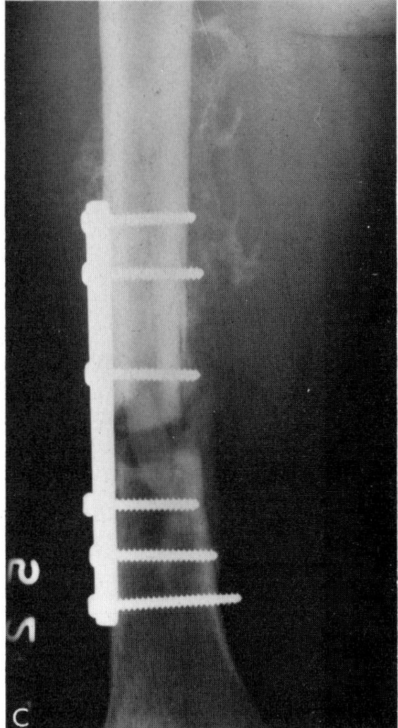

Figure 19–4 *A*, This 18-year-old white male was thrown from his motorcycle and received a fracture of the left femur which was open through a 10-inch wound over the anteromedial thigh. Three to four inches of the femoral shaft is missing. The foot was cold and pulseless. *B*, In addition, there was in the same extremity the severely comminuted fracture of the upper third of the tibia. Exploration of the femoral artery through the large thigh wound revealed the artery to be intact. An arteriorgram showed the artery disrupted at the trifurcation. *C*, Stabilization by means of internal fixation must be carried out if at all possible where arterial injury must be repaired in the presence of major long bone fractures. Either plate and screw fixation or intramedullary nail fixation can be used.

the extremity immobilized. Antibiotics and tetanus immunization are started at this time, and when replacement therapy is well on its way, the patient should be under control and the physician should have a good working diagnosis.

Once resuscitation is accomplished, each physician who manages trauma must ask himself a searching question: Are he and other members of the staff competent to care for all the patient's problems and can this care be accomplished in that institution? If the answer is no, then the patient should immediately be transferred to the nearest facility so prepared. Under no circumstances should wounds be closed while awaiting transfer, and there is no need to submit the patient to the trauma of extensive x-ray. I cannot emphasize this point too much, for it is one of the major reasons for poor results in trauma management. All too frequently, therapy is begun and wounds are closed either without thorough cleaning or when they should be left open. Sometimes, despite considerable effort and time devoted to fracture reduction, it is deemed advisable, for one reason or another, to send the patient to another hospital. Be honest with the patient and yourself and decide what is best for him. If it is going to be necessary to transfer him elsewhere, do it at once.

The factors that determine success or failure of wound treatment are: (1) the virulence of the organism contaminating the wound, (2) the number of these organisms, (3) the length of time they remain in the wound, (4) the health of the tissue contaminated, and (5) the resistance of the host.

The physician has no control over the number of organisms that get into the wound at the time of injury. He can decrease the number of organisms that subsequently get into the wound by immediate application of sterile dressing and protection of the wound while the extremity is being prepared for wound surgery. Early administration of antibiotics will tend to lessen virulence. Although we are not aware of definite experimental evidence that indicates that organisms remain as contaminants for six hours and then suddenly begin to grow, from a clinical standpoint at least it seems that there is about this much grace period, but this is not always true. So that the earlier debridement is done the better the chances of a clean wound. With the possible exception of small puncture wounds and wounds caused by low-velocity missiles, all open fracture wounds must have a debridement. There is no substitution for good wound surgery. For it is this treatment that reduces the number of organisms, shortens the time they remain in the wound and is a vital factor in determining the health of the tissue contaminated. The fifth factor, the resistance of the host, is augmented by blood replacement, antibiotics and diet.

Let's look at the wound itself. With the initial cellular damage there are released into the wound, probably as by-products of the injured cell, leukotoxins, necrosin, thyroxin and perhaps a leukopenic factor. In all probability, these substances promote the invasion of the damaged area by leukocytes, plasma cells and mast cells, and may contribute to the destruction of damaged but not entirely killed cells. A hematoma forms and is clotted with a fine meshwork of interwoven fibrin strands. In the first 24 hours there accumulates in the wound material with the staining properties of an acid mucopolysaccharide which is water-soluble and contains hexosamine. It is likely that this material is derived from plasma glycoprotein. Dunphy[12] found that hexosamine increases rapidly in the wounds, appearing as early as six hours after wound infliction, and usually reaches a peak after about 48 hours, returning to normal on the eighth or ninth day. Between 16 and 36 hours, there is a proliferation of mesenchymal cells and fibroblast, and by the third day there is active invasion of the clot by fibroblasts which are followed by vascular buds so that slowly the clot is organized into a highly vascular network. In the first 24 hours the pH of the hematoma may drop quite low, in the neighborhood of 5.6, which is likely due to a decreased oxygen tension and the damaged cells. Inorganic phosphorus levels are increased within the first 24 hours, and there is usually a second rise at the end of the first week. Alkaline phosphatase in wound fluid remains about the same as in the blood for the first week and then gradually rises. There is increased sulphur uptake by the fibroblasts, apparently to form sulphated polysaccharides, and after about three weeks this tagged sulphur shifts to an extracellular position. Somewhere between the fourth and sixth day, evidence of collagen formation is apparent with the appearance of hydroxyproline, and this rapidly increases to a peak about the twelfth day. It is assumed that this same type of reaction takes place in wounds which are associated with fracture. But so far as we know, no one has made a study of wound healing when a fracture is also present.

Wound fluid in the first week has a lower concentration of sodium, potassium, calcium and phosphorus than in the plasma. Early in the wound period the protein is also less. The chlorides remain about equal to the plasma concentration. Alkaline phosphatase moves from cells to matrix during the healing, and it has been suggested that the energy required for differentiation in cellular activity in the repair of a wound is by way of the Krebs cycle. In those wounds which are associated with a fracture, by somewhere around the eighth to the fourteenth day, the mesenchymal cells which have been actively proliferating to repair the injury differentiate into osteoblasts and chondroblasts with the early production of cartilage and osteoid, and several days later the osteoid matrix begins to be calcified.

The operation described as debridement has changed but little since it was described by Hugo of Lucca about 1200 B.C., and we quote from Whipple,[41] "In the first place the sides of the wound should be debrided or abraded, and then the wound should be completely cleansed of fuzz, hair, or anything else, and let be wiped dry with lint moistened with warm wine."

During the preparation and draping of the surrounding skin, the wound is protected, after which it is thoroughly irrigated, hopefully from within out. Except in the hand where it is so important to identify all structures, debridement is best done without a tourniquet, as we find it easier to determine viability of tissue. In certain instances it may be advisable to use a tourniquet to prevent excess blood loss, but if used, complete hemostasis is accomplished at the end of the procedure by removing the compression before final dressing. Then the margins of the skin and all dead and devitalized structures are excised continuing to extend the wound usually in a longitudinal direction until the most remote recess is thoroughly opened and in clear view. All foreign substances within the wound are removed. When the wound is thoroughly open, it is again irrigated with Ringer's solution, again removing strands of tissue floated up by the irrigating solution. After the teaching of Dr. J. Albert Key, we have used a sulfa crystal in the irrigating solution, at first sulfanilimide, and when manufacture of this was discontinued, sulfathiazole crystals. When sulfa was no longer available, we changed to a solution of polymixin, bacitracin and neomycin.

When the wound is thoroughly explored and revised, attention should turn to the bone. Small pieces of bone completely detached from soft tissue should be removed. However, large detached fragments, even if contaminated, are best cleaned and replaced in most instances.

At this stage the physician knows

the extent of soft tissue and bone damage and has a pretty good idea of the wound health. Damaged major vessels should be repaired; in certain instances this is mandatory. Where major artery repair has been accomplished, internal fixation of the fracture offers a better chance for function and healing of the vessels.[35] The vessels should be covered by soft tissue (muscle) if possible, but there is no other contraindication to packing the wound open (Fig. 19–4).

Nerve repair is probably not advisable but may be loosely brought together to facilitate future exposure and repair. Major tendons in certain instances may be repaired, but, for the most part, soft tissue structures are best treated by delayed repair.

What to do with the bone? We stated that the treatment of open fractures is the treatment of the wound so that it could early be converted to a closed fracture. The fracture, therefore, is not important and should not be treated except (1) as mentioned above when major vessels have been repaired, and (2) where there is extensive soft tissue loss associated with a very unstable fracture, such as both bones of the leg. In this situation secondary procedures, perhaps several, will be required to close the wound and stability of the fracture facilitates wound management. In all other situations the fracture usually can be controlled either by traction or external fixation and the bone should not be fixed. If internal fixation is indicated, intramedullary fixations should be employed if possible, for the more foreign bodies left in the wound, the greater the chance of wound infection.

What should be done with the wound? An occasional case will be seen early in which it appears that a careful and complete debridement has been done leaving healthy tissue and in which it is possible to bring the wound edges together without tension and obliterating dead spaces. In such a patient it may be permissible to close the wound but even here perhaps over continuing suction. In all other situations the wound should not be closed but packed open. In fact, it is far safer to pack all wounds open, for it does no harm, and if clean, they may then be closed in five days by delayed suture or appropriate skin grafts or flaps.

We have found that fine mesh gauze saturated with glycerine is best for the wound pack as this affords good drainage, does not macerate the tissue, and one may remove it and apply a skin graft without first wet-dressing the wound.

Once the wound is closed and healed without infection, then in about four weeks internal fixation may be used if indicated.

In those patients with multiple injuries about the anus, perineum and pelvis, conservative treatment is indicated in order to avoid the risk of infection. Infections resulting from internal fixation require prolonged skilled surgical care or they may result in amputation (Fig. 19–5). With conservative treatment one accepts the increased hospital cost, the increased risk from thromboembolic disease, residual permanent stiffness of joints, particularly the knee, the increased risk of decubiti and prolonged inactivity of the patient. The advantages of this form of treatment are decreased chance of infection, low mortality, infrequent delayed union and maintenance of length. Hip and knee motion are usually satisfactory although less than normal. This form of treatment is recommended for all children over four years of age and for extensively comminuted fractures at any level. The advantages of internal fixation by either an intramedullary nail or one or two plates are early ambulation, shortened hospital stay and early active motion of joints. Moreover, sedentary workers can be returned to work at a significantly earlier date.

Supracondylar and intracondylar fractures present difficult problems due to comminution, persistent displacement of fragments and disorganization

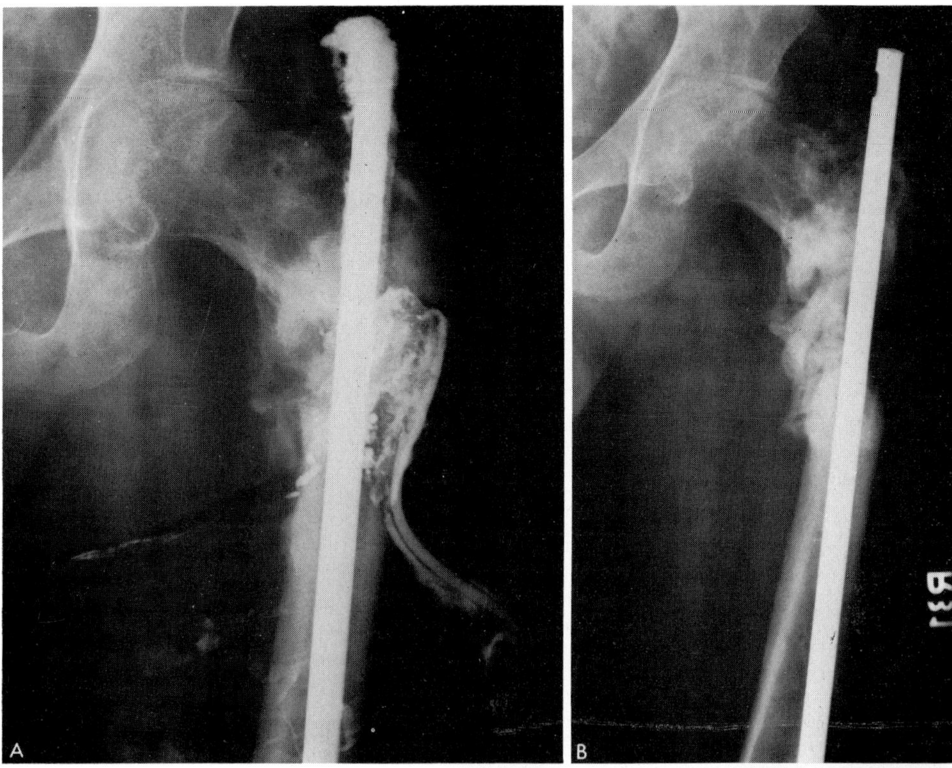

Figure 19–5 Open reduction and internal fixation of femoral shaft fractures complicated by wound infection, portend many months of incapacitation for the patient. *A* is the x-ray of a man two and a half years after intramedullary fixation of a femoral shaft fracture complicated by infection and non-union. The sinogram shows the extensive abscess cavity. In this instance, wide excision of the entire abscess cavity with extensive sequestrectomy was carried out. The nail was left in place for stability and the wound remained packed open for months. *B*, Six months after sequestrectomy there is evidence of new bone formation and some fracture healing. *C*, One and a half years after sequestrectomy bony union had occurred, the nail had been removed and the drainage from the wound had ceased.

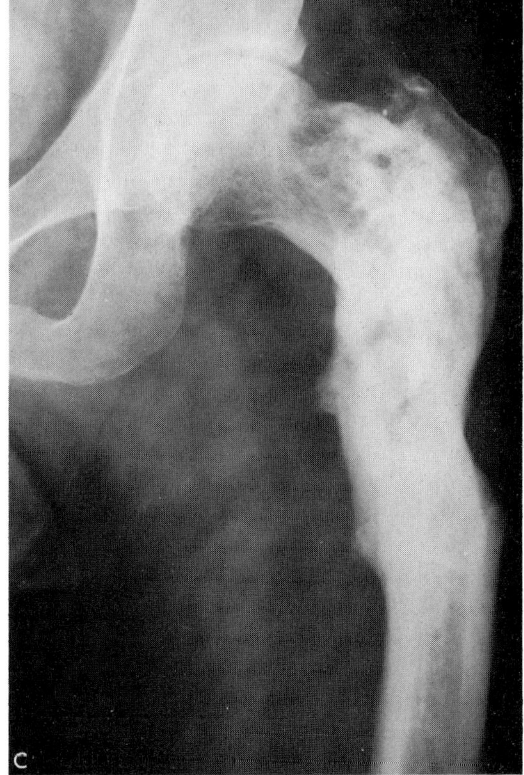

of the articular surface. Manipulation combined with skeletal traction applied to the tibia is frequently successful in obtaining and maintaining a functional position. At times it is necessary to apply skeletal traction to the distal fragment to bring it up into alignment. Occasionally, restoration of the articular surface and re-alignment of the condyles of the femur cannot be obtained without open reduction. Once obtained, often a single Webb bolt is adequate to maintain the position. Various other types of internal fixating devices have been used. However, caution is indicated as there seems to be a direct relationship between the incidence of infection and the magnitude and amount of metal employed to secure fixation (Fig. 19–6). If the articular surface and alignment can be restored without surgical violation of the fascial envelope of the thigh, maximum knee motion may be maintained.[36] It is our experience, however, that open reduction and secure internal fixation with Webb bolt or blade plate is often required to restore joint surfaces.

INJURIES TO THE KNEE

The position and architecture of the knee joint and the functional demands placed upon it result in frequent knee injuries. The exact number that occurs in the country each year is unknown. Certainly, a large number occur in sports. Reported injuries by professional football for the American and National Conferences in the year 1967 were 55 knee injuries occurring in preseason practice, 62 in regular practice sessions, and 91 during the course of the regular season. These 208 injuries were sufficiently severe to incapacitate the player for at least one week. Thirty of these players had surgery for torn cartilages. Nineteen players had surgical repair for torn ligaments, and 13 of these 19 involved a collateral ligament and one or both cruciates. Sixty-nine of the 208 players receiving knee injuries in 1967 gave a history of prior injury to the involved knee. There were 83 other injuries to the knee that were considered to be reasonably minor and did not incapacitate the player. It would appear that for the year 1967 in professional football, approximately 10 per cent of the participating athletes received a knee injury. Some years ago in an effort to determine knee injury proneness, 137 athletes were examined prior to their participation in football at Washington University and were thereafter followed through their college career.[28] We found that there was a significantly greater chance of re-injury to a knee that had suffered a prior injury and also that there was a significantly greater chance of injury to a loose knee as compared to a tight knee. These findings have recently been substantiated by Nicholas.[21]

Stability of the knee joint is provided both by ligaments and surrounding muscles, the muscles augmenting and reinforcing the ligamentous system. Within this system the ligaments are called upon to support the knee against stress for that fraction of a second before muscle contraction occurs. Therefore, although large, strong muscles surrounding the knee joint are a help in support, they do not prevent serious ligament damage.

The aim in the treatment of injuries to the knee is to establish an anatomically accurate diagnosis as soon as possible and then to carry out appropriate treatment. It is a great help to know the status of the knee prior to the injury. This, however, can only be done where it is possible to examine athletes prior to their participation in sport. It is also helpful to be present at the sports activity and to examine the injured knee immediately following the injury. However, we do not believe that impressions obtained from examination on the field should constitute the final assessment. This examination, however, can give the physician some idea of the degree of severity

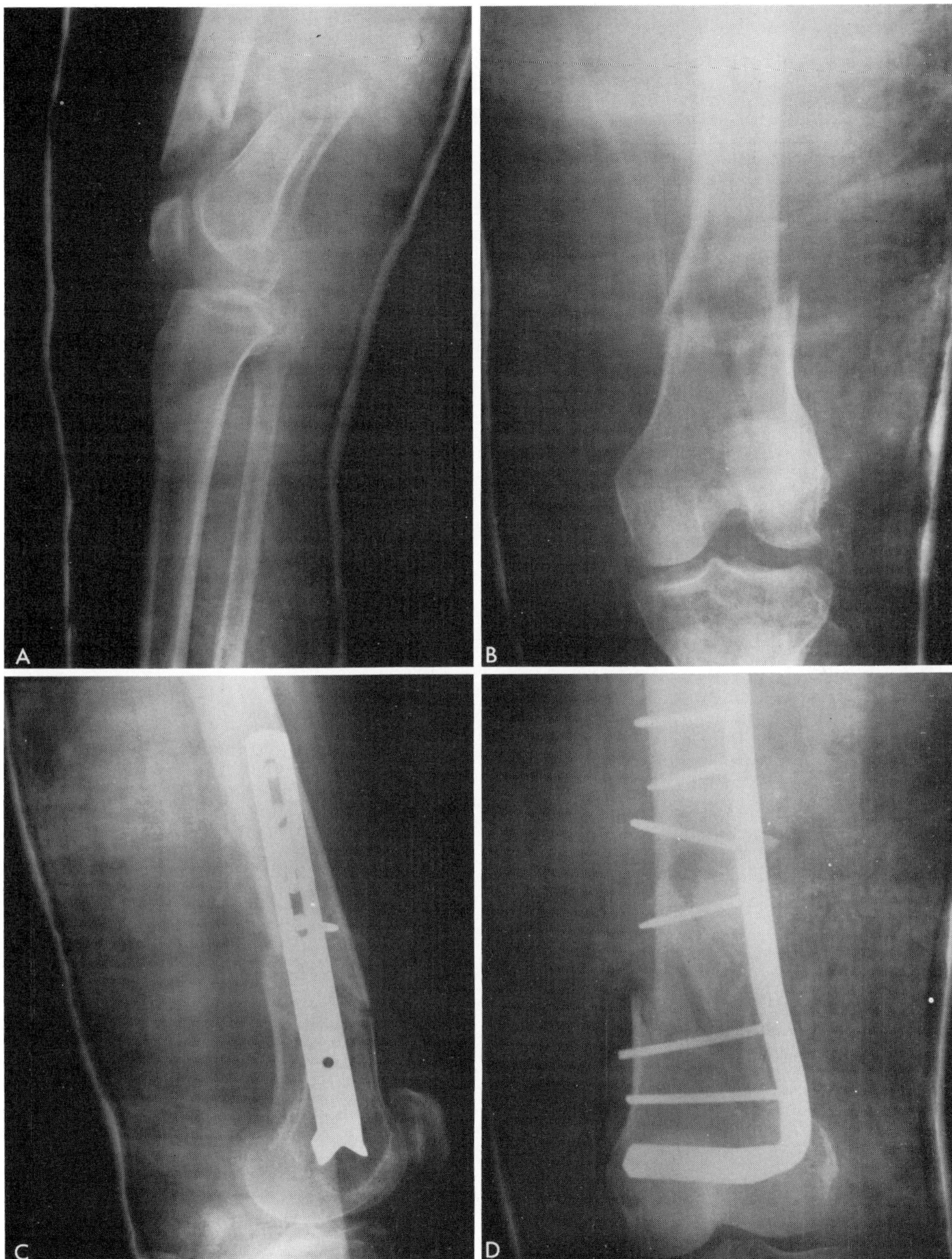

Figure 19–6 *A* and *B*, These are anteroposterior and lateral views of the left knee in a 65-year-old woman which show a markedly displaced intracondylar and supracondylar fracture of the left femur. This patient had a comparable injury of the right femur along with rib fractures resulting in a bilateral flail chest. Closed manipulation and traction failed to achieve a satisfactory reduction of these fractures. *C* and *D*, Open reduction and internal fixation was required but could not be done for approximately one month, which was the amount of time required for stabilization of the thoracic injuries.

of the injury and a judgment can be made as to whether or not the player should return to that particular activity. It has been our observation that the severity of the injury seems to be greater or less when examined immediately on the field than it does after the game when inspection and observation can be carried out comparing both knees in the dressing room. We, therefore, see no great advantage to being in a hurry to make a final decision or rushing into a surgical repair, as repeated observations have given us a clearer view of the anatomical damage.

When the physician is not present at the time of the injury and sees the patient at a later time, history can be helpful in that with a severe ligamentous injury, the player will not be able to continue in the sport because of pain and loss of function in the knee joint. With a less severe ligament or cartilage injury, pain may subside rapidly so that he is able to return to the game without trouble for the remainder of the day. However, that evening there will be a steadily increasing amount of pain and swelling.

Whether the examination is carried out early or some time later, prior to the examination an effusion should be aspirated and, of course, the character of this effusion examined. After this the injured knee is systematically examined, always comparing the findings with the uninjured, opposite knee. Immediately after the injury, even after a serious ligament injury, the patient has the power of full active extension. Active or passive block in extension at this time indicates an associated cartilage tear. However, in a few days even a minor ligament injury may prevent both active and passive extension and be confused with a cartilage tear. Rarely is it possible for the patient to fully flex the knee in the presence of significant ligament damage, even after the effusion has been removed.

When dealing with severe ligament ruptures, interpreting the physical findings usually is not too difficult. If the knee joint readily opens on either abduction or adduction stress, as the case may be, the supporting ligaments on the medial or lateral side of the knee have been torn as well as one or both cruciates. There may, in addition, be damage to one or both menisci. Excess internal rotation of the tibia on the femur suggests lateral structural rupture, while excess external rotation of the tibia on the femur indicates medial capsular tear. In both of these situations there may be an associated cruciate tear. A posterior drawer's sign indicates posterior cruciate rupture and there frequently is damage to the posterior capsule. The anterior drawer's sign suggests tear or stretch of the anterior cruciate ligament together with capsular tear. But an absence of the anterior drawer's sign does not rule out damage to the anterior cruciate ligament. Rupture of the anterior cruciate ligament is a rotational injury and may occur without damage to any other structure of the knee. It is more commonly ruptured from its femoral attachment and drops into the front of the joint, thus blocking extension more commonly to the lateral side, and the true nature of the lesion, found only after a diagnosis of a meniscus tear, has been made and the knee explored. This injury frequently is associated with a marked bloody effusion, pain being referred to the posterior lateral aspect of the knee joint.

Another indication of rupture of the anterior cruciate ligament is hyperextension in the injured knee as compared with the uninjured knee. At times an arthrogram can be of help in arriving at this specific diagnosis.

The location of tenderness and swelling as well as the location and degree of instability will as a rule allow for an anatomical diagnosis. The ordinary x-ray in these injuries is usually negative, although at times when the lateral ligaments are ruptured, the lateral collateral ligament and the biceps tendon will pull off a piece of bone from the upper end of the fibula and this then affords con-

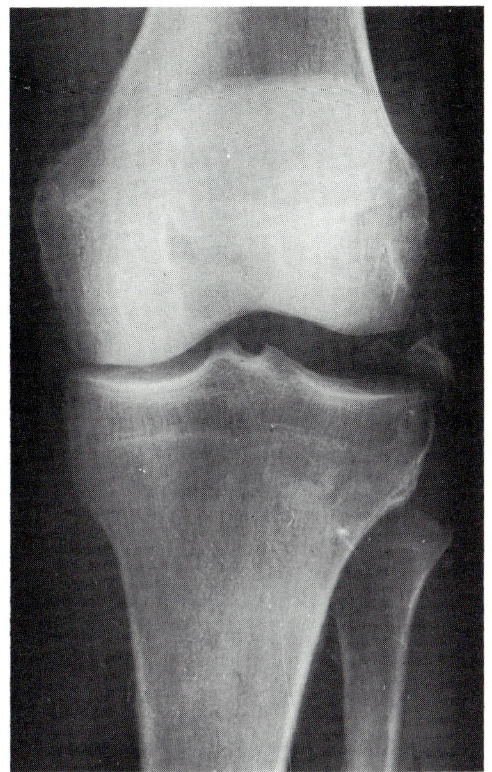

Figure 19–7 Avulsion of the lateral collateral ligament and biceps tendon with a portion of the upper fibula. (Courtesy of Dr. Bernard Rineberg.)

siderable conformation to your diagnosis (Fig. 19–7). Occasionally, a fleck of bone will also come off of the medial side of the joint and, of course, the tibial spine is at times pulled away from the cruciate ligament. Except for illustrative purposes, the stress films are of no great help, nor has the arthrogram been revealing in recent collateral ligament injuries. In dealing with youngsters before the epiphyses have closed, one has to constantly keep in mind the possibility of epiphyseal displacement masquerading as a ligament injury (Fig. 19–8). In these circumstances the ordinary x-ray plus the stress film may be most helpful. For the most part, however, diagnosis depends on the history and physical findings, and once this diagnosis has been established, one must then assess the degree or severity of injury for the purpose of treatment which is to allow the patient the best chance to reconstitute his ligaments. If the collateral ligaments are cut or torn and fall back into apposition, there is an excellent chance that the ligament will be reconstituted. If, however, they are not in apposition, the gap will fill with scar and the ligament will not be reconstituted, thus, functional instability will remain. In injuries in which one or more of the ligaments are completely severed, diagnosis usually is not difficult as the instability is profound. The decision on treatment is also not difficult in that the likelihood that these ligaments will fall back into apposition is not sufficiently great to justify conservative treatment. These ligaments, therefore, need to be explored surgically and brought together by suture, but not sutured so tightly that circulation is impaired. This will prevent reconstitution of the ligament. Diagnosis of a partially torn ligament is, as a rule, not too difficult. While there is disability, tenderness, swelling, pain and some instability, the instability is not of great magnitude and for the most part these can be treated non-surgically. Unfortunately, a large number of injuries fall in between these two categories. In these circumstances trying to make a decision as to which one to repair and which one not to repair is extremely difficult. We believe, therefore, that the wise policy to adopt is that once the diagnosis of a ligament tear has been established, if there is doubt as to its severity, it should be exposed surgically rather than to take a chance that the torn ligament is in apposition. If surgical repair is decided upon, we believe it is advisable to carry out this procedure within the first ten days.

When the cruciate ligaments are torn either from their attachments or in the body of the ligament, they will never fall back into apposition except in an occasional rare circumstance when one or both of the cruciate ligaments are torn from the tibia without significant displacement. In such a

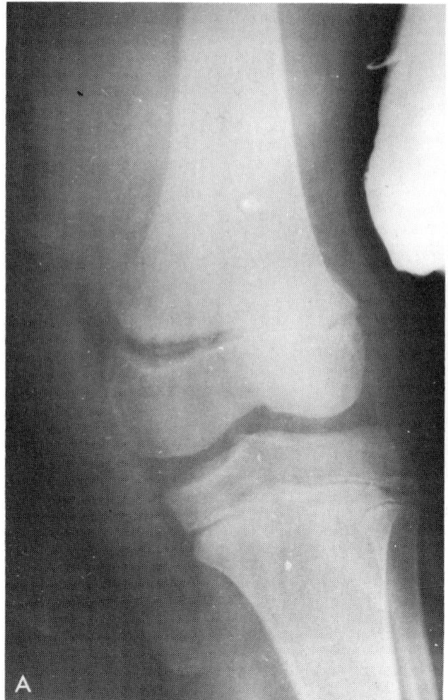

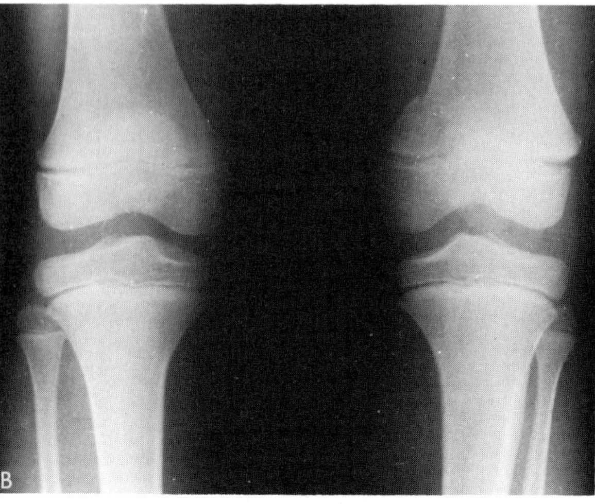

Figure 19–8 *A,* AP of right knee with epiphyseal injury. *B,* AP of right knee. Epiphyseal injury simulating tibial collateral ligament rupture.

case, they may re-attach, although we have never personally seen an instance of this type proved by later re-operation. The cruciate ligaments, therefore, need surgical repair. When they are avulsed from either the femur or the tibia with a piece of bone, chances of success are good. However, when the ligament ruptures close to its attachment on either side or in its substance, the chances of success are very poor indeed. Since the cruciates are fan-shaped compound ligaments, virtual mirror images of each other and so arranged that some segments of the cruciate ligaments are tight in all positions of the knee, it is almost always impossible following rupture to re-align and re-attach the ligament in its anatomical position. The repair is further hampered by the technical problem of trying to re-attach the shortened ligament to bone as the excess tension placed on the ligament may result in a necrosis rather than in a repair. However, we do not believe that the effort is entirely hopeless and that they should be excised rather than repaired. We believe that an attempt should be made to repair all the damaged structures when it is possible to do so.

Ligamentous injuries which are not sufficiently severe to require surgery, in our opinion, are best treated by a period of non-weight-bearing exercises rather than by plaster fixation. Weight-bearing may be permitted as soon as range of motion and muscle function have returned and the effusion has disappeared. Following surgery, we believe that immobilization is necessary for a variable period of time, depending upon the number of ligaments torn, the repair and the muscle control of the individual. Some will be out of the plaster in a few days and started on a program of non-weight-bearing exercises, while others may require plaster fixation for three to four weeks before such a program can be instigated.

The menisci are torn somewhat more frequently than are the major ligaments about the knee. An abnormal meniscus may be found at all ages and in various occupations. In the young child it is more apt to be a discoid lateral meniscus. In the athlete one or both menisci may be torn with rotational injuries, while a similar stress of considerably less degree in the older person may tear a meniscus already undergoing degenerative changes. Tears in the menisci that are very close to the capsule and also apparently close to the anterior or posterior attachment to bone may heal. Other tears, however, do not and result in some alteration of the normal function of the joint, and, therefore, should be removed. Once the meniscus is torn, even when removed, the knee is not normal and a certain percentage of these will go on to degenerative changes. This is particularly apt to happen when both menisci are removed. In an effort to reduce the likelihood of degenerative arthritis occurring following meniscal tears, we do not attempt to remove the entire meniscus but leave a rim attached to the capsule when this part of the meniscus appears normal. We have also found it next to impossible to remove the posterior attachment of the medial meniscus even when a posterior medial incision has been made. It is indeed rare that this posterior fragment has caused trouble requiring subsequent surgery. Perhaps the posterior one-third could be left without too much difficulty. Follow-up studies by Tapper and Hoover[38] indicated that the best results from medial meniscectomy were in those in which there was a bucket handle tear in which the displaced portion was detached, leaving the outer rim intact. There is, however, some hazard to leaving a rim of cartilage in that it may subsequently be torn loose from its lateral attachments and displace into the joint, resulting in further locking and necessitating a second operative procedure. This has occurred in about three per cent of our patients. It is, of course, difficult for the patient and relatives to understand and perhaps of some embarrassment to the surgeons. However, we have felt that leaving the rim resulted in a better functioning joint than when the entire meniscus was removed. We, therefore, feel that we would rather do a second procedure than to take it all out. Here again, postoperative immobilization seems to have little to offer and, therefore, we prefer early active non-weight-bearing exercises and weight-bearing as soon as muscle function and support has returned.

In 1927, Galeazzi[14] described the frequent firm attachments of the anterior horn of the lateral meniscus to the anterior cruciate ligament as well as the attachment of the posterior horn of the lateral meniscus to the anterior cruciate ligament (Fig. 19–9). In addition, he called attention to the attachment of the posterior horn of the lateral meniscus to the medial condyle of the femur when the ligaments of

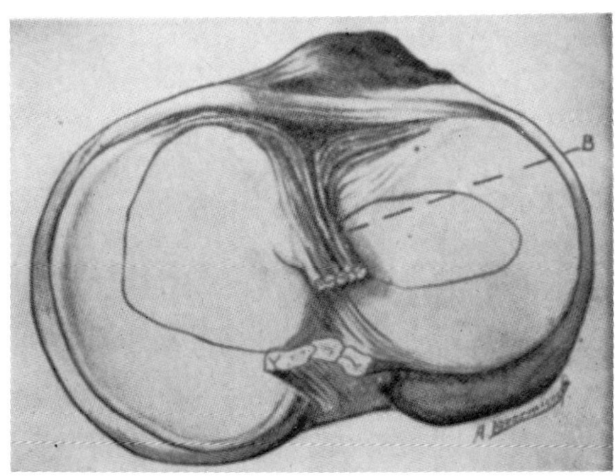

Figure 19–9 Attachments between cruciate ligament and menisci. (From Galeazzi, R., J.B.J.S., 9:515, 1927.)

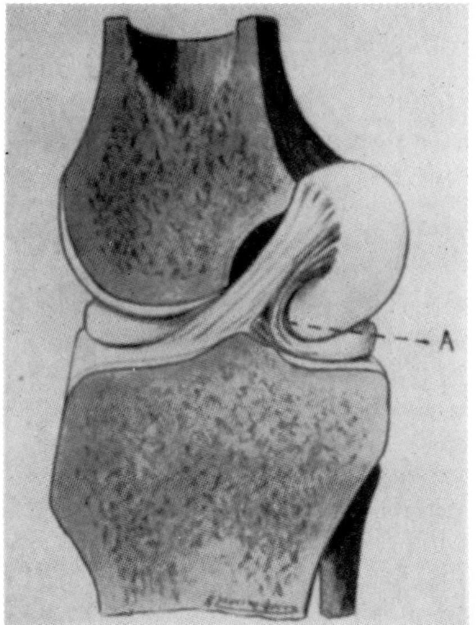

Figure 19–10 Lateral dissection showing connection of lateral menisci to anterior cruciate. (From Galeazzi, R., J.B.J.S., 9:515, 1927.)

Wrisberg and Humphry were present (Fig. 19–10). He also found that at times there was a strong attachment from the posterior horn of the lateral meniscus to the anterior horn of the medial meniscus, the so-called Barkow's ligament (Fig. 19–11), and stressed the importance of the transverse ligament that connects the anterior horn of the medial and the lateral meniscus and their firm attachments to the tibia by the coronary ligaments. Professor Galeazzi felt that the menisci were an integral part of the cruciate ligament system and that both were important in guiding the joint in flexion, extension and rotation. Helfet,[16] in 1959, agreed with the mechanisms and the relationship of the cruciates and the menisci described by Galeazzi and postulated that the medial meniscus would be torn when the normal rotary motions of the knee were forcefully prevented. Incidentally, he also explained chondromalacia of the patella and degenerative changes in the articular surface of the medial condyle of the femur on this same mechanism; that is, utilization of the leg while normal rotary motions were prevented by something blocking the joint.

In recent years the diagnosis of internal derangement of the knee has been facilitated by the improved technique of arthrography. Reliability depends upon the skill of the radiologist performing the test, his experience in interpreting the films and consultation with the examining physician.

Other injuries about the knee involve the quadriceps mechanism, the quadriceps tendon, the patella and the patella tendon. The quadriceps tendon is more prone to rupture in individuals 30 years of age or older and it usually occurs as a result of sudden severe contraction of the quadriceps mechanism against a

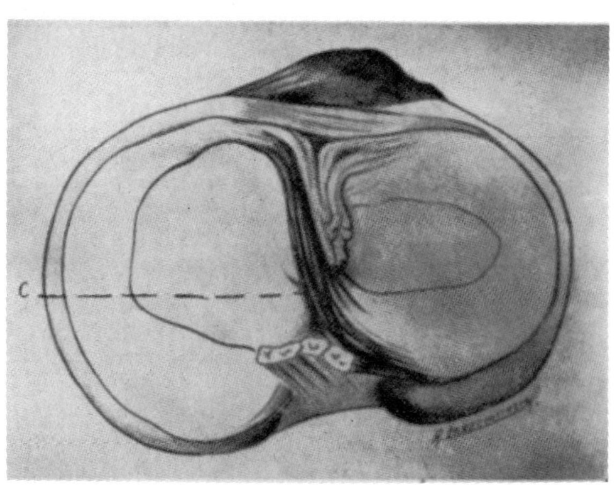

Figure 19–11 Barkow's ligament. (From Galeazzi, R., J.B.J.S., 9:515, 1927.)

fixed lower extremity. It may also occur in falls and other injuries. There is immediate pain and local swelling and impairment of knee extension. As a rule, the patella can be palpated intact with a defect in the soft tissue just superiorly to the patella. Although from the history and physical findings one may be confused with a fracture of the patella, the x-rays reveal that the patella is intact. The diagnosis, therefore, is not difficult. The treatment is surgical repair followed by plaster immobilization for six weeks and the instigation of a system of resistant exercises.

Rupture of the patella tendon may also occur in like manner followed by inability to extend the knee against gravity, frequently a palpable defect in the tendon, and when compared with the opposite side, the patella is found to lie caudal toward the head. Again, the diagnosis is not difficult and the treatment is surgical repair of the tendon with the postoperative management the same as for the quadriceps tendon.

Fractures of the patella are much more common than ruptures of the ligament on either side and are usually associated with a direct blow, although occasionally they occur from indirect violence. The fractures may be of any configuration but tend to be somewhat transverse, involving the junction of the middle and lower third of the patella. These fractures are important to the future function of the knee joint in that complete fracture of the patella disrupts the quadriceps mechanism with loss of extension of the knee, and unless the damaged patella heals with a smooth joint surface, degenerative changes in the knee will occur. Nondisplaced fractures that are associated with no loss of function of the quadriceps mechanism may be treated by simple plaster immobilization. All displaced fractures must be treated surgically. A major fragment of the patella may be left and the patella tendon reconstituted. However, if the fragments are small or if there is extensive comminution, total excision of the patella with suture of the tendon as well as the lateral expansion to the knee joint gives a better result than attempting to restore the fracture fragments. The surgical approach we prefer for correction of fractures of the patella is a horseshoe-shaped incision placed in the transverse creases under the knee about an inch below the normal position of the patella. This gives a much better cosmetic result than another incision about the knee.

FRACTURES OF THE TIBIA

The crest of the tibia is subcutaneous for its entire length. Fractures of the shaft of the tibia may penetrate this thin tissue. Any suspect fracture of the leg should be immediately splinted, immobilizing the knee and the ankle. Proper initial treatment of a closed fracture will prevent it from becoming an open fracture due to skin necrosis and slough. Initial treatment of an open fracture should be with a dressing over the wound and an adequate splint. No attempt should be made to push an exposed piece of bone back under the skin, and no real attempt should be made at reduction unless there is a grotesque deformity of the leg. In that case, the leg should be straightened and splinted.

Fractures of the proximal tibia can result from a varus or valgus stress on the knee. A direct blow, such as that from an automobile bumper, is a frequent cause of these injuries. Any fracture involving the articular surface of either the medial or lateral tibial plateau can result in traumatic arthritis. In common with most fractures near the end of a long bone, these fractures do unite readily. However, late changes in the articular surface may cause difficulties in the future.

Minimally displaced fractures of the proximal end of the tibia involving the articular surface can be managed by elevating the leg and beginning early motion in a few days in balanced suspension. Once the acute symptoms have subsided, usually in one or two weeks, the patient can be started on non-weight-bearing exercises. Weight-bearing can begin as soon as radiologic evidence of union occurs. More extensively displaced or depressed fractures are managed by either traction and early motion or open reduction and reassembly of the fracture fragments. If this latter course is chosen, the depressed fragments are elevated and held in position with supplemental bone grafts and fixed internally. Usually, wires in the form of either a Webb bolt or Kirschner wires, or sometimes pins, are necessary. Fixation should be secure enough to allow early active motion before fracture healing. In any fracture or surgery involving the tibial articular surfaces, early motion in the post-injury period is essential in restoring as nearly normal knee action as possible.[30] Immobilization of these fractures until union occurs inevitably results in some loss of motion.

Fractures of the shaft of the tibia may occur from a direct blow, a twisting force or a penetrating wound. If the fibula remains intact, the fracture will be stable and can be managed by a cast and early weight-bearing once the swelling subsides. Isolated fractures of the tibia are rarely significantly displaced, although occasionally the fracture will be angulated toward the fibula. This position can rarely be altered without open reduction, and is usually acceptable.

Fractures of both bones of the leg are serious injuries. The older literature is filled with cases of tibial fractures treated by open reduction with resulting non-union and/or infection. Most of the complications of fractures of the shaft of both bones of the leg are the result of the fracture being open. Definite risk of infection occurs with any open fracture, whether the fracture is opened by the injury or by a surgeon. Infection is probably the single most common factor in the development of non-union, resulting frequently in shortening as well as extensive scarring of the leg. In the past ten years, considerable data have been accumulated on the advantages of closed reduction and early weight-bearing in the management of tibial fractures.[9, 33] This technique is now recommended for the vast majority of these injuries. Open reduction and fixation with plates or nails is rarely indicated in non-segmental fractures of both bones of the leg.

Proper x-rays are mandatory before beginning treatment. These must include both ends of the bone; occasionally a rotary injury will produce a spiral fracture of the middle or distal third of the tibia and a fracture of the neck of the fibula. This latter injury will be missed on an x-ray showing only the suspected tibial fracture. Once the nature of the injury is appreciated, the patient should be hospitalized. With a reasonably stable fracture, the limb is placed in a long leg cast and elevated. Unstable fractures should be held in traction. No attempt to reduce the fracture should be made in the acute state. Generally, it will take a week to ten days for the swelling to subside so that manipulation can be done. Manipulation can be performed successfully without anesthesia in a well-sedated, cooperative patient, although many surgeons prefer general anesthesia. The leg is bent at the knee and allowed to dangle unsupported over the side of the table. A layer of stockinette followed by a thin layer of cotton padding is rolled on, and, using gravity and traction, the fracture is manipulated. Any angulation of malrotation is corrected and the cast applied in sections. We agree with Watson-Jones[40] that under no circumstances should a non-padded cast be applied to a fresh fracture of both bones of the leg. X-rays are obtained as soon as the cast is set. Minor angular deformities can be corrected by wedging, but any major misalignment requires remanipulation. If a short-leg patellar tendon-bearing cast is applied, it must be molded carefully around the tibial condyles and patellar tendon and popliteal fossa and then, with the knee in 0 degrees, brought up to mid-thigh. A walking heel is attached and the patient allowed to bear weight on crutches as soon as the plaster is hard.

Once weight-bearing begins, further x-rays are obtained. Some shortening may occur when weight-bearing starts but, if the cast is properly applied, does not progress. The patient is encouraged to bear full weight on the fractured limb and can be discharged from the hospital once he is comfortable. The patient should then be seen at frequent intervals, particularly if there are any complaints of discomfort. If the cast becomes loose or breaks down in spots, it should be replaced. The cast is routinely changed at five weeks, and, if a long-leg cast has been used initially, a short-leg patellar tendon-bearing cast is applied at this time. Cast support should continue until radiologic evidence of fracture healing occurs, usually about three months from the time of injury (Fig. 19–12).

Open fractures of the tibia can be managed like open fractures elsewhere in the body. The wound should be explored in the operating room under anesthesia and then debrided as necessary, although little skin debridement is usually indicated. The wound is dressed, the fracture is aligned and a cast applied. Five days later the cast and dressing are removed, the wound is closed or covered with a skin graft, and the fracture is manipulated and recasted. Once the wound is closed, the fracture is managed as a closed fracture. Occasionally, the wound is small and clean. In such instances, the surgeon may elect to close the wound primarily and then initiate treatment as a closed fracture. However, if the slightest doubt exists as to the cleanliness or viability of the wound edges, the wound should be left open at the initial debridement and sutured by delayed closure five days later.

Internal fixation is rarely necessary in open tibial fractures. If associated injuries are present which would require multiple handling of the patient, then the fracture might better be held in position with internal fixation. Fractures of the tibial shaft can rarely be kept in proper alignment by a cast in a recumbent patient, and associated injuries remain one of the primary indications for considering open reduction and internal fixation of an unstable fracture of both bones of the leg (Fig. 19–13). However, the surgeon who performs this procedure must bear in mind that open reduction and fixation of a tibial shaft fracture is a particularly hazardous procedure with associated risks of infection and nonunion. If internal fixation with an intramedullary nail is decided upon, once the nail has been inserted and the fracture reduced, weight-bearing can begin in a long leg cast with the knee straight as soon as the patient's condition permits, and with continued cast support until the fracture has united. Frequently, the nail will require removal because of tenderness at its insertion underneath the tibial tubercle. This should not be done before a year has elapsed from the time it was inserted. If internal fixation with plates and screws is decided upon, these should be placed on either the lateral or posterior portion of the tibia, never over the crest. Frequently, plates can be left after the fracture unites, unless they cause discomfort to the patient.

FRACTURES INVOLVING THE ANKLE JOINT

The types of fractures and ligamentous injuries about the ankle joint are determined by the mechanism of the injury, i.e., inversion of the foot in relation to the tibia, eversion of the foot, rotation of the foot about the distal tibia, forceful plantar flexion of the foot, direct blow, or a combination of the above. The magnitude and direc-

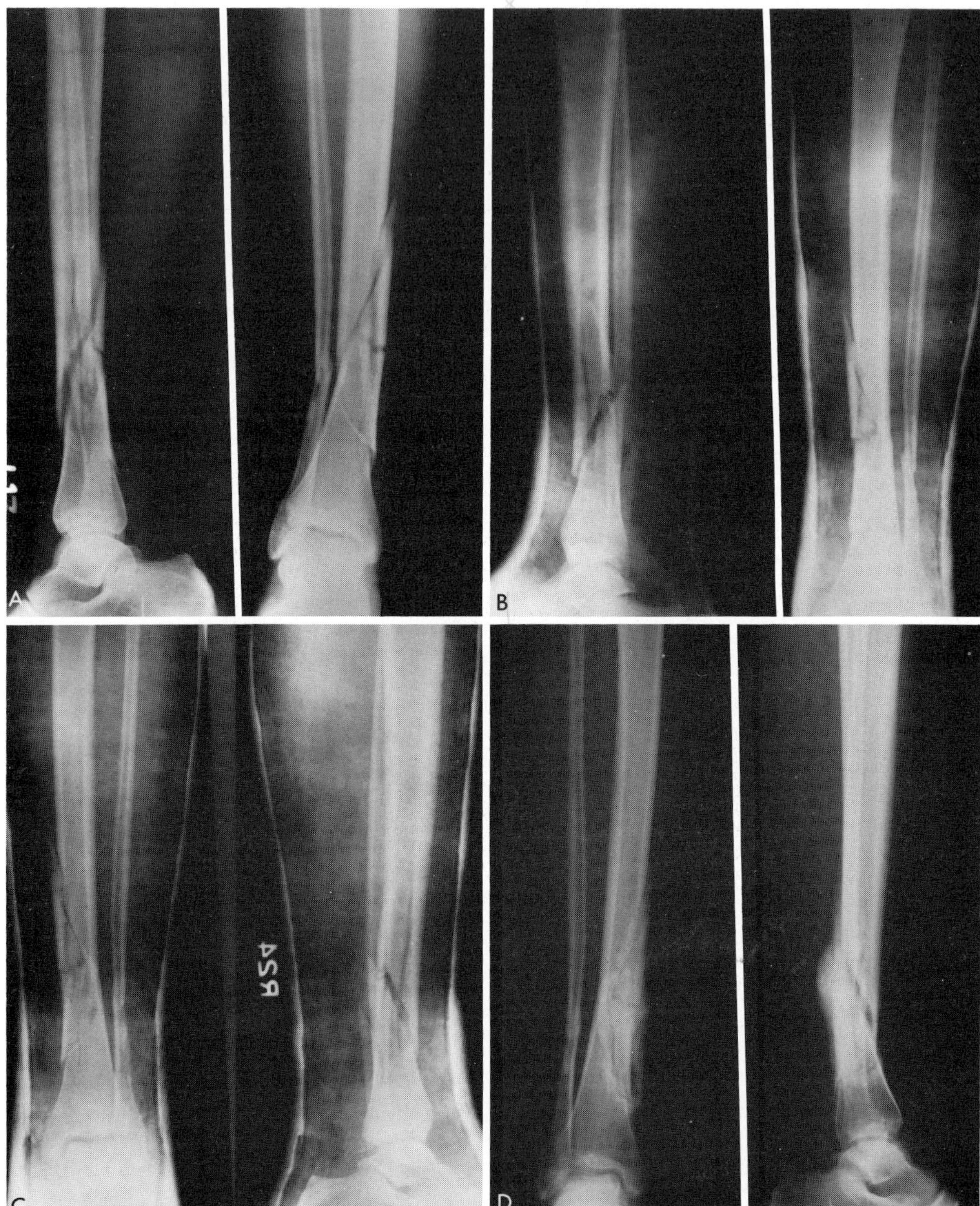

Figure 19–12 A closed fracture of the shaft of the tibia and fibula in a 19-year-old college girl, sustained in a twisting injury while ice skating. *A*, X-rays of the leg on admission to the hospital. A spiral, comminuted fracture is apparent, with lateral angulation of the distal fragment. *B*, The patient was hospitalized for a week, and under general anesthesia the fracture manipulated. Appearance of the limb immediately after manipulation and application of a long leg patellar tendon bearing cast. The angular deformity has been corrected and the alignment restored. *C*, After application of the cast the patient was begun on weight bearing. Appearance of the limb after weight bearing for four days. Some minimal posterior angulation of the fracture fragments, otherwise no change in position. *D*, Three months after injury. The fracture is united. The position is not changed since weight bearing began.

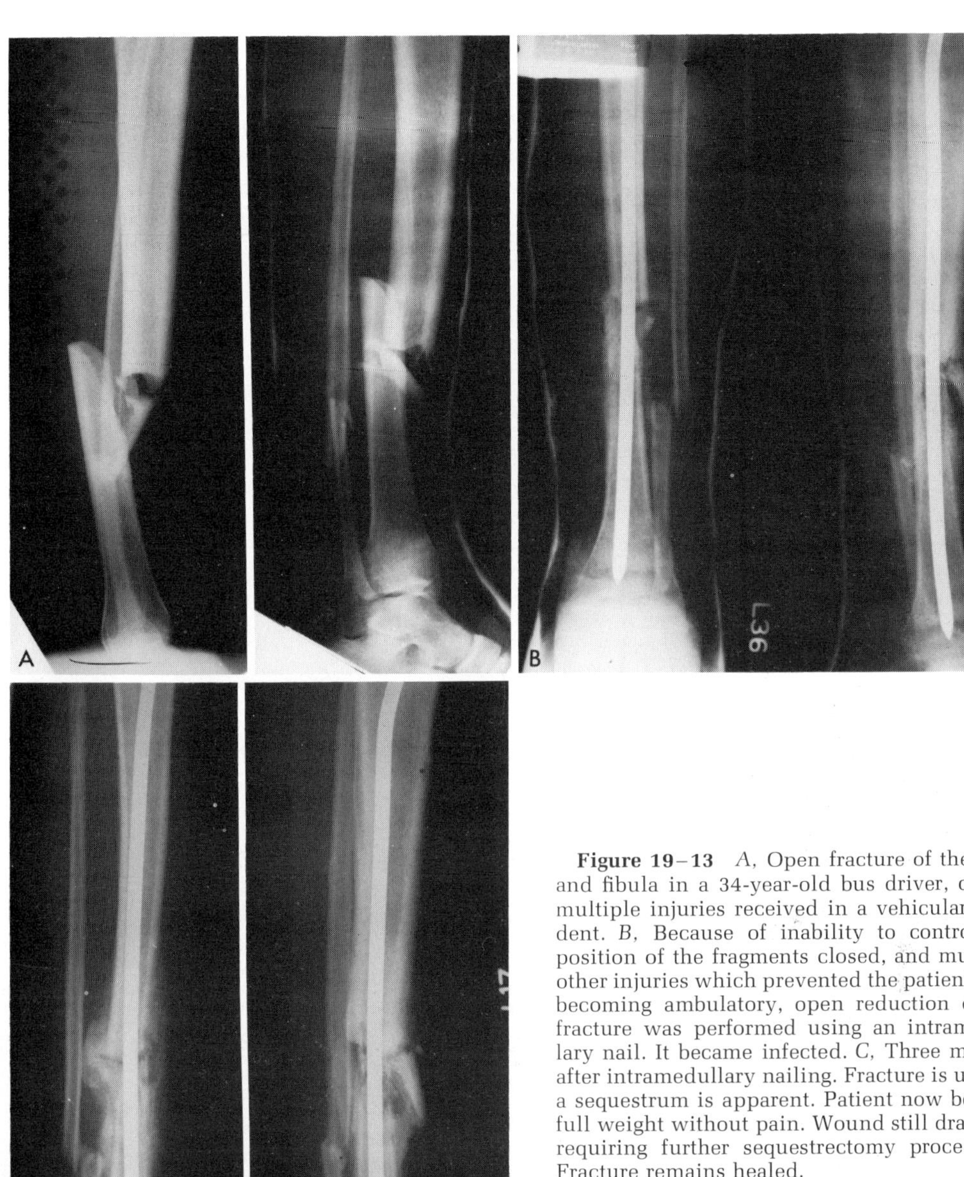

Figure 19–13 *A*, Open fracture of the tibia and fibula in a 34-year-old bus driver, one of multiple injuries received in a vehicular accident. *B*, Because of inability to control the position of the fragments closed, and multiple other injuries which prevented the patient from becoming ambulatory, open reduction of the fracture was performed using an intramedullary nail. It became infected. *C*, Three months after intramedullary nailing. Fracture is united, a sequestrum is apparent. Patient now bearing full weight without pain. Wound still draining, requiring further sequestrectomy procedures. Fracture remains healed.

tion of the forces applied are also an important factor, i.e., twisting injury during football or a high-speed vehicular accident. With an understanding of the mechanism of the injury, the extent of ligamentous injury should be suspected, though radiographic examination may be negative for bone pathology. Further radiographic examination may then be necessary, consisting of stress films of the tibiotalar-fibular joint with or without anesthesia.

In evaluating the fracture roentgenograms, the surgeon must first decide whether the fracture is stable or unstable. In general, closed stable fractures and ligamentous injuries are adequately treated by external means —splint or cast. Unstable fractures are made stable by open reduction and internal fixation of fracture fragments and suture of ligaments followed by adequate external support. Generally, these are surgical emergencies only if the neurovascular status is impaired.

Open fractures or fracture-dislocations about the ankle constitute surgical emergencies. (See Management of Open Fractures.)

Innocent-appearing lateral malleolar fractures, usually the result of a fall and a twisting injury, may also involve injury to the medial side of the ankle. X-rays showing the ankle mortise are necessary. The space between the medial malleolus and the talus should be equal to the space between the dome of the talus and the distal tibial articular surface (plafond) on the x-ray, and, if any widening is not immediately apparent but suspected, x-rays of the normal ankle should be taken for comparison. If the medial space is widened, a tear of the deltoid ligament should be suspected. If closed manipulation of the lateral malleolar fragment does not succeed in restoring the normal medial distance, then foreign tissue must be trapped in the space and must be removed by open operation and direct suture of the deltoid ligament. Occasionally, in such an injury, the lateral malleolus requires open reduction and internal stabilization (Fig. 19–14).

Bimalleolar fractures usually can be reduced closed and maintained in anatomical position by external fixation (cast) if the medial malleolar fragment is distal to the tibial plafond. With fractures at the level of the plafond or proximal, loss of reduction is common

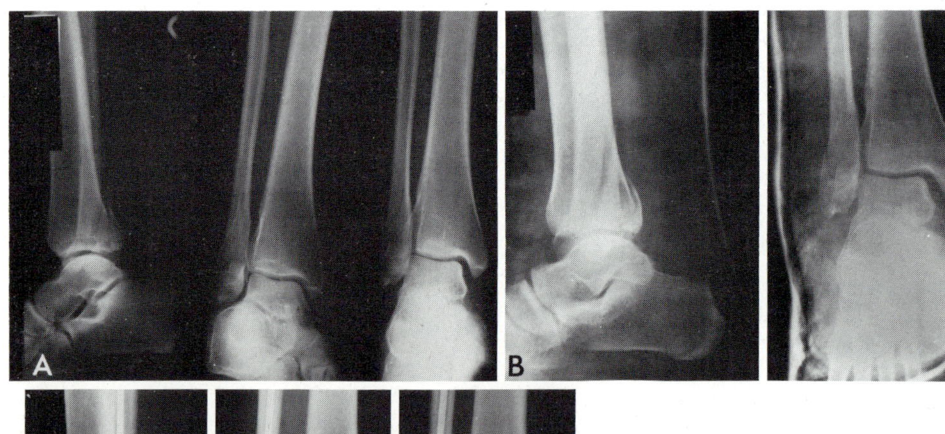

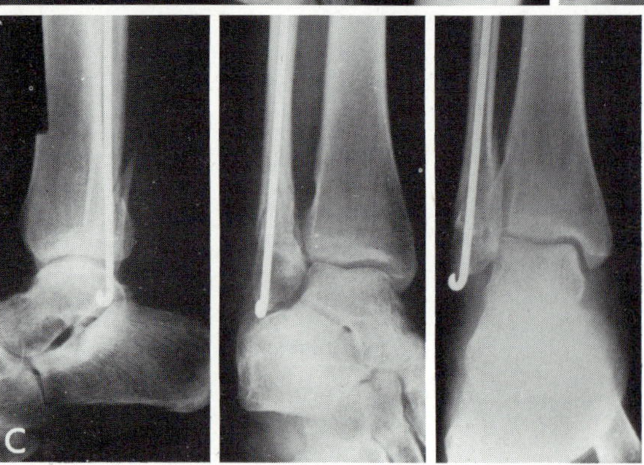

Figure 19–14 Eversion injury: fracture of the lateral malleolus with deltoid ligament tear. *A*, Closed reduction attempted. *B*, Persistent widening of the talomedial malleolar joint space indicating entrapped deltoid ligament. *C*, Open reduction: ligament disengaged and repaired and fibula fixed with Rush rod.

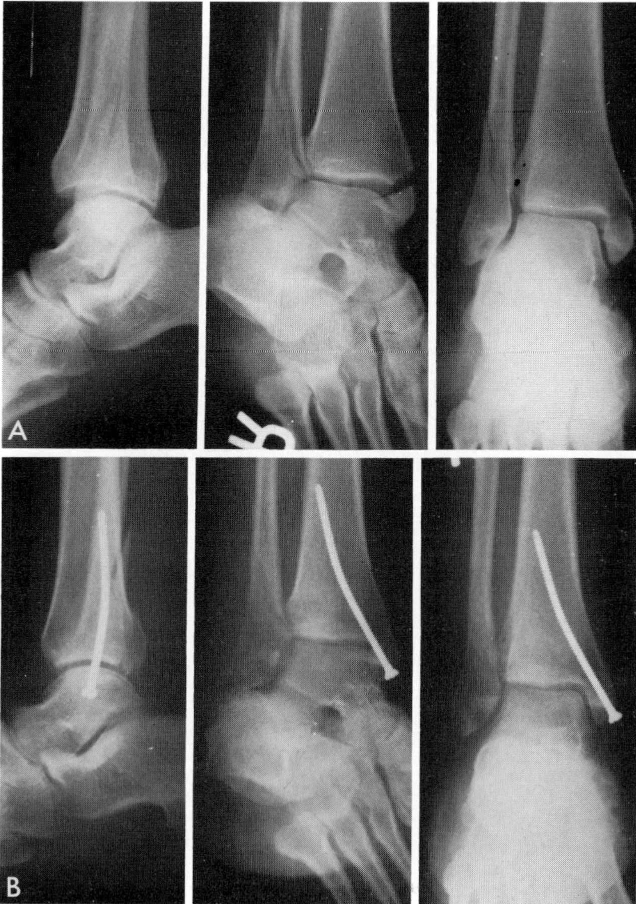

Figure 19–15 Bimalleolar fracture—inversion injury. *A*, Initial injury with minimal displacement. *B*, Two months after injury: malunion of fracture fragments.

(Fig. 19–15). For these fractures, elective medial malleolar internal fixation is recommended, followed by closed reduction of the lateral malleolus by manipulation and maintenance of the reduction in a plaster cast. Fractures of the lateral malleolus proximal to the joint line may also coincide with disruption of the distal tibial fibular ligament and subsequent widening of the ankle mortise. Operative reduction of this ligament is necessary, usually by a transverse screw or bolt across the tibia and fibula, which must be removed after the ligament has healed.

Trimalleolar fractures and fracture-dislocations are produced by severe trauma to the ankle joint. The size of the posterior malleolar fragment, the size of the medial malleolar fragment and any evidence of disruption of the tibial fibular ligament must all be evaluated. If the posterior malleolus (posterior articular surface of the tibia) involves more than a third of the joint surfaces, then open reduction and internal fixation of this fragment is necessary to restore the major weight-bearing surface of the ankle (Fig. 19–16).

In falls from a height, not only may the ankle mortise be disrupted, but the distal tibia may be fractured as well (Fig. 19–17). Closed manipulation under anesthesia is first indicated, and if the ankle mortise and alignment of the knee and ankle can be satisfactorily restored, open reduction is not indicated. Open reduction may be advisable if a fairly large fragment is

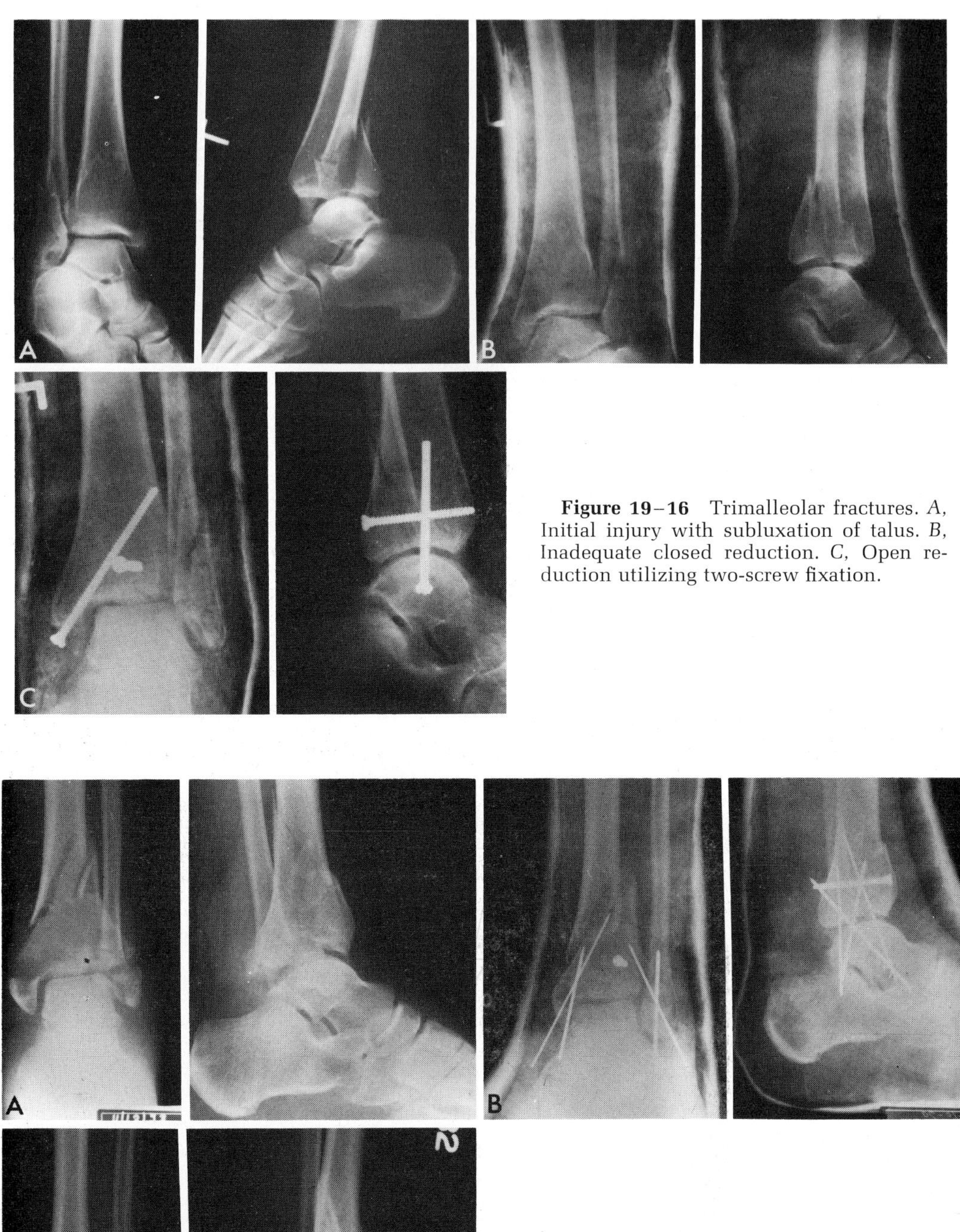

Figure 19–16 Trimalleolar fractures. *A*, Initial injury with subluxation of talus. *B*, Inadequate closed reduction. *C*, Open reduction utilizing two-screw fixation.

Figure 19–17 Trimalleolar fracture with fracture of the distal tibia. *A*, Original injury. *B*, Method of internal fixation. *C*, One-year follow-up: traumatic arthritis.

present, in which case screw fixation and attempt at restoration of the anatomical surface are indicated. This may prove to be extremely difficult technically, particularly if the articular surface is comminuted, and the patient must be advised preoperatively that traumatic arthritis is a common accompaniment of any extensive injury about a joint and that future procedures in the form of arthrodesis, for pain relief, may be necessary.

Open fracture-dislocations may be evaluated at surgery and internally stabilized only if necessary to protect the neurovascular supply to the foot. The chances of chronic osteomyelitis can be minimized only by meticulous wound toilet, gentle manipulation of tissues and adequate immobilization. Even then, the complication rate is high (Fig. 19–18).

An increasingly common source of open injury about the ankle is the power lawnmower, i.e., when an individual backs into its rotating blade with resulting open fracture of the malleoli and contamination of the ankle joint. Meticulous debridement is necessary in these wounds with subsequent delayed primary closure. Missile wounds of the ankle should be treated by adequate debridement of entrance and exit, removal of intra-articular missile fragments, or fragments that would result in pain on weight-bearing. Again, the status of the missile (low-velocity) will determine the extent of debridement (Fig. 19–19).

In summary, ankle joint injuries must be classified as to stability; stable fractures can be treated by closed means. Unstable fractures require open reduction, internal fixation and external support. Open fractures and/or

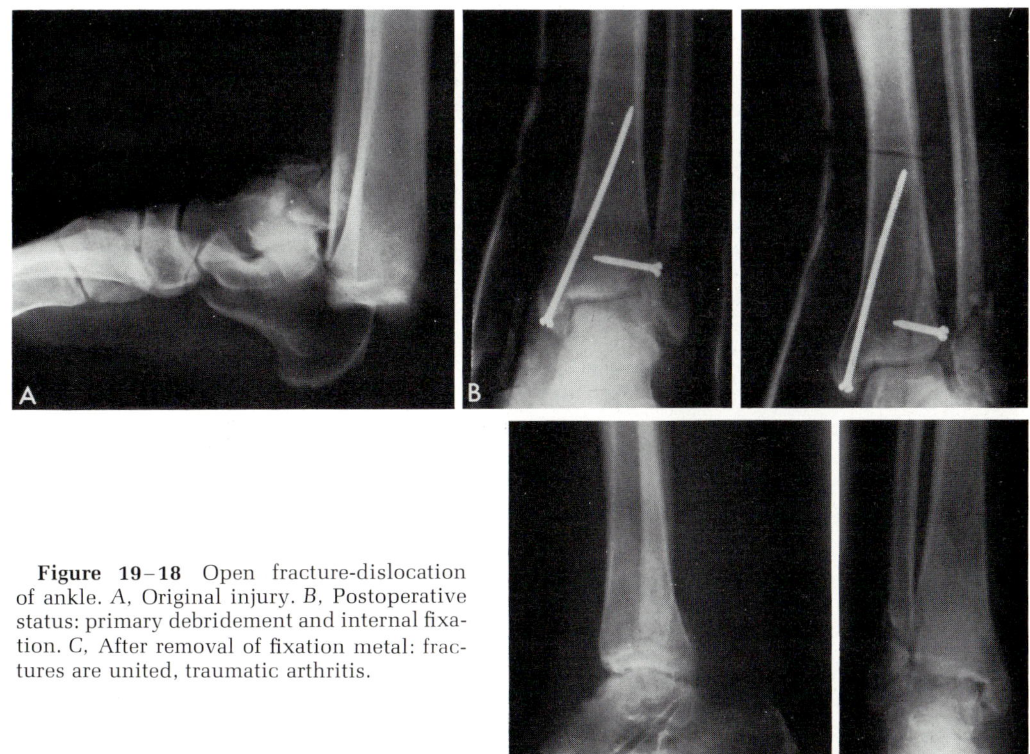

Figure 19–18 Open fracture-dislocation of ankle. *A*, Original injury. *B*, Postoperative status: primary debridement and internal fixation. *C*, After removal of fixation metal: fractures are united, traumatic arthritis.

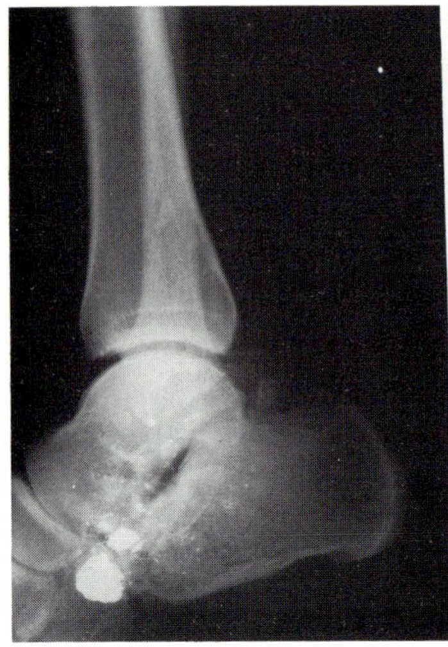
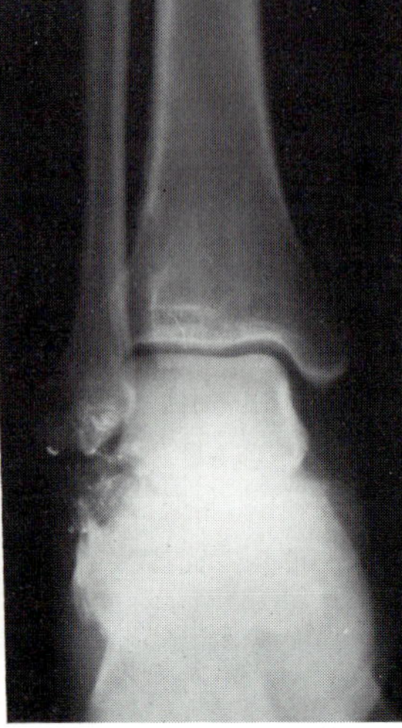

Figure 19–19 Low-velocity missile wound to ankle and subtalar joints.

fracture-dislocations are surgical emergencies and should be treated in the operating suite. Severely contaminated wounds, such as from lawn mowers or weapons, should be debrided and managed by delayed primary closure.

FRACTURES AND DISLOCATIONS OF THE FOOT

Most injuries to the foot are the result of a direct blow. Many are crush injuries with resulting injury to the thin skin on the dorsum of the foot. Swelling is a common sequel of any major trauma to the foot, not only because of the thin skin but because of the foot's usually dependent position. A good deal of the venous drainage of the foot and toes occurs across the dorsum of the foot; this drainage can be compromised by an extensive crush or laceration injury. Initial management of any significant foot injury is with a moderate pressure dressing and elevation of the limb until the swelling subsides. Once this has occurred, reduction of displaced fractures should be done.

Fractures about the mid-foot, fracture-dislocations of the mid- and forefoot, and displaced metatarsal shift fractures will frequently require open reduction and internal fixation.[3] The heads of the metatarsals must be aligned on the weight-bearing portion of the foot in order for the patient to walk painlessly and to wear shoes. Frequently, open reduction is necessary to satisfactorily achieve this alignment (Fig. 19–20). Such surgery should not be done through edematous, torn skin or excessive tension on the operative suture line will result with skin slough and infection as a possible consequence.

Fractures of the base or the shaft of the fifth metatarsal usually result from an inversion injury to the ankle. These injuries should be suspected when pain over the lateral aspect of the foot follows an inversion sprain or fracture of the lateral malleolus.[26] Fractures of the base of the fifth metatarsal are rarely displaced, although they usually are sufficiently painful that a short-leg walking cast is necessary for about two weeks until the acute symptoms subside. Fractures of the fifth metatarsal shaft, even if partly displaced, can frequently be treated with a stiff-soled shoe without immobilization, as they are frequently not particularly painful. These fractures unite readily. If there is excessive discomfort, a short-leg walking cast can be applied for two weeks until the pain goes down. Once the cast is removed from

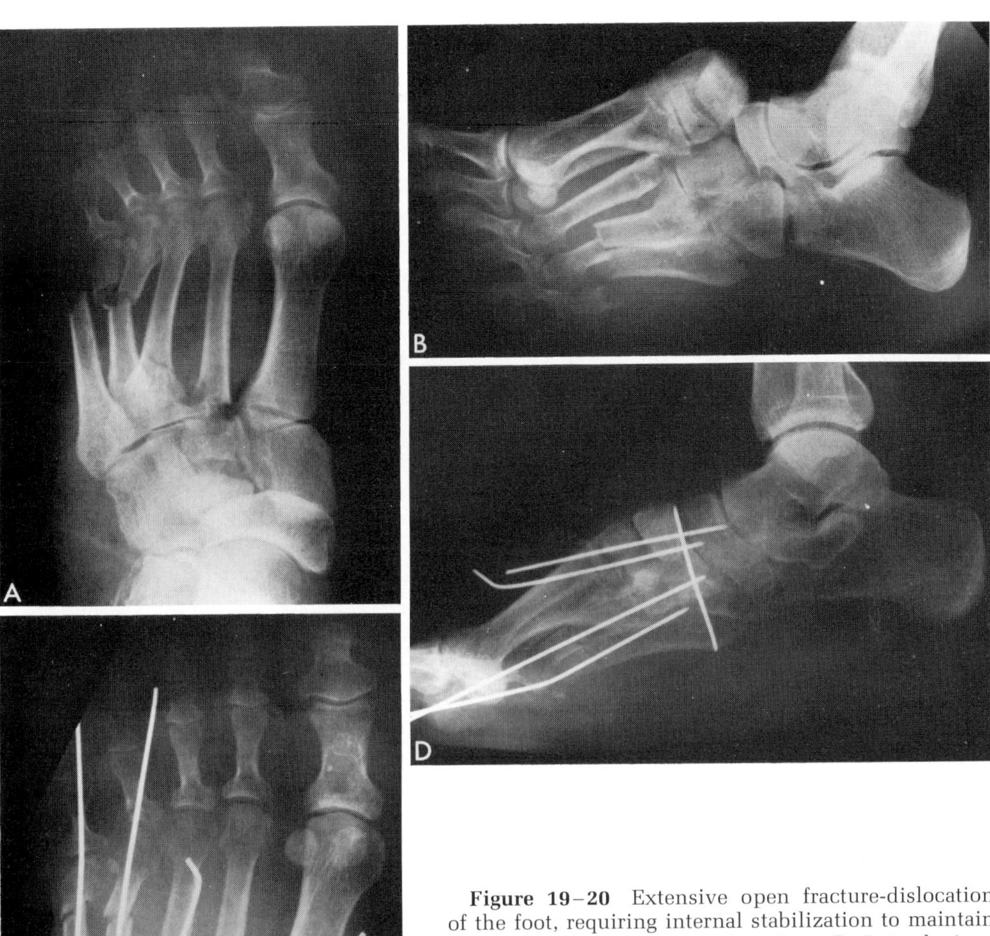

Figure 19–20 Extensive open fracture-dislocation of the foot, requiring internal stabilization to maintain alignment. *A*, Anteroposterior view. *B*, Lateral view: the midfoot dislocation is apparent on this view. *C*, Anteroposterior view after reduction. *D*, Lateral view after reduction.

either of these two fractures, the foot should be protected in a stiff-soled shoe for three or four weeks more.

Stress fractures of the metatarsal shaft should be kept in mind in any patient with obscure metatarsalgia. Tenderness, heat, redness and swelling over the distal metatarsals may mimic cellulitis, particularly in the absence of a good history of trauma. Initial x-rays will be normal, although eventually, x-ray changes will be visible and the diagnosis of a healing fracture can be made. Early treatment is with a short-leg walking cast if the patient is particularly uncomfortable. This is rarely necessary for more than a few weeks. A major consequence of a stress fracture of a metatarsal is over-diagnosis and over-treatment. Once the healing fracture callus is seen on x-ray, it could be mistaken for osteosarcoma by the unwary doctor and the fracture subjected to open biopsy. However, careful inspection of the x-rays will show a fracture line to be almost always visible, the tip-off to the diagnosis.

Fractures of the phalanges and dislocations of the interphalangeal joints usually result from stubbing the toe or from a heavy object being dropped on it. Any injury to a toe with resulting ecchymosis should be highly suspect, and x-rays should be taken. Minimally or non-displaced fractures of the phalanges are best treated by taping the injured toe to its neighbor until the acute symptoms subside, usually in a week, and then protecting it with a stiff-soled shoe for a few weeks more. Dislocations and displaced fractures should be reduced. Occasionally, an anesthetic is necessary; this is conveniently done by an ankle block. Direct pressure over the dislocation with traction in line with the foot will usually effect reduction easily, and angulated fractures of the phalanges may be corrected likewise by traction and pressure in the opposite direction of the angulation. Once the dislocation or fracture has been reduced, the toe should be taped to its neighbor and treated as a closed fracture. Phalangeal fractures generally take several weeks to heal solidly, although the toe usually is symptom-free by two weeks or so from the time of injury.

FRACTURES IN CHILDREN

The general principles which form the basis of the treatment of fractures are as applicable to children as to adults. Most fractures in children are closed fractures and, wherever possible, are best handled by closed methods. With certain notable exceptions, internal fixation is to be avoided.

The x-ray diagnosis of fractures in infants and children is frequently difficult because, depending on the age of the patient, some portion of the growing bone is composed of cartilage and, of course, cannot be visualized on the routine x-ray examination. Growth centers appear at predictable ages and have been charted. Such a chart must be available to the surgeon and the radiologist in order to adequately interpret the x-ray. In the older child, epiphyseal plates are visualized as translucent lines which may be confused with a fracture line, and epiphyseal injuries are frequently difficult to appreciate. A cardinal rule in this connection should be that a diagnostic x-ray examination in a child should always include the corresponding uninjured part and, of course, at least two projections should always be obtained.

Treatment should be directed at achieving the best possible alignment, in most cases, that which can be achieved by closed means. Gross angulation, however, should never be accepted. Rotational deformities must always be corrected at the time of initial treatment. A certain amount of persistent angulation at the fracture site may be acceptable and may be compatible with a perfectly satisfactory end result, depending on the location of the fracture as related to growth centers and the amount of growth potential present (i.e., the age of the child).

Some general rules are herewith listed which are useful in evaluating the acceptability of reduction and in establishing a prognosis for the final result. The amount of residual angulation which can be accepted and the degree of remodeling which can be expected are dependent on several factors:

A. General considerations include: (1) the age of the child, (2) the location of the fracture with relationship to the end of the bone, and (3) the severity of the angulation. In a very young child or infant with a fracture close to the epiphysis, the more residual angulation may be accepted. Conversely, in an older patient with a fracture near the middle of the long bone, an accurate reduction is demanded.

B. The greatest degree of angular

deformity can be accepted when the apex of the deformity is in the direction of motion of neighboring hinge joints. Lateral angulation, on the other hand, is more likely to persist to some extent, and rotational deformities are not completely corrected by the growth and remodeling process.

C. An important exception to the foregoing rules involves fracture of the proximal femur or femoral neck. The remodeling process will correct local irregularities but any abnormality of the angle of the femoral neck relationship to the shaft of the femur will be permanent, as will rotational deformities.

End-on reduction of fractures in long bones of children is of little importance. These fractures may be allowed to unite with bayonet apposition in most patients, with an excellent prognosis. Indeed, bayonet apposition with some degree of overriding is desirable in fractures of the long bones to compensate for the acceleration of longitudinal growth resulting from the injury. Fractures of long bones resulting in overgrowth and leg length inequality for whatever reason result in a permanent difference in leg length for which there is no spontaneous compensation.

As a general rule, an excellent result may be obtained by traction or closed reduction and plaster immobilization. Certain fractures of long bones (i.e., the shaft of the femur) are best treated by traction followed by plaster immobilization (Fig. 19–21). Bryant's traction should not be used except occasionally in infants because of the possibility of vascular damage (Fig. 19–22). There are certain notable exceptions to this rule which will be described in detail below. Except for specific instances, open reduction and the use of metallic fixation devices are never justified. Even though, for whatever reason, unnecessary operative treatment may have been carried out, in many instances without serious complications, even one unnecessary catastrophe is sufficient reason to condemn the practice.

The ability to accurately predict the ultimate outcome of a fracture in a child is of the utmost importance. The amount of growth potential remaining in each individual case is one of the most important factors which make fractures in children different from those in adults. The growth and remodeling process can frequently be depended upon to correct the deformities or shortening; conversely, growth may be an inexorable force which produces increasing deformity in certain epiphyseal injuries.

Fractures through the end of a long bone in a child quite frequently involve the epiphyseal plate and sometimes the epiphyseal center itself. These injuries are quite common and because of the involvement of the epiphyseal plate may, in some instances, cause premature closure of the involved epiphysis in whole or in part, resulting in inequality of the length of the limbs or progressive angular deformities. Long bones are preformed in cartilage with a primary ossification center and usually two or more secondary ossification centers appearing at either end of the long bone. In most cases, the secondary ossification centers are apparent at birth or shortly thereafter, although the ossification of some may be delayed until later years. Longitudinal growth occurs in the epiphyseal plate between the diaphysis and the epiphysis of the secondary ossification center at either end of the long bones. The weakest area of the epiphyseal plate is in the zone of provisional ossification and it is through this area that most of the epiphyseal fractures occur. In the majority of instances, the injury will result from a shearing force applied across the epiphyseal plate with disruption of the plate and displacement of the epiphysis. These injuries are best treated by closed reduction with replacement of the displaced epiphyseal in as nearly anatomic a position as can be achieved and plaster immobilization (Fig. 19–8). Rarely, the fracture will be sufficiently unstable that some form of internal

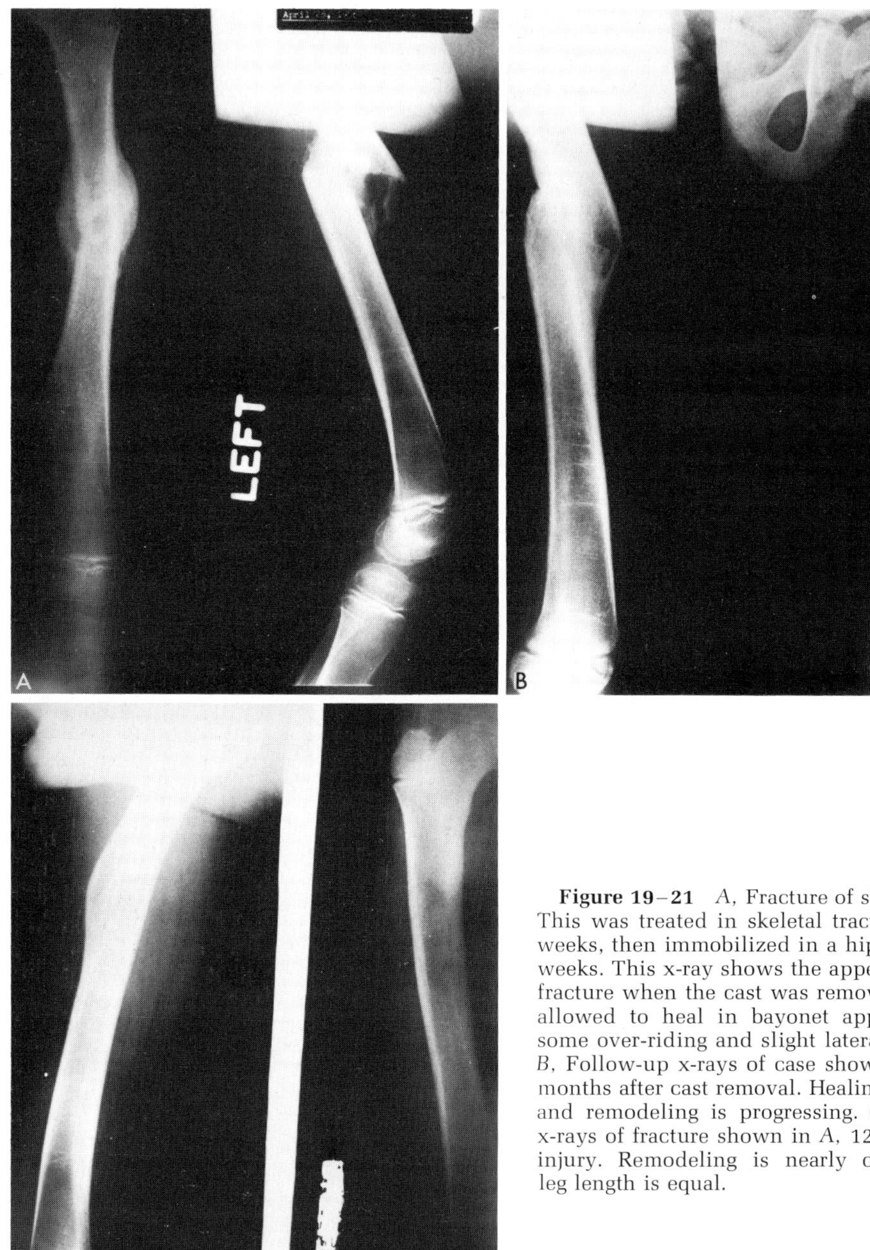

Figure 19–21 *A*, Fracture of shaft of femur. This was treated in skeletal traction for three weeks, then immobilized in a hip spica for 11 weeks. This x-ray shows the appearance of the fracture when the cast was removed. This was allowed to heal in bayonet apposition with some over-riding and slight lateral angulation. *B*, Follow-up x-rays of case shown in *A*. Four months after cast removal. Healing is complete and remodeling is progressing. *C*, Follow-up x-rays of fracture shown in *A*, 12 months post injury. Remodeling is nearly complete and leg length is equal.

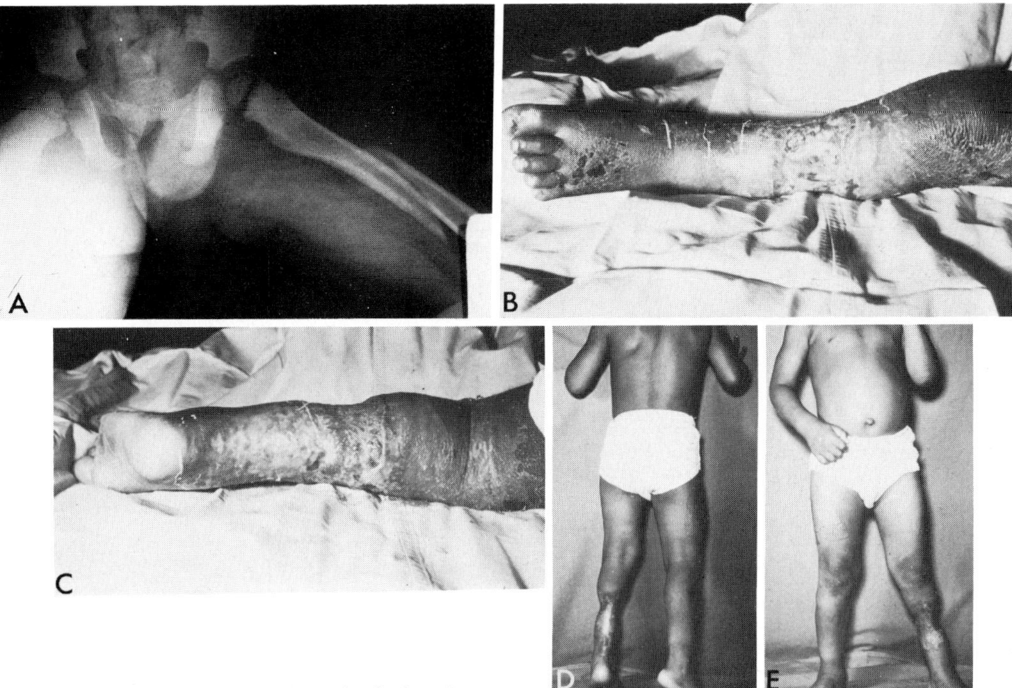

Figure 19–22 *A*, Fracture of shaft of femur in a 2-year-old. Treated initially in Bryant's traction. This x-ray shows the spiral fracture in good position and alignment. This ultimately healed with a good result on the right. *B* and *C*, Front and back views of the uninjured leg. He developed a Volkman's ischemic contracture with skin slough from the Bryant's traction. *D* and *E*, Front and back views of the final result of the injury shown in *A*. This required skin graft and resulted in loss of all of the muscles in the left leg below the knee. Lengthening of the tendo-Achilles and triple arthrodesis was done later.

fixation is necessary temporarily to maintain position while healing takes place. If the trauma which produces the injury is applied in such a way that it results in a crushing injury to the epiphyseal plate with or without a fracture or displacement of the epiphysis itself, the prognosis becomes much worse since premature closure of the epiphyseal plate may result. Several authors have attempted to classify epiphyseal injuries according to their x-ray appearance as related to the probable mechanism of injury—Aitken,[2] Salter and Harris,[32] most notably. Such classifications are helpful to the surgeon by providing some indication of the ultimate prognosis and also some indication as to the best method of treatment. Injuries involving a shearing force with displacement of the epiphysis with or without a fragment of metaphysis can usually be managed by closed reduction and plaster immobilization. These injuries are at the very extremity of the long bones where the effects of future growth and remodeling will be the greatest, and provided reasonable alignment can be obtained, anatomic reduction is not always necessary. Occasionally, these injuries, particularly those involving the distal femoral and distal tibial epiphyses, may be sufficiently unstable that some form of temporary internal fixation is necessary until healing provides stability. This fixation should always be minimal and should be removed as early as possible. The more severe types in which a vertical fracture line runs through the epiphysis and frequently the articular surface of the joint demand accurate reduction and maintenance of reduc-

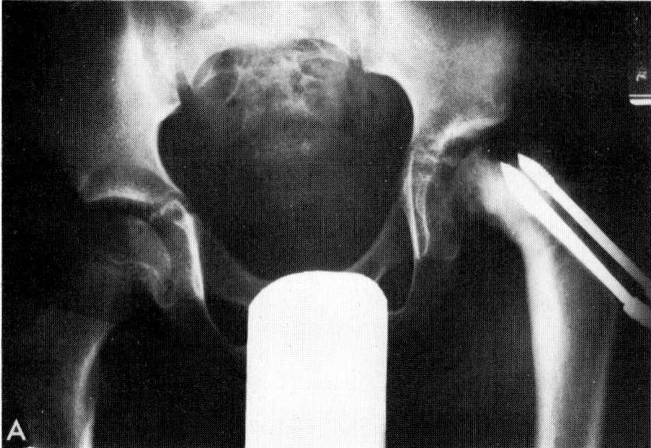

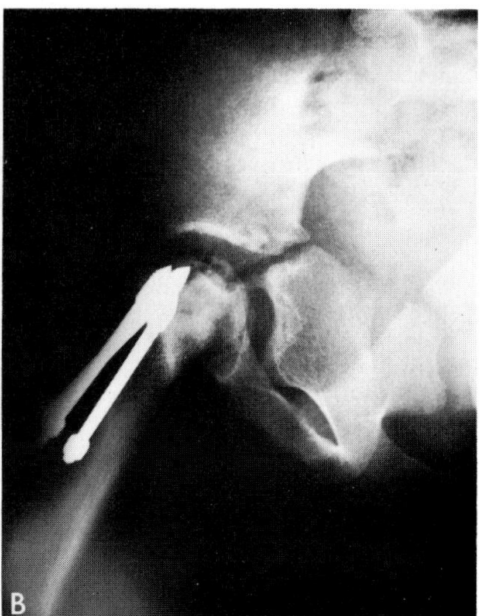

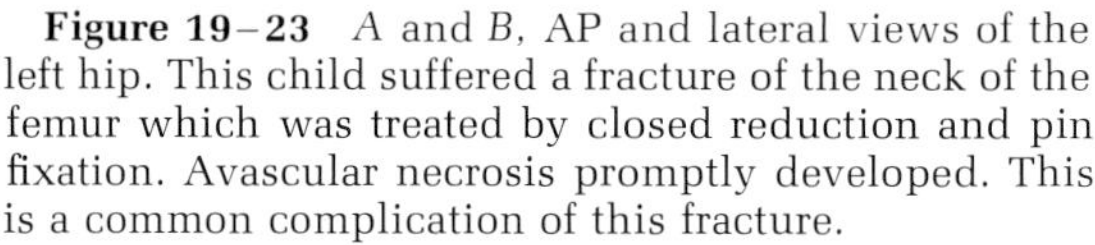
Figure 19–23 *A* and *B*, AP and lateral views of the left hip. This child suffered a fracture of the neck of the femur which was treated by closed reduction and pin fixation. Avascular necrosis promptly developed. This is a common complication of this fracture.

tion and frequently require surgical treatment. Since it is not always possible to be certain as to the degree of damage to the epiphyseal plate, regardless of the x-ray appearance of the injury, the prognosis must always be guarded and the parents must always be alerted to the possibility of growth disturbance in the future.

The basic principles described above apply to injuries involving the distal femoral, proximal tibial and distal tibial epiphysis. Injury to the capital femoral epiphysis demands special mention. This injury characteristically occurs between the ages of 10 and 16, is usually gradual in onset and is thought to be due to some hormonal or metabolic condition as yet unknown. Acute displacement of the femoral capital epiphysis does occur, however, and is best handled by gentle manipulative reduction, closed if possible, and internal fixation until healing is complete (Fig. 19–23).

As stated previously, fractures of the long bones in children are best treated by closed reduction and casting. Satisfactory position and alignment should be obtained and rotational deformities must be corrected. Except in a few special instances, open reduction is not necessary and internal fixation is rarely indicated.

REFERENCES

1. Abbott, L., Saunders, J. De C., Bost, F. C., and Anderson, C.: Injuries to ligaments of the knee. J. Bone Joint Surg. *26*:503, 1944.
2. Aitken, A. P.: Fractures of the epiphyses. Clin. Orthop. *41*:19, July-August 1965.
3. Aitken, A. P., and Poulson, D.: Dislocations of the tarsometatarsal joint. J. Bone Joint Surg. *45A*:246, 1963.
4. Appel, Helge: Late results after meniscectomy in the knee joint. Acta Orthop. Scand. (Suppl. 133) 1970.
5. Blount, Walter P.: Fractures in Children. Baltimore, The Williams and Wilkins Co., 1955.
6. Brantigan, O. C., and Voshell, A. F.: The mechanics of the ligaments and menisci of the knee joint. J. Bone Joint Surg. *23*:44, 1941.
7. Brantigan, O. C., and Voshell, A. F.: The tibial collateral ligament: its function, its bursae, and its relation to the medial meniscus. J. Bone Joint Surg. *25*:121, 1943.
8. Brantigan, O. C., and Voshell, A. F.: Ligaments of the knee joint: the relationship of the ligament of Humphry to the ligament of Wrisberg. J. Bone Joint Surg. *28*:66, 1946.
9. Brown, P. W., and Urban, J. G.: Early weight-bearing treatment of open fractures of

the tibia. J. Bone Joint Surg. *51A*:59, 1969.
10. Bryan, R. S., Dickson, J. H., and Taylor, W. F.: Recovery of the knee following meniscectomy. An evaluation of suction drainage and cast immobilization. J. Bone Joint Surg. *51A*:973, 1969.
11. DeLorme, T. L.: Influence of progressive resistive exercises on knee function following femoral fractures. J. Bone Joint Surg. *32A*:910, 1950.
12. Dunphy, J. E., and Udupa, K. N.: Chemical and histochemical sequences in the normal healing of wounds. New Eng. J. Med. *253*:847, 1955.
13. Edwards, L. C., Pernokas, L. N., and Dunphy, J. E.: The use of a plastic sponge to sample regenerating tissue in healing wounds. Surg. Gynec. Obstet. *105*:303, 1957.
14. Galeazzi, R.: Clinical and experimental study of lesions of the semilunar cartilages of the knee. J. Bone Joint Surg. *9*:515, 1927.
15. Hallin, L. G., and Lindahl, O.: Rotation in the knee joint in experimental injury to the ligaments. Acta Orthop. Scand. *36*: 400, 1965.
16. Helfet, A. J.: Mechanism of derangements of the medial semilunar cartilage and their management. J. Bone Joint Surg. *41B*: 319, 1959.
17. Jack, E. A.: Experimental rupture of the medial collateral ligament of the knee. J. Bone Joint Surg. *32B*:396, 1950.
18. Kaplan, E. B.: Injuries and afflictions of the menisci of the knee. Instructional Course Lectures, Amer. Acad. Orthop. Surgeons, *16*:161, 1959.
19. Keon-Cohen, B. T.: Function and malfunction of the coronary ligaments of the knee. Paper presented at a meeting of the American Academy of Orthopaedic Surgeons, Chicago, 1966.
20. Kirkup. J.: Mechanism of femoral shaft fractures. J. Bone Joint Surg. *46B*:571, 1964.
21. Nicholas, J. A.: Injuries to knee ligaments. Relationship to looseness and tightness in football players. J.A.M.A. *212*:2236, June 29, 1970.
22. Nicholas, J. A., Freiberger, R. H., and Killoran, P. J.: Double-contrast arthrography of the knee. J. Bone Joint Surg. *52A*:203, 1970.
23. Odell, R. T., and Leydig, M.: The conservative treatment of fractures in children. Surg. Gynec. Obstet. *92*:92, 1951.
24. O'Donoghue, D. H.: Surgical treatment of fresh injuries to the major ligaments of the knee. J. Bone Joint Surg. *32A*: 721, 1950.
25. Palmer, I.: On the injuries of the ligaments of the knee joint: A clinical study. Acta Chir. Scand. *81*:(Suppl. 53) 1938.
26. Pearson, J. R.: Combined fracture of the base of the fifth metatarsal and the lateral malleolus. J. Bone Joint Surg. *43A*:513, 1961.
27. Rancels, R. J., and Noble, N. L.: Connective tissue; a technic for its isolation and study. Arch. Pathol. *59*:553, 1955.
28. Reynolds, F. C.: Injuries of the knee. Clin. Orthop. No. 50, January-February 1967.
29. Rhoads, J. E., and Howard, J. M.: The Chemistry of Trauma. Springfield, Ill., Charles C Thomas, Publisher, 1963.
30. Roberts, J. M.: Fractures of the condyles of the tibia. J. Bone Joint Surg. *50A*:1505, 1968.
31. Russell, R. H.: Fracture of the femur: A clinical study. Brit. J. Surg. *11*:491, 1924.
32. Salter, R. B., and Harris, W. B.: Injuries involving the epiphyseal plate. J. Bone Joint Surg. *45A*:587, 1963.
33. Sarmiento, A.: A functional below-the-knee cast for tibial fractures. J. Bone Joint Surg. *49A*:855, 1967.
34. Schilling, J. A., Milch, L. E., et al.: Fractional analysis of experimental wound fluid. Proc. Soc. Exper. Biol. Med. *89*: 189, 1955.
35. Stein, A. H.: Diagnosis of arterial injury in the extremities. Instructional Course Lectures, Amer. Acad. Orthop. Surgeons, *17*:47, 1960.
36. Stewart, M. J., Sisk, T. J., and Wallace, S. L.: Fractures of the distal third of the femur. J. Bone Joint Surg. *48A*:784, 1966.
37. Struthers, A. M., Grindlay, J. H., and Figi, F. A.: An experimental study of formation of autogenous bone within polyvinyl sponge. Proc. Mayo Clinic *30*:462, 1955.
38. Tapper, E. M., and Hoover, N. W.: Late results after meniscectomy. J. Bone Joint Surg. *51A*:517, 1969.
39. Taylor, L. W.: Principles of treatment of fractures and non-union of the shaft of the femur. J. Bone Joint Surg. *45A*:191, 1963.
40. Watson-Jones, R.: Fractures and Joint Injuries. Baltimore, Williams and Wilkins Co., 1946.
41. Whipple, A. O.: The Story of Wound Healing and Wound Repair. Springfield, Ill., Charles C Thomas, Publisher, 1963.

chapter

20

CARE OF THE BURNED PATIENT

Thomas J. Krizek, M.D., Mark C. Robson, M.D. and Robert C. Wray, Jr., M.D.

Thermal destruction of the skin produces local and systemic alterations so severe and so diverse that burn injury forms the prototype for the study of all major trauma. The initial and continued systemic hemodynamic, metabolic and nutritional changes and an altered host defense mechanism against infection are merely a reflection of the profound changes in the local wound. The management of the systemic changes is the means of sustaining the patient; the therapeutic imperative, however, is closure of the wound. No matter how elegant the treatment, ultimate survival, convalescence and functional recovery can occur only when the local wound is healed. An understanding of burn injury must begin and end with the burn wound.

Success in treatment is not necessarily reflected in survival statistics. Hideous deformity, limiting contractures and scarred personalities may all reflect well in data which report only mortality. Functional rehabilitation and social acceptance should constitute our measure of success. Our challenge is not how well we treat burns but how well we treat burned patients.

Functional Anatomy of the Skin

The skin is by size and weight the largest organ in the body. It is also a vital organ; loss of a substantial area is, if unreplaced by the patient's own skin, incompatible with life. So too, invasive bacterial infection, limited to the skin and subcutaneous tissue, may be lethal without visceral spread. Despite wrinkles, we are not possessed of any excess skin. Moreover, it has only limited powers of regeneration and lacks much of the functional reserve characteristic of visceral organs.

Skin has the obvious functions of protection from the environment, sensibility and heat regulation. It is also that of ourselves which we present to the world and may, therefore, be a source of visual beauty. If scarred, it is a physical and potential social handicap.

Skin Area

The skin of an adult has a surface ranging from 1.5 to 1.9 square meters (average 1.7 sq. m.). More exact calculations can be obtained from the formula:[153]

$$\text{Area of skin sq. cm.} = \text{height in cm.}^{0.725} \times \text{weight in kg.}^{0.425} \times 71.84.$$

In actual weight the skin represents from 14 to 17 per cent of our total body weight. For practical purposes, however, and in particular for assessing thermal injury, it is customary to think in terms of percentage of total surface area and the functional significance of the area, rather than the actual area or weight.

Anatomy

An understanding of functional disturbances and reparative processes of the skin requires consideration of its anatomy (Fig. 20–1). The skin is a two-layered covering resting on a subcutaneous padding of fat. The outer, highly cellular epidermal layer measures 0.06 to 0.8 mm. in thickness and is in contact with the dermis by way of multiple, irregular, interpapillary ridges, often inappropriately called rete pegs (in three-dimension they

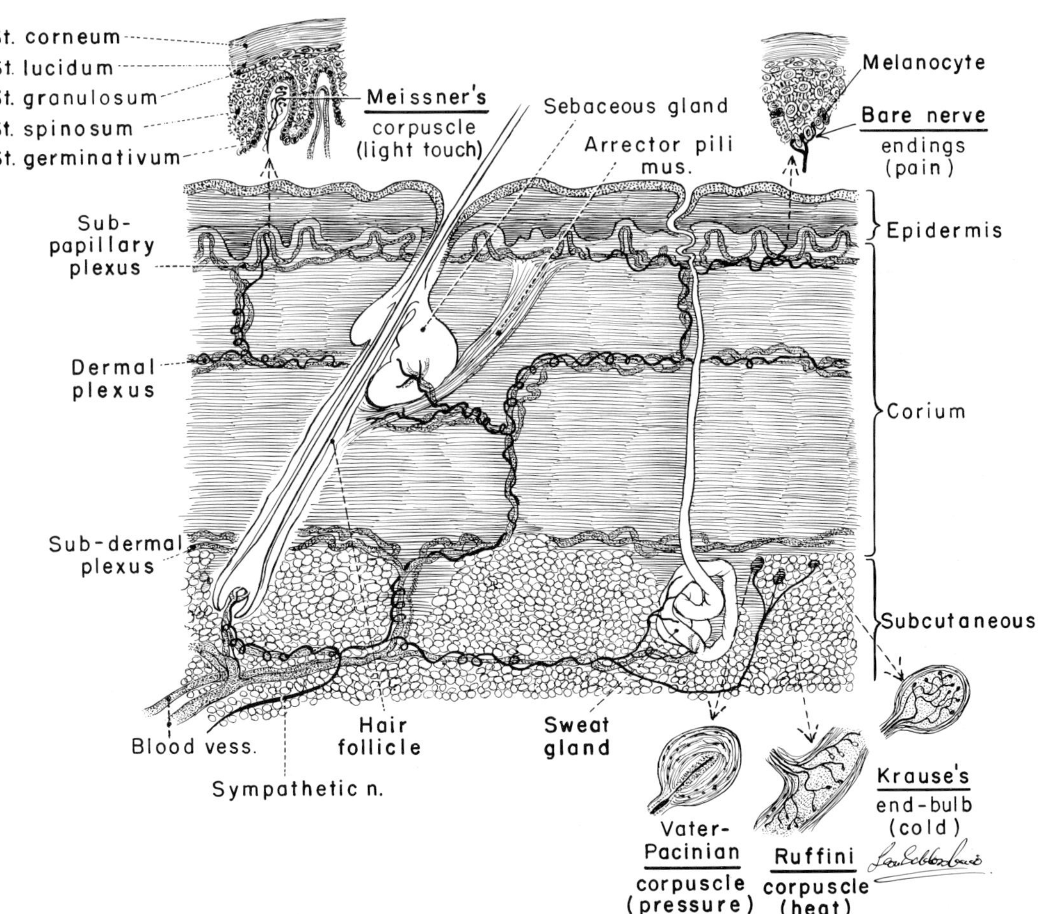

Figure 20–1 Normal cross-sectional anatomy of the skin.

are ridges not pegs). These ridges result in increased surface contact between the two layers; they provide much of the resistance of normal skin to tangential stress. The innermost layer of the epidermis is the basal or germinal layer (stratum germinativum) containing the cells destined for keratin production (95 per cent of total cells) and melanocytes (5 per cent of total). This layer is the total epidermal contact with a neurovascular supply. Injury through this layer may spare sufficient keratin-producing cells to allow regeneration; melanocytes, however, are of neural origin and do not regenerate.

Cells generated from this layer are gradually extruded toward the surface, forming first the prickle-layer (stratum spinosum), characterized by prominent, interlocking cell wall projections which further aid the skin's ability to withstand shearing forces. The next layer of evolution is the granular layer (stratum granulosa) which merges imperceptibly with the clear zone (stratum lucidum). These layers have a high, transferable water content (70 per cent) which is intimately concerned with water retention and heat regulation. These cells finally die and form the outer, nonliving, waterproof, fibrous protein which is keratin (stratum corneum). Keratin contains only 15 per cent water, which when increased by immersion causes softening and "wrinkles," whereas decreased water content results in calluses.

The underlying dermis is 20 to 30 times thicker and contains the nervous, vascular, lymphatic and supporting structures for the epidermis as well as harboring the epidermal appendages. Dermal fibrocytes produce the fibrous proteins, collagen and elastin and give skin its strength. Mastocytes (mast cells) containing histamine and heparin also probably produce the mucopolysaccharides of hyaluronic and chondroitin sulfuric acid which form the interfibrillary matrix of the dermis. Histiocytes or tissue macrophages are distributed around blood vessels and hair follicles. The appendages of the skin include hair follicles and their associated sebaceous glands, the eccrine sweat glands which enter through interpapillary ridges, and the apocrine glands located in the axillary and inguinal regions.

Functions

Sensibility. The various nerve endings in the skin provide for major sensory contact with the environment, and for protection from it as well. Naked nerve endings, insinuated between cells of the basal layer, enable us to perceive pain and to discriminate pinprick. Meissner's corpuscles lie just beneath the epidermis, particularly in the fingers and lips, and provide the sensation of light touch. Corpuscles of Ruffini (heat), Krause's end bulbs (cold) and Vater-Paccini's corpuscles (pressure) all lie deep in the dermis or even in the subcutaneous tissues. Sympathetic nervous system fibers are distributed to blood vessels and the arrector pili muscles of the hair follicles and allow hair to "stand on end." The anatomical location of these various endings is important in understanding the symptom complex of burns of various depths.

Heat Regulation. Body heat is generated by the metabolic oxidative processes and is added to by the environment from conduction (the transfer of heat from one molecule to another), convection (transfer of heat through a moving liquid or gas) and radiation (via electromagnetic waves).

To maintain thermal equilibrium, heat is dissipated by evaporation, conduction, radiation, convection and, in trifling amounts, via excreta. To be lost, internal heat must be brought to the surface. There is a rich dermal network which sends branches outward to form a subpapillary plexus. Characterized by multiple arteriovenous shunts, this vascular bed, if need be, can accept up to one-sixth or one-fifth of the cardiac output. Thus, in addition to its obvious nutritional function for the skin, it has great capacity for delivering blood for heat dissipation. Normally, man loses 70 per cent of the body heat load via conduction, 25 per cent by evaporation and the rest by convection or radiation.

Heat moves by molecular conduction and is dependent upon the specific conductivity of the tissues, with the physiological gradient (hotter to cooler) being toward the surface. The heat exchange is accomplished by thermal gradients obeying physical laws and varying not only with body but also with ambient air temperature and moisture. When the air temperature exceeds the body temperature, the gradient is reversed and heat can be dissipated from the body only by evaporation.

Sweating will occur at 37° C. air temperature at 0 per cent humidity. When the air is saturated and has a temperature exceeding body temperature, heat cannot be lost and fever will result (heat stroke). The eccrine sweat glands are capable of excreting 10 liters per day. Since water vapor molecules have a higher kinetic energy than molecules in water, thermal energy is required to convert sweat to water vapor. Five hundred and eighty calories of energy are required to convert one liter of water to vapor at 37° C. This energy is provided by the oxidative processes and normally accounts for 20 to 30 per cent of our total metabolic heat production.

Thermal equilibrium is, therefore, primarily a problem of delivery to the vascular system (dilatation or constriction), conductivity, convection and radiant loss supplemented, when necessary, by evaporative loss and the expenditure of energy.

Protection. The continuity of the skin and an intact sensibility are the major factors in protection. In addition to being an obvious barrier against mechanical and chemical trauma, it protects against thermal injury by heat dissipation and against cold injury by heat conservation. It is nearly waterproof, so that immersion in water does not cause swelling of tissues. Perhaps of major importance is the barrier it presents to bacterial invasion. The skin is never sterile, nor can it be easily sterilized. It is colonized by two major groups of organisms, its resident flora and a transient flora (Fig. 20–2). The bacteria are not normally recoverable from the surface or from the sweat glands, but rather are harbored in the hair follicles, particularly near the orifices of the sebaceous glands. The quantitative distribution of bacteria is related to the distribution of hair, and in levels ranging from 5

Bacteriology of Normal Skin

I. Resident flora
- A. Aerobic bacteria
  1. Micrococcus Group
     - a. *M. albus*
     - b. *M. epidermis*
     - c. *M. candidus*
     - d. *M. flavus*
  2. Corynebacterium
     - a. Lipophilic species
- B. Lipophilic fungi
  1. Pityrosporon
     - a. *P. ovale*
     - b. *P. orbiculare*
- C. Anaerobic bacteria
  1. *Propionibacterium acnes*
  2. *Micrococcus saccharolyticus*

II. Transient flora
- A. Aerobic bacteria
  1. Streptococci
  2. *Micrococcus (Staphylococcus) aureus*
  3. Enteric bacteria
     - a. *Pseudomonas aeruginosa*
     - b. *Escherichia coli*
     - c. *Aerobacter aerogenes*
     - d. *Proteus vulgaris*

Figure 20–2 Resident and transient bacterial flora of the skin. Any of the transient flora may appear on random cultures.

to 865,000 aerobic bacteria and 50 to 200,000 anaerobic bacteria per sq. cm.[173]

The skin exists in a nicely balanced state with its resident flora but actively resists the presence of its transient flora. The exposure to streptococci, staphylococci and enteric bacteria is frequent, and random cultures may recover any of these on occasion. The antibacterial qualities of the skin are related to active and passive activities. The secretion of sebaceous glands, sebum, contains high levels of fatty acids, particularly oleic acid. In addition to lubricating the skin surface, sebum actively destroys streptococci and, less effectively, staphylococci.[91] However, any break in the skin or any inflammation results in serum accumulation which inactivates sebum and streptococci may colonize rapidly.[188] Staphylococci are also susceptible to dessication on the normally dry skin surface; the application of a wet dressing with an impervious outer layer will both remove sebum and provide moisture, and staphylococcal furunculosis may rapidly appear. The enteric bacteria are not affected by sebum but are readily killed by dessication on dry skin. The presence of moisture or maceration can result in colonization of enteric bacteria. Pseudomonas, particularly, is susceptible to dessication and can be recovered from only 5 to 10 per cent of random skin cultures. Since bacteria tend to colonize in hair follicles, random skin swabs may often be sterile, and special techniques are necessary to accurately identify the bacteria.

Regeneration. The often presented concepts of wound healing are not totally applicable to thermal injury. The cleanly incised, coapted wound heals by a lag or inflammatory stage followed by the laying down of new collagen, realignment of fibers and the return of structural integrity. Implicit though not stated in this description is an intact epithelial covering. The understanding of healing in burns requires some conceptual alterations since burns constitute horizontally as well as vertically directed wounds. Loss of epidermal continuity requires ingrowth of new epidermis from the margin, or re-epithelialization from remaining epidermal elements. For practical purposes, this means regrowth from remaining basal cells or hair follicle epithelium since the glands contribute very little. Until epidermal continuity is reestablished by this regeneration or marginal ingrowth (or artificially, by applying a graft), there will be no healing. There will be little progress beyond the lag or inflammatory stage, characterized grossly and histologically by granulation tissue. Perhaps the greatest single advance in burn therapy is the realization and acceptance of the fact that a wound lacking epidermal covering cannot heal.

MECHANISMS OF THERMAL INJURY

At an internal temperature of 37° C. we are only 6° C. below our thermal death point (43 to 44° C. for visceral cells). Our ability to rapidly dissipate heat is related to blood supply, thermal conductivity and evaporative water loss from the skin. The amount of external heat energy delivered to the skin is related to the intensity of the heat and the time of exposure. The skin can maximally dissipate heat at the rate of 0.04 cal./sec./sq. cm.; however, since a flash exposure may deliver 30 cal./sec./sq. cm., the ability to dissipate this falls short by a factor of almost 1000.

Experimentally, the time of exposure and intensity of the heat are easily measured and controlled. Although the response of the skin follows the same basic laws of physical energy, it is also subject to great biologic variability. The water content of the skin, its varying thickness within a given area, pigmentation, the presence of hair, oil and dirt, as well as the rapid changes in peripheral circulation, all influence the tissue response to heat. These variations occur not only among

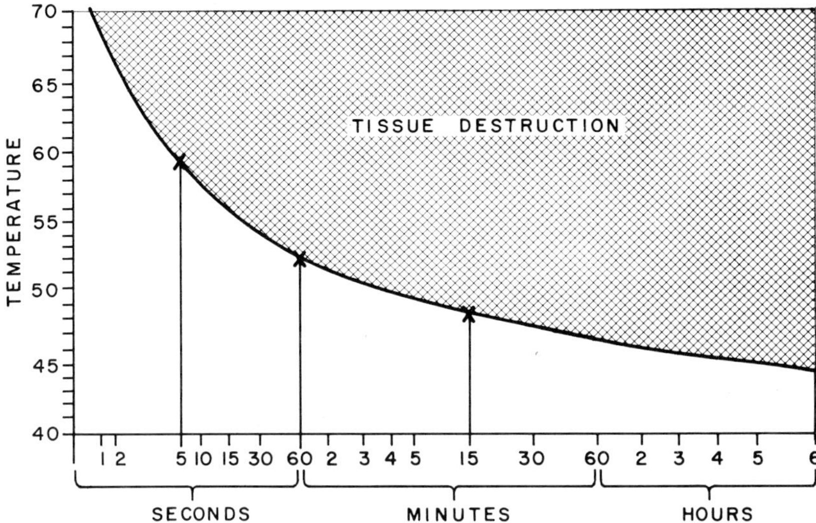

Figure 20–3 Tissue destruction as a function of time and temperature (in degrees Centigrade). Exposure of the skin to 70° C. for one second results in damage. At lesser temperatures, increasing length of exposure is necessary, such as that at 45° C. exposure for six hours is required to cause damage. (Based on data of Moritz and Henrique.[149])

species but also within very limited areas of the skin itself. The uniform application of heat to the surface does not result in a biologically uniform injury.

Within the limits of biologic variability, skin will tolerate temperatures up to 40° C. if the time of exposure is short. Thereafter, increased temperatures result in a logarithmic increase in tissue damage irrespective of time of exposure; fleeting exposure to 70° C. will produce epidermal necrosis (Fig. 20–3). The rate of damage at 60 to 65° C. is ten million times greater than it is at 45° C.[87]

Short of incineration, thermal injury will destroy cells by interference with necessary biological function. The mechanics of injury are the result of denaturation of cell protein, interference with cell metabolism and secondary interference with vascular supply.

LOCAL RESPONSE TO THERMAL INJURY

The body reacts to thermal injury with a series of responses which are not unique for burns; rather, it is the intensity and magnitude of the responses which differentiate the burn injury. The severity of the injury is related to both depth and spatial distribution. The alterations result from the initial injury and, more significantly, the subsequent loss of skin function.

Although totally interrelated, the local reaction to burning may be artificially divided into: (1) the response of the thermally injured cell; (2) the local vascular response to injury; (3) local response related to depth of injury and (4) burn wound sepsis.

Response of the Thermally Injured Cell

The depth of thermal injury is determined by the combination of the burning agent, temperature, time of exposure, and the series of events set in motion by the injury. There is a direct, vertical decrease in the severity of injury from the surface to the depth of the wound. Some cells are immediately destroyed, some are irrevocably injured, and some cells although injured are capable of surviving under suitable conditions.

The earliest cytologic evidence of injury is a redistribution of the fluid and solid components of the cell nuclei. Imbibition of fluid results in nuclear swelling, membrane rupture and pyknosis. Cell cytoplasm first becomes granular and finally homogeneously coagulated. Progressive denaturation of cell protein occurs as temperatures rise. These latter changes in the thermally injured cell are theoretically reversible since protein is constantly being denatured by the body and being replaced. Only at temperatures in excess of 45° C. does this denaturation exceed the reparative ability of the cell.[149] Therefore, reducing the temperature should reduce the denaturation of protein. Indeed, experimentally this has proved to be the case.

Cells are also injured and destroyed by interference with vital metabolic processes. Thermolabile enzyme systems are blocked at approximately the same temperatures that effect protein denaturation.[47] The metabolic response of an individual cell is quite variable, even within a homogeneous cell population. A decrease in enzyme activity below 50 per cent of normal results in cell death, whereas lesser degrees of injury may be reflected in altered survival.

The specialized functions of the various types of cells comprising the skin are affected differently. In deeper injuries the dermal collagen and elastic fibers show coagulation and dissolution. Hair follicles show pyknosis of nuclei and rupture of the follicle from basal cell attachments. Lysis of epithelium of the sebaceous and sudoriferous glands may occur.

The response to thermal injury on the cellular level is neither uniform nor static. Much of the result will be determined by the vascular supply and the local environment of the wound. Additional heat, mechanical or chemical trauma or bacterial invasion will further destroy the injured cell which had a potential for survival.

Local Vascular Response to Injury

The local vascular response can be divided into immediate and delayed fluid and cellular phases. This is the normal inflammatory response and in mild thermal injuries (51 to 60° C. for 20 seconds) is indistinguishable from that following mechanical trauma.[159] Longer or more severe exposure brings about more characteristic changes due to the heat itself.

Fluid Response. The cardinal feature of thermal injury is accumulation of fluid within the injured area. This fluid and electrolyte shift within the wound is related to the type and magnitude of injury. There is an immediate and reversible vascular response to burning. It is characterized by spasm of venules and dilatation of capillaries. An initial arterial and arteriolar vasoconstriction is followed by vasodilatation.[131] Capillaries and venules in the burned area become immediately permeable to plasma proteins of a molecular weight of 125,000 or below.[143] This capillary permeability occurs throughout the vascular tree in patients with greater than 30 per cent body burns. This type of response is transient, reversible and stimulated experimentally by histamine, serotonin and other vasoactive substances. It may be prevented experimentally by antihistamines and delayed by previous serotonin depletion.

The initial response is followed in one to six hours by a delayed response.[13] This delayed response is not endogenously mediated and is indistinguishable from the response to injection of bacteria. The response may be initiated by histamine (although not preventable by antihistamines) but is probably sustained by slower-acting vasoactive substances in the kinin system.[6] It appears to develop at the capillary rather than the venule level. The greatest loss of both plasma and fluid occurs in the first 12 hours postburn. After this period, platelets and red cells marginate on the vessel wall and plugging of the capillaries takes place.

Fluid and electrolyte changes occur in the thermally injured tissue by other mechanisms than capillary permeability. If capillary permeability alone accounted for fluid accumulation, externally applied pressure in excess of hydrostatic pressure could prevent it. This is not the case. In fact, fluid will accumulate in uninjured tissue around the site of pressure in almost equal amounts. Nor does it explain loss of fluid into areas of the body not involved by burns. Experimentally, burned tissue, even if immediately transplanted and devoid of a direct vascular supply, accumulates fluid far in excess of unburned, transplanted tissue.[157]

Normal protein (macromolecules) of the skin has an adsorption coefficient for water and electrolytes which may be very high. For comparison, the adsorption coefficient for a simple system such as water-charcoal is 37,000 atmospheres. These normal coefficients may be disturbed by burning and cause cellular tissue swelling irrespective of vascularity, and would theoretically occur at pressures far in excess of hydrostatic pressure. It would also tend to explain the more marked fluid and electrolyte accumulations in cell populations of injured and recovering cells, as opposed to areas where all cells are dead.[75]

This fluid and electrolyte shift is related to the type of injury. Thermal injury breaks down cell membrane, and potassium is released into the extracellular space. The concentration gradient between arteries and veins in the burned area may reach 0.72 mEq. per liter within a few hours.[145] Fox demonstrated that after a severe flash burn with immediate death of cells, the water, sodium and potassium content was less than in normal skin, although the underlying muscles showed increased water and sodium concentration.[75] In contrast, a low-intensity scald burn with severe injury to cells but less immediate cell necrosis results in increased water (three times greater than flash burn), sodium and potassium in both the burned tissue and the underlying muscle. This sequestering of fluid has been shown to be due to an uptake of water and sodium by injured collagen.[139,157] In addition, an abnormality of the sodium pump exists with the intracellular sodium content increasing and a potassium efflux.[50]

The fluid-electrolyte-protein loss described is obligatory. It enters a functional "third-space" and represents an overall hemodynamic deficit. Those vascular alterations are an integral part of the response to burning. In milder injury, the response may be limited to subpapillary vessels; whereas, in full-thickness skin destruction the vascular response will occur in the subcutaneous tissue and at the margins of the wound.

Cellular Response. The cellular response is characterized by neutrophil emigration from vessels to the tissues. This begins on a small scale immediately, but progresses to a peak over five to six hours. The stimulus for emigration is not known, although it is probably related to a decreased expulsion force between the endothelial cell and the leukocyte. It is an integral part of the basic inflammatory response to any injury and may be stimulated by any substance that increases vascular permeability.

Once the neutrophil emerges through the permeable capillary membrane, it is attracted by chemotaxis to the site of injury. At that point phagocytosis of the bacteria which have broached the burned portal of entry occurs. Phagocytosis proceeds normally in burned patients, but once phagocytized the bacterial intracellular kill ratio is decreased.[4]

Monocytes enter the injured area with the neutrophils, although in much smaller numbers. Because of their longer life span, they predominate in the wound after the first few days. These monocytes evolve into tissue macrophages and are effective against the remaining bacteria.

Red blood cells are affected in proportion to the severity of the vascular injury in the burn area. Loss of red cells into the tissue is not a part of the burn injury. However, a variable number of red cells in the area of the injury will be destroyed immediately and others will die prematurely. Decrease in blood flow, agglutination, sludging and eventual thrombosis will add to red cell loss.[103] Platelets are removed from the circulatory system in a similar fashion and an initial thrombocytopenia develops.

Although the cellular losses are an integral part of the early response to burning, the functionally important response is the noncellular fluid and electrolyte loss.

Local Response Related to Depth of Injury. The ultimate significance of depth of injury is not what has been lost, but rather the functional capacity of that which remains—whether there is adequate capacity in the injured skin to withstand bacterial invasion and to provide regeneration. Although clues to depth may be obtained by clinical observation, the true extent of injury is usually determined only in retrospect. Although, in any given area, the depth will vary tremendously, it is conceptually easier to view burns as a uniform injury.

Superficial Burn. FIRST DEGREE. In low-intensity–prolonged exposure injury, the damage is superficial (Fig. 20–4). The local response is characterized by erythema due to the vascular response in subpapillary vessels. Edema will occur in basal layers, irritating naked nerve endings at this

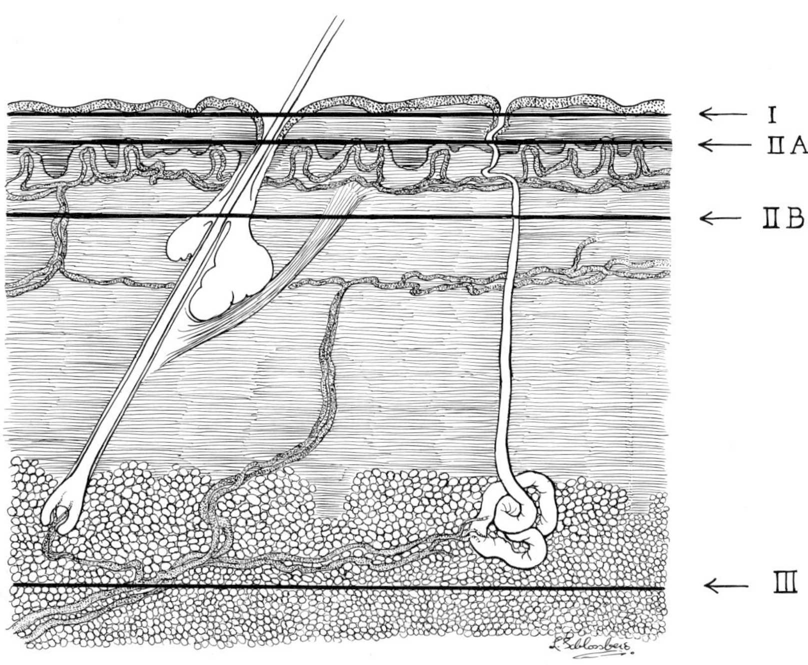

Figure 20–4 Depth of injury from burns. *I*, Superficial burn, involves only subcorneal level. *IIA*, Partial thickness—superficial: involves some but not all the basal layer. Healing should occur spontaneously but perhaps with some depigmentation due to loss of melanocytes. *IIB*, Partial thickness—deep: loss of basal layer is complete. Only potential for spontaneous healing lies in the viable epidermal elements present in the skin appendages. *III*, Full thickness: by definition, all epidermal elements have been destroyed and spontaneous healing is impossible other than from the margins of the wound.

level and causing discomfort, although clinical swelling and blistering are not seen. Denaturation of the outer nonliving keratin layer does occur, accompanied by some cellular destruction, often delayed, in the underlying stratum granulosa. Premature cell death may result in desquamation at this level, which is noted as "peeling" a few days after the burn. Other than discomfort, there is no clinical significance to injury at this level. All germinal cells of the basal layer survive. Healing occurs by evolution of cells to the surface and is not accompanied by scarring or discoloration.

Partial-Thickness Burn. SUPERFICIAL, SECOND DEGREE—A. As intensity of heat or time of exposure is increased, there is increased tissue destruction. Since any injury short of full-thickness loss is "partial thickness," this injury requires further subdivision. Included in superficial partial thickness is any injury that does not totally destroy the basal layer. This injury is clinically and histologically characterized by fluid accumulation. Erythema is seen but the distinguishing finding is blistering. When the edema of burning is close to the surface, it is easily visible. The same vascular response occurs with edema formation either at the dermal-epidermal junction or within the epidermis itself. Cells of stratum granulosa are destroyed and, together with the stratum corneum, form the covering of the blister. Intercellular processes of "prickle cells" dissolve; edematous separation and often destruction of these cells are seen. Marked dilatation of the subpapillary plexus occurs, but the structural integrity of the dermis remains intact. Basal cells may be destroyed in part and nerve endings at this level irritated.

Intact blisters maintain a sterile, waterproof covering of the wound, and healing occurs by continued growth of the remaining basal cells. Removal or breaking of blisters results in a weeping wound and loss of "membrane-barrier" of the skin. Stripping this layer of epidermis results in an increase in evaporative water loss, attended by the necessary metabolic expenditure of thermal injury.[68] Loss of the blister also exposes naked nerve fibers and increases discomfort. Once the blister is broken, the edema fluid forms a coagulum or "crust," under which healing will also usually proceed uneventfully.

Blistering is not a phenomenon limited to superficial burns but can also be seen in full-thickness loss when the intensity of the heat is sufficient to cause "steam" within the epidermis. In these cases, it appears promptly in conjunction with the fluid phase of the injury (first eight hours). The appearance of blisters after this time is suggestive of bacterial invasion and should be investigated in this light.

Since basal cells are not destroyed in quantity, regeneration is usually prompt and complete without scarring. Temporary discoloration may occur, and some permanent changes toward a lighter color may be related to loss of melanocytes. The cellular barrier to bacterial invasion is generally intact at this level, although the presence of plasma inactivates the antistreptococcal potency of sebum and streptococcal invasion may be a danger.

DEEP, SECOND DEGREE —B. This level of injury is characterized by disruption of epidermal continuity and loss of much of the basal cell layer, but with survival of viable, epidermal elements in hair follicles and glands.

The major histological changes occur in the subpapillary plexus. The initial fluid and cellular phases of vascular response occur with edema accumulation at the dermal-epidermal junction. Coagulation necrosis of epidermal cells occurs as vascular injury progresses to vascular blockage, thrombosis and dissolution of endothelial cells. An inflammatory leukocyte response beneath the basal layer occurs.

There may be blistering in this injury but more often there is the development of dry coagulum of plasma and necrotic cells—an eschar. Fluid loss is quantitatively similar to weeping or blistered superficial wounds but is deceptively hidden beneath the coagulum. Since naked nerve endings in the basal layer are destroyed, the wound is not responsive to pinprick, although pressure sensation remains intact. The membrane barrier to water is lost and evaporation through coagulum is 15 to 20 times that of normal skin.[39] This wound is clinically indistinguishable from full-thickness loss.

The cellular barrier to bacterial invasion is also lost, and wound sepsis is the major clinical determinant of healing of this wound.

Injury at this level, if not further traumatized or subjected to bacterial invasion, has the potential for spontaneous regeneration. Undamaged epithelial cells in hair follicles and the margins of the wound will proliferate and resurface the wound. If the eschar is removed prematurely, the clinical appearance will be that of a granulating wound with multiple punctate epithelial islands. These will progressively enlarge and coalesce to form a new surface. When coverage is complete, underlying collagen fibers degenerate. New collagen is laid down and remodeling will occur over a period of time. The new epithelium is thin and lacks sebaceous secretions to lubricate the surface, sensation is diminished and since most melanocytes are destroyed, it will be lighter than surrounding tissue. Failure to redevelop interpapillary ridges results in prolonged susceptibility to even minor, tangentially directed stress forces.[105]

Full-Thickness Burn. THIRD DEGREE. As the depth of injury increases in more severe trauma, all epidermal elements and dermal supporting structures are destroyed. Whereas the more superficial injuries are characterized by increased vascularity, this is an avascular injury. The fluid and cellular response to injury occurs at the margins, in normal viable tissue and in the depths of the subcutaneous tissue. Coagulation necrosis of cells, thrombosis of vessels, accumulation of fluid and cellular infiltrate in the margins of the wound characterize the injury. Fluid accumulation is related to the initial intensity of the heat. It is as great as in superficial injuries or injuries from lower-intensity exposure, in which cell death is more gradual.

Clinically characterized by the same eschar as deep partial-thickness burns, third-degree burns are also insensitive to pinprick. The leathery eschar also permits evaporative water loss to an excess degree and forms no functional barrier to bacterial invasion.

This injury cannot heal itself. There will be a natural progression of increased marginal and subcutaneous inflammatory response, development of granulation tissue and autolysis at the junction of viable and nonviable tissue with eventual slough of eschar. Resurfacing can occur only from the margins of the wound or by application of skin graft.

FOURTH DEGREE. Occasional severe incineration injuries occur in which the depth of injury extends through the subcutaneous tissue to involve fascia, muscle, periosteum or bone. The natural history of the wound is not dissimilar to other full-thickness injury, except for the individual problems of skin coverage that they present. Extensive destruction of muscle will also impose a myoglobin load on the renal tubules.

The burn wound, therefore, represents an injury of mixed severity and depth. The vascular and cellular response is more representative of the nonspecific inflammatory response than unique to thermal injury. The natural history of the wound is related to the amount of cellular destruction and the capacity for regeneration. These concepts, however, are presented as though they occur in the germ-free patient. Such is not the case and, clinically, the major determinant in the healing of burns and the survival of patients relates to the altered functional capacity of the skin to resist bacterial invasion. Although theoretically a "complication," wound sepsis is part of the natural history of the burn wound.

Burn-Wound Sepsis

The local cutaneous defense against bacterial invasion is a function of an intact membrane barrier, antibacterial substances in sebum, dessication on dry skin and a natural competition with the normal flora of the skin. Each of these is altered following thermal trauma. Contributing to the altered local defense mechanisms are modifications in systemic response such as hypovolemia and an altered immune mechanism.

Bacteria of the resident flora of the skin are resistant to heat injury in approximately the same proportions as are the skin cells. Those on the surface are heat-killed as are the surface cells, and initial swab cultures are usually sterile.[236] The bacteria in the hair follicles and glands, however, survive and quantitative counts of *biopsy* specimens show the same 10^3 bacteria per gram of tissue as found in the tissue prior to burning.[14] These organisms (*Staph. epidermidis*, etc.) we would now classify as "amphibionts." Not normally prime invaders, they do, indeed, have the potential for becoming the infecting organisms.

The initial danger to the burned patient is most often the *B-hemolytic Streptococcus*, the most common of the transient flora, and present in most patients. The rich vascularity of the inflammatory phase of early injury, the edema, and the neutralization of the bacteriocidal defense mechanisms of sebum all render the burn particularly prone to streptococcal invasion. Historically, the recognition of "burn shock" and its management in the early 1940's resuscitated patients only to have them succumb to streptococcal invasion in the first few days after burning. The introduction of penicillin provided both effective treatment and prophylaxis against streptococcal burn sepsis. Although streptococci remain exquisitely sensitive to penicillin and its use in the early phases of burn care remains appropriate today, it proved to be no panacea.[14]

Shock controlled and streptococcal sepsis prevented, the 1950's recorded only prolonged rather than increased survival. Opportunistic, ubiquitous, penicillin-resistant *Staphylococcus aureus* replaced streptococci as the offender.[180] Unchecked by competition with normal skin flora, and flourishing in the warm, moist environment of the fresh burn wound, staphylococci were able to colonize the wound. A quantitative increase in staphylococci resulted in microabscesses in and around hair follicles, then showering bacteria into the blood stream, resulting in secondary abscesses. The aerobic nature of the staphylococci and their dependence on a good blood supply made the development of penicillinase-resistant antibiotics both timely and effective. Their apparent disappearance has been deceptive and a 900 per cent increase in *Staphylococcus aureus* septicemia between 1968 and 1970 was noted at the U.S. Army Institute of Surgical Research.[49]

The control of staphylococci did not produce a "germ-free" patient. Indeed, the first of the true "amphibiont" organisms, *Pseudomonas aeruginosa*, appeared as a major threat in the 1960's. The "amphibionts" are those organisms previously classified as "non-pathogens," which under conditions of altered host resistance and disturbed bacterial ecology can become predominant in a wound and reach sufficient quantitative levels to be truly pathogenic. Previously thought to be a harmless saprophyte, pseudomonas was encountered in only 8 per cent of burned patients in 1948; by the early 1960's it was encountered in 70 per cent of burned patients within one week after burning and was the leading cause of death.[122]

Indigenous to man, pseudomonas can be identified in 15 to 20 per cent of random nasopharyngeal and stool cultures. It is now ubiquitous in most hospitals; isolation has been ineffective prophylaxis. In mixed full- and partial-thickness injury, early pseudomonas colonization occurs within the lumen of hair follicles and glands; in full-thickness wounds it may not gain access until the eschar cracks.[167] Lodgement and quantitative growth to levels not exceeding 10^5 bacteria per gram, as determined by biopsy techniques, are compatible with survival and healing of deep dermal elements in partial-thickness injury. If the count exceeds 10^5 bacteria per gram, the bacteria spread from the hair follicles and colonize along the dermal-subcutaneous interface.[223, 224, 225, 230] Perivascular growth is accompanied by thrombosis of vessels, necrosis of any remaining dermal elements, converting partial-thickness burns to full-thickness loss. Levels of growth in excess of 10^5 bacteria per gram of tissue constitute "burn-wound sepsis," and levels of 10^8 to 10^9 bacteria per gram may be associated with lethal burns.[168] Since the process occurs in a subeschar plane, surface swabs may be deceptive. So too, lethal burn-wound sepsis may occur with no spread of viable organisms into the blood stream and without secondary visceral lodgement; negative blood cultures provide no security.[148]

The vascular changes of full-thickness burns with local occlusion of small vessels isolate the wound from many normal host defense mechanisms. So too, they prevent the adequate delivery of potent systemic antibiotics to the foci of bacterial growth. The use of topical antibacterial agents applied directly to the wound has been both rational and effective. Quantitative bacterial cultures of biopsy specimens have been a useful guide to management. The mere presence of bacteria is not so critical as the quantitative level of bacterial growth.

Evidence suggests that pseudomonas burn sepsis is yielding to a variety of topical antibacterial agents and techniques. The repetition of history suggests, however, that this is leading to the emergence of the opportunistic growth of new and different "amphibiont" organisms. Prominent among these is *Candida.* Mycotic infection from *Candida* was not recognized in one series in the period from 1953–1959, appeared in 24 cases in the next eight-year period, and in the three years 1967–1970 there were *50* cases of candida septicemia identified.[53] Candida, although part of the normal bowel flora, is clearly a secondary invader. Predisposition is provided by decreased host resistance seen in the chronic burn patient, and potentiated by the disturbance in the bacterial ecology resulting from antibiotic therapy. Long-standing indwelling catheters may provide a portal of entry, but more often it is the bowel. Candida septicemia is heralded by hypothermia, leukopenia, agitation and later vasculitis with purpura. There are no specific features to distinguish it from bacterial infection. Its presence in the gut, burn wound, or even the blood stream can be misinterpreted as "harmless" contamination. The finding of candida in the urine, however, particularly in the non-catheterized patient, is ominous and should be considered an indication for antifungal therapy.[113, 130, 163]

In addition to candida, mycotic burn-wound sepsis has been associated with Phycomycetes and the *Aspergillus* species. Infection with these species is identified by a change in the clinical appearance of the wound, development of purplish or black spots, ulceration of the burn wound, unexplained fever or unusual tenderness. Biopsy and histologic identification are mandatory. Cultures are positive in only 30 per cent of histologically proved cases and follow only after a three-to-five day lag for growth on culture media.[34] Pathologically, all produce fat necrosis, ischemia of underlying muscle, vascular invasion and systemic dissemination. Of 30 cases reported in one series, 22 were of the Phycomycetes class (two were *Rhizopus* and the remainder probably *Mucor*) and the other eight from Aspergillus.[34]

Among the bacterial species emerging as threats to the burned patient, most prominent are the gram-negative bacteria, particularly the Enterobacteriaceae family.[52] Among these are *Serratia marcescens*, the *Klebsiella-Enterobacter* group, *Erwinia* species and, of particular note, the *Providencia* species. Providencia species, formerly known as *Proteus inconstans*, are gram-negative rods which fall into the general category of paracolon bacteria. *Providencia stuartii* has been identified with increasing frequency in the burn population, and in 1970 at the U.S. Army Institute of Surgical Research, it supplanted Pseudomonas as the predominant fatal blood stream pathogen.[49] Whereas staphylococcal septicemias were identified more frequently in 1970, only 37.2 per cent died. The mortality with Providencia or Pseudomonas bacteremia was 70 to 75 per cent. During the four-year period 1967–1970, there was a 700 per cent increase recovery rate of Providencia from sputum cultures and a 61.8 per cent mortality rate in those with positive cultures.[49] Of particular concern was the observation that only 12 per cent of isolates were sensitive to antibiotics at the usual therapeutic blood levels achieved. An epidemic of totally antibiotic-resistant Providencia has been reported by Zawacki.[240] Rather than invasive burn sepsis as such, much of the mortality seems to be associated with pulmonary complications.

Fortunately of more academic than practical interest thus far has been the frightening reports of viral burn sepsis, particularly, a report of six cases of herpes virus infection with two fatalities.[71] A single case of cytomegalic virus (CMV) with disseminated cytomegalic inclusion disease has been reported.[162]

Finally, not peculiar to burn wounds but common to all ischemic injuries with large masses of devitalized tissue, is clostridial infection.

Clostridia welchii and others of this group (*Cl. septique* and *Cl. novyi*) can manifest themselves in burn injury as either a crepitant cellulitis or a more lethal myositis. The cellulitis form spreads rapidly along fascial planes, does not involve muscle, and is clinically manifest by a sudden increase in pain prior to appearance of swelling, erythema or crepitus. Slough of overlying skin may occur and is associated with variable systemic toxicity. Clostridial myositis is a more highly lethal infectious gangrene of the underlying muscle. It also tends to appear early (24 to 48 hours after injury) and is ushered in with sudden increase in pain, pallor, listlessness and, eventually, circulatory collapse. Crepitation may be a late finding. Overlying normal skin may develop a dusky appearance and, later, vesicles; drainage of the area is productive of a foul-smelling, brown discharge.

Tetanus may occur from any wound, even if apparently insignificant. Proper tetanus prophylaxis is mandatory.

SYSTEMIC RESPONSE TO THERMAL INJURY

The function of all organ systems will eventually be altered due to the effects of a major burn. Some of the changes are in response to the stress of injury; some are related to burning itself; most, however, are due to the altered functional capacity of the skin. Although interrelated and interdependent, the systemic response is presented by organ systems and functions rather than in a chronological fashion.

Hemodynamics. Hemodynamic instability ("burn shock") was for centuries the major cause of death in burned patients. Buhl in 1855 noted that burn patients looked like those dying from cholera and reported their need for fluid. Yet as late as 1943, fully 50 to 75 per cent of burn deaths occurred in the first 48 hours from shock.[13] Blalock in 1930 observed that burn fluid was qualitatively similar to plasma and quantitatively sufficient to cause shock.[25]

Fully 60 per cent of the extracellular fluid volume may be lost in a major burn. Most of the loss occurs within the first 8 to 12 hours, but fluid loss continues for 48 hours after injury.[18] Patients may easily gain 10 per cent of their body weight during the course of replacement. This massive fluid loss is a combination of loss through the wound and a translocation into a "functional third space" which is lost to the circulating blood volume.

Added to this volume loss into the burn is an obligatory loss by respiration and urine, plus a suddenly increased evaporation from the burn surface. Loss of the stratum corneum increases the evaporative water loss 10 to 70 times over the loss from intact skin. Roe and Kinney have demonstrated that there may be a loss of six to eight liters of fluid per day by evaporation alone.[190] Blood flow is further reduced by rising hematocrit, increased viscosity and sludging of cellular elements.

Compensation for these hemodynamic changes occurs at the expense of adequate perfusion. Hypovolemia results in splanchnic vasoconstriction, decreased renal, hepatic and intestinal perfusion, and subsequent compromised function of these organs.

Cardiac Function. Cardiac alterations originally thought to be in response to hemodynamic changes are now known to precede them. A precipitous drop in cardiac output occurs before any significant change in blood volume.[55] This may amount to as much as a 50 per cent decrease. This initial decrease suggests a direct myocardial "toxic" effect of thermal injury. As blood volume and plasma fall, the cardiac output decreases further and may reach a low of 20 per cent of normal.[143] Experimentally in lethal burns, the cardiac output continues to decrease until death occurs. However, in surviving animals the cardiac output returns toward normal—reaching preburn levels by 36 hours. Plasma volume, however, does not return as rapidly—again suggesting a direct myocardial effect. Evidence for this myocardial "toxin" has been accumulated from cross-perfusion studies between burned and unburned animals.[142]

Pulmonary edema is difficult to produce in a patient with a normal heart. However, in the elderly or in a patient with previous cardiopulmonary embarrassment, fluid overload may become a problem. This becomes increasingly important because of the increase in pulmonary blood volume and pulmonary vascular resistance which has been demonstrated in the immediate post-burn period.[42]

Renal Function. Renal function is altered in the burned patient as a direct effect of the stress of injury and secondarily as the result of the loss of extracellular fluid volume.

In response to the stress of trauma itself the posterior pituitary releases antidiuretic hormone (ADH) and maximum reabsorption of water occurs. So, too, aldosterone is released from the adrenal cortex and maximum sodium reabsorption results. In the untreated burn under the ADH–aldosterone influence, the kidney will excrete only an amount of urine necessary to handle the normal solute load, represented largely by urea. The result is oliguria (15 to 25 ml./hr.), increased urine concentration and decreased urine sodium concentration.[238]

Early destruction of red cells may present free hemoglobin in the urine. This situation may result in tubular necrosis only if accompanied by prolonged renal ischemia.

As volume loss is replaced in kind, renal blood flow is reestablished. This results in an increased glomerular filtration rate and increased urine volume. Normally in this situation the urine volume reflects solute load and glomerular filtration rate, and changes are not the result of fluctuating ADH levels. The ADH response to stress will continue for variable periods of time, and the high urine specific gravity continues. This cannot be lowered by hydration, and a large free-water load will cause water intoxication without changing the urine concentration. An osmotic diuretic, such as mannitol, will increase urine volume as a result of the increased solute load.

Renal function, therefore, is altered in the burn patient in a manner similar to that in any injured patient. Decreased renal function is almost inevitably a result of inadequate fluid and electrolyte replacement. Sodium and chloride are lost into the injured tissue in the same proportion as their plasma levels. An isotonic depletion results and, unless adversely influenced by treatment, alterations in serum concentration are not seen.

Respiratory Function. The response of the respiratory system to thermal injury may be violent and may of itself prove lethal. It is not, however, due to "burning." Mortiz et al. demonstrated that application of a blow torch at 550° C. through an endotracheal tube caused minimal injury beyond the carina.[150] The pulmonary tree is thus protected by the cooling produced by rapid vaporization. Only the inhalation of live steam results in true "burning" of the trachea or bronchi.

Edema of the epiglottis and larynx with burns of the face may endanger the upper airway. More commonly, particularly in burns sustained in close spaces, inhalation of products of incomplete combustion (including carbon monoxide, sulfides, aldehydes, acid anhydrides, or even phosgenes) may lead to chemical pulmonary irritation, edema and pneumonitis. The pathological changes include congestion and edema of the respiratory tree, particularly small bronchi, with denudation of respiratory mucosa and obstruction from the denuded epithelial cells. Alveoli similarly may be filled with edema fluid and cellular debris. Scattered atelectasis and emphysema are early signs followed by evidence of bacterial invasion, septic microemboli and focal or diffuse bronchopneumonia.

Pulmonary function studies show that minute ventilation increases in the post-burn period. This increase peaks at about five days and appears to be related to the size of the burn more than to any other measurable parameter. Oxygen consumption has shown a similar rise after thermal injury. Vital capacity may show a decrease up to 35 per cent of the predicted normal. Hypoxemia has been demonstrated in the initial period but usually returns to normal during the first week if severe inhalation injury has not accompanied the burn. The blood gas changes seen following the thermal injury are not dissimilar to those following other major nonthermal injury.[177] Most of these changes are due to impairment of diffusion and uneven distribution of alveolar gas and blood.[64]

Metabolic and Nutritional Response. The metabolic rate of a patient with a major burn is greatly accelerated. Oxygen consumption is increased and nitrogen losses are magnified. Urinary excretion of nitrogen (normally 10 to 15 grams per day) may increase to 30 grams per day in the first week post-injury. The water-holding lipid in skin is destroyed by the burn so that up to four times the normal amount of water vapor is transmitted by burned skin.[99] Since it requires 580 kcal. per liter to convert water to vapor, the loss of 5 liters per day would result in an expenditure of 2880 kcal. per day just for the increased evaporative loss.

The increased evaporative water loss (and accompanying heat loss) results in cooling of the body. This produces shivering and a further increase in the metabolic rate (30 to 300 per cent). Increasing the environmental temperature in which a burned patient is maintained has been shown to decrease his catabolism. The critical temperature appears to be about 34° C.[12] A decrease in urinary excretion of nitrogen has been found in burns of 10 to 50 per cent treated in environments of 32° C. compared to those treated at 22° C.

Nitrogen loss occurs into the burn wound itself in addition to the urinary losses. These losses are proportional to the size and depth of the burn and have been calculated by Nylen and Wallenius to reach levels of 2 to 3 grams for each per cent body burn per day.[164] The amount of nitrogen per square meter that is necessary for equilibrium varies with the phase of wound recovery after burning.[210] Prolonged protein depletion is associated with lowered serum proteins, weight loss (up to a pound a day), decreased muscle tone, poor appetite, decreased pain threshold, depression, poor resistance to infection and possibly delayed wound healing.[27] Granulation tissue may enter a chronic phase in which the pink color is lost and it becomes pale, gray, fibrotic and accepts grafts poorly.

Vitamin metabolism has been poorly studied. Vitamin C is obviously necessary for collagen formation and maintenance. Recently the role of vitamin A in collagen has been demonstrated.[63] B-complex vitamins are assumed to be necessary in normal doses. There is some evidence to suggest that alphatocopheral (vitamin E) may be useful in wound healing.[92]

Trace metals may become depleted in major burns. Zinc deficiency has been found to cause indolent-chronic wounds with minimal epithelialization and poor skin-graft acceptance.[112] Cohen has demonstrated decreased taste acuity with low zinc levels.[38] This contributes to further lack of appetite, thus deterring correction of the zinc deficiency by dietary means. These changes can be reversed with zinc administration.

Blood Elements. Progressive anemia occurs during the first week post-injury. Whereas previously this had been attributed to direct thermal damage to the erythrocyte itself and sequestration in the burn wound, newer findings suggest that an extrinsic mechanism produces the observed reduction in red cell survival.[20] Red blood cells from nonburned patients have decreased survival when injected into burned patients. Conversely, red cells from burned patients survive normally in nonburned patients.

Platelet changes after thermal injury are biphasic. Immediately post-burn a thrombocytopenia exists.[93] This is accompanied by a decrease in fibrinogen levels and a brief episode of diffuse intravascular coagulation.[65] By 24 to 36 hours, the platelet count and fibrinogen levels rise and remain elevated for up to three weeks.

Liver Function. Liver function is measurably altered following thermal injury, but frank liver necrosis is unusual. Changes are probably due more to altered circulation and hypoxia in the early stages; later alterations may be the result of toxic waste products. Liver biopsies have shown early cloudy swelling and evidence of glycosis at three hours post-burn. Later changes may include some hepatocellular necrosis, vacuolization and fatty degeneration. After four weeks, reparative proliferation may still be present. Necropsy specimens show congestion, periportal necrosis or other changes indicating shock or sepsis.[21] Almost all liver function tests are abnormal at some time after a severe burn.[213]

Neuroendocrine Response. Epinephrine and norepinephrine release are increased greatly by all forms of trauma, including burns, as quantitatively reflected in urinary excretion. The amount of epinephrine excreted seems to parallel the size of the injury; norepinephrine responds out of proportion to other types of trauma, and levels may be seen comparable to those observed with pheochromocytomas.[86]

Although the resynthesis of both

hormones is quite rapid, fatal burns may be accompanied by evidence of severe depletion. Such sympathetic depletion has been noted in up to 70 per cent of lethal burns. Although not the cause, this depletion may help to explain the mechanism of death.

Adrenal Cortical Response. Studies of the adrenal cortical response have revealed initially high and sustained levels of plasma 17-hydroxy-corticosteroids which return to normal with healing. Higher levels develop in patients with infected burns. Patients with burns of less than 40 per cent respond adequately and continuously to stress; it is doubtful that any burn ever becomes depleted of its adrenal steroids.[13]

The increased secretion of aldosterone seen in response to injury is principally due to the renin-angiotensin stimulus. However, its secretion is enhanced in situations which result in a falling serum sodium and rising potassium such as seen with burns. The effect of the aldosterone is to conserve the sodium as a compensatory mechanism for combating hypovolemia.[95]

Gastrointestinal Tract Function. The initial response to thermal trauma is similar to the response to any major trauma. As a result of severe splanchnic vasoconstriction, an early and sustained reflex ileus may occur. Acute gastric dilatation may occur early and be accompanied by abdominal distention, regurgitation and possible aspiration.

Although gastroduodenal mucosal ulceration is frequently seen following burns, it does not appear to be due to gastric hyperacidity. O'Neill has shown that Pavlov and Heidenhain pouches in dogs do not secrete increased levels of acid following burning.[165] When hyperacidity does occur, it appears to be related to hypercarbia and not to the thermal injury per se.[166] The amount of gastric mucus is decreased, and it may be this lack of protection to normal or even decreased amounts of acid which is responsible for mucosal ulceration.

Immune Response. The systemic immune response is altered by thermal injury. The presence or absence of a "burn toxin" has not been completely defined in humans. However, immunity relative to bacterial invasion has both theoretical and practical importance. Munster has documented that most mechanisms active in normal host defenses are affected in patients with severe burns.[159]

BURN TOXINS. Although survival chances after burning appear to be related to the area and depth of the body surface involved, the mortality is not a direct function of the per cent of body burn. Instead, a plot of mortality versus per cent of burn yields a sigmoid-chaped curve characteristic of a dose-mortality plot for a drug or toxic substance.[156]

Early reports on burn toxins, antitoxins, and convalescent burn sera have proved not to be due to any generalized toxic product but instead related to bacteria and their products. Sera and vaccines have been developed in several centers specifically to supplement the immune mechanisms against *Pseudomonas aeruginosa*. This is not to be construed as evidence for a generalized "burn toxin."

Recent isolation of a lipid-protein complex from thermally treated mouse skin fulfills criteria postulated for a true "burn toxin."[7] This substance is lethal when injected into recipient mice. The same physico-chemical and biological activity was obtained for this complex when germ-free donor and recipient animals were used, thus eliminating the bacterial role previously confusing the issue. Also the toxic effect was demonstrated in genetically identical animals, proving that immunological incompatibility was not responsible for the toxicity. Preliminary animal data show that antitoxic serum can be produced to this substance which markedly increases survival.

ALTERATIONS IN IMMUNE RESPONSE. Immunological changes in response to burning have received a great deal of interest.[161] It has now been generally accepted that (1) serum immunoglobulins become depleted, (2) rejection of skin allografts is delayed in proportion to the severity of the burn, and (3) patients with burns show anergy when challenged with certain agents to test delayed cutaneous hypersensitivity.

Other changes in host defense mechanisms, although not entirely immune in nature, affect the ability of the burned patient to withstand bacterial invasion.[193] Most important is the loss of integrity of defenses at the portal of entry because of the obvious mechanical injury to the skin. The inflammatory reaction is less than optimal because of venular stasis, microthrombosis and impaired margination of the leukocytes. Alexander has shown that neutrophil phagocytosis progresses normally but the intracellular killing is decreased.[4] He has related this to decreased levels of three hydrolases within the neutrophil (beta glucuronidase, lysozyme and acid phosphatase). Phagocytosis within the R-E system is impaired. Together with the immunological deficiencies, these responses result in an overall deficit in host defense mechanisms.

Skeletal Changes. Localized as well as generalized skeletal abnormalities accompany burns and are not usually reflected in altered urine or blood biochemical changes.

Bone may be involved directly in deep thermal injury causing necrosis of periosteum and outer cortex.[115] Also it may be involved with either local or generalized osteoporosis related to local disease or immobilization. Periosteal new bone growth is not uncommon in children, particularly near areas of open granulation tissue. Recent reports of heterotopic calcification around joints following burns have appeared.[160] Articular destruction with fibrosis and even bony ankylosis can appear in children. These changes do not necessarily occur near areas involved in the burn wound; other changes are more directly related to exposure from burning or to sepsis.[66]

PSYCHIATRIC IMPLICATIONS

Patients adjust to the burn situation in a manner reflecting their total personality adjustment prior to injury.[118] Pain, helplessness, change in appearance and potential deformity all tend to bring about a situational depression aggravated by some very real financial and social adjustments. Sleeplessness, restlessness, loss of libido, or a sensation of being "closed-in," and increasing acuity to lesser degrees of discomfort are normal in the burned patient. It is tempting to attribute all such personality changes to "psychological factors", however, psychoses are rare unless the patient was previously psychotic. Such manifestations are more often toxic in origin.

Evidence of delirium should be a danger signal. Alterations in perception are manifest as hallucinations; disturbed interpretation results in illusions and delusions. There may be altered activity patterns with over-talkativeness, tremors, restlessness, laughing and crying. Moods may suddenly swing from euphoria to fear and temper tantrums. More progressive disturbances occur in the form of disorientation, diminished sensibility and coma.

The most common causes of these toxic psychotic symptoms in the burned patient are shock, hypoxia, altered water load (water excess and hypotonicity) and electrolyte disturbances and sepsis. Later in the burn course there may occur vitamin deficiencies and protein and glucose intoxication from forced feedings. Excessive alcoholic intake, epilepsy and drug addiction may all have preceded the burning and may result in withdrawal symptoms.

Drug administration must be cautious; narcotics and barbiturates may easily become necessary to the patient. Many of the phenothiazine tranquilizers will cause toxic symptoms, including twitching, nystagmus and other extrapyramidal signs.

The presence of wound sepsis and fever result in a wide variety of toxic manifestations including restlessness, decreased emotional control, inability to concentrate and vivid dreams. These may precede, accompany or follow an acute febrile episode and, in children, may be accompanied by convulsions and postictal depression.

Toxic psychotic disturbance in burns is rare after the first week except with sepsis. Multiple dressing changes and persistent, chronic pain tend to produce a very real situation disturbance characterized by detachment despondency, crying and lack of patient cooperation.

CLINICAL AND THERAPEUTIC IMPLICATIONS

Etiology and Incidence

Each year there are approximately 2,000,000 people in the United States burned seriously enough to require medical attention. The 8,000 deaths per year reflect the tragic mortality. The 80,000 hospitalized patients with total or partial disability and problems in rehabilitation reflect the tremendous cost in time, money and suffering. Almost 50 per cent of major burns occur during growing and formative years (under age 20) and 30 per cent occur in children under 10 years of age.[26] People over the age of 65 years (9 per cent of the population) experience 28 per cent of the deaths from fire and explosion.[14]

In general, for children up to the age of three years, scalds are the most common form of burns. From three to 15 years, flame burns from ignition of clothing are most common. For those over the age of 60 years, smoking in bed and house fires predominate. Hot bath water (above 115° F.) is a serious cause of burns in young children, the disabled and the aged. Fully 80 per cent of burn accidents occur within the home.

Important studies by Lawson[116] and Zuidema et al.[241] on the inflammability of certain types of material used in clothing provided an opportunity for meaningful advances in prevention. The most critical garments are loose-fitting children's nightwear. It is now practical and commercially feasible to treat clothing chemically to make them flame-retardant. Legislation has now been implemented requiring such treatment of children's night clothes in sizes 0 to 6X.

Mortality

Meaningful data are extremely difficult to acquire. A great many burned patients die before reaching a hospital. Many patients with minor burns never seek professional care. Inclusion of either group would obviously influence the statistics. Thorough probit analyses of burn mortality are available and demonstrate that the most important criteria influencing survival are the size of the burn and the age of the patients (Fig. 20–5).[35, 126, 182]

There have been two distinct trends in the last 30 years. The incidence of death in the early period from shock has almost disappeared. This has been reflected more in prolonged rather than increased survival. Secondly, with prolonged survival, sepsis has become the major cause of death, particularly burn-wound sepsis.[228] In recent years, however, respiratory complications have caused more deaths than burn-wound sepsis.[208]

In the first 24 hours following burn injury, the major causes of death are incineration and respiratory failure. From two to 21 days post-burn infec-

	PER CENT OF BODY SURFACE BURNED									
	10	20	30	40	50	60	70	80	90	100%
2 Years	0	5	17	40	63	80	92	98	100	100
4 Years	0	5	16	39	63	79	92	98		
8 Years	0	4	14	37	60	78	91	97		
12 Years	0	4	13	36	59	77	91	97		
16 Years	0	3	13	35	59	77	90	97		
20 Years	0	3	13	35	59	77	90	97		
24 Years	0	4	14	37	60	78	91	97		
28 Years	0	4	15	38	62	78	92	97		
32 Years	0	5	17	40	63	80	92	98		
36 Years	1	6	19	44	66	81	94	98		
40 Years	1	7	22	47	69	84	94	98		
44 Years	2	9	27	52	71	87	95	99		
48 Years	3	11	32	56	75	89	96	99		
52 Years	4	15	39	62	79	92	97	100%		
56 Years	6	20	45	67	83	94	98			
60 Years	9	27	53	72	87	96	99			
64 Years	13	36	59	77	91	97	100%			
68 Years	19	45	67	83	94	98				
72 Years	29	54	73	88	96	99				
76 Years	40	63	80	92	98	100%				
80 Years	51	71	86	95	99					
84 Years	61	78	92	97	100%					
88 Years	71	86	95	99						
90 Years	75	89	97	99%						

Figure 20–5A Predicted mortality in males. (Modified and reprinted by permission from Lynch, J. B.: Thermal burns. *In* Grabb, W. C., and Smith, J. C. (eds.): Plastic Surgery. Boston, Little, Brown, 1968.[126])

	PER CENT OF BODY SURFACE BURNED									
	10	20	30	40	50	60	70	80	90	100%
2 Years	0	5	17	40	64	80	93	98	100	100
4 Years	0	5	16	39	63	79	93	98		
8 Years	0	4	14	38	61	78	91	97		
12 Years	0	4	14	36	60	77	91	97		
16 Years	0	4	13	36	59	77	90	97		
20 Years	0	4	14	36	59	77	90	97		
24 Years	0	4	14	37	60	78	91	97		
28 Years	0	4	15	39	62	79	92	97		
32 Years	0	5	17	40	64	80	92	98		
36 Years	1	6	19	45	66	81	94	98		
40 Years	1	7	22	48	69	84	94	98		
44 Years	2	9	27	52	72	87	95	99		
48 Years	3	12	33	56	75	89	97	99		
52 Years	4	15	39	62	79	92	97	100%		
56 Years	6	20	46	67	83	94	98			
60 Years	9	27	53	72	87	96	99			
64 Years	14	36	60	77	91	97	100%			
68 Years	20	45	67	83	94	98				
72 Years	29	57	74	88	96	99				
76 Years	40	63	80	92	98	100%				
80 Years	51	71	87	95	99					
84 Years	62	79	92	98	100%					
88 Years	71	86	95	99						
90 Years	75	89	97	99%						

Figure 20–5*B* Predicted mortality in females. (From Lynch, *ibid.*)

tion is the major cause of death. Included with infection beyond three weeks are stress ulcers and from 10 to 12 weeks, hepatitis.[232] Except in hospitals particularly interested in burn care, autopsies tend to be cursory, and unless there is some striking finding such as a perforated ulcer, the death is attributed solely to "burns."

EVALUATION OF THE BURNED PATIENT

History. A careful history is as important in caring for the burned patient as in any other patient. Often done hurriedly, it should nevertheless be thorough and include the circumstances of the injury.

Pre-existing cardiovascular, renal respiratory or metabolic diseases will complicate care and increase mortality. Epilepsy and alcohol or drug intoxication tend to predispose patients to burns, and the subsequent withdrawal symptoms or convulsions complicate treatment. Specific inquiries regarding previous tetanus immunization and drug allergies should be made.

Careful questioning of the patient as well as the firemen, police or ambulance emergency medical technicians who bring the patient to the hospital must ascertain the circumstances of the burning. A history of the burns being sustained in confined areas, accompanied by considerable smoke inhalation, will alert the physician to possible respiratory damage better than x-ray or physical findings. Evidence of suicide attempt and, in children, the battered child syndrome will indicate problems in later social adjustment.

Extent of Injury. The ultimate determinant in burn injury is the volume of tissue destroyed. Although it is difficult to determine depth, the extent of the burn can be assessed by careful observation and is important from a therapeutic, statistical and prognostic point of view. It is customary to record burns in terms of per cent of body surface area. Original estimates of surface area by location were introduced by Berkow[22] and have since been modified by Lund and Browder to make them applicable for all age groups[125] (Fig. 20–6). Although rapid estimates may be made using the Lynch-Blocker rule of fives[26] and the rule of nines introduced by Pulaski,[183] they are of value primarily for triage; more accurate assessment should be made on individual patients. A more direct and quantitative estimate of volume of burned tissue has been introduced by Klein et al.[102] Hydroxyproline, a degradation product of collagen, is serially measured in urine; the level indicates the volume of tissue destroyed by burn.

The extent of the burns in terms of per cent of surface is meaningless in discussing burns of special areas including the face, neck, hands, feet and genitalia as it is in burns in young children and the elderly. These are all serious burns.

Any burn in excess of 20 per cent of surface area (5 to 10 per cent in children), burns in special areas, those with associated injuries and all electrical and acid burns are major burns and require special care in hospitals. Any burn in excess of 30 per cent of surface area should be considered critical. Minor burns that may in selected cases be treated on an outpatient basis include partial-thickness burns of less than 15 per cent of the body surface area. An intelligent and dependable patient or family is a prerequisite for successful outpatient care.

Depth of Injury. As emphasized before, the biological response to thermal injury is exceedingly variable within even a limited area. Superficial burns can be ascertained from the history and the appearance of erythema without blistering, and the patient can be dismissed from the office or emergency room with topical analgesics and the reassurance that heal-

BURN SHEET

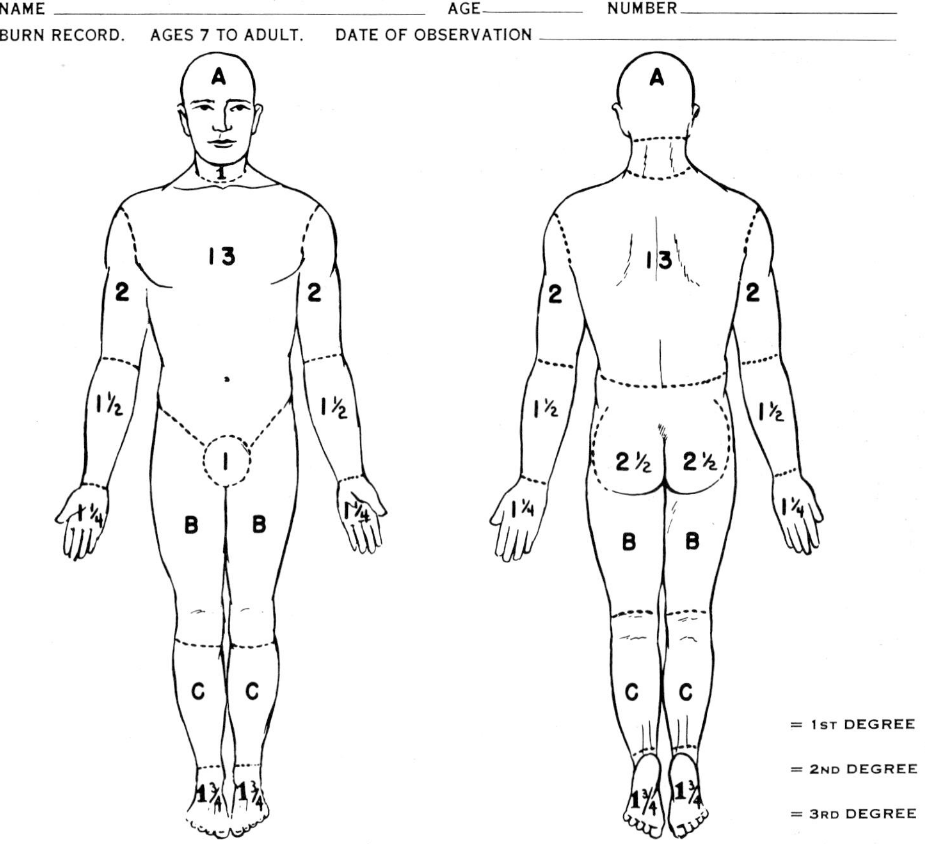

RELATIVE PERCENTAGES OF AREAS AFFECTED BY GROWTH

AREA	AGE 10	15	ADULT
A ½ OF HEAD	5½	4½	3½
B ½ OF ONE THIGH	4¼	4½	4¾
C ½ OF ONE LEG	3	3¼	3½

% BURN BY AREAS

PROBABLE 3RD° BURN	HEAD____	NECK____	BODY____	UP. ARM____	FOREARM____	HANDS ____
	GENITALS____	BUTTOCKS____	THIGHS____	LEGS____	FEET ____	
TOTAL BURN	HEAD____	NECK____	BODY____	UP. ARM____	FOREARM____	HANDS ____
	GENITALS____	BUTTOCKS____	THIGHS____	LEGS____	FEET ____	

Figure 20–6 Chart for estimating body surface area in burned adults based on Lund-Browder figures.[125]

ing will occur inevitably and without noticeable sequelae.

A careful history will also prove valuable in assessing deeper burns. Flash and flame burns are all at least partial-thickness and often full-thickness injuries. Scald burns in adults tend to be superficial partial thickness but they may well be full thickness in children and in the elderly.

Attempts at differentiation on clinical grounds are also misleading. Sensation is deceptive since even full-thickness burns have pressure sensation. Pinprick is more accurate, but even here partial-thickness burns may be anesthetized by loss of naked nerve fibers in the basal layer.

Blistering is characteristic of superficial burns but may also occur with very deep burns from steam accumulation in the epidermis or, later, from infection. The appearance of a tough, leathery, anesthetic eschar is seen in full-thickness injury but also is seen frequently in deep partial-thickness injury as well.

Although many elaborate tests have been proposed for differentiating depth of burn, none has been reliable. All studies assume that (a) the injury is uniform, at least within a given area, (b) that the depth of the injury remains the same, and (c) that if we knew the depth exactly, we would somehow change our treatment. However, the injury is not uniform, nor is it static. Infection or further trauma may well convert superficial injury to full-thickness loss. So, too, deep burns thought to be full-thickness injury may later re-epithelialize from viable epidermal islands if infection is prevented. The important triage concept is to differentiate the patients with deep burns from those with superficial burns who may be treated as outpatients. Further classification into numerical "degrees" is difficult, often incorrect, and does not materially affect the course of treatment.

Hemodynamic Evaluation. The hemodynamic response is a direct systemic manifestation of the type of injury and magnitude of tissue destruction in the local burn wound. Attention to the burn wound should not take precedence over the lifesaving hemodynamic support of the burned patient any more than this phase of treatment should assume exclusive importance in burn care. The various new topical agents introduced in burn therapy result in profound fluid and electrolyte alterations in addition to changes imposed by the wound itself. Proper patient care demands that the burn wound, the accompanying systemic changes, and the alterations produced by treatment be conceptually viewed as a dynamic interrelated process, not as isolated phenomena.

TREATMENT

Immediate Care. The burned patient demands the same thorough attention to cardiorespiratory function, hemorrhage and associated injuries as any other emergency trauma victim. Immediate treatment of his impending shock is begun by introducing a large-bore needle or catheter into the central venous system, preferably through unburned skin. Antibiotic ointment and a sterile dressing should be placed around the site of catheter entry. If an intraluminal catheter is used, suppurative thrombophlebitis must be watched for throughout the treatment period.[181] Blood is drawn for typing, complete blood count, serum electrolytes, glucose and urea nitrogen. Arterial blood gases are obtained if there is any evidence of smoke inhalation or pulmonary dysfunction. An infusion of Ringer's lactate or other buffered isotonic fluid is begun at a brisk rate. A urinary catheter is inserted, attached to a closed drainage system. Tetanus immunization should be provided as recommended by the American College of Surgeons Committee on Trauma.

Initial Volume Replacement. The weight of the patient, the type of burn wound (scald versus flame) and the extent of the initial injury in per cent of body area provide the initial guide to thinking. Rigid applications of formulas ignore the variability of patients. The greatest loss of plasma and fluid occurs during the first 12 hours after burning and then continues much more slowly for another 12 hours. Replacement therefore must be most rapid immediately and then can be slowed to correspond with the rate of loss.

Formulas have been advanced to predict the amount and type of fluid correction needed. Originally replacing suspected plasma loss with plasma to maintain a normal hematocrit, they have evolved into a volume/weight scale in relation to the percentage of body surface burn. A realization of the need for crystalloid replacement as well as plasma has resulted in the change in proportion and type of fluid used in resuscitation. Critical analysis of the various popular formulas reveal that the total volume replacement recommended varies only two per cent over 48 hours and the total milliequivalents of sodium vary only six per cent during the same period.[141]

The problem with formulas, besides their inherent rigidity, is that their adequacy of fluid replacement has been measured by survival alone. This has led to erroneous conclusions since it can be demonstrated that survival is compatible with a cardiac output as low as 25 per cent of normal and a plasma or blood volume deficit of 30 to 50 per cent.[143]

Simultaneous measurements of cardiac output, plasma volume and extracellular fluid have shown that plasma volume replacement during the first 24 hours post-burn is dependent only upon the rate of fluid replacement.[179] The type of fluid, whether colloid or crystalloid electrolyte solution, does not matter. Sodium ion seems to be most important in the replacement. Therefore, a sodium-containing electrolyte solution is now recommended as the sole replacement for the first 24 hours. The obligatory loss of fluid from the vascular compartment has been shown to remain uncompensated until the replacement rate of administration exceeds 4.4 milliliters per kilogram of body weight per hour.[143] Above this rate plasma volume is not only maintained but actually expanded. Extracellular fluid volume replacement requires 3 to 4 milliliters per kilogram per cent body burn. Therefore, it can be predicted that this volume of fluid will be required and the rate of administration will have to exceed 4.4 milliliters per kilogram per hour. The rate will have to be greatest during the first few hours after injury.

Because of the capillary permeability occurring after thermal injury, colloid administration is of no benefit in the immediate post-burn period. Osmotic pressure cannot be built up over a freely permeable membrane; Starling's law is negated. Edema fluid will not be pulled back into the vascular compartment; rather, the colloid will leak into the extravascular spaces.

Some proponents of electrolyte-containing fluids only for resuscitation have suggested the use of hypertonic sodium-containing fluids to decrease the amount of fluid given. It is known that 0.5 mEq. of sodium per kg. per per cent body burn is required for adequate resuscitation. A mixture containing 300 mEq. of sodium, 200 mEq. of lactate and 100 mEq. of chloride per liter has been recommended as an alternative to more isotonic solutions.[138] However, measurements of cardiac output during resuscitation with hypertonic solution reveal that it remains up to 40 per cent less than cardiac output seen with isotonic replacement. Extracellular fluid volume replacement occurs at the expense of intracellular volume loss. Even so, a persistent deficit in extracellular fluid volume has been documented. Occasionally, hypertonic solutions may be desirable despite the persistent deficits in cardiac output, plasma volume and extracellular fluid volume. Such an example may be the very elderly or the patient with previous cardiopulmonary disease in whom the volume of fluid given is of paramount importance.

Just as it has been demonstrated that a sodium-containing electrolyte solution alone should be given during the first 24 hours and that colloid is of no demonstrable benefit, the reverse is true during the next 24 hours.[143] Capillary integrity returns and Starling's Law appears to be restored. Colloid is now effective in maintaining plasma volume, and further administration of sodium tends to aggravate the edema. Therefore, the only non-colloid required during this period is that to cover insensible obligatory losses.

MONITORING REPLACEMENT. In monitoring the adequacy of fluid and electrolyte replacement, one must assess the patient carefully by clinical observation, vital signs, hematocrit, serum electrolytes and urine output. The adequacy of fluid and electrolyte replacement is determined neither by ability to fulfill a previously outlined formula, nor by any single clinical or laboratory finding. However, a urine output of 30 to 50 milliliters per hour is the best single guide to adequacy of fluid replacement. If the urine output decreases, the rate of intravenous fluid administration must be increased.

The patient should remain alert; evidence of confusion may suggest hypoxia, fluid deficit or improper drug administration. Blood pressure and pulse rate are of value, but insufficient alone; arterial pressure remains compensated until late in shock and a tachycardia of 100 to 120 per minute may be quite compatible with adequate replacement.

The hematocrit will gradually rise in the first 24 hours to levels of 55 to 60 per cent, even in the presence of adequate fluid replacement and excellent clinical response. Attempts to lower it may lead to dangerous over-replacement of fluid. Moreover, there is no information to suggest that the implied dangers of a high hematocrit have any correlation in fact.

Central venous pressure has been of debatable use in burns. Reports of its lack of value in the acute stage suggest that reliance on CVP readings may be dangerous.[197] If urine output is maintained, there is far greater tendency to give too much rather than too little fluid. The central venous pressure frequently does not reflect this overload. As shown by Achauer et al., with a falling cardiac output, the left ventricle can become transiently overloaded and go in and out of failure for brief periods.[2] This results in a left atrial pressure exceeding 25 mmHg, thus causing pulmonary transudation. This increase in interstitial water in the lung can occur without causing gross change in the right atrial pressure which would be reflected in CVP readings. A more reliable guide in the acute post-burn period would be pulmonary artery pressure.

After stabilization of the capillary membrane and the return to normal of cardiac output, central venous pressure monitoring may be indicated in patients with inhalation injury and in children or elderly patients with pre-existent cardiopulmonary disease.

Treatment of an isotonic fluid loss with balanced electrolyte solution should maintain normal serum electrolyte values. Hypernatremia and hyperchloremia may result from either excess saline administration or lack of water; hyponatremia and hypochloremia can occur only with the administration of excess water relative to electrolytes. Treatment of hyponatremia with hypertonic saline solution will expand the entire extracellular fluid to isotonicity but may overload the patient. Such a situation is best treated by restriction of water or by administration of a solute diuretic (mannitol 50 gm. as a 10 per cent solution in saline infused over a few hours). All fluid replacement in the early burn stage is administered intravenously. Attempts at oral replacement in other than the most minor burns are discouraged by evidence of gastric dilatation and ileus.

Renal Failure. In the burn patient acute renal failure can occur only after prolonged and profound shock from unrecognized or untreated hypovolemia. The patient seen for the first time a few hours after burning who has oliguria and perhaps hemoglobinuria should not be assumed to have renal failure. To assume this diagnosis and to delay needed volume replacement will only insure the accuracy of the diagnosis. Acute renal failure is properly diagnosed by exclusion and with great reluctance.

In the initial evaluation it should be assumed that oliguria reflects the presence of hypovolemia. Ten to 15 gm. of mannitol should be infused rapidly in order to provide an osmotic load that will insure urine output if the mannitol can be filtered and the tubules are intact. However, osmotic diuresis will result in obligatory increase in urine volume even at the expense of dehydrating a hypovolemic patient, so volume replacement must begin rapidly. After an initial load of balanced salt solution (4.4 ml./kg./hr.) in an hour, plasma may have some particular value. By virtue of the large molecular protein components, it remains in the vascular compartment for slightly longer periods than crystalloids. The adequacy of volume replacement is assessed only on the basis of therapeutic results, namely, the appearance of adequate urine output. There is little guide to overload during this test. Central venous pressure may reflect only the rapidity of the fluid administration if elevated and not the increased interstitial lung water if normal or depressed.[2] Pulmonary artery pressure monitoring is very useful in this situation. Only the absence of urine output and an elevated pulmonary pressure suggest acute renal failure.

Later Fluid Changes. Major loss after the initial sequestration (48 hours post-burn) is from evaporative water loss from the wounds. These losses are not entirely free of electrolytes, and the administration of large amounts of free water may induce hyponatremia. Measurement of the serum sodium should guide therapy. Urine output is not an accurate guide to the patient's state of hydration after the initial 48- to 72-hour post-burn period.

Use of Blood and Blood Products. BLOOD. The initial hematocrit readings deceptively understate the amount of red cell loss that occurs, both at the time of injury and with delayed hemolysis (up to 40 per cent of the total red cell mass).[158] As the hematocrit falls, the need for blood transfusion becomes obvious (fourth to seventh day). Multiple transfusions to maintain a hematocrit between 35 and 40 per cent are indicated. Approximately 1 ml. of blood for each per cent of body area burned is needed daily. The advisability of blood administration in the first 48 hours is open to considerable doubt; however, the maintenance of a hematocrit near normal in the later stages is accepted as beneficial.

PLASMA. The use of plasma or other colloids was discussed under initial volume replacement. Its use should be in the form of stored plasma, Plasmanate, or albumin to reduce the dangers of serum hepatitis. Plasma has been documented to have value in children, but perhaps on an immunologic rather than a hemodynamic basis.[132, 133]

GAMMA GLOBULIN. Gamma globulin has been suggested in children in a dose of 1 milliliter per kilogram of body weight on the first, third and fifth post-burn days.[44, 101] Its value has not been totally documented.

HYPERIMMUNE AND CONVALESCENT SERUM. Definite benefit from hyperimmune and convalescent serum has not been adequately demonstrated in humans. Passive immunization has been shown by Jones in animals.[100] However, he warns that immunization by antiserum causes risk of allergic reactions and occasionally anaphylactic shock. The benefits of any antibacterial resistance may be overshadowed by these hazards.

VACCINES. Vaccination against *Pseudomonas aeruginosa* has been used to decrease the incidence of Pseudomonas sepsis.[5, 172] When used, it must be a polyvalent variety made from numerous strains of Pseudomonas. Regardless of the number of strains used to develop the vaccine, new strains of *Pseudomonas aeruginosa* continue to emerge, limiting its usefulness. Therefore, vaccination still is not used in most burn centers.

However, the further development of immunotherapy may be the most important means to decrease mortality from burns.

Respiratory System. Pulmonary dysfunction after burns may be divided into two general categories, that due to inhalation of smoke and those complications secondary to burn injury, such as pneumonitis, pulmonary edema and thromboembolism. Patients with a history of flash burns or being burned indoors and having burns of the face (especially if deep) have a much increased incidence of pulmonary dysfunction. A combination of the above factors resulted in an 88 per cent chance of respiratory problems. Respiratory problems have been reported to eventually occur in 67 per cent of all patients with greater than 40 per cent burns.[169, 170, 171] Hoarseness, dyspnea, restlessness, agitation and carbon particles in the sputum may all indicate that the patient has significant smoke inhalation; however, the most sensitive indicator is blood gas determination. Carbon monoxide inhalation may result in a deceptively healthy appearance. The initial treatment for smoke inhalation is humidification of inspired air and careful tracheobronchial toilet.

If hypoxemia develops despite the use of an oxygen mask, then tracheostomy and assisted respiration or possibly positive pressure is indicated. Tracheostomy is accomplished in the standard fashion, but the use of silicone tracheostomy tubes is recommended. After tracheostomy, frequent effective suctioning using extreme precautions with sterile technique is required. Antibiotic coverage is no substitute for good technique, and antibiotics should only be employed in response to specific cultured bacteria. A constant moist atmosphere is best applied by a "T" adapter. By adherence to the above techniques, the incidence of complications from tracheostomy in burn patients may be reduced below the reported 40 per cent rate.[89] In addition to the above treatment, corticosteroids in the form of ACTH or hydrocortisone are often administered. Evidence for their effectiveness is not conclusive.

Another problem of the respiratory system caused by burns is that caused by the restrictive unyielding eschar in burns of the thorax.[184] This causes restriction of rib motion and thoracic excursion with resultant impaired ventilatory function and CO_2 accumulation. Early and adequate escharotomy or primary excision of the eschar is indicated as an emergency measure.

Metabolic and Nutritional Needs. Negative nitrogen balance and increased metabolic needs begin abruptly and continue progressively until the wound is closed. Protein loss into the wound, loss of muscle from disuse and increased metabolic rate from evaporative water loss are all aggravated by poor oral intake.

Arguments are occasionally raised that malnutrition does not reduce the rate of wound healing or increase the incidence of infection. Vast clinical experience, however, has demonstrated the increased morbidity in the nutritionally depleted burn patient. Recovery of intestinal motility allows oral intake usually by the fifth post-burn day. As lack of appetite is typical in the post-burn patient, attention should be directed toward attractively presented and tastefully prepared foods. Total caloric needs are about 60 cal./kg. per day in the average adult.[154]

Vitamin needs are not defined but probably should include 1 gm. of ascorbic acid, 50 mg. of thiamine, 50 mg. of riboflavin and 500 mg. of nicotinamide as well as twice the usual amounts of vitamins A and D daily.

Tube feedings may occasionally be required. Diarrhea may develop during tube feedings and is usually due to inadequate water intake. If oral or tube feedings are not tolerated, intravenous hyperalimentation can be used. Up to 5000 calories per day can be provided by vein with resultant positive nitrogen balance, weight gain and even normal growth in children.[237]

Pseudodiabetes. A syndrome of hyperglycemia, glycosuria without acetonuria, acute dehydration, shock, coma and renal failure was described originally by Evans and Butterfield and has been called burn-stress pseudodiabetes.[67] Hyperglycemia resulting from the stress of trauma is well known and includes a diabetic-type glucose tolerance curve and decreased sensitivity to insulin. Arney et al. studied two cases carefully and noted that hyperglycemia followed high carbohydrate, high caloric forced feedings.[9] They also noted a high urine specific gravity and intense solute diuresis with subsequent dehydration and a rising BUN, hematocrit, serum sodium and serum chloride accompanied by a brisk urine flow. The severe hyperglycemia probably reflects an inability to utilize large amounts of glucose.[196] These patients had intakes of four to five times normal amounts of glucose. Experience with intravenous hyperalimentation suggests that a tolerance to these extreme solute loads can be developed and that insulin needs will be decreased.

Gastrointestinal System. Due to loss of peristalsis, initial therapy of most major burns should include nasogastric intubation for 24 to 48 hours. No oral feeding should be given until evidence of active peristalsis is present.

CURLING'S ULCERS. Curling's ulcers develop clinical significance in 12 to 25 per cent of patients with major burns.[89, 147] The exact mechanism is unknown, but the ulcers are not accompanied by hyperacidity. The incidence of the ulcers increases with increasing burn size and are more common in patients who develop sepsis. The ulcers may be gastric or duodenal, and 15 per cent of the patients will have both gastric and duodenal ulcers. Duodenal ulcers are twice as frequent in children as in adults.[202] Bleeding is the usual manifestation and may be very brisk. Perforation occasionally occurs and is an indication for surgery. Indications for surgery in a patient with bleeding are shock unresponsive to blood replacement and loss of 2500 cc. of blood over a 12-hour period in an adult (or a proportional amount in a child). Patients surviving such a major bleeding episode and not operated upon have a 30 per cent chance of having a subsequent bleed.[178] The incision may on occasion necessarily be made directly through eschar. Most authors feel that the ulcer-bearing portion of the gastrointestinal tract should be removed; subtotal gastrectomy alone or combined with a vagectomy, are equally successful. In children under age 15, vagectomy, over-sewing of the ulcer and an adequate drainage procedure have resulted in increased survival.[58] The incision should undergo delayed primary closure.

SUPERIOR MESENTERIC ARTERY SYNDROME. Compression of the distal duodenum at the level of the superior mesenteric artery may result in partial or complete duodenal obstruction. Reckler et al. have reported 19 cases of such obstruction.[187] This obstruction causes problems in the burned patient both because of the intestinal obstruction complications and the interference with alimentation at the time of increased metabolic needs. Post-feeding fullness, bile-stained vomitus, or excessive nasogastric drainage suggests the need for barium studies. The diagnosis can best be made by cinefluorography. The syndrome may require operative intervention by means of a duodeno-jejunostomy but conservative means should be tried. These include feeding in the prone position, attempting to pass a long intestinal tube beyond the obstruction for feeding, and/or intravenous hyperalimentation.

Fever. Because of the inability of the burned patient to regulate temperature in the area of his burn, small environmental changes in the wound may be reflected in markedly fluctuating body temperature recordings. The appearance of sustained fever, however, demands systematic evaluation of the patient. Investigation should begin and end with the burn wound. Dressings clogged with coagulum or wet dressings that have dried out may prevent heat exchange, and a dressing change itself may eliminate the fever. The development of wound sepsis may independently increase the metabolic rate and, unaccompanied by heat loss, result in increased body temperature.

Smears of the wound drainage should be stained and cultures performed. The smear is vital for identification of clostridia. The pulmonary status of the patient must be carefully evaluated by sputum smear and culture as well as by chest x-ray, particularly if the patient has a tracheostomy. The urinary tract, especially if an indwelling catheter is being used, is a common site of infection. Cellulitis or phlebitis secondary to the use of an intravenous catheter is a possibility. Repeated blood cultures may be necessary to identify causative organisms.

The patient's state of hydration should be carefully reconsidered and electrolytes checked, since either dehydration or salt excess may produce fever. Many drugs may also cause fever as a result of allergic reactions (e.g., penicillin) or as a side effect (e.g., atropine and derivatives).

Systemic Antibiotics in Burns

Although there is ample evidence that systemic antibiotics fail to reduce the incidence of burn-wound sepsis, this does not mean that they are totally ineffective.[140] There is, for instance, documentation that streptococcal infection, a major threat in the early post-burn period, can be prevented by prophylactic administration of penicillin. Although topical antibacterials may be antistreptococcal, most burned patients should receive intravenous penicillin in dosages of one to five million units every six hours. It should be continued through the edema phase of 48 to 72 hours and then stopped to reduce chances of emergence of resistant organisms.[8] Since the goal of therapy is specifically antistreptococcal, the alternate choices in the patient allergic to penicillin are lincomycin or erythromycin rather than broad-spectrum coverage.

Beyond the first few days no systemic antibiotics are used without specific indications and documentation of burn sepsis on quantitative cultures of the wound or blood stream isolates. Although staphylococci were not a major problem of the last decade, increased identification of staphylococcus bacteremias has been noted in the last few years.[49] Quantitative cultures of staphylococci exceeding 10^5 bacteria per gram of burn-wound tissue or positive blood cultures require systemic penicillinase-resistant antibiotics and possible alteration in the topical antibacterial regimen.

The key to pseudomonas burn sepsis is clearly prophylaxis with topical antibacterial agents. Identification of greater than 10^5 pseudomonas per gram of burn tissue demands intensive local wound care and probable change of topical agents. Although lethal pseudomonas burn-wound sepsis may indeed occur without visceral spread, systemic coverage with gentamicin or carbenicillin is indicated when quantitative levels exceed 10^5 bacteria per gram or positive blood cultures are obtained.

The plethora of strains of pseudomonas has resulted in an increasing incidence of resistance to systemic antibiotics. The other gram-negative infections, particularly *Providencia stuartii*, have been disturbingly resistant to all antibiotics.[240] So too, futile efforts to provide the patient with a broad spectrum of "blanket" prophylactic coverage only seems to predispose to their emergence. This is particularly true of the mycotic infections.

In a recent survery of 233 patients with candidiasis, only eight had not been on systemic antibiotics and 140 had been receiving multiple drugs.[130] Since the source of infection is usually the bowel, oral mycostatin is administered. Systemic antibiotics also should be discontinued in an effort to allow the normal bacterial flora to return.

If total antibacterial control is to be attempted, the aggressive approach of Collentine[40] and Waisbren[229] is perhaps most reasonable. Meticulous wound care and topically applied antibiotics (neomycin, polymyxin B and nystatin) are supplemented by massive amounts of penicillin, methicillin, polymyxin and chloramphenicol. Results are comparable to those obtained with topical antibacterial agents in other institutions. The use of such an antibacterial "potpourri," however, is not without hazard and demands vigilance to potential toxicity and exquisite supervision of management.

As with antibiotics in any other phase of surgical practice, the agent must be chosen with precision and administered at a time, by a route and in a dosage most likely for it to be effective.

Pain. All burns are initially painful. The amount of discomfort thereafter is related to the depth and area of the burn, the method of treatment and the individual response of the patient himself.

All analgesics administered in the acute period should be given intravenously and in small amounts. Morphine 4 mg. or meperedine (Demerol) 20 mg. may be given initially and repeated as needed to insure comfort. Other routes of administration are contraindicated because of the dangers of delayed absorption. Long-term analgesia in a chronically painful injury is a difficult problem, and every effort should be made to avoid making the patient drug-dependent.

Aspirin has a lytic effect on gastric and duodenal mucus; repeated and prolonged administration should be avoided, particularly on this already ulcerogenic situation. Large amounts of tranquilizers may cause hepatotoxicity and may produce neurologic aberrations. A mild antidepressant such as Elavil may be of value.

Dressing changes should be accomplished without the necessity of general anesthesia whenever possible; moderate amounts of appropriately timed analgesia will usually be sufficient. Ketamine has been of particular value in children both for dressing changes and grafting procedures.

Hypnosis may be of value in long-term management, particularly during manipulation of the wounds. Constant reassurance, full explanation of procedures and conversational diversion are forms of hypnosis used by all surgeons when the services of trained hypnotherapists are not available.

LOCAL CARE OF THE BURN WOUND

The principles of local care must be directed to:

1. *Primo non nocere* ("do not harm").
2. Prevent infection and allow survival of all remaining viable tissue.
3. Obtain the best functional and aesthetically attractive coverage as quickly as feasible.

Superficial Burn. FIRST DEGREE. Clinically, superficial burns are usually due to minimal exposure to flash, contact or scalding. There is evidence to suggest that immediate cooling, by immersion in ice water for 15 to 20 minutes, will diminish the amount of edema and subsequent discomfort. Since discomfort is aggravated by air currents over the injured area, application of any ointment or cream will reduce discomfort. Application of thick layers of gauze saturated in oil-base materials or use of any impermeable material will prevent proper drainage of sebaceous glands, lead to maceration and may result in staphylococcal furunculosis. Thin layers of water-soluble creams, which may be readily washed off, are probably best. Healing without scarring will occur in three to seven days, perhaps accompanied by "peeling."

Partial-Thickness Burns. SUPERFICIAL, SECOND DEGREE—A. Unless complicated by infection or treatment, this injury also heals spontaneously and promptly, with minimal discoloration. Blistering is usually present and if left intact will provide a barrier to infection and allow prompt healing. In practice, however, the patient rarely finds it possible to keep a blister intact. Once broken, serum and desquamated cells form a crust which is more susceptible to bacterial invasion, particularly streptococcus. Except in the palm of the hand, where a very tough blister is often present, blisters are best trimmed away and the wound gently cleansed with bland soap and dressed. Blisters which appear for the first time after 48 hours usually mean infection; they should be opened and the contents smeared and cultured. Dressings should be inspected frequently and changed promptly when dirty, dislodged, or saturated with exudate. Healing should occur in seven to 14 days.

Any superficial burn of this type in excess of 15 per cent in adults, any in areas of special importance (face, hands, etc.), or any occurring in geographical areas in which dependable follow-up care is not possible should be treated initially in the hospital. These burns are usually of major significance only if neglected.

Deeper Burns. PARTIAL THICKNESS, DEEP; SECOND DEGREE—B; AND FULL THICKNESS, THIRD DEGREE. It has been repeatedly emphasized that differentiation into degrees is artificial since the initial treatment of these burns is similar whether or not they are full thickness. Except for limited area injuries in highly intelligent, dependable people, all patients burned to this degree should be cared for in a hospital.

The initial local care of these injuries is directed to removing dirt, debris, charred clothing and any grease or ointment applied as an emergency measure on the scene.

A decision must then be made in the emergency room as to the best form of local care. The choices available include: (1) occlusive dressing technique, (2) exposure, (3) semiopen, including topical therapy, and (4) excision.

Occlusive Dressings ("Closed")

Choice of the occlusive dressing technique should be based on definite indications and must be done properly if it is to be effective. The reason for an occlusive dressing is not to reduce edema; nothing short of that pressure which will result in ischemic necrosis will affect the fluid accumulation. Rather, the functions of a proper dressing are: (1) to protect the wound from further mechanical or bacterial contamination, (2) to absorb any external drainage, and (3) to immobilize the injured part. The classic indication is the burned extremity. Burns of the trunk, face and perineum lend themselves poorly to this technique.

To accomplish these purposes, the dressings should be carefully constructed from a variety of materials and thoughtfully applied. The inner layer, in contact with the wound, should be fine-meshed gauze, either plain or impregnated. The purpose of impregnating gauze is not to prevent sticking to the wound, since macerating amounts of impregnate are necessary to accomplish this; rather, it provides a coating to the fibers and therefore promotes drainage through to absorptive layers. Plain gauze tends to entrap the drainage and form a coagulum at the innermost layer. Commercially impregnated gauze must be "wrung out" since its heavy impregnation tends to prevent drainage and to macerate tissue.

The rest of the dressing consists of bulky, absorptive materials; however, cotton-containing gauze should not be applied next to a weeping wound, since later removal is difficult. The dressing is completed by the application of firm, even compression using roller bandage or Kling. Kerlix does not provide firm or regular compression, being much too distensible. The use of Ace or elastic bandages is mentioned only to be condemned. An even, controllable amount of compression is not possible and dangerously constrictive dressings may result as the wound swells with fluid. The dressing is completed only by positioning and immobilizing in the appropriate position, which often requires the use of plaster splints. The functional position of the burn differs from the position of function often described. Except for the hand, all burns involving the flexor aspects of extremities or neck should be splinted in full extension.

Dressing should be changed when necessary, a nonspecific recommendation, but based on the variability of wounds. Actively weeping wounds may require changes two or three times per day; dry wounds may not require altering the dressing for four to five days. Evidence of odor, pain or unexplained fever are absolute indications for prompt inspection of the wound.

Exposure Method ("Open")

Exposure therapy was reintroduced by Wallace in 1949 in an attempt to reverse the practice of applying noxious compounds, such as tannic and picric acids, to the burn wound.[231] The basis for this form of therapy is the formation of a coagulum of protein and debris on the surface of the wound (an eschar) which will theoretically protect against mechanical and bacterial trauma. It sustains the principle that we should actively "do no harm"; but it violates another well-known principle of surgery—that an open wound should be covered with a sterile dressing or skin. The classic indications have included burns of the perineum, the face and those limited to one aspect of the trunk.

If such a method is chosen, the room is prepared and reverse isolation techniques (gowns, masks and gloves when touching the patient) should be instituted. Clean sheets (not necessarily sterile) are placed under and cradled over (not touching) the patient. In 24 to 48 hours burned tissue and coagulum will form a thick, leathery surface, a process which may be hastened by use of fans. In superficial burns, a spontaneous regeneration of epithelium will occur beneath the crust or eschar, which will then separate in 14 to 21 days, a process which is unfavorably altered by mechanical trauma or bacterial invasion. In full-thickness injuries, the eschar will also separate in 14 to 21 days, leaving a granulating bed suitable for the application of grafts.

The objections to this form of therapy are numerous and valid. It is not a particularly good mechanical barrier and this function is lost when the eschar cracks. Nor is it a barrier to the increased heat and the water lost by evaporation; Cohen noted evaporation to occur at a rate 10 to 12 times that of normal skin through even the toughest, driest eschar.[39] It also seems to have little value in preventing bacterial proliferation. The bacteria are either beneath it from the beginning, arrive endogenously through the blood stream, are autogenously deposited by the patient, or enter exogenously by a break in technique. Whatever the source, the natural history of exposure therapy is all too often burn-wound sepsis.

Semiopen (Topical Therapy)

Somewhere between the occlusive dressing technique and exposure are a variety of techniques which include continuous wet dressings (0.5 per cent silver nitrate) and topical antibacterials. The application of topical agents to burn wounds is hardly a new approach; the wide variety of agents used (and discarded) in the past reflects the surgeon's innate urge to "do something" to the burn. The particularly tenacious resistance of Pseudomonas to systemic manipulation stimulated reinvestigation of topical therapy.

Of the topical agents readily available commercially, petrolatum may effectively control pain in superficial burns but is macerating and inhibitory to drainage in deep burns. It has no bactericidal qualities and has no place in treating deep burns. Furacin is antigenic and only weakly antibacterial; its only advantage is that it is water soluble. Xeroform (tribromophenol-bismuth, beeswax and petrolatum) suffers the same limitations and also tends to macerate if applied as packaged. Topical antibiotics such as penicillin, bacitracin, or most sulfa creams are highly antigenic or ineffective. Combinations of polymyxin B with other antibiotics (Neosporin) have had enthusiastic trials in Great Britain but have gained no widespread acceptance in the United States. Many inorganic salts and organic chemicals are toxic or bacteriologically inert.

Silver Nitrate. The continuous wet dressing technique, employing 0.5 per cent silver nitrate, evolved from Moyer's efforts to develop a method of burn care that would simultaneously reduce the nutritional and metabolic deficit related to evaporative water loss and control burn-wound sepsis.[155] Discarded 25 years ago as toxic (then used in a 10 per cent solution) silver nitrate was reintroduced in a 0.5 per cent concentration. This level is bacteriostatic against *Pseudomonas aeruginosa*, *Staphylococcus aureus* and *Escherichia coli* (although less effective against Klebsiella and Providencia species).[29] At the same time, this concentration seems to be nontoxic when absorbed and appears to be innocuous to healing epithelial cells.[137]

The patient to be treated is carefully cleansed of debris and particularly of any previously applied ointment, which will prevent diffusion. The wounds are wrapped in six to eight layers of coarse-mesh gauze that has been saturated in 0.5 per cent silver nitrate; it is covered with Kerlix or bias-cut stockinette. The treated areas are then covered with two layers of sheeting or blankets. This soggy complex is then saturated with 0.5 per cent silver nitrate every two to three hours and the entire dressing is changed twice a day. The meticulous removal of debris and separating eschar carried out with each dressing change and the frequent rubbing result in a scrupulously clean wound.

The apparent benefits include a markedly diminished evaporative water loss which is accomplished by reducing conductive and convective heat loss by confining it to the surface of the dressing, by blocking air currents and by establishing a heat reservoir between the dressings and overlying sheets.[155] Covering the wet dressing with an impervious outer layer creates the danger of possible hyperthermia and lessens the concentration of silver nitrate. (As silver nitrate is precipitated at wound-dressing interface, some water loss from the dressing is necessary to maintain the concentration near 0.5 per cent). If the dressing is not covered with the blankets or sheets, heat loss is not prevented.

The use of silver nitrate is not without hazard and should be approached with great care. Silver nitrate in 0.5 per cent solution contains 29.4 mEq./liter and is thus hypotonic. The permeable nature of the burn wound requires prompt equilibration, and sodium, chloride and other ions are drawn into the dressings as deposits of silver chloride, carbonate and proteinate are formed. Such osmolar dilution can rapidly produce severe electrolyte deficits and cause hyponatremia and hypochloremia. Potassium is also lost but the gradient (5 mEq./liter in serum to 0 in dressing) is less. Careful salt replacement, initially intravenously and later orally, is necessary. Careful monitoring of serum electrolytes is vital and should be done initially every three to four hours in children and every 12 hours in adults and continued until oral supplements are being tolerated well and serum electrolytes are stable.

Silver may be absorbed through granulation tissue and has been identified in the visceral organs of experimental animals. However, clinical argyria has not been described, and the physiologic significance of what absorption there is remains to be seen.

The margins of error in silver nitrate solutions are also rather limited since a one per cent solution is necrobiotic for epithelial cells. The vagaries of evaporation from the dressing and the difficulties in determining the exact concentration at the wound-dressing interface render the entire method fairly inexact.

From a technical viewpoint the presence of grease, ointments or dead tissue will interfere with diffusion; these must be carefully removed. Although relatively painless, the presence of raw areas (without eschar) or donor sites may result in considerable discomfort during dressing changes. Silver nitrate, of course, causes permanent discoloration of linen, floors and walls and is removed from the skin only with some difficulty.

The silver ion precipitates on the surface and therefore penetrates eschar poorly. A singular limitation observed in the experimental animal[104, 106, 107] and confirmed clinically is its relative ineffectiveness in established infection;[137] to be most valuable it must be begun immediately as the definitive form of treatment.[189]

Several large series have documented silver nitrate as being effective in managing major burns, particularly when begun early.[175] The problems of methemoglobinemia seem related to the infrequent appearance of *Aerobactor cloacae* which will convert the nitrate to nitrite.

The course of healing of the local burn wound confirms the absence of bacterial invasion. Deep partial-thickness burns heal spontaneously from multiple epithelial islands which have been preserved from a bacterial death (Fig. 20–7). No full-thickness injury, of course, ever heals spontaneously, even with silver nitrate therapy, except by marginal ingrowth, and therefore must be grafted. Deep partial-thickness burns tend to heal with hypertrophic scars, particularly in flexor areas and the hands; resurfacing with split grafts is an integral part of the rehabilitation. The surface of these spontaneously healed wounds tends to be thin and susceptible to minor abrasive trauma (Fig. 20–8). So too, erysipelatous-type inflammatory reactions seem to develop in apparently healed tissue. Care must be taken to avoid applications of cocoa butter or other emolients which definitely aggravate these complications.

Sulfamylon. Used by the German Army in World War II as a prophylaxis against gas gangrene, mafenide or Sulfamylon (para-amino methyl benzene sulfonamide acetate) is not a new drug. It was introduced to this country by Mendelsohn and Lindsey, who were also studying gas gangrene and who suggested its use in burns.[135] After prolonged experimental trial,[121] using the excellent Walker burn-wound model, Lindberg and Moncrief introduced it for clinical trial in 1963.

Sulfamylon is available as a 10 per cent concentration of mafenide acetate in a water-soluble base. It is applied as a thin layer to the burn surface twice daily, and the wound is allowed to remain exposed to the air. If the drug is accidentally removed by the patient while turning in bed, it is promptly reapplied. Prior to application, the wound is gently cleansed of previously applied drugs and any loose eschar by washing or immer-

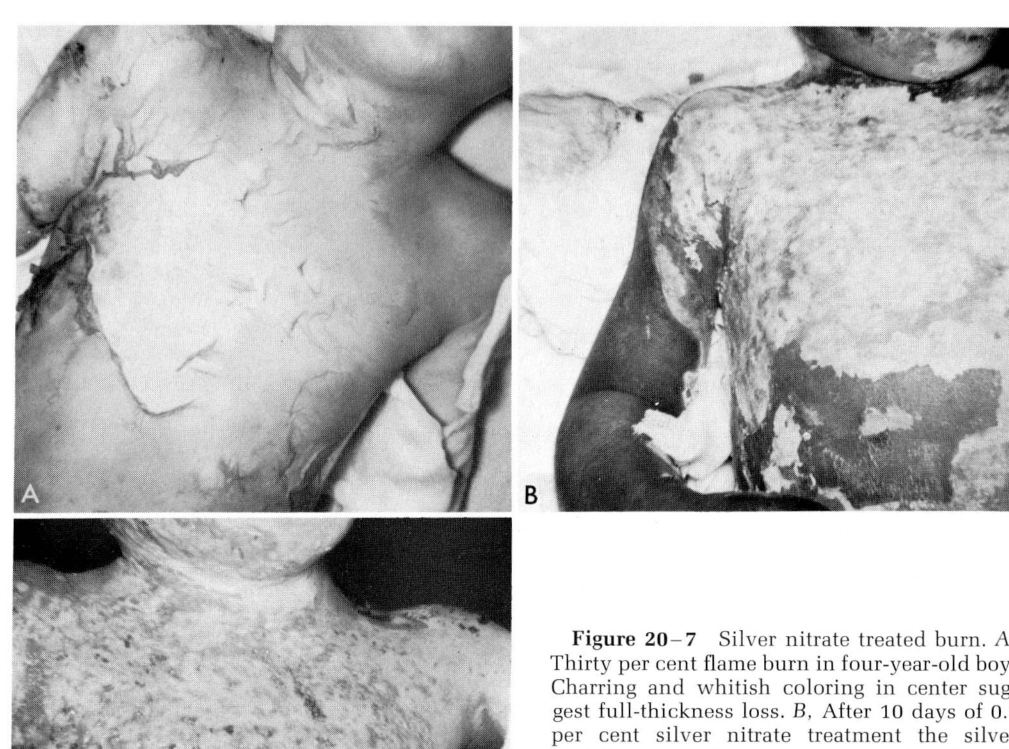

Figure 20–7 Silver nitrate treated burn. *A*, Thirty per cent flame burn in four-year-old boy. Charring and whitish coloring in center suggest full-thickness loss. *B*, After 10 days of 0.5 per cent silver nitrate treatment the silver proteinate coagulum makes evaluation of depth difficult. *C*, After three weeks of treatment considerable spontaneous re-epithelialization has occurred and multiple islands of granulation tissue are rapidly being covered. Bacterial cultures fail to grow pathogenic bacteria.

sions of the patient in a whirlpool tank.

Applied in this fashion, Sulfamylon effectively penetrates intact eschar and experimentally and clinically reduces the flora to less than 10^4 bacteria per gram, a level compatible with survival of epithelial islands and "take" of skin grafts.[88, 123, 146] Particularly effective against *Pseudomonas aeruginosa*, its spectrum includes also the other major burn pathogens.

Sulfamylon is considerably easier to use than silver nitrate. However, it also causes discomfort to the patient when applied. It shares with all sulfa drugs incidence of topical antigenicity that may require that it be temporarily or permanently discontinued. Of particular importance, it has greater value in controlling established burn-wound sepsis than has silver nitrate. Although Sulfamylon generally seems to be nontoxic when absorbed, it may produce severe physiologic alterations. Sulfamylon is metabolized by monamide oxidase to paracarboxybenzene sulfonamide, a carbonic anhydrase inhibitor with a Diamox-like effect. Sodium is not exchanged for hydrogen in the renal tubules, and increased secretion of sodium bicarbonate occurs, producing an alkaline urine and a tendency to metabolic acidosis. The compensatory pulmonary buffering mechanism of a normal lung

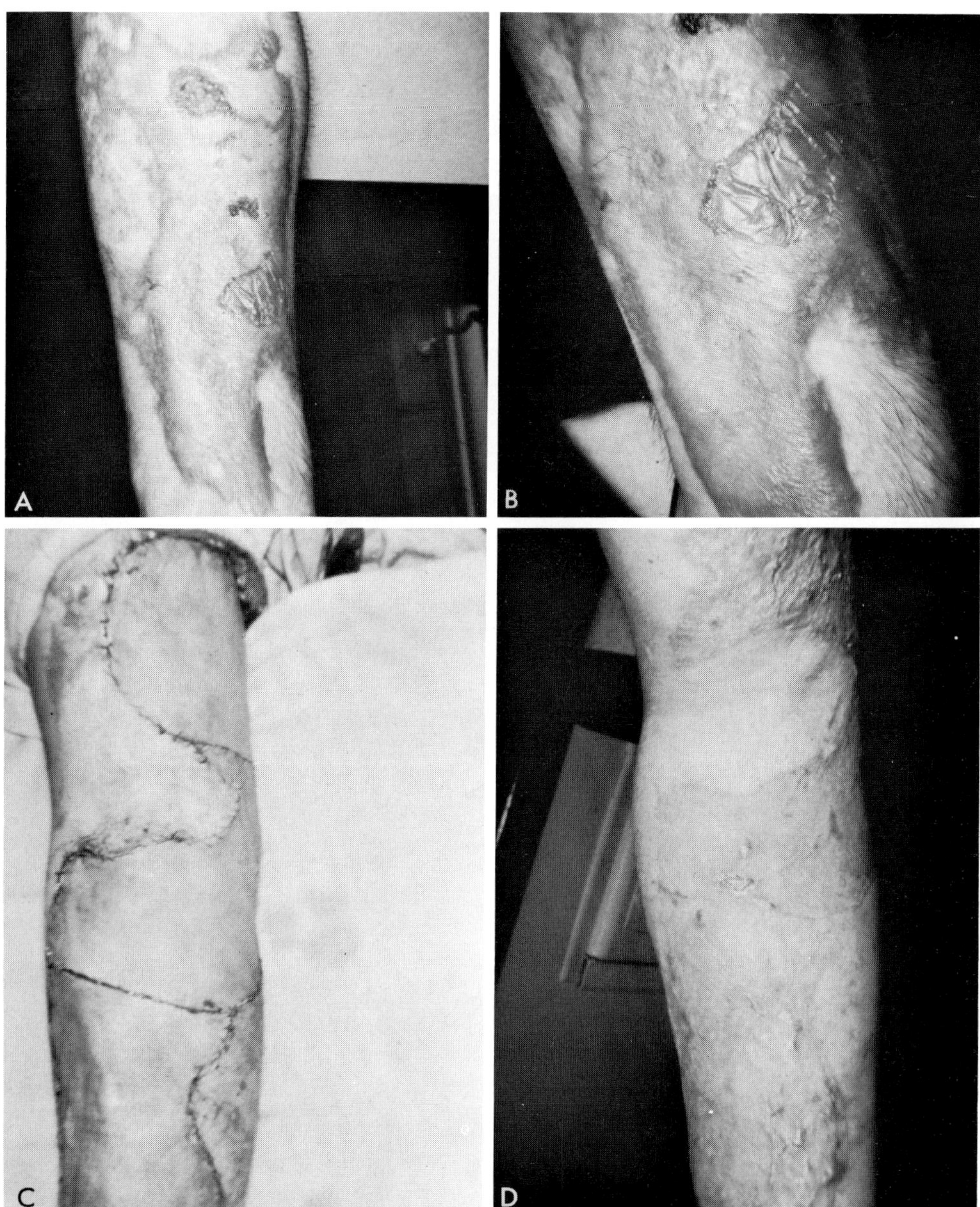

Figure 20–8 Hypertrophic scarring. *A*, Deep partial-thickness burn of right forearm healed spontaneously with 0.5 per cent silver nitrate therapy. Photographs at four months indicate hypertrophic scarring and blistering. *B*, Close-up of *A*. Epithelium very susceptible to minor abrasive trauma, tending to be "wiped-off." *C*, Entire area excised and split-thickness grafts applied. *D*, Result two months later.

handles this without difficulty. However, with the development of pulmonary irritation from smoke inhalation, atelectasis or pneumonia, the addition of carbonic anhydrase blockade may interfere with pulmonary carbon dioxide exchange and result in a characteristic clinical picture including tachypnea, falling pH, severe acidosis and even cardiac arrest. Careful observation with monitoring of pulmonary function and blood gases may provide the warning that the drug should be discontinued and blood buffering with intravenous sodium bicarbonate begun.

Sulfamylon is commercially available and experience has been wide and acceptable.[134, 144, 176, 204] Significant reduction in mortality, particularly in burns ranging from 40 to 60 per cent of body surface area, has been reported. Boswick reports a reduction of mortality of burns in the 30 to 50 per cent body surface area from 70 to 34 per cent with mafenide (from 49 to 32 per cent in all burns).[28] Clearly, Sulfamylon is the agent against which any new agent must be measured.

Gentamicin. Gentamicin sulfate (Garamycin) is a broad-spectrum antibiotic structurally similar to Neomycin and Kanamycin, with an unusual bacteriocidal potency against *Pseudomonas aeruginosa*.[23, 217] Clinical application has been best in the 0.1 per cent cream form (the ointment penetrates eschar poorly), applied in fine-mesh gauze and either by semi-open or occlusive dressing technique. Dressing changes are variously recommended from twice a day to twice a week.[214] Although the drug is absorbed, at a 0.1 per cent concentration the amounts rarely reach 10 per cent of toxic levels.[215] In the presence of sepsis, it should be supplemented by systemic gentamicin therapy.[219]

Stone has reported a drop in mortality in burns under 50 per cent surface area from seven per cent before gentamicin to 0.3 per cent.[215] In the 50 to 59 per cent body surface area burns mortality was reduced from 96 to five per cent and over-all from 16 to 2.3 per cent. A major disadvantage of topical gentamicin, which has limited even its availability, is the rapid emergence of resistant strains of pseudomonas.[216] Toxicity and side-effects remain minimal. Its effectiveness and resistance patterns suggest its very important selective value but caution against indiscriminate use.

Silver Sulfadiazine. The best of silver nitrate, the silver ion, has been compounded with sulfadiazine as a one per cent cream for use as a topical antibacterial agent.[74, 77, 211] The binding with silver apparently prevents inactivation of the sulfonamide by altered pH or para-amino-benzoic acid.[19] The release of the sulfa is apparently slow and systemic toxicity has not been a problem. The silver apparently binds with the DNA of the bacteria, thus releasing the sulfadiazine.[77] Its use has included semi-open and closed dressing techniques, usually with a once daily application. Its use is not associated with unusual discomfort and local skin allergies have been surprisingly few. The eschars become soft and a thick creamy discharge is seen on the wound; however, this represents drug, some leukocytes and amorphous protein material, but not necessarily bacteria. Bacterial control is measured by quantitative cultures rather than the deceptive purulent-appearing wound.

Serial biopsy cultures in one large series confirm its wide antibacterial spectrum.[19] *Pseudomonas aeruginosa* organisms were the most common isolate followed by *Enterobacter aerogenes. E. coli, Proteus, Serratia* and candida were seen less frequently. Early colonization (15 per cent of patients) with penicillinase-producing *Staphylococcus aureus* was seen but easily controlled systemically.

Early reports of reduced mortality have been encouraging, and comparative studies indicate that its effectiveness is comparable to Sulfamylon but without the side effects.[73, 76, 77] Silver sulfadiazine, however, remains an investigational drug, not available for widespread use.

Silver Lactate. Silver lactate is a silver-lacto-allantoin complex prepared in a hydrophylic ointment. It is 0.9 per cent silver and has a pH of 5.5. It shares with silver sulfadiazine the advantage of the silver ion. It is easily applied, may be incorporated into a dressing and preliminary clinical data suggest that it deserves further trial.[43, 94, 108]

Silver Nitrate Cream. A water-soluble cream incorporating silver nitrate has been investigated experimentally and clinically. It has the advantage of not leaching out electrolytes since it is not hypotonic. It also does not require the bulky dressings like the liquid. Its neatness compares favorably to other creams. Its ability to penetrate eschar has not yet been totally evaluated.[60]

Betadine Ointment. Betadine (povidone iodine) is an antibacterial agent of documented value in skin preps and surgical scrubs. Its effective ingredient is iodine; however, its use on intact skin has not been accompanied by a high incidence of allergenicity or toxic side effects. Betadine is effective in dilutions of 1:400 or even greater against most common burn pathogens as well as fungi and viruses. Its use in burns includes the aerosal spray and the solution full-strength as a wet dressing. Most interest has been in 10 per cent Betadine ointment.[81, 115] It should be applied at least every six hours and may be used either semi-open or in dressings. It shares with Sulfamylon a discomfort to the patient with application. Skin sensitivity and systemic side effects have not been recorded.

Experimental and early clinical data suggest that like silver nitrate it is not effective against established burn sepsis, and to be effective, it should be used early as prophylaxis. Although commercially available, its efficacy in the management of major burns has not yet been documented.

COMPARATIVE STUDIES

Experimental Comparisons. The topically-seeded experimental full-thickness scald burn in the rat has been an invaluable model for studying Pseudomonas burn-wound sepsis. Pseudomonas organisms colonize in hair follicles, spread to adjacent dermis and are lethal when concentrations of bacteria exceed 10^8 organisms per gram.[223, 224, 225] Against this model, Sulfamylon was demonstrated to effectively control pseudomonas burn-wound sepsis leading to its clinical trial.[122] These studies formed the basis for evaluation of other new agents. However, it is clear that all strains of pseudomonas are not lethal in this model and it has not been useful for the study of other pathogens.[108] The model is truly one of established sepsis and only gentamicin and silver sulfadiazine, experimentally, have been as effective as Sulfamylon.[59] Silver nitrate (0.5 per cent), silver lactate and Betadine are not therapeutic and, indeed, clinical data support the observation that these agents, to be effective, must be given prior to development of established wound sepsis (greater than 10^5 bacteria per gram of tissue).

Experimental data have varied depending on the time of infecting after burning, the type of organism or the strain employed, and the method and frequency of drug applications. Moreover, a variety of other experimental models, using different size and methods of burning and employing a variety of other experimental animals have made comparisons difficult.

Clinical Comparisons. Any agent, to be suitable for application to a burn wound, should ideally be comfortable when applied, innocuous to the viable cells of the wound or to the patient if (and when) absorbed, nonallergic and most importantly, bactericidal. It would be nice if it were simple to apply and cheap, and even more salutory if it would both allow drainage and prevent evaporative water-heat loss. No agent yet available fulfills all these criteria. The history of topical therapy has been the introduction of new agents, attended by initial success, and abandonment when they have become obviously toxic, ineffective or both. The introduction of any new agent or form of treatment is enthusiastically received by physicians and hospital personnel, who, in their curiosity, render meticulous and diligent patient care that this agent might be properly evaluated. One must be careful lest the apparent benefit be the result of this new interst in the burned patient rather than the agent or the form of therapy. There is also a tendency to evaluate results uncritically in comparison to what was accomplished in the years prior to the introduction of the new treatment, ignoring other factors, including a changing bacterial ecology, which would influence results.

Some comparative studies have appeared including MacMillan's comparison of four agents in 354 children.[96, 127] The largest group (192) was gentamicin (0.1 per cent) cream, but also compared were silver nitrate (0.5 per cent), Sulfamylon and silver sulfadiazine (one per cent). All received systemic penicillin in the first few post-burn days. A group treated previously with occlusive dressings and Polysporin ointment formed the control group. The data suggest that all the topical agents had a role in decreasing the expected incidence of burn-wound sepsis. Sulfamylon was the most effective in containing invasive sepsis from Pseudomonas, but gentamicin resulted in the best overall mortality rate. Superinfection with other gram-negative infections was not seen, but *candida* did emerge as a threat, particularly in patients treated with sulfamylon or gentamicin.

No comparative study yet published has established any one of these agents as the single best method of treating the burned patient.

PRIMARY EXCISION AND GRAFTING

The burned patient is never in better shape to tolerate an operation than moments after he has been burned. His course thereafter is downhill until the wound is closed.

Many studies have been undertaken to test the feasibility of early excision of major burns.[16 45, 129] Although burns of less than 10 per cent of body surface area can be readily excised and skin grafted, attempts at removing larger areas have been attended by excessive blood loss.[41] Most studies have failed to document a reduced mortality from such an approach.[129, 221] However, new grafting techniques, the availability of biologic dressings for temporary wound coverage, and hypotensive anesthesia have stimulated new interest in this approach.

Law and MacMillan have recently performed 52 excisional procedures on 35 patients with a mean body surface area of 35 per cent full-thickness burn, usually at about the tenth post-burn day.[114] Coverage was obtained with meshed skin grafts expanded from 3:1 to 6:1 in large areas. Blood loss in such massive excisions can be minimized by use of a CO_2 laser for dissection[69, 212] or by the use of controlled hypotensive anesthesia. Burke recently reported successful excision of burns in three patients with full-thickness loss extending over 75 per cent of body surface area.[36] Closure was obtained with matched and typed allograft from parental donors and "take" maintained with Imuran immunosuppression. As donor sites healed, they were used again until all allograft had been replaced.

SKIN GRAFTING

Over 100 years ago, George David Pollock performed the first skin graft on a burned patient and speculated that employing grafts early would promote healing and reduce contractures.[78] A century later, wound closure remains the therapeutic imperative. Large areas of the body should be covered as the first priority in efforts to reduce the size of the wound. Second priority is given to areas of great functional importance, particularly the hand and flexion areas.

The preservation of epidermal

islands by prevention of burn-wound sepsis may result in spontaneous healing in many deep burns. However, the process is often prolonged and depleting to the physical and emotional resources of the patient. So too, the quality of healing from these wounds is often disappointing with unstable epithelium, hypertrophic scarring and contractures.

Preparation of the Wound

Historically, eschar separation occurred predictably between the tenth and fourteenth post-burn days. Clearly, much of this pattern was due to bacterial growth and autolysis of necrotic tissue and even destruction of remaining viable dermal tissue in deep burns. Successful control of burn wound sepsis by topical antibacterial agents has been attended by prolonged adherence of eschar, delay in preparing of the wound for grafting and even retardation of normal wound healing. Preparation of the wound requires persistence in mechanical debridement and perhaps, enzyme therapy.

Mechanical Methods

Physical removal of necrotic debris may take the form of early, total excision of the burn or, more commonly, daily surgical cleansing of loosening eschar. This tedious approach is accompanied by minimal blood loss and discomfort and may be performed by paramedical personnel. Efforts to speed this process have included tangential excision. By this technique a freehand dermatome blade is used to separate off the outer debris down to a layer of punctate bleeding. Performed deftly and early it is not associated with pain and reportedly prepares the bed for grafting quickly.[137] Its disadvantages include destruction of viable epidermal elements in partial-thickness areas, bleeding, and opening portals of infection in the presence of sepsis. More classical use of electric or air-driven dermatomes is simply a technique for widely excising areas of full-thickness loss.

The frequent changing of dressings and the use of tub baths are additional mechanical methods of removing necrotic debris. The use of tub baths has additional salutory effects of providing patient comfort and an opportunity to maintain muscle tone and joint motion by subaqua exercises. Previous drug applications are washed away, debris is softened and loosened, and this presents an appropriate time for trimming away eschar prior to reapplying topical antibacterials. Prolonged immersion in hypotonic bath water will tend to leach out electrolytes from the wound, and salt should be added to the water if prolonged tubbing is employed. It is recognized that anything added to the immersate may also be absorbed, interdicting the use of pHisoHex or other hexachlorophene compounds in the tank.

Enzymes

Enzymes of many types have been introduced to dissolve the necrotic tissue. Each new agent has been later abandoned as uncontrollable, ineffective or potentially dangerous by allowing bacterial proliferation. A newer agent, Travase, is currently being investigated.[80, 209] A product of *Bacillus subtilis*, the enzyme works only in a moist environment and is inactivated by any of the silver- or iodine-containing topical antibacterials (although apparently compatible with silver sulfadiazine and Sulfamylon). Applied every six to eight hours in a moist dressing, it will dissolve eschar within hours and often debride a wound completely within two to three days. However, it will often expose the subcutaneous fat layer, which it will not debride, and which forms granulation tissue slowly and presents a difficult bed for skin grafting. More importantly, unless combined with continued antibacterial therapy, its use may dispose the wound to rapid bacteria proliferation.

TEMPORARY WOUND COVERAGE

In a 50 per cent full-thickness burn in an adult, the amount of skin necessary to obtain coverage has been estimated at 6000 square centimeters. Such large amounts of donor areas are not readily available. Temporary biologic dressings applied to the burn wound render it less painful, reduce fluid and protein loss, and will preserve bacteriologic control of the wound while awaiting donor sites to re-epithelialize prior to re-use.

Allografts

The first allograft on a burn patient was performed by Pollock on the same patient receiving the first autograft using his own arm as a donor.[78] Until Brown demonstrated that postmortem allografts could be used,[32, 97] the necessity of using live donors limited the favor of the technique. Although the depressed immune response of the burned patient leads to prolonged survival of allografts, permanent take has been realized only in identical twins. Burke has prolonged allograft survival in selected patients with immunosuppressives,[36] and recent work suggests that temporary storage of allograft in tissue culture reduces the antigenicity of the skin and may lead to indefinite and perhaps permanent survival when transplanted. Such a breakthrough, if confirmed, could lead to fulfillment of the burn surgeon's dream, an inexhaustible and readily available bank of skin.

At the present time, allografts are customarily used only as a temporary cover.[90, 128, 152, 203, 205, 206, 239] Harvested within six to 12 hours after death, allograft may be stored up to two weeks at 4° C. Applied to a bacteriologically receptive wound, the allograft will clearly establish a vascular connection with the bed and truly "take." A bacterial flora containing more than 10^5 organisms per gram of tissue will usually prevent "take" and under such circumstances the allograft should be changed every 24 to 48 hours until "take" occurs. Such frequent changes will, of themselves, reduce the bacterial counts. Successful "take" of the allografts documents potential receptiveness of the bed to autografts. The allografts should be changed every 48 hours lest complete vascularization make later removal difficult and attended by profuse bleeding. Allowing the graft to reject only reproduces the necrotic surface that was presented by the burn eschar itself.

In practice, allografts are not readily available in the general hospital and require that a surgical team be kept on hand ready to procure the grafts if a suitable cadaver donor presents.

Xenografts

To substitute for the scarce allograft supply, a variety of xenograft tissues have been employed. Canine xenografts seemed to provide adequate temporary coverage but are tedious to obtain and not aesthetically pleasing.[220] Because of certain structural similarity to human skin, porcine xenografts have become popular and most successfully distributed commercially.[30]

Porcine xenografts are provided fresh, frozen and in a lyophilized form. Sterility is maintained by irradiation or by antibiotics. Their size is limited by the dermatome used to obtain the tissue, but they are aesthetically acceptable and easy to use, albeit quite expensive. As with allografts, porcine xenografts should be changed every 48 hours. There is controversy regarding take, and although vascular continuity has been occasionally seen on histologic sections, injection of India ink fails to penetrate the graft. The biologic adherence by fibrin clot, however, may be more important to effectiveness than actual take.

Xenografts reduce evaporative water loss, reduce exudation of protein from the wound and promote patient comfort.[186] They are neither experimentally nor clinically as effective as allografts in reducing or maintaining a low bacterial wound flora. A most disturbing report has identified toxicity to the Neomycin used as the preservative antibiotic in fresh xenograft.[218]

Amniotic Membranes

Introduced by Sabella in 1912 as a cover for burn wounds,[198] amniotic membranes have found minimal favor in reported trials.[51, 54, 56] The histologic similarity to skin and a presumed immunologic immaturity led to hopes of permanent take and coverage. Although vascularization clearly occurs, autolysis and rejection are inevitable as with any allograft tissue.[57] The realization that temporary biologic dressings should be changed frequently has led to a rebirth of interest in fetal membranes.

Fresh amniotic membranes are obtained from sero-negative mothers with no history of endometritis or premature rupture of the membranes. The membranes are aseptically passed through four rinses of saline, one of 0.025 per cent hypochlorite and an additional four rinses of saline prior to storage at 4° C. Cultures confirm sterility prior to application and storage time up to six weeks has been identified. The membranes are applied with the amnion (shiny) side up and the chorion in contact with full-thickness wounds and are changed every 48 hours until the time of autografting.

In vitro experiments demonstrate no inherent bacteriocidal substance in amnion.[194] However, applied as a membrane to infected burn and other open wounds in the experimental animals, it was superior to both allograft and xenograft skin and the equal of the animal's own skin in reducing the bacterial flora of their monocontaminated wounds. In a series of 100 clinical cases, amniotic membranes provided bacteriologic control that was the equivalent of allograft and superior to xenograft.[194] They are readily available, come in large sizes and at no cost to the patient.

Other Covers

No synthetic skin substitute has proved the equal of the biological adherence achieved with biologic dressings. Although many materials will reduce water loss and protein exudation, none provides suitable bacterial protection and all tend to allow bacterial proliferation and potential wound sepsis at the interface with the wound.

Predicting Skin Graft Survival

There are certain conditions that must prevail to insure the successful application of a skin graft to an open wound. However, each surgeon tends to establish his own criteria to a wound which are largely subjective and in reported series have resulted in a failure rate as high as 21 per cent.[124]

More objective data may be obtained by serial quantitative cultures of biopsy specimens of the open wound.[62, 192] It has been observed that a graft take of 94 per cent was achieved in wounds containing 10^5 or fewer bacteria per gram of tissue.[109] When the bacterial counts exceeded 10^5 bacteria per gram, the survival rate for grafts fell to 19 per cent. It has also been observed that when allografts are applied, an apparent take is associated with take of subsequently applied autografts.

In a series of 30 patients these two test methods were compared.[195] Allografts were changed until a take was observed; an average of 3.7 applications was necessary before this occurred. Simultaneous quantitative cultures of biopsy specimens indicated that such allograft take was associated in all cases with a bacterial flora of 10^5 or fewer organisms per gram. In 77 of 81 failures of allograft take, a bacterial flora exceeding 10^5 organisms per gram was identified. Successful autografting proceeded in 29 of 30 cases as predicted by these two tests.

TECHNIQUES OF SKIN GRAFTING

Donor Sites

In extreme situations, any and all available skin can be and has been used as a donor site, including the scalp and soles of the feet. However, when lesser amounts of skin are needed, consideration should be given to the long-term results; an unsightly donor site may later be of more concern to the patient than the original injury. Although no area of the body is immune to exposure, the buttocks and lower abdomen should be used first, particularly in young girls. The thighs provide more accessible donor sites, but are more visible postoperatively and the skin is less thick. Donor sites should be dressed with fine-mesh gauze, and spontaneous re-epithelialization will occur in 10 to 14 days. If thin grafts are used and the donor site heals kindly, the donor sites may be re-used every two to three weeks.

Obtaining a Graft

It is rarely possible to cover more than 20 to 30 per cent of the body area at one time. In general, it is best to cover the anterior or posterior trunk at separate times. Grafts may be obtained with a freehand knife or any of the standard dermatomes. The Reese dermatome takes an even graft and is very useful on irregular surfaces, but it has the disadvantage of the necessity for changing the dermatome tape after each drum of skin. The Padgett dermatome also requires reapplication of tape after each drum of skin. The infant Padgett dermatome is of great value in children and in inaccessible areas. Reese or Padgett dermatomes are particularly useful in obtaining a large uniform sheet to cover the hands or an aesthetic unit of the face. The Brown air-driven or electric-driven dermatomes have great value in burns, particularly for obtaining long sheets of skin quickly and easily. However, Brown dermatomes require a flat surface (which may be obtained by ballooning the skin with saline injections) and produce a graft of irregular thickness.

Due to variations in skin thickness, a graft of 10/1,000 of an inch may produce a thin split graft when taken from the back, but may result in full-thickness loss when taken from the medial aspect of the thigh. In general, grafts should be 0.008 inch to 0.010 inch thick in children and 0.012 to 0.014 inch thick in adults. Where insufficient donor skin is available, thin grafts are used as the take is more predictable and donor sites may be re-used quickly. In areas of great functional stress, such as the hand, a thicker graft is probably preferable. Full-thickness grafts require an ideal recipient site and have little place in the treatment of acute burns. Pinch grafts offer no advantage and produce full-thickness loss at the donor sites.

"Postage-stamp" grafts are of value if it is necessary to cover large areas with small amounts of skin; these grafts will also allow drainage in contaminated areas. The graft is cut into sections, laid raw side up on wet fine-mesh gauze and implanted as a unit. The raw areas between the small grafts rapidly re-epithelialize from the graft margins. A more elegant modification is the Tanner mesh graft (Figs. 20–9 and 20–10) which produces multiple slices in the graft allowing it to be opened to three to nine times its original size. The interspersed raw areas heal by marginal ingrowth from the many edges of the graft. Mesh grafts should not be used

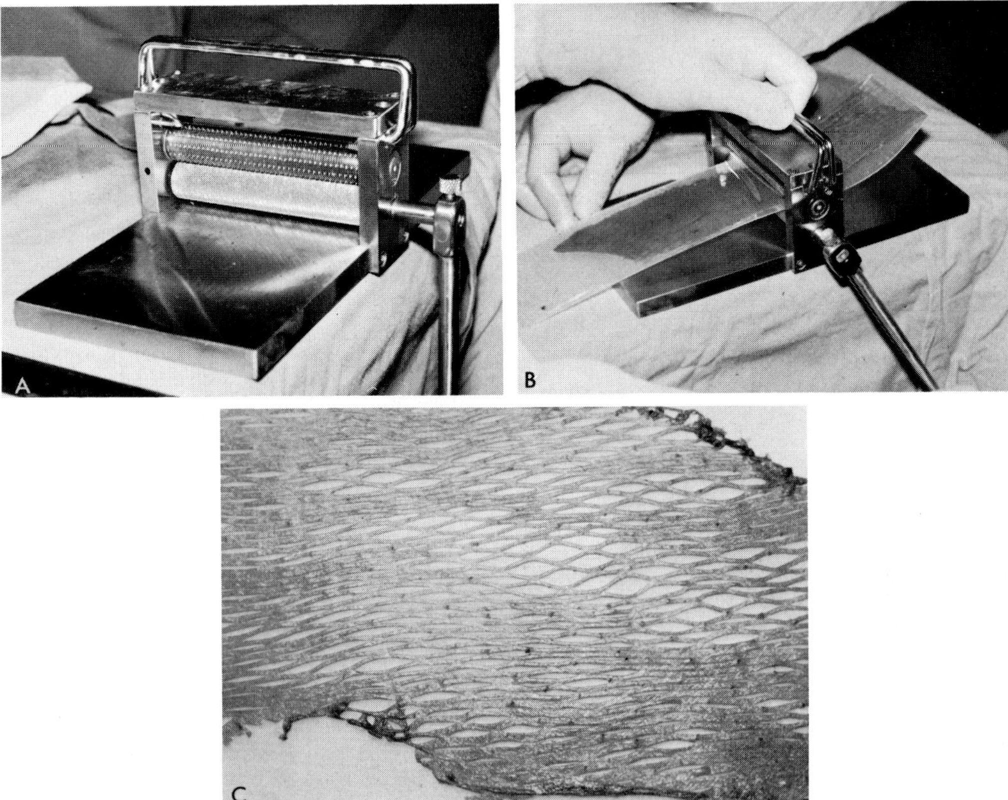

Figure 20-9 Tanner-Vanderput mesh graft. *A,* Zimmer Dermatome. *B,* Split-thickness graft is placed against backing and run through "mesh grafter." *C,* Multiple linear perforations enable the graft to be expanded to three times its original width. Intervening areas spontaneously re-epithelialize.

on the face, hands, feet or flexor aspects of the body. When large sheets of skin are laid on the trunk, neither sutures or dressings will be required. Dressings are useful on the extremities for compression and immobilization, but open grafting is suitable if skeletal traction is used to elevate the limb and allow circumferential grafting. It should be reemphasized that any open area, not covered with graft, can only heal by scar.

Special Groups of Patients

Children. The tragedy of the burned child is that the injury was usually preventable. Children are the innocent victims of their own curiosity and ignorance and the carelessness and lack of supervision of their guardians. A small but significant number represent the effects of deliberate injury—"the battered child." Fully 70 per cent of burns occur in the home and more than 50 per cent occur in the formative years of life. Thermal burns are the number-one cause of fatal accidents in the preschool child.[1] Mortality figures do not cover the social significance of the burn-scarred child.

The etiology of these injuries is about equally divided between scalds and flash burns. The thinner skin of the child predisposes him to full-thickness loss from hot liquids. The overturning of coffee pots and other containers on the stove results in a

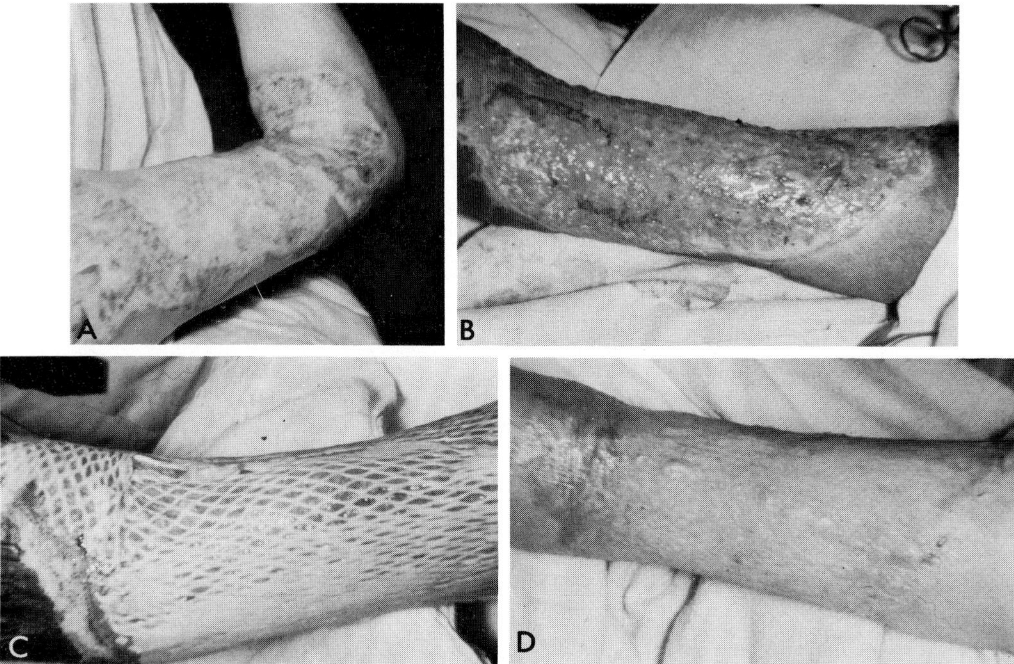

Figure 20–10 Use of mesh graft. *A*, Full-thickness burn, upper extremity. *B*, After treatment with 0.5 per cent silver nitrate, a clean granulating bed is present. *C*, Mesh graft applied and silver nitrate occlusive dressings continued. *D*, Result at two months shows complete re-epithelialization with minimal cosmetic deformity and good functional skin.

high incidence of burns of the face, neck, shoulders and arms. The curious child is also highly subject to burns of the palm of the hand. Hot bath water can produce full-thickness loss in areas difficult to treat, including the soles of the feet and perineum.

Children are not small adults, and their initial and continued therapy should be appropriately altered. Special charts should be consulted to determine the size of the burn (Fig. 20–11), which is usually overestimated, whereas depth is usually underestimated. There is an even greater danger of fluid overload in children than in adults, and fluids should be administered with the same caution. The use of large amounts of colloid has demonstrated value in children if not in adults and may be more important immunologically than hemodynamically. The same interdiction against early oral replacement applies in children; gastric dilatation may be even more common. Indwelling catheters for urine measurement are used reluctantly in small children, but the need exceeds the dangers. Tracheostomy, a management problem in the young, is indicated on the same terms as in the adult.

Orthopedic complications are more common in children, and ankylosis may occur in joints remote from the burn. The local response to thermal injury, burn-wound sepsis and appropriate local therapy are no different in children from adults. Current experience would suggest the use of some form of topical therapy.

Hospitalization is often prolonged and the diversionary value of "play ladies" and the facilities for continued schooling in the hospital are important. Early psychiatric and social

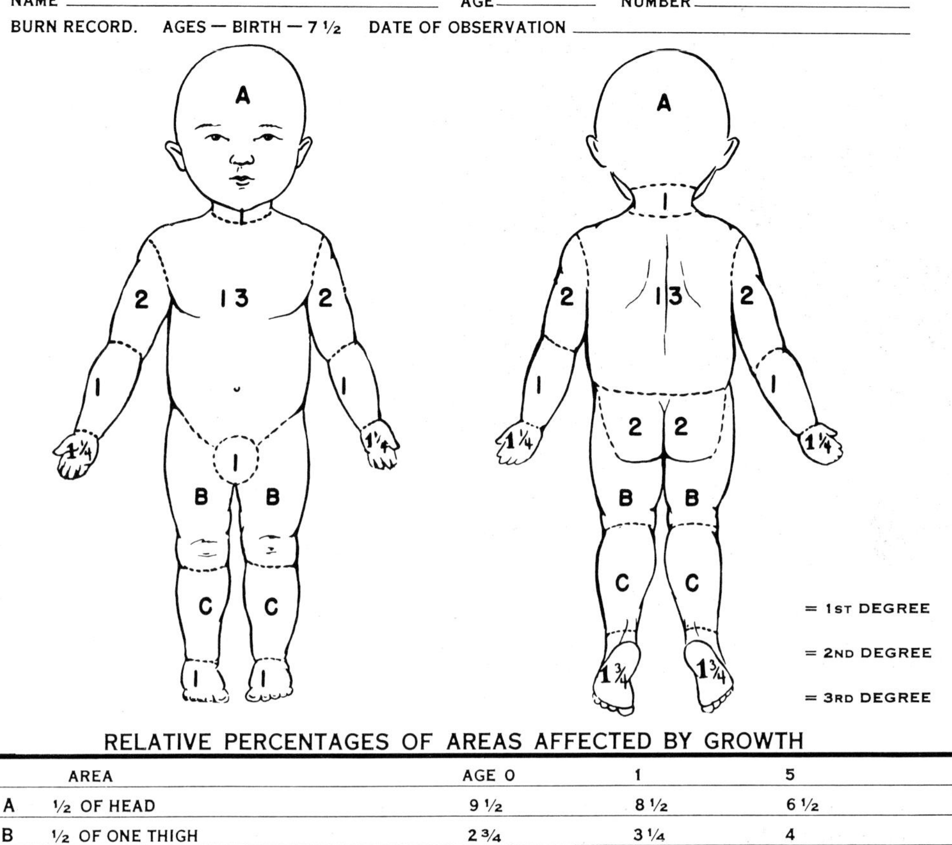

RELATIVE PERCENTAGES OF AREAS AFFECTED BY GROWTH

	AREA	AGE 0	1	5
A	½ OF HEAD	9 ½	8 ½	6 ½
B	½ OF ONE THIGH	2 ¾	3 ¼	4
C	½ OF ONE LEG	2 ½	2 ½	2 ¾

% BURN BY AREAS

PROBABLE 3RD° BURN { HEAD____ NECK____ BODY____ UP. ARM____ FOREARM____ HANDS____ GENITALS____ BUTTOCKS____ THIGHS____ LEGS____ FEET____

TOTAL BURN { HEAD____ NECK____ BODY____ UP. ARM____ FOREARM____ HANDS____ GENITALS____ BUTTOCKS____ THIGHS____ LEGS____ FEET____

SUM OF ALL AREAS____ PROBABLY 3RD°____ TOTAL BURN____

Figure 20–11 Chart useful in estimating body surface area in burned children, based on Lund-Browder figures.[125]

consultation and support for the family will do much to relieve some of the anxiety and profound guilt the parents experience following the burning of a child. Prophylactic measures devoted to safety education of the parents concerning flammability of clothing and thermostatic control on hot water fixtures are all steps in the proper direction.

The Elderly. The elderly patient faces a dismal prognosis, far out of proportion to other age groups. The attenuation of the skin, diminished reflexes and the lack of agility which attend the aging process render this group prone to thermal injury. Scald burns have the same propensity for full-thickness loss as those in infants and similarly may be sustained in the bathtub.

Associated cardiovascular, renal, pulmonary and metabolic derangements in this age group render resuscitation difficult. The principles are the same, but the execution must necessarily be altered, depending on the circumstances. The tendency to overload the circulation is perhaps the most common early mistake.

Local burn-wound care is similar to other groups. Thin skin makes split grafts difficult to obtain. Healing is slow and even minor injury or infection in the donor site will result in full-thickness loss. The ultimate goals of treatment must be altered. The healed wound is vital, even to the extent of accepting some functional limitation. Prolonged bed rest presents problems of its own, and efforts at continued ambulation or wheelchair use are attempted even during the course of treatment of the semiacute burn.

Others. Other frequently encountered groups of patients present unique problems. The obese patient is a particularly poor surgical risk for many reasons, including pulmonary problems and the difficult mechanical task of postoperative mobilization. The burn wound itself tends to be different, often demonstrating exceedingly slow separation of eschar and a tendency to develop a thin, collagenous film over the fatty wound rather than healthy granulation tissue. This results in poor graft take and prolonged disability. The application of a dry dressing to this wound, normally a poor surgical maneuver, may result in irritation and stimulation of granulation tissue.

The alcoholic, the drug addict, the epileptic and the suicide-prone all tend to be subject to thermal injury and present both therapeutic and social problems of rehabilitation.

Burns in Special Areas

Burns in areas of significant functional or aesthetic importance often require reconstruction. However, the prompt recognition of the unique problems of these areas, accompanied by aggressive attention to small detail, may prevent many of the deformities which are so resistant to later reconstruction. Consideration of these areas must begin immediately; a delay of a few days while efforts are directed toward the more dramatic systemic alterations may result in irreparable damage. The responsibility rests with the physician initially in charge of the patient, not with the reconstructive surgeon, who may not be consulted until some days, weeks or months later.

Hands. The hands represent to most patients the key to functional rehabilitation. The goals of treatment are preservation of a functional range of motion and adequate resurfacing as the prime area of skin grafting.

Initial care is directed to evaluation of the vascular status. Circumferential burns either of the hand or more proximally in the forearm or arm can result in ischemia, as an obligatory fluid accumulation occurs beneath an often unyielding eschar. Surgical decompression of the eschar should be done at first suggestion of vascular compromise and should often include not only the eschar but the underlying fascial compartments as well. It may be of particular importance to decompress the intrinsic musculature of the hands as well.

The hand should be splinted in a position of advantage from which motion can be most easily regained and which most completely neutralizes the forces tending to produce deformity. The wrist should be extended, thumb abducted and the metacarpal phalangeal joints placed in complete flexion to avoid shortening of the collateral ligaments. The interphalangeal joints should be placed in a position near full extension. Since no position is functional if the fingers can't move, it is imperative that early and persistent efforts be made to maintain a full active and passive range of motion. Elevation helps reduce the contribution of gravity to edema formation. Topical antibacterials are equally indicated to prevent burn-wound sepsis.

Most burns of the hands occur on the dorsum as the hands are thrown up to protect the face against flashes of flames. So too, most burns are superficial and will be sufficiently healed within two weeks that topical medications may be discontinued. All burns which heal spontaneously within two weeks will be accompanied by acceptable skin cover and a good functional result. Another small group of patients have burns limited to the hand, whose depth is obviously deep as a result of contact with hot objects. In this group of patients, primary excision of the entire burn wound is indicated, with either immediate or delayed (24–48 hours) application of skin grafts.

A disturbing group of patients fail to heal spontaneously within two weeks. The depth of their wounds may have been initially unclear or systemic problems may have prevented definitive early surgery. These wounds are often characterized by healed epithelium at the margins and islands of epithelium dotting an ill-defined granulating bed. It is tempting to allow these wounds to proceed to delayed healing; it is among this group that occur the most disastrous complications of unstable epithelium, contracture and deformity. So too, application of skin graft to the surface of the granulating bed does not prevent contraction of the already healed margin or underlying bed. Even successful graft takes may be followed by deforming contractures.

Burns unhealed in two weeks should be considered for delayed primary excision of the entire area of the original injury and skin grafting (Fig. 20–12). Bacteriologic control by topical

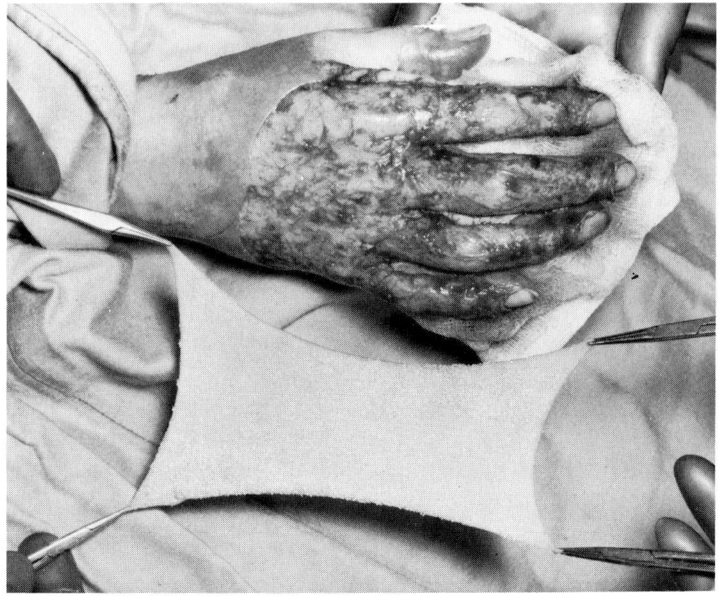

Figure 20–12 Primary excision and grafting of a full-thickness dorsal burn of the hand. A definite effort is made to preserve the venous network. (Courtesy of John E. Hoopes, M.D.)

antibacterial agents makes this procedure feasible even weeks after injury. The biology of wound healing and contraction makes excision of the entire wound reasonable and appropriate.

Sheets of skin should be employed. Adequate skin should be dressed into web spaces and adequate attention paid to abduction of the fingers as part of the physiotherapy. Burn syndactyly is a common complication requiring later z-plasty release or further grafting. Postoperative splinting is also in the position of advantage and early motion is paramount.

Early and successful treatment of the burned hand has functional and psychological importance; a useful hand gives the patient needed reassurance of recovery and allows him to participate in his own care.

Face. Fortunately, the nature of burning and the vascularity of the facial skin usually prevent full-thickness loss. However, explosions, flash burns and scalds in children may indeed result in significant skin loss. The initial wound is often covered with grease, oil, dirt and other debris, which should be meticulously removed. Burned hair should be shaved (except the eyebrows). Blisters tend to break early and are best opened surgically and the devitalized epithelium meticulously trimmed away. The wound should then be gently cleansed with a bland soap and choice of treatment made.

These initial maneuvers require considerable intellectual discipline since they are to be done at a time when all efforts are normally expended in resuscitation. Immediate care, however, is the most appropriate; it is the least uncomfortable and avoids the development of a thick, dirty coagulum, which is present the next morning.

Vigorous scrubbing is to be avoided since it may destroy injured cells. Bacterial wound sepsis will be a determinant in conversion to full-thickness skin loss, as in other areas of the body. The use of silver nitrate is technically unsatisfactory, but the other topical antibacterials are suitable.

Eyes. The eyes are usually protected in other than chemical burns, but often at the expense of the eyelids. Burns of the eyelids are often full thickness and will result in ectropion and corneal ulcers unless grafts are applied. Initial therapy includes liberal irrigation of eyes, tarsorrhaphy and skin grafting as an area of major priority. Contracture, even to separating a healed tarsorrhaphy, will occur unless sufficient skin is applied.

Ears. The ears are particularly exposed to thermal injury. The skin is thin and when lost results in perichondritis and avascular dissolution of cartilage. Such a complication presents an exceedingly difficult reconstructive problem since surrounding tissue is usually injured as well.

Particularly gratifying results may be obtained with the application of topical creams to the ear. Bacterial invasion is resisted, and skin may well be salvaged. Exposed cartilage, usually of the helix, should be trimmed away promptly until skin coverage can be obtained.

Neck. The neck is an area of priority because of its propensity to early and severe flexion deformity. Such contracture is not only disabling but it renders anesthesia for any other procedure difficult and dangerous. The neck should be splinted in full extension and skin grafts applied early and in sufficient quantity to prevent this deformity. Postoperative splinting is also of value and may reduce the contraction of split-thickness grafts applied in this area.

Team Care

One of the great advances in burn care has been the team concept of management. In addition to surgical and nursing care, the physical and occupational therapists have assumed a proper role in the early and continued management of the patient.

It does not seem as important that all patients be localized in a special area ("burn unit") as that they be cared for by a single team of interested personnel. Distribution of patients in several areas of the hospital is not as convenient as a unit but has the psychological advantage of allowing recovering patients to mingle with other than burned patients. An as yet unresolved danger of the "unit" concentrating all patients with major open wounds in a single area is cross-contamination. The appearance of a resistant organism, such as Providencia, may rapidly spread to involve the other equally susceptible patients.

QUALITY OF HEALING AND REHABILITATION

The criterion of success is how well we treat burned patients.

Prevention of invasive burn-wound sepsis sustains lives. It also preserves epidermal elements in deep partial-thickness injuries. Such wounds reepithelialize from the follicles and glands, usually over prolonged periods of time. Such healing is attended by problems.[105] Pruritis is frequent and persistent for many months. Lack of adequate skin oils to lubricate the surface and regenerating sensory fibers contribute to this irritating problem. Spontaneously healed burns also are covered by a thin, fragile epithelium which tends to crack and be easily abraded by minor tangential stress. In important functional areas, resurfacing may be required. So too, spontaneously healed deep burns are prone to infection. Lacking the protective antibacterial qualities of the sebaceous glands, these wounds are susceptible to streptococcal infection and may require long-term prophylaxis with penicillin.

The normal biology of normal healing includes contraction. The duration and intensity of the inflammatory stage of healing, prior to coverage, will help determine the amount of scar and the amount of contraction. Skin grafts applied to granulating beds retard but do not prevent such contraction. If sufficient, the clinical correlate of contraction, which is contracture, will develop.

Prevention of contracture is both more desirable and more effective than correction of deformity. The principles include splinting at all times in the optimal position to avoid contracture. Adequate resurfacing of areas lost to burn injury is the *sine qua non.* Prolonged pressure of healing tissue seems to reduce hypertrophic scarring, increase pliability and preserve contouring. Finally, the greatest enemy and ally of the reconstructive surgeon is time; an enemy because all patients are desirous of early definitive correction of scarring and deformity, and an ally since time will mature scar and reduce disfigurement.

Marjolin's Ulcers

Originally noted by Celsus and accurately described by Marjolin in 1828, these ulcers are carcinomas arising in scars, particularly burn areas.

An estimated two per cent of all squamous cell carcinomas arise in old burn scars;[227] the incidence of burn scars becoming malignant is unknown. The presumed cause is persistent stimulation to marginal epithelialization for repeated growth and repair in irritated areas. Scar tissue is particularly liable to trauma since it is raised, tense, relatively avascular and unable to glide over underlying tissue.[11] Glover and Kiehn have failed to identify carcinoma developing in skin areas properly grafted.[82]

The age of the scar is more important than the age of the patient, with a median time interval of about 35 years, although acute carcinomas have been noted as early as two to 12 months post-burning. Marjolin's ulcers have a prevalence for the lower extremities and scalp and have a high incidence of regional metastasis (35 per cent) when first seen. Although the true incidence is unknown, the major hospitals treating burns report a frequency of about one new case a year.[10]

It is readily apparent from the reported cases that the neglected burn scar is the one prone to carcinoma. Evidence of skin breakdown or constant irritation makes proper skin coverage imperative.

ELECTRICAL INJURIES

Robert C. Wray, Jr.

ELECTRICAL BURNS

Electricity causes 1100 deaths annually in the United States. Lightning accounts for one-fourth of this number. The remainder are accidents from defective electrical equipment, momentary carelessness on part of the workers on high-tension lines and the curious child exploring electric outlets and wires. Although the number of deaths is great, serious and disabling injuries are more frequent.

EFFECTS OF ELECTRICITY

The most important factors in determining the extent of injury are intensity of current and duration of contact. Resistance at points of contact, efficiency of grounding and the pathway of current through the body also affect the severity of the injury. Low-voltage direct current is less dangerous than alternating current. In general, the higher the voltage and the longer the contact, the more severe the injury. Skin resistance is increased by thick skin and oil or grease and is decreased by thin skin and moisture. The larger the area of grounding, the greater the current flow. The current probably follows a direct line between the points of grounding. If the pathway of the current includes the heart or brain, cardiac or respiratory arrest is much more likely than if the path involves only the limbs.[33] Ineffective cardiac action may be due to asystole or fibrillation.

Local Tissue Effects

It is unclear whether the local tissue effects of electricity are due to the heat generated or cellular damage from electricity itself. The local lesion is quite characteristic and almost always consists of three concentric areas: (1) a charred black center, (2) a middle zone of gray-white coagulation necrosis, and (3) an outer bright red zone of partial coagulation. The area of coagulation may increase over a period of several days following the injury; this is thought to be due to progressive vascular thrombosis.

Blood Vessel Reactions

Intravascular thrombosis often leads to extensive ischemic destruction of tissue surrounding the initial injury. Furthermore, the extensive destruction of arteries may lead to secondary hemorrhage hours or days after the initial accident. Electrical injury is said to result in friability of the vessels, making control of hemorrhage difficult or impossible.

Experimental arterial lesions were produced in dogs by using 110- and 220-volt alternating and direct currents.[98] Lesions resulted only when the vessel was occluded and the circulation was stopped. From this observation it was concluded that the destructive effect of electricity on the vascular wall resulted from overheating. During free circulation heat was dissipated by the flow of blood and damage to the vascular wall was prevented. The arterial lesions that were produced in this experimental model were similar to those observed clinically. The involved wall was grossly thin and friable. The media was most strikingly involved, with marked destruction of the individual muscle cells. The internal elastic lamina was in time disrupted. In the most extensive injury, the endothelial cells were swollen and destroyed. Thrombosis was not a feature of these acute, sharply localized, experimental lesions, but widespread thrombosis is frequently observed clinically.

Bone Destruction

Extensive destruction of bone is common in electrical injuries. Grossly, the bone is avascular and appears whitened. Histologic section shows the cells to be swollen and destroyed. The gradual sequestration and discharge of devitalized areas of bone results in prolonged delay in healing.

Nervous System Injury

In addition to the fairly common respiratory paralysis, other temporary paralyses may occur (particularly in the lower limbs). Ill-defined pain syndromes are often observed in addition to serious and persistent headache. Although these sequelae may subside spontaneously over the course of days, permanent residual disability has been reported.[207] Hemiplegia, aphasia, cerebellar dysfunction and epilepsy have all been reported following electrical injuries. Similarly, late evidence of localized neurological injury may be reflected by the appearance of Parkinsonism and a variety of cranial nerve defects including auditory and vestibular dysfunction, facial paresis and optic atrophy. A few instances of mononeuritis, with permanent loss of function of one or more peripheral nerves, have been observed. Among the more common sequelae of electrical injury is the occurrence of post-traumatic psychoneurosis, which may be prolonged and disabling.

Eye Injuries

The occurrence of cataracts following electrical injuries is of particular importance since their appearance may develop many months after the initial injury.[3] Cataracts usually follow accidents in which electrical contact was made near the eyes and may be unilateral or bilateral. In the majority of cases, the first changes appear in the anterior capsule as punctate opacities and vacuoles; this may proceed to complete opacification of the lens. Although electrical cataracts are relatively rare, patients with evidence of electrical contact near the eyes should be followed by an ophthalmologist.

Renal Dysfunction

Abnormalities of the urine sediment are commonly observed in electrothermal injuries. The problem of anuria following these accidents has only recently been emphasized. Taylor and his co-workers[222] noted seven instances of prolonged renal complications in a consecutive series of 22 electrical injuries treated at the Brooke Army Medical Center. Six of these seven patients expired and at autopsy acute tubular necrosis was observed in each. Shock undoubtedly plays a significant role in the production of this lesion. Fischer[70] has emphasized the importance of myoglobinuria and hemoglobinuria in predisposing the kidney to acute failure following electrical injuries. Significant hemoglobinemia may be observed following electrical accidents as a result of electrothermal injury and lysis of red cells. Similarly, the release of myoglobin from destroyed muscle may further increase the levels of circulating chromoprotein. Most authorities agree that precipitation of myoglobin and hemoglobin in the renal tubules, if not the cause of, is certainly contributory to the development of acute renal failure.[37]

Gastrointestinal Tract Abnormalities

Nausea, vomiting and prolonged paralytic ileus are common following electrothermal injuries as they are after thermal burns and other major trauma. Although the ileus is usually brief, other gastrointestinal tract problems are more severe. Pancreatic necrosis as well as necrosis and perforation of the gallbladder and intestine have been observed following electrical injuries.[17] The etiology of these intra-abdominal lesions is uncertain; however, diffuse vascular injury seems the most likely cause.

Fluid and Electrolyte Disturbances

The coexistence of electrical and thermal injuries is relatively common when clothing is ignited by arcing in high-tension injuries. Fluid loss in most of these patients is proportional to the area of the thermal burn. However, in severe electrical injuries with death of large volumes of muscle, extremely large fluid loss may occur.[199] Significant blood loss may occur as a consequence of vascular injury or from associated fractures and chest and abdominal trauma. Shock must not be accepted as a manifestation of the uncomplicated electrical injury; the possibility of associated hemorrhage or perforation of an intra-abdominal viscus must always be considered.

Associated Injuries

The violent, tetanic muscular contraction that results from contact (particularly with alternating-current sources) may result in a variety of fractures and dislocations. Furthermore, falls resulting from electrical contact frequently produce associated injuries.

TREATMENT

Resuscitation

Immediate first aid involves mouth-to-mouth respiration and external cardiac massage if cardiorespiratory arrest has occurred. Prolonged respiratory support may be required as coma is occasionally observed following electrical injury. The associated injuries mentioned above must be treated. Continuous nasogastric suction for 24 to 48 hours is required following major electrical injuries. The fluid and electrolyte requirements are usually due to any associated thermal injury, but in massive electrical injuries large volumes of fluid must be administered. No formula is available for calculating the requirement, but sufficient lactated Ringer's solution to produce an adequate urine output is recommended. Due to the possibility of renal failure from precipitation of myoglobin and hemoglobin urine output should be

40 to 50 cc. per hour. Alkalinization of the urine with intravenous sodium bicarbonate is probably helpful, although its value is not proven. If urine output decreases despite apparently adequate volume loading, solute diuresis with mannitol is indicated.

Surgical Treatment

Both primary excision and watchful waiting have their place in the management of electrical burn wounds.[191] The proper choice is determined by the nature and location of the initial wound. The progressive necrosis that occurs with electrical injuries often leads to underestimation of the severity in the early stages. Difficulty with early excision lies in determining the depth of injury. Attempts at early primary closure may fail as a result of extension of the necrosis. On the other hand, the irretrievably damaged limb may serve as a source for the absorption of substances that destroy the kidneys and provide a culture medium for bacteria. In massive injury, early open amputation may be lifesaving. Injuries involving the volar surface of the forearm and the hand are among the most challenging. Although the tendon and nerve may not be involved in the primary wound, they may be jeopardized when subsequently exposed by tissue slough. Early excision and closure by pedicle flap have been used to prevent secondary involvement but loss of the tendon still occurs in the majority of cases.

It is generally agreed that the conservative approach is preferred in children with electrical burns about the mouth.[174] Delayed reconstruction appears to provide the most satisfactory results. Similarly, delayed debridement seems most satisfactory in electrical burns of the head. Large areas of the calvarium may be exposed and devitalized in these injuries. This devitalized bone should be allowed to sequestrate spontaneously before a program of reconstruction is begun.

CHEMICAL BURNS

Robert C. Wray, Jr.

Most chemical burns are due to contact with acid or alkali. The most important step in the care of these burns is the removal of the noxious agent. Copious irrigation with water is the best initial treatment for all chemical burns.[31] If the patient has come into contact with hydrofluoric acid of greater than 20 per cent concentration, subcutaneous injection of a 10 per cent solution of calcium gluconate (about 0.5 $cc./cm.^2$ of burn) is the second step in treatment. The second step in the treatment of white phosphorus burns is irrigation with one per cent copper sulfate; re-irrigation with water and debridement of the particles should follow.[48] Other acid and alkali burns require only water irrigation for about 24 hours. Tissue repair cannot proceed until the agent has been inactivated by combination with tissues, neutralization or disposal. Following initial management, the basic principles utilized in thermal injury are applicable. Early excision and grafting usually cannot be employed because of uncertainty regarding the depth of injury. Definitive wound closure awaits the appearance of healthy granulation tissue.

COLD INJURY

Robert C. Wray, Jr.

CLINICAL FEATURES

The impression that trench foot and frostbite are distinct clinical entities has caused considerable confusion. Although the thermal conditions that lead to trench foot or frostbite may be quite different in degree, the common factor is cold.

TRENCH FOOT

Trench foot develops slowly over a period of hours or days due to exposure to moisture and cold (at temperatures usually above freezing). The extremity first becomes anesthetic; pain is noted only during extremes of motion and during weight-bearing. Considerable swelling later develops and the skin appears white and cold. As the lesion progresses, blisters filled with serous or serosanguineous fluid appear; eventually, the overlying skin desiccates and becomes gangrenous. The limb is never actually frozen.

In the late stage, the skin overlying the digits or indeed the whole lower limb may appear nonviable. It is difficult to estimate the depth of injury since the nonviable skin may separate, leaving pink, newly formed underlying skin or granulation tissue. If there is more severe damage, the deeper tissues are involved. These extensive injuries ultimately become shrunken and there is a sharp line of demarcation between the viable and nonviable parts.

FROSTBITE

Frostbite occurs rapidly and as a consequence of exposure to extreme cold; in the past this was frequently due to exposure at high altitudes while flying. The skin becomes blanched, and a stinging sensation is noted. The involved part becomes numb and a sensation of clumsiness is often reported. The member is firm to the touch and is, in fact, frozen. However, swelling is not an early manifestation. Thawing is attended by severe, dull, aching pains; the limb rapidly becomes hypermic and swelling and blister formation are soon observed. Vesicles are filled with straw-colored or blood-tinged fluid. In time, the involved areas of skin become black and firm, producing the appearance of gangrene. Again, it is impossible to determine the depth of injury since the blackened skin may peel off, revealing healthy granulation tissue or newly formed skin. In the most severe injuries, however, gangrene may involve the entire substance of the extremity.

In the usual nonmilitary practice, most cold injuries involve both exposure to cold and water.

PREDISPOSING FACTORS TO INJURY

The most important environmental factors which influence the effects of cold are humidity and wind. Increase in the humidity or wind velocity increases the rate of heat loss from tissues. Anything which decreases local tissue perfusion (e.g., atherosclerosis, arteritides, constriction due to tight clothing, etc.) will increase the susceptibility of tissue to cold injury.

PATHOPHYSIOLOGY OF COLD INJURY

The application of cold produces an immediate and marked arteriolar vasoconstriction.[119] Profound tissue anoxia results from the disturbance of blood flow that accompanies arteriolar vasoconstriction, and the derangement in oxygen transport that is produced by the influence of cold upon the dissociation of oxyhemoglobin.

With thawing, the arterioles reopen and blood flow returns to the involved vascular bed, changing the white frozen appearance to that of hyperemia. This "flare" is soon accompanied by swelling which results from the loss of intravascular fluid into the interstitial spaces as edema. Lewis[119, 120] related the occurrence of this wheal and flare response to the local release of a tissue substance (possibly histamine). After mild cold injury, this may be the only consequence; with more severe degrees of injury, however, an additional sequence is observed. Coincident to the development of interstitial edema, blood flow again slows and the dilated vessels become engorged with masses of erythrocytes.[110] For an undetermined period of time, these masses of erythrocytes can be broken up by gentle manipulation and only later are true occlusive thrombi formed. The importance of thrombotic arterial occlusions in cold injury seems often to have been overlooked.[79, 185]

Weatherley-White and his coworkers[235] reported the results of an instructive experiment that defines the importance of the vascular lesions in the pathogenesis of cold injury. Injury was produced in one rabbit ear by its immersion in a mixture of solid carbon dioxide and ethanol. A circular full-thickness skin graft was then removed from both ears and each graft was reimplanted on the opposite ear—frozen skin on the normal ear and normal skin on the frozen ear. Uniformly, the frozen skin survived when transplanted to the normal ear, whereas normal skin necrosed on the frozen ear. Undoubtedly, cell death can be produced by the direct effects of cold, but tissue loss in the clinical circumstances appears to be more dependent upon the status of the local circulation following cold exposure. The anatomy of the vascular lesions apparently determines the eventual extent of tissue necrosis.

Since the extent of ischemic tissue loss following cold injury seems ultimately related directly to vascular occlusion, arteriography should afford a useful means of evaluating the extent of these injuries. Although Leriche and Kinlin[117] published in 1940 the results of Thorotrast arteriography in extremities injured by cold, there seems to have been little subsequent interest in their observations.

TREATMENT

Local Therapy

Since cold exerts its influence from exposure of the body surface and human tissues are imperfect thermal conductors, the extent of injury diminishes from the surface toward the deeper tissue levels. The superficial layers of skin are most strikingly involved; therefore, it is difficult to assess the eventual extent of tissue loss from the early appearance of the part. Consequently, it is expedient to avoid premature excision of apparently nonviable extremities after cold injury. A few days' to weeks' delay will allow a clear demarcation between viable and nonviable tissues and obviate the risk of removing salvageable and potentially useful tissue.

Rapid warming of the injured area is the most important step in treatment.[136, 233] The frozen extremity is placed in water having a temperature of 40 to 44° C. Dry heat should never be used and the application of blankets alone results in slow warming. The injured area should be cleansed carefully, and if injury involves the lower limbs, the toes should be separated by gauze. The area is then allowed exposure to air as bacterial proliferation in the tissue is not a common problem. Tetanus prophylaxis is given. Prophylactic antibiotics are usually administered, although proof for their effectiveness is lacking. Early amputation is indicated only in the face of uncontrolled or gas-producing sepsis. As a clear line of demarcation between viable and nonviable tissues becomes apparent, surgical debridement is undertaken. The normal vascularity of tissues immediately proximal to those destroyed provides the opportunity for a variety of reconstructive procedures. Useful limbs can, as a rule, be salvaged. In planning these procedures as well as in evaluating the eventual extent of tissue loss, arteriography may have considerable value.

The unpredictability of the eventual extent of tissue loss makes evaluation of the measures that have been proposed to diminish the tissue loss difficult.

Sympathectomy

Enthusiastic reports from Europe concerning the results of sympathetic block and of sympathectomy in the treatment of cold injuries during World War II were soon followed by reports of similar experiences in this country. Controversy continues about the precise role of sympathectomy in the acute lesion. This is based partly on the lack of an adequate means of assessing the results of treatment and partly on a lack of general agreement concerning the rationale of sympathectomy in the treatment of cold injury. It seems significant, however, that the precise role remains poorly defined more than 25 years after Ducuing[61] reported the results of sympathetic nerve interruption in some 300 patients.

It has been suggested that the vascular stasis that is observed after cold injury reflects the presence of arterial vasospasm. It has also been suggested that arteriovenous shunting may reduce effective tissue perfusion after cold injury. In support of this latter suggestion, it has been observed that the venous oxygen content is increased during recovery from cold injury. Fontaine and his co-workers[72] observed a rapid rise in the venous oxygen content during cooling of the canine limb. This rise in venous oxygen content, to a level nearly equal to arterial blood, apparently reflects the diminished metabolism of the limb occasioned by cooling as well as the influence of cold upon the oxygen dissociation curve of hemoglobin. With warming, the venous oxygen difference never returned to the control level. In the absence of direct measurements of blood flow in the limb or of a quantitative measure of tissue damage in the limb, these data cannot be conclusively interpreted to support the suggestion that arteriovenous shunts are opened by cold injury.

If an influence of the sympathetic nervous system is primarily concerned in the pathophysiology of cold injury, it seems reasonable that early sympathectomy should protect against tissue loss. On the contrary, experimental evidence indicates that sympathectomy performed within the first few hours of injury increased the edema formation and accelerated the pathologic process of tissue destruction.[85, 234] It is difficult, therefore, to assign the sympathetic nervous system a primary role in the production of cold injury. It has been demonstrated in an experimental cold injury involved in the rabbit ear, however, that sympathectomy performed 24 to 48 hours after thawing hastens the resolution of edema and reduces the extent of tissue loss.[85] These experimental findings coincide with the clinical observation of the many proponents of sympathectomy.[83, 84, 200] The apparent beneficial effects of sympathectomy seem to reflect an increase in collateral circulation in the injured limb. The prominent element of arterial occlusion in relationship to cold injury has been emphasized. Sympathectomy apparently effects an increase in collateral circulation about these vascular occlusions.

In summary, sympathectomy 36 to 72 hours after injury is recommended only in those patients who may be anticipated to have a significant loss of a portion of the limb.

Anticoagulants

It has been noted that vessels shortly after thawing are dilated and filled with clumps of erythrocytes. In this early stage there is no evidence that thrombosis has occurred, since the erythrocyte clumps can easily be dislodged by gentle manipulation. The mechanism that leads to clumping is not known, but it may reflect the presence of a cold-induced increase in blood viscosity. This possibility suggests that low-molecular-weight dextran might be useful in the early treatment of cold injury. No controlled clinical study of the influence of this substance on the natural history of cold injury has been reported. Experimentally, however, treatment with low-molecular-weight dextran in doses of one gm./kg./day has been demonstrated to protect against tissue loss in rabbits.[234] Therefore, 1,000 cc. of six per cent dextran should be given on the day of injury and 500 cc. of the same solution every day for five days.

It is generally agreed that thrombi eventually form in the dilated, erythrocyte-filled vessels, possibly as late as 72 hours after thawing. This observation led to the suggestion that heparin might be useful in treatment of cold injury. The early favorable clinical experimental results were reported by Lange and his co-workers.[111] Subsequent workers,[46, 201] however, have been unable to substantiate these findings, and at the present time there is no evidence that heparin alters the natural history of the disease. Due to the aforementioned and the dangers of the use of heparin, I do not recommend the administration of heparin in the treatment of cold injury.

LATE SEQUELAE

A particularly informative study of the late sequelae to cold injury was reported by Blair et al.,[24] who observed a group of 100 veterans of the Korean conflict four years after their injuries. They found that the late symptoms, in order of decreasing frequency, included excessive sweating, pain, coldness, numbness, abnormal skin color and pain and stiffness of the joints. In addition, frequent asymptomatic abnormalities of the nails, including ridging and inward curving of the edges, were observed.

It is likely that hyperhydrosis is both a cause and result of cold injury. Hyperhydrosis suggests the presence of an abnormality involving the sympathetic nervous system induced by cold injury and, indeed, hyperhydrosis is abolished by appropriate sympathetic denervation. Sensitivity to cold and the predisposition to recurrent cold injury are, in some respects, analagous to the consideration of hyperhydrosis. Blanching and pain upon subsequent cold exposure may be quite troublesome and at times so dramatic as to suggest a diagnosis of Raynaud's phenomenon. These symptoms are commonly dramatically relieved by sympathetic interruption. It seems quite unjustified, however, to imply that hyperhydrosis or cold sensitivity is necessarily the manifestation of an abnormality of the sympathetic nervous system or of an abnormal vascular response to sympathetic vasoconstrictor impulses. Hyperhydrosis and cold sensitivity may both proceed and follow cold injury.

The late abnormalities of change in skin color, including depigmentation in the Negro and an appearance resembling erythrocyanosis in the white patient, are most likely the result of ischemia. Similarly, the abnormalities of the nails are comparable to those seen with ischemia, regardless of its cause. Neither of these abnormalities usually requires specific treatment.

Late symptoms of joint stiffness and pain on motion are relatively common and undoubtedly are often related to overlying scars and to mechanical problems occasioned by the variety of amputations required. Blair and his co-workers,[24] however, frequently observed "punched-out" defects in the subchondral bone of the involved limbs. These localized areas of bone resorption generally appear within five to 10 months after injury and may heal spontaneously. Vascular occlusion was felt to represent the most likely cause of these lesions. These bone changes, in close proximity to joint surfaces, help explain the joint symptoms.

REFERENCES

1. Abramson, D. J.: The care of severely burned children. Surg. Gynec. Obstet. *122*:855, 1966.
2. Achauer, B. M., Allyn, P. A., Furnas, D. W., and Bartlett, R. H.: Pulmonary complications of burns: The major threat to the burn patient. Ann. Surg. *177*:311, 1973.
3. Adam, A. L., and Klein, M.: Electrical cataract: Notes on a case and a review of the literature. Brit J. Ophthal. *29*:169, 1945.
4. Alexander, J. W.: Serum and leukocyte lysosomal enzymes. Derangements following severe thermal injury. Arch. Surg. *95*:482, 1965.
5. Alexander, J. W., Fisher, M. W., and MacMillan, B. G.: Immunological control of *Pseudomonas* infection in burn patients: A clinical evaluation. Arch. Surg. *102*:31, 1971.
6. Alexander, J. W., and Meakins, J. L.: Natural defense mechanisms in clinical sepsis. J. Surg. Res. *11*:148, 1971.
7. Allgöwer, M., Cueni, L. B., Stadtler, K., et al.: Burn toxin in mouse skin. J. Trauma *13*:95, 1973.
8. Altemeier, W. A., MacMillan, B. G., and Hill, E. O.: The rationale of specific antibiotic therapy in the management of major burns. Surgery *52*:240, 1962.
9. Arney, G. K., Pearson, E., and Sutherland, A. B.: Burn stress pseudodiabetes. Ann. Surg. *152*:77, 1960.
10. Arons, M. S., Lynch, J. B., Lewis, S. R., and Blocker, T. G., Jr.: Scar tissue carcinoma. Part I. A clinical study with special reference to burn scar carcinoma. Ann. Surg. *161*:170, 1965.
11. Arons, M. S., Rodin, A. E., Lynch, J. B., Lewis, S. R., and Blocker, T. G., Jr.: Scar tissue carcinoma. II. An experimental study with special reference to burn scar carcinomas. Ann. Surg. *163*:445, 1966.
12. Arthurson, G.: Evaporation and fluid replacement: Research in burns. *In* Matter, P., et al. (eds.): Transactions of the Third International Congress on Research in Burns. Berne, Hans Huber Publishers, 1971, p. 520.
13. Artz, C. P.: Understanding thermal burns and principles of management. *In* Davis, J. H. (ed.): Current Concepts in Surgery. New York, McGraw-Hill Book Co., 1965.
14. Artz, C. P., and Moncrief, J. A.: The Treatment of Burns. Philadelphia: W. B. Saunders Co., 1969.
15. Asch, M. J., Curreri, P. W., and Pruitt, B. A., Jr.: Thermal injury involving bone: Report of 32 cases, J. Trauma *12*:135, 1972.
16. Backdahl, M., Liljedahl, S. O., and Troel, L.: Excision of deep burns. Acta Chir. Scand. *123*:351, 1962.
17. Baldwin, W. M., and Dondate, M.: High frequency current burns in rats. Proc. Soc. Exper. Biol. Med. *27*:65, 1929.
18. Baxter, C. R.: Burns. *In* Shires, G. T. (ed.): Care of the Trauma Patient. New York, McGraw-Hill Book Co., 1966.
19. Baxter, C. R.: Topical use of 1.0% silver sulfadiazine. *In* Polk, H. C. and Stone, H. H. (eds.): Contemporary Burn Management. Boston, Little, Brown, 1971, pp. 217–225.
20. Baxter, C. R., Loebl, E. C., and Curreri, P. W.: Mechanism of erythrocyte destruction in the early post-burn period. Presented, fifth annual meeting of The American Burn Association. Dallas, Texas, April 7, 1973.
21. Benain, F., Pattin, M., and Rappaport, M.: Puncture biopsies of the liver in critical burns. *In* Artz, C. P. (ed.): Research in Burns. Philadelphia, F. A. Davis Co., 1962, pp. 185–193.
22. Berkow, S. A.: A method for estimating the extensiveness of lesions (burns and scalds), based on surface area proportions. Arch. Surg. *8*:138, 1924.
23. Black, J., Calesnick, B., Williams, D., and Weinstein, M. J.: Pharmacology of Gentamicin, a new broad-spectrum antibiotic. Antibiot. Chemother. 138–147, 1963.

24. Blair, J. R., Schatzki, R., and Orr, N. D.: Sequelae to cold injury in one hundred patients: Follow-up study four years after occurrence of cold injury. J.A.M.A. *163*:1203, 1957.
25. Blalock, A.: Experimental shock. VII. The importance of the local loss of fluid in the production of the low blood pressure after burns. Arch. Surg. *22*: 610, 1931.
26. Blocker, T. G., Jr.: Burns. *In* Converse, J. M. (ed.): Reconstructive Plastic Surgery. Philadelphia, W. B. Saunders Co., 1964.
27. Blocker, T. G., Lewis, S. R., Kirby, E. J., Levin, W. C., Perry, J. H., and Blocker, V.: The problem of protein disequilibrium following severe thermal trauma. *In* Artz, C. P. (ed.): Research in Burns. Philadelphia, F. A. Davis Co., 1962, pp. 121–124.
28. Boswick, J. A., Jr.: Topical therapy of the burn wound with mafenide acetate. *In* Polk, H. C., and Stone, H. H. (eds.): Contemporary Burn Management. Boston, Little, Brown, 1971, pp. 193–202.
29. Brentano, L., Moyer, C. A., Grovens, D. L., and Monafo, W. W.: Bacteriology of large human burns treated with silver nitrate. Arch. Surg. *93*:456, 1966.
30. Bromberg, B. E., and Song, I. C.: Homografts and heterografts as skin substitutes. Am. J. Surg. *112*:28, 1966.
31. Bromberg, B. E., Song, I. C., and Walden, R. H.: Hydrotherapy of chemical burns. Plast. Reconstr. Surg. *35*:85, 1965.
32. Brown, J. B., Fryer, M. P., Randall, P., and Lu, M.: Postmortem homografts as "biological dressings" for extensive burns and denuded areas. Ann. Surg. *138*:618, 1953.
33. Brown, K. L., and Moritz, A. R.: Electrical injuries. J. Trauma *4*:608, 1964.
34. Bruch, H. M., Nash, G., Foley, F. D., and Pruitt, B. A.: Opportunistic fungal infection of the burn wound with Phycomycetes and *Aspergillus*. Arch. Surg. *102*:476, 1971.
35. Bull, J. P., and Squire, J. R.: A study of mortality in a burns unit: Standards for the evaluation of alternative methods of treatment. Ann. Surg. *130*: 160, 1949.
36. Burke, J. F.: The use of skin transplantation and immunosuppression in the treatment of extensive full thickness thermal burns. Presentation, American Burn Association, Dallas, Texas, April 1973.
37. Bywaters, E. G. L.: Ischemic muscle necrosis; crushing injury, traumatic edema, crush syndrome, traumatic anuria, compression syndrome; type of injury seen in air raid casualties following burial beneath debris. J.A.M.A. *124*:1103, 1944.
38. Cohen, I. K., Schecter, P. J., and Henkins, R. I.: Decreased taste acuity and zinc loss following thermal injury. Presentation, American Society of Plastic Surgeons, Las Vegas, September 1972.
39. Cohen, S.: An investigation and fractional assessment of the evaporative water loss through normal skin and burn eschars using a microhydrometer. Plast. Reconstr. Surg. *37*:475, 1966.
40. Collentine, G. E., Waisbren, B. A., and Mellender, J. W.: Treatment of burns with intensive antibiotic therapy and exposure. J.A.M.A. *200*:939, 1967.
41. Conizaro, P. C., Sawyer, R. B., and Switzer, W. E.: Blood loss during excision of third degree burns. Arch. Surg. *88*:800, 1964.
42. Cook, W. A., Baxter, C. R., and Ferrell, J. M., Jr.: Pulmonary circulation after dermal burns. Vasc. Surg. *2*:1, 1968.
43. Cossman, D. V., and Krizek, .T. J.: Effect of silver lactate and silver sulfadiazine on experimental burn wound sepsis. Surg. Forum *22*:495, 1971.
44. Craig, R. D. P.: Immunotherapy for severe burns in children. Plast. Reconstr. Surg. *35*:263, 1965.
45. Cramer, L. M., McCormack, R. M., and Carroll, D. B.: Progressive partial excision and early grafting in lethal burns. Plast. Reconstr. Surg. *30*:595, 1962.
46. Crismon, J. M.: Science in World War II. Advances in Military Medicine. Boston, Little, Brown, 1948, p. 176.
47. Cruickshank, G. N. D., and Hershey, F. B.: The effect of heat on the metabolism of guinea pigs' ear skin. Ann. Surg. *151*:419, 1960.
48. Curreri, W. P., Asch, M. J. and Pruitt, B. A.: The treatment of chemical burns; specialized diagnostic, therapeutic and prognostic considerations. J. Trauma *10*:634, 1970.
49. Curreri, P. W., Bruck, H. M., Lindberg, R. B., Mason, A. D., Jr., and Pruitt, B. A.: *Providencia stuartii* sepsis: a new challenge in the treatment of thermal injury. Ann. Surg. *177*:133, 1973.
50. Curreri, P. W., Wilmore, D. W., Mason, A. D., Jr., et al.: Intracellular cation alterations following major trauma: Effect of supranormal caloric intake. J. Trauma *11*:390, 1971.
51. Dahinterova, J., and Dobrkovsky, M.: Treatment of the burned surface by amnion and chorion grafts. Sborn. Ved. Prac. Lek. Fak. Karlov. Univ. (Suppl.) *11*:513, 1968.
52. Davis, B., Lilly, H. A., and Lowbury, E. J. L.: Gram-negative bacilli in burns. J. Clin. Path. *22*:634, 1969.
53. Dennis, D. L., and Peterson, C. G.:

Candida and other fungi. *In* Polk, H. C., and Stone, H. H. (eds.): Contemporary Burn Management. Boston, Little, Brown, 1971, pp. 329–338.

54. Dino, B. R., Eufemio, G. G., and DeVilla, M. S.: Human amnion: The establishment of an amnion bank and its practical applications in surgery. J. Phillip Med. Assoc. *42*:357, 1966.
55. Dodson, E. L., and Warner, G. E.: Early circulatory disturbances following experimental thermal trauma. Circ. Res. *5*:69, 1957.
56. Douglas, B.: Homografts of fetal membranes as a covering for large wounds—especially those from burns. J. Tenn. Med. Assoc. *45*:230, 1952.
57. Douglas, B., Conway, H., Stark, R. B., Jeslin, D. and Nieto-Cano, G.: The fate of homologous and heterologous chorionic transplants as observed by the transparent tissue chamber technique in the mouse. Plast. Reconstr. Surg. *13*:125, 1954.
58. Dorr, L. D., Asch, M. J., and Zawacki, B. E.: Re-evaluation of surgical therapy of Curling's ulcer in children: Report of five patients with four survivors. Presented at the fifth annual meeting, American Burn Association, Dallas, Texas, April 6, 1973.
59. Dressler, D. P., and Skornick, W. A.: Silver sulfadiazine and Sulfamylon cream in the burned rat model: A comparative evaluation. Surgery *67*:644, 1970.
60. Dressler, D. P., and Skornick, W. A.: The laboratory evaluation of topical silver nitrate in experimental burn wound sepsis. J. Trauma *12*:791, 1972.
61. Ducuing, J., D'Harcourt, J., Folch, A., and Bofill, J.: Les troubles trophiques des extremité produits par de froid sec en pathologie de guerre. J. Chir. *55*:385, 1940.
62. Eade, G. G.: The relationship between granulation tissue, bacteria, and skin grafts in burned patients. Plast. Reconstr. Surg. *22*:42, 1958.
63. Ehrlich, H. P., Tarver, H., and Hunt, T. K.: Effects of vitamin A and glucocorticoids upon inflammation and collagen synthesis. Ann. Surg. *177*:222, 1973.
64. Epstein, B. S., Hardy, D. L., Harrison, H. N., Teplitz, G., Villareal, Y., and Mason, A. D.: Hypoxemia in the burned patient. A clinical-pathologic study. Ann. Surg. *158*:924, 1963.
65. Eurenius, K., McManus, W. F., McEuen, D. D., et al.: Coagulation dynamics after thermal injury. Presented, fifth annual meeting of The American Burn Association, Dallas, Texas, April 7, 1973.
66. Evans, E. B., and Blumel, J.: Bone and joint changes following burns. *In* Artz, C. P. (ed.): Research in Burns. Philadelphia, F. A. Davis Co., 1962, pp. 26–32.
67. Evans, E. I., and Butterfield, W. J. H.: The stress response in the severely burned patient. Ann. Surg. *134*:588, 1951.
68. Fallon, R. H., and Moyer, C. A.: Rates of insensible perspiration through normal, burned, tape-stripped and epidermally denuded living human skin. Ann. Surg. *158*:915, 1963.
69. Fidler, J. P., MacMillan, B. G., Law, E. J., et al.: CO_2 laser excision of acute burns with immediate autografting. Presentation: American Burn Association, Dallas, Texas, April 1973.
70. Fischer, H.: Pathological effects and sequelae of electrical accidents. J. Occupat. Med. *7*:564, 1965.
71. Foley, F. D., Greenawald, K. A., Nash, G., and Pruitt, B. A., Jr.: Herpesvirus infection in burned patients. New Eng. J. Med. *282*, 652, 1970.
72. Fontaine, R., Klein, M., Bollack, C., Kuhlman, N., and Sapicas, I.: Clinical and experimental contribution to the study of frostbite. J. Cardiovasc. Surg. *2*:449, 1961.
73. Fox, C. L., Jr.: Clinical experience with silver sulfadiazine: a new topical agent for control of pseudomonas infection in burns. J. Trauma, *9*:377, 1969.
74. Fox, C. L., Jr.: Silver sulfadiazine—a new topical therapy for *Pseudomonas* in burns. Arch. Surg. *96*:184, 1968.
75. Fox, C. L., and Lasker, S. E.: Response to fluid therapy and tissue electrolyte changes in scalded and flash burned monkeys. Surg. Gynec. Obstet. *112*:274, 1961.
76. Fox, C. L., Jr., Rappole, B. W., and Stanford, W.: Control of *Pseudomonas* infection in burns by silver sulfadiazine. Surg. Gynec. Obstet. *128*:1021, 1969.
77. Fox, C. L., Jr., Sampath, A. C., and Stanford, J. W.: Virulence of *Pseudomonas* infection in burned rats and mice: comparative efficacy of silver sulfadiazine and mafenide. Arch. Surg. *101*:508, 1970.
78. Freshwater, M. F., and Krizek, T. J.: Skin grafting of burns: A centennial. J. Trauma *11*:862, 1971.
79. Friedman, N. B.: The pathology of trench foot. Am. J. Path. *21*:387, 1945.
80. Garrett, T. A.: *Bacillus subtilis* protease: A new topical agent for debridement. Clin. Med. *76*:11, 1969.
81. Georgiade, N. G., and Harris, W. A.: Open and closed treatment of burns with Povidone-iodine. *In* Polk, H. C.,

and Ehrenkranz, N. J. (eds.): Medical and Surgical Antisepsis with Betadine Microbicides. Purdue Frederick and Co., 1972.

82. Glover, D. M., and Kiehn, C. L.: Marjolin's ulcer; a preventable threat to function and life. Am. J. Surg. *78*:722, 1949.

83. Golding, M. R., deJong, P., Sawyer, P. N., Nehhigar, G. R., and Wesolowski, S. A.: Protection from early and late sequelae of frostbite by regional sympathectomy. Mechanism of "cold sensitivity" following frostbite. Surgery *53*:303, 1963.

84. Golding, M. R., Martinez, A., deJong, P., et al.: The role of sympathectomy in frostbite with a review of 68 cases. Surgery, *57*:774, 1965.

85. Golding, M. R., Mendoza, M. F., Hennigar, G. R., Fries, C. C., and Wesolowski, S. A.: On settling the controversy on the benefit of sympathectomy for frostbite. Surgery *56*:221, 1964.

86. Goodall, McC., and Moncrief, J. A.: Sympathetic nerve depletion after severe thermal injury. Ann. Surg. *162*:893, 1965.

87. Hardy, J. D.: Summary: Physiology. *In* Artz, C. P. (ed.): Research in Burns. Philadelphia, F. A. Davis Co., 1962, pp. 385–392.

88. Harrison, H. N., Bales, H., and Jacoby, F.: The behavior of mafenide acetate as a basis for its clinical use. Arch. Surg. *103*:449, 1971.

89. Haynes, B. W.: Current problems in burns. Arch. Surg. *103*:454, 1971.

90. Haynes, B. W., Jr.: Skin homografts—a lifesaving measure in severely burned children. J. Trauma *3*:217, 1963.

91. Hellat, A.: Studies on the self-disinfecting power of the skin. Ann. Med. Exper. Biol. Fenniae *26*:1, 1948.

92. Hellstrom, J. G.: Vitamin E—A general review of the literature with assessment of its role in the healing of burns and wounds. Med. Serv. J. Canada *17*:238, 1961.

93. Hergt, K.: Blood levels of thrombocytes in burned patients: Observations on their behavior in relation to the clinical condition of the patient. J. Trauma *12*:599, 1972.

94. Hoopes, J. E., Butcher, H. R., Margraf, H. W., et al.: Silver lactate burn cream. Surgery *70*:29, 1971.

95. Hume, D. M.: Endocrine and metabolic responses to injury. *In* Schwartz, S. I. (ed.): Principles of Surgery. New York, McGraw-Hill Book Co., 1969, p. 17.

96. Hummel, R. P., MacMillan, B. G., and Altmeier, W. A.: Topical and systemic antibacterial agents in the treatment of burns. Ann. Surg. *172*:370, 1970.

97. Ivanova, S. S.: The transplantation of skin from dead body to granulating surface. Ann. Surg. *12*:354, 1890.

98. Jaffe, R. J., Willis, D., and Backem, A.: The effect of electric currents on the arteries. Arch. Path. *7*:244, 1929.

99. Jelenko, C. III, and Ginsburg, J. M.: Water-holding lipid and water transmission through homeothermic and poikilothermic skins. Proc. Soc. Exp. Biol. Med. *136*:1059, 1971.

100. Jones, R. J.: Passive immunization against gram-negative bacilli in burns. Brit. J. Exp. Path. *51*:53, 1970.

101. Kefalides, N. A., Arana, J. A., Bazan, A., and Stastny, P.: Clinical evaluation of antibiotics and gamma globulin in septicemias following burns. *In* Artz, C. P. (ed.): Research in Burns. Philadelphia, F. A. Davis Co., 1962, pp. 219–228.

102. Klein, L., Curtiss, P. H., and Davis, J. H.: Collagen breakdown in thermal burns. Surg. Forum *13*:459, 1962.

103. Knisley, M. H.: Post burn pathologic circulatory physiology. *In* Artz, C. P. (ed.): Research in Burns. Philadelphia, F. A. Davis Co., 1962, pp. 51–57.

104. Koehnlein, H. E., and Lemperle, G.: Experimental studies on local treatment of pseudomonas-infected burn wounds. Plast. Reconstr. Surg. *45*:558, 1970.

105. Krizek, T. J.: Topical therapy of burns—Problems in wound healing. J. Trauma *8*:276, 1968.

106. Krizek, T. J., and Davis, J. H.: Experimental Pseudomonas burn sepsis—evaluation of topical therapy. J. Trauma *7*:433, 1967.

107. Krizek, T. J., Davis, J. H., DesPrez, J. D., and Kiehn, C. L.: Topical therapy of burns—experimental evaluation. Plast. Reconstr. Surg. *39*:248, 1967.

108. Krizek, T. J., and Cossman, D. V.: Experimental burn wound sepsis: variations in response to topical agents. J. Trauma *12*:553, 1972.

109. Krizek, T. J., Robson, M. C., and Kho, E.: Bacteria growth and skin graft survival. Surg. Forum *18*:518, 1967.

110. Lange, K., and Boyd, L. J.: The functional pathology of frostbite and the prevention of gangrene in experimental animals and humans. Science *102*:151, 1945.

111. Lange, K., and Loewe, L.: Subcutaneous heparin in the Pitkin menstruum for the treatment of experimental human frostbite. Surg. Gynec. Obstet. *82*:256, 1946.

112. Larson, D. L., Maxwell, R., Abston, S., and Dobrkovsky, M.: Zinc deficiency in burned children. Plast. Reconstr. Surg. *46*:13, 1970.

113. Law, E. J., Kim, O. J., Stieritz, D. D., and MacMillan, B. G.: Experience with systemic candidiasis in the burned patient, J. Trauma *12*:543, 1972.
114. Law, E. J., and MacMillan, B. G.: Excision of acute burns with immediate meshed autografting. Presentation, American Burn Association, Dallas, Texas, April, 1973.
115. Law, E. J., and MacMillan, B. G.: Topical treatment of small burn wounds with Povidone-iodine. *In* Polk, H. C., and Ehrenkranz, N. J. (eds.): Medical and Surgical Antisepsis with Betadine Microbiocides. Purdue Frederick and Co., 1972.
116. Lawson, D. I.: The propagation of flame over textiles. Brit. J. Plast. Surg. *9*:186, 1956.
117. Leriche, R., and Kunlin, J.: Pathologic physiology and frostbite illness. Mem. Acad. Chir. *66*:196, 1940.
118. Lewis, S. R., Goolishian, H. A., Wolf, C. W., Lynch, J. B., and Blocker, T. G.: Psychological studies in burn patients. Plast. Reconstr. Surg. *31*:323, 1963.
119. Lewis, T.: The Blood Vessels of the Human Skin and their Responses. London, Shaw and Sons, Ltd., 1927, p. 51.
120. Lewis, T., and Love, W. S.: Observations upon the regulation of blood flow through the capillaries of the human skin. Heart *13*:1, 1926.
121. Lindberg, R. B., Brame, R. E., Moncrief, J. A., and Mason, A. D., Jr.: Prevention of invasive *Pseudomonas aeruginosa* infection in seeded burned rats by use of a topical sulfamylon cream. Fed. Proc. *23*:388, 1964.
122. Lindberg, R. B., Moncrief, J A., and Mason, A. D., Jr.: Control of experimental and clinical burn wound sepsis by topical application of Sulfamylon compounds. Ann. N.Y. Acad. Sci. *150*: 950, 1968.
123. Lindberg, R. B., Moncrief, J. A., Switzer, W. E., Order, S. E., and Mills, W.: The successful control of burn wound sepsis. J. Trauma *6*:407, 1966.
124. Lowry, K. F., and Curtis, G. M.: Delayed suture in the management of wounds: analysis of 721 traumatic wounds illustrating the influence of time interval in wound repair. Am. J. Surg. *80*:280, 1970.
125. Lund, C. C., and Browder, N. C.: The estimation of areas of burns. Surg. Gynec. Obstet. *79*:352, 1944.
126. Lynch, J. B.: Thermal burns. *In* Grabb, W. C., and Smith, J. C. (eds.): Plastic Surgery. Boston, Little, Brown, 1968.
127. MacMillan, B. G.: Comparison of topical antimicrobial agents. *In* Polk, H. C., and Stone, H. H. (eds.): *In* Contemporary Burn Management. Boston, Little, Brown, 1971.
128. MacMillan, B. G.: Homograft skin—a valuable adjunct to the treatment of thermal burns. J. Trauma *2*:130, 1962.
129. MacMillan, B. G., and Altemeier, W. A.: Massive excision of the extensive burn. *In* Artz, C. P. (ed.): Research in Burns. Philadelphia, F. A. Davis Co., 1962.
130. MacMillan, B. G., Law, E. J., and Holder, I. A.: Experience with *Candida* infections in the burn patient. Arch. Surg. *104*:509, 1972.
131. Majno, G., and Palade, G. E.: Studies on inflammation. I. The effect of histamine and serotonin on vascular permeability: An electron microscopic study. J. Biophys. Biochem. Cytol. *11*:571, 1961.
132. Markley, K., Boconegra, M., Bazan, A., Temple, R., Chiaporri, M., Morales, G., and Carrion, A.: Clinical evaluation of saline solution therapy in burn shock. II. Comparison of plasma therapy with saline solution therapy. J.A.M.A. *170*:1633, 1959.
133. Markley, K., and Kefalides, N.: Further studies in the evaluation of saline solutions in the treatment of burn shock. *In* Artz, C. P. (ed.): Research in Burns. Philadelphia, F.. A. Davis Co., 1962, pp. 81–88.
134. Mason, A. D., Jr., Pruitt, B. A., Jr., Lindberg, R. B., et al.: Topical sulfamylon chemotherapy in the treatment of patients wilth extensive thermal burns. *In* Matter, P., Barclay, T. L., and Konicfova, Z. (eds.): Research in Burns: Transactions of Third International Congress of Research in Burns, Prague, September 20–25, 1970. Berne, Hans Huber Publishers, 1971, pp. 120–123.
135. Mendelson, J. A., and Lindsey, D.: Sulfamylon (mafenide) and penicillin as expedient treatment of experimental massive open wounds with *C. perfringens* infection. J. Trauma *3*:239, 1962.
136. Merryman, H. T.: Tissue freezing and local cold injury. Physiol. Rev. *37*:233, 1957.
137. Monafo, W. W.: The Treatment of Burns: Principles and Practice. St. Louis, Warren H. Greene, 1971.
138. Monafo, W. W.: Hypertonic balanced saline solutions in the treatment of burn shock. *In* Fox, C. L., and Nahas, G. G. (eds.): Body Fluid Replacement in the Surgical Patient, New York, Grune and Stratton, 1970, p. 237.
139. Monafo, W. W.: Hypertonic sodium solutions for the treatment of burn shock. *In* Polk, H. C., and Stone, H. H. (eds.): Contemporary Burn Management. Boston, Little, Brown, 1971, pp. 33–42.

140. Monasterio, F. O., Serrano, R. A., Barrera, G., Araico, J., Gutierrez-Bosque, R., Escobosa, J. E., and Barreto, F. R.: Comparative study in treatment of extensive burns with and without antibiotics. *In* Artz, C. P. (ed.): Research in Burns. Philadelphia, F. A. Davis Co., 1962, pp. 229–234.
141. Moncrief, J. A.: Editorial: Burn formulae. J. Trauma *12*:538, 1972.
142. Moncrief, J. A.: Effect of various fluid regimens and pharmacologic agents on the circulatory hemodynamics of the immediate postburn period. Ann. Surg. *164*:723, 1966.
143. Moncrief, J. A.: Medical progress—Burns. New Eng. J. Med. *288*:444, 1973.
144. Moncrief, J. A.: The status of topical antibacterial therapy in the treatment of burns. Surgery *63*:862, 1968.
145. Moncrief, J. A.: Thermal and radiation injuries. *In* Zimmerman, L. M., and Levine, R. (eds.): Physiologic Principles of Surgery. Philadelphia, W. B. Saunders Co., 1964, pp. 62–85.
146. Moncrief, J. A., Lindberg, R. B., Switzer, W. E., et al.: Use of topical antibacterial therapy in the treatment of the burn wound. Arch. Surg. *92*:558, 1966.
147. Moncrief, J. A., Switzer, W. E., and Teplitz, C.: Curling's ulcer. J. Trauma *4*:481, 1964.
148. Moncrief, J. A., and Teplitz, C.: Changing concepts in burn sepsis. J. Trauma *4*:233, 1964.
149. Moritz, A. R., and Henrique, F. C., Jr.: Studies of thermal injury; the relative importance of time and surface temperature in the causation of cutaneous burns. Am. J. Path. *23*:695, 1947.
150. Moritz, A. R., Henrique, F. C., Dutra, F. R., and Weisiger, J. R.: Studies of thermal injury. IV. An exploration of the casualty producing attributes of conflagrations; local and systemic effects of general cutaneous exposure to excessive circumambient air and circumradiant heat of varying duration and intensity. Arch. Path. *43*:466, 1947.
151. Morris, A. H., and Spitzer, K. W.: Pulmonary pathophysiologic changes following thermal injury. U.S. Army Institute of Surgical Research. Annual Research Progress Report. Brooke Army Medical Center, Ft. Sam Houston, Texas. Section 52, 1, 1971.
152. Morris, P. J., Bondoc, C., and Burke, J. F.: The use of frequently changed skin allografts to promote healing in the non-healing infected ulcer. Surgery *60*:13, 1966.
153. Moyer, C. A.: Burns. *In* Harkins, H., Moyer, C. A., Rhoads, J. E., and Allen, J. G. (eds.): Surgery, Principles and Practice. Philadelphia, J. B. Lippincott Co., 1961.
154. Moyer, C. A.: The metabolism of burned mammals and its relationship to vaporizational heat loss and other parameters. *In* Artz, C. P. (ed.): Research in Burns. Philadelphia, F. A. Davis Co., 1962, pp. 113–120.
155. Moyer, C. A., Brentano, L., Grovens, D. L., Margraf, H. W., and Monafo, W. W.: Treatment of large human burns with 0.5 per cent silver nitrate. Arch. Surg. *90*:812, 1965.
156. Moyer, C. A., and Butcher, H. R., Jr. (eds.): Burns, Shock and Plasma Volume Regulation. St. Louis, C. V. Mosby, 1967, p. 355.
157. Moyer, C. A., Margraf, H. W., and Monafo, W. W.: Burn shock and extravascular sodium deficiency—treatment with Ringer's solution with lactate. Arch. Surg. *90*:799, 1965.
158. Muir, F. K.: Red cell destruction in burns with particular reference to the shock period. Brit. J. Plast. Surg. *14*:273, 1961.
159. Munster, A. M.: Alterations of the host defense mechanisms in burns. Surg. Clin. N. Amer. *50*:1217, 1970.
160. Munster, A. M., Bruck, H. M., Johns, L. A., et al.: Heterotopic calcification following burns: A prospective study. J. Trauma *12*:1071, 1972.
161. Munster, A. M., Eurenius, K., Katz, R. M., et al.: Cell-mediated immunity after thermal injury. Ann. Surg. *177*:139, 1973.
162. Nash, G., Asch, M. J., Foley, F. D., and Pruitt, B. A., Jr.: Disseminated cytometalic inclusion disease in a burned adult. J.A.M.A. *214*:587, 1970.
163. Nash, G., Foley, F. D., and Pruitt, B. A.: *Candida* burn wound invasion: a cause of systemic candidiasis. Arch. Path. *90*:75, 1970.
164. Nylen, B., and Wallenius, G.: The protein loss via exudation from burns and granulating wound surfaces. Acta Chir. Scand. *122*:97, 1961.
165. O'Neill, J. A., Jr.: The influence of thermal burns on gastric acid secretion. Surg. *67*:267, 1970.
166. O'Neill, J. A., Jr., Pruitt, B. A., Jr., Monerret, J. A., et al.: Studies related to the pathogenesis of Curling's ulcer. J. Trauma *7*:275, 1967.
167. Order, S. E., Mason, A. D., Jr., Walker, H. L., et al.: Vascular destructive effects of thermal injury and its relationship to burn wound sepsis. J. Trauma *5*:62, 1965.
168. Order, S. E., and Moncrief, J. A.: The Burn Wound. Springfield, Ill., Charles C Thomas, 1965.
169. Phillips, A. W., and Cope, O.: Burn therapy.

II. The revelation of respiratory tract as principal killer. Ann. Surg. *155*:1, 1962.

170. Phillips, A. W., and Cope, A.: Burn Therapy, III. Beware the facial burn. Ann. Surg. *156*:759, 1962.
171. Phillips, A. W., Tanner, J. W., and Cope, O.: Burn therapy. IV. Respiratory tract damage (an account of the clinical, x-ray and post mortem findings) and the meaning of restlessness. Ann. Surg. *158*:799, 1963.
172. Pierson, C., and Feller, I.: A reduction of Pseudomonas septicemias in burned patients by the immune process. Surg. Clin. N. Amer. *50*:1377, 1970.
173. Pillsbury, D. M., Shelley, W. B., and Kligman, A. M.: Dermatology. Philadelphia, W. B. Saunders Co., 1956.
174. Pitts, W., Pickrell, K., Quinn, G., et al.: Electrical burns of lips and mouth in infants and children. Plast. Reconstr. Surg. *44*:471, 1969.
175. Polk, H. C., Monafo, W. W., Jr., and Moyer, C. A.: Human burn survival: study of the efficacy of 0.5% aqueous silver nitrate. Arch. Surg. *98*:262, 1969.
176. Pruitt, B. A., and Curreri, P. W.: The burn wound and its care. Arch. Surg. *103*:461, 1971.
177. Pruitt, B. A., Jr., DiVincenti, F. C., Mason, A. D., Jr., et al.: The occurrence and significance of pneumonia and other pulmonary complications in burned patients: comparison of conventional and topical treatments. J. Trauma *10*:519, 1970.
178. Pruitt, B. A., Jr., Foley, F. D., and Moncrief, J. A.: Curling's ulcer: a clinical-pathological study of 323 cases. Ann. Surg. *172*:523, 1970.
179. Pruitt, B. A., Jr., Mason, A. D., Jr., and Moncrief, J. A.: Hemodynamic changes in the early postburn patient: The influence of fluid administration and of a vasodilator (Hydralazine). J. Trauma *11*:36, 1971.
180. Pruitt, B. A., and Moncrief, J. A.: Current trends in burn research. J. Surg. Res. *7*:280, 1967.
181. Pruitt, B. A., Jr., Stein, J. M., Foley, F. D., et al.: Intravenous therapy in burn patients: Suppurative thrombophlebitis and other life-threatening complications. Arch. Surg. *100*:399, 1970.
182. Pruitt, B. A., Tumbusch, W. T., Mason, A. D., and Pearson, E.: Mortality in 1100 consecutive burns treated at burns unit. Ann. Surg. *159*:396, 1964.
183. Pulaski, E. J., and Tennison, C. W.: Quoted in Artz, C. P., and Reiss, E. (eds.): The Treatment of Burns. Philadelphia, W. B. Saunders Co., 1957, p. 9.
184. Quinby, W. C.: Restrictive effects of thoracic burns in children. J. Trauma *12*:646, 1972.
185. Quintanilla, R., Krusen, F. H., and Essex, H. E.: Studies on frost-bite with special reference to treatment and the effect on minute blood vessels. Am. J. Physiol. *149*:149, 1947.
186. Rappaport, I., Pepino, A. T., and Dietrick, W.: Early use of xenografts as a biologic dressing in burn trauma. Am. J. Surg. *120*:144, 1970.
187. Reckler, J. M., Bruck, H. M., Munster, A. M., et al.: Superior mesenteric artery syndrome as a consequence of burn injury. J. Trauma *12*:979, 1972.
188. Rickells, L. R., Squire, J. R., Topley, E., and Lilly, H. A.: Human skin lipids with particular reference to the self-sterilizing power of the skin. Clin. Sci. *10*:89, 1951.
189. Richetts, C. R., Lowbury, E. J. L., Lawrence, J. C., et al.: Mechanism of prophylaxis by silver compounds against infection in burns. Brit. Med. J. *1*:444, 1970.
190. Roe, C. F., and Kinney, J. M.: The caloric equivalent of fever. II. Influence of major trauma. Ann. Surg. *161*:140, 1965.
191. Robinson, N. W., Masters, F. W., and Forest, W. J.: Electrical burns: A review and analysis of 33 cases. Surgery *57*:385, 1965.
192. Robson, M. C., and Heggers, J. P.: Bacterial quantification of open wounds. Mil. Med. *134*:19, 1969.
193. Robson, M. C., Krizek, T. J., and Heggers, J. P.: Biology of surgical infection. Current Problems of Surgery, March 1973.
194. Robson, M. C., and Krizek, T. J.: The effect of human amniotic membranes on the bacterial population of infected rat burns. Ann. Surg. *177*:144, 1973.
195. Robson, M. C., and Krizek, T. J.: Predicting skin graft survival, J. Trauma *13*:213, 1973.
196. Rosenberg, S. A., Brief, D. K., Kinsley, J. M., Herrera, M. G., Wilson, R. E., and Moore, F. D.: The syndrome of dehydration, coma and severe hyperglycemia without ketosis in patients convalescing from burns. New Eng. J. Med. *222*:931, 1965.
197. Rubin, L. R., and Bongiovi, J., Jr.: Central venous pressure: Unreliable guide to fluid therapy in burns. Arch. Surg. *100*:269, 1970.
198. Sabella, N.: Use of fetal membranes in skin grafting. Med. Rec. N.Y. *83*:478, 1913.
199. Sachatello, C. R., and Stephenson, S. E., Jr.: High voltage burns. Am. Surg. *31*:807, 1965.
200. Schumacker, H. B., Jr., and Kilman, J. W.:

Sympathectomy in the treatment of frostbite. Arch. Surg. *89*:575, 1964.

201. Schumaker, H. B., White, B. H., Wrenn, E. L., Cordell, A. R., and Sanford, T. F.: Studies in experimental frostbite—The effect of heparin in preventing gangrene. Surgery *22*:900, 1947.
202. Sevitt, S.: Duodenal and gastric ulceration after burning. Brit . J. Surg. *54*:32, 1967.
203. Shuck, J. M., Bedeau, G. W. and Thomas, P. R. S.: Homograft skin for the early management of difficult wounds. J. Trauma *12*:215, 1972.
204. Shuck, J. M., and Moncrief, J. A.: The management of burns. Part I: General considerations and the sulfamylon method. Curr. Prob. Surg. February 1969.
205. Shuck, J. M., Moncrief, J. A., and Monafo, W. W.: The management of burns. Curr. Probl. Surg. 38–41, 1969.
206. Shuck, J. M., Pruitt, B. A., Jr., and Moncrief, J. A.: Homograft skin for wound coverage: A study in versatility. Arch. Surg. *98*:472, 1969.
207. Silversides, J.: The neurological sequelae of electrical injury. Can. Med. Assoc. J. *91*:195, 1964.
208. Silverstein, P., and Dressler, D. P.: Effect of current therapy on burn mortality. Ann. Surg. *171*:124, 1970.
209. Silverstein, P., Helmkamp, G. M., Walker, H. L., and Pruitt, B. A., Jr.: Laboratory evaluation of enzymatic burn wound debridement *in vitro* and *in vivo*. Surg. Forum *23*:31–33, 1972.
210. Soroff, H. S., Pearson, E., and Artz, C. P.: An estimation of the nitrogen requirements for equilibrium in burned patients. Surg. Gynec. Obstet. *112*:159, 1961.
211. Stanford, W., Rappole, B. W., and Fox, C. L., Jr.: Clinical experience with silver sulfadiazine, a new topical agent for control of *Pseudomonas* infection in burns. J. Trauma *9*:377, 1969.
212. Stellar, S., Levine, N., Ger, R., and Levenson, S. M.: Laser excision of acute third-degree burns followed by immediate autograft replacement: An experimental study in the pig. J. Trauma *13*:45, 1973.
213. Stenberg, T., and Hogeman, K. E.: Experimental and clinical investigations on liver function in burns. *In* Artz, C. P. (ed.): Research in Burns. Philadelphia, F. A. Davis Co., 1962, pp. 171–176.
214. Stone, H. H.: Review of pseudomonas sepsis in thermal burns. Verdoglobin determination and Gentamicin therapy. Ann. Surg. *163*:297, 1966.
215. Stone, H. H.: Wound care with topical gentamicin. *In* Polk, H. C., and Stone, H. H. (eds.): Contemporary Burn Management. Boston, Little, Brown, 1971, pp. 203–216.
216. Stone, H. H., and Kolb, L. D.: The evolution and spread of gentamicin-resistant pseudomonads. J. Trauma *11*:586, 1971.
217. Stone, H. H., Martin, J. D., Huger, W. E., and Kolb, L.: Gentamicin sulfate in the treatment of pseudomonas sepsis in burns. Surg. Gynec. Obstet. *120*:351, 1965.
218. Sugarbaker, P., Sabath, L., and Morgan, A.: Neomycin toxicity from porcine skin xenografts. Presentation, American Burn Association, Dallas, Texas, April 1973.
219. Summerlin, W. T., and Artz, C. P.: Gentamicin sulfate therapy of experimentally induced pseudomonas septicemia. J. Trauma *6*:233, 1966.
220. Switzer, W. E., Moncrief, J. A., Mills, W., Order, S. E., and Lindberg, R. B.: The use of canine heterografts in the therapy of thermal injury. J. Trauma *6*:391, 1966.
221. Taylor, P. H., Moncrief, J. A., Pugsley, L. G., Rose, L. R., and Switzer, W. E.: The management of extensively burned patients by staged excision. Surg. Gynec. Obstet. *115*:347, 1962.
222. Taylor, P. H., Pugsley, L. Q., and Vogel, E. H., Jr.: The intriguing electrical burn: A review of thirty-one electrical burn cases. J. Trauma *2*:309, 1962.
223. Teplitz, C.: Pathogenesis of pseudomonas vasculitis and septic lesions. Arch. Path. *80*:297, 1965.
224. Teplitz, C., Davis, D., Mason, A. D., and Moncrief, J. A.: Pseudomonas burn wound sepsis. I. Pathogenesis of experimental pseudomonas burn wound sepsis. J. Surg. Res. *4*:200, 1964.
225. Teplitz, C., Davis, D., Walker, H. L., Raulston, G. L., Mason, A. D., and Moncrief, J. A.: Pseudomonas burn wound sepsis. II. Hematogenous infection at the junction of the burn wound and the unburned hypodermis. J. Surg. Res. *4*:217, 1964.
226. Ternberg, J. L., and Luce, E.: Methemoglobinemia: Complication of the silver nitrate treatment of burns. Surgery *63*: 328, 1968.
227. Treves, N., and Pack, G. T.: Development of cancer in burn scars. Surg. Gynec. Obstet. *51*:749, 1930.
228. Tumbusch, W. T., Vogel, E. H., Butkiewicz, J. V., Graber, C. D., Larson, D. L., and Mitchell, E. T.: Septicemia in burn injury. J. Trauma *1*:22, 1961.
229. Waisbren, B. A.: Antibiotics in the treatment of burns. Surg. Clin. N. Amer. *50*:1311, 1970.
230. Walker, H. L., Mason, A. D., Jr., and Raulston, G. L.: Surface infection

with pseudomonas aeruginosa. Ann. Surg. *160*:297, 1964.
231. Wallace, A. B.: Treatment of burns; a return to basic principles. Brit. J. Plast. Surg. *2*:232, 1949.
232. Wartman, W. B.: Mechanisms of death in severe burn injury: The need for planned autopsies. *In* Artz, C. P. (ed.): Research in Burns. Philadelphia, F. A. Davis Co., 1962, pp. 6–13.
233. Washburn, B.: Frost-bite—what it is—how to prevent it. Emergency treatment. New Eng. J. Med. *266*:974, 1962.
234. Weatherley-White, R. C. A., Paton, B. C., and Sjöstrom, B. L.: Experimental studies in cold injury. III. Observations on the treatment of frostbite. Plast. Reconstr. Surg. *36*:10, 1965.
235. Weatherley-White, R. C. A., Sjöstrom, B. L., and Paton, B. C.: Experimental studies in cold injury: II. The pathogenesis of frostbite. J. Surg. Res. *4*:17, 1964.
236. Wickman, K.: Studies on burns. XIV. Acta Chir. Scand. 140 (suppl.) 408, 1970.
237. Wilmore, D. W., Curreri, P. W., Spitzer, K. W., et al.: Supranormal dietary intake in thermally injured hypermetabolic patients. Surg. Gynec. Obstet. *132*:881, 1971.
238. Wright, H. K., Gann, D. S., and Drucker, W. R.: Current concept of therapy for derangements of extra-cellular fluid. *In* Davis, J. H. (ed.): Current Concepts in Surgery. New York, McGraw-Hill Book Co., 1965.
239. Zaroff, L. I., Mills, W., Jr., Duckett, J. W., et al.: Multiple uses of viable cutaneous homografts in the burned patient. Surgery *59*:368, 1966.
240. Zawacki, B. E., and Pearson, H. E.: Epidemic nosocomial infection by antibiotic-proof Providencia: Its origin, course and relation to topical chemotherapy on a large burn ward. Presentation, American Burn Association, Dallas, Texas, April 1973.
241. Zuidema, G. D., Clarke, N. P., Prine, J. R., and Salzman, E. W.: An experimental study relating fabric types with severity of burns. Surg. Gynec. Obstet. *103*:581, 1956.

chapter

21

TRAUMA AND THE CHILD

J. Alex Haller, Jr., M.D.
and
James L. Talbert, M.D.

In 1963 four out of every ten children who died in the United States were victims of trauma.[36] The same was true in Europe; in 1964 Stolowsky (Germany) estimated that one-third of all childhood deaths were a direct or indirect result of trauma with little chance of survival. It is now estimated that for the United States in 1970, one out of every two children who dies between the ages of one year and 14 years will die as a result of major injuries![12]

A majority of accidents in childhood occur between the ages of two and seven years.[36] One-fourth of the accidents of 17,000 children seen at the Sick Children's Hospital in Toronto in a single year occurred between the ages of two and three years; one-half occurred between two and seven years.[22] Thus, from the standpoint of public health and accident prevention, the greatest problem exists in the transition years between total parental protection and adequate education for self-preservation; the greatest risk is encountered during this period of transfer of responsibility from the parent to the child.

Although the death rate from serious accidents is higher in young children than in adults, the hospital morbidity and the long-term sequelae of these injuries have even greater medical and social significance. It has been conservatively estimated that approximately 50,000 children are permanently crippled by accidents every year and that another two million are incapacitated.[7] This enormous rehabilitation problem will increase each year simply on the basis of the increase in size of this segment of our population.

No evaluation of the expense and grief to the individual family can be meaningful. From a more objective viewpoint, however, this carnage represents an inestimable loss in potential earning power which could be coldly calculated in dollars and cents. If this fact were not sufficient to document the economic problem, a consideration of the actual years lost by the death of a child further emphasizes the tragedy of trauma in childhood. Ten adults of 50 years lose an additive 150 years by sudden death, but ten young children lose 600 years. Trauma in childhood differs qualitatively from adult trauma but quantitative differences are more strikingly apparent.

GENERAL PRINCIPLES IN THE CARE OF THE INJURED CHILD

In the management of major trauma, the necessity for immediate, accurate evaluation of the extent of injury is not unique to the child. The margin for error in this age group is far less, however, and some aspects merit special emphasis.

The responses of young children to serious trauma are qualitatively, as well as quantitatively, different from those of adults. For example, abdominal distention and diaphragmatic elevation from post-traumatic ileus are greater threats to the limited chest volume of children than to adults. Any blood loss assumes dramatic importance with the tiny blood volume of a young child. Increased surface area in a child allows excessive and rapid heat loss, especially in situations of multiple injuries and prolonged exposure during emergency management. Transfusion of large quantities of cold blood and fluids may lead to further serious loss of body heat. Associated congenital defects are much more likely to complicate the management of serious injury in children, especially those related to congenital heart abnormalities. The characteristic ability of a young child in his response to stress demands the utmost vigilance in detecting subtle signs of inadequate response to ongoing treatment. Blunt trauma is responsible for probably 80 to 90 per cent of serious injuries in children. External evidence of internal injury may be misleading and result in serious delay in operative treatment. This is especially true of multiple injuries which involve the head, and head injuries are associated with multiple trauma in children in a much higher percentage than in adults. Associated with these head injuries is a much higher incidence of subdural hematoma in children. Head injuries greatly increase the difficulty of evaluating generalized trauma in children, for it is similar to blunt trauma in a drunken adult. A young child may be unable to express his pain and to localize his symptoms, even when he is conscious; this fact places multiple trauma in childhood almost in the category of veterinary medicine. Finally, serious injuries in an immature child may have disastrous effects upon his emotional well-being at this impressionable age. The terror of separation from familiar faces is greatly magnified by the usual busy and impersonal environment of a major emergency room. Serious emotional aftereffects are not uncommon from even minor injuries which are treated under threatening circumstances by physicians who are not aware of this important additional insult to a child.[13]

Each patient deserves his physician's maximal kindness and compassion. Unfortunately, this truism meets its most stringent challenge in a busy emergency treatment room. The few moments required to win the confidence and trust of a child, however, reward the doctor by facilitating his examination and by ensuring the validity of his observations. There are few more difficult tasks than attempting to evaluate the abdomen of an apprehensive, struggling child.

After major injuries have been excluded, sedation is an important and useful adjunct in the treatment of minor trauma in children. Pentobarbital in a dosage of 5 mg. per kg. of body weight or the popular "lytic cocktail" may be employed for this purpose. The standard lytic cocktail used on the Pediatric Surgical Service of The Johns Hopkins Hospital is composed of Demerol (2 mg. per kg.), Phenergan (2 mg. per kg.) and Thorazine (2 mg. per kg.). These drugs are administered intramuscularly, 45 to 60 minutes prior to painful procedures. This regimen should not be employed in infants less than one year of age. The total dosage of Phenergan and Thorazine should not exceed 50 mg. each, and the dosage of Demerol should not exceed 150 mg. It must be remembered that any contraindication to general anesthesia is equally applicable to heavy sedation. Standard formulas are useful only as baselines and must be adapted by the physician to the individual child and situation.

Both preoperative sedation and local anesthesia require a critical delay period before their maximal effect is realized. Haste may obviate any reward that might otherwise be expected.

Positioning and restraint of children is particularly important for minor surgical procedures. Details of the techniques of restraining children (Fig. 21–1) as well as other forms of specialized treatment are ably presented by Dr. Walter T. Hughes, Jr., in his book, *Pediatric Procedures*.[19]

Most techniques in management of local trauma are no different in the child than in the adult. The physician should be encouraged, however, to use fine suture material in the younger patient, both for technical and cosmetic reasons.

Serious trauma in the young child presents the classic "raison d'etre" for a trauma unit directed by a general surgeon. In a few medical centers, new children's trauma units, distinct from but closely coordinated with adult trauma units, have been developed and offer innovative approaches to emergency care for this special group of patients. In such centers the children's trauma unit may be directed by a pediatric surgeon who is, in essence, a general surgeon for children. The need for command decisions cutting across specialty fields and the high incidence of injuries to multiple organ systems makes the injured child a clear example of the need for a team approach to trauma.

The following cases illustrate the multiplicity of systems that may be involved in severe trauma and the importance of appointing a surgeon with a diversity of experience—in most instances a general surgeon—as the coordinator of patient care.

Case History No. 1. K. B., JHH #111 65 97. A four-year-old girl was brought to the Emergency Room in a semicomatose state shortly after being struck by an automobile. The remainder of the history was sketchy, but it was subsequently learned that the patient had been thrown into the air by the initial impact only to fall back on the hood of the car, thereby suffering a second blow.

The vital signs on admission were surprisingly stable. Although she was semiconscious, the child's mental status appeared to stabilize under observation. In the course of the next hour a thorough evaluation, including multiple x-ray studies, revealed the following injuries:

1. Multiple fractures of the right pelvis.
2. Fractures of the left mandible.
3. Vaginal tear from a bone spicule of the pelvic fracture.
4. Contusion of the left cerebral hemisphere as manifested by decreased level of consciousness, right hemiparesis and clonus of the right leg.
5. Fracture of the right first rib.
6. Right pulmonary contusion.
7. Abrasion of right cornea.
8. Laceration of lip.
9. Multiple contusions and abrasions of the body.

Although mild hematuria was evident initially, an intravenous pyelogram failed to demonstrate any significant renal injury. The urethra and bladder were demonstrated to be intact on cystogram, although a large right retroperitoneal hematoma from the pelvic fracture distorted the lateral bladder wall.

Despite some localization of cerebral signs, the absence of any significant deterioration combined with actual stabilization of the patient's condition appeared to allow further observation. The question of coexistent, unrecognized intra-abdominal trauma was another contraindication to immediate craniotomy. Accordingly, the patient was admitted to the Intensive Care Unit of The Children's Medical and Surgical Center where close monitoring of the vital signs, with fluid and colloid replace-

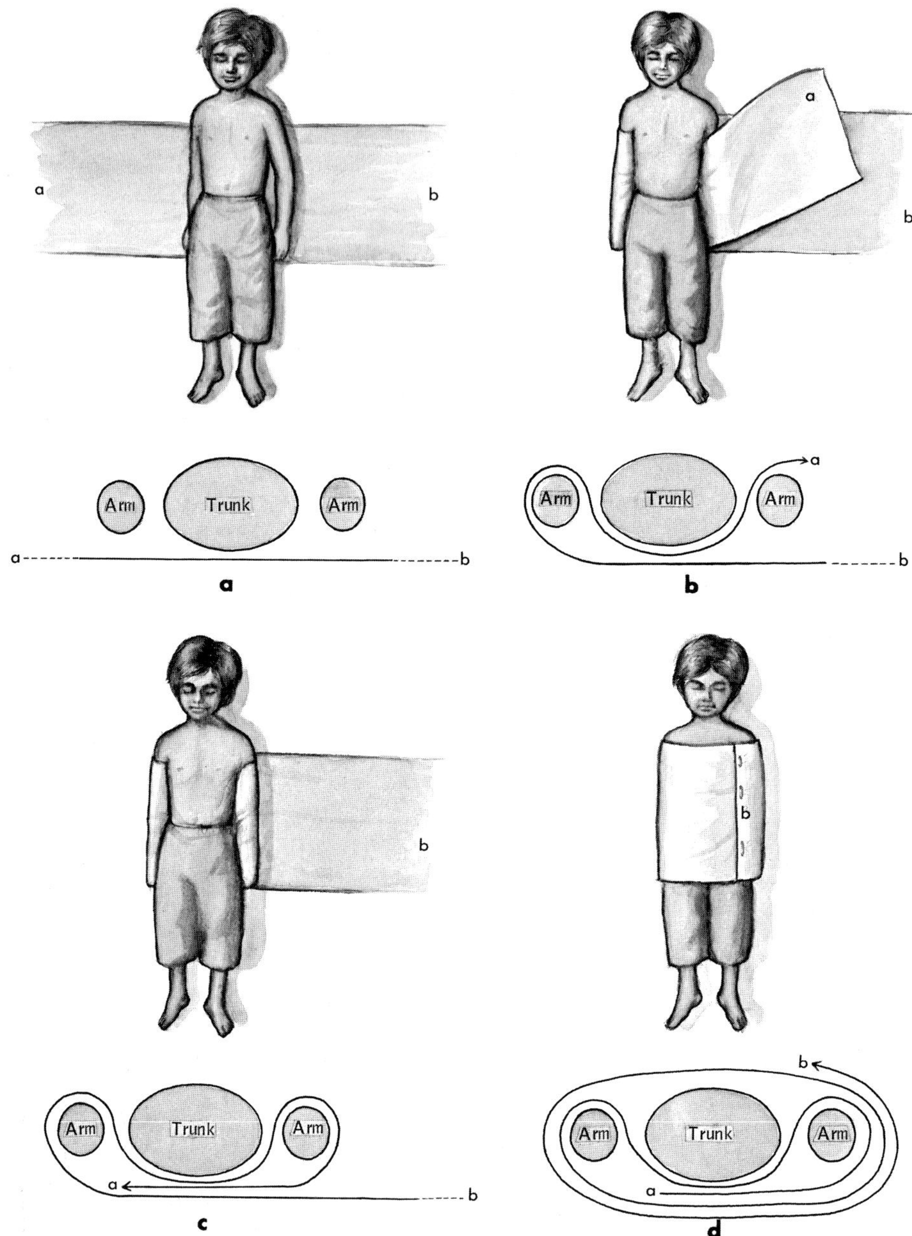

Figure 21–1 A technique of body restraint for the infant and young child. (From Hughes, W. T., Jr.: Pediatric Procedure.)

ment was undertaken. The pulmonary congestion secondary to the right lung contusion progressed, resulting in an acute episode of respiratory embarrassment. Tracheal intubation and positive pressure respiration were instituted. (We would now use continuous positive pressure breathing with a volume ventilator and with an end expiratory pressure of 5–10 cm. H_2O.) Subsequently it was elected to perform a tracheostomy while the endotracheal tube was in place. The tracheostomy tube was attached to a Mörch type respirator, modified by Benson.[2]* See

*Currently manufactured as the Emerson Piston Respirator, J. H. Emerson Company, Cambridge 40, Massachusetts.

Chapter 4 for details of positive pressure ventilation.

The patient's general picture was one of gradual improvement. The positive pressure respirator was discontinued after four days because of clearing of the right lung. The level of consciousness also improved to the point that the patient responded to verbal stimuli by 12 days. A cerebral arteriogram obtained during this period confirmed the absence of a subdural hematoma. After 30 days the patient spoke her first words. In six months she had recovered completely from her injuries and had no evidence of either physical or mental retardation.

It can be easily understood how associated serious injuries might escape detection in the natural concern that arises during treatment of any one of the many systems involved. Only with the appointment of a single coordinator of therapy can such errors of omission be minimized. Although some cases appear to involve only one specialty service, the importance of having all cases of pediatric trauma seen by the general surgeon is again emphasized by the following example.

Case History No. 2. W. B., JHH #114 93 74. A three-year-old boy was admitted to the Accident Room with a history of having been struck by an automobile. There was no suggestion that the patient had been crushed or run over. He had lost consciousness for several minutes, but his sensorium was relatively clear on admission. There was no subsequent deterioration in his mental state. Admission examination revealed a large contusion and smaller laceration of the left fronto-occipital area of the skull. There were no localizing neurologic signs. The remainder of the examination was within normal limits except for minimal contusions of the left flank. Specifically, there was no evidence of abdominal tenderness; bowel sounds were active.

The hematocrit was 34 per cent on admission, the white blood cell count was 22,000 and urinalysis revealed 25 to 30 red blood cells per high powered field. Skull x-rays demonstrated a large depressed skull fracture, but abdominal and chest x-rays were interpreted as normal. An intravenous pyelogram subsequently demonstrated good bilateral renal function.

Approximately one and a half hours following admission, at the termination of the work-up just outlined, the patient was first noted by the general surgical consultant to have developed left upper quadrant abdominal tenderness. The hematocrit was rechecked and remained 35 per cent. The central venous pressure was also stable. In view of the strong possibility of intra-abdominal injury and the necessity for elevation of the depressed skull fracture, simultaneous exploratory laparotomy and craniotomy were performed.

This decision was clearly justified by the physical signs of peritoneal irritation and was substantiated by the finding of a ruptured spleen at laparotomy. Splenectomy and an open reduction of multiple skull fractures were performed. The postoperative course was uneventful, and the patient was discharged 13 days later.

The recognition of coexistent abdominal and cerebral trauma and the prompt institution of treatment avoided the confusion that inevitably results when a patient undergoing craniotomy for a head trauma develops hypotension at the time of surgery. Hidden bleeding from a ruptured spleen or other organ may pass unrecognized in these situations and may prove fatal. Screening of trauma cases by a general surgeon helps to decrease the frequency of such problems. There can be no substitute for immediate total evaluation of the seriously injured patient. This fact is strongly underlined in the pediatric age group.

SPECIAL CONSIDERATIONS IN THE TREATMENT OF TRAUMA IN INFANTS

Size. The small size of the injured child is the single most influential factor differentiating his management from that of the adult. The margin for error is diminished correspondingly and may seem infinitesimal in the newborn and premature infant. Seemingly trivial details, which assume importance only in complicated cases of adult trauma, demand routine attention in the management of children.

The obvious discrepancies in physical size of adults and children are reflected in alteration of physiologic function. The importance of a tiny blood volume is immediately apparent. In the newborn infant a single blood-soaked sponge may represent the difference between circulatory stability and shock.

Respiratory Reserve. From both an anatomic and physiologic standpoint, the infant has a much lower respiratory reserve than the adult.[17] The vital capacity at one week of age is approximately 140 ml. and the tidal volume is 15 ml. The trachea may be only 4 cm. in length and 6 mm. in diameter. These factors coupled with a weak thoracic musculature, flexible rib cage and narrow air passages all complicate the movement of tracheobronchial secretions.

Heat Loss. The increased surface area of the infant relative to his weight allows excessive heat loss under circumstances of debility. The thermal regulatory mechanism of children often is unable to meet the requirements of such situations, and great care must be taken to monitor and support the temperature of all infants. This inadequacy is magnified by the transfusion of large quantities of cold blood, a circumstance that may lead to rapid loss of body heat and even significant cardiac arrhythmias.

Fluid and Electrolyte Balance. Fluid and electrolyte balance presents an additional problem in these small patients. Although numerous formulas have been devised for the routine maintenance of fluid and electrolytes in children, they are usually inadequate in situations leading to rapid internal or external losses of fluids. The physiologic maturity of the baby may play an important role in such circumstances. Renal immaturity in the newborn is reflected in an inability to concentrate and conserve fluid and electrolytes. There is a concomitant limitation in glomerular filtration rate. The combination of these two factors restricts the infant's ability to respond to conditions of stress and increased metabolic demand.

Drug Therapy. The general physiologic immaturity of the infant also may exert its influence in other areas. Any physician caring for such patients must have a thorough knowledge of possible drug idiosyncrasies as well as proper dosages for this age group. Chloramphenicol, vitamin K, sulfonamides, atropine, aspirin, succinylcholine, novobiocin and digitalis are particularly hazardous for the newborn if administered improperly.[8, 28] Chloramphenicol, of course, has been implicated in the production of aplastic anemia in children; but, in neonates, it may also be responsible for a picture of acute vascular collapse which has been descriptively labeled the "gray baby syndrome." Vitamin K toxicity may be reflected in hyperbilirubinemia. This complication is related to the administration of the water-soluble derivatives of menadione (Hykinone, Synkayvite) and may be prevented either by the limitation of dosage or substitution of vitamin K_1 (Mephyton, Konakion). The administration of sulfonamides has been associated with an unusual incidence of kernicterus in premature infants. Overdosage of atropine may result in central nervous system involvement in newborns. Extensive discussions of these and other hazards are presented in the accompanying references.[8, 28]

The necessity for adjusting medication dosages in infants to the variables of weight and surface area is immediately apparent. However, other factors such as alterations in rate of absorption and excretion, differences in distribution and, finally, variables in metabolism and detoxification are equally important in newborn and premature infants. It is recommended that any group caring for an injured child include a physician who is conversant with these problems.

Congenital Defects. Another potential source of complications in the management of injured children is the coexistence of congenital anomalies. Cardiac defects are of particular significance. A unique example of a complicating anomaly was seen recently in a small child hospitalized for a supracondylar fracture of the elbow. There was no evidence of coexistent abdominal trauma. However, the child subsequently developed signs and symptoms of partial intestinal obstruction and was found to have a partial malrotation with volvulus of the small intestine.

Response to Trauma. Lability often is cited as the outstanding characteristic of the response of infants and children to trauma. *The smaller the size of the patient, the briefer the transition from health to illness and illness to death.* The utmost vigilance is demanded in detecting the subtle signs that suggest alterations in the infant's condition. Fortunately, the elasticity of the healthy child's response seems boundless, allowing a rapid compensation for potential catastrophes if corrections can be instituted promptly.

SPECIAL TECHNIQUES IN THE MANAGEMENT OF TRAUMA IN CHILDHOOD

Fluid and Electrolyte Balance. As indicated, the single most difficult task in the management of a small infant or child may involve adequate fluid and electrolyte replacement. To the physician who infrequently handles children the maintenance of such a patient on prolonged parenteral replacement itself poses a formidable challenge. Knowledge of fluid and electrolyte therapy in infants and children has advanced tremendously in recent years, with an increased understanding of the physiologic mechanisms that are involved.

Many formulas have been devised for the calculation of maintenance fluids in children, but the most rational ones appear to be those based on the rate of metabolic turnover. The use of this factor enables one to consolidate his thinking in terms of a single variable, that is, allows an integration of the basal requirements with the additional influences of activity and environmental temperature. With this approach, one is furnished simultaneously with the caloric requirements of his patient. This figure becomes increasingly important in situations demanding long-term parenteral alimentation.

CALORIC REQUIREMENTS. Table 21–1 is a brief outline of basal caloric requirements in children varying in weight from 3 to 31 kg. The maintenance supply of water for the average patient varies from 110 to 120 ml. per 100 calories metabolized.[27] Thus, the maintenance fluid requirements of

TABLE 21–1 STANDARD BASAL CALORIES*

WEIGHT (kg.)	CALORIES/24 HOURS MALE AND FEMALE	
3	140	
5	270	
7	400	
9	500	
11	600	
13	650	
15	710	
17	780	
19	830	
21	880	
25	1020	960
29	1120	1040
33	1210	1120
37	1300	1190
41	1350	1260
45	1410	1320
49	1470	1380
53	1530	1440
57	1590	1500
61	1640	1560

Increments or decrements

1. Add or subtract 12 per cent of above for each degree C. (8 per cent for each degree F.) above or below rectal temperature of 37.8° C. (100° F.)
2. Add 0 to 30 per cent increments for activity.

*From Cooke, R. E., *In* Nelson, W. E. (ed.): Textbook of Pediatrics. 8th Ed.

a child may be obtained easily by multiplying this last figure (110–120) by the calculated caloric requirement divided by 100 (the latter having been obtained by adjusting the standard basal caloric requirement [Table 21–1] to conditions of temperature and activity). The postoperative patient, of course, will have a tendency to retain water and certain electrolytes, and maintenance fluids should not exceed 80 to 90 cc. per 100 calories metabolized.

FLUID RETENTION. The tendency of pediatric patients to retain fluids postoperatively seems to vary directly with age. An infant, for instance, has a much briefer period of water retention postoperatively than an older child. There is also an individual variation in fluid and electrolyte excretion in children, especially during infancy. However, the average sodium requirement for parenteral fluid therapy is 2 to 4 mEq., and the potassium requirement is 2 to 3 mEq. for each 100 calories metabolized. A solution of 5 or 10 per cent glucose containing 30 mEq. of sodium and chloride and 20 mEq. of potassium per liter represents an adequate maintenance fluid which meets the usual requirements when administered intravenously at the rate of 110 to 120 ml. per 100 calories metabolized.

MASSIVE REPLACEMENT. The difficulties of fluid maintenance in infants and small children are compounded in situations demanding massive volume replacement. Little effort has been made to simplify this problem in the small patient, although great strides have been taken in monitoring similar shifts of fluids in adults.[38] Fortunately, the elasticity of the child is such that he will often weather prolonged episodes of relative hyper- or hypovolemia without lasting damage. Even so, inaccuracies in replacement therapy may spell the difference in ultimate survival. In an effort to consolidate the various monitoring factors into a simplified, readily available scheme, the following approach has been adopted by the Pediatric Surgical Service of the Children's Medical and Surgical Center in The Johns Hopkins Hospital.

USE OF FLOW CHART. All patients admitted for major surgery or with severe trauma are monitored on a fluid and electrolyte flow chart with minimum six-hour calculations of balance. Important features of this system include measurements of central venous pressure, total serum solids, hematocrit, urinary specific gravity and serum electrolytes, with precise calculations of all fluid intake and output. The patient's vital signs and clinical response remain the most important criteria of adequate return of homeostasis. Such signs may be misleading, however, under certain situations, and the addition of the supplemental information outlined above allows a more controlled approach to patient management.

URINARY OUTPUT. Urinary output in the child is a sensitive index of volume expansion and renal perfusion, but here, again, one may be mislead. The newborn infant, for instance, may be limited in both his ability to increase volume and to concentrate urine.[29] As a result, urinary specific gravity in these patients may remain relatively low in the face of inadequate fluid intake. On the other hand, congestive failure may rapidly ensue from overhydration, since a diminished glomerular filtration rate limits the renal response in such situations. Older children present the same problems evident in the adult, in that the antidiuretic response of the immediate postoperative period may limit urinary output even with maximal hydration. Urinary output, then, is a valuable index of homeostasis only if intrinsic pitfalls are recognized.

CENTRAL VENOUS PRESSURE. The use of central venous pressure has found increasing advocates in recent years since its first application in the field of cardiac surgery.[3, 41] Again, this is not necessarily an absolute value. Rather, in the absence of a coexistent cardiorespiratory problem, this indicator provides an excellent index of functional intravascular volume. In essence, the central venous pressure is a direct reflection of the effective cardiac filling pressure. If there is decreased central venous pressure one may assume that additional fluids may be administered; whereas elevations of pressure, in the absence of local venous obstruction, indicate that the cardiac filling pressure is adequate for the state of cardiac function at that particular moment. In such circumstances other means of increasing cardiac output must be sought.

One reason central venous pressure has not been applied so widely in the infant as in the adult is the seeming sparsity of satisfactory sites through which central venous cannulation may be achieved.[37] Experience has indicated that catheterization of the inferior vena cava may be unfavorable in some children because of interference by abdominal pressure changes. Such situations may be particularly frequent in the infant and small child, in whom the changes in intra-abdominal pressure associated with distention, crying or breathing are much more pronounced than in adults. The sites for cannulation, therefore, are limited. Routes that have been chosen include the basilic vein in the antecubital fossa, and the external and internal jugular veins in the neck (Fig. 21–2). In infancy, such cannulation usually necessitates a cutdown. The internal jugular particularly is a sizable vein in infancy and offers a readily accessible spot for introduction of a large-bore catheter *when other routes are inadequate.* Such cannulation conceivably may be performed percutaneously, but direct exposure appears surer and possibly safer (Fig. 21–3). Percutaneous puncture of the subclavian vein, however, via the subclavicular route offers an alternate route, although there is a definite hazard of producing pneumothorax with this method and it is chosen only when other sites seem poorer. Such a situation did arise recently in a severely burned three

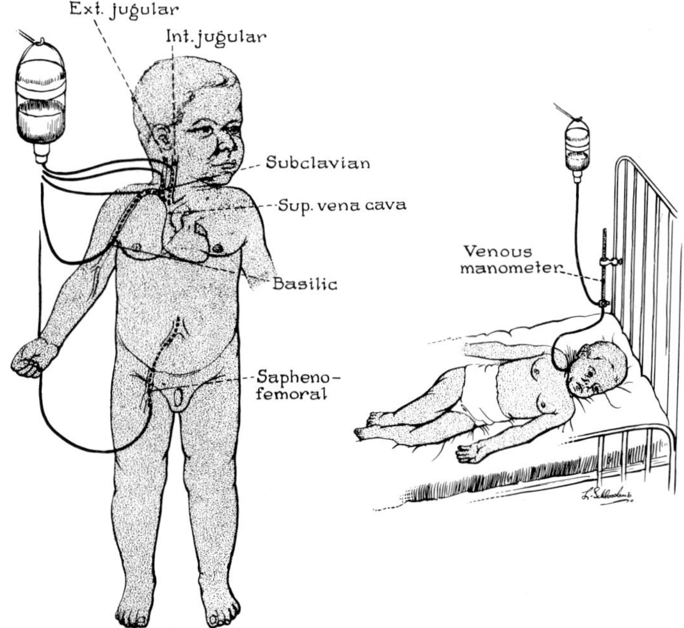

Figure 21–2 Sites for central venous pressure monitoring in the infant. (From Talbert, J. L., and Haller, J. A., Jr.: Amer. Surg. *32*:767, 1966.)

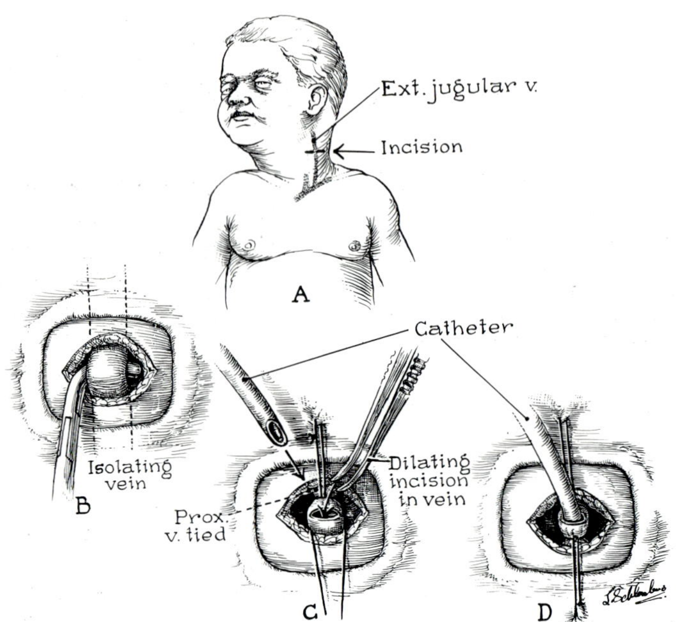

Figure 21–3 Catheterization of the external jugular vein as performed in the infant (*A* and *B*). The vein is isolated with a small curved clamp through a short, transverse skin incision. (*C*) A 4-0 plain catgut ligature is tied about the cephalic end of the vein. A second ligature is placed distally, with traction exerted in opposite directions by clamping the ties to the adjacent drapes. A transverse incision is made in the anterior wall of the vein. This opening is then enlarged by inserting and spreading the tips of a small curved forceps. (*D*) While the vein lumen is exposed in this manner, a beveled cannula may be introduced with relative ease. When the catheter has been positioned at the level of the innominate vein or superior vena cava, the second ligature is secured. The use of fine, plain catgut avoids any necessity for subsequent removal of these ligatures. The skin incision is closed with a single vertical mattress suture of fine silk. This same suture may be tied about the cannula with a separate knot at a point 1.5 cm. from the skin. By dividing this distal knot, subsequent withdrawal of the catheter is possible and removal of the skin suture itself may be avoided. Finally the cannula should always be carefully taped to the skin of the neck as an additional safeguard against accidental dislodgment. (Talbert, J. L., and Haller, J. A., Jr.: Amer. Surg. *32*:767, 1966.)

month old infant whose only area of uninvolved skin lay in the shoulder. Subclavian catheterization allowed fluid and antibiotic administration through this route for more than four weeks.

The importance of placing the monitoring catheter in a central position has been emphasized repeatedly. The effects of either venous spasm or valves interposed between the central and peripheral venous systems may lead to discrepancies if pressures are monitored peripherally.[41] When measured correctly, however, venous pressure provides an accurate guide to fluid volume, especially under conditions of massive replacement or hidden losses.

USE OF SERUM SOLIDS. The use of total serum solids as an indication of serum protein levels has become increasingly popular with the introduction of small, accurate refractometers (Fig. 21–4).[32] The measurements are particularly useful in situations associated with such massive fluid and concomitant protein losses as might occur in burns. The measurement has also been employed in monitoring major surgical and traumatic cases, however, and has been equally applicable in these instances. The losses incurred following major surgical dissections often consist primarily of protein rich fluid. Again, the measurement of total serum solids, coupled with simultaneous determi-

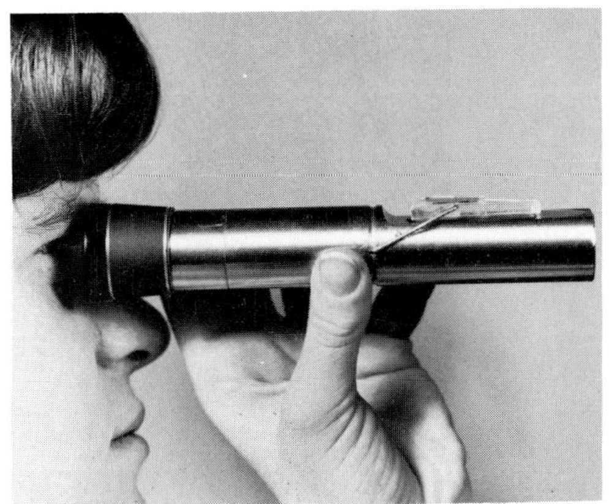

Figure 21–4 A total solid meter. This visual refractometer provides accurate measurements (maximum error 0.1 per cent TS) of urinary specific gravity, total serum solids and total serum proteins when one drop of test solution is placed between the measuring prisms on top of the instrument. In general, the serum contained in two small microhematocrit tubes is sufficient for such determinations. (TS Meter Model 10400. American Optical Company, Instrument Division, Buffalo 15, New York.)

nations of the hematocrit and venous pressure, allows considerable insight as to whether the patient requires water, plasma or blood replacement at any particular moment.

ADDITIONAL PROBLEMS. A flow chart, as outlined previously, coupled with daily determinations of body weight gives a continuing picture of the patient's condition. These data on the state of hydration and intravascular volume are particularly valuable in situations in which one is uncertain whether the oliguria (or anuria) that so often follows severe trauma is a reflection of primary renal damage or of inadequate replacement. The flow chart also serves as a valuable indicator of unusual trends in therapy and may allow the physician to anticipate and avoid complications prior to their development. The danger of overhydration and excessive transfusion in small infants may thus be obviated. Since none of these observations requires elaborate equipment, they should be readily accessible to the physician and, when coupled with determinations of serum electrolytes, offer a precise guide to therapy.

An additional hazard of massive fluid replacement in infants and small children is encountered in the administration of cold blood or plasma. These solutions must be warmed prior to their administration, if by no other means than coiling plastic intravenous tubing in a container of warm water. The warming water should not be hotter than 110 to 115°F. Relatively inexpensive equipment is available which is designed specifically for this purpose. Large quantities of citrated blood may necessitate calcium replacement in small infants. This practice has been followed for many years in adults but is relatively unimportant in this group as compared to infants whose calcium stores are more quickly expended and whose compensatory mechanisms are less able to respond to potential calcium depletion. A final complication of massive colloid replacement in children is the potentiation of the metabolic acidosis of shock by the infusion of stored blood or plasma. The seriousness of this problem is proportional to the size of the patient and the rapidity of replacement therapy. Administration of bicarbonate or tris buffer may be necessary in such circumstances.[19]

Another significant problem encountered in infants is the administration of small, precise quantities of parenteral fluids over prolonged periods. The use of a constant infusion pump, such as the Holter Pump, for this purpose has proved extremely useful (Fig. 21–5). Carefully measured volumes may be given at low flow rates with these units without fear of clotting in the intravenous tubing.

Although hypodermoclysis has proved helpful as a method of fluid administration in the past, the indica-

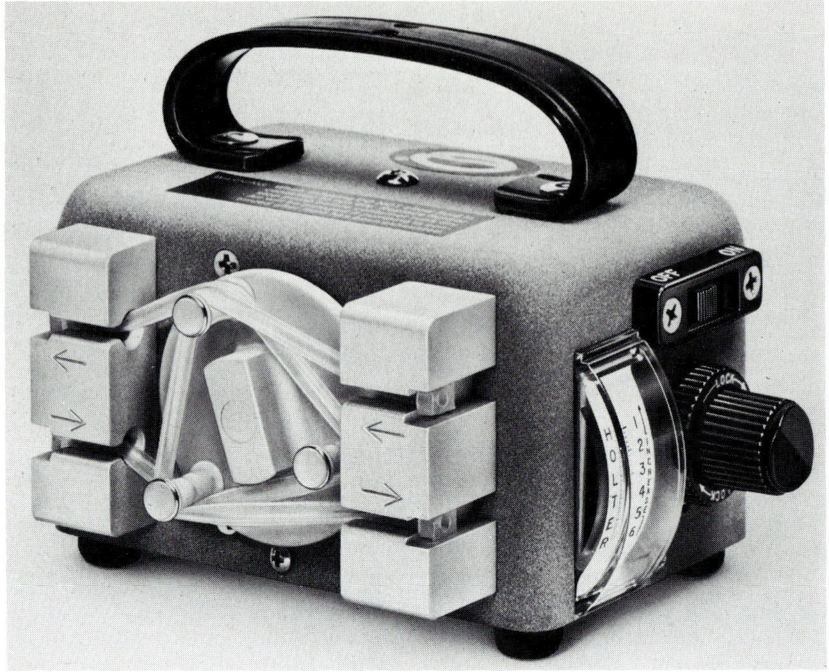

Figure 21–5 The Holter[R] Series 900 Infusion Pump provides a means of administering an exact amount of fluid at a controlled rate of infusion, thus avoiding many of the problems inherent in regulating intravenous drips in small infants. (Courtesy of Extracorporeal Medical Specialties, Inc., Royal and Ross Roads, King of Prussia, Pa.)

tions for its use on a trauma service are few indeed. Other routes of administration such as intra-arterial, intraperitoneal or intraosseous infusions are not necessary. There is no situation in which the indications for these approaches would obviate the potential hazards of their use.

Airway Provision. The establishment of an adequate airway in a child may also present special problems. The older child should be managed as an adult. That is, when prolonged respiratory support is demanded, a tracheostomy should be performed, using an adapter tube for the respirator. Tracheostomies in infants, however, are notorious for their accompanying complications. There are difficulties in the management of tiny tracheostomies and sometimes removal of the tube may be a problem. To obviate this problem some pediatric surgeons have resorted to prolonged use of endotracheal tubes.[39] Many of these physicians have been enthusiastic about this technique, but we have found that it also creates difficulties, especially increased problems with tracheobronchial secretions and damage to delicate laryngeal tissues. The concomitant use of steroids may help to diminish any laryngeal edema resulting from prolonged irritation by such tubes but, in general, we have continued to employ tracheostomies, attempting to remove them within three to five days to avoid the troublesome dependence on the tube which may develop and to decrease scarring and stricture of the tracheal wall.

Tracheostomy in infants and children should *not* be performed like an adult tracheostomy (see Chapter 9). Three salient features of the operative technique of tracheostomy in an infant need emphasizing:

1. Tracheostomy should never be

attempted in a baby without first intubating the patient to ensure an adequate, temporary airway.

2. No tracheal tissue should be exised. A vertical incision through two or three cartilages will provide a quite adequate opening, and the elastic tracheal rings will subsequently reconstitute the airway cylinder on tube removal. Traction on stay sutures on either side of the vertical incision can restore the airway and allow easy, controlled replacement of the tube, should it be inadvertently dislodged (Fig. 21–6).[14,40] The adult technique of excising a window promotes tracheal instability in an infant, in view of the proportionately larger amount of the central part of the cartilaginous rings exised. The poorly supported trachea may collapse, and the soft tissues of the neck can fall into the lumen, narrowing it considerably during healing.

3. Finally, the infant's tracheostomy tube must be securely and snugly sutured or tied in position, since dislodgement occurs very easily, and reinsertion may be more difficult than in adults.

Proper nursing care is as critical to successful tracheostomy as the technical procedure itself. Several items deserve emphasis:

1. Because of his short neck, a baby must be positioned with his neck extended by a small roll under his shoulders, to prevent obstruction by his fat neck or chin.

2. Suctioning must be a sterile procedure using a fresh, sterile catheter and clean glove each time.

3. Adequate suctioning past the tip of the catheter is essential to prevent plugs. (Even the relatively inert Silastic tubes will plug at the tip if inadequately suctioned). Adequate humidification is, of course, mandatory.

Failure to recognize significant anatomic difference between an infant's and an adult's tracheal anatomy has led to inappropriate miniaturization

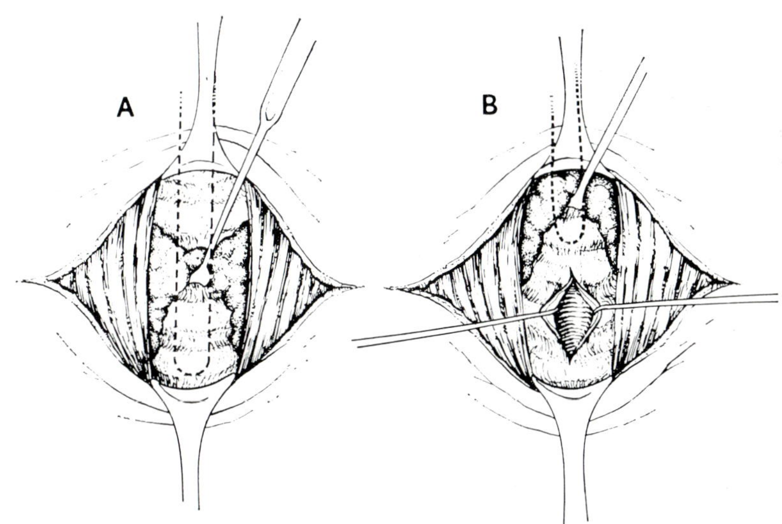

Figure 21–6 Tracheostomy technique: A transverse skin incision has proved preferable for use of the Silastic tube which is equipped with an inferior "tracheostomy incision shield" that prevents angulation and erosion of the edge of the tube into the lower margin of the skin wound. The strap muscles are separated vertically by blunt dissection and the thyroid isthmus is reflected cephalad after division of the pretracheal fascia (*A*). The anterior tracheal wall is then incised vertically, dividing the second, third, fourth and, if needed, the fifth tracheal cartilages in the midline. No transverse counter incision is employed and no tracheal flap or window is ever removed in infants. The endotracheal tube is then withdrawn into the proximal tracheal, the tracheotomy margins are retracted laterally by small hooks, and an appropriate Silastic tube is inserted (*B*).

of adult metal tracheostomy tubes, which can prove unsatisfactory in size, length and configuration. Taking into account the narrow tracheal lumen of a child, the extreme flexibility of his cartilages and the increased activity and movement of his body, head and neck, a relatively larger tube lumen is required for an infant than an adult in order to achieve satisfactory air exchange and avoid additional airway resistance. Rigid tubes which cannot conform to the length and shape of the trachea can encourage mucosal ulceration and all its attendant morbidity, particularly if the constant movement of a mechanical ventilator is added.[40]

Over the past four years, we have explored the use of flexible, synthetic tracheostomy tubes for our infants and children. We have been quite pleased with the basic tracheostomy tube designed by Aberdeen. We have used such tubes manufactured by Dow Corning and constructed of Silastic, the very inert and well-tolerated silicone rubber, in well over 100 patients with no unusual complications, no permanent strictures and ready extubation in all babies who survived their original disease.[14, 40]

Attention to several factors is important:

1. The period of initial nasotracheal or orotracheal intubation before tracheostomy should be sufficiently brief to avoid subglottic inflammation and subsequent scarring and stenosis. Two to three days appears to be relatively innocuous.

2. Careful tracheostomy technique suited to children, such as previously described, can prevent scarring and narrowing at the tracheostomy site itself.

3. The use of flexible, inert tracheostomy tubes, such as the Silastic tubes (Aberdeen design), can help avoid inflammation and scarring of the distal trachea.

4. Finally, the tracheostomy tubes should be progressively diminished in caliber to the narrowest size over several days prior to extubation. The patient can become accustomed to breathing through the relatively wider trachea and pharynx, and the surgeon can observe how well the patient tolerates the normal ventilatory path. When this is accomplished, the small tube is simply removed with the child in a high humidity atmosphere. "Corking" of a tracheostomy tube prior to removal may be dangerous, particularly in a child who may not be able to remove the cork if the trachea becomes obstructed around the tube.[40] A special Morch respirator, as modified by Benson, has been used for respiratory support of these children.[2] This machine has an excellent humidifying system and is a low-volume ventilator.

Gastrointestinal Decompression. A final area demanding special consideration in children is that of gastrointestinal decompression following abdominal trauma and surgery. The objections to nasogastric tubes are compounded in children, particularly because of their infringement on an already marginal airway. To decrease this problem we have resorted increasingly to the use of gastrostomy in infants and children. Not only can gastrointestinal decompression be achieved during the initial stages of convalescence, but also early feeding may be administered through these tubes, thus conserving the strength of the patient during a critical phase of recovery. To avoid overdistention in infants during these initial feedings, a Y-tube arrangement has been employed which allows excessive pressure to be vented. In this way the frequent complications of regurgitation and aspiration of feedings in infants are avoided. A greater degree of freedom and mobility is also allowed the older child, resulting in a much happier convalescence. It should be emphasized, however, that nasogastric tube satisfactory for short-term decompression in older children should be used when indicated.

Temperature Regulation. As mentioned previously, the thermal regulatory mechanism of pediatric patients often seems immature, and great care must be taken to monitor temperatures frequently and to provide some means of external warmth. Warming blankets can be employed for this purpose in older children. For infants, Isolettes are an ideal means of providing both warmth and moisture, and their use is encouraged in this age group. It should be emphasized, however, that all connections with intravenous tubes, drainage tubes and ancillary equipment should be arranged so that ready access to the Isolette is preserved. There is no more frustrating situation than that presented by a critically ill infant who requires instant attention but who is enclosed by a cage of tangled tubes and plastic walls.

Other facets of management in children are not unlike those employed for older patients. The use of extensive monitoring equipment, including electrocardiograms and pressure recorders, may become necessary and should be readily available. The radial artery at the wrist in older children and the femoral artery in the groin in infants are the most frequent sites for positioning of catheters for monitoring arterial pressures.[11]

TRAUMA PECULIAR TO CHILDHOOD

Much of the trauma encountered in children is similar in both etiology and treatment to that seen in adults. Particular types, however, are distinguished by their predominance in infancy and childhood. Included in this latter group are neonatal trauma, the "battered child" syndrome, and certain forms of home accidents.

Neonatal Trauma

Neonatal trauma constitutes an important percentage of birth mortality. Any practicing surgeon may be confronted with a seriously injured newborn and should be prepared to handle the varied aspects of such situations.

The most frequent area of traumatic birth injury in the neonate is the head. Superficial molding, erythema, abrasions, ecchymoses or even fat necrosis are not uncommon.[27] The caput succedaneum with passive edema of the presenting part is well recognized. Such injuries are usually of no consequence. A cephalohematoma with subperiosteal hemorrhage or actual skull fractures occasionally may be encountered. The neophyte may have difficulty in interpreting skull x-rays in these patients and, on palpation, may confuse suture lines with depressed fractures. Routine needle aspirations should be avoided and, in the absence of a depressed fracture or localizing neurological signs, close observation should be the only treatment necessary. The usual source of intracranial injury is the molding of the skull that occurs in the birth process rather than an actual impact force. Overriding of the sutures may lead to tearing of small veins and sinuses on the tentorium, producing subarachnoid or subdural bleeding.

Traumatic damage to the vertebrae and spinal cord may result from traction or forced movements of the neck during the delivery, producing compression or laceration of the vertebral arteries, tears in cervical joint capsules, dura or nerve roots, or compression of the spinal cord.[1] The premature infant is particularly susceptible to such damage. Injuries of this type may be more common than realized, since the signs are usually obscured by associated cerebral damage.

Peripheral nerve damage is another well recognized product of traumatic delivery, with a classic Erb-Duchenne paralysis (C 5-6), Klumpke's paralysis (C 7-8 and T 1), phrenic nerve paralysis and facial nerve paralysis the most frequent forms of this type of injury.

The skeletal injuries most commonly observed in newborns are clavicular fractures and fractures and dislocations of the extremities.[1] Of this group, clavicular fractures are most frequent and should always alert the physician to the possibility of an associated brachial plexus, pulmonary or phrenic nerve injury. A common manifestation of these last two complications is respiratory distress, induced either by pneumothorax or diaphragmatic paralysis.

Although figure-of-eight shoulder bandages are useful in treating clavicular fractures in older children, it may be extremely difficult, and probably unnecessary, to employ this technique in newborns. In tiny infants there is a tendency for such bandages to exert maximum pressure immediately over the fracture site rather than at an optimal point on the distal shoulder. Certainly, as emphasized by Dr. Schmeisser in Chapter Sixteen, Velpeau dressings and arm slings are contraindicated for treatment of this problem in any age group. In the neonate the easiest, and safest, treatment is to avoid lifting the affected extremity. Maintaining the infant in the usual prone position achieves a result comparable to splinting with a figure-of-eight dressing and permits excellent healing.

Fractures and dislocations of the extremities are commonly associated with neurological and developmental anomalies such as meningomyelocele or arthrogryposis multiplex congenita. Detailed treatment of these fractures is outlined in Chapter Sixteen.

Respiratory embarrassment following delivery may result from injuries that compromise the nasal airway, from dislocations of the cricothyroid or cricoarytenoid articulations or pneumothorax.[1, 27] Dislocation of the cricothyroid or cricoarytenoid articulations may necessitate immediate tracheostomy. A tension pneumothorax may present a critical emergency necessitating immediate decompression by needle aspiration, with subsequent drainage for persistent leaks (Fig. 21–7). Minor degrees of pneumothorax in infancy may be treated expectantly, since rapid absorption of air in the pleural or peritoneal cavities will occur within 24 to 48 hours, especially in the presence of high oxygen concentrations. There should be no hesitancy, however, in inserting a small intercostal chest catheter attached to underwater seal drainage in those instances in which a continuing air

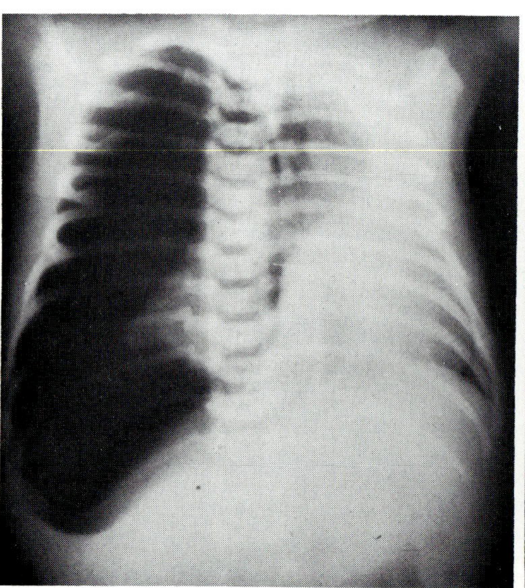
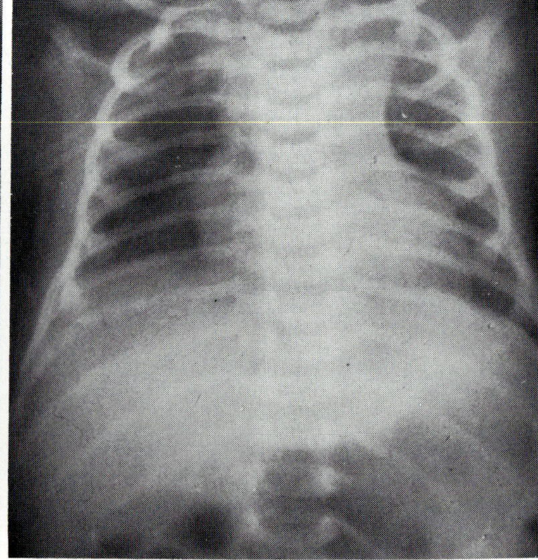

Figure 21–7 Tension pneumothorax of the newborn relieved by tube drainage.

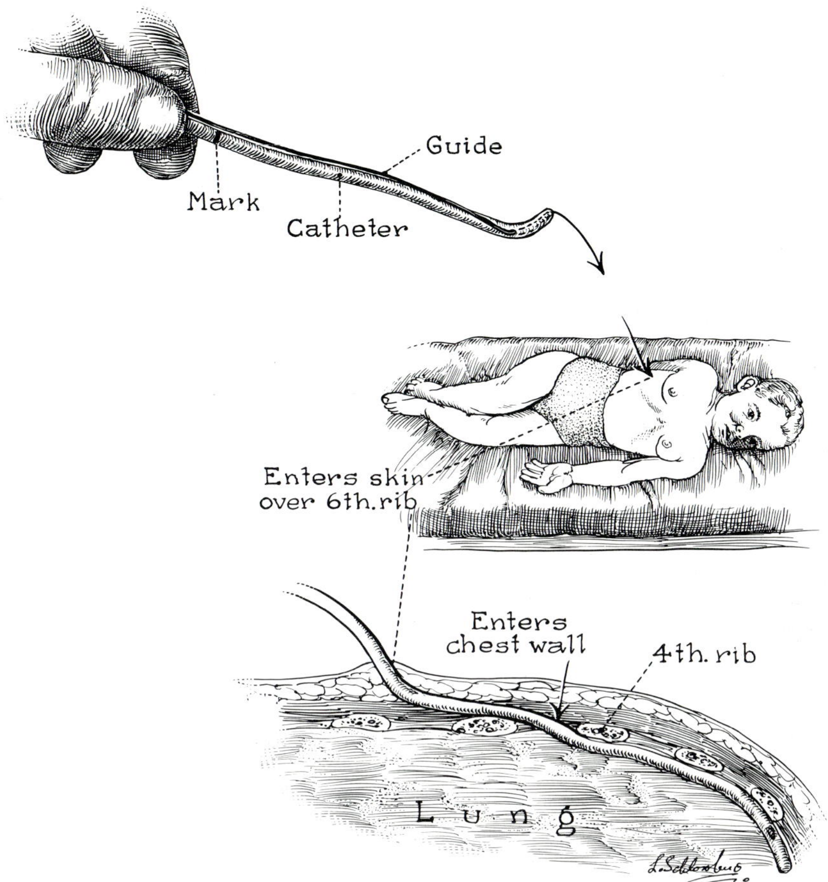

Figure 21–8 A technique for chest tube insertion in the infant. A short skin incision is made over the 6th rib in the midaxillary line following infiltration with 0.5 per cent procaine. A subcutaneous tract is then dissected bluntly with a small curved clamp over the superior margin of the 5th rib and through the intercostal muscles into the pleural cavity. A malleable probe is then inserted as a stylet into the proximal side-hole of a small French catheter (Nos. 10 to 12). The tip of the stylet is curved in order to facilitate introduction of the catheter through the skin incision and subcutaneous tract into the chest cavity. The catheter has been marked previously at the optimum depth of insertion in order to prevent excessive penetration into the thorax and possible injury to apical or mediastinal structures. The use of a stylet facilitates placement of the drainage tube in an optimum position along the lateral thoracic wall. Once positioning is achieved, the probe may easily be withdrawn. A lateral insertion site is preferable in infants, even in the treatment of pneumothorax. Introduction of a catheter through the second intercostal space anteriorly, as recommended in adults, is excessively difficult and hazardous in view of the limited pleural space and the close proximity of vital structures. In infants, direct insertion of the catheters into the chest, rather than tunneling through the subcutaneous tissues, as described, may result in a significant delay in healing of the tube tract.

leak is encountered (Fig. 21–8). Suction is rarely needed. In general, these tubes are best inserted laterally under direct vision, with care taken to prevent excessive medial protrusion into the mediastinum, either displacing the latter structure or preventing complete pulmonary expansion. A small removable stylet inserted through the catheter has been found to facilitate insertion of these tubes through lateral stab wounds. The use of a trocar is prohibitively dangerous in a small patient in whom deviations of a fraction of an inch may lead to major injuries.

Abdominal trauma is unusual in the neonate. Injury of the liver comprises the more frequent form. Adrenal hemorrhage has been attributed to trauma but it is questionable whether this is not a secondary rather than a primary condition.

Battered Child Syndrome

The so-called battered child represents another large category of injuries peculiar to this age group.[9, 35] These children are victims of maltreatment, either neglect or abuse, which usually occurs within the home environment. This type of injury is characterized by the subtleness with which it may present and in the medicolegal complications which it may produce. Nearly all these patients are under three years of age and the majority less than one year old. The history is often of no help, either through apparent ignorance of the parents of any foul play or through careful attempts at concealment of the injury. The incidence of this injury syndrome appears to be directly proportional to the alertness of the physician. The frequency of reports in recent medical literature attests to the fact that physicians are more aware of the entity, and many states have now undertaken active legislation to insure accurate reporting and follow-up. Although the medical treatment in such situations is not necessarily unique, a failure to follow through with adequate investigation of the home environment and prevention of future recurrences all too often leads to a final fatal outcome when the child is readmitted later with lethal injuries. If continuing trauma seems probable after careful investigation, the child should be removed from the home environment. Many progressive communities have aided the physician by requiring reports to legal authorities when any suspected instances of willfully inflicted trauma are encountered.

An excellent example of the battered child syndrome is provided in the following case report:

W. B., JHH, 102 10 55. A three-year-old white male child was admitted through the Emergency Room with complaints of "throwing up for four days." Except for previous admissions to The Johns Hopkins Hospital for repair of a cleft lip and palate, the child had remained asymptomatic until three days prior to admission. At that time he was noted to vomit on several occasions, the symptoms persisting with increasing frequency. The mother denied all knowledge of possible trauma until the patient was seen by a local physician who inquired as to the etiology of numerous contusions over the abdomen and extremities.

The family and social history were pertinent, since the mother was divorced and the child had not been the product of the marriage.

On examination, the patient was obviously an acutely ill, dehydrated child with evidence of multiple areas of old bruising, particularly over the right abdomen (Fig. 21–9). Diminished bowel sounds were present, although there were no signs of peritoneal irritation. There was tenderness to direct palpation in the right lower quadrant of the abdomen, but no masses were evident. X-rays of the abdomen, chest and right arm revealed Colles' fracture of the right wrist and an adynamic ileus. The hematocrit was 30 per cent (the hematocrit on discharge one month previously had been 34 per cent), the white blood count was 17,000, and the urinalysis revealed 4+ proteinuria and numerous red blood cells. Serum chemistries revealed a serum urea nitrogen of 75 mg. per cent; sodium, 127 mEq./L.; potassium, 7.2 mEq./L.; carbon dioxide, 18 mEq./L.; and amylase, 900 mg. per cent (reducing substance).

The clinical impression was one of generalized blunt trauma resulting in a fracture of the right wrist and right renal damage associated with retroperitoneal hematoma. An intravenous pyelogram confirmed the presence of a nonfunctioning kidney on the right. The blood pressure was noted to be normal on admission and remained so throughout the course of hospitalization.

The patient was admitted to the Intensive Care Unit of The Children's Medical and Surgical Center under the immediate supervision of the Pediatric General Surgical Service with consultant services supplied by Pediatrics, Orthopedics and

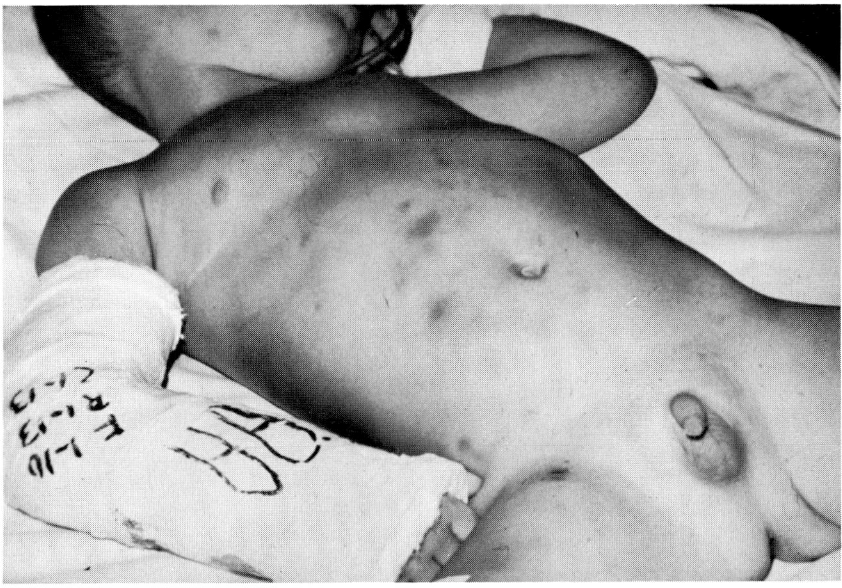

Figure 21–9 The "battered child syndrome" as exemplified by abdominal ecchymoses and fracture of the right arm.

Urology. Fluid and electrolyte replacement was instituted immediately and all chemistries, including the serum amylase, had returned to normal by the fourth hospital day. A gastrointestinal series demonstrated continuity of the intestinal tract. A retrograde pyelogram revealed evidence of dye extending out from the superior calyx into the renal parenchyma, suggesting a traumatic fracture. Renal scan showed no evidence of uptake of the radioactive material by the right kidney. Several repeat pyelograms during the subsequent months continued to reveal absence of function of the right kidney. The hematuria cleared during this time, however. Since there was no evidence of developing hypertension or localized abdominal mischief, a conservative, watchful approach was directed toward the renal injury.

The social problem was quite involved and required a thorough evaluation of the home situation, both by the police and the social service division. The patient was finally discharged to the mother's care after the latter was cleared completely of any possible complicity in the child's injury. A third person was implicated by the investigation and was removed from all contact with the patient. Further steps in management have included efforts to improve the family's socioeconomic situation.

O'Neill and associates have presented an excellent review of the patterns of injury seen in battered children.[30] In their series of 110 battered children, the types of injuries in the order of frequency were soft tissue injuries, fractures and head injuries. Eight of the patients died from head injuries. Combined injuries were common. Evidence of chronic or prior injury was the rule.

Home Injuries

Any classification of injuries unique to childhood includes those occurring in the home. Such injuries may result from falls; from entanglements with various types of vehicles, including automobiles, wagons, bicycles, skateboards and skates; from body burns, either electrical or thermal; from ingestion of caustic substances and foreign bodies; or from so-called wringer injuries.

Body Burns. The treatment of body burns is particularly difficult in the infant and young child. This problem is reflected in the high mortality encountered in this age group. The body surface area of these patients is large in relation to their weight and differs in distribution from that observed in adults. As a result, standard charts which have been prepared for estimation of extent of burns in adults are useless when applied to infants or small children.[5]

Certain complications of burn therapy are encountered more frequently in children than adults. Airway obstruction due to laryngeal edema is a greater hazard because of the smaller structures. Alterations in metabolic response may also prove troublesome in these patients. Excessive sodium replacement is much more likely to occur in infants. Colloid loss in the adult may be balanced by normal physiologic responses, whereas any serious burn in the young child usually will necessitate some form of extrinsic colloid replacement.[26] The introduction of topical therapy with either 0.5 per cent silver nitrate solution or Sulfamylon cream has proved both a tremendous boon and a potential hazard. Serious electrolyte dilution may develop within six hours in infants when Moyer's silver nitrate method of treatment is employed.[24] Severe hyperchloremic acidosis, particularly with a respiratory burn, may be a complication of Moncreif's method of Sulfamylon therapy.[23] Careful monitoring and electrolyte replacement are mandatory under these circumstances.

Although basic replacement formulas are useful in projecting fluid and colloid losses in burn patients, the addition of the monitoring routine outlined previously for management of other forms of surgical trauma may be particularly helpful in the infant or young child during the first four to five days of treatment. Other details of routine therapy are discussed in Chapter Eighteen.

Ingestion of Caustic Materials. The accidental ingestion of strong acids or alkalies by children is largely limited to the preschool age group. This serious injury is a result of gross carelessness in leaving caustic substances within reach of one to five year old children. The material most often swallowed is lye, either in crystalline form or as a liquid cleaner.[6] Strong solutions of ammonia may cause serious burns, but ammonia solutions have usually been diluted before use in the home. The ingestion of ammonia, therefore, is seldom a cause of significant esophageal burns. Concentrated acids are usually not found in the home and so are seldom swallowed by children.

Unlike the adult who swallows lye to commit suicide, the young child immediately tries to rectify his painful mistake by spitting and regurgitating any residual material. For this reason, gavage will not yield enough caustic solution in a child to make it worthwhile. In most lye ingestion suspects, only the mouth and pharynx will be burned but the minority with esophageal burns have a potentially grave injury.

Lye, which is practically pure sodium hydroxide, destroys tissue by producing a liquefaction necrosis.[4] This process results in deep penetration through the wall of the esophagus and may produce esophageal perforation. Acids, on the contrary, produce a coagulation necrosis which prevents deep penetration. Thus, the ingestion of acids usually does not result in serious injury.

The immediate problems are airway obstruction by epiglottal edema and esophageal perforation. Fortunately, both occur rarely. The most common complication is the dense scar tissue which circumferentially constricts the esophagus at the burn site and produces significant obstruction or total occlusion of the esophagus. Most of our intensive treatment is directed toward the prevention of this serious complication of caustic burns.

The first step in the examination of a child suspected of lye ingestion is a careful evaluation of the history. Usually the person who arrives with the child will bring the evidence and relate the exposure to the substance. If the material is a corrosive agent and the story of ingestion is plausible, an immediate examination of the mouth and pharynx is imperative. Often the lips and mucous membranes will be reddened and occasionally partially coagulated. Any evidence of pharyngeal edema or erythema raises the question of epiglottal edema and airway obstruction. This finding requires immediate hospitalization because the period of maximal edema and danger is between six and 24 hours.

All children with evidence of oral or pharyngeal burns must be assumed to have esophageal burns as well. It is our practice to esophagoscope all such children within 24 hours of the lye ingestion to document the presence or absence of the burn. There is no increased danger of instrumental perforation if the operator stops *when he sees the burn and does not attempt to visualize the extent of the burn.* Numerous authors, especially Kaplan and associates in this country and Palva in Finland, have pointed out that the best way to make a positive diagnosis of an esophageal burn is by immediate esophagoscopy.[21, 31] Certainly it is important to determine if a significant caustic burn has occurred before initiating any regimen of intensive therapy which will require close observation and expensive hospitalization.

High humidity and systemic steroids are the basic ingredients of treatment for airway edema. Prophylactic antibiotics, preferably penicillin or methicillin, are necessary only when a serious burn is suspected and esophageal perforation may be impending.

In most hospitals the time-honored treatment for prevention of esophageal stricture has been early and frequent dilation of the acutely burned esophagus. This therapy was introduced by the Austrian, Hans Salzer, in 1920 and bears his name.[33] It is usually carried out blindly, using tapered bougies, and is then repeated once a day for several weeks, then every other day for two to three weeks and, finally, once a week for many months. Bougie dilatation alone has been reasonably effective in preventing complete stricture but has not prevented significant areas of serious stenosis in some patients.

Because of inherent difficulties with prolonged bougienage and many unsatisfactory long-term results, intensive short-term adrenal steroid therapy has been tried recently in many medical centers in an attempt to decrease the inflammatory reaction associated with the burn. The steroid therapy is entirely nonspecific and its use is based only on the antiphlogistic effect of these drugs. If the inflammatory response is largely prevented, the subsequent scar tissue will be much less extensive.

Based on these theoretical considerations, Haller and Bachman studied comparative effects of bougienage and steroid treatment in experimental caustic burns of the cat's esophagus.[10] Their data strongly support the recent clinical experience that steroids are more effective than bougienage in preventing late stricture formation. Bougienage is currently being used in The Johns Hopkins Hospital only when a barium swallow shows evidence of beginning stenosis of the esophagus. Preliminary clinical experience would suggest that a steroid dosage of 1 to 2 mg. of prednisone per kg. of body weight per day in young children is adequate to control edema at the burn site.[15] The steroid is continued for a minimum of three weeks, at the end of which period a repeat esophagram is obtained. If there is no evidence of stricture formation at this time, the steroids are discontinued and the patient followed closely with repeat studies of the esophagus at three-month intervals for a year. If, on the other hand, stricture formation is apparent at the completion of this initial treatment, the steroids are discontinued and a regimen of esophageal bougienage is instituted.

We have recently reviewed our long-term results with this type of treatment protocol for caustic burns of the esophagus. The conclusions of this study were as follows:

Two hundred eight-five children with possible caustic burns of the esophagus have been managed at two university hospitals using similar protocols. Of these, 235 (82 per cent) had immediate esophagoscopy and 69 (29 per cent) had demonstrated esophageal burns. They were treated with steroids and antibiotics. Eight (12 per cent) with proven burns developed strictures that responded to prolonged dilatations and none has required esophageal replacement. The remainder are free of swallowing symptoms. By contrast, eight patients from other hospitals who were not treated by this protocol were referred for esophageal replacement and prolonged dilatation.[10, 16] Our strong impression is that immediate steroid-antibiotic therapy greatly decreases the incidence of esophageal stricture but does not completely eliminate it. Those children who develop strictures on this treatment regimen seem to have milder esophageal scarring, which usually responds to dilatation rather than requiring esophageal replacement.[16]

Only more extensive experience will ultimately define the comparative roles of bougienage, steroids and antibiotics in the treatment of caustic burns of the esophagus. The need for good preventive therapy cannot be disputed, because a severe stricture of the esophagus is a major problem. Repeated dilatations with calibrated bougies may give adequate relief for the chronic stricture. If the stricture becomes too narrow and too dense, some type of resectional surgery becomes necessary. It is beyond the scope of this discussion to consider these operative procedures, but none is entirely satisfactory, for the esophagus is an organ which cannot be easily replaced.

Foreign Bodies. Young children test many small objects with their lips and mouth. This inquisitiveness explains most of the cases of aspiration and ingestion of foreign bodies. Aspiration, because it endangers the airway, usually presents a real emergency, but ingestion of a foreign body seldom requires immediate surgical intervention.

Aspiration probably occurs because a child becomes choked while attempting to swallow and, on vigorous inhalation, sucks the object into the larynx and trachea. The foreign body initiates a sudden spasm of coughing and wheezing, with varying degrees of cyanosis. Fortunately, most objects produce acute symptoms and proper treatment is instituted at once. Occasionally, smooth objects, especially food such as a peanut or bean, becomes lodged in a bronchus, with only transient acute symptoms. These children present later with recurrent pneumonia and lung abscesses due to bronchial obstruction.

Acute respiratory obstruction from a foreign body in a young child requires immediate bronchoscopy by the most skillful endoscopist available. Even diagnostic bronchoscopy in infants is a treacherous examination because of the small structures and tiny airway, but endoscopy to remove foreign bodies is more difficult. It is best done under very light anesthesia and requires great skill and experience. Dr. Paul H. Holinger has repeatedly emphasized that it is essential to use small caliber bronchoscopes to decrease instrumental trauma, and it is best to expose the larynx first with a small laryngoscope and then insert the bronchoscope under direct vision.[18] Aspirated foreign bodies are usually *not* radiopaque so that x-ray studies are not so helpful as in the diagnosis of objects in the esophagus or stomach.

Once the foreign body has been grasped and removed, the child should be kept in high humidity and given a brief course of steroid therapy for three to five days. Fortunately, after removal there are very few acute or chronic complications from an impacted foreign body.[18]

Swallowed objects may become lodged anywhere in the gastrointestinal tract, but unless it has sharp points any foreign body that passes the esophagus can be expected to pass out the rectum. The most frequent sites of lodgment in the esophagus are at the level of the cricopharyngeal muscle (beneath the clavicle) and at the esophagogastric junction, with the upper site being much more common. The initial symptoms of coughing, choking and gagging strongly suggest the presence of a foreign body, but if it becomes fixed in the esophagus, the symptoms may disappear and give a false sense of security. If the history and symptoms are suspicious, an x-ray examination, including a thin barium swallow, will usually confirm the diagnosis.

Coins and discs are most common, but any object or toy can be found in the esophagus. All sharp-pointed objects should be removed with reasonable speed, but esophagoscopy can be delayed for 12 to 24 hours if the object is smooth and there is no significant symptomatology. Often repeated attempts at swallowing will dislodge round foreign bodies, and they will pass on through the gastrointestinal tract. In a very young child general anesthesia, administered via an endotracheal tube, is desirable for the endoscopy, but older children tolerate the procedure quite well under moderate sedation and topical anesthesia.

The round or smooth foreign body that reaches the stomach can be followed expectantly without x-ray studies by carefully examining the stools until the object is passed. If the object is pointed or has sharp edges, such as an opened safety pin or a nail, a single abdominal x-ray should be taken two to three times a week to document its progressive passage. Operative intervention is indicated if the foreign body fails to move down the gastrointestinal tract. This lodgment implies penetration into the intestinal wall and may represent impending perforation.

The rectum and vagina occasionally harbor foreign bodies which have been inserted by the ever-inquisitive fingers of young children. Foreign bodies in the rectum are one of the commonest causes of rectal bleeding in childhood; the foreign body is always palpable on rectal examination. A remarkable assortment of small foreign bodies have been removed from the vaginas of little girls. A persistent vaginal discharge, especially if it is purulent, should prompt a thorough x-ray and/or digital examination. When the diagnosis is made, the treatment is simple removal. (See Chapter Thirteen.)

Wringer Injuries. The wringer injury represents a particular type of crush injury that occurs almost exclusively in childhood. In spite of the introduction of spin dryers, there still remain an astounding number of the old type wringer washers judging by the persistent frequency with which this type of injury is encountered in an accident room population. With the recognition of potential seriousness of such trauma the morbidity has diminished greatly. All children with wringer injuries extending above the midarm are immediately hospitalized. The extremity is wrapped in a bulky pressure dressing and suspended in an upright position for 24 hours, with close monitoring of sensation and circulation during this time (Fig. 21–10). The dressing is changed in 24 hours, and if any significant degree of swelling is evident, hospitalization is prolonged and treatment continued. If there is minimal swelling, the bulky dressing is reapplied and the patient discharged home with continuation of suspension of the extremity for 48 hours. Subsequent treatment in each case is adapted to individual evidence of ancillary damage such as skin loss or nerve paralysis.

Although this regimen probably represents overtreatment in the major-

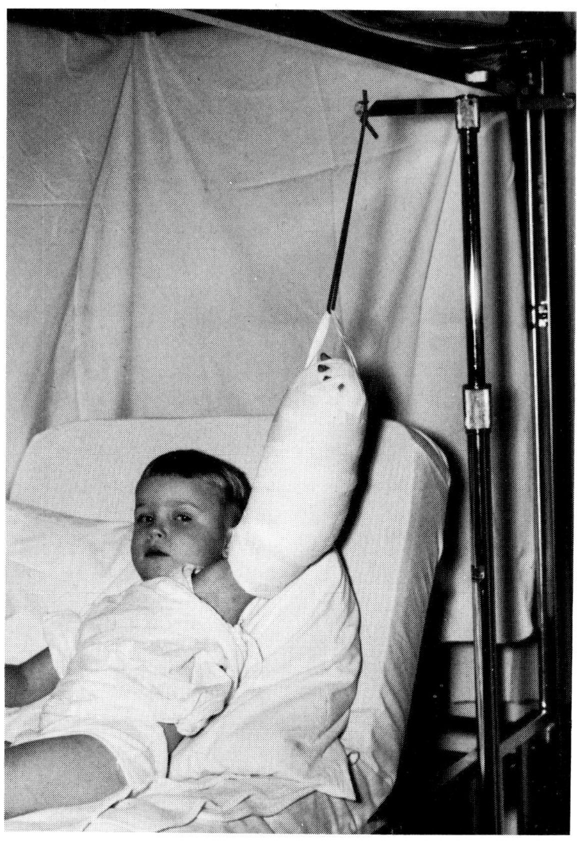

Figure 21–10 A demonstration of the technique of treating "wringer injuries" of the arm with a bulky pressure dressing and suspension. Exposure of the finger tips allows hourly checks of sensation and circulation. Any evidence of impaired capillary filling or anesthesia may indicate compression of the nerves and vessels in the fascial compartment of the forearm by an expanding hematoma. The dressing should be removed immediately under such circumstances, and the arm should be carefully examined. Prompt performance of a fasciotomy may be necessary to prevent the progression of this process.

ity of cases, the infrequency of serious residual damage has led to its perpetuation. Under this program the only instances of persistent morbidity in recent years have involved those cases of skin loss that required grafting. There have been no cases in which increasing edema has led to impairment of blood supply to the distal extremity. Although fasciotomies have been recommended for patients with swelling and progressive vascular embarrassment, no such cases have been encountered since the above treatment was instituted.

The "Accident-Prone" Child

Many children seem to suffer recurrent injuries and may be described as "accident prone."[27] At times, particularly in older children, such injuries appear to result from deliberate flirtation with danger. In younger children, the patient often appears to be a tense, high strung individual who seems under pressure to be active—the type who must take a dare and who rushes headlong into situations without considering the risks. This behavior may be described as counterphobic, because a child attempts to cope with his unconsciously determined fear by exposing himself to the very danger of which he is afraid. Most of the resulting injuries are not unique and are handled in a standard way.

SUMMARY

Trauma in childhood is not fundamentally different from serious injuries at any age, but the potential earning power and social contributions make the injured child a trauma problem of special significance. The basic principles of rapid, careful evaluation and sequential correction of altered physiology are the backbone of successful therapy. The unique metabolic demands and miniature anatomic relationships of the infant or young child present the physician with a special challenge and great responsibility. However, the rewards are high; the younger the injured child, the greater is our total investment.

REFERENCES

1. Benson, C. D., Mustard, W. T., Ravitch, M. M., Snyder, W. H., Jr., and Welch, K. J.: Pediatric Surgery. Chicago, Year Book Medical Publishers, Inc., 1962.
2. Benson, D. W.: Unpublished data.
3. Borrow, M., Aquilizan, L., Krausy, A., and Stefanides, A.: The use of central venous pressure as an accurate guide for body fluid replacement. Surg. Gynec. Obstet. *120*:545, 1965.
4. Bosher, L. H., Burford, T. H., and Ackerman, L.: Pathology of experimentally produced lye burns and strictures of the esophagus. J. Thoracic Surg. *21*:483, 1951.
5. Conway, H.: Management of burns in children. Am. J. Surg. *107*:537, 1964.
6. Crowe, J. T.: Poisoning due to lye. Am. J. Dis. Child. *68*:9, 1944.
7. Dietrich, H. F.: Prevention of childhood accidents, J.A.M.A. *156*:929, 1954.
8. Done, A. K.: Developmental pharmacology. Clin. Pharmacol. Therapeutics *5*:432, 1964.
9. Fontana, V. T.: The Maltreated Child. Springfield, Ill., Charles C Thomas, 1964.
10. Haller, J. A., Jr., and Bachman, K.: The comparative effect of current therapy on experimental caustic burns of the esophagus. Pediatrics *34*:236, 1964.
11. Haller, J. Alex, Jr.: Monitoring of arterial and central venous pressure in infants. Pediat. Clin. N. Amer. *16*:637, 1969.
12. Haller, J. Alex, Jr.: Problems in children's trauma. J. Trauma *10*:269, 1970.
13. Haller, J. Alex, Jr., and Talbert, James L.: Trauma workshop report: Trauma in children. J. Trauma *10*:1052, 1970.
14. Haller, J. Alex, Jr., and Talbert, James L.: Clinical evaluation of a new silastic tracheostomy tube for respiratory support of infants and young children. Ann. Surg. *171*:915, 1970.
15. Haller, J. Alex, Jr., and Andrews, H. Gibbs: Pathophysiology and management of acute corrosive burns of the esophagus. Modern Treatment *7*:1182, 1970.
16. Haller, J. Alex, Jr., Andrews, H. Gibbs, White, John J., Tamer, M. Akram, and Cleveland, William W.: Pathophysiology and management of acute corrosive burns of the esophagus: Results of treatment in 285 children. J. Pediat. Surg. *6*:578, 1971.
17. Holder, T. M.: Problems peculiar to infants. *In* Gibbon, J. H., Jr. (ed.), Surgery of the Chest. Philadelphia, W. B. Saunders Co., 1962.
18. Holinger, P. H., and Johnston, K. C.: Foreign bodies in the air and food passages. Pediat. Clin. N. Amer. *1*:827, 1954.
19. Hughes, W. T., Jr.: Pediatric Procedures. Philadelphia, W. B. Saunders Co., 1964.
20. Iritani, R. I., and Siler, V. E.: Wringer injuries of the upper extremity. Surg. Gynec. Obstet. *113*:677, 1961.
21. Kaplan, J., Gandhi, K., Elsen, J., and Oppenheimer, P.: Early esophagoscopy for diagnosis of esophageal burns. Arch. Otol. *73*:52, 1961.
22. Keddy, J. A.: Accidents in childhood. Canad. Med. Assoc. J. *91*:675, 1964.
23. Lindberg, R. B., Moncrief, J. A., Switzer, W. E., Order, S. E., and Mills, W.: The successful control of burn wound sepsis. J. Trauma *5*:601, 1965.
24. Monafo, W. W., and Moyer, C. A.: Effectiveness of dilute aqueous silver nitrate in the treatment of major burns. Arch. Surg. *91*:200, 1965.
25. Moore, D., Bernhard, W. F., and Kevy, S. V.: Method for control of hydrogen ion concentration in stored heparinized blood prior to use in cardiac surgery. Am. Surg. *158*:1000, 1963.
26. Moyer, C. A., Margraf, H. W., and Monafo, W. W., Jr.: Burn shock and extravascular sodium deficiency—treatment with Ringer's solution with lactate. Arch. Surg. *90*:799, 1965.
27. Nelson, W. E.: Textbook of Pediatrics. 8th Ed. Philadelphia, W. B. Saunders Co., 1964.
28. Nyhan, W. L., and Lampert, F.: Response of the fetus and newborn to drugs. Anesthesiology *26*:487, 1965.
29. Odell, G. B.: The magnitude of volume and solute disturbances in the neo-natal period associated with fasting and thirsting. J. Saint Barnabas Medical Center *2*:92–98, 1964.
30. O'Neill, J. A., Meacham, W. F., Griffin, P. O. and Sawyers, J. L. Patterns of injury in the battered child syndrome. J. Trauma *13*:332, 1973.
31. Palva, T.: Corrosions of the esophagus. Acta Otolaryng. Suppl. *158*:44, 1960.
32. Rubini, M. E., and Wolf, A. V.: Refractometric determination of total solids and water of serum and urine. J. Biol. Chem. *255*:869, 1957.
33. Salzer, H.: Early treatment of corrosive

esophagitis. Wien. Klin. Wschr. *33*: 307, 1920.

34. Stolowsky, H. J.: Blunt abdominal trauma and intestinal perforation in childhood. Chirurg. *36*:4, 1965.
35. Storey, B.: The battered child. Med. J. Australia *2*:789, 1964.
36. Tabulations Prepared by the Childrens Bureau, Welfare Administration, Based on Data of the National Center for Health Statistics, Public Health Service, Department of Health, Education, and Welfare.
37. Talbert, J. L., and Haller, J. A., Jr.: The optimal site for central venous measurement in newborn infants: A critical comparison of superior versus inferior caval pressures with increasing abdominal distention. J. Surg. Res. *6*:168, 1966.
38. Thal, A. P., and Wilson, R. F.: Shock. Current Prob. Surg. September, 1965.
39. Thomas, D. V., Fletcher, G., Sunshine, P., Schafer, I. A., and Klaus, M. H.: Prolonged respirator use in pulmonary insufficiency of newborn. J.A.M.A. *193*: 183, 1965.
40. White, John J., and Haller, J. Alex, Jr.: An improved technique for tracheostomy in infants and children. Resident Staff Physician, p. 11s, February 1972.
41. Wilson, J. N.: The management of acute circulatory failure. Surg. Clin. N. Amer. *43*:469, 1963.

chapter

22

WOUND SEPSIS: PREVENTION AND CONTROL

John F. Burke, M.D.

GENERAL CONSIDERATIONS

The successful management of an injured patient rests on an accurate understanding of the physiologic disturbances caused by trauma and their timely repair. Repair, in the medical sense, not only involves the restoration of anatomic continuity and alignment of soft tissue or fracture but, equally important, rests on the maintenance of this restoration and alignment while the processes of healing are carried out. Sepsis is the major stumbling block to this completion of accurate healing. Over the past twenty years, the considerable increase in physiologic knowledge and its application to the traumatically injured patient have considerably improved his chance for immediate survival. Too often, however, the dramatic rescues of the emergency ward and operating room are lost in the ensuing weeks on the hospital ward through bacterial infection. It is clear that the successful management of trauma depends not only on the early repair of physiologic and anatomic defects but, equally important, on the prevention or successful treatment of a septic complication. In assessing the overall problems of sepsis in trauma, it appears that prevention is easier to accomplish and far more likely to lead to a satisfactory result than is the treatment of an infection once established. This chapter will be divided into two sections— the first and most important section will deal with the problems and techniques useful in preventing infection, and the second section will deal with the problems and techniques of dealing with established sepsis in traumatically injured patients.

PREVENTION OF SEPSIS

As already noted, it is almost always easier to prevent sepsis than it is to treat a bacterial lesion once established in the tissue. This concept is particularly important in the patient following trauma for tissue injury, and the surgical manipulations required for restoration of normal anatomy seriously decrease the patient's usual resistance to bacterial invasion, particularly in the localized area of trauma itself. Post-traumatic swelling, relative ischemia, areas of hematoma and direct soft tissue damage all combine with the systemic derangements of circulatory volume and cardiovascular instability to make the seriously injured patient an easy mark for bacterial invasion. This extensive defect in the patient's ability to defend himself against bacteria begins immediately after injury and is perhaps at its lowest ebb immediately before resuscitation in the emergency room. With this in mind, it is obvious that if sepsis is to be avoided, preventive measures must begin as shortly after injury as possible (i.e., along with the life-saving measures instituted to establish an airway, halt blood loss or repair circulatory volume). In general, these preventive measures may be divided into several categories for the purpose of discussion. The categories are: (1) reestablishment of physiologic stability, (2) prevention of further bacterial contamination of tissue, (3) elimination of the tissue bacterial contamination inflicted at the time of trauma, and (4) preventive antibiotics. Although these points are easiest to discuss separately, it is important to understand that they should not be carried out sequentially but simultaneously as early as possible in the post-injury period.

Establishment of Physiologic Stability

In the overall treatment of the trauma patient, including those measures designed to prevent sepsis, the rapid and effective use of measures to bring the patient to the state of near normal physiology is perhaps the cornerstone on which all other measures must rest. The most extensive debridement, the most timely and accurate repair of vascular occlusion, or the most extensive use of antibiotics will accomplish little without the simultaneous resumption of normal physiologic function. In addition to seriously compromising the function of the brain, heart and kidney, low cardiac output and systemic hypoperfusion produce other more subtle but nevertheless as potentially lethal effects. These effects are seen, in particular, on the bacterially contaminated, traumatic wound. It is widely recognized that immediate correction of circulatory failure is essential to prevent death from CNS or cardiac failure. It is not widely recognized that immediate correction of circulatory failure is an essential ingredient in the prevention of wound sepsis. The effects of hypotension on the ability to defend against bacterial invasion have been adequately documented.[1, 2] Therefore, both for the immediate and the long-term wellbeing of the injured patient, particularly those with open wounds or compound fractures, timely reestablishment of adequate circulation is indispensable. Unfortunately, the operational definition of "adequate circulation" is at times considered to be clinically achieved with the resumption of urine flow or the recording of a nearly normal central arterial pressure. It is important to realize that in this situation the peripheral muscle mass and skin may remain seriously underperfused. This defect in circulation in the area of a contaminated wound is a steppingstone for sepsis. It is not sufficient to prevent the patient's death from shock in the immediate post-injury period; the trauma surgeons must also prevent the development of sepsis in the area of the injury itself. Although sepsis may not be manifest for a few days or a week following trauma, the bacterial contamination causing suppuration occurs during or close to the time of injury, and prevention of infection is impossible without "adequate circulation" to the soft tissue injuries themselves. Restoration of circulation, therefore, includes not only the restoration of the central but also the restoration of the peripheral circulation, if wound infection is to be avoided. In this context, the peripheral hypoperfusion produced by vasoconstrictive agents provides a further reason to avoid their use in traumatic shock.

The exact method of repairing circulatory volume and near normal peripheral as well as central circulation has been outlined in detail elsewhere in this book. It is, however, important to recognize that the physiologic defects caused by red cell loss are, at this time, most effectively repaired by red cell replacement.

In addition to the problems of circulatory volume and level of vascular perfusion, there are further systemic abnormalities that must be corrected before physiologic equilibrium and near normal antibacterial defenses can be expected. Normal respiratory function and adequate gas exchange are vital; acid-base equilibrium, electrolyte concentration and hydration are important areas to bring to balance. In addition, pre-existing disease states, such as diabetes, must be carefully controlled. It is well to remember that the patient's own bacterial defenses are the most important in preventing sepsis.

Prevention of Further Bacterial Contamination

Although for practical purposes bacterial contamination of a traumatically inflicted, open wound occurs at the time of injury, further bacterial contamination continues until the wound is closed or otherwise protected through medical intervention. It is important to recognize that this further bacterial contamination of an open wound can be largely eliminated by the efficient use of dressings and sterile technique well known to all surgeons. In assessing the need to protect the wound from further contamination as early as possible following injury, it is particularly important to note that although the bacterial species likely to contaminate a wound at the time of injury may, on rare occasion, produce serious, if not lethal, infection, they are also likely to be sensitive to the available antibiotic agents. On the other hand, the bacterial species found in hospitals are perhaps, on the whole, more virulent; but, even more important, are much more likely to be resistant to the antibiotic therapy. Therefore, infection generated by bacterial contamination of a traumatic wound in the factory, on the farm, or at the roadside almost always responds to active antibiotic therapy, but infection produced by hospital bacterial strains resulting from contamination in the hospital itself is likely to be antibiotic-resistant and difficult to treat successfully.

The preventive measures used to protect the patient from further contamination are simply those involved in accurate sterile techniques and the prevention of cross infection. Unfortunately, many injured patients are thoroughly contaminated by hospital strains of bacteria in the emergency ward because accurate attention to the details of sterile technique and prevention of cross infection are temporarily pushed to the background by urgent measures which are required to deal with massive hemorrhage, respiratory insufficiency or cardiovascular collapse. Too often, intravenous catheters, tracheostomy tubes, foley catheters, instruments and dressing sponges are contaminated in the hurry of emergency resuscitation of a seriously injured patient. Again, too often, the life saved by emergency resuscitation is lost later through the consequences of bacterial contamination during resuscitation but not manifest as sepsis for days or weeks later on the ward.

The wound does not provide the only portal of entry for bacterial invasion of the traumatically injured patient. The respiratory tract, the urinary tract, the blood stream, as well as the wound, are often infected, as noted above, by bacteria carried on catheters, tubes and instruments placed in the emergency situation without proper precautions for maintenance of sterility.

As in the restoration of normal physiology, the protection of the patient from further contamination must begin immediately on the patient's admission to the emergency ward and continue unabated until the wound is closed and all catheters, tubes and drains have been removed.

Elimination of Contaminating Bacteria and Devitalized Tissue

Ranking in importance close behind the establishment of near normal physiology in preserving life and preventing wound infection are the measures which are taken to eliminate the bacteria, foreign bodies and devitalized tissue from the patient's wound when he is presented for medical care. These measures may be loosely collected under the title of "debridement." This is a simple and relatively clear-cut concept, but in clinical application it is likely to present considerable judgment and technical difficulties. The maneuvers of debridement have their basis in experience gained in the First World War through the attempts by the French army surgeons to reduce the incidence of sepsis and gas gangrene in the wounded. In brief, debridement implies the removal of all foreign material, devitalized tissue and contaminating bacteria from a wound as early as possible following injury. Although the idea of removing dead tissue is simple enough, the actual problems faced in carrying out these concepts may be very difficult, as noted above. The problems lie, on the one hand, in the difficulties of accurately separating tissue which has been injured and is destined to die from tissue that is injured but destined to recover, and, on the other hand, on the reluctance of the surgeon to sacrifice skin, muscle, bone, or tendon (and along with it useful function) which he cannot be sure does not have the ability to recover. For these reasons, debridement is often incomplete, leaving devitalized tissue and bacteria in the wound and thereby producing the disasters of suppuration. Experience has therefore taught that following the debridement of a traumatic wound, unless the total removal of actual and potentially devitalized tissue can be ascertained with certainty, the wound must be left open to be closed after secondary debridement, if necessary, in three to seven days. This technique is known as delayed primary or secondary closure.

Using the combination of early debridement, thorough irrigation with saline and delayed primary closure, both the risk of suppuration and of loss of function secondary to removal of potentially viable tissue can be held to a minimum. In the classic application of the principles of delayed primary closure, the edges of the wound are held apart by a thin layer of gauze covered by an occlusive dressing preventing further bacterial contamination. The wound is then splinted in a position of rest to prevent motion and strain. If pain, exudate, fever, or other systemic reaction demands, the wound can be examined at any time without difficulty and further debridement carried out. If there is no sign of suppuration, the wound is prepared for closure, usually on the ward with supplemental local anesthesia. The gauze is removed, the wound edges examined, and, if necessary, further debridement is carried out. If the wound edges are clean and beginning to granulate, the wound is closed by opposing the edges as in a primary closure. If suppuration is present, the gauze is replaced and a further delay is carried out.

The use of a thin layer of gauze between the wound edges in a delayed primary closure prevents pocketing of exudate and ensures drainage of purulent material if it occurs. It allows the wound to be examined on clinical demand without seriously interrupting the time schedule of healing. The amount of scar tissue, however, is increased if a foreign body such as gauze is allowed to remain in a wound a matter of days, and the loss of fluid, electrolyte and protein from large wounds is considerable. Recently, the use of split-thickness cadaver skin allografts have been substituted for a thin layer of gauze holding the wound apart.[3] The skin provides physiologic closure of the wound edges while maintaining all of the advantages of delayed primary closure. Fluid, electrolyte and protein losses are reduced to zero, and scar tissue formation is not in excess of that seen in the usual primary healing. The technique of delayed primary closure and the use of split-thickness allografts as temporary primary closure are demonstrated in Figures 22–1 and 22–2.

Occasionally, soft tissue wounds, because of their size or because of the natural immobility of the skin, such as that found in the lower leg, may be impossible to close using the simple expedient of advancing the skin edge to repair the defect. Plastic surgical procedures, such as the swinging of a flap or the harvesting and transfer of a split-thickness autograft, may be required. In the emergency operative situation, these plastic surgical procedures further complicate the technical problems at hand and considerably prolong the operative procedure and the anesthesia time. Here again, the use of previously harvested, split-thickness skin allografts, stored in the operating room, may be employed.[3] The cadaver skin allograft supplies all of the benefits of primary closure without the additional surgical problem or time required to harvest an autograft. This method has proved far superior to the use of gauze dressings in the management of wounds such as open fractures or open reduction of the lower third of the tibia and fibula, where soft tissue protection of the bony structures is largely absent if the leg skin cannot be primarily closed.

Along with the techniques of debridement, delayed primary closure and special wound management using skin allograft, it is essential to employ impeccable surgical technique. The use of foreign bodies should, in general, be avoided. Accurate hemostasis, general tissue management and precise use of sutures without tension, along

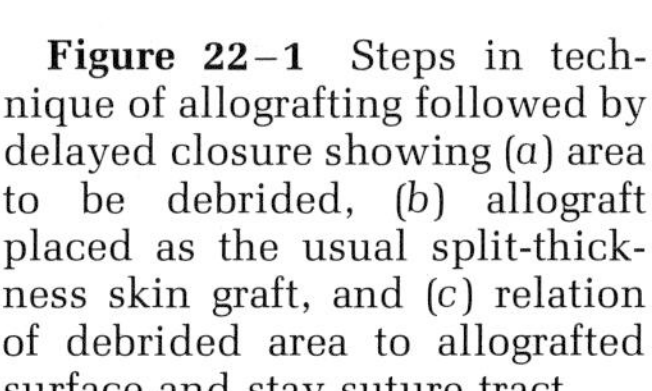

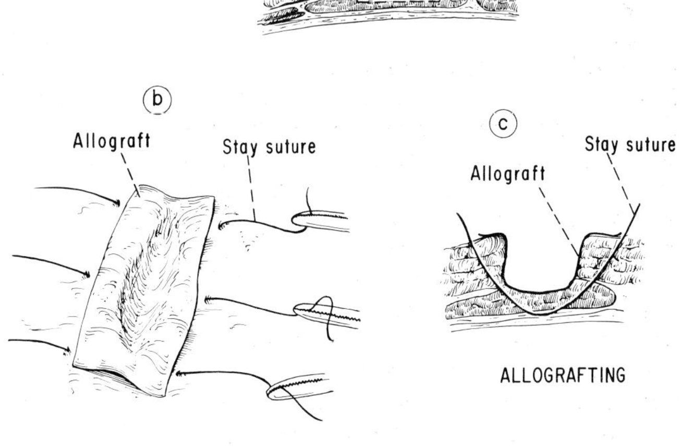

Figure 22–1 Steps in technique of allografting followed by delayed closure showing (*a*) area to be debrided, (*b*) allograft placed as the usual split-thickness skin graft, and (*c*) relation of debrided area to allografted surface and stay suture tract.

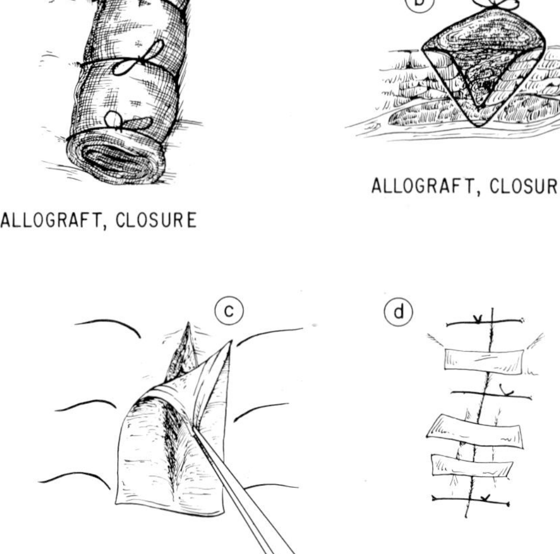

Figure 22–2 Steps in the technique of allografting followed by delayed closure showing (*a*) and (*b*) stent holding allograft in place on debrided surface, (*c*) removal of allograft at time of definitive closure, and (*d*) appearance of wound following definitive closure.

with accurate anatomic reconstruction, will provide the optimum functional result with the least danger of wound sepsis.

Preventive Antibiotics

The restoration of normal physiology and the preparation of the wound by removal of contaminating bacteria, foreign body and devitalized tissue, followed by a means of physiologic closure, are the most important components of the therapeutic regime leading to timely healing without suppuration. Unfortunately, it is not always possible to accurately achieve the goals stated above, and in these clinical instances it is reasonable to consider supplementing the patient's sagging resistance to bacteria with antibiotic substances. In this instance, the term *preventive antibiotics* is used, for, to be effective, the antibiotics must be delivered before infection begins with the idea of preventing bacterial invasion, not with the idea of treating an already established lesion.

Over the past few years, considerable experimental and clinical evidence has been amassed, documenting the effectiveness of preventive antibiotics in both elective and emergency surgery.[4, 5, 6, 7] This experience has demonstrated a number of points important to the prevention of sepsis in seriously injured patients. First, preventive antibiotics can markedly decrease the risk of postoperative sepsis if they are delivered at a time when they can supplement the activity of the tissue to prevent bacterial invasion. Second, preventive antibiotics are most effective when the antibiotic substance is in the tissue before the bacteria arrive and are progressively less effective over the next four hours.

Using these concepts as guidelines, it is clear that antibiotics must be delivered to the injured patient at risk as soon after injury as possible. In fact, if indicated, antibiotics should be given with the initial fluid requirement at the same time that shock or acidosis is being reversed. It is again pointed out that preventive measures designed to allow healing without sepsis, if they are to be effective, cannot wait until the more dramatic activities related to repair of shock or respiratory insufficiency calm down. Antibacterial measures must be among the initial therapeutic measures in the resuscitation of a seriously injured patient.

The choice and dose level of antibiotic to be used cannot be easily categorized. Because of the danger of less than normal perfusion of traumatized areas, if renal function is intact, daily doses of antibiotic probably should range toward the upper end of the recommended dose of the antibiotic chosen. The intravenous route of administration is perhaps the most useful because of the unreliability of the gastrointestinal tract and of intramuscular absorption in a patient with an unstable cardiovascular system. Further, it is urgently necessary to deliver antibiotic substance to the injured tissue as soon as possible. The choice of antibiotic must rest with the clinical judgment and experience of the surgeon. In general, a single antibiotic with low toxicity should be chosen. Multiple antibiotics should be used only in clinical situations where risk of life-threatening infection is extensive. Oxacillin, cephalothin, ampicillin and tetracycline have been used with success. The combinations of kanamycin and oxacillin, or penicillin and tetracycline have also been used.

CONTROL OF WOUND INFECTIONS

The important first step in dealing with an established infection in a traumatic wound is establishing the diagnosis of infection itself. The earlier this can be accomplished on indirect clinical grounds, the less likely generalized infection is to occur and the smaller the tissue damage secondary to local bacterial invasion. The final level of function of a joint or an extremity may well depend on the early recognition and prompt, effective treatment of developing infection in a traumatic wound. In small wounds, the diagnosis can easily be made by observing the cardinal signs of inflammation—pain, heat, redness and swelling. In large wounds complicating extensive trauma, which may extend into body cavities or deeply into the intramuscular spaces, the diagnosis of deep sepsis is far more difficult to make at an early time. The patient may complain of local pain, tightness, or tenderness in the region of the wound, but these signs are not universally present. The systemic evidence of inflammation, consisting of spiking fevers, leukocytosis, malaise and, in extreme cases, shock, are those which must be carefully evaluated. Occasionally, a rapidly spreading cellulitis may be seen, often indicating a beta-hemolytic streptococcal infection, and, rarely, gas may be noted in the tissue, indicating infection caused by gas forming organisms.

Once the diagnosis of infection is established, treatment must be begun immediately in order to confine the advance of the infection to as small an area of tissue as possible. The general principles of treatment of established infection in traumatic wounds are the same in small wounds treated as outpatient problems as they are for major life-threatening injuries. The principles are:

1. Establishing and maintaining drainage of loculated, purulent material;
2. Debridement of tissue devitalized by the septic process;
3. General systemic support of the patient, including antibiotics if the bacterial invasion of the tissue surrounding the wound is present.

The exact technical method chosen for drainage and debridement, the need for systemic support and the decision to use or not to use antibiotics depends on the extent of the wound and its anatomic location. Wound infections involving abdominal or thoracic cavities or the brain cannot be handled in the same manner as sepsis following a compound fracture of the femur, or in a small, soft tissue wound of the forearm. In all cases of sepsis requiring medical treatment, cultures and identification of bacteria and their antibiotic sensitivities should be carried out. Although the treatment of wound infection in the anatomic or physiologic special areas of the body is detailed elsewhere in this volume, there are several general principles which are worth mentioning here. For practical purposes, the varying difficulty of bringing a post-traumatic wound infection under control is related directly to the possibility, or impossibility, of (1) establishing open, continuous drainage of the infection site, and (2) the ability, or impossibility, of wide debridement of the bacterially involved tissue. In a soft tissue wound of an extremity, it is physiologically and functionally feasible to open an infected area widely for drainage and maintain this adequate drainage until infection has been overcome by maintaining the wound open. In the same wound, the sacrifice of skin, subcutaneous tissue and muscle is not limited by devastating loss of function. On the other hand, for physiologic reasons, it is impossible to establish, much less maintain, wide-open drainage of an infection in the peritoneal or pleural cavities, and, for reasons of maintenance of function, it is impossible to debride wide areas of the brain in order to remove all bacteria-laden tissue. These special cases should be recognized and special methods of management employed.

The Treatment of Specific Infection

Although the principles of treatment of bacterial infection in a traumatic wound are broadly similar no matter what species of bacteria is involved, there are important differences in the pathophysiologic evolution of infection caused by certain bacteria; and, perhaps more important, the life-threatening alterations produced by specific bacteria are worth special note.

Beta-Hemolytic Streptococcus Infections. Infections caused by beta-hemolytic streptococcus are notable for their early onset, rapid invasion of tissue and frequent production of life-threatening bloodstream invasion. These infections usually produce a rapidly evolving cellulitis, or lymphadenitis, at times called erysipelas, which may begin hours after the traumatic contamination of a wound and progress to fatal septicemia in a day or two. Fortunately, the beta-hemolytic streptococcus is exquisitely sensitive to antibiotic therapy, particularly to penicillin and, for practical purposes, does not develop resistance to the antibiotic. Because of its sensitivity and inability to develop resistance, beta-hemolytic streptococcal infections are easily preventable by the early use of preventive antibiotics; or, if an infection develops, they are easily eliminated by the early use of therapeutic antibiotics. The danger in this infection lies in its ability to produce a rapidly evolving systemic infection, raising the possibility of extensive bacterial invasion before diagnosis and treatment is carried out.

Tetanus. Tetanus,[8] usually called lockjaw, is a clinical syndrome caused by a toxin produced by Clostridium tetani, a spore-forming, strictly anaerobic, gram-positive bacillus. The bacteria are found widely distributed in nature, being commonly found in the gastrointestinal tract of domestic animals and in soil. Unlike bacterial infections which produce clinical difficulties by direct invasion as well as by intoxication, the tetanus bacillus produces disease by elaborating a toxin which diffuses throughout the tissue. Severe or even lethal tetanus can be caused by minor bacterial growth with little inflammation in the most minor of wounds. Natural tissue resistance to the tetanus bacillus is high, so that under ordinary circumstances contamination of tissue with this bacillus, or its spores, does not result in bacterial growth or invasion. However, if devitalized tissue and/or foreign bodies are allowed to remain in a wound, anaerobic conditions may be produced and tetanus infection established. *Puncture wounds*[9] have particular importance in this context, for the depth of the wound and the narrowness of the opening to the surface prevent efficient cleaning of the wound at time of injury, and foreign bodies, such as dirt, rust and bits of clothing, are not easily removed. In addition, purulent exudate resulting from inflammation in a puncture wound tends to pocket, for the external opening of the wound is soon sealed by a protein coagulum and a closed-space infection produced. For this reason emergency treatment of puncture wounds should have special attention and for the most part should be opened widely in order to insure adequate cleaning, debridement and drainage.

Tetanus is, perhaps, one of the easiest diseases to prevent, for active immunization using toxoid has proved to be effective in its prevention, and the preventive effect is long-lasting. However, the civilian public health measures attempting to produce a uniformly immunized population have not been effective, and there are many patients who come to the emergency ward following trauma without adequate tetanus immunization. Although the clinical disease of tetanus is rare today, it is seen sporadically throughout the country so that its development must be considered and measures for its prevention routinely taken. Prophylaxis against tetanus is usually carried out using alum-precipitated toxoid in three subcutaneous doses of 0.5 ml. each. The second is given four to six weeks following the initial infection, and the third is given six to 12 months following the second dose. This regime produces effective, active immunization for at least a year, and a repeat booster dose of 0.5 ml. tetanus toxoid subcutaneously within the following 10 years produces a rapid rise in antitoxin titer. This response to a booster dose may occur for as long as 25 years after active immunization and in many patients may last throughout the patient's life.

For minor injuries in a patient who has a clear history of tetanus immunization within the last five years, a booster dose is all that is required. In the immunized patient who has had a booster dose within the year, no specific antitetanus treatment is indicated. However, when the wound is more serious, with extensive destruction of tissue and contamination, penicillin or tetracycline should be given in addition. In the unimmunized patient, passive immunity can be established using human antitetanus globulin by intramuscular injection. The usual recommended dose is 250 units, although larger doses have occasionally been recommended. In addition to the administration of antibody for passive immunity, active immunity, according to the above schedule, should be begun immediately.

The diagnosis of tetanus may be suspected in a patient who suffers insomnia, irritability, tremor, spasms and rigidity of muscles adjacent to a wound. The incubation period varies from four to 21 days, but is usually between seven and 10 days. The severity of the clinical disease and the mortality rate are inversely proportional to the length of incubation. The shorter the incubation period, the more serious the disease.

The major objectives of treatment of tetanus are removal of the sources of tetanus toxin production and the neutralization of the circulating toxin already produced. The former is accomplished by thoroughly debriding any traumatic wound by wide excision. Anaerobic conditions must be prevented at all cost, and the wound, therefore, is usually left open following debridement. Circulating tetanus toxin is destroyed by administering 500 units of immune human globulin daily for about 10 days. Antibiotics, usually in the form of penicillin, cephalosporin, or tetracycline,[10] are given to the patient in large doses in order to further prevent elaboration of the toxin by growth of the tetanus bacillus. Because the main symptoms are muscle spasms, sedation with valium and a quiet, dark environment are essential. In severely ill patients with pharyngeal spasm, tracheostomy should be performed and muscle relaxants used as necessary to ensure adequate respiration. Nutrition may be maintained with a nasogastric tube, and constant nursing care will be required.

Patients being treated for tetanus should have active immunization begun using tetanus toxoid. The clinical disease does not uniformly confer immunity.

Gas Gangrene (Clostridial myositis). Gas gangrene[11] is a life-threatening infection involving destruction of muscle and must be clinically separated from gas-forming infections which do not carry the grim prognosis of Clostridial myositis. Gas gangrene usually develops early after traumatic injury, often within 12 hours. It is characterized by extreme pain, rapid pulse, restlessness, a thin brownish discharge and a profound toxemia. There is swelling and edema of the affected tissue, crepitus may be present, and bubbles are occasionally seen in the discharging serosanguinous exudate.

For clinical success, treatment must be immediate and thorough. Early excision of the entire involved muscle mass should be carried out. If the wound is in an extremity, immediate amputation may be necessary. Antibiotics should be given by the intravenous route in large doses. Penicillin or, in the case of sensitivity to penicillin, tetracycline has proved effective. The use of gas gangrene endotoxin is not clearly established but, if used, should be administered early and in doses consisting of 10,000 to 15,000 units per kilogram of body weight. Hyperbaric oxygen treatment has been used and, in some cases, has proved beneficial.[12]

REFERENCES

1. Miles, A. A., Miles, E. M., and Burke, J. F.: The value and duration of defense reactions of the skin to the primary lodgement of bacteria. Brit. J. Exp. Path. *38*:1, 1957.
2. Miles, A. A.: Nonspecific defense reactions in bacterial infections. Ann. N.Y. Acad. Sci. *66*:356, 1956.
3. Burke, J. F., and Bondoc, C. C.: A method of secondary closure of heavily contaminated wounds providing "physiologic primary closure". J. Trauma *8*:228, 1968.
4. Burke, J. F.: The effective period of preventive antibiotic action in experimental incisions and dermal lesions. Surgery *50*:1, 161–168; 184–185, 1961.
5. Burke, J. F.: Preoperative antibiotics. Surg. Clin. N. Amer. *43*:665, 1963.
6. Burke, J. F.: The significance of time between injury and treatment. Conn. Med. *29*: 110, 1965.
7. Bernard, H. R., and Cole, W. R.: The prophylaxis of surgical infection: The effect of prophylactic antimicrobial drugs on the incidence of infection following potentially contaminated operations. Surgery *56*:151, 1964.
8. Robles, N. L., et al.: Tetanus prophylaxis and therapy. Surg. Clin. N. Amer. *48*:799, 1968.
9. Committee on Trauma, American College of Surgeons: Prophylaxis against tetanus. *In* The Management of Fractures and Soft Tissue Injuries. 2nd Ed. Philadelphia, W. B. Saunders Co., 1965.
10. Goodman, L. S., and Gilman, A.: Pharmacological Basis of Therapeutics. 4th Ed. New York, MacMillan, 1970.
11. Altemeier, W. A., and Furste, W. L.: Collective review—gas gangrene. Surg. Gynec. Obstet. *84*:507, 1947.
12. Boerema, I.: An operating room with high atmospheric pressure. Surgery *49*:291, 1961.

chapter

23

MASS CASUALTY MANAGEMENT

Jack M. Zimmerman, M.D.

The occurrence of a sizeable number of casualties in a localized area in a brief period of time creates special problems. Though in dealing with such a disaster many principles of patient management remain unchanged from ordinary practice, certain modifications must be made if optimal results are to be achieved.

Experience in handling large numbers of injured patients is relatively limited, and much of the accumulated experience has been military rather than civilian. In addition, there are virtually no controlled studies on the handling of mass casualties. Since the essence of the problem is too much work for too few people provided with inadequate facilities, it is unlikely that we will ever have much carefully controlled data on which to base our management of this type of problem. Nonetheless, from military experience[1] and from civilian disasters such as the Cocoanut Grove fire and the Texas City explosion,[2, 6, 7] some lessons have been learned which have given rise to certain principles of mass casualty management that, at this point, seem reasonably sound.

The most important and generally agreed upon principle which has emerged from the experience of the medical profession in handling disasters is the need for realistic advanced *planning*. The importance of planning is the major theme of this chapter.

In spite of the importance and wide acceptance of this principle, there can be little doubt that, with few exceptions, there has been less thoughtful planning for handling mass casualties than there should. It seems that there are two principal factors which impede proper disaster planning. The first is a subconscious "it can't happen here" philosophy. By their very nature these disasters have occurred infrequently and, as a consequence, we are prone to assign realistic planning for a disaster rather low priority in our daily concern with urgent problems. There is no completely satisfactory antidote to this "poison"; the most reasonable is a healthy "it can and perhaps will happen here" attitude among those who will bear the responsibility for dealing with a mass casualty situation.

The other factor that interferes with adequate planning for handling massive numbers of casualties is the fact that it is difficult to develop plans that will be suitable to apply to the limitless types and sizes of disasters that may occur. Some disasters cause a general disruption in the community and others are localized to a building or two. Some damage and disrupt the hospital itself, others do not. Some involve fire; some, collision; some, exposure to dangerous chemicals. All this makes for a feeling of frustration once a community or a hospital has decided to embark on a course of disaster planning. The critical point here is that there are certain features that are sufficiently common to enough different types and sizes of disasters to justify the effort involved in planning.

In all mass casualty situations the demands always exceed the capacities of the personnel and facilities. The purpose of advanced planning is, therefore, to establish a system that will assure the optimum utilization of personnel and facilities for the particular situation at hand.

The fundamental unit for handling the medical aspects of a disaster is, of course, the hospital. This is not to say that the hospital alone should be involved in mass casualty planning. On the contrary, the community at large and its various elements are vitally concerned in this planning. However, the focus in this chapter is on the hospital and its activities in mass casualty management. Clearly, there are differences among hospitals and it follows that each hospital should have its own particular Disaster Plan. Our aim here will be to try to lay down some basic guides for developing and executing these plans. It is evident that during a massive disaster those responsible for medical care could not sit down to read about mass casualty management. When the first casualty arrives, the decisions will already have been made that will determine whether the institution is prepared to cope adequately with the chaos and confusion that will follow.

Those who undertake development of a disaster plan may find helpful not only the references listed at the end of this chapter but a series of publications on disaster planning which are available, from the Division of Health Mobilization of the Department of Health, Education and Welfare.

GENERAL PRINCIPLES

In mass casualty management well-established guidelines are hard to come by because there has been limited experience with, and even more limited study of, such management. Hopefully, as the occurrence of future disasters forces increasing experience upon us, we will gain an increasing understanding of the best means of handling such problems. For example, a careful retrospective look at the results of triage decisions in a disaster or two might be quite helpful to future triage officers.

The difficulty in establishing guidelines for civilian practice is accentuated by the fact that so much of past experience with mass casualties has been in a military setting. The problems involved in transferring lessons learned in military practice to civilian practice do not need to be belabored. As in all of medicine, we must be prepared to change our guidelines as new knowledge enables us to do so. The guidelines that are laid down today may become outmoded as a consequence of new concepts in casualty care. Nonetheless, at this point in time, certain principles in the handling of mass casualties seem to have emerged from our prior experience and to be reasonably well grounded.

As already noted, the key to effective handling of disaster situations is realistic advance planning. A second principle is that, within broad limits, the number and type of casualties that will occur in various types of disasters can be predicted. For example, in a thermonuclear explosion one will probably see relatively few missile injuries in patients without hopeless radiation damage. Also, in most civilian disasters as contrasted with military situations, a large percentage of the injured population will have multiple injuries. Bowers and Hughes[3] have discussed in some detail the estimation of the injuries likely to occur in various types of disasters. Such estimates, although crude, can be of help in disaster planning.

A third principle is that certain maneuvers that are quite economical or personnel, facilities and time can produce a marked decrease in mortality, early morbidity and long-term functional loss. Such steps as relief of airway obstruction, wide debridement of devitalized tissue and control of hemorrhage by pressure can be carried out quickly, in many instances by individuals with limited training, and are thus an efficient use of resources in mass casualty circumstances. Conversely, certain more sophisticated techniques which require the prolonged services of highly trained individuals using complex equipment and many supplies, though extremely valuable in ordinary practice, are not a wise investment of resources in handling large numbers of injured people in a brief period of time. Precisely how much of a shift from more extensive procedures to simpler and more efficient ones must be made in the mass casualty situation will depend upon the circumstances of the particular situation.

A corollary of this principle is that the way in which we handle specific types of injuries in ordinary practice must often be modified when we are dealing with casualties from a disaster. This shift in thinking and action is extremely difficult for many physicians to make—a fact which should not be underestimated by those responsible for mass casualty management. Experience with civilian disasters has revealed that strong-willed physicians thoroughly familiar with their own particular specialty but unaware of the modifications that must be made in a mass casualty situation are likely to continue to utilize conventional techniques in such a situation unless there is foreceful direction from those in charge.

This brings us to a fourth principle of mass casualty management: teamwork. In ordinary practice each physician is accustomed to working in a more or less independent capacity. The effective management of large numbers of casualties in a short time demands a totally different organizational structure. There must be someone in charge who is capable of giving orders, and others must be able and willing to follow directions. The individual in charge, referred to in this chapter as the Disaster Plan Director, should have control as close to absolute authority as is ever seen in medical practice. Although this is, indeed, an environment which is quite different from that in which most physicians ordinarily function, repeated experience with civilian casualties has demonstrated conclusively that it is essential to optimal mass casualty management.

Special attention should be given to the readjustment of thinking—literally of philosophy—that is necessary if the best possible results are to be obtained from the medical care of disaster victims. The physician is ordinarily committed to the highest quality of care for his individual patient. When a hospital is flooded with tremendous numbers of seriously injured individuals, an abrupt modification of this philosophy is essential. For example, certain individuals will arrive at the hospital in such condition that, under the disaster circumstances, there is no hope of salvaging them, though had they arrived as isolated casualties, aggressive treatment might have permitted their survival. In the disaster situation we have no reasonable choice but to regard these individuals as hopelessly injured and to turn the bulk of our efforts to those less seriously wounded.

The problems involved in this can run quite deep and deserve more discussion than can be devoted to them here. In most mass casualty situations decisions must be made regarding which patients should receive the attention of physicians. Difficult as the concept may be to entertain and to decide upon, those responsible for disaster planning in a community should give thought to the matter of whether usefulness to the community should be a criterion in selecting patients for the limited medical care that may be available. The handling of this problem in the event of a massive thermonuclear war or other major catastrophe could vitally affect the community in the months and years following the disaster. Though this idea may seem unattractive, it simply reflects the immense change in philosophy that is sometimes called for when we must shift from the ordinary practice of medicine to the care of casualties from a massive disaster.

PLANNING FOR MASS CASUALTY MANAGEMENT

Community Planning

The hospital is the basic unit of medical care in the management of disaster victims, but planning for a disaster is the responsibility of the entire community. The hospital cannot function in isolation in a disaster any more than it can in its usual activities. Physicians, and most particularly surgeons, should play an active role in community disaster planning. If such planning is not already under way, the first role of physicians must be to initiate community activity in this regard. Other elements of the community, of course, must be included in the development of disaster plans: the police and fire departments, the press, the clergy, the legal profession and lay people should participate actively.

In community planning thought must be given to several matters. Each community should establish means of transportation for casualties from the disaster area to hospitals. A disaster of any size is likely to create casualties far in excess of the capabilities of the ordinarily available ambulance services. The possibility of converting other vehicles to use as ambulances should be considered. Furthermore, certain types of disasters will damage roadways; consequently, in outlining transportation facilities to be used in a disaster situation, availability of bulldozers and other equipment to clear debris is significant.

Since often in a catastrophe the number of casualties will greatly exceed the available transportation equipment even if special vehicles are converted to ambulance use, it is probably worthwhile to consider how casualties will be sorted at the scene of the disaster, and how priority for ambulance usage will be established. One approach to this is, of course, to establish a program whereby physicians will be dispatched to the disaster scene to make this priority selection. There are two principal disadvantages to this approach. There is, inevitably, a considerable time lapse between the occurrence of a disaster and the arrival of physicians at the disaster area. Also, this system draws a certain number of physicians away from the hospital where the need for them may be even greater. The alternative approach is to have those driving the ambulances carry out this priority selection; in the absence of physicians at the scene they will obviously do this. Far better, then, that they be trained to do it as well as possible. Each community should see that there is a course of instruction for those who will drive ambulances in a disaster situation, and one of the primary aims of this course should be to provide the drivers with some guidelines for making priority selection. Incorporated into this course should be instruction in certain measures of first aid that can be applied readily at the disaster scene.

In many disaster situations, a number of victims will have to remain at the scene of the disaster for a period of time. Accordingly, in addition to expediting the transportation of patients from the disaster area, community planning should include the provision of supplies such as tarpaulins and blankets at the scene of the disaster.

One of the critical factors both in and out of the hospital at the time of a disaster is, of course, communication. The most carefully conceived programs will fail if they depend upon communications systems that are not available. Each community should see to it that its communications network is geared to the handling of a disaster situation, but must take into account in its planning the possibility that in a major catastrophe involving large portions of the city the normal communications network may be disrupted. The liberal use of sturdy two-way radio systems is probably the most reliable approach to the communication problem. However, the establishment of a messenger or courier system should also be considered.

In some relatively small disasters it is quite acceptable to channel all patients to a single nearby hospital, but planning that prepares only for this type of disaster is inadequate. Provision must be made by each community for the distribution of patients to several hospitals. The way in which this is done will depend upon the particular community, but the important point is that it must be done. A comprehensive community disaster plan should include a program for initial distribution of casualties and for subsequent interhospital transfer if necessary.

Another area in which the community at large bears the responsibility in disaster planning is in teaching first aid. The curriculum for first aid courses must be carefully conceived so that the techniques taught do not call for the use of supplies, equipment and presence of mind that are not likely to be available in the mass casualty situation.

In any mass casualty situation availability of supplies and equipment is one of the critical determinants of the success of medical care. Drugs, dressings, blankets and other items will be needed in abundance. There are some advantages to community stockpiling of these materials for use in a disaster. If such stockpiling is employed, plans must be made in advance for distribution of supplies and equipment where needed.

Just as periodic disaster exercises are helpful for individual hospitals, a community-wide exercise may be of considerable benefit to a community in originating and modifying its disaster plan.[11]

HOSPITAL PLANNING

Supplies, Equipment and Physical Facilities

In bulding, equipping and supplying new hospitals, care of mass casualties should be a factor in the plans. Similarly, already established hospitals must give attention to changes in physical plant, equipment and supplies to achieve a reasonable level of preparedness for a disaster.

There are, unquestionably, practical limitations to the level of preparedness that can be achieved in any particular hospital. Nonetheless, in setting up its disaster plan one of the first matters a hospital should consider are the physical facilities, supplies and equipment that will be available in the event that large numbers of casualties arrive at the hospital in a short span of time.

Certain physical facilities are essential to adequate handling of the disaster situation. The first is a triage area; this should be a room of ample size near the point of arrival of patients. A large conference room or entry-way is quite acceptable; separate entrances and exits are desirable, but numerous accesses will make it difficult to bar unnecessary individuals.

Locations at which minor and major surgery may be performed should be selected. Generally, hospitals in disaster situations have a sufficient number of regular operating rooms to handle the amount of major surgery that is necessary and for which there are sufficient personnel to carry out the procedures. However, simpler types of surgery such as wound debridement will be utilized extensively in a major disaster, and it may be desirable to select certain areas that can be set up especially for this purpose.

Facilities for preoperative, postoperative and nonoperative care must be provided. The simplest approach is to shift patients already in the hospital to other areas. Insofar as possible the extra-operative care of mass casualties should be conducted in large open "ward-type" rooms. Since in major disasters even the largest hospital's facilities of this type may be saturated, thought should be given to other open areas that may be utilized, such as dining rooms and auditoriums. High priority should be given to the convenience of those caring for patients in moving rapidly from one patient to another and the ability of a small number of medical personnel to observe a large number of patients expeditiously.

A facility should exist to which families and friends of victims can be directed to wait and to be informed of the status of those about whom they inquire.

An area should be set up in which a responsible member of the hospital staff can communicate periodically with the press. Providing a room for this and making it entirely plain to members of the press that this is the only area of the hospital to which they are allowed access during the emergency will reduce confusion appreciably. The provision of such a room is the responsibility of the hospital; provision of communication from this room to the press representatives' particular agencies is the responsibility of the press.

Some type of morgue will be needed in almost every disaster. An important point to remember in selecting the room for this is that it will be used for more than the storage of corpses; families and friends will be coming to it to identify bodies.

In all the planning relating to physical facilities it should be remembered that most of the areas selected for various functions during a mass casualty situation will require some rearrangement from their pattern during normal usage. This rearrangement should be minimized but, above all, provisions should be made in the disaster plan for personnel to move furniture and in other ways prepare rooms for their emergency use.

Careful thought must be given to the stocking of supplies for a disaster situation. Maintaining an inventory of unused supplies is an expensive undertaking, particularly for supplies that deteriorate under storage conditions. Furthermore, storage space is quite limited in most hospitals. Finally, the particular types of supplies that will be needed will depend upon the particular disaster that occurs and can be anticipated in only a crude way. Minor surgical equipment and supplies such as scalpels, blades, tissue forceps, suture materials and dressings should be stocked in some reasonable quantity. When circumstances genuinely demand it, most physicians can get along with fewer of these materials than they ordinarily use in their practices.

Certain drugs useful in the traumatized patient should be stored in as ample quantity as practical. Narcotics and antibiotics should clearly be included; decisions on other drugs should be made in accordance with the judgment of the individual hospital. As indicated, it may be more practical for the community rather than the individual hospital to undertake the storage of supplies for a catastrophe. Those responsible should be aware that lack of oxygen and anesthetic agents can be paralyzing in the care of large numbers of casualties and that the storage of these items presents particular problems. Finally, with respect to supplies, some provision must be made for maintenance and periodic check on the condition of stored supplies and for the delivery of these supplies to the area in which they will be used.

Equipment presents a particular problem in disaster planning since the expense of storing equipment against the day when it may be used places practical restrictions on preparedness in this regard. In the final analysis, most hospitals possess about the amount of equipment that their personnel would be able to use in the event of a mass casualty situation. Those responsible for disaster planning should consider this matter, and where exceptions to this general principle are found, some provision must be made to obtain additional equipment.

Finally, the disaster planning in a hospital must take into account the possibility that the hospital itself will be damaged in the disaster. Obviously, not every contingency can be anticipated through advanced planning; the triage area may be wrecked, the stored supplies may be ruined by flood or the nonoperative care area may be burned out by fire. An endless succession of alternative plans would be necessary to prepare adequately for all possibilities. A sensible substitute for such an unmanageable group of plans is for the Disaster Plan Director to have sufficient knowledge of the institution under his command and sufficient flexibility in his thinking to adopt alternatives to prearranged programs as the circumstances dictate.

Communications and Transportation

As with the community at large, the most carefully conceived hospital disaster plan can be rendered completely ineffectual if there is no provision for communication throughout the hospital during the disaster situation. From the first moment a catastrophe occurs there must be a means for notifying all of those who will have responsibilities in the hospital, whether or not they are in the hospital at the time, of the occurrence of a disaster. If this communication depends upon telephones inside and outside the hospital, chaos will prevail in the event of a widespread electrical failure.

Again, the use of durable two-way radios and messengers or couriers can make the difference between a workable plan and hopeless disorganization. Even if all communication systems are in order, it is most helpful if the Disaster Plan Director and his associates know of the location of most members of the staff during the execution of a disaster plan. If the Disaster Plan Director and several others are familiar with the assignments of various individuals, communications will be greatly facilitated.

The Disaster Plan Committee

Planning for mass casualty management in a hospital is best done by a committee. Though the committee should probably not exceed six to eight members, it should be broadly representative of various areas of the hospital that will be concerned in disaster management. Hospital divisions that are not represented directly on the committee should be carefully consulted as the disaster plan is developed. It is important that the Disaster Plan Director be a member, if not the chairman, of the committee; it is further desirable that his alternates be invited to review the plan prior to its adoption and be invited periodically to sit in on the committee's deliberations if they are not members of the committee.

It may be desirable, particularly in larger hospitals, to have several types or levels of disaster plans to meet different sorts and sizes of mass casualty situations. Whatever programs are decided upon, the Disaster Plan Committee should be certain that necessary information regarding the plan is distributed to hospital personnel and that it is understood by them. In order to assure the latter, the role that each individual will play in the plan should be presented to him as simply as possible; also information about the Disaster Plan should be included in the orientation of new employees and rehearsals should be conducted regularly.

Once the plan has been established, the committee's responsibility does not end. It must constantly monitor the program and from time to time make such modifications in it as seem desirable. Medical progress and changes in personnel and the physical plant of the hospital may make it advisable for the committee to alter its disaster plan. The committee should see to it that periodic disaster rehearsals are held and should review the results of these rehearsals. If the hospital is called upon to cope with a disaster situation, the committee should oversee the evaluation of the performance of the plan.

The Disaster Plan Director

It is important that one individual be placed in overall charge of managing the mass casualty situation in a particular hospital. The selection of the particular individual will, of course, depend upon local circumstances; but, in any event, he should be an experienced physician—almost certainly a surgeon—interested in trauma and mass casualties and possessing sound judgment and some administrative skill. He will, of course, require assistance and support, and the extent of this must be determined on the basis of the size of the hospital. Several alternates should be appointed for the Director, since it is entirely possible that he will not be available, cannot reach the hospital or will be incapacitated in the event of a disaster.

The Disaster Plan Director should be charged with the responsibility of determining, if a catastrophe of some type occurs, whether the disaster plan should be placed in effect. If there are several levels of plans for the hospital, it is he who will determine which level will be activated. It is he who determines how personnel, facilities and supplies will be utilized and it is he who is responsible for shifting assignments and making changes in the physical arrangements of the hospital in accordance with the specific characteristics of the disaster situation.

Triage

One thing which has been evident from all experience in handling mass casualties is that execution of triage is one of the critical determinants of the success of a disaster plan. It is at the triage point that many of the irretrievable decisions regarding care are made.

The triage officer should, like the Disaster Plan Director, possess superb judgment and experience in the management of injured patients. He, and his alternates, must be selected with the utmost care.

Two approaches commonly used in hospital disaster plans deserve comment here. One is the tendency to utilize the most experienced and able surgeons as members of operating teams, assigning triage duties to less experienced and knowledgeable individuals. For the reasons already outlined, this is an unacceptable arrangement. The other, and perhaps more frequently utilized, approach is to combine the jobs of triage officer and Disaster Plan Director. Except in the small institution dealing with a small disaster, this is not a desirable arrangement. When the triage officer is busiest sorting casualties, the demands are greatest on the Disaster Plan Director to determine details of the execution of the disaster plan. Both individuals will become somewhat less busy, though still perhaps quite frantic, after the initial rush of casualty arrivals has abated. It is perhaps at this point that the Disaster Plan Director can conveniently take over what remaining triage activities there are, releasing the triage officer for responsibilities elsewhere. However, as a rule, the initial triage should be conducted by someone other than the Disaster Plan Director.

The details of sorting will, of course, depend upon the particular circumstances. Generally, patients arriving at the hospital should be classified into one of four major categories by the triage officer. These categories are as follows:

I. Patients with minimal injuries who will do well on self-care or "buddy" care.

II. Patients whose injuries are less trivial and will require medical attention but are not of a terribly serious nature and will not require intensive care.

III. Patients whose injuries will require major medical attention. This group may be subdivided into the following:
   A. Require early operation
      1. Immediate
      2. After an interval
   B. Do not require operation or operation will be performed only later in their course.

IV. Patients who are either dead on arrival or so hopelessly wounded that under the circumstances of the disaster there is no reasonable chance of saving them.

Considerable surgical sophistication is required in making the judgments that must be executed in the triage area. It is not simply a question of recognizing quickly the severity of various injuries and the urgency with which they must be tended to, though this is an important aspect. In addition, the triage officer must be familiar with the extent of the overall disaster as this will influence the categorization of patients. For example, in a limited disaster that will not tax resources extensively, few patients who arrive at the hospital alive will be placed in Category IV. On the other hand, in a major catastrophe that nearly wipes out an entire city, a triage officer who carelessly assigns patients who should be in Category IV to Category III will jeopardize many legitimate Category III patients. The triage officer knows the number and status of arriving casualties; the Disaster Plan Director knows the conditions in the hospital. Each, then, has information that is essential for the decisions that the other must make; obviously, they should be in close communication.

In addition to sorting patients into these four categories, the triage officer may or may not be assigned two additional responsibilities. The first is the establishment of priorities in Category III patients. In other words, the triage officer may determine which patients most urgently need surgical attention, blood transfusions and other care. Except for those hospitals that are relatively small and have relatively limited staffs, it is probably not desirable for the triage officer to have responsibility for priority assignment on Category III patients. It is better for the most part, for the triage officer simply to assign the patient to a category, send the patient on his way to the appropriate area and leave the determination of priority of management to those in the area to which the patient goes. The reasons for this are evident; the triage officer's judgment must be made hastily and on the basis of an exceedingly brief period of observation, while those in the area to which the patient goes will have a longer period of observation and perhaps better facilities with which to make a judgment.

The other responsibility sometimes assigned to triage officers is the institution of certain measures of immediate care such as the relief of airway obstruction and the control of hemorrhage. There are strong arguments for carrying out this type of care in the triage area since it usually requires only a few moments and may be lifesaving. In most disasters, however, few patients reach the hospital alive for whom postponement of lifesaving measures from the triage to the treatment area would be fatal. The ideal would be for those who are transporting patients to the hospital to institute these measures when they are called for; to some extent this ideal can be approached with proper planning on a community-wide basis.

If it is elected to assign to the triage officer the responsibility of priority determination for Category III patients or the responsibility for execution of some immediate care measures, provisions must be made for this in the disaster planning by assigning to the triage officer adequate assistance in his work.

In the triage area some identification should be attached to each patient. The way in which this is done will depend upon the particular hospital and its plan, but in any case account needs to be taken of this in designing a disaster program.

Patient Care

Each category should be cared for in a separate location. The segregation of patients on this basis—what in ordinary hospital practice is called progressive patient care—is probably the most efficient means of handling large numbers of casualties in a brief period of time with limited resources. Other methods may be employed, but this seems to be the most effective for the variety of disaster situations that may be encountered by a hospital. No triage officer is infallible, and conditions may change after a patient is assigned to a category; consequently, someone should be given the authority to shift patients from one category to another after their initial assignment.

Category I—Minimal Care. Almost no medical personnel are necessary to handle patients in this category. Some responsible individual should be present in the area to be sure that order is maintained and if possible to supervise the administration of self-and "buddy" care.

Category II—Light Medical Attention. Again, very little medical talent needs to be expended. The principal duties to be carried out are perhaps the administration of tetanus shots, the application of light dressings and other chores that can safely be performed by interns, senior medical students and nurses. The alert triage officer may assign to this category a few individuals whom he thinks probably have trivial injuries but in whom he suspects a more serious injury; consequently, some of these patients will require rather close observation.

Category III—Major Medical Attention. It is this category that will utilize most of the personnel, equipment and supplies. The specific organizational structure of Category III care is best determined by the individual hospital on the basis of its particular resources. The designation of a Deputy Disaster Plan Director to supervise this large portion of the mass casualty management is probably advisable in most hospitals. Patients with burns and other injuries that will not require initial operative care during the emergency situation (Category III-B patients) can be attended by internists, pediatricians and other nonsurgical personnel, though it is desirable to have in the area in which these patients are being handled a member of the surgical staff who is familiar with the care of trauma patients. Many of the patients in this area will have blood volume problems that require attention.

Patients who require early operative treatment must, if priority has not already been determined by the triage officer, be sorted with respect to the urgency of operative intervention. The decision regarding the timing of operation will, of course, depend in large measure upon the nature and size of the disaster. For example, in a relatively limited disaster, several patients with moderately severe head injuries may require decompression quite early. On the other hand, in the event of a major catastrophe with hundreds of soft-tissue injuries to be cared for by a few surgeons, the talents of the neurosurgeon and his associates may be much better utilized in the performance of 30 or 40 wound debridements than in the performance of three or four cranial decompressions. This goes back to a principle outlined earlier, namely that there are certain procedures that are rather simply performed but have a high yield in terms of reducing mortality and morbidity. In a major catastrophe it is wise for most medical attention to be directed at these. The Disaster Plan Director should aid those attending Category III patients in making these decisions. He contributes a comprehension of the overall size and nature of the disaster and the demands it is placing upon personnel, facilities and supplies.

A problem that merits mention is the question of whether Category III patients in whom there is initially some doubt regarding the need for operation should be assigned to Category III-A or III-B. This decision must be based largely upon the personnel and facilities available for tending these subcategories but, in general, since it will usually be non-surgeons who are caring for Category III-B patients and surgeons who are caring for Category III-A patients, it is probably preferable for patients in whom a decision regarding need for surgical management must be made to be placed in Category III-A.

It is probably desirable for a relatively high-ranking member of the surgical staff to serve as a Deputy Disaster Plan Director in charge of Category III patients. His major responsibility will be to keep the workload reasonably well distributed among the personnel caring for these patients. These decisions will depend upon his assessment of the nature and extent of the disaster and upon his observation of conditions in his area.

The nonoperative care of patients in Category III-A—both preoperative and postoperative—can be carried out by relatively junior surgeons and by some nonsurgical physicians, though they should be supervised by one of the more senior members of the hospital's surgical staff.

Teams should be designated for the operative management of surgical cases. There is a strong temptation on the part of disaster planners to place the most senior, experienced and able surgeons in charge of operating teams and then to assign patients for surgical care in harmony with the talents of these surgeons. This may not result in the greatest good for the greatest number of patients. As already emphasized, there are certain procedures such as debridement and control of hemorrhage that yield excellent results in large numbers of patients with minimal expenditure of talent. Again and again in disasters, the soundness of this principle has been demonstrated. In other words, it is a mistake to tie up one operating room and three or four physicians for several hours while an arterial reconstruction is carried out on an extremity when during this time the same individuals could have performed 10 to 20 debridements which might have saved several lives and markedly decreased long-term morbidity. This is not to say that arterial reconstruction, thoracotomy and craniotomy have no place in mass casualty management. The point is simply that the optimum deployment of personnel, facilities and supplies must be utilized to achieve the best possible results for the most patients, and how this is done will depend upon the nature and size of the disaster and the facilities and the personnel of the hospital.

The best talent should be utilized to fill the positions of Disaster Plan Director, triage officer, Deputy Disaster Plan Directors and other "non-operating" positions. In the latter stages of the mass casualty situations, as patients held for subsequent surgery come to the operating room, it may be possible to free individuals from these chores to head operating teams. When patients are assigned to operating teams with little training and experience, it is quite worthwhile for a senior member of the surgical staff to supervise the selection of operative procedures. The maximum use can often be made of an able and experienced surgeon by having him circulate among operating teams of less experienced surgeons, utilizing his judgment as to the procedure to be carried out and utilizing the hands of less thoroughly trained individuals to execute the operative technique.

Other factors besides the availability and talent of surgeons will determine the type of surgical care that can be carried out in a disaster situation. As already suggested, anesthetists, anesthetic agents and oxygen may be limiting factors. It has been estimated that the average operating team in a disaster can handle about 15 cases every 24 hours. Naturally, this figure will vary, depending upon the type of operative procedures that are carried out, but this does give a rough guide to the Disaster Plan Director.

Category IV—Hopelessly Injured and D.O.A. The emotional difficulty involved in and the importance of assigning some patients who arrive at the hospital alive to this category has already been discussed. Without question, patients in Category IV should be made as comfortable as possible with the facilities at hand. A few nurses equipped with drugs can ordinarily do this. As the initial stages of a mass casualty situation pass, it may become evident that personnel, supplies and equipment will permit the care of additional patients in Category III and a physician may be assigned to screen surviving Category IV patients for transfer to Category III.

Other Considerations

The extent to which X-ray and laboratory facilities can be employed in managing patients in a mass casualty situation will depend upon the particular circumstances. Both facilities are likely to be quickly saturated. Fortunately, few laboratory tests are ordinarily essential in handling the acutely traumatized patient. On the other hand, X-rays can be of immense help. Consequently, the senior radiologist on the hospital staff will have a critical responsibility in determining how the hospital's X-ray facilities are to be used. When differences of opinion arise between surgeon and radiologist regarding the value of x-rays, the decision will have to be made by the Disaster Plan Director after discussion with both parties.

Keeping adequate records on emergency patients is always a problem but is magnified many times in the mass casualty situation. One approach has been to dispense completely with any record-keeping whatsoever in the event of a major disaster except for the crudest records on the most seriously injured patients. This is not an acceptable solution. In the wake of most disasters, there follows a long succession of legal repercussions, and experience has shown that in spite of almost unbelievable and superhuman effort in coping with a situation far beyond their capacities, hospitals and physicians are not immune from involvement in these legal matters. Furthermore, we will hopefully learn something from each mass casualty situation; our only opportunity to learn what we ought to rather than what we expect to is the availability of reasonable records and a careful retrospective review of these. For these and other reasons, some compromise must be found for keeping records in the disaster situation. Certainly, the compromise does not lie in doctors, nurses and other personnel attempting to keep their own records. In a disaster situation, there will be numerous hospital personnel who will be displaced from their normal activities. With a little planning and instruction they can be productively used as stenographers and can be of great assistance in this capacity.

In the confusion that goes with handling a disaster, it is essential that the hospital be adequately patrolled by authoritative individuals responsible for maintaining order and for directing ambulatory patients, relatives, friends, press and spectators to the appropriate locations. This function can be combined with a messenger function, and again hospital personnel displaced from their normal activities can be used.

It has already been mentioned that an area should be set aside for providing information to the relatives and close friends of patients. It is equally important that an experienced individual from the hospital staff be assigned the responsibility for handling this matter. This individual should be selected carefully and should be provided with the assistance and support necessary to carry out his job. A nonmedical person or a junior member of the medical staff can be assigned here if he possesses the requisite qualities. If the hospital has a chaplain, he is often an excellent choice. It is important in setting up a disaster plan that a means be provided whereby information can be easily relayed to the area in which families will receive information about patients. In the disaster situation the possibilities for mass hysteria among the minimally injured and among the relatives and friends of the seriously injured are very real. A little advanced planning about the handling of these seemingly trivial problems can avert much serious trouble. Furthermore, it may be necessary to have friends and relatives identify seriously injured and deceased patients; this needs to be taken into account in setting up the disaster plan.

Much of what has been said about dealing with families also applies to relations with the news media. Here again a tactful individual with sound judgment and some knowledge of the nature of the situation is necessary and can avert much misunderstanding and confusion. A rather senior member of the hospital staff should be assigned this responsibility; many lay hospital directors are well suited to this job. It is desirable, however, if a layman is to serve as press relations officer, that at periodic meetings with the press he have in attendance either the Disaster Plan Director or one of his immediate assistants.

Throughout the emergency situation the Disaster Plan Director must be fully cognizant of developments both outside and inside the hospital. He must know something of the continuing arrival of further casualties and he must know the status of his personnel and their supplies. Provisions should be made in disaster planning for such information to reach the Disaster Plan Director. He cannot, however, hope to gain all of the information he needs by remaining in one spot and having information brought to him. He must periodically tour the hospital and talk with his deputies and others who are involved in the care of patients and related activities.

Aftermath

Most mass casualty situations develop suddenly and without warning, but their effects go on for weeks, months and years. We have been concerned above with the early handling of the medical aspects of a disaster. These are the ones that require the greatest advanced planning because there is the least time to prepare for them when they occur. Subsequent events can be dealt with in a somewhat more orderly fashion.

In handling any mass casualty situation there is an initial flurry of exhausting activity that may last from a few hours to a few days. However, thought must be given to the "secondary" care of the casualties who survive and to the orderly return to normal hospital routine and normal community function. The amount of "secondary" care required of victims of a disaster will depend upon a number of factors. If the immediate situation has required that vast numbers of wounds be left open and a sizeable number of fractures left unreduced, then soon after the initial stage of disaster management will follow another period of high activity in caring for disaster victims. Further rehabilitation may go on for months or years. The point to be emphasized here is that there is less need and less possibility for planning in this, though some attention needs to be directed to it in establishing a disaster plan.

Special Consideration—Riots

Because civil disturbances rank among the more probable mass casualty problems for urban hospitals, and because they raise some special problems,[14] particular attention should be directed in community and hospital planning to the handling of such disturbances.

Unlike most other mass casualty situations, injuries tend to occur in clusters over a period of several days. During this time the peak load is likely to be at night. Since the demands on hospital personnel are likely to occur somewhat erratically over a period of time, careful thought must be given by the Disaster Plan Director to the optimal use of such personnel and the provision of adequate rest for them.

The nature of the disturbance is likely to disrupt not only the transportation of casualties but of personnel to and from the hospital. Ample provision must be made by the community to assure that both casualties and personnel will reach the hospital as expeditiously as possible.

In addition, this is one type of disaster in which the security of the hospital itself is jeopardized. Community and hospital planning must provide protection for the hospital building and its occupants. A further complication is the presence in the hospital of large numbers of casualties who are likely also to be prisoners. Again, planning for this type of disaster must include some means of guarding such individuals.

By and large, the types of injuries seen do not differ greatly from those in other disaster situations. Usually, individuals exposed to the riot control gases, CN (including chemical Mace) and CS, require no special care other than removal to an area of clean air. Exposure to these agents initially leads to a burning sensation in the eyes with considerable lacrimation and usually some rhinorrhea; heavier exposure is likely to produce cough and a sensation of tightness in the chest; dense concentrations of the agents may cause nausea and vomiting. All of these symptoms also are ordinarily relieved upon removal to an uncontaminated atmosphere. Contact with the agents over a prolonged period, particularly in warm weather, may produce irritation of the skin. Since these "gases" are in actuality particulate solids in a finely divided state, heavy contamination of the body or clothing is best dealt with by removal of the clothing and washing the individual with water or a 5 per cent sodium bisulphite solution. If eye irritation is not relieved by removal of the individual to clean air, the eyes should also be washed out with water or physiological salt solution. As nearly as can be determined, these riot control agents produce no adverse effect on pre-existing respiratory, cardiac, or other conditions.

CARE OF SPECIFIC DISORDERS

In the mass casualty situation, certain modifications must often be made in the handling of various types of injuries and disorders in order to achieve the maximum benefit for the most patients. As already suggested, these modifications do not come easily to some surgeons, but they are essential if the limited resources at hand are to be utilized effectively.

Obviously, the ways in which ordinary care is altered for the disaster situation will depend upon the casualty load, the size of the hospital, the personnel present, the availability of supplies and equipment, whether there is damage to the hospital itself and a variety of other factors. A precise determination of these modifications must be made on the basis of the particular situation. Since in making these modifications various areas of the hospital must be coordinated, the ultimate responsibility in deciding how particular injuries are to be handled must rest with the Disaster Plan Director. It is he who knows the casualty load, the availability of dressing materials, the supply of oxygen and anesthetic gases, the fatigue factor in his personnel and other items that must enter into the decisions.

Because of the need for individualization to the specific circumstances of a particular disaster, it is not possible here to do any more than suggest some of the ways in which ordinary care may be modified in a disaster situation in an effort to obtain optimal utilization of resources. These suggestions are based upon military and civilian experience and emphasize the principle that certain relatively simple maneuvers yield rich dividends in decreasing mortality and long-term functional loss.

Blood Volume Deficit

Blood volume deficit has been a major source of morbidity and mortality in past disasters.

As in dealing with individual patients, the first step in coping with massive acute blood loss is to do everything possible to stop the loss. In mass casualty situations, however, it may be feasible to attempt to stanch bleeding only in those patients in whom this can be done rather readily. The application of a pressure dressing to an extremity or the clamping of a lacerated jugular vein can be carried out quickly; however, except in quite limited disasters, patients who are bleeding rapidly from intrathoracic or intra-abdominal injuries may have to be assigned to Category IV.

In disaster planning, the need for volume replacement in massive amounts must be taken into consideration. The stockpiling of materials to combat blood volume deficits in large numbers of patients is necessary. Precisely what substances should be available is at present subject to some debate. Certainly, some plasma substitute should be included, but recent work suggests that large volumes of saline and Ringer's lactate will be valuable. Since some patients will have dangerous deficits in red cell mass, some blood will be needed. The utilization of deceased patients as exsanguination donors has been suggested; frozen blood,[9] perhaps, offers some promise. Developments in the field of replacement in patients with volume deficits are occurring at a rapid rate; some of these developments may provide some solutions to the difficult problem of coping with hypovolemia in the mass casualty situation. They should, therefore, be followed closely by those responsible for disaster planning.

The administration of intravenous fluids of any type requires certain supplies, and there is no value in having available solutions to combat blood volume deficits unless there are also available sufficient supplies of intravenous therapy equipment.

Excellent judgment is required of those responsible for care of Category III patients in dealing with utilization of available materials for the treatment of hypovolemia. Optimal decisions require the exercise of critical thought. It has been pointed out[8] that if there are five liters of solution available, it is generally preferable to divide them among five patients who will be salvaged by the administration of one liter rather than to give all five liters to one patient. However, it requires superb clinical acumen to determine which patients will indeed be salvaged by the administration of one liter of blood.

In almost every major disaster that has occurred in the past, hypovolemia has been a major cause of death among patients who arrive at the hospital alive. Proper handling of the hypovolemia problem by advance planning and the execution of sound clinical judgment with regard to managing blood volume deficits in the disaster situation will be important determinants of the success of the medical operation in the disaster.

Metabolic Disturbances

Following severe trauma, a variety of metabolic disturbances including renal shut-down and respiratory acidosis may occur. It is evident that in the mass casualty situation the facilities for coping with these disorders will be limited. Laboratory studies to follow metabolic disorders will usually not be readily available. Since metabolic derangements cannot be dealt with optimally in most disaster situations and may result in the shift of patients from Category III to Category IV, everything possible should be done to prevent their development. Again, experience has shown that the removal of crushed and damaged tissue—including amputation if necessary—can often decrease substantially the likelihood of development of acute renal failure. Consequently, these measures should have a high priority in the handling of injuries.

Infections

Wound infection has often been a major problem in mass casualty situations. Just as they are in ordinary practice, keystones in the management of infection once it has developed are adequate drainage and the administration of antibiotics. However, in a major catastrophe the available supply of antibiotics may be limited even a few days after the catastrophe when infection becomes a problem. This gives infection prophylaxis a high priority. However, infection prophylaxis is not easy in the disaster situation. On one hand, many wounds are deep and contain large amounts of devitalized tissue and foreign material providing a superb medium; and on the other, it is quite difficult to maintain adequate sterility.

Two measures that experience has shown are quite valuable in infection prophylaxis in mass casualty situations are the wide debridement of wounds and the postponement of wound closure.

Though one cannot say with finality that prophylactic antibiotics are not useful in preventing infection following trauma, the bulk of evidence available today suggests that they are not. Furthermore, the limited supply of antibiotics is a practical curb on their use for prophylactic purposes even if one concedes their value. Burke[4] has suggested on the basis of his work relating to primary lodgment that there is a critical period at the time a wound is inoculated during which it is determined whether infection will develop. His evidence suggests that when the risk of infection is high, the administration of antibiotics in massive dosage at the time of wounding and immediately thereafter may act as an effective prophylaxis against infection. If antibiotics are available in some quantity, then patients who are otherwise salvageable and who arrive at the hospital soon after sustaining extensive wounds with much devitalized tissue, which cannot all be removed and in which there is heavy contamination, might profitably be treated by the administration of massive doses of antibiotics immediately upon arrival at the hospital and for a short period thereafter.

Burns

The number of burns occurring in a mass casualty situation will, of course, depend upon the nature of the disaster. The amount of care that can be rendered to burns will depend upon the number of burn and other victims and the status of facilities at the hospital. In limited disasters the majority of burns can be cared for quite adequately. However, in major catastrophes burns over a certain percentage are best placed in Category IV if the maximum number of patients are to be salvaged. Conversely, patients with minimal burns (i.e., less than 20 per cent of body surface) would be assigned to Categories I and II. This is a decision to be made by the Disaster Plan Director on the basis of his assessment of the situation.

The first aid use of local hypothermia[10] in burn cases might be of immense help in the mass casualty situation; thus in disaster planning thought should be given to the instruction of those who will be manning the ambulances in the value and techniques of local hypothermia. Few patients will arrive at the hospital sufficiently soon for local hypothermia to be of any benefit there.

The bulk of medical attention in major catastrophes will be directed toward those patients with 20 to 50 per cent body surface burns. Whatever the relative merits of open and closed dressing of burns in ordinary practice, there can be little doubt that in the mass casualty situation open treatment is generally preferable. Silver nitrate and sulfamylon therapy may be utilized, but with both techniques metabolic derangements present a problem and the facilities for following and handling these may be limited.

Fluid therapy in burns of more than 20 per cent will present a challenge. It is not simply a question of available solutions but also of time and equipment required for proper administration. The use of oral electrolyte solutions may offer some assistance in this regard.

Though the decisions regarding burn management in a mass casualty situation hinge on particular circumstances, some advanced thought during the disaster planning stage concerning the techniques to be employed is valuable. If the Disaster Plan Director knows at the time of arrival of the first burn victim what resources will be at his disposal for burn therapy and has an idea of the alternatives that will be available to him, much time can be saved at a period when time is at a premium.

Cold Injuries

During a major disaster in frigid weather, cold injury may present a problem, but it does not usually do so in the initial rush of casualties. Individuals displaced and homeless as a consequence of the disaster may have protracted periods of exposure to freezing outdoor temperatures. Adequate first aid instruction of the population in the prevention of cold injuries will be helpful here. Once such an injury has occurred, watchful waiting for demarcation is usually all that can be employed in the disaster situation. However, as emphasized previously, large areas of necrosis should be debrided promptly to circumvent the problems of infection and metabolic derangement.

Chemical Injuries

Chemical injuries will usually be associated with mechanical and thermal injuries. In the mass casualty situation, antidotes are not likely to be plentiful. Consequently, efforts must be directed primarily toward the associated mechanical and thermal injuries. If antidotes are available, they obviously should be administered.

Radiation Injuries

Some continue to feel that a thermonuclear explosion would so demolish a community and render it so helpless that planning for such an event is useless. It is possible that a thermonuclear holocaust would completely destroy vast areas of civilization so that no amount of planning and preparedness would be effective. However, it is conceivable that one nation might launch against another a limited thermonuclear attack creating a limited focus of damage. Furthermore, scattered throughout the world are industrial plants in which limited disasters involving radiation can occur. For these reasons, it is advisable to prepare for the eventuality of sizeable number of radiation injuries.

These injuries create special problems; most surgeons, though familiar to varying extents with the other types of injuries encountered in a disaster, are unfamiliar with the problems that arise from radiation damage. It is essential that someone familiar with radiation be included in the disaster plan development and be available for its execution.

Essential to proper disaster planning is a trained decontamination team headed by someone familiar with the procedures to be employed. In the event that radiation injuries are included in the mass casualties, the decontamination team should be stationed at the entrance of the hospital just ahead of the triage team. Two monitors can handle patients about as rapidly as the ordinary triage team. Beta-gamma instruments provided with an audio amplifier should be available to eliminate the necessity for watching a meter or wearing earphones. Since batteries may fail early, a spare set of batteries should be available for each instrument. Instruments should be of a type that do not saturate (return to zero) in a high radiation field, or areas of high-level activity will be missed.

In the mass casualty situation with radiation injuries, the decontamination team screens patients before they arrive at the triage area. If patients are contaminated, removal of clothing will usually take care of a major portion of the radiation activity. Therefore, the team should have a container for contaminated clothing and some covering for the patients whose clothing is removed.

Patients who are minimally contaminated after removal of their clothing may be divided into two groups. Those who require no emergency medical attention for other injuries need not be decontaminated. If emergency care is needed, the contaminated areas of the body may be wrapped in plastic or paper and medical attention provided.

For patients severely contaminated, decontamination should be carried out by the decontamination team prior to the administration of any but the most urgent and simple care. If a segregated area for contaminated patients including locations for nonoperative and operative treatment can be provided, decontamination can be conducted simultaneously with other emergency care. Only in the largest hospitals will this be feasible, however.

In addition to his responsibilities in directing the decontamination team, a member of the disaster force familiar with radiation should assist the triage officer by determining those patients who have obviously had a lethal radiation exposure. If the consignment of patients to Category IV is emotionally difficult for the surgeon, it is even more so for the radiologist or other individual who holds the position of disaster radiation officer. Nonetheless, this individual must appreciate the importance of the proper utilization of personnel and facilities so that valuable time, effort and supplies are not expended in the medical care of a patient who will ultimately die of total body radiation. Whether the patient has received a lethal amount of radiation will not be an easy determination but, as with decisions of the triage officer, it must be based upon the best available evidence.

Soft-Tissue Injuries

Extensive injuries to the soft tissue will be seen in rather large numbers in most disasters. The value of early and wide debridement of these wounds has already been emphasized. Crushing injuries involving extensive areas of soft tissue present a special problem because of the frequent development of acute renal failure following such injuries. In dealing with the individual case of crush injury, a certain degree of conservatism is doubtless in order; however, in the mass casualty situation a more radical approach to these patients is appropriate. Early removal of the crushed tissue may provide the only means of avoiding later renal shut-down which, as already noted, cannot be adequately managed very often in the mass casualty situation. In the extremities wide debridement may mean amputation. This decision in an individual case will require the exercise of careful judgment and indicates again the need for having in charge of Category III care one of the senior members of the hospital's surgical staff.

Bone and Joint Injuries

Early and careful reduction, with open reduction as required, is ordinarily the approved method of therapy for most fractures and dislocations. In the mass casualty situation, such treatment often will not represent the optimal utilization of personnel, supplies and equipment during the most hectic stage of the emergency. Immobilization of closed fractures by the simplest means at hand is ordinarily called for. For compound fractures adequate debridement plus immobilization should be carried out in the mass casualty situation. Reasonably satisfactory long-term results can be achieved through reduction of fractures and dislocations by closed and open methods after the initial patient load has been handled.

Injuries to the Nervous System

Generally, patients with severe cranial and spinal cord injuries have a poor prognosis and require a heavy expenditure of operative and nonoperative care. In limited disasters in which the facilities of a neurosurgeon are available and adequate postoperative care can be provided without jeopardizing other patients, decompression of the brain and spinal cord may be warranted. However, in a major catastrophe most of these patients will have to be assigned to Category IV if optimal use is to be made of personnel and facilities to gain the best results for the largest number of individuals.

The fact that a disaster is of sufficient size to require institution of a disaster plan is generally an indication that peripheral nerve injuries should all be treated by delayed repair.

Injuries to the Cardiovascular System

Injuries to the heart and great vessels seldom present a problem in the mass casualty situation. With the difficulties of transportation from the area of injury in such circumstances, few of these patients reach the hospital alive. Those who do will often have disorders that can be handled definitively after the initial stages of the disaster have ended. As with other intrathoracic injuries, aggressive treatment of the few patients with injuries of the heart and great vessels who arrive at the hospital alive may be possible in a limited disaster with proper personnel and facilities available. However, in most disasters of any size this will simply be out of the question if reasonable utilization of resources is to be achieved.

Peripheral vascular injuries also will have a high pre-hospital mortality. However, a percentage of these patients will arrive at the hospital alive, and some of them will be in otherwise reasonably good condition. The nature and extent of the disaster and the personnel and facilities of the hospital will determine whether vascular reconstruction should be carried out on such patients.

Abdominal Injuries

Most surgeons feel that in ordinary practice all penetrating wounds of the abdomen should be explored unless other injuries demand more immediate attention. Those who do not subscribe to this philosophy stress careful observation of the patient and the performance of certain relatively sophisticated diagnostic tests to determine whether laparotomy is necessary. Except in relatively limited disasters, neither approach is feasible; the resources are simply not available. The precise compromise to be made with this ideal will depend upon the circumstances of the particular situation. In the most massive catastrophe all patients with significant intra-abdominal injuries may very well have to be placed in Category IV; in less devastating situations, careful selection of appropriate patients for exploratory laparotomy may be possible. If laparotomy is carried out in patients with abdominal injuries, the operating surgeon should usually perform the simplest procedure to save the patient's life. This means exteriorization of any but the most trivial colon injuries, for example.

Injuries to the Genitourinary System

In disasters that do not thoroughly exhaust the resources of the hospital, it may be possible to handle injuries of the genitourinary tract in a fashion somewhat similar to ordinary practice. However, as with cranial, thoracic and abdominal injuries, significant trauma to the kidneys, renal pedicles, ureters, bladder and urethra require the expenditure of considerable personnel, time and talent. Here again, however, the prognosis for patients is considerably better than with cranial injuries. As with thoracic injuries, certain simple measures such as the insertion of a catheter may provide reasonable temporary treatment until definitive care can be given after the initial stages of the disaster have passed. Decisions regarding the handling of individuals with this type of disorder will have to be made by a physician familiar not only with genitourinary tract trauma but with the overall disaster situation.

Injuries to Eyes, Face and Ears

Maxillofacial injuries are of significance in the early stages of a mass casualty situation because they present a hazard to respiratory function that can often be removed by the execution of simple maneuvers such as stopping bleeding and providing a patent airway. For those patients with maxillofacial injuries who arrive at the hospital alive, these maneuvers can often be carried out in the triage area; if not, they should be given high priority as soon as the patient reaches the Category III treatment area since they are extremely efficient maneuvers in the sense of giving a high yield for little input. However, in a mass casualty situation many patients with maxillofacial injuries will arrive at the hospital after airway obstruction has already done its damage, and many others will have very significant associated injuries.

Little care can usually be given to patients with ear injuries in the mass casualty situation. The preservation of as much viable tissue about the external ear as possible is advisable if debridement of injuries in this area is carried out.

The nature and frequency of eye injuries will depend upon the type of disaster; the care that can be rendered in the initial stages of the emergency will depend upon local factors. Whatever duties the hospital's ophthalmologists are assigned in the disaster plan, a member of the ophthalmology staff should be free to render opinions regarding eye injuries. The decision as to whether enucleation should be carried out in a particular patient will require even greater clinical skill than it does in ordinary practice. The possibility of the development of infection must be weighed carefully against the problem of permanent total loss of vision. Patients with minor eye injuries can be given tremendous relief by the application of relatively simple measures. The practice of bandaging both eyes in the presence of a relatively severe injury to one eye is seldom the wisest course in a disaster of any extent because it converts a casualty with an injured eye to a patient totally dependent upon others.

Hand Injuries

Though the operative technique utilized in ordinary practice for the restoration of an injured hand to optimal function will seldom be practical in the mass casualty situation, a few relatively simple techniques can markedly reduce the long-term functional impairment of patients with hand injuries. Cleansing with soap and water is helpful. This is one of the few areas of the body in which a conservative debridement is often the best course. Two principal factors are responsible for this. The first is that a few cubic centimeters of skin, subcutaneous tissue, muscle and bone can make a much greater difference in ultimate functional result than in most other areas of the body. Second, because the muscle mass is less extensive, the hazards to the kidney from damaged muscles in the hand are less than in other areas. If this sort of conservatism is exercised for hand injuries in the early stages of a disaster situation, hand wounds must be observed very carefully over the next few days. If evidence of spreading infection appears, it can be quickly taken care of with further debridement or possibly amputation.

If sufficient supplies and appropriate personnel are available, wounded hands should be dressed in the position of function. In the mass casualty situation in which there are a large number of hand injuries, personnel familiar with proper hand dressing techniques may not be available to dress all hands. In this case, temporary open treatment until proper dressings can be applied is likely the most sensible course.

Multiple Injuries

In ordinary practice a patient with multiple serious injuries presents an interesting challenge to the physicians who care for him. In the mass casualty situation of any but the most modest size, patients with multiple injuries will generally have to be given a relatively low priority for care. They cannot be automatically assigned to Category IV, of course, since some of them will have one major injury for which relatively expedient treatment may be lifesaving. However, in a major disaster most of them will be so severely injured that the expenditure of the amount of effort, time and supplies needed to attend to them will not be justified by the chances of a successful result. The triage officer and those in charge of Category III care will find that even the proper evaluation of these patients will require considerable time and care. In many disasters it is more time and care than can be expended if other more productive activities are to be carried out.

Anesthetic Problems

In mass casualty situations, anesthetists and the materials they use are likely to be quite scarce. The shortage of anesthesiologists may be handled to some extent by the use of those available in a supervisory capacity with the administration of anesthesia itself turned over to individuals with less training. Some thought should be given to this in establishing a hospital or community disaster plan. The same general rules regarding safe anesthesia apply in the mass disaster situation as in ordinary practice. The anesthetic with the least hazard should be selected; availability of agents will have to be added to familiarity of the anesthetist with these agents as prime factors in determining which agents are to be employed.

In general, it is wise to make the necessary compromises with the ideals of normal practice in the area of selection of patients for operative procedures rather than in the technique of administering anesthetic agents.

Thought may be given to the use of local and spinal anesthesia. Both have the disadvantage of an awake and emotionally as well as physically traumatized patient, but if sedatives are available and can be used safely, they may make it possible for some patients to be operated upon under local and spinal anesthesia. Regional block requires considerable skill and time to execute, and in most institutions it will probably have little role in the disaster situation.

Psychiatric Disorders

In the chaos, heartbreak, pain and anxiety that accompany every major disaster, the mental stability of everyone involved is challenged. Individuals who might otherwise have gone through life without any significant psychological difficulty may break under the strain. Those who break may be moderately injured patients, those with trivial wounds, close relatives of injured individuals or the lucky ones who escape physical damage. Though intensive psychotherapy in the mass casualty situation can hardly be seriously considered, simple measures such as adequate sedation and tranquilization may be helpful. Closely connected with, in fact perhaps truly a part of, the psychiatric disorders that occur in disaster situations is the potential for mass hysteria.

In a community already disrupted by extensive damage and partly decimated by physical injuries, the occurrence of minor and major riots may seriously interfere with recovery of normalcy. To some extent the handling of problems of mass hysteria is the responsibility of the community at large rather than the hospital. However, in its relationship with minimally injured patients, anxious families and the press, the hospital is likely to influence the degree to which group misbehavior interferes with those who are attempting to cope with the consequences of the disaster.

CONCLUSION

Optimal medical care in disasters of all sizes and types is dependent upon realistic advance planning by the community and its hospitals. The type of catastrophe that will occur in a particular community cannot be anticipated, but planning can assure that when a disaster occurs, appropriate individuals will be in a position to deal effectively with the specific problems which arise. The fact that planning cannot be complete is no justification for the absence of preparation. This chapter has proposed some guidelines for those who will design and execute disaster plans; these guidelines are based upon what has been learned from previous experience with mass casualty management.

REFERENCES

1. Beebe, G. W., and DeBakey, M. E.: Battle Casualties. Springfield, Ill., Charles C Thomas, 1953.
2. Blocker, T. V.: Texas City disaster: Pattern of injury in 300 casualties. Am. J. Surg. *78*:756, 1960.
3. Bowers, W. F., and Hughes, C. W.: Surgical Philosophy in Mass Casualty Management. Springfield, Ill., Charles C Thomas, 1960.
4. Burke, J. F.: Preoperative antibiotics. Surg. Clin. N. Amer. *43*:665, 1963.
5. Conrad, M. B., and Klippel, A. P.: Disaster planning in a metropolitan area. Bull. Am. Coll. Surg., May, 1972.
6. Cope, O., et al.: Management of the Cocoanut Grove burns at the Massachusetts General Hospital. Ann. Surg. *117*:801, 1943.
7. Emergency Medical Care in Disasters: Summary of Recorded Experience. Disaster Study 6, National Research Council Publication 457. Washington, D.C., U.S. Government Printing Office, 1958.
8. Emergency War Surgery. U. S. Armed Forces, NATO Handbook, 1958.
9. Huggins, C. E.: Frozen blood—Clinical experience. Surgery *60*:77, 1966.
10. King, T. C., and Zimmerman, J. M.: First aid cooling of the fresh burn. Surg. Gynec. Obstet. *120*:1271, 1965.
11. Menczer, L. F.: The Hartford disaster exercise. New Eng. J. Med. *278*:822, 1968.
12. Principles of Disaster Planning for Hospitals. Chicago, American Hospital Association, 1957.
13. Readings in Disaster Planning for Hospitals. Chicago, American Hospital Association, 1966.
14. Walt, J. W., Wilson, R. F., Rosenberg, I. K., Arbula, A., Gufka, T. J., Kobold, E. F., and Lucas, C. E.: The anatomy of a civil disturbance. J.A.M.A. *202*:394, 1967.
15. Ziperman, H. H.: Principles in surgical management of mass casualties. Arch. Surg. *77*:1, 1958.

INDEX